Contents

ELSEVIER

evolve

Get the latest evolution in health assessment...
Health Assessment Online.

In addition to your text and Student CD-ROM, you can purchase **Health Assessment Online** with interactive study tools, such as video clips, audio clips, animations, and interactive exercises, that will enhance your physical examination skills.

HEALTH ASSESSMENT ONLINE GIVES YOU:

280 interactive exercises to help you learn key points from every chapter.

800 electronic images that allow you to review key visual concepts.

Practice tests to ensure that you've mastered the material in each chapter before moving on.

28 audio clips that allow you to hear actual heart and lung sounds.

60 animations that bring anatomic and physiologic processes to life.

180 video clips that allow you to view demonstrations of key examination techniques and procedures on multiple patients.

65 lab and diagnostic tests that serve as a reference to help you understand the lab values that can affect assessment findings.

1800 WebLinks to pertinent Internet sites that offer the opportunity for further research.

A **glossary** that helps you understand key terms and concepts.

The **User's Guide** gives you a unique access code to get you started on this one-of-a-kind learning adventure! An enclosed CD-ROM contains all *Health Assessment Online* video clips to decrease download time.

For a preview of this study tool, go to **http://evolve.elsevier.com**

MORE WAYS TO LEARN

STUDENT CD-ROM

Includes in-depth case studies with critical thinking questions, new printable health promotion handouts, and a complete head-to-toe adult video examination. Packaged with each book!

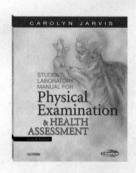

STUDENT LABORATORY MANUAL

Provides multiple-choice, matching, and short-answer questions, as well as anatomy and physiology review. Plus, this resource offers assessment video critical thinking questions, clinical objectives, regional write-up sheets, and student performance checklists.
Sold separately. (0-7216-9775-5)

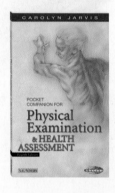

POCKET COMPANION

Offers convenient, full-color access to health history points, examination steps for each body system, normal versus abnormal findings, lifespan and cultural considerations, nursing diagnoses, and summary checklists for each chapter.
Sold separately. (0-7216-9774-7)

Available at your local campus bookstore,
via the web at www.elsevierhealth.com,
or by calling toll-free 800-545-2522.

CAROLYN JARVIS, PhD, APN, CNP

Family Nurse Practitioner
Chestnut Health Systems
Bloomington, Illinois

~ and ~

Adjunct Assistant
 Professor of Nursing
Illinois Wesleyan
 University
Bloomington, Illinois

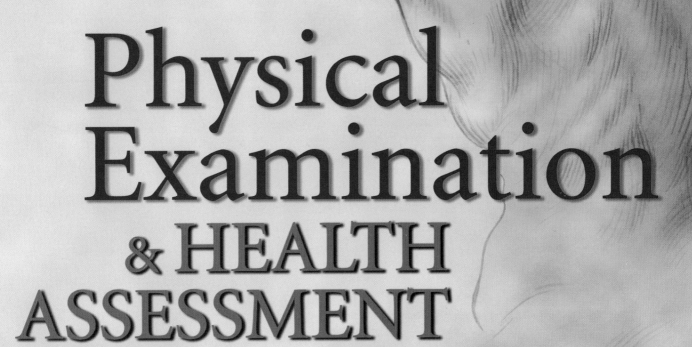

Physical Examination
& HEALTH
ASSESSMENT

Fourth Edition

Original Illustrations by **Pat Thomas, CMI, FAMI**
Oak Park, Illinois

Assessment Photographs by **Kevin Strandberg**
Associate Professor of Art
Illinois Wesleyan University
Bloomington, Illinois

SAUNDERS
An Imprint of Elsevier

Saunders
An Imprint of Elsevier

11830 Westline Industrial Drive
St. Louis, Missouri 63146

Physical Examination and Health Assessment

NOTICE

Nursing is an ever-changing field. Standard safety precautions must be followed, but as new research and clinical experience broaden our knowledge, changes in treatment and drug therapy may become necessary or appropriate. Readers are advised to check the most current product information provided by the manufacturer of each drug to be administered to verify the recommended dose, the method and duration of administration, and contraindications. It is the responsibility of the licensed health care provider, relying on experience and knowledge of the patient, to determine dosages and the best treatment for each individual patient. Neither the publisher nor the author assumes any liability for any injury and/or damage to persons or property arising from this publication.

Previous editions copyrighted 2000, 1996, 1993.

Library of Congress Cataloging-in-Publication Data

Jarvis, Carolyn.
   Physical examination and health assessment / Carolyn Jarvis; original illustrations by
Pat Thomas ; assessment photographs by Kevin Strandberg.—4th ed.
      p.; cm.
   Includes bibliographical references and index.
   ISBN-13: 978-0-7216-9773-4   ISBN-10: 0-7216-9773-9
   1. Physical diagnosis. 2. Nursing assessment. I. Title.
   [DNLM: 1. Physical Examination—methods. 2. Medical History Taking—methods.
3. Nursing Assessment—methods. WB 205 J38p 2004]
RC76.J37 2004
616.07′54—dc21

                                                                2003045490

ISBN-13: 978-0-7216-9773-4
ISBN-10: 0-7216-9773-9
Executive Vice President, Nursing and Health Professions: Sally Schrefer
Executive Publisher: Robin Carter
Developmental Editor: Kristin Geen
Editorial Assistant: Jamie Randall
Publishing Services Manager: Catherine Jackson
Senior Project Manager: Jeff Patterson
Senior Designer: Kathi Gosche
Cover Art: Max Fischer
Cover Designer: Kathi Gosche

Printed in Canada

Last digit is the print number: 9   8   7   6

To

Donald *and* **Frances**, *for charting and steering the course,*

Paul, *for steadfast love and support,*

Sarah *and* **Julia** *for truth, beauty, trust, joy.*

About the Author

Carolyn Jarvis received her B.S.N. cum laude from the University of Iowa in 1968 and her M.S.N. from Loyola University (Chicago) in 1974. She has taught physical assessment and critical care nursing at Rush University (Chicago), University of Missouri (Columbia), and University of Illinois (Urbana), and she has taught physical assessment, pharmacology, and pathophysiology at Illinois Wesleyan University (Bloomington). Ms. Jarvis is a recipient of the University of Missouri's Superior Teaching Award and has taught physical assessment to hundreds of baccalaureate students and nursing professionals, has held 150 continuing education seminars, and is the author of numerous articles and textbook contributions. Ms. Jarvis has maintained a clinical practice in advanced practice roles—first as a cardiovascular clinical specialist in various critical care settings and, for the last 20 years, as a certified family nurse practitioner in primary care. She is currently a nurse practitioner at Chestnut Health Systems, Bloomington, Illinois, and is licensed as an advanced practice nurse in the state of Illinois.

Ms. Jarvis is currently a doctoral candidate at the University of Illinois in Chicago, with a research interest in the physiologic effect of alcohol on the cardiovascular system.

Contributors

CHAPTER 3

MARGARET M. ANDREWS, PhD, RN, CTN

The contributor for Chapter 3, Transcultural Considerations in Assessment, is Chairperson and Professor in the Department of Nursing at Nazareth College of Rochester, New York, and is certified by the Transcultural Nursing Society. In addition to her teaching experience, she is the author of many articles and books on transcultural nursing, has practiced nursing worldwide, and is a respected authority in that field.

CHAPTER 5

JACQUELYN C. CAMPBELL, PhD, RN, FAAN

The contributor for Chapter 5, Domestic Violence Assessment, is the Anna D. Wolf Endowed Professor and Associate Dean for Faculty Affairs in the Johns Hopkins University School of Nursing with a joint appointment in the Bloomberg School of Public Health. Her BSN, MSN, and PhD are from Duke University, Wright State University, and the University of Rochester Schools of Nursing. She has been conducting advocacy policy work and research in the area of domestic violence since 1980. Dr. Campbell has been the PI of 9 major NIH, NIJ, or CDC research grants and published more than 120 articles and five books on this subject. She is an elected member of the Institute of Medicine and the American Academy of Nursing, a member of the congressionally appointed U.S. Department of Defense Task Force on Domestic Violence, and on the Board of Directors of the Family Violence Defense Fund and the House of Ruth Battered Women's Shelter.

DANIEL J. SHERIDAN, PhD, RN, CNS

The co-contributor for Chapter 5, Domestic Violence Assessment, is an Assistant Professor in the Johns Hopkins University School of Nursing where he coordinates a forensic clinical nurse specialist graduate degree program. Dr. Sheridan also works as a forensic Clinical Nurse Specialist in the Johns Hopkins Hospital Department of Emergency Medicine. Dr. Sheridan has almost 20 years of experience working with survivors of family abuse and sexual assault and lectures and consults nationally and internationally on these topics.

CHAPTER 8

JOYCE K. KEITHLEY, DNSc, RN, FAAN

The contributor for Chapter 8, Nutritional Assessment, is Practitioner-Teacher and Professor, Rush-Presbyterian—St. Luke's Medical Center and Rush University College of Nursing in Chicago. Because she has worked in both clinical and instructional settings, she is an experienced and well-known practitioner, teacher, researcher, and author in the area of clinical nutrition.

CHAPTER 11

JEANNINE FORREST, PhD, RN

The contributor for Chapter 11, Pain Assessment: The Fifth Vital Sign, is Research Assistant Professor in the Department of Medical Surgical Nursing at the University of Illinois at Chicago College of Nursing. In addition to her teaching and clinical instruction experience, she has a research interest in pain in cognitively impaired older adults.

CHAPTER 27

DEBORAH E. SWENSON, BSN, ARNP

The contributor for Chapter 27, The Pregnant Female, is a Perinatal Nurse Practitioner with OBSTETRIX Medical Group of Washington, Inc., P.S. in Seattle, Washington. She holds certification from the NCC as a Women's Health Care Nurse Practitioner. She is the author of *Telephone Triage for the Obstetric Patient: A Nursing Guide* and contributing author for *All-In-One Care Planning Resource*. She is an Editorial Advisory Board Member for *Advance* Magazine for Nurse Practitioners and a Certified Medical-Legal Nurse Consultant.

Reviewers

KITTY CASHION, RN, BC, MSN
Clinical Nurse Specialist
Department of OB/GYN
University of Tennessee Health Science Center
Memphis, Tennessee

LINDA MEADE HARRIS, RN, MSN
Instructor
Nursing and Allied Health Division
Cuesta Community College
San Luis Obispo, California

D. ELIZABETH JESSE, PHD, CNM
Assistant Professor
School of Nursing
Purdue University
West Lafayette, Indiana

GEORGINA JORDAN, MSN, MPH, RN
Lecturer
School of Nursing
San Jose State University
San Jose, California

NANCY A. PRINCE, RN, MSN, WHNP, FNP
Assistant Professor
Department of Nursing
Eastern Michigan University
Ypsilanti, Michigan

RACHEL E. SPECTOR, RN, PHD, CTN, FAAN
Associate Professor
Department of Community Health
Boston College School of Nursing
Chestnut Hill, Massachusetts

DEBORAH E. SWENSON, ARNP
Perinatal Nurse Practitioner
OBSTETRIX Medical Group of Washington
Seattle, Washington

Preface

It is important to me that students develop, practice, and then learn to trust their health history and physical examination skills. In this book, I give you the tools to do that. Learn to listen to the patient—most often he or she will tell you what is wrong (and right) and what you can do to meet the health care needs. Then learn to inspect, examine, and listen to the person's body. The data are all there and are accessible to you by using just a few extra tools. "High-tech machinery" is a smart and sophisticated adjunct, but it cannot replace your own bedside assessment of your patient.

Whether you are a beginning examiner or an advanced-practice student, this book holds the content you need to develop and refine your clinical skills. The fourth edition of *Physical Examination and Health Assessment* continues to be a comprehensive textbook of health history–taking methods, physical examination skills, health promotion techniques, and clinical assessment tools. This text presents a firm foundation in these subjects and continues to be an excellent clinical reference.

I am grateful for the enthusiastic response of instructors and students to the earlier editions of *Physical Examination and Health Assessment*. I am also grateful for your encouragement and for your suggestions, which are incorporated wherever possible. In preparing this fourth edition, I have worked hard to build on the strengths of *Physical Examination and Health Assessment* while updating information and adding timely features.

NEW TO THE FOURTH EDITION

Three new chapters are presented in this edition. Chapter 5, **Domestic Violence Assessment**, defines and describes this important range of health problems. Health effects of domestic violence include acute injury, chronic medical problems, mental health problems, sexually transmitted disease, injury during pregnancy, and isolation from family and friends. Your health care visit may be the victim's only chance to talk alone to a health care provider. Thus you must learn to ask *all* patients if they are in a relationship that includes violence or control. Routine screening includes health history questions, assessment tools, and examination of physical injuries. Assessing for the risk of homicide, including the Danger Assessment tool, is presented, because women in this country are more often killed by an intimate partner (especially one who has abused them in the past) than by anyone else.

Chapter 11, **Pain Assessment**, is presented as **The Fifth Vital Sign** that nurses should assess as routinely as we assess the standard vital signs. The neuroanatomic pathways of pain are detailed and illustrated, as well as nociception and neuro-pathic pain. For all age groups, health history questions are presented that assist the person to describe pain. Pain assessment tools and scales are defined and illustrated, as well as physical effects of pain.

Chapter 1, **Critical Thinking in Health Assessment**, presents new content on critical thinking skills. Including this content in the opening chapter is important so that you as students can integrate clinical judgment as you learn physical examination and health assessment. The descriptions of expanded health assessment, the four types of data bases, frequency of assessment, and transcultural considerations are retained and updated from previous editions.

All chapters are revised and updated, with expanded coverage in anatomy and physiology, physical examination, and assessment tools.

Abnormal Findings tables, located at the end of the chapters, are fully revised with 80 new full-color photographs of abnormalities. The goal for this section is to form a selected illustrated atlas of frequently encountered conditions.

Transcultural Considerations are revised and updated in each chapter. Together with a revised Chapter 3 on Transcultural Considerations in Assessment, this content reflects the importance of diversity and cultural awareness.

Full-color art includes over 114 newly redrawn illustrations. All the art in Chapter 11, Pain Assessment: The Fifth Vital Sign, is new.

Examination illustrations contain over 80 new full-color photographs located in Chapter 22, Musculoskeletal System, Chapter 23, Neurologic System, and others.

Chapter bibliographies are thoroughly updated to include the best of clinical practice readings as well as basic science research and nursing research, with an emphasis on scholarship from the last 5 years.

Physical examination skills continue to be refined as the clinician notes what works in his or her own setting and then validates it through research.

Assessment video critical thinking questions are included in each body systems chapter. These questions provide a connection to the *Saunders Physical Examination and Health Assessment Video Series*, which is developed from this textbook.

DUAL FOCUS AS TEXT AND REFERENCE

As mentioned, *Physical Examination and Health Assessment*, 4th edition, is a text for beginning students of physical examination as well as a text and reference for advanced practitioners. The chapter progression and format permit this scope without sacrificing one use for the other.

Chapters 1 through 8 focus on health assessment of the whole person, including developmental tasks and health promotion for all age groups, cultural assessment, nutritional assessment, interviewing and complete health history gathering, and mental status assessment.

In Chapters 9 through 27, the focus turns to physical data–gathering techniques. The physical examination and related health history are presented in a body systems approach, the most efficient method of performing the examination and, thus, the most logical method for student learning and retrieval of data. Each chapter has four major sections: Structure and Function, Subjective Data (History), Objective Data (Examination and Findings), and Abnormal Findings. The beginning student can review anatomy and physiology in the Structure and Function sections and learn the skills, expected findings, and common variations for generally healthy people and selected abnormal findings in the Objective Data sections.

Students may continue to use this text in subsequent courses throughout their education and into advanced practice. As each course demands more advanced skills and techniques, students can review the detailed presentation and the Additional Techniques in the Objective Data sections as well as variations for different age levels. Students can also study the extensive pathology illustrations and detailed text in the Abnormal Findings sections.

This text is valuable to both advanced practice students and experienced clinicians because of its comprehensive approach. *Physical Examination and Health Assessment* can help clinicians learn the skills for advanced practice, refresh the memory, review a specific examination technique when confronted with an unfamiliar clinical situation, and compare and label a diagnostic finding.

Continuing education students who are learning or refining assessment techniques can appreciate the clear and orderly presentation, excellent full-color artwork, and use of space.

CONCEPTUAL APPROACH

Physical Examination and Health Assessment, 4th edition, is written with the belief that practitioners must have a current and thorough knowledge base and highly developed examination skills to function effectively in a demanding, multidisciplinary inpatient setting, as well as in an independent, sometimes isolated, outpatient setting.

This book reflects commitment to:

- Holism, in the focus on the individual as a whole, both in wellness needs and illness needs
- Health promotion, in the health history questions that elicit self-care behaviors, the age-specific charts for periodic health examinations (Chapter 2), and the self-examination teaching presented for skin, breast, and testicles, and for nutrition
- Contracting with the person as an active participant in health care, by encouraging discussion of what the person

currently is doing to promote health and by engaging the person to participate in self-care
- Transcultural considerations that take into account this global society in which culturally diverse people seek health care
- Individuals across the life cycle, supported by the belief that a person's state of health must be considered in light of developmental stage. Chapter 2 presents a baseline of developmental tasks and topics expected for each age group, and subsequent chapters integrate relevant developmental content. Developmental anatomy, modifications of examination technique, and expected findings are given for infants and children, adolescents, pregnant females, and aging adults.

FEATURES FROM EARLIER EDITIONS

Physical Examination and Health Assessment, 4th edition, is built on the previous edition strengths designed to engage students and enhance learning:

1. **Method of examination** (Objective Data section) is clear, orderly, and easy to follow. Hundreds of original examination illustrations are placed directly with the text to demonstrate the physical examination in a step-by-step format.
2. **Two-column format** begins in the Subjective Data section, where the running column highlights the rationales for asking history questions. In the Objective Data section, the running column highlights selected abnormal findings to show a clear relationship between normal and abnormal findings.
3. **Abnormal Findings tables** organize and expand on material in the examination section. The atlas format of these extensive collections of pathology and original illustrations helps students recognize, sort, and describe abnormal findings. When applicable, the text under a table entry is presented in a Subjective Data–Objective Data format.
4. **Developmental approach** in each chapter presents prototypical content on the adult, then age-specific content for the infant, child, adolescent, pregnant female, and aging adult so that students can learn common variations for all age groups.
5. **Transcultural considerations** are extensive throughout and present the expected variations for culturally diverse people. In addition to Chapter 3, the organizational chapter on cultural content, this includes cultural customs to consider when planning the interview, cultural variations to consider when reviewing examination findings, and a Cultural Assessment Guide.
6. **Stunning full-color art** shows detailed human anatomy, physiology, examination techniques, and abnormal findings.
7. **Health history** (Subjective Data) appears in two places: The Complete Health History in Chapter 6, and pertinent history questions that are repeated and expanded in

each regional examination chapter, including history questions that highlight health promotion and self-care. This presentation helps students understand the relationship between subjective and objective data. Considering the history and examination data together, as you do in the clinical setting, means that each chapter can stand on its own if a person has a specific problem related to that body system.

Chapter 4, The Interview, has the most complete discussion available on the process of communication, interviewing skills, techniques and traps, and transcultural considerations (for example, how nonverbal behavior varies crossculturally and the use of an interpreter).

8. **Chapter outlines** on the first page of each chapter show the contents at a glance.

9. **Summary checklists** toward the end of each chapter provide a quick review of examination steps to help develop a mental checklist.

10. **Sample recordings** of normal findings show the written language you should use so that charting is complete yet succinct.

11. **Focused assessment/clinical case studies** of frequently encountered situations show the application of assessment techniques to patients of different ages in differing clinical situations. These case histories, in SOAP format ending in diagnosis, are presented in language actually used in recording.

12. **Nursing Diagnosis boxes** in NANDA format show how nursing diagnoses are derived from assessment data by demonstrating the relationship between medical and nursing diagnoses. A list of nursing diagnoses commonly used with function or dysfunction of each body system is presented.

13. **Integration of the complete health assessment** for the adult, infant, and child is presented as an illustrated essay in Chapter 28. This approach integrates all the steps into a choreographed whole. Included is a complete write-up of a health history and physical examination.

14. **User-friendly design** makes the book easy to use. Frequent subheadings and instructional headings assist in easy retrieval of material.

15. **Spanish language translation chart** highlights important phrases for communication during the physical examination and appears on the inside back cover.

SUPPLEMENTS

• The free *Student CD-ROM* presents realistic patient scenarios—including a variety of developmental and cultural variables—to help you apply your health assessment skills and knowledge. It includes 16 in-depth case studies with critical thinking questions and answer guidelines, as well as **new printable health promotion handouts** (cross-referenced with an icon 〈 〉 in relevant chapters of the text).

Also included is a complete head-to-toe video examination of the adult that can be viewed in its entirety or by systems.

• A dynamic new *Instructor's Resource Kit* contains annotated learning objectives; key terms; teaching strategies for classroom, skills laboratory, and clinical setting; critical thinking exercises; as well as a test manual of over 1000 multiple-choice questions with coded answers and rationales. The critical thinking exercises comprise 8 to 10 case studies per chapter in which students study and discuss the developmental, age, socioeconomic, and transcultural considerations that are addressed during the gathering of subjective and objective data and the implications for the provision of health care. Also included are reproducible worksheets with critical thinking questions related to the video series that accompanies this text (see below).

• *Online Faculty Course Resources* available to instructors contain a computerized test manual, an electronic image collection with approximately 300 color images from the text, and more than 200 text-based PowerPoint slides.

• The *Pocket Companion for Physical Examination and Health Assessment*, **4th edition**, continues to be a handy clinical reference that provides pertinent material in full color and 100 illustrations from the textbook.

• The *Student Laboratory Manual*, **4th edition**, with physical examination forms, is a workbook that includes for each chapter a student study guide, glossary of key terms, clinical objectives, regional write-up forms, and review test questions. All are on perforated pages so that students can use the regional write-up forms in the skills laboratory or in the clinical setting and turn them in to the instructor.

• The all-new *Health Assessment Online* is an innovative and dynamic teaching and learning tool with over 4000 assets, including video clips, animations, audio clips, lecture materials, interactive exercises, laboratory/diagnostic tests, practice tests, test bank, glossary, and WebLinks to accompany each chapter.

• *Saunders Physical Examination and Health Assessment Video Series* is a 17-tape package developed in conjunction with this text. There are 12 body-system videos and 5 head-to-toe videos, the latter containing complete examinations of the neonate, child, adult, older adult, and pregnant female.

• The *EVOLVE Website* for this book (located at http://evolve.elsevier.com/Jarvis/) contains Content Updates, WebLinks, and Data Gathering Checklists.

Throughout all stages of manuscript preparation and book production, every effort has been made to develop a book that is readable, informative, instructive, and vital. Your comments and suggestions have been important to this task and continue to be welcome for this fourth edition.

Carolyn Jarvis
c/o Nursing Editorial
Saunders
11830 Westline Industrial Drive
St. Louis, MO 63146

Acknowledgments

It is my pleasure to recognize the many wonderful friends and colleagues who helped make the revision of this textbook possible. For their help and support I send my gratitude:

To my colleagues, who were a willing resource of information and constructive comments. I am particularly grateful to Joyce Keithley, RN, DNSc, who contributed the chapter on nutritional assessment and who was always willing and responsive to my queries about content and photographs. Margaret Andrews, PhD, RN, contributed the chapter on transcultural considerations in assessment, sharing a wealth of pertinent content on diversity and a global perspective. Jacquelyn Campbell, PhD, RN, FAAN, and Daniel Sheridan, PhD, RN, CNS, provided a thoughtful and important chapter on domestic violence assessment. I am grateful to Jeanine Forrest, PhD, RN, who wrote a timely and worthwhile chapter on pain assessment. These last two topics are new to this edition—it is my belief that they will become a standard part of every complete health assessment. Finally, my thanks to Deborah Swenson, BSN, ARNP, who brought her knowledge and years of experience to the revised chapter on The Pregnant Female, and to Constance Sinclair, MSN, CNM, CEN, who contributed the in-depth pregnancy content to the previous edition.

To my colleagues who provided advice on specific topics in this edition: David Chow, MD; Donna Hartweg, RN, PhD; Paul Jarvis, PhD; Mariann Piano, RN, PhD; Marilyn Prasun, RN, PhD; Lawrence Raines, MD; and Diane Clemons, RN, C, MSN.

To my artistic colleagues, who made this book the vibrant visual display it is. Pat Thomas, medical illustrator, is a gifted artist with an eye for detail and clarity. Kevin Strandberg is a clever and careful photographer, who has endless patience for capturing the images of children and adults in just the right moment of the examination. Our team has worked together for four editions, providing an artistic unity and clarity to this latest textbook.

To my research assistants, whose tireless help enabled me to survive and proceed through manuscript preparation and revision. Marsha Van Etten read and reread endless copies of galley and page proofs, making astute suggestions and correcting errors. Marie Watts, RN, BSN, retrieved countless articles.

To the faculty and students who took the time to write letters of encouragement and suggestions—your comments are gratefully received and are very helpful. To the reviewers who spent considerable time in reading the chapter manuscript and filling out response questionnaires—your suggestions and ideas are very important for this fourth edition.

Thank you to the remarkable professional team at Saunders. I am grateful to Sally Schrefer, Executive Vice President for Nursing and Health Professions, for her guidance and support for the book and its ancillaries. Sally knows the text well and has been personally involved in its advancement and promotion. Robin Carter, Executive Publisher, has been a beacon of support for me and for the book. Robin always has sound suggestions for new ideas for the book and is everlastingly prompt and positive. Jamie Randall, Editorial Assistant, has spent countless research hours in our quest for fresh new photographs for examples of abnormalities in the book. Jamie has shuffled an enormous number of texts from office to office and has been responsible for so many other tasks in editorial support.

I am grateful to Catherine Jackson, Publishing Services Manager, for supervising the schedule for book production and making all the contacts to keep everyone on schedule. My thanks go to Jeff Patterson, Senior Project Manager, who has been a great point man in our day-to-day production schedule. He has solved countless situations in style and format. I am grateful to Kathi Gosche, Senior Designer, for the beautiful interior design. The design draws the reader into the book and guides one through all the subsections. The dramatic cover is the work of Kathi and Max Fischer as well. The individual page layout is the wonderful work of Leslie Roesler, Illustrator/Designer. Leslie crafts every page, always planning how the page can be made even better. I will always be grateful to Robin Richman, Senior Developmental Editor, who guided me through production of three previous editions with patience, hard work, and friendship. Finally, I am so fortunate to have the support of Kristin Geen, Senior Developmental Editor. Kristin has worked tirelessly and efficiently to keep the manuscript moving. Kristin has answered so many questions and seen to so many details that I could not work without her. Thank you for everything, Kristin.

Most important are the members of my wonderful family for their help, love, and complete support. Their constant belief in me and their encouragement have kept me going throughout this process.

CAROLYN JARVIS

Contents

Reference Guide
for Student CD-ROM

Case Studies

CASE STUDY	RELATED CLINICAL CHAPTERS*	TRANSCULTURAL AND DEVELOPMENTAL VARIABLES
Case study #1	Chapter 8: Nutritional Assessment Chapter 21: Abdomen	Nikki White Age: 16
Case study #2	Chapter 18: Thorax and Lungs	Tommy White Age: 4
Case study #3	Chapter 10: General Survey, Measurement, Vital Signs Chapter 15: Ears	Molly and Maggie Native American Ages: 2 months and 11 years
Case study #4	Chapter 22: Musculoskeletal System Chapter 6: The Complete Health History Chapter 15: Ears Chapter 14: Eyes	Mrs. Emerson African American Age: 68
Case study #5	Chapter 19: Heart and Neck Vessels Chapter 18: Thorax and Lungs	Mrs. Lee Asian American Age: 80
Case study #6	Chapter 7: Mental Status Assessment	Mr. Fletcher White Age: 77
Case study #7	Chapter 17: Breasts and Regional Lymphatics	Mrs. Reynaldo Hispanic Age: 40
Case study #8	Chapter 19: Heart and Neck Vessels Chapter 20: Peripheral Vascular System and Lymphatic System	Mr. Madison African American Age: 49
Case study #9	Chapter 18: Thorax and Lungs Chapter 12: Skin, Hair, and Nails	Joe White Age: 30
Case study #10	Chapter 26: Female Genitalia Chapter 27: The Pregnant Female	Rosie Native American Age: 25
Case study #11	Chapter 5: Domestic Violence Assessment Chapter 27: The Pregnant Female	Sue Li Asian American Age: 20

*Content in Chapters 1-11 is integrated throughout the case studies.

Case Studies

Case Study	Related Clinical Chapters*	Transcultural and Developmental Variables
Case study #12	Chapter 12: Skin, Hair, and Nails Chapter 24: Male Genitalia	Jason White Age: 26
Case study #13	Chapter 11: Pain Assessment: The Fifth Vital Sign Chapter 19: Heart and Neck Vessels	Esperanza Vasquez Hispanic Age: 39
Case study #14	Chapter 18: Thorax and Lungs Chapter 16: Nose, Mouth, and Throat	Daniel Little Bear Native American Age: 14
Case study #15	Chapter 14: Eyes Chapter 19: Heart and Neck Vessels	Ruby Jones African American Age: 78
Case study #16	Chapter 23: Neurologic System Chapter 20: Peripheral Vascular System and Lymphatic System	Kurt White Age: 48

Health Promotion Guides

Depression *(relates to Chapter 6)*
High Blood Pressure *(relates to Chapter 9)*
Skin Cancer *(relates to Chapter 10)*
Breast Cancer *(relates to Chapter 15)*
Heart Disease *(relates to Chapter 17)*
Smoking Cessation *(relates to Chapter 18)*
Testicular Cancer *(relates to Chapter 22)*
Colon and Rectal Cancer *(relates to Chapter 23)*
Prostate Cancer *(relates to Chapter 23)*
Cancer of the Cervix *(relates to Chapter 24)*

Adult Head-to-Toe Exam Video

- Complete full-length video
- Video clips organized by body system

Critical Thinking in Health Assessment

*E*llen K. is a 23-year-old white unemployed female who entered a substance abuse treatment program because of numerous drug-related driving offenses. After her admission, the examiner collected a health history and performed a complete physical examination. The actual preliminary list of significant findings looked like this:

- High school academic record strong (A−/B+) in first 3 years, grades fell senior year but did graduate
- Alcohol abuse, started age 16, heavy daily usage × 3 years PTA (prior to admission), last drink 4 days PTA
- Smoked 2 PPD (packs per day) × 2 years, prior use 1 PPD × 4 years
- Elevated BP (blood pressure; 142/100 at end of exam today)
- Diminished breath sounds, with moderate expiratory wheeze and scattered rhonchi at both bases
- Grade ii/vi systolic heart murmur, left lower sternal border
- Resolving hematoma, 2 to 3 cm, R (right) infraorbital ridge
- Missing R lower first molar, gums receding on lower incisors, multiple dark spots on all teeth
- Well-healed scar, 28 cm long × 2 cm wide, R lower leg, with R leg 3 cm shorter than L (left), sequela of auto accident age 12
- Altered nutrition—omits breakfast, daily intake has no fruits, no vegetables, meals at fast food restaurants most days
- Oral contraceptives for birth control × 3 years, last pelvic exam 1 year PTA
- Unemployed × 6 months, previous work as cashier, bartender
- History of physically abusive relationship with boyfriend, today has orbital hematoma as a result of being hit; states, "it's OK, I probably deserved it"
- History of sexual abuse by father when Ellen was 12 to 16 years of age
- Relationships—estranged from parents, no close women friends, only significant relationship is with boyfriend of 2 years whom Ellen describes as physically abusive and alcoholic

The examiner analyzed and interpreted all the data; clustered the information, sorting out which data to refer and which to treat; and identified the diagnoses. Although the diagnostic process is discussed later, it is interesting now to note how many significant findings are derived from data the examiner collected. Not just physical data but cognitive, psychosocial, and behavioral data are significant for an analysis of Ellen's health state. Also, the findings are interesting when considered from a life cycle perspective; that is, Ellen is a young adult who normally should be concerned with the developmental tasks of emancipation from parents, building an independent lifestyle, establishing a vocation, and choosing a mate (see Chapter 2, p. 25). Many factors are important for a complete health assessment.

ASSESSMENT—POINT OF ENTRY IN AN ONGOING PROCESS

Assessment is the collection of data about the individual's health state. Throughout this text, you will be studying the techniques of collecting and analyzing **subjective data** (i.e., what the person *says* about himself or herself during history taking) and **objective data** (i.e., what you as the health professional *observe* by inspecting, percussing, palpating, and auscultating during the physical examination). Together with the patient's record and laboratory studies, these elements form the **data base.**

From the data base, you make a clinical judgment or diagnosis about the individual's health state or response to actual or risk health problems and life processes, as well as diagnoses about higher levels of wellness. Thus, the purpose of assessment is to make a judgment or diagnosis.

An organized assessment is the starting point of all models of clinical reasoning. Discussed below are these clinical reasoning models: diagnostic reasoning, the nursing process, and critical thinking.

DIAGNOSTIC REASONING IN CLINICAL JUDGMENT

The step from data collection to diagnosis can be a difficult one. Most beginning examiners perform well in gathering the data, given adequate practice, but then treat all the data as being equally important. This makes decision making slow and labored.

One way of collecting and analyzing information is the model of *diagnostic reasoning* based on the scientific method. It has four major components: (1) attending to initially available cues; (2) formulating diagnostic hypotheses; (3) gathering data relative to the tentative hypotheses; and (4) evaluating each hypothesis with the new data collected, thus arriving at a final diagnosis. A cue is a piece of information, a sign or symptom, or a piece of laboratory data. A hypothesis is a tentative explanation for a cue or a set of cues that can be used as a basis for further investigation.

For example, consider Ellen K, who presents with a number of initial cues, one of which is the resolving hematoma under her eye. (1) You can recognize this cue even before history taking begins. Is it significant? (2) Ellen says she ran into a door, although she mumbles as she speaks and avoids eye contact. At this point, you formulate a hypothesis of trauma. (3) During the history and physical examination, you gather data to support or reject the tentative hypothesis. (4) You synthesize the new data collected, which support the hypothesis of trauma but eliminate the accidental cause. The final diagnoses are resolving right orbital contusion and risk for trauma.

Diagnostic hypotheses are activated very early in the reasoning process. This helps diagnosticians adapt to large amounts of information because it clusters cues into meaningful groups and directs subsequent data collection.

Once you complete data collection, develop a preliminary list of significant signs and symptoms and all patient health needs. This is less formal in structure than your final list of diagnoses will be and is in no particular order. (Such a list for Ellen is found above). In some institutions, it is easier to generate such a list if you use a conceptual model. Examples of conceptual models are described later in this chapter.

Cluster or group together the assessment data that appear to be causal or associated. For example, with a person in acute

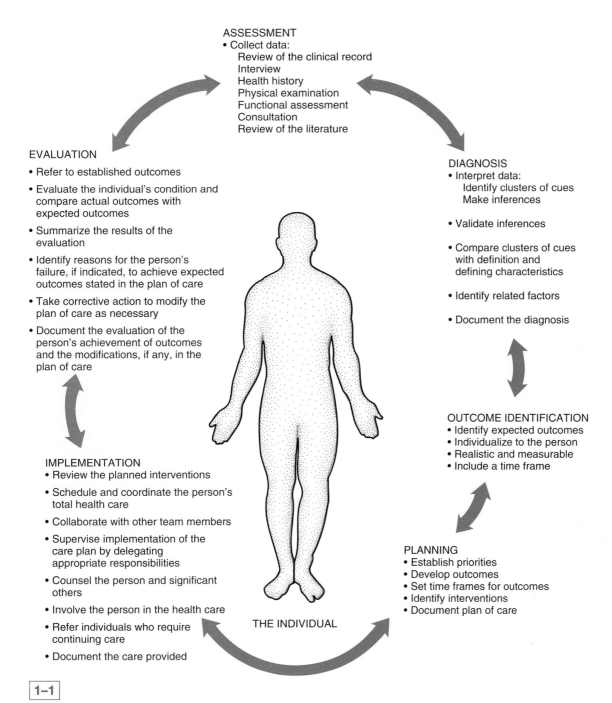

ASSESSMENT
• Collect data:
    Review of the clinical record
    Interview
    Health history
    Physical examination
    Functional assessment
    Consultation
    Review of the literature

EVALUATION

• Refer to established outcomes

• Evaluate the individual's condition and compare actual outcomes with expected outcomes

• Summarize the results of the evaluation

• Identify reasons for the person's failure, if indicated, to achieve expected outcomes stated in the plan of care

• Take corrective action to modify the plan of care as necessary

• Document the evaluation of the person's achievement of outcomes and the modifications, if any, in the plan of care

DIAGNOSIS
• Interpret data:
    Identify clusters of cues
    Make inferences

• Validate inferences

• Compare clusters of cues with definition and defining characteristics

• Identify related factors

• Document the diagnosis

OUTCOME IDENTIFICATION
• Identify expected outcomes
• Individualize to the person
• Realistic and measurable
• Include a time frame

IMPLEMENTATION
• Review the planned interventions

• Schedule and coordinate the person's total health care

• Collaborate with other team members

• Supervise implementation of the care plan by delegating appropriate responsibilities

• Counsel the person and significant others

• Involve the person in the health care

• Refer individuals who require continuing care

• Document the care provided

THE INDIVIDUAL

PLANNING
• Establish priorities
• Develop outcomes
• Set time frames for outcomes
• Identify interventions
• Document plan of care

1–1

pain, associated data are rapid heart rate and anxiety. Organizing the data into meaningful clusters is slow at first; experienced examiners cluster data more rapidly because they recall proven results of earlier patient situations. Use of a conceptual model helps to organize data.

Validate any data you need to make sure they are accurate. Again, this depends on experience. If you are sure of the blood pressure, validate it by repeating it yourself. Eliminate any extraneous variables that could influence BP results, such as recent activity or anxiety over admission. If you have less experience analyzing breath sounds or heart murmurs, ask an expert to listen. Even with years of clinical experience, some signs always require validation (e.g., a breast lump).

NURSING PROCESS IN CLINICAL JUDGMENT

Also based on the scientific method, the **nursing process** includes six phases: assessment, diagnosis, outcome identification, planning, implementation, and evaluation (ANA, 1998). In the 1970s and 1980s, the nursing process was considered a clear, stepwise, linear approach that started with assessment and ended with evaluation. Now we consider it to be a more dynamic, interactive process; in today's complex clinical setting, practitioners move back and forth within the steps (Fig. 1–1).

Although the nursing process is a problem-solving approach to clinical judgments, it seems that expert nurses vault over the steps and arrive at a judgment in one leap (Benner et al., 1997). This is true particularly with expert nurses in critical care situations in which patient status changes rapidly and accurate decisions are paramount. The stakes are high, and nursing autonomy is strong. In these cases, the expert focuses on patient responses and prevents complications with vigilant monitoring (Hanneman, 1996). The expert has well-developed physical assessment skills and trusts these physical assessment skills, even if this conflicts with technologically driven data. For example, consider the expert's actions in assessing a woman with a drug overdose who had an endotracheal tube and was receiving mechanical ventilation.

> The expert nurse examined the woman's posterior chest during medical rounds. She said to the medical team, "Mrs. Potter has bronchial breath sounds and dullness to percussion here and here (pointing to an area the size of a nickel and to another area the size of a quarter over the right lower lobe). Do you think she aspirated?" The physicians said, "No, her chest x-ray is normal." Three physicians took turns auscultating and percussing Mrs. Potter's chest. None of them could hear the changes, even when the expert drew circles around the areas. The medical conclusion was that Mrs. Potter had not aspirated. Undaunted, the expert nurse initiated a regimen of pulmonary interventions. On rounds the next day, the medical team ordered antibiotics and frequent pulmonary treatments based on the early morning chest x-ray findings of right lower lobe consolidation (Hanneman, 1996, p. 332).

Functioning at the level of expert in clinical judgment includes using intuition—that is, knowledge received as a whole. Intuition is characterized by immediate recognition of patterns—expert practitioners learn to attend to a pattern of assessment data and act without consciously labeling it. Whereas the beginner operates more from a set of defined, structured rules, the expert practitioner uses intuitive links, has the ability to see salient issues in a patient situation, and knows instant therapeutic responses (Benner et al., 1997). The expert has a storehouse of experience about which interventions have been successful in the past.

For example, compare the actions of the nonexpert and the expert nurse in the following situation of a young man with *Pneumocystis carinii* pneumonia.

> He was banging the side rails, making gurgling sounds, and pointing to his endotracheal tube. He was diaphoretic, gasping, and frantic. The nurse put her hand on his arm and tried to ascertain whether he had a sore throat from the tube. While she was away from the bedside retrieving an analgesic, the expert nurse strolled by, hesitated, listened, went to the man's bedside, reinflated the endotracheal cuff, and accepted the patient's look of gratitude because he was able to breathe again. The nonexpert nurse was distressed that she had misread the situation. The expert reviewed the signs of a leaky cuff with the nonexpert and pointed out that banging the side rails and panic help differentiate acute respiratory distress from pain (Hanneman, 1996, p. 333).

CRITICAL THINKING

The way of moving from novice to becoming an expert practitioner is through the use of critical thinking. We all start as novices, when we need the familiarity of clear-cut rules to guide actions. Critical thinking is the means by which we learn to assess and modify, if indicated, before acting.

Critical thinking is required for sound diagnostic reasoning and clinical judgment. During your clinical career, you will need to sort through vast amounts of data and information in order to make the sound judgments to manage patient care. This data will be dynamic, unpredictable, and ever changing. There will not be any one protocol you can memorize that will apply to every situation.

Critical thinking enables you to (Oermann, 1999):

- Analyze complex data about patients
- Make decisions about the patients' problems and alternate possibilities
- Evaluate each problem to decide which applies
- Decide on the most appropriate interventions for the situation

What is critical thinking? Paul (1993) calls it "thinking about your thinking while you're thinking in order to make your thinking better." This sounds like circular feedback, but it means that a critical thinker is simultaneously problem-solving while self-improving his or her thinking ability.

> The ideal critical thinker is habitually inquisitive, well-informed, trustful of reason, open-minded, flexible, fair-minded in evaluation, honest in facing personal biases, prudent in making judgments, willing to reconsider, clear about issues, orderly in complex matters, diligent in seeking relevant information, reasonable in the selection of criteria, focused in inquiry, and persistent in seeking results that are as precise as the subject and the circumstances of the inquiry permit. (American Philosophical Association, 1990, p. 3)

Picture critical thinking ability as having three overlapping dimensions (Fig. 1–2). Your critical thinking ability grows as you develop (1) a critical thinking character (a commitment to learning critical thinking characteristics, attitudes, and dispositions); (2) the theoretical and experiential knowledge (what to do, when to do it, why to do it); and (3) the intellectual and manual skills (assessing systematically and psychomotor skills) (Alfaro-LeFevre, 1999). Watson and Glaser (1991) have a similar definition of the three dimensions of critical thinking: an attitude of inquiry, knowledge of the subject, and skills in using this knowledge in problem situations.

Alfaro-LeFevre (1999) presents the following 17 critical thinking skills, organized in the logical progression of the ways the skills might be used in the nursing process. Although each skill here is described separately, they are not used separately, or even linearly, in the clinical area. Rather than a step-by-step linear process, critical thinking is a multidimensional thinking process. With experience, you will be able to apply these skills in a rapid, dynamic, and interactive way.

1. **Identifying assumptions.** That is, recognize that you could take information for granted or see it as fact when actually there is no evidence for it. In every clinical situation, you must get the facts. Ask yourself, what am I taking for granted here? For example, in Ellen's situation, you might have assumptions of a "typical profile" of a person

1-2

with alcohol abuse, based on your past experience or exposure to media coverage. However, the facts of Ellen's situation are unique.

2. Identifying an **organized and comprehensive approach** to assessment. This depends on the priority needs of the individual, and your personal or institutional preference. Ellen has many problems, but at her time of admission, she is not acutely physically ill. Thus you may use any organized format for assessment that is feasible for you: a head-to-toe approach, a body systems approach (e.g., cardiovascular, gastrointestinal), a regional area (e.g., pelvic examination), or the use of a preprinted assessment form developed by the treatment facility.

3. **Validation,** or checking the accuracy and reliability of data. For example, in substance abuse treatment, a clinician will arrange a corroborative interview with a family member in order to verify the accuracy of Ellen's history data. In Ellen's particular case, her significant others are absent or nonsupportive, and the corroborative interview may need to be with another social service worker.

4. Distinguishing **normal from abnormal** when identifying signs and symptoms. This is the first step to problem identification, and your ease will grow with study, practice, and experience. Increased BP, wheezing, and heart murmur are among the many abnormal findings in Ellen's case.

5. **Making inferences,** or drawing valid conclusions. This involves interpreting the data and deriving a correct conclusion about the health status. This presents a challenge for the beginning examiner, because it needs a baseline amount of knowledge and experience. Is Ellen's increased BP due to the stress of admission or a chronic condition? Is the heart murmur innocent or due to heart valve pathology?

6. **Clustering** related cues, which will help you see relationships among the data. For example, heavy alcohol use, so-

cial consequences of alcohol use, academic consequences, and occupational consequences are a clustering of cues that suggest a maladaptive pattern of alcohol use.

7. Distinguishing **relevant from irrelevant.** A complete history and physical exam furnishes a vast amount of data. Look at the clusters of data, and consider which data are important for a health problem or a health promotion need. This skill is also a challenge for beginning examiners, and one area where a clinical mentor can be invaluable.

8. **Recognizing inconsistencies.** When Ellen gives the explanation that she ran into a door (subjective data), it is at odds with the location of the infraorbital hematoma (objective data). With this kind of conflicting information, you can investigate and further clarify the situation.

9. **Identifying patterns.** This helps to fill in the whole picture and discover missing pieces of information. You need to know usual function of the heart, characteristics of innocent murmurs, and risk factors for abnormal or pathologic murmurs in order to decide if the systolic murmur is a problem for Ellen.

10. Identifying **missing information**, gaps in data, or a need for more data to make a diagnosis. Ellen will need more interviewing regarding any increasing tolerance to alcohol, any withdrawal signs or symptoms, and laboratory data regarding liver enzymes and blood count, in order to name a diagnosis.

11. **Promoting health** by identifying risk factors. This applies to generally healthy people and concerns disease prevention and health promotion. To accomplish this skill, you need to identify and manage known risk factors for the individual's age group and cultural status. This will drive your wellness diagnosis. For example, counseling for injury prevention is an important intervention for Ellen because motor vehicle and other unintentional injuries are a leading cause of death for this age group.

12. Diagnosing **actual and potential (risk) problems** from the assessment data. A full list of diagnoses (both medical and nursing) derived from Ellen K.'s health history and physical examination is found in Chapter 28.

13. **Setting priorities** when there is more than one diagnosis. In the hospitalized, acute care setting, the initial problems are usually related to the reason for admission. However, the acuity of illness often determines the order of priorities of the person's problems (Table 1–1).

For example, **first-level priority problems** are those that are emergent, life threatening, and immediate, such as establishing an airway, supporting breathing and ventilation, maintaining circulation, and monitoring severely abnormal vital signs.

Second-level priority problems are those that are next in urgency—those requiring your prompt intervention to forestall further deterioration, for example, mental status change, acute pain, acute urinary elimination problems, untreated medical problems, abnormal laboratory values, risks of infection, or risk to safety or security. Ellen has abnormal physical signs that fit in the category of untreated medical problems. For example, Ellen's adventitious breath sounds are a cue to further assess respiratory

TABLE 1–1: A Common Approach to Identifying Immediate Priorities

Treatment for first- and second-level priorities is usually initiated in rapid succession or simultaneously. At times, the order of priority might change, depending on the seriousness of the problem and relationship between the problems. For example, if abnormal laboratory values are life threatening, they become a higher priority; if the patient is having trouble breathing because of acute pain, treating the pain might become the highest priority. It is important to consider the relationship between the problems; for example, if *Problem Y* causes *Problem Z*, *Problem Y* takes priority over *Problem Z*.

1. **First-level priority problems** (immediate priorities; remember the ABCs):
   - **A**irway problems
   - **B**reathing problems
   - **C**ardiac/circulation problems
   - **S**igns (vital **signs** concerns)
2. **Second-level priority problems** (immediate, after treatment for first-level problems is initiated).
   Note: To help you remember, the mnemonic MAA-U-AR provides the first letter of each of the second-level priority problems):
   - **M**ental status change
   - **A**cute pain
   - **A**cute urinary elimination problems
   - **U**ntreated medical problems requiring immediate attention (e.g., a diabetic who hasn't had insulin)
   - **A**bnormal laboratory values
   - **R**isks of infection, safety, or security (for the patient or for others)
3. **Third-level priority problems** (later priorities):
   - Health problems that do not fit into the above categories (e.g., problems with lack of knowledge, activity, rest, family coping)

From Alfaro-LeFevre R: *Critical thinking in nursing: a practical approach,* ed 2, Philadelphia, 1999, W.B. Saunders.

status to determine the final diagnosis. Ellen's mildly elevated blood pressure needs monitoring also.

Third-level priority problems are those that are important to the patient's health but can be addressed in a more deliberate manner. In Ellen's case, the data indicating diagnoses of knowledge deficit, altered family processes, and low self-esteem fit in this category. Interventions to treat these problems are more long term, and the response to treatment is expected to take more time.

Collaborative problems are those in which the approach to treatment involves multiple disciplines. Collaborative problems are certain physiologic complications in which nurses have the primary responsibility to diagnose the onset and monitor the changes in status (Carpenito, 2002). For example, the data regarding alcohol abuse represent a collaborative problem. With this problem, the nurse must be aware of the profound implications that the sudden withdrawal of alcohol has on the central nervous and cardiovascular systems. The nurse must manage Ellen's response to the rebound effects of these systems during detoxification.

14. Determining **patient-centered expected outcomes.** What specific, measurable results will you expect to observe that will show an improvement in the person's problem after treatment is complete? The outcome statement should include a specific time frame. *After 5 days, Ellen will demonstrate how to manage balanced nutrition by keeping a food diary and by stating which food groups are present/absent in her diary.*

15. Determining **specific interventions** that will achieve your outcomes. These interventions aim to prevent, manage, or resolve health problems. This is the health care plan. For specific interventions, state who should perform the intervention, when and how often, and the method used.

16. **Evaluating and correcting thinking.** Look at the expected outcomes, and apply them as criteria for evaluation. Do the stated outcomes match the individual's actual progress? Then, analyze whether your interventions were successful or not. Continually think, "what could I be doing differently or better?"

17. Determining **a comprehensive plan**/evaluating and updating the plan. Record the revised plan of care and keep it up to date. Communicate the plan to the multidisciplinary team. Be aware that this is a legal document, and accurate recording is important for evaluation, insurance reimbursement, and research.

USING A CONCEPTUAL FRAMEWORK TO GUIDE NURSING PRACTICE

The *organization* of assessment data—the data base—varies depending on the conceptual model that is used by the institution. A model provides the framework in determining what to observe, how to organize the observations or data, and how to interpret and use the information. Many different conceptual models exist, but they all deal with the same concepts: human beings, environment and society, health and illness, and nursing.

Although all nursing models describe the same four concepts, each one has a different focus or emphasis. For example, the focus of Orem's model (2001) is self-care. The focus of Roy's model (1998) is adaptation. The focus of Leininger's model (1995) is cultural diversity. The focus of Gordon's structural framework (1994) involves functional health patterns.

If you were using Orem's model to collect data, you would focus on the abilities and limitations of the individual for self-care. In using Roy's model, you would focus on data about stimuli in the environment and the individual's adaptation to those stimuli. In using Leininger's model, you would focus on factors that influence care and health patterns for individuals, families, and cultural groups. Although each route is different, all three nursing models should lead to similar nursing diagnoses.

A nursing model is used along with, not in place of, a medical model. Nurses use the medical model when they work interdependently with the physician in the diagnosis and treatment of disease. A concurrent nursing model is needed to focus assessment on core nursing concerns, such as nutrition, activity, hygiene, skin problems, coping problems, or self-care limitations.

Numerous nursing models exist, some of which are more appropriate in various settings or with certain types of patients. Nursing models currently are being tested in clinical practice and refined. Although subject to refinement, a model is useful as a framework for assessment and is useful because it leads to the formulation of nursing diagnoses. Although a detailed discussion of conceptual models is beyond the scope of this text, you should become familiar with the one in use at your institution. Use this framework to cluster the assessment data and to prioritize the diagnoses. The use of nursing diagnoses and the companion classification systems for interventions and outcomes give nurses a common language with which to communicate nursing findings.

Nursing diagnoses are clinical judgments about a person's response to an actual or potential health state, which are amenable to primarily independent nursing interventions (North American Nursing Diagnosis Association [NANDA], 1990). The most recent approved NANDA list is given in Appendix A. Note that the list includes three types of nursing diagnosis: (1) *actual diagnoses,* existing problems that are amenable to independent nursing interventions, (2) *risk diagnoses,* potential problems that an individual does not currently have but is particularly vulnerable to developing, and (3) *wellness diagnoses,* which focus on strengths and reflect an individual's transition to a higher level of wellness. Throughout this book, appropriate diagnoses from this list are presented and developed as they pertain to related content in each chapter. In Chapter 28, "The Complete Health Assessment," the list of findings for Ellen K. are analyzed and rewritten as diagnoses.

The medical diagnosis is used to evaluate the etiology (cause) of disease. The nursing diagnosis is used to evaluate the response of the whole person to actual or potential health problems. For example, both the admitting nurse and later the physician auscultate Ellen's lung sounds and determine that they are diminished and that wheezing is present. This is both a medical and a nursing clinical problem. The physician listens to diagnose the cause of the abnormal sounds (in this case, asthma) and to order specific drug treatment. The nurse listens to detect abnormal sounds early, to monitor Ellen's response to treatment, and to initiate supportive measures and teaching; for example, the nurse may teach Ellen which behavioral measures may help her to quit smoking and may recommend that Ellen initiate a walking program.

The medical and nursing diagnoses are independent but interrelated; they should not be seen as isolated from each other. It makes sense that the medical diagnosis of asthma be reflected in the nursing diagnoses, as interpreted by the nurse's knowledge of the person's response to asthma. In this book, common nursing diagnoses are presented along with medical diagnoses to illustrate common abnormalities. Please observe how these two types of diagnoses are interrelated.

EXPANDING THE CONCEPT OF HEALTH

Assessment is the collection of data about an individual's health state. A clear idea of health is important because this determines which assessment data should be collected. In general, the list of data that must be collected has lengthened as our concept of health has broadened.

The **biomedical model** of Western tradition views health as the absence of disease. Health and disease are opposites, extremes on a linear continuum. Disease is caused by specific agents or pathogens. Thus, the biomedical focus is the diagnosis and treatment of those pathogens and the curing of disease. Assessment factors are a list of biophysical symptoms and signs. The person is certified as healthy when these symptoms and signs have been eliminated. When disease does exist, medical diagnosis is worded to identify and explain the cause of disease.

The accurate diagnosis and treatment of illness is an important part of health care. But the medical model has limiting boundaries. The public's concept of health has expanded since the 1950s. Now we view health in a wider context. We have an increasing interest in lifestyle, personal habits, exercise and nutrition, and the social and natural environment. **Wellness** is a dynamic process, a move toward optimal functioning. Different levels of wellness exist; optimal health is high-level wellness. Wellness is a direction of progress. Health care providers serve to maximize the person's potential, to assist the person to grow toward high-level wellness.

Consideration of the whole person is the essence of **holistic health.** Holistic health views the mind, body, and spirit as interdependent and functioning as a whole within the environment. Health depends on all these factors working together. The basis of disease is multifaceted, originating both from within the person and from the external environment. Thus, the treatment of disease requires the services of numerous providers.

A natural progression to **health promotion and disease prevention** now rounds out our concept of health. Guidelines to prevention emphasize the link between health and personal behavior. The Report of the U.S. Preventive Services Task Force (1996) asserts that the majority of deaths among Americans under age 65 are preventable. Prevention can be achieved through counseling from primary care providers designed to change people's unhealthy behaviors related to smoking, alcohol and other drug use, lack of exercise, poor nutrition, injuries, and sexually transmitted diseases. This is a wider, more dynamic concept of health. Health promotion is a set of positive acts the consumer can take. In this model, the focus of the health professional is on teaching and helping the consumer choose a healthier lifestyle.

Nursing includes many aspects of the holistic model—the interaction of the mind and body, the oneness and unity of the individual. Both the individual human and the external environment are open systems, which are dynamic and continually changing and adapting to each other. Each person is responsible for his or her own personal health state and should be considered an active participant in health care. Health promotion and disease prevention form the core of nursing practice.

In a holistic model, assessment factors must be expanded to include such things as culture and values, family and social roles, self-care behaviors, job-related stress, developmental tasks, and failures and frustrations of life. All are significant to health.

COLLECTING FOUR TYPES OF DATA

The amount of the assessment data varies depending on the patient's needs, the health care setting, and the nurse's role in that setting. Every examiner needs to collect four different kinds of data base depending on the clinical situation: complete, episodic or problem-centered, follow-up, and emergency.

1. COMPLETE (TOTAL HEALTH) DATA BASE

This includes a complete health history and a full physical examination. It describes the current and past health state and forms a baseline against which all future changes can be measured. It yields the first diagnoses.

In primary care, the complete data base is collected in a primary care setting, such as a pediatric or family practice clinic, independent or group private practice, college health service, women's health care agency, visiting nurse agency, or community health agency. When you work in these settings, you are the first health professional to see the patient and have primary responsibility for monitoring the person's health care. For the well person, this data base must describe the person's health state, perception of health, strengths or assets such as health maintenance behaviors, individual coping patterns, support systems, current developmental tasks, and any risk factors or lifestyle changes. For the ill person, the data base also includes a description of the person's health problems, perception of illness, and response to the problems.

For well and ill people, the complete data base must screen for pathology as well as determine the ways people respond to that pathology or to any health problem. You must screen for pathology because you are the first, and often the only, health professional to see the patient. You will screen for pathology in order to refer the patient to another professional, to help the patient make decisions, and to perform appropriate treatments. But this data base also notes the human responses to health problems. This factor is important because it provides additional information about the person that leads to nursing diagnoses.

In acute hospital care, the complete data base also is gathered following admission to the hospital. In the hospital, data related specifically to pathology may be collected by the admitting physician. You will collect additional information on the patient's perception of illness, functional ability or patterns of living, activities of daily living, health maintenance behaviors, response to health problems, coping patterns, interaction patterns, and health goals. This approach completes the data base from which the nursing diagnoses can be made.

2. EPISODIC OR PROBLEM-CENTERED DATA BASE

This is for a limited or short-term problem. Here, you collect a "mini" data base, smaller in scope and more focused than the complete data base. It concerns mainly one problem, one cue complex, or one body system. It is used in all settings—hospital, primary care, or long-term care. For example, 2 days following surgery, a hospitalized person suddenly has a congested cough, shortness of breath, and fatigue. The history and examination focus primarily on the respiratory and cardiovascular systems. Or, in an outpatient clinic, a person presents with a rash. The history and examination follow the direction of this presenting concern, such as whether the rash had an acute or chronic onset, was associated with a fever, and was localized or generalized. History and examination must include a clear description of the rash.

3. FOLLOW-UP DATA BASE

The status of any identified problems should be evaluated at regular and appropriate intervals. What change has occurred? Is the problem getting better or worse? What coping strategies are used? This type of data base is used in all settings to follow up short-term or chronic health problems.

4. EMERGENCY DATA BASE

This calls for a rapid collection of the data, often compiled concurrently with lifesaving measures. Diagnosis must be swift and sure. For example, in a hospital emergency department, a person is brought in with suspected substance overdose. The first history questions are "What did you take?," "How much did you take?," and "When?" The person is questioned simultaneously while his or her airway, breathing, circulation, level of consciousness, and disability are being assessed. Clearly, the emergency data base requires more rapid collection of data than the episodic data base.

FREQUENCY OF ASSESSMENT

The interval of assessment varies with the person's illness and wellness needs. Most ill people seek care because of pain or some abnormal signs and symptoms they have noticed. This prompts an assessment—gathering a complete, an episodic, or an emergency data base.

But for the well person, opinions are changing about assessment intervals. The term *annual checkup* is vague. What does it constitute? In practice, its extent varies considerably among physicians, nurses, and agencies. Is the annual checkup necessary? Is it cost effective? Does it sometimes give an implicit promise of health and thus provide false security? Many health professionals are aware of the classic situation of a person suffering a heart attack 2 weeks after a routine checkup and normal findings on electrocardiogram. The timing of some formerly accepted procedures is now being questioned—for example, the annual Papanicolaou test for cervical cancer in women. The same annual routine physical examination cannot be recommended for all persons because health priorities vary among individuals in different age groups and risk categories and because some preventive services are effective only in certain populations (Report, 1996).

The Age-Specific Charts for the Periodic Health Examination are one example of a positive approach to health assessment (Report, 1996). These charts define a lifetime schedule of health care, organized into packages for four specific age groups (see tables in Chapter 2). Each chart lists a frequency schedule for periodic health visits and preventive services for that age group. These services include screening factors to gather during the history, and age-specific items for physical examination and laboratory procedures, counseling topics, and immunizations. The charts focus on *major risk factors specific for each age group* based on lifestyle, health needs, and problems. These charts move away from an annual physical ritual and toward rational and varying periodicity. The charts incorporate health promotion and disease prevention at *every* health visit, not just at one annual physical examination. Health education and counseling are highlighted as the means to deliver health promotion.

For example, the routine periodic examination for Ellen K.'s age group (11 to 24 years old) would be recommended to include the following services for preventive health care:

1. **Screening history** for dietary intake, physical activity, tobacco/alcohol/drug use, and sexual practices
2. **Physical examination** for height and weight, blood pressure, and Papanicolaou test for sexually active females
3. **Counseling** for injury prevention (lap/shoulder belts, bicycle/motorcycle/ATV [all terrain vehicle] helmets, smoke detector, safe storage/removal of firearms), substance use (avoid tobacco, avoid underage drinking and illicit drug use, avoid alcohol/drug use while driving, swimming, boating), sexual behavior (STD [sexually transmitted disease] prevention, abstinence, avoidance of high-risk behavior, use of condoms or female barrier with spermicide, unintended pregnancy, contraception), diet and exercise (limit fat and cholesterol; maintain caloric balance; emphasize grains, fruits, vegetables; adequate calcium intake for females; regular physical activity), dental health (regular visits to provider, floss, brush with fluoride toothpaste)
4. **Immunizations** for tetanus-diphtheria (11 to 16 years); hepatitis B, MMR (measles-mumps-rubella), and varicella (11 to 12 years); and rubella (females over 12 years)
5. **Chemoprophylaxis** to include multivitamin with folic acid (females capable of or planning pregnancy)

Additionally, the **leading causes of death** in Ellen K.'s age group are listed as motor vehicle/other injuries, homicide, suicide, malignant neoplasms, and heart disease.

Obviously, Ellen's individual health problems demand immediate intervention and preclude a strict adherence to this preventive list. Indeed, many of Ellen's findings are seen as "red flags" based on predictable risk factors from this list.

ASSESSMENT THROUGHOUT THE LIFE CYCLE

It makes good sense to consider health assessment from a life cycle approach. First, the health professional must be familiar with the usual and expected developmental tasks for each age group (see Chapter 2). This alerts you to which physical, psychosocial, cognitive, and behavioral tasks are currently important for each person. For example, an adult in Ellen K.'s age group should have developmental tasks that include growing independent from the parents' home and care, establishing a career, forming an intimate bond with another, making friends, and establishing a social group (see complete lists on pp. 25-26).

Next, once assessment skills are learned, they are more meaningful when considered from a developmental perspective. Your knowledge of communication skills and health history content is enhanced as you consider how they apply to individuals throughout the life cycle. The physical examination also is more relevant when you consider age-specific data about anatomy, method of examination, normal findings, and abnormal findings. For example, an average normal blood pressure for a woman Ellen K.'s age is 116/70 mm Hg (see Fig. 10–18 on p. 198).

For each age group, a holistic approach to health assessment arises from an orientation toward wellness and health maintenance. One learns to capitalize on the person's strengths. What is the person already doing that promotes health? What other areas are ripe for health teaching so that the person can further build his or her potential for health?

TRANSCULTURAL CONSIDERATIONS

In a holistic model of health care, assessment factors must include culture. An introduction to transcultural concepts follows in Chapter 3. These concepts are developed throughout the text as they relate to specific chapters.

Metaphors such as *melting pot, mosaic,* and *salad bowl* have been used to describe the cultural diversity that characterizes the United States. According to the U.S. Census Bureau, close to 50% of the population of the United States soon will consist of people from racial, ethnic, and cultural groups sometimes referred to as minorities (Fig. 1–3). Because the term *minority* is perceived to connote inferiority, members of some groups object to its use and prefer terms such as *ethnicity* and *cultural diversity.*

If current demographic trends continue, the following cultural diversity is expected in the United States in the 21st century: Hispanics, 24.3%; blacks, 13.2%; Asian/Pacific Islander, 8.9%; and Native American, 0.8% (U.S. Bureau of the Census, 2000). Hispanic and Asian populations are expected to double between now and 2050.

In these first years of the 21st century, there is a steady flow of immigrants and refugees into the United States. Because the United States is sometimes perceived as the center of advanced health care and technology, foreign nationals who return home after treatment have been inflating the census reports at many U.S. hospitals, with the more popular types of U.S. interventions being cardiovascular, neurological, and cancer treatments. For example, 35% of kidney transplant recipients at some U.S. hospitals have come from other countries. At the same time, U.S. health care providers go abroad to work in a wide variety of health care settings in the international marketplace. Furthermore, international interchanges are increasing among nurses and physicians, making attention to the cultural aspects of health and illness an even greater priority.

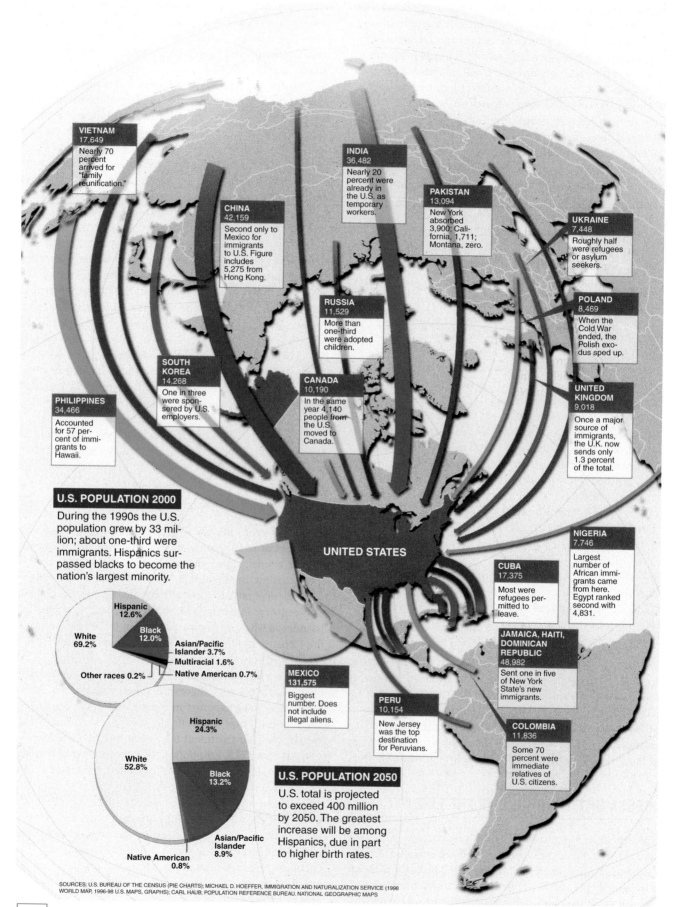

VIETNAM
17,649
Nearly 70 percent arrived for "family reunification."

CHINA
42,159
Second only to Mexico for immigrants to U.S. Figure includes 5,275 from Hong Kong.

INDIA
36,482
Nearly 20 percent were already in the U.S. as temporary workers.

PAKISTAN
13,094
New York absorbed 3,900; California, 1,711; Montana, zero.

UKRAINE
7,448
Roughly half were refugees or asylum seekers.

POLAND
8,469
When the Cold War ended, the Polish exodus sped up.

RUSSIA
11,529
More than one-third were adopted children.

SOUTH KOREA
14,268
One in three were sponsored by U.S. employers.

CANADA
10,190
In the same year 4,140 people from the U.S. moved to Canada.

UNITED KINGDOM
9,018
Once a major source of immigrants, the U.K. now sends only 1.3 percent of the total.

PHILIPPINES
34,466
Accounted for 57 percent of immigrants to Hawaii.

U.S. POPULATION 2000

During the 1990s the U.S. population grew by 33 million; about one-third were immigrants. Hispanics surpassed blacks to become the nation's largest minority.

Hispanic 12.6%
Black 12.0%
White 69.2%
Asian/Pacific Islander 3.7%
Multiracial 1.6%
Other races 0.2%
Native American 0.7%

UNITED STATES

NIGERIA
7,746
Largest number of African immigrants came from here. Egypt ranked second with 4,831.

CUBA
17,375
Most were refugees permitted to leave.

JAMAICA, HAITI, DOMINICAN REPUBLIC
48,982
Sent one in five of New York State's new immigrants.

MEXICO
131,575
Biggest number. Does not include illegal aliens.

PERU
10,154
New Jersey was the top destination for Peruvians.

COLOMBIA
11,836
Some 70 percent were immediate relatives of U.S. citizens.

U.S. POPULATION 2050

U.S. total is projected to exceed 400 million by 2050. The greatest increase will be among Hispanics, due in part to higher birth rates.

Hispanic 24.3%
White 52.8%
Black 13.2%
Asian/Pacific Islander 8.9%
Native American 0.8%

SOURCES: U.S. BUREAU OF THE CENSUS (PIE CHARTS); MICHAEL D. HOEFFER, IMMIGRATION AND NATURALIZATION SERVICE (1998 WORLD MAP, 1996-98 U.S. MAPS, GRAPHS); CARL HAUB, POPULATION REFERENCE BUREAU. NATIONAL GEOGRAPHIC MAPS

1-3

During your professional career, you may be expected to assess short-term foreign visitors, international university faculty, students from abroad studying in U.S. high schools and universities, family members of foreign diplomats, immigrants, refugees, members of more than 106 different ethnic groups, and Native Americans from 510 federally recognized tribes. A serious conceptual problem exists in that nurses and physicians are expected to know, understand, and meet the health needs of people from culturally diverse backgrounds without any formal preparation for doing so.

The inclusion of cultural considerations in health assessment is of paramount importance to gather data that are accurate and meaningful and to intervene with culturally sensitive and appropriate care. Members of some cultural groups are demanding culturally relevant health care that incorporates their specific beliefs and practices. An increasing expectation exists among members of certain cultural groups that health care providers will respect their "cultural health rights," an expectation that frequently conflicts with the unicultural, Western, biomedical world view taught in U.S. educational programs that prepare nurses and other health care providers.

Given the multicultural composition of the United States and the projected increase in the number of individuals from diverse cultural backgrounds anticipated in the future, a concern for the cultural beliefs and practices of people is becoming increasingly important. Nursing is inherently a transcul-tural phenomenon in that the context and process of helping people involves at least two persons who generally have different cultural orientations or intracultural lifestyles.

HIGH-LEVEL ASSESSMENT SKILLS

This attention to life cycle, holism, and culture does not detract from the importance of assessment skills themselves. Assessment skills must be practiced and refined to a high level. In many community settings, the nurse is the first and often the only health professional to see an individual. In the hospital, the nurse is the only health professional continually present at the bedside.

Current efforts of cost containment result in a hospital population composed of people who have increased acuity, a shorter stay, and an earlier discharge than in the past. This situation requires faster, more efficient assessments from the nurse. Procedures that used to require a standard hospital stay of several days (e.g., surgery for inguinal hernia, insertion of a central intravenous line for total parenteral alimentation) now are done on an outpatient basis. As a result, nurses often go to people's homes for follow-up assessment and diagnosis. These situations require first-rate assessment skills that are grounded in a holistic approach and a knowledge of age-specific problems.

BIBLIOGRAPHY

Alfaro-LeFevre R: *Critical thinking in nursing: a practical approach,* ed 2, Philadelphia, 1999, W.B. Saunders.

American Nurses Association: *Standards of clinical nursing practice,* ed 2, Washington, DC, 1998, American Nurses Association.

American Philosophical Association: *Critical thinking: a statement of expert consensus for purposes of educational assessment and instruction.* The Delphi Report: Research Findings and Recommendations Prepared for the Committee on Pre-College Philosophy. ERIC Document Reproduction Service. No. ED315-423. Millbrae, Calif, 1990, American Philosophical Association.

Benner P, Tanner C, Chesla C: *Expertise in nursing practice,* New York, 1996, Springer.

Benner P, Tanner CA, Chesla CA: Becoming an expert nurse, *Am J Nurs* 97(6):16BBB-16DDD, June, 1997.

Carpenito LJ: *Nursing diagnosis: application to clinical practice,* ed 9, Philadelphia, 2002, Lippincott-Raven.

Colucciello ML: Critical thinking skills and dispositions of baccalaureate nursing students: a conceptual model for evaluation, *J Prof Nurs* 13(4):236-245, 1997.

Daly WM: Critical thinking as an outcome of nursing education. What is it? Why is it important to nursing practice? *J Adv Nurs* 28(2):323-331, 1998.

Elstein A, Shulman L, Sparfka S: *Medical problem solving: an analysis of clinical reasoning,* Cambridge, Mass, 1978, Harvard University Press.

Facione NC, Facione PA: Assessment design issues for evaluating critical thinking in nursing, *Holist Nurs Pract* 10(3):41-53, 1996.

Gordon M: *Nursing diagnosis: process and application,* ed 3, St Louis, 1994, Mosby.

Hanneman SK: Advancing nursing practice with a unit-based clinical expert, *Image* 28(4):331-337, 1996.

Jones SA, Brown LN: Alternative views on defining critical thinking through the nursing process, *Holist Nurs Pract* 7(3):71-76, 1993.

Leininger M: *Transcultural nursing: concepts, theories, and practice,* ed 2, New York, 1995, McGraw-Hill.

May BA et al: Critical thinking and clinical competence: a study of their relationship in BSN seniors, *J Nurs Educ* 38(3):100-110, 1999.

North American Nursing Diagnosis Association: News, *Nurs Diagn* 1(3):124, 1990.

Oermann MH: Critical thinking, critical practice, *Nurs Manage* 30(4):40C-40I, 1999.

Orem DE, Taylor SG, Renpenning KM: *Nursing: concepts of practice,* ed 6, St Louis, 2001, Mosby.

Paul R: *Critical thinking: how to prepare students for a rapidly changing world,* Santa Rosa, Calif, 1993, Foundation for Critical Thinking.

Paul RW, Heaslip P: Critical thinking and intuitive nursing practice, *J Adv Nurs* 20:40-47, 1995.

Pender N, Murdaugh CL, Parsons MA: *Health promotion in nursing practice,* ed 4, Paramus, NJ, 2001, Prentice Hall.

Pesut DJ, Herman J: *Clinical reasoning: the art and science of critical and creative thinking,* Albany, 1999, Delmar.

Report of the U.S. Preventive Services Task Force: *Guide to clinical preventive services,* ed 2, Baltimore, 1996, Williams & Wilkins.

Roy C: *The Roy adaptation model: the definitive statement,* ed 2, Englewood Cliffs, NJ, 1998, Prentice Hall.

U.S. Bureau of the Census: *General population characteristics.* Washington, DC, 2000, U.S. Government Printing Office.

Watson G, Glaser EM: *Critical thinking appraisal manual,* Kent, England, 1991, Psychological Corporation.

ntal Tasks and Health
Across the Life Cycle

*M*uch of this book details the method of collecting subjective and objective data about a person to construct a data base. The **data base** is used to assess the health state; to applaud health strengths and assets; and to uncover, diagnose, and treat health problems. To fit this data base into a meaningful frame, one must consider the developmental stage of that individual at that particular time. Appraising the life tasks that currently absorb the individual lets one appreciate the holistic frame of reference.

Consider Walt, a 66-year-old man who seeks health care for recurrent early morning insomnia: He falls asleep easily at night but awakens around 3:00 A.M. and spends hours unable to fall back asleep, sitting in his armchair, watching television. Among the data revealed in the interview is that 7 months ago Walt was forced to retire from a powerful position as sales director for an appliance firm, a position he valued highly. The diagnosis and treatment of this presenting symptom are affected by the knowledge that the suicide rate among forced retirees is markedly greater than that for others in the same age group. Also, suicide rate peaks in later life, being highest among people age 65 and older, and men account for 83% of suicides among people age 65 and older (Centers for Disease Control, 2002). Walt is experiencing the loss of a valued occupational role and social isolation, which increase his risk. Ask yourself—what interventions would you use had this same symptom been presented by a 38-year-old man who is considering whether to stay with his company or to set up his own business?

Growth is continuous and change is perpetual throughout the life cycle. Development is lifelong, not only in biologic growth but also in maturation of the physiologic systems, in cognitive development, and in personality development. Developmental stages are "qualitative changes in thinking, feeling, and behaving that characterize particular time periods of development" (Berk, 2001). During each of the stages, certain issues are dominant and consume more of the individual's attention and energy. The stages are not precisely distinct; transitions occur and overlap exists between stages.

A full consideration of developmental stages is beyond the scope of this text. You must refer to texts on child, adolescent, and lifespan development for a complete overview of the field. However, as you study health assessment, it helps to consider a few of the major frameworks of developmental theory to construct a holistic view of health assessment.

DEVELOPMENTAL STAGES

This section combines data from biologic growth and development and from the developmental theories to give a general portrayal of the individual in each age period of the life cycle. Each portrayal considers the physical, psychosocial, cognitive, and behavioral development of the person. Although they are not intended to be limiting, these portrayals offer a general framework. The stages are:

1. Infancy (birth to 1 year)
2. Early childhood: Toddler (1 to 3 years)
3. Early childhood: Preschooler (3 to 5 or 6 years)
4. School child (6 to 10 or 12 years)
5. Preadolescent (10 to 12 or 13 years)
6. Adolescent (12 or 13 to 19 years)
7. Early adult (20 to 40 years)
8. Middle adult (40 to 64 years)
9. Late adult (65+ years)

INFANCY (BIRTH TO 1 YEAR)

The first year is the most dramatic and rapid period of growth and development. The baby changes from a totally dependent being into a person who interacts with the environment and forms close relationships with other people (Fig. 2–1).

Physical Development
GROWTH

Weight, height, and head circumference reflect physical growth and are sensitive indicators of the infant's general health.

The average normal term infant weighs 3.4 kg ($7^{1}/_{2}$ lb), with 95% of full-term infants ranging from 2.5 to 4.6 kg ($5^{1}/_{2}$ to 10 lb). During the first few days, the baby loses a little weight but regains the birth weight by 10 days. Growth spurts double the birth weight by 4 to 6 months and triple the birth weight by 1 year. Length increases 50% by 1 year.

Head circumference reflects brain size; head growth shows brain growth. At birth, the average head circumference is 35 cm ($13^{1}/_{2}$ inches), with about 95% of infants within the range of 32.6 to 37.2 cm. Brain growth occurs rapidly during the first 2 years. Nutrition is essential, with the proper type and amount of fat calories and essential fatty acids required for brain development (see Chapter 8).

PHYSIOLOGIC DEVELOPMENT

The development of each organ system through the life cycle is described in the corresponding physical examination chapter. But the central nervous system is worth mentioning here because during infancy it makes the most dramatic gains. Tremendous brain growth occurs during this period. Also, the baby has numerous primitive reflexes that are present at birth or soon after and persist for specific time periods. These are under subcortical control; as the cerebral cortex

2–1

grows and matures, it inhibits their expression. In a normal infant, these reflexes should disappear at specific times during the first year (see Chapter 23, Neurologic System). Certain protective reflexes (cough, gag, sneeze, eye-blink) are always present. Visual acuity is very poor at birth (about 20/800) and for the first few months because of immature and widely spaced foveas (i.e., the area on the retina of keenest vision). But acuity develops rapidly and is close to adult levels by the end of the first year (Barnard and Edgar, 1996).

Psychosocial Development

STAGES OF EGO DEVELOPMENT

Erik Erikson (1902 to 1994) focused on cultural and societal influences as determinants of behavior. Erikson was concerned with the growth of the **ego,** the conscious, organized, rational part of the personality. He described eight stages of ego development that encompass the life span (Erikson, 1963).

Each stage is characterized by a distinct conflict relating to the person's physiologic maturation and to what society expects of a person at that age. Each conflict is a bipolar issue, a point at which personality development may go one way or another through the choices made by the infant's caregivers, or later, by the individual. The bipolar aspect means that the conflict can be resolved along a continuum, and have a more positive or a more negative outcome.

ERIKSON'S THEORY OF TRUST VERSUS MISTRUST

Erikson's first stage has a broad psychosocial dimension. The crucial element in this stage is the *quality* of the parent-child relationship. The infant is completely helpless and depends on the parent for food, warmth, comfort, and companionship. When the parent is responsive and consistent in nurturing, the psychological conflict is resolved on the positive side and the infant learns **trust.** The security from this trust extends to trust in others and in the self. The infant learns that the world is a safe and reliable place and that he or she is welcome in it. If the parent is unresponsive, unnurturing, haphazard, or abusing, the infant learns **mistrust.** Since the infant never feels secure, he or she experiences anxiety and alienation and may protect him- or herself by withdrawing. Without a trusting foundation, this individual will flounder in attempts to resolve future crises.

Absolute trust actually is not the healthy goal of this conflict. When resolution of this crisis is successful, the infant holds *relatively* more trust than mistrust. Total trust would impede survival in later years because not everyone or everything in the world *should* be trusted.

Cognitive Development

Jean Piaget (1896 to 1980) described stages of cognitive development in the growing child. Cognition is defined as how the individual perceives and processes information about the world; it is the ability to know. Piaget believed that a child's thinking develops progressively from simple reflex behavior into complex logical and abstract thought. This development is biologically inherent in each maturing child and occurs independently of any special training.

The child's cognitive development proceeds through four definite and sequential stages. Each stage demonstrates a *qualitative* change, representing a new way of thinking and behaving. Although the ages of reaching the stages are approximate, the sequence of stages never varies. All children move through the same stages in the same order; no stage is skipped. Each stage is the foundation for the next, and the next stage builds on the stage before it. At each stage, the child's *scheme* (how the child views the world) becomes more intricate and complex.

According to Piaget, the first stage of **sensorimotor skills** (birth to 2 years) is a time of intelligent activity, although full language skill has not yet developed. Infants perceive information through the five senses and learn to modify their behavior in response to these environmental stimuli. At birth, the only response is an array of reflexes (crying, rooting, sucking, grasping) that occur automatically. Gradually, the infant learns the important concept of **object permanence,** that objects and people continue to exist even when they are no longer in sight. Piaget believed that this begins around 7 months, when the infant searches for an object that is partly hidden but does not search for one completely out of sight. By 9 to 10 months, the infant looks behind a screen for an object, but only if it was seen to be hidden there. By 18 to 24 months, the concept is fully developed and the child conducts a true search in many places for objects hidden from sight. As this concept develops, the infant also learns that he or she is *separate* from objects in the environment. Last, by age 2 the infant has acquired **mental representation** (or thought) and can think of an external event without actually experiencing it.

Piaget's work stimulated tremendous research on infant cognition, and it formed the base of our practice of providing developmentally stimulating environments for children. However, recent research indicates Piaget underestimated the cognitive capacity of infants and toddlers, perhaps because he lacked the sophisticated experimental techniques of today (Berk, 2001). Infants as young as 3 months old appear to have an abstract understanding of the world as a real and predictable place. Spelke (1992) showed that babies acted surprised and looked longer at "magical" events, such as an object disappearing through a hidden trapdoor, or an object stopping in midair without support. Spelke concluded that infants know that objects continue to exist even when you do not look at them, and they know that objects cannot pass through barriers. Infants have an awareness of real physical events even though they lack the motor coordination to demonstrate this.

Behavioral Development

GROSS MOTOR SKILLS

These skills include posture, head balance, sitting, crawling, and walking. Their development is predictable because it follows the direction of myelinization (laying down of myelin) in the nervous system; cephalocaudal (head-to-foot direction) and proximodistal (central-to-peripheral direction, or midline before extremities).*

Some head balance already is present at birth for protection; when prone, the baby can turn the head to the side to

---

*Tables summarizing growth and development milestones for infancy and for other age groups can be found in *Student Laboratory Manual for Physical Examination and Health Assessment,* 4th ed.

avoid suffocation. Otherwise there is marked head lag, as when pulled to a sitting position from a lying position. By 3 months of age, the baby can raise the head *and* chest from a prone position with the arms extended for support. By 4 months of age, the head and chest are raised 90 degrees, and only slight head lag is demonstrated when the child is pulled to a sitting position. Sitting alone without support occurs at 6 to 7 months of age.

After 7 months, the baby ventures from the sitting position to explore the environment. Crawling usually begins around 7 months. At 8 months, the baby pulls to a stand and stands while holding onto an object for support. Between 9 and 11 months, the baby starts to "cruise" the room, walking upright while holding onto the furniture. Usually, the child can stand independently around 11 months, and by 12 months the child walks alone.

FINE MOTOR SKILLS

The development of fine motor skills involves using the hands and fingers for **prehension,** or the act of grasping. The infant is born with a grasp reflex; it fades at 2 months of age and is absent at 3 months of age. At 3 months the infant expresses interest in an object more with the eyes than with the hands. At 4 months, the infant inspects his or her hands, looks from object to hands and back, and may try to grasp an object with the hands but overshoots the mark. The voluntary two-handed grasp is present at 4 to 5 months.

Further distal refinement follows at 8 to 10 months with a crude pincer grasp using the index, fourth, and fifth fingers. By 10 months, the index finger is an apposition with the thumb for a neat pincer grasp, and the baby is absorbed in picking up raisins, finger foods, and toys (Fig. 2–2). By 11 months the baby puts objects into a container and removes them. And at 13 months the baby builds a tower of two blocks.

LANGUAGE SKILLS

Crying is the infant's first means of communication. Cries are undifferentiated at first, but by 1 month of age the infant alters the pitch and intensity of the cry to communicate different needs, such as hunger, discomfort, or loneliness. Vocal sounds build rapidly; the baby laughs out loud at 3 months, coos when he or she awakens or when someone talks to him or

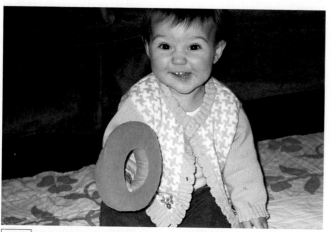

2–2

her at 2 to 4 months, and babbles at 6 months. At 9 to 10 months, the baby can imitate the sounds of others, although he or she may not necessarily understand them. At 12 months, a baby usually can say the first recognizable word with meaning.

PERSONAL-SOCIAL SKILLS

Throughout the 1st year, the infant learns more and more social ties that bind her or him to other people. Early on, the baby shows a visual preference for the human face, and even in the first 30 to 60 minutes following birth watches the mother intently (see Fig. 2–1). The social smile erupts at 6 to 8 weeks, to the family's delight and continual reinforcement. At 4 months, the baby laughs and enjoys other people, and at 6 months extends arms to the parent to be picked up.

Imitation, or the copying of another person's behavior, is present in a limited way in newborns. Even the young baby will copy adult facial expressions such as opening the mouth, protruding the tongue, and pursing the lips. As the neurologic system develops, at 7 months, the baby imitates others' actions, at 9 months their sounds, and at 10 months waves bye-bye and enjoys interactive games such as pat-a-cake and peek-a-boo. At 11 months, the baby can help with feeding and dressing and follows simple directions. Emotions develop during the 1st year, and by 12 months the baby will give a hug or kiss and show jealousy, fear, or anger.

Infant's Periodic Health Examination

Table 2–1 lists the services that you as health care provider should address during the infant's well-baby checkups. Note the aspects of screening at birth, the immunization schedule, and the parent counseling items regarding diet and injury prevention. Screening measures include those for high-risk groups, such as hearing impairment, and screening for lead poisoning. Note also that these tables are not intended to be a complete list of all the steps that *should* be included in the examination checkup. Instead, the table lists preventive services that were studied and shown to be clinically effective (U.S. Preventive Services Task Force, 1996).

SUDDEN INFANT DEATH SYNDROME (SIDS)

One important parent counseling measure is the "Back to Sleep" campaign that promotes sleeping on their backs for healthy infants as a way of decreasing the risk of SIDS (Gilbert-Barness and Barness, 1996; American Academy of Pediatrics, 1994). About 6000 infant deaths each year in the United States are attributed to SIDS, with the peak incidence occurring between 2 and 4 months. Although research has not identified the exact causes of SIDS, studies in multiple countries reported striking reductions in SIDS deaths of over 50% after media campaigns that urged avoidance of prone (abdomen) sleeping. The mechanism of sudden death in a prone position may be an increased resistance to airflow, obstruction from displacement of the mandible, compression of the nose in soft bedding, or compromised blood supply to the brain stem (Gilbert-Barness and Barness, 1996). Although the new recommendations will not prevent all SIDS deaths, placing the baby on the back to sleep will decrease the risk of SIDS. Additional parent counseling strategies to help reduce SIDS risk include avoiding smoking around the infant, avoiding drugs and alcohol while preg-

TABLE 2-1: Periodic Health Examination: Birth to 10 Years

INTERVENTIONS CONSIDERED AND RECOMMENDED FOR THE PERIODIC HEALTH EXAMINATION	LEADING CAUSES OF DEATH
	Conditions originating in perinatal period
	Congenital anomalies
	Sudden infant death syndrome (SIDS)
	Unintentional injuries (nonmotor vehicle)
	Motor vehicle injuries

INTERVENTIONS FOR THE GENERAL POPULATION

Screening

Height and weight
Blood pressure
Vision screen (age 3–4 yr)
Hemoglobinopathy screen (birth)[1]
Phenylalanine level (birth)[2]
T_4 and/or TSH (birth)[3]

Limit fat and cholesterol; maintain caloric balance; emphasize grains, fruits, vegetables (age ≥2 yr)
Regular physical activity
Substance use
    Effects of passive smoking
    Antitobacco message
Dental health
    Regular visits to dental care provider
    Floss, brush with fluoride toothpaste daily
    Advice about baby bottle tooth decay

Counseling

Injury prevention
    Child safety car seats (age <5 yr)
    Lap-shoulder belts (age ≥5 yr)
    Bicycle helmet; avoid bicycling near traffic
    Smoke detector, flame retardant sleepwear
    Hot water heater temperature <120–130°F
    Window/stair guards, pool fence
    Safe storage of drugs, toxic substances, firearms, and matches
    Syrup of ipecac, poison control phone number
    CPR training for parents/caretakers
Diet and exercise
    Breastfeeding, iron-enriched formula and foods (infants and toddlers)

Immunizations

Diphtheria-tetanus-pertussis (DTP)[4]
Oral poliovirus (OPV)[5]
Measles-mumps-rubella (MMR)[6]
H. influenzae type b (Hib) conjugate[7]
Hepatitis B[8]
Varicella[9]

Chemoprophylaxis

Ocular prophylaxis (birth)

INTERVENTIONS FOR HIGH-RISK POPULATIONS

POPULATION	POTENTIAL INTERVENTIONS
Preterm or low birth weight	Hemoglobin/hematocrit
Infants of mothers at risk for HIV	HIV testing
Low income; immigrants	Hemoglobin/hematocrit; PPD
TB contacts	PPD
Native American/Alaska Native	Hemoglobin/hematocrit; PPD; hepatitis A vaccine; pneumococcal vaccine
Travelers to developing countries	Hepatitis A vaccine
Residents of long-term care facilities	PPD; hepatitis A vaccine; influenza vaccine
Certain chronic medical conditions	PPD; pneumococcal vaccine; influenza vaccine
Increased individual or community lead exposure	Blood lead level
Inadequate water fluoridation	Daily fluoride supplement
Family h/o skin cancer; nevi; fair skin, eyes, hair	Avoid excess/midday sun, use protective clothing

[1]Whether screening should be universal or targeted to high-risk groups will depend on the proportion of high-risk individuals in the screening area, and other considerations. [2]If done during first 24 hr of life, repeat at age 2 wk. [3]Optimally between day 2 and 6, but in all cases before newborn nursery discharge. [4]2, 4, 6, and 12–18 mo, once between ages 4–6 yr (DTaP may be used at 15 mo and older). [5]2, 4, 6–18 mo, once between ages 4–6 yr. [6]12–15 mo and 4–6 yr. [7]2, 4, 6, and 12–15 mo, no dose needed at 6 mo if PRP-OMP vaccine is used for first 2 doses. [8]Birth, 1 mo, 6 mo; or, 0–2 mo, 1–2 mo later, and 6–18 mo. If not done in infancy: current visit, and 1 and 6 mo later. [9]12–18 mo; or older child without hx of chickenpox or previous immunization. Include information on risk in adulthood, duration of immunity, and potential need for booster doses.
CPR, Cardiopulmonary resuscitation; *HIV,* human immunodeficiency virus; *TB,* tuberculosis; *PPD,* purified protein derivative; *STDs,* sexually transmitted diseases; *BCG,* bacille Calmette-Guérin.
Adapted from U.S. Preventive Services Task Force: *Guide to clinical preventive services,* ed 2, Baltimore, 1996, Williams & Wilkins.
For detailed high-risk definitions, see complete table at http://evolve.elsevier.com/Jarvis/.

nant, using a firm, flat mattress, avoiding overheating, avoiding crib bumpers, stuffed animals, waterbeds, and pillows, and continuing to breast feed the baby as long as possible.

EARLY CHILDHOOD, TODDLER (1 TO 3 YEARS)

With successful completion of 1st-year tasks, the child enters the 2nd year secure in a basic sense of trust. That security plus maturing muscles and developing language enable the child to launch into the process of exploring the environment (Fig. 2–3). The toddler explores everything, inhaling the world with the zeal of all first-time adventurers. Developmental tasks of this next stage include:

1. Differentiating self from others, particularly the mother
2. Tolerating separation from mother or parent

2–3

3. Withstanding delayed gratification
4. Controlling bodily functions
5. Acquiring socially acceptable behavior
6. Acquiring verbal communication
7. Interacting with others in a more empathic way (i.e., understanding another person's emotional state)

The child does not master all tasks during the toddler years, but a good foundation at this stage will facilitate successful completion of other tasks later.

Physical Development

GROWTH

The rate of growth decelerates during the 2nd year, with the child gaining an average of 2.5 kg (5$^1/_2$ lb) in body weight and 12 cm (4$^3/_4$ in) in length.

APPEARANCE

Toddler lordosis describes the normal upright posture of the toddler, with the potbelly; sway back; and short, slightly bowed legs. The increase in head circumference slows, and the head circumference equals the chest circumference between 1 and 2 years. After the 2nd year, the chest circumference exceeds individual head and abdominal measurements, and the extremities grow faster than the trunk.

PHYSIOLOGIC SYSTEMS

Maturation of the physiologic systems is detailed in the corresponding physical examination chapters. Some neurologic advances are cited now because they permit developmental changes during the toddler years. For example, most brain growth occurs during the first 2 years, and changes in certain cortical areas permit language and motor development. In the spinal cord, myelination is almost complete by age 2, matching the gross motor achievements in locomotion. Visual acuity is close to 20/40 at 2 years and close to 20/30 by age 3 (Barnard and Edgar, 1996). The maturing convergence-accommodation mechanism matches the toddler's fascination with minute objects.

Psychosocial Development

Autonomy is the goal of all daily activities. The pursuit of independence occupies the toddler. For example, muscle matura-

tion allows walking, exploring, and some self-care in feeding and dressing; refined visual acuity enhances close scrutiny and attention span; and language advances so the child can make known independent demands, such as "me do," "mommy way," or "me out." Between 12 and 18 months, the toddler ventures away from the parent to explore the immediate environment, still using her or him as a home base to come back to for support. Practice builds confidence, which encourages more exploration. Between 18 months and 3 years, it occurs to the child that he or she really has become quite separate from the parent. This creates some anxiety, which is manifested in the negativism, or the "terrible twos" behavior, normally seen at this age.

AUTONOMY VERSUS SHAME AND DOUBT (1 TO 3 YEARS)

The quest for autonomy characterizes the psychologic conflict of Erikson's second stage. The toddler wants to be autonomous and to govern his or her own body and experiences. The child wants to apply newly attained skills to explore the world. However, the child has not yet attained any sense of discrimination or judgment. The parent lives in the balance of letting the child explore but also firmly protecting the child from experiences that are dangerous or frustrating for the child's current ability level. This conflict is resolved favorably when the parent uses patience and appropriate guidance and has reasonable expectations of the toddler's capabilities and attention span. A parent who is overcontrolling or undercontrolling may foster a negative outcome. Then the child may feel shame and experience doubts about his or her own ability.

Erikson believed that toilet training symbolizes this stage. The toddler's muscle maturation has progressed to the "holding on" and "letting go" of things; this naturally extends to the sphincter muscles.

Cognitive Development

During the 2nd year, the toddler is still considered to be in Piaget's **sensorimotor period.** The readiness for independence is demonstrated between 12 and 18 months as the child now tries out new activities and new experiments to reach a goal. To reach a desired toy in her toybox, a girl at this age may try the various routes of taking out each object one by one, overturning the box and dumping the contents out, or climbing into the box herself. Learning comes by trial and error.

Between 18 and 24 months, the child develops **mental representation** for external events. This is a major achievement because the toddler can *think* through plans to reach a goal rather than merely perform them and observe the results by trial and error.

The concept of **object permanence** now is fully developed. The toddler comprehends both visible and invisible *displacements.* That means the child can search for an object in several places, even though it was not seen as it was hidden.

Around age 2, Piaget's **preoperational** stage begins. This use of symbols to represent objects and experiences is discussed in the next section on preschoolers.

Behavioral Development

GROSS MOTOR SKILLS

Locomotion advances as the toddler usually walks alone at 12 months, runs stiffly at 18 months, and runs well without falling at 2 years. At 2 years, the child also can walk up and down stairs. The child jumps with both feet by 2 years.

FINE MOTOR SKILLS

Fine motor development shows increasing manual dexterity. At 15 months, the child can drop a pellet into a narrow-neck container and can hurl and retrieve objects. Fourteen-month-old hands can hold a pencil and make scribbles, whereas by 2 years, the child can reproduce a vertical line from a demonstration.

LANGUAGE SKILLS

Language progresses from a vocabulary of about two words at 1 year to a spurt of about 200 words by 2 years. Then the 2-year-old combines words into simple two-word phrases—"all gone," "me up," "baby crying." This is called **telegraphic speech,** which is usually a combination of a noun and a verb and includes only words that have concrete meaning. Interest in language is high during the 2nd year, and a 2-year-old seems to understand all that is said to him or her. A 3-year-old uses more complex sentences with more parts of speech.

PERSONAL-SOCIAL SKILLS

Toddlers are usually compliant and cooperative with parents who are warm and sensitive and have reasonable expectations (Berk, 2001). However, parents often are surprised at the swift transformation of their loving affectionate child into a determined toddler who resists requests. Toddlers want their parents' approval but also want to assert themselves and do as many things for themselves as they can. As they test their powers, they sometimes clash with parents' restrictions, and a battle of wills results. "No" seems to be their favorite word.

This **negativism** is a normal part of the quest for autonomy. Although they protest vigorously, toddlers seem to fare better with firm, consistent limits. The thought of a limitless world and of personal untested powers is disabling to the child. Knowing where they stand, even if they disagree, is reassuring to toddlers.

Ritualism emerges along with the negativity. A 2-year-old wants things done in the same way; any change in schedule or habit is upsetting. A consistent routine assures the child that the world is predictable and orderly. Ritualism is heightened at age $2^{1}/_{2}$, especially at bedtime, when the child insists on the same order of nighttime tasks or the same order of colored blankets on the bed.

Although attachment to the parent is still strong, the toddler begins to play alone. Children 1 and 2 years of age venture away to explore but still need the reassurance of the parent's being there. Play with peers can be comical to the observer. Toddlers engage in **parallel** play—that is, playing the same thing side by side without interaction and without trying to influence each other's behavior. The two children seemingly ignore each other yet unobtrusively check the other out to note what is happening. Imitation in play is apparent, both of peer activities and especially of parent activities such as sweeping, lawn mowing, or cooking. As the toddler is increasingly able to form mental images, play reveals increased imagination.

Toddler Periodic Health Examination

Study Table 2–1 for the immunization schedule, examination, screening measures, and parent counseling measures to address with parents of young children. Note the screening measures for high-risk categories of lead poisoning, tuberculosis exposure, and anemia.

EARLY CHILDHOOD, PRESCHOOL (3 TO 5 OR 6 YEARS)

Successful mastery of the toddler tasks plus a highly energized state make the preschooler ready for this time of developing initiative and purpose. Although parental relationships are still the most important, the preschooler begins to turn to other children and adults to broaden learning and play. Tasks during this period include:

1. Realizing separateness as an individual
2. Identifying sex role and its functions
3. Developing a conscience
4. Developing a sense of initiative
5. Interacting with others in socially acceptable ways
6. Growing use of language for social interaction
7. Developing readiness for school

Physical Development

The rate of growth continues at a slower pace, and the average child gains about 2 kg ($4^{1}/_{2}$ lb) in weight and 7 cm ($2^{3}/_{4}$ in) in height per year. The appearance changes as the "baby face" matures, the potbelly slims, and the legs elongate more than the trunk does. The preschooler looks taller, slimmer, and more graceful.

Most physiologic systems are now mature, but the musculoskeletal system is still developing. Muscles are growing, and cartilage is changing to bone at a faster rate than before. Nutrition is crucial for bone growth. A serious nutrient loss at this age alters the shape, thickness, and growth of bones.

Psychosocial Development

Although still primarily egocentric, the preschooler now broadens the scope to include some awareness of other people's interests, needs, and values. As this happens, the **conscience** or **superego** develops. The child learns right from wrong and their corresponding rewards and punishments.

IDENTIFYING THE GENDER ROLE

As children become aware of their separateness, they also learn that they belong to a further differentiated category—male or female. They are learning **gender,** or how males and females *do* differ. As early as age 2, children label themselves as "girl" or "boy" and assign their family members and pets to these basic gender categories. Then children begin to develop gender roles by a process called **gender typing,** or how society says males and females *should* differ. Children learn the behaviors and attitudes that their culture says are right for a man or a woman. The parents have a strong influence in gender typing, as is seen, for example, as a preschool girl imitates words and actions she has observed in her mother. But her social circle is enlarging, and the girl also picks up important messages from peers, teachers, books, and television about how girls and boys should differ. These messages can forge strong gender stereotyping, and the preschooler often develops rigid rules about what boys and girls should wear and about what roles they can "be" when they play make-believe (Berk, 2001).

Learning at this stage has a broader scope, though, than just learning the appropriate gender role. As the girl mentioned earlier identifies with her mother, she assimilates and internalizes the mother's ideals and values. She learns the standards of society presented to her by the words and deeds of the mother. This is the development of the conscience, which now will direct the girl's behavior. Interaction with peers helps to develop the conscience too, as in play where children construct notions of justice and fair play.

INITIATIVE VERSUS GUILT (4 TO 5 YEARS)

For this stage of ego development, Erikson believed that the child's chief task is to develop a sense of initiative. With increasing locomotor and mental power, the child now has an energy surplus, resulting in determination and enterprise. The child plans and attacks a new task with gusto and wants to stay with it. Any failures are easily forgotten in the quest to test the world. When the parent encourages, reassures, and cheers the child on (while protecting him or her from harm), the child learns self-assertion, spontaneity, self-sufficiency, direction, and purpose. But if the parent ridicules, punishes, or prevents the child from following through on tasks that could be done, the child feels guilty. The guilt exists not only when the child acts inappropriately but also when he or she is thinking of goals that the child would like to accomplish.

By nurturing successes and promoting a healthy self-image, the parents help the preschooler develop *self-esteem.* Self-esteem is the judgment the child makes about his or her own worth as well as any feelings about the judgment (Berk, 2001). Self-esteem is most important because it becomes the way we value our own competence. Our self-esteem affects our emotional experiences, future behavior, and long-term psychological adjustment (Berk, 2001).

Cognitive Development

Piaget's **preoperational stage** covers age 2 to 7 years, a longer span than the preschool years. It is characterized by **symbolic function,** because the child now uses symbols to represent people, objects, and events. This process is liberating. Now the child can conjure up thoughts of the father, for example, without actually seeing him or hearing his voice. The symbolic function is revealed in child's play, as in **delayed imitation.** That means a child can witness an event, form a mental representation of it, and imitate it later in the absence of the model. For example, a little boy watches his father dress and leave for work, then later in the day the boy wraps a tie around his neck, packs his "briefcase," and heads for the door.

Although representational thought is a great milestone, the preschooler's thinking continues to be limited. Thinking is concrete and literal. The preschooler focuses on only one aspect of a situation at a time and ignores others, a characteristic known as **centration.** For example, given a pile of blocks, a preschooler will sort by color (red, blue,

yellow), or by shape (square, triangle, circle), but not by both. According to Piaget, a child in the preoperational stage is **egocentric.** This child cannot see another's point of view and feels no need to elaborate his or her own point of view, because the child assumes everyone else sees things as he or she does (Piaget, 1968). More recent research suggests that 4-year-olds can have an awareness of another's view (Berk, 2001).

Behavioral Development

MOTOR SKILLS

The physical bumbling of the toddler fades, and the preschool child demonstrates admirable gross motor and fine motor control (Fig. 2–4). A 4-year-old child can hop on one foot. A 5-year-old child can skip on alternate feet and jump rope and may begin to swim and skate. Girls often achieve fine motor milestones ahead of boys of the same age. A 3-year-old child can draw a circle; a 4-year-old child can cut on a line with scissors, draw a person, and make crude letters. A 5-year-old can string beads, control a crayon well, and copy a square and letters and numbers, and has demonstrated preference for the right or left hand.

2–4

LANGUAGE SKILLS

Between 3 and 4 years of age, the child uses three- to four-word **telegraphic** sentences containing only essential words. By 5 to 6 years, the sentences are six to eight words long, and grammar is well developed.

Piaget labeled the earlier speech pattern as egocentric (Piaget, 1975). Children at this age talk incessantly. They are wrapped up in their own thoughts and talk to themselves merely for the pleasure of hearing their own voices say the words. Piaget believed speech here is in the form of a *monologue* to the self, or a *collective monologue* between two children, in which they talk at each other but are still absorbed in themselves, and no communication has occurred.

However, more recent research challenges Piaget's views and demonstrates that this **private speech** is a problem-solving tool that is beneficial to all children as they try new tasks or work through unfamiliar situations (Berk, 1994). Children chatter to themselves between the ages of 4 and 6; this chatter becomes inaudible muttering during early elementary school, and then it mostly drops away. Researchers noted that when a child undertakes a new task, an adult usually explains the steps needed to perform the task, often in detail, as directions or strategies. When the child next works through the task alone, he or she uses private speech as a way of repeating the adult's expert advice as his or her own independent guidelines. This evolves into muttering because one often uses verbal shorthand with one's own self; that is, the child omits saying the words that refer to familiar steps and verbalizes only the words that refer to the still-confusing steps. Finally, as the child has mastered the skill, the air is silent because the mind has internalized the private speech into thinking inner speech. Private speech reemerges throughout life as we confront new tasks or unfamiliar or stressful situations (Berk, 1994).

PERSONAL-SOCIAL SKILLS

The preschooler is self-assertive, but the negativism of the toddler years has diminished. This child wants to please others. By taking on the values of the family and developing a conscience, the child monitors his or her own behavior to maximize acceptance. The preschooler is proud of his or her self-sufficiency and accomplishes everyday self-care (dressing, feeding, toileting) almost completely. The world enlarges because the child's anxiety toward strangers and fear of separation decreases; the at-home preschooler is able to tolerate brief separations from the parents to enjoy visiting peers or preschool. Some preschoolers have already been in day care from an early age, and parental separations are less of an issue.

With their growing social regard, preschoolers enjoy **cooperative play** with each other. This means that they play the same game and interact while doing it. The child's imagination runs rampant, and this factor shows in the play. Preschoolers love to dress up and imitate the sex role behaviors of their parents as well as admired adult models, such as nurses, doctors, media heroes, firefighters, or police officers. Often this make-believe or fantasy play is a coping strategy: a sheltered workshop in which the preschooler can work out conflicts and fears or master life experiences.

It is easy for fantasy and reality to blur. Children experience the greatest number of new fears between 2 and 6 years of age. Visions of ghosts and monsters, fear of the dark, fear of being lost—all arise from the child's increased imagination as well as from some frightening experiences that the child really has had. Also, beginning around age $2^1/_2$ or 3 years, children often invent imaginary playmates. The imaginary friend often serves as an alter ego and tries out behaviors that the child yearns to try or takes the blame when the child misbehaves. Although it is important for a time, the imaginary friend is easily given up when the child enters school.

MIDDLE CHILDHOOD, SCHOOL-AGE CHILD (6 TO 10 OR 12 YEARS)

The best preparation for this age is a firm foundation in trust, autonomy, and initiative (Fig. 2–5). Secure in these attributes, the child is able to move into a larger world and tackle these tasks:

1. Mastering skills that will be needed later as an adult
2. Winning approval from other adults and peers

2–5

3. Building self-esteem and a positive self-concept
4. Taking a place in a peer group
5. Adopting moral standards

Physical Development

Physical growth is slow but steady during the school years. The average child gains about 3 kg ($6^1/_2$ lb) and grows about 5.5 cm (2 in) per year. The growth rates in boys and girls are basically the same, with boys only slightly heavier and taller than girls. Black children are slightly larger and Asian children slightly smaller than white children of the same age. The preadolescent growth spurt occurs earlier in girls, at about age 10, as compared with age 12 for boys.

The physical appearance of the school-age child is relatively slimmer than that of the younger child because of the older child's proportionately longer legs, diminishing body fat, and a lower center of gravity. Although the cranium achieved most of its growth in the early years, now the bones of the face and jaw grow faster. During these years, primary teeth are lost, which the child hails as a big event and developmental milestone. The eruption of large permanent teeth into a mouth and face that looks too small for them gives this child the ungainly, so-called ugly duckling appearance.

Body carriage is more agile and graceful. Bones continue to ossify during these years, and bone replaces cartilage. Muscles are stronger and more developed, though not yet fully mature. Neuromuscular control is more coordinated. All these refinements ready the school child for repetitive pursuit of activities requiring fine motor skills, such as writing, drawing, needlework, small model building, and playing instruments, and large muscle activities, such as running, throwing, jumping, biking, and swimming.

Psychosocial Development

Erikson highlighted the directing of energy into learning skills when he characterized middle childhood as a period focused on **industry versus inferiority**. In this stage, age 6 to 11 years, the child focuses much of the time at school. Now, the approval and esteem of people outside the immediate family become important. The child wins this recognition by working and producing. Play and fantasy give way to mastering the skills that the child will need later to compete in the adult world. This child values independence in tackling a new task and takes pleasure in carrying it through to completion. The young worker is eager, diligent, and absorbed. Also, the value of social relationships emerges as the child sees the benefits of working in an organized group. Children learn to divide labor and to cooperate to achieve a common goal.

Real achievement at this stage builds a feeling of confidence, competence, and industry. The child is rewarded by his or her own inner sense of satisfaction in achieving a skill and, more importantly at this age, by external rewards such as approval from teachers, parents, and peers in the form of grades, allowance, or special gifts. Problems arise when the child feels inferior. If the child believes that he or she cannot measure up to society's expectations, the child loses confidence and does not take pleasure in the work. A gnawing feeling of inferiority and incompetence grows and will continue to haunt this child.

The reality is that no one can master everything. There is bound to be something at which each child will feel inferior. Caring parents and teachers will try to balance these weaker skills with areas in which the child can excel. The problem is that, in some cultures, success in certain areas has a higher social value, particularly among peers. For example, in Western cultures, team sports are admired more than playing chess, or success in reading may be rewarded more than in drawing. The challenge to adults is to provide the successful experiences and positive reinforcement so that each child can achieve.

At this age, peer approval is beginning to be significant. During middle childhood, it is important to belong to a peer group. The peer group is a key socializing agent. Group solidarity is enhanced by secret codes or strict rules. The child conforms to group rules because acceptance is paramount. The child begins to prefer peer group activities to activities with the parents.

Cognitive Development

Piaget labels the stage of middle childhood, age 7 to 11 years, as the period in which the child focuses on **concrete operations**. At this age, the child can use symbols (mental representations) of objects and events in more logical ways. This means a child can experience mentally what she or he would have had to do physically before. For example, to describe the classic hopscotch maneuvers to you, a girl now can articulate them ("first you hop on one foot . . .") rather than merely performing them.

Armed with the ability to use thinking to experience things or events, the school child can:

- *Use numbers.* While counting with numbers begins in preschool years, the school-age child has the combinational skill to add and subtract, multiply and divide.
- *Read.* By using printed symbols (words) for objects and events, the child can process a significant amount of information. Also, reading fosters independence in learning.

- *Serialize.* While this begins in preschool years, the school-age child can order objects by an increasing or decreasing scale, such as according to number size (smallest to largest) or weight (lightest to heaviest).
- *Classify.* This is the ability to sort objects by something they have in common. While young children can do this, the school-age child is able to organize a hierarchy of classes and subclasses. It shows in the school-age child's penchant for collections: rocks, shells, novelty cards, cars, and dolls. A child spends many hours sorting the collections, and the logic of the classification system gets more complex as the child grows.
- *Understand conservation principles.* Understanding conservation of matter is the ability to tell the difference between how things seem and how they really are. It is the ability to see that mass or quantity stays constant even though shape or position is transformed. For example, the child who can conserve sees that two equal amounts of water remain the same even if one is poured into a beaker with a different shape.

At this age, thinking is more stable and logical. The school-age child can *decenter* and consider all sides of a situation to form a conclusion. The school-age child is able to reason, but this reasoning capacity still is limited because he or she cannot yet deal with abstract ideas.

PREADOLESCENCE (10 TO 12 OR 13 YEARS)

This period covers fifth to eighth grades, ending with puberty (Fig. 2–6). Although this stage is still part of childhood, children in this group have common skills and interests that set them apart. It becomes more difficult now to typify characteristics of a single year. Because of rapid growth, the age levels start to blend and overlap. A child may be at one level physically and intellectually but at another level socially. Children of the same age show diverse development levels.

Physical Development

Physical growth is markedly different at this stage; boys show slow and steady growth, whereas girls have rapid growth. On the average, the growth spurt begins in girls at age 10 years and reaches its greatest velocity at 12, whereas in

2–6

boys the growth spurt begins at 12 and attains its maximum velocity at 14 years.

Even among girls, growth is varied. In a group of 11-year-old girls, each girl looks different from the others. Some look like children, and some are starting to look like adolescents. At 10 years, some girls have begun their growth spurt and have begun to grow pubic hair and to have breast development. At 12 years, girls demonstrate the most rapid growth in height and weight. The breasts enlarge, the areolae darken, growth of axillary hair begins, and menarche occurs.

Physical size among 11-year-old boys is fairly uniform. At 12 years, boys show a wider range of growth. Most demonstrate the onset of secondary sex characteristics with initial genital growth, appearance of pubic hair, and the occurrence of erections and nocturnal emissions.

Boys and girls both exhibit a great amount of physical restlessness. Their activity is well directed into individual and team sports. Their percolating energy makes it hard for them to sit still, and it shows by tapping the foot or drumming the finger.

2–7

Psychosocial Development

Parent-child ties exhibit some strain as the child gradually starts to drift away from the family. The parents continue to set standards and values, but the child begins to challenge authority and to reject their standards. Parents decrease in stature in the child's eyes as the child learns that parents are not perfect and do not know everything. Yet the child loves the parents. He or she needs and wants some restrictions. Making up one's own rules is too frightening.

At 9 to 10 years, the child demonstrates a new ability to love by establishing a relationship with a best friend. This is important because the best friend is the first one outside the family that the child loves as being as important as himself or herself. By sharing interests, goals, and secret ideas with the best friend, the child learns a lot about himself or herself. This is comforting because the child realizes that he or she is not so different from other children after all. This yields a valuable lesson in self-acceptance.

Preadolescents demonstrate social interest outside the family. There is strong identity with the peer group by a small *clique* or a larger, more loosely organized *crowd* formation. Girls and boys stay within their own sex group. The clique has an exclusive membership, and one is privileged to belong. The code of the clique is important, with rules for dressing, speaking, and behaving in common. The child merges his or her identity with that of the peer group. The child is substituting conformity with the family to that with the peers because he or she needs the security of a temporary identity before formulating a clear sense of self (Berk, 2001).

Despite the fact that peer groupings are composed of the same sex, some preadolescents show an emerging interest in mixed groups, an interest that will flourish in adolescence.

ADOLESCENCE (12 OR 13 TO 19 YEARS)

This is a transition stage between childhood and adulthood (Fig. 2–7). Beginning at puberty and extending through the teenage years, the most important task of adolescence is the **search for identity**—"who I really am." With successful mas-

tery of skills from the previous stage, childhood ends. Now the adolescent must process the information from earlier stages and assume a personal identity that is more than just the sum of childhood experiences. The search for identity is the motive behind all the other tasks of the period:

1. Searching for one's identity
2. Appreciating one's achievements
3. Growing independent from parents
4. Forming close relationships with peers
5. Developing analytic thinking
6. Evolving one's own value system
7. Developing a sexual identity
8. Beginning to choose a career

Physical Development

Adolescence begins with puberty. Puberty is a time of dramatic physiologic change. It includes the growth spurt—rapid growth in height, weight, and muscular development; development of primary and secondary sex characteristics; and maturation of the reproductive organs.

A changing body affects a person's self-concept. With bodies that are changing so rapidly, it is difficult for boys and girls to adjust. Their self-awareness peaks; they continually compare how their body looks with that of their peers and to some ideal standard of attractiveness. They are keenly attuned to the appearance of secondary sex characteristics but are embarrassed if these appear too early or too late. It is best when their own development parallels that of close friends and peers. Being an early maturer or, especially, a late maturer adds to normal self-doubts that they experience.

Physical health is generally good. Childhood illnesses are behind them, and the risks of adult illnesses are not yet present. What does place their health at risk are episodes of poor or immature judgment resulting in accidents, drug or alcohol abuse, sexually transmitted disease (STD), and unwanted pregnancy. Psychologic dysfunction may occur, such as anorexia nervosa or depression. Suicide acts and attempts affect an increasing number of adolescents. Suicide is a leading cause of death in this age group. Its incidence would probably be higher if more accidental deaths were investigated.

Adolescent's Periodic Health Examination

Study Table 2–2 for screening procedures and counseling measures. The physical examination now should include self-care on skin self-examination, breast self-examination or testicular self-examination, and frequency of pelvic examina-

tions (see Chapters 12, 17, 24, and 26 for details). It is particularly important to include counseling on substance use, unwanted pregnancy prevention, and STD risk reduction.

Psychosocial Development

Erikson believed the main psychologic conflict of adolescence (the fifth stage in his theory) to be **ego identity versus identity confusion.** The adolescent is preoccupied with how he or she looks to others, and how that image fits with his or

TABLE 2–2: Periodic Health Examination: Ages 11–24 Years

INTERVENTIONS CONSIDERED AND RECOMMENDED FOR THE PERIODIC HEALTH EXAMINATION	LEADING CAUSES OF DEATH
	Motor vehicle/other unintentional injuries Homicide Suicide Malignant neoplasms Heart diseases
INTERVENTIONS FOR THE GENERAL POPULATION	
Screening	

Height and weight
Blood pressure[1]
Papanicolaou (Pap) test[2] (females)
Chlamydia screen[3] (females <20 yr)
Rubella serology or vaccination hx[4] (females >12 yr)
Assess for problem drinking
	Diet and exercise
	  Limit fat and cholesterol; maintain caloric balance;
	    emphasize grains, fruits, vegetables
	  Adequate calcium intake (females)
	  Regular physical activity
	Dental health
	  Regular visits to dental care provider
	  Floss, brush with fluoride toothpaste daily

Counseling	**Immunizations**

Injury prevention
  Lap/shoulder belts
  Bicycle/motorcycle/ATV helmets
  Smoke detector
  Safe storage/removal of firearms
Substance use
  Avoid tobacco use
  Avoid underage drinking and illicit drug use
  Avoid alcohol/drug use while driving, swimming, boating, etc.
Sexual behavior
  STD prevention: abstinence; avoid high-risk behavior; use condoms
    female barrier with spermicide
  Unintended pregnancy: contraception
	Tetanus-diphtheria (Td) boosters (11–16 yr)
	Hepatitis B[5]
	MMR (11–12 yr)[6]
	Varicella (11–12 yr)[7]
	Rubella[4] (females >12 yr)
	
	Chemoprophylaxis
	
	Multivitamin with folic acid (females planning/capable of
	  pregnancy)

INTERVENTIONS FOR HIGH-RISK POPULATIONS	
POPULATION	**POTENTIAL INTERVENTIONS**
High-risk sexual behavior	RPR/VDRL; screen for gonorrhea (female), HIV, chlamydia (female); hepatitis A vaccine
Injection or street drug use	RPR/VDRL; HIV screen; hepatitis A vaccine; PPD; advice to reduce infection risk
TB contacts; immigrants; low income	PPD
Native Americans/Alaska Natives	Hepatitis A vaccine; PPD; pneumococcal vaccine
Travelers to developing countries	Hepatitis A vaccine
Certain chronic medical conditions	PPD; pneumococcal vaccine; influenza vaccine
Settings where adolescents and young adults congregate	Second MMR
Susceptible to varicella, measles, mumps	Varicella vaccine; MMR
Blood transfusion between 1978–1985	HIV screen
Institutionalized persons; health care/lab workers	Hepatitis A vaccine; PPD; influenza vaccine
Family h/o skin cancer; nevi; fair skin, eyes, hair	Avoid excess/midday sun, use protective clothing
Prior pregnancy with neural tube defect	Folic acid 4.0 mg
Inadequate water fluoridation	Daily fluoride supplement

[1]Periodic blood pressure for persons aged ≥21 yr. [2] If sexually active at present or in the past: q ≤3 yr. If sexual history is unreliable, begin Pap tests at age 18 yr. [3]If sexually active. [4]Serologic testing, documented vaccination history, and routine vaccination against rubella (preferably with MMR) are equally acceptable alternatives. [5]If not previously immunized: current visit, 1 and 6 mo later. [6]If no previous second dose of MMR. [7]If susceptible to chickenpox. *ATV,* All-terrain vehicle; *STD,* sexually transmitted disease; *MMR,* measles-mumps-rubella; *TB,* tuberculosis; *HIV,* human immunodeficiency virus; *RPR,* rapid plasma reagin; *VDRL,* Venereal Disease Research Laboratories; *PPD,* purified protein derivative; *BCG,* bacille Calmette-Guérin.

her own view of the self. If this process is successful, a sense of ego identity emerges, culminating in what Erikson terms a *career choice*. If unsuccessful—if the teen is unsure of his or her skills, self-worth, or sexual identity—identity confusion results. The adolescent feels cut adrift and experiences anxiety about being a social outcast.

Finding one's own identity is stressful. In the search for identity, teens often form cliques; wear fad clothing; and follow rock singers, movie stars, or charismatic heroes in an attempt to siphon identity from them. Falling in love also feeds the quest for personal identity; the teen projects his or her own ego qualities onto another person and tries to understand them as they are reflected by the loved one.

Cognitive Development

Adolescence corresponds to Piaget's fourth stage, in which the person focuses on **formal operations** and the ability to develop abstract thinking, deal with hypothetical situations, and make logical conclusions from reviewing evidence. Now, thinking is no longer confined to the concrete or the real but encompasses all that is possible. Abstract thinking is liberating. The adolescent is no longer limited to the present but can ponder the lessons of the past and the possibilities of the future. The adolescent now can analyze and use scientific reasoning. One can imagine hypotheses and then set up experiments to test them. One learns to use logic and solves problems by methodically eliminating each possibility, one by one. This opens the doors to new academic achievements such as mastering advanced mathematical concepts, chemistry, physics, or logic (Fig. 2–8).

This analytic thinking extends to values. Developing personal values is a part of the search for identity. The adolescent does not accept packaged values of parents or institutions but can reason through his or her inconsistencies and recognize injustices. The adolescent is sensitive to hypocrisy and notes when an adult professes a value (such as honesty) and then acts counter to it (such as cheating on income tax).

Behavioral Development

Socially, the adolescent is in limbo, because he or she rejects identity with the parents but is not yet sure of his or her own

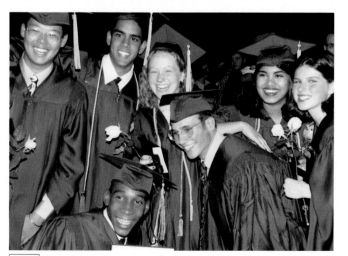

2–8

individual identity. The perfect solution to this dilemma is immersion in a peer group. Pressure to belong to a peer group intensifies at this age. The adolescent is influenced strongly by the group's norms for dress and behavior. By identifying with peers, the adolescent joins a sheltered workshop in which he or she feels safe and can experiment with various roles. Group members are allies in the universal goal of seeking freedom from parental domination.

Group identity means the adolescent spends more time away from home and the parents. Adolescents often feel ambivalent toward the parents. They desperately want to be independent from the parents but realize that economically, and even emotionally, this is impossible. Their stated desire to escape from parental dominance conceals their anxiety about leaving the safety of the family. The conflict is exacerbated when the parents try to maintain rigid control and use the protective stance that worked during earlier childhood. Often, things go smoother when the parents are not as strict; allow privacy; respect the adolescent's budding identity; and, above all, take the adolescent seriously.

Developing close friendships is important to personal identity. In preadolescence the experience of the relationship with the best friend is valuable in teaching intimacy, trust, and regard for another person. These lessons become a link in the new quest of developing close relationships with the opposite sex. Finding a girlfriend or boyfriend enables the adolescent to learn his or her own sex role identity. In many settings, group dating (youth groups, teen dances) is the norm at first. This decreases stress from paired dating. When adolescents do pair off, they usually have a monogamous relationship involving affection and fidelity.

Most adolescents worry that an occasional homosexual thought or act means that they are homosexual. These adolescent experiences are common and do not turn a person into a gay or lesbian. Of course, some teenagers do discover that they have a homosexual orientation and that this lifestyle feels natural for them.

The end of adolescence is more difficult to define. Some societies have recognized rites of passage, usually at puberty, when the young person earns a place in the adult world with its attendant responsibilities. But in complex Western societies, the adolescent remains dependent on the parents through the teen years and into the 20s for economic and educational reasons. This extends the period of adolescence. Consequently, the role is not well defined in our society, and this is a source of conflict.

EARLY ADULTHOOD (20 TO 40 YEARS)

The young adult is concerned with emancipation from his or her parents and building an independent lifestyle. The young adult has finished most formal schooling and is ready to embark on a chosen path (Fig. 2–9). The tasks of this era include:

1. Growing independent from the parents' home and care
2. Establishing a career or vocation
3. Forming an intimate bond with another and choosing a mate

2-9

4. Learning to cooperate in a marriage relationship
5. Setting up and managing one's own household
6. Making friends and establishing a social group
7. Assuming civic responsibility and becoming a citizen in the community
8. Beginning a parenting role
9. Forming a meaningful philosophy of life

Physical and cognitive developments now are steady and do not affect the young adult as much as they have before. Rather, sociocultural factors and values buffet the novice adult.

Physical Development

By early adulthood, the body reaches its maximum potential for growth and development. All body systems now operate at peak efficiency. The young adult enjoys maximum muscle tone and coordination, a high energy level, and optimum mental power. This person exudes freshness and vitality.

Since growth is finished, nutritional needs depend on maintenance and repair requirements and on activity levels. If activity decreases from its level during adolescence, calories must be reduced. Sensible nutrition is a major problem for many adults, and this is not confined to persons with low incomes. The diet should be high in fruits, vegetables, and grain but all too often is high in sugar, salt, and fat. A sedentary lifestyle adds further problems. However, more adults are learning that frequent steady exercise maintains weight, muscle strength, and joint flexibility; builds heart and lung capacity; and reduces stress. Table 2–2 lists these and other preventive counseling measures to address during health care visits.

Cognitive Development

During adolescence, cognitive functioning reached the new level of formal operations, or the capacity for abstract thinking. This level continues, but the young adult's thinking is different from the adolescent's. The young adult is less egocentric and operates in a more realistic and objective manner. Now the young adult is close to maximum ability to acquire and use knowledge. The potential for sophisticated problem solving and creative thinking is at a new height.

Education continues for many young adults, from formal courses in college to on-the-job training, military service, and continuing education classes. Usually, this education prepares the young adult to do some type of work. Work is an important factor in the young adult's life because it is tied closely with ego identity. A person with job satisfaction feels challenged, rewarded, and fulfilled. One who is frustrated with work feels bored and apathetic.

However, other young adults cannot find work. Those from dysfunctional families, those from low-income households, and those who have recently immigrated to the United States lack the resources to obtain the education they need. Because the United States has become an increasingly technologic society, fewer jobs are available for people with little schooling. Unemployment has profound social implications, and one of them is a lack of money for health care. A frustrating clinical paradox arises for the health care provider. That is, nurses and physicians can assess a person, diagnose health problems, and treat or make appropriate referrals, but the individual may fail to comply when he or she does not have the money.

Psychosocial Development

Erikson's sixth stage covers the first years of early adulthood, from 20 to 24 years. He believed the major psychologic conflict to be resolved is that of **intimacy versus isolation.** Once self-identity is established after adolescence, it can be merged with another's in an intimate relationship. During the early 20s, the adult seeks the love, commitment, and intimacy of an intense lasting relationship. This mature relationship includes mutual trust, cooperation, sharing of feelings and goals, and complete acceptance of the other person. Although Erikson had a heterosexual union in mind, this intimacy could be satisfied through a homosexual relationship or through a bond with a cause or an institution.

Erikson believed that without a secure personal identity, a person cannot form a love relationship. The result is the negative outcome of a person who is isolated, withdrawn, and lonely. This person may fill the void with numerous transient liaisons or promiscuity, but Erikson believed that these experiences will be found to be shallow and the person will feel remote and alone.

Daniel Levinson's (1986, 1996) time frame of early adulthood is much broader than Erikson's. It encompasses 22 to 40 years. Levinson believes that an adult's life alternates between periods of **structure building,** in which a lifestyle is fashioned, and periods of **transition,** in which this lifestyle is evaluated, appraised, and modified.

The era of Early Adulthood has two structure-building periods. In the 20s (about 22 to 28 years), the novice adult establishes the "entry structure," a first provisional lifestyle linking him or her to adult society. He or she is building a home base. During this time, the first set of important choices are made concerning a mate, friends, an occupation, values, and lifestyle. In making these choices, the person must juggle the conflicting drives of (1) *exploring* many possibilities and keeping options open on the one hand, and (2) securing some *stability* on the other hand (Levinson et al., 1986).

The Age Thirty Transition, age 28 to 33 years, is a time of self-reflection. Questions asked include "Where am I going?" and "Why am I doing these things?" This is the first major reassessment in life. A person ponders aspects that he or she wants to add, exclude, or modify in life. The person feels, "If there is anything I want to change I better start now, or it will be too late" (Levinson et al., 1986).

According to Levinson, the rest of the 30s (33 to 40 years) is characterized by settling down. A person takes the reforms or the reaffirmations established during the transitional period of the 30s and fashions a culminating life structure, one that realizes his or her youthful aspirations. During these years, the adult strives to establish a niche in society and to build a better life in all the choice points. This person is building a nest, using deliberation and seeking order and stability.

Sometimes, the reforms include having children. The addition of children brings a major readjustment to the couple's relationship. Roles are reshaped in the new family unit. For some couples, the father is more involved in child care than most fathers were in past generations. The mother's role may include a choice between full-time parenting or a return to employment outside the home. More women are in the work force now. Although the opportunities are wider, the risk for stress exists because choices often must be made. The tension shifts from having no choice in a former traditional role to whether or not the right decision is being made now.

However, for many women, the luxury of having options does not exist. Single parents struggle to support themselves and their children. Often they have neither the time nor the financial resources to provide the basic needs for their children or for themselves.

MIDDLE ADULTHOOD (40 TO 64 YEARS)

At some point around or after age 40, the realization dawns and grows that life is half over. No longer does the dream of young adulthood seem fully attainable. To some, it seems that there is more time to look back on than to see ahead. How the person deals with these feelings and builds a meaningful life structure is the task of middle adulthood (Fig. 2–10). Its composite tasks include:

1. Accepting and adjusting to the physical changes of middle age
2. Reviewing and redirecting career goals
3. Achieving desired performance in career
4. Developing hobby and leisure activities

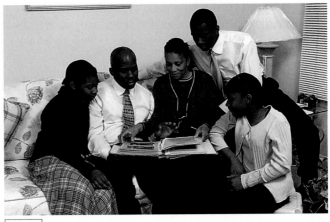

2–10

5. Adjusting to aging parents
6. Helping adolescent children in their search for identity
7. Accepting and relating to the spouse as a person
8. Coping with an empty nest at home

Physical Development

A look in the mirror brings rueful recognition of the beginning of aging effects on the body. The skin loses its taut surface and forms wrinkles around the eyes, mouth, and forehead. Some notice pouches under the eyes and sagging jowls. The hair thins a little, starts to lose pigment, and turns gray, and in men the hairline often recedes. An abdominal paunch grows from increased fat deposits and decreased physical activity. Internally, most organ systems hold constant, with some small decrease in respiratory capacity and cardiac function. Sensory function remains intact except for some visual changes (e.g., decreased accommodation for near vision, or presbyopia).

In the late 40s and early 50s, females experience **menopause,** the decreasing frequency and finally the cessation of menstruation. This involves a decrease in the female hormones, estrogen and progesterone, which brings attendant symptoms such as atrophy of reproductive organs, vasomotor disturbances, and mood swings (see Chapter 26). Although men do not have such an abrupt halt to reproductive ability, they experience a decrease in the production of testosterone, which causes decreased sperm and semen production and less intense orgasms.

Middle-aged adults are suddenly aware of the occasional death of their peers. This is a rude reminder of their own mortality. The leading causes of death during middle adulthood are cancer, heart diseases, and injuries (Table 2–3). Morbidity also is increased, probably caused most often by obesity. Obesity is associated primarily with hypertension and also with cardiovascular disease, diabetes, and mobility dysfunction such as arthritis. Chronic smoking leads to health problems in middle adulthood.

Cognitive Development

Intelligence levels remain generally constant during middle adulthood. Intelligence is further enhanced by the

TABLE 2–3: Periodic Health Examination: Ages 25–64 Years

INTERVENTIONS CONSIDERED AND RECOMMENDED FOR THE PERIODIC HEALTH EXAMINATION	LEADING CAUSES OF DEATH
	Malignant neoplasms
	Heart diseases
	Motor vehicle and other unintentional injuries
	Human immunodeficiency virus (HIV) infection
	Suicide and homicide
INTERVENTIONS FOR THE GENERAL POPULATION	
Screening	
Blood pressure	Injury prevention
Height and weight	Lap/shoulder belts
Total blood cholesterol (men age 35–65, women age 45–65)	Motorcycle/bicycle/ATV helmets
Papanicolaou (Pap) test (women)[1]	Smoke detector
Fecal occult blood test[2] and/or sigmoidoscopy ($\geq$50 yr)	Safe storage/removal of firearms
Mammogram $\pm$ clinical breast exam[3] (women 50–69 yr)	Sexual behavior
Assess for problem drinking	STD prevention: avoid high-risk behavior; use condoms/
Rubella serology or vaccination hx[4] (women of childbearing age)	female barrier with spermicide
	Unintended pregnancy: contraception
Counseling	Dental health
Substance use	Regular visits to dental care provider
Tobacco cessation	Floss, brush with fluoride toothpaste daily
Avoid alcohol/drug use while driving, swimming, boating, etc.	**Immunizations**
Diet and exercise	Tetanus-diphtheria (Td) boosters
Limit fat and cholesterol; maintain caloric balance; emphasize	Rubella[4] (women of childbearing age)
grains, fruits, vegetables	**Chemoprophylaxis**
Adequate calcium intake (women)	Multivitamin with folic acid (women planning or capable of
Regular physical activity	pregnancy)
	Discuss hormone prophylaxis (peri- and postmenopausal
	women)

INTERVENTIONS FOR HIGH-RISK POPULATIONS

POPULATION	POTENTIAL INTERVENTIONS
High-risk sexual behavior	RPR/VDRL; screen for gonorrhea (female), HIV, chlamydia (female); hepatitis B vaccine; hepatitis A vaccine
Injection or street drug use	RPR/VDRL; HIV screen; hepatitis B vaccine; hepatitis A vaccine; PPD; advice to reduce infection risk
Low income; TB contacts; immigrants; alcoholics	PPD
Native Americans/Alaska Natives	Hepatitis A vaccine; PPD; pneumococcal vaccine
Travelers to developing countries	Hepatitis B vaccine; hepatitis A vaccine
Certain chronic medical conditions	PPD; pneumococcal vaccine; influenza vaccine
Blood product recipients	HIV screen; hepatitis B vaccine
Susceptible to measles, mumps, or varicella	MMR; varicella vaccine
Institutionalized persons	Hepatitis A vaccine; PPD; pneumococcal vaccine; influenza vaccine
Health care/lab workers	Hepatitis B vaccine; hepatitis A vaccine; PPD; influenza vaccine
Family h/o skin cancer; fair skin, eyes, hair	Avoid excess/midday sun, use protective clothing
Previous pregnancy with neural tube defect	Folic acid 4.0 mg

[1]Women who are or have been sexually active and who have a cervix: q $\leq$3 yr. [2]Annually. [3]Mammogram q1–2 yr, or mammogram q1–2 yr with annual clinical breast examination. [4]Serologic testing, documented vaccination history, and routine vaccination (preferably with MMR) are equally acceptable alternatives.
ATV, All-terrain vehicle; *STD,* sexually transmitted disease; *TB,* tuberculosis; *RPR,* rapid plasma reagin; *VDRL,* Veneral Disease Research Laboratories; *HIV,* human immunodeficiency virus; *PPD,* purified protein derivative; *MMR,* measles-mumps-rubella.

knowledge that comes with life experience, self-confidence, a sense of humor, and flexibility. The middle-aged adult is interested in how new knowledge is applied, not just in learning for learning's sake. Continuing education courses meet the need to keep knowledge current in occupational and personal interest areas. Many middle-aged adults are seeking college degrees for the first time or are pursuing advanced degrees.

Psychosocial Development

Physical, personal, and social forces all interact during the era of middle adulthood. How a person reacts to the physical cues of aging affects his or her personality and self-perception. A success or disappointment in the career affects a person's self-image, stress level, and interpersonal relationships.

Erikson believed that the most important task for personality development is resolution of the conflict of **generativity versus stagnation.** Erikson believed that during the middle years adults have an urge to contribute to the next generation. This need can be fulfilled either by producing the next generation or by producing something to pass on to the next generation. Thus, middle-aged adults want to rear their own children or to engage in other creative, socially useful work. The motivation is to create and/or nurture those who will follow.

The middle-aged adult needs to be needed, to leave something behind, to leave his or her mark on the world. Generativity is sharing, giving, contributing to the growth of others. If this need is not fulfilled, the negative outcome is stagnation. Stagnation means experiencing boredom and a sense of emptiness in life, which leads to being inactive, self-absorbed, self-indulgent, and a chronic complainer.

Levinson (1986) describes the era of middle adulthood as beginning with a mid-life transition. Roughly between 40 and 45 years, the person starts a major reassessment: "What have I done with my life?"

The rest of the 40s, according to Levinson, involves making choices and building a new life structure. The person confronts reality; some goals simply cannot be met. This must be accepted and goals adjusted. The person takes stock and emerges with a new perception of the self and the environment. For those who have come through the mid-life transition and have found inner meaning, life will be "less tyrannized by the ambitions, passions, and illusions of youth" (Levinson et al., 1986).

For women, the mid-life transition includes the issue that the biologic boundary of childbearing is now in sight. Women feel a time pinch that forces a survey of their life. Aging and biology force women to review options that were set aside and that will be closed off in the now-foreseeable future. Even those satisfied with the number of children that they have or those without children will face this review.

Whatever the central issue, all those in mid-life transition explore the meaning of their career, their family, and their personal identity. In terms of career, a person who spent the 30s searching for power and responsibility now may crave inner meaning (Levinson, 1986). Also, the middle-aged adult is aware of the time left until retirement. This may result in a reordering of career goals or in a new career path.

Career reassessment is intertwined with personal and family reassessment. New roles emerge as the middle-aged adult deals with growing children and aging parents. This popularly is termed the "sandwich generation." The adult often is caught in a "squeeze" between the simultaneously changing needs of adolescent children and aging parents.

Role realignment occurs in the individual's relationship with aging parents. Even if the parents are healthy and active, a role reversal occurs. The middle-aged adult gradually starts to take the parent's place as the one in charge. When one of the parents dies, the middle-aged adult is confronted with loss of the protective myth that "Death cannot happen to me or my loved ones" (Gould, 1979). The parent was a shield between the self and death. Once the parent dies, the middle-aged adult is more vulnerable and realizes the limited quantity of time left.

Another family task facing the middle-aged adult is to help the adolescent child in his or her search for identity. The parent must adjust to the adolescent's desire to be independent and less involved in the family activities and the need for increased responsibility. Some parents nurture the independence and delight in the budding individual. Others tend to be overprotective and controlling. They may feel that their adolescent is too immature. Or they do not want the adolescent to make the same mistakes that they did. The adolescent resents this attempt to relive the parent's life through his or her own. Also, some parents dread the empty nest.

Once the youngest child does leave home, the parent faces the empty nest. If the parent (often the mother) has focused only on the children, she may feel left with little to live for. Will she find something as important as the children to replace them? This dilemma is more poignant now than it was in the past when adult children stayed fairly close to home. With society's current mobility, the grown child often starts a new nuclear family at a faraway location.

The empty nest leaves parents alone as a couple again. They may face a relationship that is devoid of meaning apart from their children. They may find themselves dissatisfied, that they do not know each other, that they have drifted apart. Divorce may result and loom as a major crisis. Other couples find this a positive and liberating phase. Their marriage is happier, with shared activities, increased freedom, and more time to travel. They look back on the shared memories of parenting with a satisfied smile.

LATE ADULTHOOD (65+ YEARS)

Although negative stereotypes exist for each age group, none is more prevalent than the one for aging adults. **Ageism** means discrimination based on age. It is a derogatory attitude that characterizes older adults as sick, senile, and useless and as a burden on the economy. It reveals our society's anxiety about aging. The attitude stems in part from our cultural emphasis on youth, beauty, and vigor. Other cultures respect and revere their aging members.

This ageist attitude is changing, partly because late adulthood now is the fastest-growing segment of our population and its members command attention. Older adults should be seen not as a homogeneous group with predictable reactions but as individuals with specific needs and widely divergent responses (Fig. 2–11). Developmental tasks of this group include:

1. Adjusting to changes in physical strength and health
2. Forming a new family role as an in-law and/or grandparent
3. Affiliating with one's age group
4. Adjusting to retirement and reduced income

2–11

5. Developing postretirement activities that enhance self-worth and usefulness
6. Arranging satisfactory physical living quarters
7. Adjusting to the death of spouse, family members, and friends
8. Conducting a life review
9. Preparing for the inevitability of one's own death

Physical Development

Everyone does not age at the same rate. One person at 60 years can look older and feel weaker than another at 75 years. The widely divergent response depends on subjective attitude, physical activity, nutrition, personal habits, and the occurrence of physical illness. Although aging is known to be a lifelong process, its mechanism is not fully understood. An inevitable decline occurs in body functions that seems to be independent of stress, trauma, and disease. The degenerative effects of normal aging are described for each organ system in the corresponding chapter on physical examination.

Illness affects aging people more than those in other age groups. Incidence of chronic disease increases, resistance to illness decreases, and recuperative power decreases. That is, after an acute illness an aging person does not recover as quickly or as completely as a younger person. Everyday body aches and pains increase. Some older people become preoccupied with their physical discomfort, whereas others adjust to a few aches with equanimity. All these events mean that the aging person is increasingly dependent on the health care system for advice, health teaching, and physical care (Table 2–4).

Cognitive Development

Aging does not have a predictable effect on intelligence. Intellectual function depends on various factors, such as motivation, interest, sensory impairment, educational level, general health, social concerns, involvement in community activities or stimulating leisure activities, as well as a compensatory tendency to conserve time and emotional energy. Older adults do have a slower reaction time. They often have decreased ability for complex decision making and decreased speed of performance, but no decrease in general knowledge occurs. Older adults experience little or no loss in verbal comprehension or in the application of experience. Age-related memory declines are usually on tasks that need deliberate processing, (i.e., problems remembering names, where they placed their keys or other objects, appointments, or medication schedules) (Berk, 2001).

Psychosocial Development

Levinson (1986) suggests a relationship between physical changes of the body and personality. By 60 years, most people are aware of some body decline. Although variations exist, most aging persons have at least one serious illness or limiting condition and are aware of the increasing frequency of death in peers. These issues, coupled with society's negative connotation of aging, lead to a fear that the person has lost all vestiges of youth, even those to which he or she had a tenuous hold during middle adulthood. The person fears "that the youth within him is dying and that only the old man—an empty, dry structure devoid of energy, interests or inner resources—will survive for a brief and foolish old age" (Levinson et al., 1986). The task, then, is to look for a new form of youthfulness, a new force of inner growth to sustain the last era.

The era of late adulthood directs this inner youthfulness toward new creative endeavors. The older adult has stepped off center stage both in formal employment and in the family clan. This can be traumatic because it means a loss of recognition and authority. But now the person can direct energy inward. When financially and socially secure, the older adult can pursue whatever activity is important. One has paid one's dues to society and now can pursue whatever is pleasing. The person creates a new balance with society; he or she is less interested in society's extrinsic rewards and more interested in using inner resources.

CONFRONTING TASKS

How an older adult responds to retirement depends largely on job satisfaction. If the job was rote and meaningless, the person may welcome the release provided by retirement. But if the job signified power and status, or had high complexity, retirement may have a devastating effect. The retired person feels the loss of title and authority. A loss of professional associates who had common interests and were intellectually stimulating also occurs, and a social outlet is lost when co-workers constituted a friendship group.

It is important to develop postretirement activities that enhance self-worth and give a feeling of usefulness. These activities may include developing a new "semiretired" career, or a hobby, sport interest, or community service activity. The transition to retirement is eased if these activities are well in place before the last formal day on the job.

Having the retired person spend more time at home affects the marriage relationship. Traditionally, it was the husband who was suddenly at home and "under foot." Now more

TABLE 2–4: Periodic Health Examination: Age 65 and Older

INTERVENTIONS CONSIDERED AND RECOMMENDED FOR THE PERIODIC HEALTH EXAMINATION

LEADING CAUSES OF DEATH

Heart diseases
Malignant neoplasms (lung, colorectal, breast)
Cerebrovascular disease
Chronic obstructive pulmonary disease
Pneumonia and influenza

INTERVENTIONS FOR THE GENERAL POPULATION

Screening

Blood pressure
Height and weight
Fecal occult blood test[1] and/or sigmoidoscopy
Mammogram ± clinical breast exam[2] (women ≤69 yr)
Papanicolaou (Pap) test (women)[3]
Vision screening
Assess for hearing impairment
Assess for problem drinking

Counseling

Substance use
  Tobacco cessation
  Avoid alcohol/drug use while driving, swimming, boating, etc.
Diet and exercise
  Limit fat and cholesterol; maintain caloric balance; emphasize grains, fruits, vegetables
  Adequate calcium intake (women)
  Regular physical activity

Injury prevention
  Lap/shoulder belts
  Motorcycle and bicycle helmets
  Fall prevention
  Safe storage/removal of firearms
  Smoke detector
  Set hot water heater to <120–130° F
  CPR training for household members
Dental health
  Regular visits to dental care provider
  Floss, brush with fluoride toothpaste daily
Sexual behavior
  STD prevention: avoid high-risk sexual behavior; use condoms

Immunizations

Pneumococcal vaccine
Influenza[1]
Tetanus-diphtheria (Td) boosters

Chemoprophylaxis

Discuss hormone prophylaxis (women)

INTERVENTIONS FOR HIGH-RISK POPULATIONS

POPULATION	POTENTIAL INTERVENTIONS
Institutionalized persons	PPD; hepatitis A vaccine; amantadine/rimantadine
Chronic medical conditions; TB contacts; low income; immigrants; alcoholics	PPD
Persons ≥75 yr; or ≥70 yr with risk factors for falls	Fall prevention intervention
Cardiovascular disease risk factors	Consider cholesterol screening
Family h/o skin cancer; nevi; fair skin, eyes, hair	Avoid excess/midday sun, use protective clothing
Native Americans/Alaska Natives	PPD; hepatitis A vaccine
Travelers to developing countries	Hepatitis A vaccine; hepatitis B vaccine
Blood product recipients	HIV screen; hepatitis B vaccine
High-risk sexual behavior	Hepatitis A vaccine; HIV screen; hepatitis B vaccine; RPR/VDRL
Injection or street drug use	PPD; hepatitis A vaccine; HIV screen; hepatitis B vaccine; RPR/VDRL; advice to reduce infection risk
Health care/lab workers	PPD; hepatitis A vaccine; amantadine/rimantadine; hepatitis B vaccine
Persons susceptible to varicella	Varicella vaccine

[1]Annually. [2]Mammogram q1–2 yr, or mammogram q1–2 yr with annual clinical breast exam. [3]All women who are or have been sexually active and who have a cervix: q ≤3 yr. Consider discontinuation of testing after age 65 yr if previous regular screening with consistently normal results.
CPR, Cardiopulmonary resuscitation; *STD*, sexually transmitted disease; *TB*, tuberculosis; *PPD*, purified protein derivative; *HIV*, human immunodeficiency virus; *RPR*, rapid plasma reagin; *VDRL*, Veneral Disease Research Laboratories.

employed women exist who face the same retirement adjustment. Some couples do find that having one or both at home more means an invasion of previously held "turf," such as the kitchen, garden, or workshop. Other couples develop a more egalitarian relationship. They are now free of earlier sex role

definitions and are able to share household tasks and leisure activities equally.

Family roles also are adjusted with the marriage of grown-up children and the addition of in-laws. How the sons- or daughters-in-law are absorbed into the family affects the older adult. This often involves a new role as grandparent. Being able to indulge and provide moral support to a grandchild is usually positive for all, unless the caretaking becomes a burden to the grandparent.

Retirement often involves financial adjustment. This may involve a reduced income, perhaps only social security and a small pension. This may be hard if the person is used to a higher standard of living. Even if the retired person owns his or her own home, the cost of maintaining it may exceed the income.

Establishing suitable living arrangements has both financial and family significance. In our culture, the extended family mostly has disappeared today. No longer do three generations live under one roof. In the past, the older adult contributed light household tasks that gave a sense of personal worth. Now, the contributions to the extended family that were made by the older family member have been replaced by advances in household mechanization, food processing, and day care centers.

Thus most older adults choose to live independently, either as couples or alone. When it becomes difficult to manage self-care, they face the choice of moving in with grown children or moving into a retirement home or nursing home. All of these choices involve some disbursement of personal belongings and the relinquishing of some privacy.

Through the late adult years, each person is reminded of one's own limited time left by the increasing frequency of death and serious illness of friends; colleagues; siblings; or other family members, perhaps including the spouse.

THE LIFE REVIEW

One important task of late adulthood is performing a life review. Older adults have finished all or most of their life's work. Their contribution to society and to their own immortality are mostly completed (Levinson et al., 1986). The life review is a cataloging of life events, a considering of one's successes and failures with the perspective of age. The objective of the task is to gain a sense of integrity in reviewing one's life as a whole (Fig. 2–12).

This period relates to Erikson's last ego stage, with its key psychological conflict of **ego integrity versus despair.** A successful resolution to this final conflict occurs when the adult accepts "one's one and only life cycle as something that had to be and that, by necessity, permitted of no substitutions" (Erikson, 1963). The adult feels content with his or her one life on earth, satisfied that if it were possible to do it over again, he or she would live it the same way. The older adult reviews events, experiences, and relationships and realizes that these have been mostly good. There are cherished memories. The person has had a meaningful part in human history and can meet death with equanimity.

Failure to resolve this last conflict leaves the person with a sense of despair, resentment, futility, hopelessness, and a fear of death. However, a successful outcome completes a cycle. The contented older adult who does not fear death serves as a role model for younger adults that life can be trusted.

Levinson believes everyone has a sense of utter despair at some point during this time. To gain a sense of integrity, one

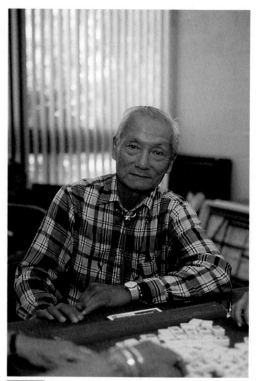

2-12

has to confront the *lack* of integrity (Levinson et al., 1986). Some goals have not been achieved, and what is worse is that the damage is done and it is too late to set it right. The person realizes that whatever values were held, he or she cannot fully live up to them. This must be reconciled; it is an imperfect world. The task is to make peace with the self.

This final sense of what life is about is a close parallel to Erikson's last stage. Levinson likens the person's perspective at this time as a "view from the bridge" at the end of the life cycle (Levinson et al., 1986). One "must come finally to terms with the self—knowing it and loving it reasonably well, and being ready to give it up."

DEVELOPMENTAL SCREENING TESTS

THE DENVER II—REVISION AND RESTANDARDIZATION OF THE DENVER DEVELOPMENTAL SCREENING TEST (DDST)

Age range: birth to 6 years
Time required: 10 to 25 minutes
Authors: W. Frankenburg, J. Dodds, P. Archer,
        B. Bresnick, H. Shapiro
Available from: Denver Developmental Materials, Inc.
        P.O. Box 6919
        Denver, CO 80206

This is a screening instrument designed to detect developmental delays in infants and preschoolers. It tests four functions: gross motor, language, fine motor-adaptive, and personal-social skills.

The Denver II is not an intelligence test; it does not predict current or future intellectual ability. It is not diagnostic; it does not suggest treatment regimens. What the Denver II does do is screen; it helps identify children who may be slow in development. This is important because early detection increases the opportunities for effective treatment.

The Denver II was revised in 1989 and restandardized for a sample including three ethnic groups, three residence categories (rural, suburban, and urban), and three levels of maternal education (less than high school, high school, and more than high school). These norms should ameliorate the limitations of the earlier DDST concerning its relevance to various population groups (Frankenburg et al., 1981). The Denver II also appears to address the limitations experienced by Olade (1984) in using the earlier DDST in developing countries. Olade's study of African children in Nigeria suggested that language differences (naming certain colors, limited use of plurals and parents' last names) and unfamiliar interactive games (peek-a-boo) affected DDST results. These items are omitted or adjusted in the Denver II. However, the culture of developing countries still must be considered when using screening tests.

The Denver II easily is incorporated into the daily professional regimen of nurses, physicians, and teachers. The 125 items are arranged in chronologic order and are displayed in groupings corresponding to recommended ages for health maintenance visits.* The clear pictorial charts aid in administering, scoring, and interpreting the test. It is reliable and economical. The materials are few in number, attractive to children, and easily maintained and replaced. The scoring avoids diagnostic labeling (such as mental retardation, language disorder, and cerebral palsy). Instead, the child's performance is scored either "normal," "abnormal," or "questionable," and includes an adjustment in scoring for premature infants.

Uses of the Denver II include (Frankenburg et al., 1981):

- Screening of infants, whose rapid rate of development makes it difficult to rely on professional opinion or on parent history alone
- Longitudinal following of a single child in health care or educational setting
- Follow-up in clinics, where a child may be seen briefly, infrequently, or by different examiners
- Prekindergarten screening

ADULT LIFE STRESS MEASURES

Some tools are available that attempt to quantify the impact of life change on a person's health. They are based on the assumption that a relationship exists between daily life stress

---

*For a copy of the Denver II, please see the *Student Laboratory Manual* that accompanies this text.

and a person's susceptibility to physical and psychologic problems. Many of the life change events are the developmental tasks discussed earlier in the chapter.

The Hassles and Uplifts Scale
Age range: adult
Author: DeLongis

This is a 53-item self-administered questionnaire whose purpose is to assess day-to-day stress (Table 2–5). Take this test yourself just before you go to bed some day. Consider each item on the list, and circle a number on the left-hand side regarding how much of a hassle the item was for you that day. On the right-hand side, circle a number regarding how much of an uplift the same item was for you that day. Total scores are obtained by summing across ratings given to all items.

Relatively minor but frequently experienced stresses, termed *Hassles* in this tool, have been found to correlate strongly with negative health status (Weinberger, Hiner, and Tierney, 1987). DeLongis, Folkman, and Lazarus (1988) found a significant relationship between daily stress and concurrent or later occurrence of physical health problems, such as flu, sore throat, headaches, and backaches. There was great individual variation, however, with one third of the respondents reporting a somewhat improved health and mood with increased stress levels! Regarding daily stress and psychologic disturbance, they found that individuals with unsupportive social relationships and low self-esteem had a greater risk of psychologic and somatic health problems, both on their stressful days and following their stressful days, than did individuals with positive social networks and high self-esteem (DeLongis, Folkman, and Lazarus, 1988).

Life Experiences Survey (LES)
Age range: adult
Authors: I.G. Sarason, J.H. Johnson, J.M. Siegel

This is a 47-item self-administered questionnaire that considers events that occurred over the past year. This test weighs the desirability or undesirability of life experiences. The assumption is that events considered *negative* by the respondent are more likely to be associated with stress. Also the respondent is allowed to rate the personal impact of the events experienced.

The respondent weighs the desirability or undesirability of each event on a 7-point scale, from extremely negative (-3) to extremely positive ($+3$) (Table 2–6). The negative and positive subscores are added to determine a total change score.

This test suggests a relationship between negative life changes and psychologic problems. The effect of stress differs depending on individual characteristics, the degree of perceived control over the events, and the degree of psychosocial assets (Sarason et al., 1978).

TABLE 2–5: The Hassles and Uplifts Scale

HASSLES are irritants—things that annoy or bother you; they can make you upset or angry. UPLIFTS are events that make you feel good; they can make you joyful, glad, or satisfied. Some hassles and uplifts occur on a fairly regular basis and others are relatively rare. Some have only a slight effect, others have a strong effect.

This questionnaire lists things that can be hassles and uplifts in day-to-day life. You will find that during the course of a day some of these things will have been only a hassle for you and some will have been only an uplift. *Others will have been both a hassle AND an uplift.*

DIRECTIONS: Please think about how much of a hassle and how much of an uplift each item was for you today. Please indicate on the left-hand side of the page (under "HASSLES") how much of a hassle the item was by circling the appropriate number. Then indicate on the right-hand side of the page (under "UPLIFTS") how much of an uplift it was for you by circling the appropriate number.

Remember, circle one number on the left-hand side of the page *and* one number on the right-hand side of the page for *each* item.

PLEASE FILL OUT THIS QUESTIONNAIRE JUST BEFORE YOU GO TO BED.

HASSLES AND UPLIFTS SCALE

HOW MUCH OF A HASSLE WAS THIS ITEM FOR YOU TODAY?	HOW MUCH OF AN UPLIFT WAS THIS ITEM FOR YOU TODAY?
HASSLES	UPLIFTS
0 = *None or not applicable*	0 = *None or not applicable*
1 = *Somewhat*	1 = *Somewhat*
2 = *Quite a bit*	2 = *Quite a bit*
3 = *A great deal*	3 = *A great deal*

DIRECTIONS: Please circle one number on the left-hand side *and* one number on the right-hand side for each item.

Hassles	Item	Uplifts
0 1 2 3	1. Your child(ren)	0 1 2 3
0 1 2 3	2. Your parents or parents-in-law	0 1 2 3
0 1 2 3	3. Other relative(s)	0 1 2 3
0 1 2 3	4. Your spouse	0 1 2 3
0 1 2 3	5. Time spent with family	0 1 2 3
0 1 2 3	6. Health or well-being of a family member	0 1 2 3
0 1 2 3	7. Sex	0 1 2 3
0 1 2 3	8. Intimacy	0 1 2 3
0 1 2 3	9. Family-related obligations	0 1 2 3
0 1 2 3	10. Your friend(s)	0 1 2 3
0 1 2 3	11. Fellow workers	0 1 2 3
0 1 2 3	12. Clients, customers, patients, etc.	0 1 2 3
0 1 2 3	13. Your supervisor or employer	0 1 2 3
0 1 2 3	14. The nature of your work	0 1 2 3
0 1 2 3	15. Your work load	0 1 2 3
0 1 2 3	16. Your job security	0 1 2 3
0 1 2 3	17. Meeting deadlines or goals on the job	0 1 2 3
0 1 2 3	18. Enough money for necessities (e.g., food, clothing, housing, health care, taxes, insurance)	0 1 2 3
0 1 2 3	19. Enough money for education	0 1 2 3
0 1 2 3	20. Enough money for emergencies	0 1 2 3
0 1 2 3	21. Enough money for extras (e.g., entertainment, recreation, vacations)	0 1 2 3
0 1 2 3	22. Financial care for someone who doesn't live with you	0 1 2 3
0 1 2 3	23. Investments	0 1 2 3
0 1 2 3	24. Your smoking	0 1 2 3
0 1 2 3	25. Your drinking	0 1 2 3
0 1 2 3	26. Mood-altering drugs	0 1 2 3
0 1 2 3	27. Your physical appearance	0 1 2 3
0 1 2 3	28. Contraception	0 1 2 3
0 1 2 3	29. Exercise(s)	0 1 2 3
0 1 2 3	30. Your medical care	0 1 2 3
0 1 2 3	31. Your health	0 1 2 3
0 1 2 3	32. Your physical abilities	0 1 2 3
0 1 2 3	33. The weather	0 1 2 3
0 1 2 3	34. News events	0 1 2 3
0 1 2 3	35. Your environment (e.g., quality of air, noise level, greenery)	0 1 2 3
0 1 2 3	36. Political or social issues	0 1 2 3
0 1 2 3	37. Your neighborhood (e.g., neighbors, setting)	0 1 2 3
0 1 2 3	38. Conserving (gas, electricity, water, gasoline, etc.)	0 1 2 3
0 1 2 3	39. Pets	0 1 2 3
0 1 2 3	40. Cooking	0 1 2 3
0 1 2 3	41. Housework	0 1 2 3
0 1 2 3	42. Home repairs	0 1 2 3
0 1 2 3	43. Yardwork	0 1 2 3
0 1 2 3	44. Car maintenance	0 1 2 3
0 1 2 3	45. Taking care of paperwork (e.g., paying bills, filling out forms)	0 1 2 3
0 1 2 3	46. Home entertainment (e.g., TV, music, reading)	0 1 2 3
0 1 2 3	47. Amount of free time	0 1 2 3
0 1 2 3	48. Recreation and entertainment outside the home (e.g., movies, sports, eating out, walking)	0 1 2 3
0 1 2 3	49. Eating (at home)	0 1 2 3
0 1 2 3	50. Church or community organizations	0 1 2 3
0 1 2 3	51. Legal matters	0 1 2 3
0 1 2 3	52. Being organized	0 1 2 3
0 1 2 3	53. Social commitments	0 1 2 3

Received March 21, 1986
Revision received July 20, 1987
Accepted August 4, 1987

From DeLongis A, Folkman S, Lazarus RS: The impact of daily stress on health and mood: psychological and social resources as mediators, *J Pers Soc Psychol* 54(3):486–495, 1988. © 1988 by the American Psychological Association. Used with permission.

TABLE 2–6: Life Experiences Survey

Listed below are a number of events that sometimes bring about change in the lives of those who experience them and that necessitate social readjustment. *Please check those events that you have experienced in the recent past and indicate the time period during which you have experienced each event.* Be sure that all check marks are directly across from the items they correspond to.

Also, for each item checked below, *please indicate the extent to which you viewed the event as having either a positive or negative impact on your life* at the time the event occurred. That is, *indicate the type and extent of impact that the event had.* A rating of −3 would indicate an extremely negative impact. A rating of 0 suggests no impact either positive or negative. A rating of +3 would indicate an extremely positive impact.

	0–6 MO	7 MO TO 1 YR	EXTREMELY NEGATIVE	MODERATELY NEGATIVE	SOMEWHAT NEGATIVE	NO IMPACT	SLIGHTLY POSITIVE	MODERATELY POSITIVE	EXTREMELY POSITIVE
1. Marriage			−3	−2	−1	0	+1	+2	+3
2. Detention in jail or comparable institution			−3	−2	−1	0	+1	+2	+3
3. Death of spouse			−3	−2	−1	0	+1	+2	+3
4. Major change in sleeping habits (much more or much less sleep)			−3	−2	−1	0	+1	+2	+3
5. Death of close family member			−3	−2	−1	0	+1	+2	+3
a. Mother			−3	−2	−1	0	+1	+2	+3
b. Father			−3	−2	−1	0	+1	+2	+3
c. Brother			−3	−2	−1	0	+1	+2	+3
d. Sister			−3	−2	−1	0	+1	+2	+3
e. Grandmother			−3	−2	−1	0	+1	+2	+3
f. Grandfather			−3	−2	−1	0	+1	+2	+3
g. Other (specify)			−3	−2	−1	0	+1	+2	+3
6. Major change in eating habits (much more or much less food intake)			−3	−2	−1	0	+1	+2	+3
7. Foreclosure on mortgage or loan			−3	−2	−1	0	+1	+2	+3
8. Death of close friend			−3	−2	−1	0	+1	+2	+3
9. Outstanding personal achievement			−3	−2	−1	0	+1	+2	+3
10. Minor law violations (traffic tickets, disturbing the peace, etc.)			−3	−2	−1	0	+1	+2	+3
11. *Male:* wife/girlfriend's pregnancy			−3	−2	−1	0	+1	+2	+3
12. *Female:* pregnancy			−3	−2	−1	0	+1	+2	+3
13. Changed work situation (different work responsibility, major change in working conditions, working hours, etc.)			−3	−2	−1	0	+1	+2	+3
14. New job			−3	−2	−1	0	+1	+2	+3
15. Serious illness or injury of close family member			−3	−2	−1	0	+1	+2	+3
a. Father			−3	−2	−1	0	+1	+2	+3
b. Mother			−3	−2	−1	0	+1	+2	+3
c. Sister			−3	−2	−1	0	+1	+2	+3
d. Brother			−3	−2	−1	0	+1	+2	+3
e. Grandfather			−3	−2	−1	0	+1	+2	+3
f. Grandmother			−3	−2	−1	0	+1	+2	+3
g. Spouse			−3	−2	−1	0	+1	+2	+3
h. Other (specify)			−3	−2	−1	0	+1	+2	+3
16. Sexual difficulties			−3	−2	−1	0	+1	+2	+3
17. Trouble with employer (in danger of losing job, being suspended, demoted, etc.)			−3	−2	−1	0	+1	+2	+3
18. Trouble with in-laws			−3	−2	−1	0	+1	+2	+3
19. Major change in financial status (a lot better off or a lot worse off)			−3	−2	−1	0	+1	+2	+3
20. Major change in closeness of family members (increased or decreased closeness)			−3	−2	−1	0	+1	+2	+3
21. Gaining a new family member (through birth, adoption, family member moving in, etc.)			−3	−2	−1	0	+1	+2	+3

From Sarason IG, Johnson JH, Siegal JM: Assessing the impact of life changes: development of life experiences survey, *J Consult Clin Psychol* 46(5):932–946, 1978. © 1978 by the American Psychological Association. Used with permission.

Continued

TABLE 2–6: Life Experiences Survey—cont'd

	0–6 MO	7 MO TO 1 YR	Extremely Negative	Moderately Negative	Somewhat Negative	No Impact	Slightly Positive	Moderately Positive	Extremely Positive
22. Change in residence			−3	−2	−1	0	+1	+2	+3
23. Marital separation from mate (due to conflict)			−3	−2	−1	0	+1	+2	+3
24. Major change in church activities (increased or decreased attendance)			−3	−2	−1	0	+1	+2	+3
25. Marital reconciliation with mate			−3	−2	−1	0	+1	+2	+3
26. Major change in number of arguments with spouse (a lot more or a lot less arguments)			−3	−2	−1	0	+1	+2	+3
27. *Married male:* change in wife's work outside the home (beginning work, ceasing work, changing to a new job, etc.)			−3	−2	−1	0	+1	+2	+3
28. *Married female:* change in husband's work (loss of job, beginning new job, retirement, etc.)			−3	−2	−1	0	+1	+2	+3
29. Major change in usual type and/or amount of recreation			−3	−2	−1	0	+1	+2	+3
30. Borrowing more than $10,000 (buying home, business, etc.)			−3	−2	−1	0	+1	+2	+3
31. Borrowing less than $10,000 (buying car, TV, getting school loan, etc.)			−3	−2	−1	0	+1	+2	+3
32. Being fired from job			−3	−2	−1	0	+1	+2	+3
33. *Male:* wife/girlfriend having abortion			−3	−2	−1	0	+1	+2	+3
34. *Female:* having abortion			−3	−2	−1	0	+1	+2	+3
35. Major personal illness or injury			−3	−2	−1	0	+1	+2	+3
36. Major change in social activities, e.g., parties, movies, visiting (increased or decreased participation)			−3	−2	−1	0	+1	+2	+3
37. Major change in living conditions of family (building new home, remodeling, deterioration of home, neighborhood, etc.)			−3	−2	−1	0	+1	+2	+3
38. Divorce			−3	−2	−1	0	+1	+2	+3
39. Serious injury or illness of close friend			−3	−2	−1	0	+1	+2	+3
40. Retirement from work			−3	−2	−1	0	+1	+2	+3
41. Son or daughter leaving home (due to marriage, college, etc.)			−3	−2	−1	0	+1	+2	+3
42. Ending of formal schooling			−3	−2	−1	0	+1	+2	+3
43. Separation from spouse (due to work, travel)			−3	−2	−1	0	+1	+2	+3
44. Engagement			−3	−2	−1	0	+1	+2	+3
45. Breaking up with boyfriend/girlfriend			−3	−2	−1	0	+1	+2	+3
46. Leaving home for the first time			−3	−2	−1	0	+1	+2	+3
47. Reconciliation with boyfriend/girlfriend			−3	−2	−1	0	+1	+2	+3
Other recent experiences that have had an impact on your life. List and rate.									
48. _____.			−3	−2	−1	0	+1	+2	+3
49. _____.			−3	−2	−1	0	+1	+2	+3
50. _____.			−3	−2	−1	0	+1	+2	+3

Application and Critical Thinking

NURSING DIAGNOSES COMMONLY ASSOCIATED WITH DEVELOPMENTAL DISORDERS

RELATED FACTORS (Etiology)	DEFINING CHARACTERISTICS (Symptoms and Signs)
CHILDHOOD **DIAGNOSIS:** Delayed Growth and Development	
Effects of physical disability Environmental and stimulation deficiencies Inadequate care-taking • Indifference • Inconsistent responsiveness • Multiple caretakers Prescribed dependence Separation from significant others	Delayed physical growth Decreased responses Delay or difficulty in performing skills that are typical of age group: • Motor • Social • Expressive Flat affect Inability to perform self-care or self-control activities appropriate for age
ADOLESCENCE **DIAGNOSIS:** Decisional Conflict	
Unclear personal values/beliefs Peer pressure Lack of experience or interference with decision making Support system deficit	Verbalized uncertainty about choices Verbalized undesired consequences of alternative actions being considered Vacillation among alternative choices Delayed decision making
ADULTHOOD **DIAGNOSIS:** Compromised Family Coping	
Isolation of family members from one another Lack of support for family members Temporary family disorganization and role changes Effects of acute or chronic illness Incompatible or differing values, beliefs, or goals Unrealistic expectations	Ineffective responses to illness, disability, or situational crises Inability to demonstrate supportive behaviors Expressed concern about significant other's response to health problem Impaired intimacy or closeness Attempted assistive behaviors with less than satisfactory results
LATE ADULTHOOD **DIAGNOSIS:** Anticipatory Grieving	
Expected loss of: • Friends • Occupation • Function • Home Multiple crises Lack of social support system	Expressed distress at potential loss Denial Guilt Sorrow Change in eating habits Change in sleep patterns Change in social patterns Decreased libido

OTHER RELATED NURSING DIAGNOSES

ACTUAL	RISK/WELLNESS
Caregiver Role Strain	**Risk**
Deficient Diversional Activity	Risk for Impaired Parent/Infant/Child Attachment
Interrupted Family Processes	Risk for Caregiver Role Strain
Disturbed Personal Identity	Risk for Delayed Development
Impaired Parenting	Risk for Falls
Relocation Stress Syndrome	Risk for Impaired Parenting
Ineffective Role Performance	**Wellness**
Chronic Low Self Esteem	Readiness for Enhanced Family Coping
Situational Low Self Esteem	Health-Seeking Behavior
Social Isolation	Readiness for Enhanced Spiritual Well-Being

BIBLIOGRAPHY

American Academy of Pediatrics Committee on Child Abuse and Neglect: Guidelines for distinguishing SIDS from child abuse fatalities, *Pediatrics* 94(1):124–126, 1994.

Arnett JJ: Emerging adulthood: a theory of development from the late teens through the twenties, *Am Psychol* 55(5):469–480, 2000.

Barnard S, Edgar D: *Pediatric eye care,* Oxford, England, 1996, Blackwell Science.

Berk LE: Why children talk to themselves, *Sci Am* 271(5):60–65, 1994.

Berk LE: *Development through the lifespan,* ed 2, Boston, 2001, Allyn and Bacon.

Centers for Disease Control and Prevention, National Center for Injury Prevention and Control: Suicide Prevention Fact Sheet. Available at www.cdc.gov/ncipc/factsheets/suifacts.htm (accessed 3/27/2002).

DeLongis A, Folkman S, Lazarus RS: The impact of daily stress on health and mood: psychological and social resources as mediators, *J Pers Soc Psychol* 54(3):486–495, 1988.

Erikson EH: *Childhood and society,* New York, 1963, WW Norton.

Erikson EH: *Identity: youth and crisis,* New York, 1968, WW Norton.

Frankenburg WK, Fandal AW, Sciarillo W: The newly abbreviated and revised Denver Developmental Screening Test, *J Pediatr* 99(6):995–999, 1981.

Gibson E et al: Infant sleep position practices 2 years into the "Back to Sleep" campaign, *Clin Pediatr* 39(5):285–289, 2000.

Gilbert-Barness E, Barness L: What we've learned about SIDS, *Patient Care* 30(5):98–118, 1996.

Gould RL: *Transformations: growth and change in adult life,* New York, 1979, Simon and Schuster.

Griffith H: Resources to put more prevention into your practice, *J Am Acad Nurs Pract* 6(6):253–256, 1994.

Jones MW, McMurray JL: "Baby Steps": neonatal developmental follow-up, *Neonatal Netw* 20(6):73–78, 2001.

Kingon YS, O'Sullivan AL: The family as a protective asset in adolescent development, *J Holist Nurs* 19(2):102–121, 2001.

Landis BJ, Brykczynski KA: Employing prevention in practice, *Am J Nurs* 97(8):40–46, 1997.

Levinson DJ: A conception of adult development, *Am Psychol* 41:3–13, 1986.

Levinson DJ: *The seasons of a woman's life,* New York, 1996, AA Knopf.

Levinson DJ, Darrow CN, Klein EB: *The seasons of a man's life,* ed 2, New York, 1986, Ballantine.

Oberklaid F: Is developmental assessment worthwhile? *Aust Fam Physician* 29(8):731–734, 2000.

Olade RA: Evaluation of the Denver Developmental Screening Test as applied to African children, *Nurs Res* 33(4):204–207, 1984.

Pender NJ: *Health promotion in nursing practice,* ed 3, Stamford, Conn, 1996, Appleton & Lange.

Piaget J: Judgment and reasoning in the child, Totowa, NJ, 1968, Littlefield, Adams.

Piaget J: The construction of reality in the child, New York, 1975, Ballantine.

Robbins LB et al: Physical activity research in nursing, *J Nurs Scholarsh* 33(4):315–321, 2001.

Sarason EG, Johnson JH, Siegal JM: Assessing the impact of life changes: development of life experiences survey, *J Consult Clin Psychol* 45(5):932–946, 1978.

Seibold ES: A practical guide to developmental screening, *Clinical Letter for Nurse Practitioners* 4(3):7–12, 2000.

Spelke ES et al: Origins of knowledge, *Psychol Rev* 99:605–632, 1992.

Steinberg L: The family at adolescence: transition and transformation, *J Adolesc Health* 27:170–178, 2000.

U.S. Department of Health and Human Services: *Healthy People 2010,* Washington, DC, U.S. Government Printing Office. (www.health.gov/healthypeople).

U.S. Preventive Services Task Force: *Guide to clinical preventive services, 2000,* ed 2, Baltimore, 1996, Williams & Wilkins.

Weinberger M, Hiner SL, Tierney WM: In support of Hassles as a measure of stress in predicting health outcomes, *J Behav Med* 10(1):19–31, 1987.

Whitmire K: Adolescence as a developmental phase, *Topics in Language Disorders* 20(2):1–14, 2000.

Woolf SH, Jonas S, Lawrence RS: *Health promotion and disease prevention in clinical practice,* Baltimore, 1996, Williams & Wilkins.

Transcultural Considerations in Assessment

*C*ultural assessment refers to a systematic appraisal of an individual's beliefs, values, and practices conducted for the purpose of providing *culturally competent* health care. Derived from the Latin root *competere*, meaning "to strive together," *cultural competence* refers to the complex integration of knowledge, attitudes, and skills, which enhance cross-cultural communication, promote meaningful interactions with patients, and enable you to provide culturally appropriate, congruent, and relevant health care. According to Campinha-Bacote (1999), there are four components to developing cultural competence: cultural awareness, cultural knowledge, cultural skill, and cultural encounter. Because you may encounter people from literally hundreds of different cultures and subcultures in your professional career, it is impossible to know about the culturally based, health-related beliefs and practices of them all. It is, however, possible to master the knowledge and skills associated with cultural assessment and learn about *some* of the cultural dimensions of care for individuals representing the groups you most frequently encounter (Fig. 3–1).

In addition to cultural competence, some experts have noted the considerable impact that linguistic competence by health care providers has on patients' access and response to health care services. *Cultural and linguistic competence* refers to an ability by health care providers and health care organizations to understand and effectively respond to the cultural and linguistic needs brought by patients to the health care encounter (Office of Minority Health, 1999).

One of the major challenges you will face in assessing people from culturally diverse backgrounds is overcoming your own *ethnocentrism*. Ethnocentrism is the tendency to view your own way of life as the most desirable, acceptable, or best, and to act in a superior manner toward another culture's lifeways. A related admonition is to beware of *cultural imposition*, the tendency to impose your beliefs, values, and patterns of behavior on individuals from another culture. These admonitions are more easily stated than lived.

Because health care providers deal with cultural values and belief systems, cultural assessments tend to be broad,

comprehensive, and holistic. Cultural assessment consists of both *process* and *content*. *Process* refers to your approach to the patient and includes professional interactions, etiquette, perceptions of space/distance, and gender considerations. Cross-cultural communication is also an integral component of the assessment process, and these points are discussed in Chapter 4. The *content* of the cultural assessment, which follows below, consists of the actual data categories in which information about patients is gathered for the history and physical examination.

BASIC CHARACTERISTICS OF CULTURE

Culture has four basic characteristics. Culture is (1) *learned* from birth through the processes of language acquisition and socialization; (2) *shared* by all members of the same cultural group; (3) *adapted* to specific conditions related to environmental and technical factors and to the availability of natural resources; and (4) *dynamic* and ever changing.

Culture is a universal phenomenon, without which no person exists. Yet the culture that develops in any given society is always specific and distinctive, encompassing all the knowledge, beliefs, customs, and skills acquired by members of the society. Within cultures, groups of individuals share different beliefs, values, and attitudes. Differences occur because of ethnicity, religion, education, occupation, age, and gender. When such groups function within a large culture, they are referred to as subcultural groups.

The term **subculture** is used for fairly large aggregates of people who have shared characteristics that are not common to all members of the culture and that enable them to be thought of as a distinguishable subgroup. Ethnicity, religion, occupation, health-related characteristics, age, and gender are frequently used to identify subcultural groups. Examples of subcultures based on *ethnicity* (those having common traits such as physical characteristics, language, or ancestry) include blacks, Hispanics, Native Americans, Korean-Americans, and Inuits; those based on *religion* include members of the more than 1200 recognized religions such as Catholics, Jews, Mormons, Muslims, and Buddhists; those based on *occupation* include individuals involved in health care professions, such as nursing or medicine, as well as the military; those based on a *health-related characteristic* include the blind, hearing impaired, or mentally retarded; those based on *age* include groups such as adolescents and older adults; and those based on *gender* or *sexual preference* include women, men, gay men, and lesbians.

When addressing the cultural dimensions of health care, some erroneously refer only to the federally defined ethnic minority groups—white, black, Hispanic, Asian/Pacific Islander, and Native American/Alaska Native. You should be mindful that hundreds of distinct cultural groups exist in the United States, not merely those identified by the U.S. government for statistical purposes. Furthermore, the federal classification system ignores unique characteristics of groups within the broad categories (e.g., more than 550 Na-

3–1

tive American nations exist, each with specific beliefs and practices).

CULTURAL VALUES

According to Leininger and McFarland (2002), the term *values* refers to a desirable or undesirable state of affairs. Values are a universal feature of all cultures, although the types and expressions of values differ widely. *Norms* are the rules by which human behavior is governed and result from the cultural values held by the group. All societies have rules or norms that specify appropriate and inappropriate behavior. Individuals are rewarded or punished as they conform to or deviate from the established norms. Values and norms are learned in childhood along with the acceptable and unacceptable behaviors associated with them.

DOMINANT VALUE ORIENTATION

Every society has what is called a *dominant value orientation,* a basic value orientation that is shared by the majority of its members as a result of early common experiences. According to Kluckhohn (1990), there are a limited number of basic human problems for which all people must find some solution and five common human problems with respect to values and norms: (1) the innate human nature of people; (2) relationship to nature; (3) time dimension; (4) the purpose of existence; and (5) relationships with others.

INNATE HUMAN NATURE

The innate human nature of people may be perceived as good, evil, or a combination. When conducting an interview, you may notice that some will indicate that human nature is unalterable or perfectible only with great discipline and effort, as people struggle to overcome a basically evil nature. For others, human nature is perceived to be fundamentally good, unalterable, and difficult or impossible to corrupt. The majority of people, however, are likely to view human nature in a mixed manner and may say, for example, "There are good people and bad people, good nurses and bad nurses; every profession has its combination or mixture."

RELATIONSHIP TO NATURE

In examining the ways in which our relationship to nature is perceived, there may be three perceptions: (1) *destiny,* in which the human person is subjugated to nature in a fatalistic, inevitable manner; (2) *harmony,* in which people and nature exist together as a single entity; and (3) *mastery,* in which it is believed that people are intended to overcome natural forces and put them to use for the benefit of humankind.

What does this values orientation have to do with health and illness? Let's examine three individuals who have been recently diagnosed with diabetes mellitus, each embracing one of the values orientations described. The person whose values orientation is destiny might say, "Why should I bother watching my diet? My diabetes is part of my genetic destiny and there is nothing I can do to change the outcome." The person whose values orientation embraces harmony might say, "If I follow the diet prescribed, I can achieve the balance and harmony necessary for health and wholeness by replacing what nature has failed to provide for me." Finally, the person whose values orientation leads to belief in active mastery might say, "I will overcome this diabetes no matter what. By eating the right foods and exercising, I will take charge of the situation and will ultimately be able to influence the course of my disease."

TIME DIMENSION

Perhaps one of the major areas in which cultural conflicts between nurses and patients from culturally diverse backgrounds occur is the failure to understand each other's perception of *time.* According to Kluckhohn (1990), there are three major ways in which people can perceive *time.*

1. The focus may be on the *past,* with traditions and ancestors playing an important role in the person's life. For example, many Asians, Native Americans, East Indians, and Africans hold beliefs about ancestors and tend to value long-standing traditions. In times of crisis, such as illness, individuals with a value orientation emphasizing the past may consult with ancestors or ask for their guidance or protection during the illness.
2. The focus may be on the *present,* with little attention being paid to the past or the future. These individuals are concerned with "now," and the future is perceived as vague or unpredictable. You may have difficulty encouraging these individuals to prepare for the future—for example, for discharge from the hospital, for future side effects or adverse reactions from the medication. In addition, they may fail to see the value of childhood immunizations or those aimed at preventing the flu, hepatitis, or other conditions afflicting adults.
3. For some people, the focus is on the *future,* with progress and change being highly valued. These individuals may express discontent with both the past and the present. In terms of health care, these individuals may inquire about the "latest treatment" and most modern equipment available for a particular problem and may express concern with nurses or physicians whom they perceive to be old-fashioned.

PURPOSE OF EXISTENCE

In examining the purpose of humankind's existence, three major views are held by people from various cultures: (1) *being,* in which the emphasis is on the spontaneous expression of impulses and desires because they are viewed as an integral component of the personality (e.g., some members of Hispanic cultures); (2) *being-in-becoming,* in which inner control, meditation, and detachment are emphasized as ways to achieve self-realization (e.g., some members of Asian cultures); and (3) *doing,* in which active striving and accomplishment are paramount as the individual competes against externally applied standards of achievement (e.g., some members of Judeo-Christian religions in Western cultures, including the United States, Canada, and Australia).

RELATIONSHIPS WITH OTHERS

Finally, let's consider the cultural values orientation concerning the relationships that exist with others. Relationships may be categorized in three ways:

1. *Lineal* relationships refer to those that exist by virtue of heredity and kinship ties. Lineal relationships follow an ordered succession and have continuity through time.
2. *Collateral* relationships focus primarily on group goals, and the family orientation is all-important. For example, some Asian-American people describe family honor and the importance of working together toward achievement of a group (versus personal) goal.
3. *Individual* relationships refer to personal autonomy and independence. Individual goals dominate, whereas group goals become secondary.

When making health-related decisions, people from culturally diverse backgrounds rely on relationships with others in various ways. If the cultural value orientation is lineal, the person may seek assistance from other members of the family and allow a relative (e.g., parent, grandparent, elder brother) to make decisions about important health-related matters. If collateral relationships are valued, decisions about the person may be interrelated with the impact of illness on the entire family or group. For example, among the Amish, the entire community is affected by the illness of a member because the community pays for health care from a common fund, members join together to meet the needs of both the person and his or her family throughout the illness, and the roles of dozens in the community are likely to be affected by the illness of a single member. Perhaps it is the value orientation toward *individual* relationships that is predominant among the majority of European Americans. Decision making about health and illness is often an individual matter, with the person being the sole decider, although members of the nuclear family may participate to varying degrees.

FAMILY

Despite the alarmingly high rate of divorce in the United States, the family remains the basic social unit. The essence of family consists of individuals living together as a unit. Although some social scientists argue that there are more than a dozen types of families, the following are commonly recognized types of families: (1) *nuclear* (husband, wife, and child[ren]); (2) *extended family* (nuclear plus blood relatives and even people who are not biologically related); (3) *blended* (husband, wife, and child[ren] from previous relationships); (4) *single parent* (either mother or father and at least one child); (5) *communal* (group of men, women, and children); (6) *cohabitation* (unmarried man and woman sharing a household with child[ren]); and (7) *gay/lesbian* (same-gender couple and child[ren]).

Each family modifies the culture of the larger group in ways that are uniquely its own. Some beliefs, practices, and customs are maintained, whereas others are altered or abandoned. You should also be aware that not all members of a cultural group behave according to the preconceived stereotype. For example, although many Chinese-American children behave in the manner congruent with the stereotype—showing respect for authority, polite social behavior, and moderate to soft voice—there are some who are disrespectful, impolite, and boisterous. Individual differences, changing norms over time, degree of acculturation, length of time the family has lived in the country, and other factors account for variation.

Relationships that may seem apparent sometimes warrant further exploration when interviewing people from culturally diverse backgrounds. For example, the dominant cultural group defines siblings as two persons with either the same mother, the same father, the same mother and father, or the same adoptive parents. In some Asian cultures, a sibling relationship is defined as one in which any infants are breast-fed by the same woman. In other cultures, certain kinship patterns, such as maternal first cousins, are defined as sibling relationships. In some African cultures, anyone from the same village or town may be called "brother" or "sister." Certain subcultures, such as members of the Roman Catholic or Orthodox religions (who may be further subdivided by ethnicity such as Italians, Polish, Spanish, Mexican, Greek, Russian, and so forth), recognize relationships such as *godmother* or *godfather* in which an individual who is not the biologic parent promises to assist with the moral and spiritual development of an infant and agrees to care for the child in the event of parental death. The godparent makes these promises during the religious ceremony of baptism.

When assessing families, it is important to identify key decision makers and the primary provider of care because this individual may or may not be the biologic parent. Among some Hispanic groups, for example, female members of the nuclear or extended family such as sisters and aunts are primary providers of care. In some black families, the grandmother may be the decision maker and primary caretaker of children. Remember that data about a person's family and social support network are useful in assessing the potential sources of psychosocial, emotional, physical, and financial support.

RELIGIOUS BELIEFS AND PRACTICES

As an integral component of the individual's culture, religious beliefs may influence the person's explanation of the cause(s) of illness, perception of its severity, and choice of healer(s). In times of crisis, such as serious illness and impending death, religion may be a source of consolation for the person and for his or her family. Religious dogma and spiritual leaders may exert considerable influence on the person's decision making concerning acceptable medical and surgical treatment, choice of healer(s), and other aspects of the illness.

RELIGION AND SPIRITUALITY

Religious concerns evolve from and respond to the mysteries of life and death, good and evil, and pain and suffering (Fig. 3–2). In health care settings, you frequently encounter people who find themselves searching for a spiritual meaning to help explain their illness or disability. Some nurses find spiritual assessment difficult because of the abstract and personal nature of the topic, whereas others feel quite comfortable discussing spiritual matters. Comfort with your own spiritual beliefs is the foundation to effective assessment of spiritual needs in others (Andrews & Hanson, 2002).

An important distinction needs to be made between spirituality and religion. *Spirituality* is borne out of each person's unique life experience and his or her personal effort to find purpose and meaning in life. While the religions of the world offer various interpretations to many of life's mysteries, most people seek a personal understanding and interpretation at some time in their lives. Ultimately, this personal search becomes a pursuit to discover a supreme being (called by names such as Allah, God, Yahweh, and Jehovah) or some unifying truth that will render meaning, purpose, and integrity to existence.

Religion refers to an organized system of beliefs concerning the cause, nature, and purpose of the universe, especially belief in or the worship of God or gods. There are more than 1500 religions in the United States. Seventy-seven percent of Americans report religious affiliation with a Christian church. Among the Christian denominations with which adults identify are Roman Catholic (25%), Baptist (16%), Methodist (7%), Lutheran (5%), Presbyterian (3%), Pentecostal (2%), Episcopal/Anglican (2%), Mormon or Church of Jesus Christ of Latter-Day Saints (1.3%), and Churches of Christ (1.2%). Those belonging to non-Christian religions total 6% of the U.S. population; of these the largest group are Jewish (2%). Those reporting no religious affiliation account for 14% of the population (American Religious Identification Survey, 2001; Pew Research Council, 2002).

Religious identification among people from different racial and ethnic groups is important because religion and culture are interconnected. The following provides an overview of religion and ethnicity among recent immigrants. In a recent Washington Post survey, 64% of Hispanic and 50% of black congregations in the United States regard their churches as a means of preserving their cultural heritage, compared with less than one third of white congregations (Broadway, 2001). During the past 2 decades there has been an unusually large group of immigrants from Asia and Latin America. The changing composition of the Asian population has resulted in fewer Christians (63% in 1990 compared with 43% in 2001), whereas those professing Asian religions (Buddhism, Hinduism, Islam, etc.) has risen from 15% to 28%. For example, there are more than three times as many Hindus in the United States today as there were in 1990. Although most of the Latin American immigrants are Catholic, there has been a 1% overall decline in the U.S. Catholic population—26% in 1990 compared to 25% in 2002 (American Religious Identification Survey, 2001; Pew Research Council, 2002).

Just as the trends in immigration have influenced our newest citizens, there has been a growing interest in the religious preferences of the oldest group, the Native Americans. The religious profile of Native Americans is similar to white, non-Hispanics: 20% identified themselves as Baptist, 17% as Catholic, and 17% indicated no religious preference. Only 3% indicated their primary religious identification as a tribal Indian religion, perhaps a reflection of the growing number of Native people who reside in nonreservation urban centers (American Religious Identification Survey, 2001).

DEVELOPMENTAL CONSIDERATIONS

Illness during childhood may be an especially difficult clinical situation. Children as well as adults have spiritual needs that vary according to the child's developmental level and the religious climate that exists in the family. Parental perceptions about the illness of their child may be partially influenced by religious beliefs. For example, some parents may believe that a transgression against a religious law is responsible for a congenital anomaly in their offspring. Other parents may delay seeking medical care because they believe that prayer should be tried first. Certain types of treatment (e.g., administration of blood; medications containing caffeine, pork, or other prohibited substances) and selected procedures may be perceived as *cultural taboos*—that is, practices to be avoided (by both children and adults).

Values held by the dominant United States and Canadian culture, such as emphasis on independence, self-reliance, and productivity, influence aging members of society. North Americans define people as old at the chronologic age of 65 and then limit their work, in contrast to other cultures in which persons are first recognized as being unable to work and then are identified as being old.

In adopting a cultural perspective in working with aging individuals from culturally diverse backgrounds, you should consider that the main task of these persons is to achieve a sense of integrity in accepting responsibility for their own lives and in gaining a sense of accomplishment (Fig. 3–3). Individuals who achieve integrity see aging as a positive experience, make adjustments in their personal space and social relationships, maintain a sense of usefulness, and begin closure and life review.

Older persons may develop their own means of coping with illness through self-care, assistance from family members, and support from social groups. Some cultures have developed attitudes and specific behaviors for older adults that may include humanistic care and identification of family members as care providers. The older adults may have special family responsibilities—for example, providing hospitality to

3-3

visitors among Amish cultures and communicating to members of younger generations skills and accrued wisdom among Filipinos.

Older immigrants who have made major lifestyle adjustments in their move from their homeland to the United States or from a rural to an urban area (or vice versa) may not be aware of health care alternatives, preventive programs, health care benefits, and screening programs for which they are eligible. These individuals may also be in various stages of *culture shock,* that is, the state of disorientation or inability to respond to the behavior of a different cultural group because of its sudden strangeness, unfamiliarity, and incompatibility to the stranger's perceptions and expectations.

HEALTH-RELATED BELIEFS AND PRACTICES

Before determining whether cultural practices are helpful, harmful, or neutral, you must first understand the logic of the belief system underlying the practice and then be certain that you fully grasp the nature and meaning of the practice from the person's cultural perspective.

HEALTH AND CULTURE

The first step in understanding the health care needs of others is to understand your own culturally based values, beliefs, attitudes, and practices. Sometimes this requires considerable introspection and may necessitate that you confront your own biases, preconceptions, and prejudices about specific racial, ethnic, religious, sexual, or socioeconomic groups.

Second, you need to identify the meaning of health to the patient, remembering that concepts are derived, in part, from the way in which members of their cultural group define health. Considerable research has been conducted on the various definitions of health that may be held by various groups. For example, some Jamaicans may define health as having a good appetite, feeling strong and energetic, performing activities of daily living without difficulty, and being sexually active and fertile. For Italian women, health may mean the ability to interact socially and to perform routine tasks such as cooking, cleaning, and caring for self

and others. On the other hand, some individuals of Mexican heritage believe that coughing, sweating, and diarrhea are a normal part of living, not symptoms of ill health—perhaps because of the high frequency of these conditions in the person's country of origin. Thus, individuals may define themselves or others in their group as healthy even though you identify them as having symptoms of disease.

ILLNESS AND CULTURE

For patients, symptom labeling and diagnosis depend on the degree of difference between the individual's behaviors and those the group has defined as normal, beliefs about the causation of illness, level of stigma attached to a particular set of symptoms, prevalence of the pathology, and the meaning of the illness to the individual and his or her family.

Throughout history, humankind has attempted to understand the cause of illness and disease. Theories of causation have been formulated based on religious beliefs, social circumstances, philosophical perspectives, and level of knowledge. You need to determine what the person believes has caused the illness.

Causes of Illness

Disease causation may be viewed in three major ways: from a biomedical or scientific, naturalistic or holistic, and magico-religious perspective.

BIOMEDICAL

The first, called the *biomedical* or *scientific* theory of illness causation, is based on the assumption that all events in life have a cause and effect, that the human body functions more or less mechanically (i.e., the functioning of the human body is analogous to the functioning of an automobile), that all life can be reduced or divided into smaller parts (e.g., the reduction of the human person into body, mind, and spirit), and that all of reality can be observed and measured (e.g., intelligence tests and psychometric measures of behavior). Among the biomedical explanations for disease is the germ theory, which posits that microscopic organisms such as bacteria and viruses are responsible for specific disease conditions. Most educational programs for physicians, nurses, and other health care providers embrace the biomedical or scientific theories that explain the causes of both physical and psychologic illnesses.

NATURALISTIC

The second way in which people explain the cause of illness is from the *naturalistic* or *holistic* perspective, found most frequently among Native Americans, Asians, and others who believe that human life is only one aspect of nature and a part of the general order of the cosmos. People from these groups believe that the forces of nature must be kept in natural balance or harmony.

Some Asians believe in the *yin/yang theory,* in which health is believed to exist when all aspects of the person are in perfect balance. Rooted in the ancient Chinese philosophy of *Tao,* the yin/yang theory states that all organisms and objects in the universe consist of yin and yang energy forces. The seat of the energy forces is within the autonomic nervous system where balance between the opposing forces is maintained during health. Yin energy represents the female and negative forces, such as emptiness, darkness, and cold, whereas yang forces are male and positive, emitting warmth and fullness. Foods are classified as hot and cold in this theory and are transformed into yin and yang energy when metabolized by the body. Yin foods are cold and yang foods are hot. Cold foods are eaten with a hot illness, and hot foods are eaten with a cold illness. The yin/yang theory is the basis for *Eastern* or *Chinese* medicine and is commonly embraced by many Asian Americans.

The naturalistic perspective posits that the laws of nature create imbalances, chaos, and disease. Individuals embracing the naturalistic view use metaphors such as the healing power of nature, and they call the earth "Mother." From the perspective of the Chinese, for example, illness is not seen as an intruding agent but as a part of life's rhythmic course and as an outward sign of disharmony within.

Many Hispanic, Arab, black, and Asian groups embrace the *hot/cold theory* of health and illness, an explanatory model having its origins in the ancient Greek humoral theory. The four humors of the body—blood, phlegm, black bile, and yellow bile—regulate basic bodily functions and are described in terms of temperature, dryness, and moisture. The treatment of disease consists of adding or subtracting cold, heat, dryness, or wetness to restore the balance of the humors.

Beverages, foods, herbs, medicines, and diseases are classified as hot or cold according to their perceived effects on the body, not on their physical characteristics. Illnesses believed to be caused by cold entering the body include earache, chest cramps, paralysis, gastrointestinal discomfort, rheumatism, and tuberculosis. Among those illnesses believed to be caused by overheating are abscessed teeth, sore throats, rashes, and kidney disorders.

According to the hot/cold theory, the individual as a whole, not just a particular ailment, is significant. Those who embrace the hot/cold theory maintain that health consists of a positive state of total well-being, including physical, psychological, spiritual, and social aspects of the person. Paradoxically, the language used to describe this artificial dissection of the body into parts is itself a reflection of the biomedical/scientific perspective, not a naturalistic or holistic one.

MAGICO-RELIGIOUS

The third major way in which people explain the causation of illness is from a *magico-religious* perspective. The basic premise is that the world is seen as an arena in which supernatural forces dominate. The fate of the world and those in it depends on the action of supernatural forces for good or evil. Examples of magical causes of illness include belief in voodoo or witchcraft among some blacks and others from circum-Caribbean countries. *Faith healing* is based on religious beliefs and is most prevalent among certain Christian religions, including Christian Scientists, whereas various healing rituals may be found in many other religions such as Roman Catholicism, and Mormonism.

Of course, it is possible to have a combination of world views, and many people are likely to offer more than one explanation for the cause of their illness. As a profession, nursing largely embraces the scientific/biomedical world view, but

some other aspects have begun to gain popularity, including a wide variety of techniques for management of chronic pain such as acupuncture, herbal therapies, hypnosis, therapeutic touch, and biofeedback. Belief in spiritual power is also held by many health care providers who may credit supernatural forces with various unexplained phenomena related to patients' health and illness states.

HEALING AND CULTURE

When self-treatment is unsuccessful, the individual might turn to the lay or folk healing systems, to spiritual or religious healing, or to scientific biomedicine. All cultures have their own preferred lay or popular healers, recognized symptoms of ill health, acceptable sick role behavior, and treatments. In addition to seeking help from you as a biomedical/scientific health care provider, patients may also seek help from folk or religious healers. Some people, such as those of Hispanic or Native American origins, may believe that the cure is incomplete unless healing of body, mind, and spirit are all carried out, although the division of the person into parts is itself a Western concept. For example, a Hispanic person with a respiratory infection may take the antibiotics prescribed by a physician or nurse practitioner (Fig. 3–4) and herbal teas recommended by a *curandero* and may say prayers for healing suggested by a Catholic priest.

The variety of healing beliefs and practices used by the many subcultural groups found in this country far exceeds the limitations of this chapter. It is important, however, that you be aware of the existence of alternative practices and recognize that, in addition to folk practices, many other alternative healing practices exist. Although it is dangerous to assume that all indigenous approaches to healing are innocuous, the majority of practices are quite harmless, whether or not they are effective cures.

Folk Healers

Although numerous folk healers exist, you may find Hispanics turning to a *curandero(ra), espiritualista* (spiritualist), *yerbo* (herbalist), or *sabedor* (healer who manipulates bones and muscles). Blacks may mention having received assistance from a *hougan* (a voodoo priest or priestess), *spiritual-*

3–4

ist, or *"old lady"* (an older woman who has successfully raised a family and who specializes in child care and folk remedies). Native Americans may seek assistance from a *shaman* or *medicine (wo)man.* Asians may mention that they have visited *herbalists, acupuncturists,* or *bone setters.* Among the Amish the term *braucher* refers to folk healers who use herbs and tonics in the home or community context. *Brauche,* a folk healing art, refers to sympathy curing, which is sometimes called *powwowing* in English. The treatments used by the braucher may be provided in conjunction with massage; foot treatments; acupressure; reflexology; or, less frequently, iridology (Andrews & Boyle, 2002; Wenger, 1995).

Each culture has its own healers, most of whom speak the person's native tongue, make house calls, and cost significantly less than healers practicing in the biomedical/scientific health care system. In addition to folk healers, many cultures have lay midwives (e.g., *parteras* for Hispanic women) or other health care providers available for pregnant women.

In some religions, spiritual healers may be found among the ranks of the ordained and official religious hierarchy and may be known by a variety of names such as priest, bishop, elder, deacon, rabbi, brother, and sister. In other religions, a separate category of healer may be found—e.g., Christian Science "nurses" (not licensed by states) or practitioners.

TRANSCULTURAL EXPRESSION OF ILLNESS

Wide cultural variation exists in the manner in which certain symptoms and disease conditions are perceived, diagnosed, labeled, and treated. You should not assume that the perceived symptoms or complaints of patients are equivalent to the names of recognized diseases or syndromes familiar to nurses, physicians, and other health care professionals (Wenger, 1993). The same disease that is considered grounds for social ostracism in one culture may be reason for increased status in another. For example, epilepsy is seen as contagious and untreatable among Ugandans, as a cause for family shame among Greeks, as a reflection of a physical imbalance among Mexican Americans, and as a sign of having gained favor by enduring a trial by God among the Hutterites.

Bodily symptoms are also perceived and reported in a variety of ways. For example, people of Mediterranean descent tend to report common physical symptoms more often than persons of Northern European or Asian heritage. Among Chinese, no translation exists for the English word "sadness," yet all people experience the feeling of sadness at some time in life. To express emotion, Chinese patients somaticize their symptoms, or convert mental experiences or states into bodily symptoms (e.g., complain of cardiac symptoms because the center of emotion in the Chinese culture is the heart). You may collect in-depth data about the cardiovascular system only to learn subsequently that all diagnostic tests are negative. On further assessment, you may determine that the person has experienced a loss and is grieving (e.g., has experienced the death of a close friend or relative, or has been divorced or separated). Although some biomedical/scientific clinicians may refer to this as a psychosomatic illness, others recognize it as a culturally acceptable somatic expression of emotional disharmony (Wenger, 1993).

A discussion of pain follows to illustrate the cultural variability that may occur with a symptom of significant concern.

TRANSCULTURAL EXPRESSION OF PAIN

To illustrate the manner in which symptom expression may reflect the person's cultural background, let's use an extensively studied symptom—pain. Pain is a universally recognized phenomenon and is an important aspect of assessment for people of various ages. Pain is a very private, subjective experience that is greatly influenced by cultural heritage. Expectations, manifestations, and management of pain are all embedded in a cultural context. The definition of pain, like that of health or illness, is culturally determined.

The word *pain* is derived from the Greek word for penalty, which helps explain the long association between pain and punishment in Judeo-Christian thought. The meaning of painful stimuli for individuals, the way people define their situation, and the impact of personal experience all help determine the experience of pain.

Much cross-cultural research has been conducted on pain. Pain has been found to be a highly personal experience, depending on cultural learning, the meaning of the situation, and other factors unique to the individual. Silent suffering has been identified as the most valued response to pain by health care professionals. The majority of nurses have been socialized to believe that in virtually any situation, self-control is better than open displays of strong feelings.

In research studies of nurses' attitudes toward pain, it was discovered that the ethnic background of patients is important in the nurses' assessment of both physical and psychological pain. For example, nurses preconceive that Jewish and Spanish patients suffer the most and that Anglo-Saxon, German, and Asian patients suffer the least. In addition, nurses who infer relatively greater patient pain tended to report their own experiences as more painful. In general, nurses from Eastern and Southern European or African backgrounds tend to infer greater suffering than do nurses of Northern European backgrounds. Years of experience, current position, and area of clinical practice are unrelated to inferences of suffering (Ludwig-Beymer, 2002).

In addition to expecting variations in pain perception and tolerance, you also should expect variations in the expression of pain. It is well-known that individuals turn to their social environment for validation and comparison. A first important comparison group is the family, which transmits cultural norms to its children.

CULTURE-BOUND SYNDROMES

Some people may have a condition that is culturally defined, known as a *culture-bound syndrome.* Some of these conditions have no equivalent from a biomedical/scientific perspective, whereas others, such as anorexia nervosa and bulimia, are examples of the cultural aspects of illness among members of a dominant group in North America. Table 3–1 summarizes selected examples from among the more than 150 culture-bound syndromes that have been documented by medical anthropologists.

TABLE 3-1: Selected Culture-Bound Syndromes

GROUP	DISORDER	REMARKS
Blacks	Blackout	Collapse, dizziness, inability to move
	Low blood	Not enough blood or weakness of the blood, which is often treated with diet
	High blood	Blood that is too rich in certain nutrients due to ingestion of too much red meat or rich foods
	Thin blood	Occurs in women, children, and old people; renders the individual more susceptible to illness in general
	Diseases of hex, witchcraft, or conjuring	Sense of being doomed by spell; part of voodoo beliefs
Caribbean and Southern U.S.	Rootwork	Refers to a set of cultural interpretations that explain illness causation in terms of hexing, witchcraft, voodoo, or the influence of an evil person
China	Shenkui	Marked anxiety or panic symptoms with dizziness, backache, general weakness, insomnia, frequent dreams, and complaints of sexual dysfunction (premature ejaculation and impotence). Believed to be caused by excessive semen loss. Feared because it represents a loss of vital essence and is believed to be life threatening.
Chinese/Southeast Asians	Koro	Intense anxiety that penis is retracting into body
Germany/Spain	Involutional paraphrenia	Paranoid disorder occurring in midlife
Greeks	Hysteria	Bizarre complaints and behavior because the uterus leaves the pelvis for another part of the body
Haitians	Boufée deliriante	Agitation, sudden outbursts, aggressive behavior, marked confusion. May be accompanied by hallucinations and paranoia. Similar to brief psychotic disorder.
Hispanics	Empacho	Food forms into a ball and clings to the stomach or intestines causing pain and cramping
	Fatique	Asthma-like symptoms
	Mal ojo ("evil eye")	Fitful sleep, crying, diarrhea in children caused by a stranger's attention; sudden onset
	Pasmo	Paralysis-like symptoms of face or limbs; prevented or relieved by massage
	Susto	Anxiety, trembling, phobias from sudden fright
India	Dhat	Semen-loss syndrome. Characterized by severe anxiety and hypochondriac concerns about semen discharge. Whitish discoloration of the urine and feelings of weakness.
Indonesians	Latah	Hypersuggestibility, trancelike behavior
	Waswas	Excessive repetition of words or gestures
Japanese	Wagamama	Apathetic childish behavior with emotional outbursts
Koreans	Hwa–byung	Multiple somatic and psychologic symptoms; "pushing up" sensation in the chest; palpitations; flushing; headache; sensation of a stomach mass; dysphoria, anxiety; irritability; and difficulty concentrating. Highest incidence in married women.
Malaysians	Amok	Dissociative episode characterized by a period of brooding followed by an outburst of violent, aggressive, or homicidal behavior directed at people and objects. Precipitated by a perceived insult or slight and occurs only among males. Similar to mal de pelea (Puerto Rico); iich'aa (Navajo); and related syndromes found in Laos, Papau New Guinea, and the Philippines.
Middle Eastern and North African groups (Ethiopia, Somalia, Egypt, Iran, Sudan)	Zar	Spirit possession, laughing, shouting, hitting the head against a wall, singing, or weeping. Apathy and withdrawal. Refusal to eat or engage in activities of daily living (ADLs)
Native Americans	Ghost	Tremor, hallucinations, sense of danger
Native Americans (Mohave American Indians)	Hi-wa-itck	Insomnia, depression, loss of appetite. Associated with unwanted separation from a loved one.
Taiwan	Hsieh-ping	Brief trancelike state during which the person is possessed by an ancestral ghost who is trying to communicate with family members. Symptoms include tremors, disorientation, and visual or auditory hallucinations.
Whites	Anorexia nervosa	Excessive preoccupation with thinness; self-imposed starvation
	Bulimia	Gross overeating, then vomiting or fasting

CULTURE AND TREATMENT

After a symptom is identified, the first effort at treatment is often self-care. In the United States an estimated 70% to 90% of all illness episodes are treated first, or exclusively, through self-care, often with significant success (Lipson and Steiger, 1996). The availability of over-the-counter medications, relatively high literacy level of Americans, growing availability of herbal remedies, and influence of the mass media in communicating health-related information to the general population have contributed to the high percentage of cases of self-treatment. Home treatments are attractive for their accessibility, especially when compared with the inconvenience associated with traveling to a physician, nurse practitioner, and pharmacist, particularly for people from rural or sparsely populated areas. Furthermore, home treatment may mobilize the person's social support network and provide the sick individual with a caring environment in which to convalesce. You should be aware, however, that not all home remedies are inexpensive. For example, urban black populations in the Southeast sometimes use medicinal potions that cost much more than the equivalent treatment with a biomedical intervention.

A wide variety of alternative or complementary interventions are gaining the recognition of health care professionals in the biomedical/scientific health care system. Acupuncture, acupressure, therapeutic touch, massage, therapeutic use of music, biofeedback, relaxation techniques, meditation, hypnosis, distraction, imagery, iridology, reflexology, herbal remedies, and others are interventions that people may use either alone or in combination with other treatments. Many pharmacies and grocery stores routinely carry herbal treatments for a wide variety of common illnesses. The efficacy of complementary and alternative interventions for specific health problems has been studied extensively (see National Center for Complementary and Alternative Medicine at http://www.nccam.nih.gov).

CULTURE AND DISEASE PREVALENCE

For the past generation, the United States and Canada have enjoyed improvement in the health status of their people. Despite this fact, there continues to be disparity in deaths and illnesses experienced by racial and ethnic minority populations, and it is well known that diseases are not distributed equally among all segments of the population but rather tend to cluster around certain racial and ethnic subgroups. Abnormal biocultural variations may be genetic or acquired. Information about disease prevalence for various racial and ethnic groups is useful because you are able to focus your assessment according to the increased statistical probability that a particular condition may occur. For example, if you are examining a black child with gastrointestinal symptoms, you may focus more on the possibility of lactose intolerance or sickle-cell anemia, while considering cystic fibrosis, known primarily among white children, a much less likely source of the problem. Thus, in your assessment, you will want to be certain that you have gathered the appropriate data needed to support or to refute your suspicions.

CULTURAL ASSESSMENT

A *cultural assessment* refers to a systematic appraisal or examination of individuals, groups, and communities in relation to their cultural beliefs, values, and practices to determine explicit health care needs and intervention practices within the cultural context of the people being evaluated (Andrews & Boyle, 2002; Leininger & McFarland, 2002). Cultural assessments tend to be broad and comprehensive because they deal with cultural values, belief systems, and ways of living now and in the recent past. However, you can learn to appraise segments of these larger areas, such as a particular cultural value, and then relate this finding to other aspects such as cultural practices. Table 3–2 summarizes major data categories pertaining to culture and offers suggested questions that you might ask the person to elicit the information.

TABLE 3–2: Cultural Assessment*

BRIEF HISTORY OF THE CULTURAL GROUP WITH WHICH THE PERSON IDENTIFIES

- With what cultural group(s) does the person affiliate (e.g., Hispanic, Polish, Navajo, or combination)? To what degree does the person identify with the cultural group (e.g., "we" concept of solidarity or a fringe member)?
- What is the person's reported racial affiliation (e.g., black, Native American, Asian)?
- Where was the person born?
- Where has the person lived (country, city) and when (during what years)? Note: If the person has recently relocated to the United States, knowledge of prevalent diseases in country of origin may be helpful.

VALUES ORIENTATION

- What are the person's attitudes, values, and beliefs about birth, death, health, illness, health care providers?

- How does the person view work, leisure, education?
- How does the person perceive change?

CULTURAL SANCTIONS AND RESTRICTIONS

- How does the person's cultural group regard expression of emotion and feelings, spirituality, and religious beliefs? How are dying, death, and grieving expressed in a culturally appropriate manner?
- How is modesty expressed by men and women? Are there culturally defined expectations about male-female relationships, including the health care relationship?
- Does the person have any restrictions related to sexuality, exposure of body parts, certain types of surgery (e.g., amputation, vasectomy, hysterectomy)?
- Are there any restrictions against discussion of dead relatives or fears related to the unknown?

Data for spiritual considerations from Andrews MM, Hanson PA: Religion, culture, and nursing, In Andrews MM, Boyle JS, editors: *Transcultural concepts in nursing care,* ed 4, Philadelphia, 2003, Lippincott Williams & Wilkins.
*Cultural Assessment is reprinted in a format intended for direct use with patients in Jarvis CM: *Student laboratory manual for physical examination and health assessment,* ed 4, Philadelphia, 2004, W.B. Saunders.

TABLE 3–2: Cultural Assessment—cont'd

COMMUNICATION

- What language does the person speak at home? What other languages does the person speak or read? In what language would the person prefer to communicate with you?
- Does the person need an interpreter? If so, is there a relative or friend whom he or she would like to interpret? Is there anyone whom the person would prefer did not interpret (e.g., member of the opposite sex, a person younger/older than the person, member of a rival tribe or nation)?
- How does the person feel about health care providers who are not of the same cultural background (e.g., black, middle-class nurse and Hispanic patient of a different social class)? Does the person prefer to receive care from a nurse or doctor of the same cultural background, gender, and/or age?

HEALTH-RELATED BELIEFS AND PRACTICES

- To what cause(s) does the person attribute illness and disease (e.g., divine wrath, imbalance in hot/cold or yin/yang, punishment for moral transgressions, hex, soul loss)?
- What does the person believe promotes health (eating certain foods, wearing amulets to bring good luck, exercise, prayer, rituals to ancestors, saints, or intermediate deities)?
- What is the person's religious affiliation (e.g., Judaism, Islam, Pentecostalism, West African voodooism, Seventh-Day Adventism, Catholicism, Mormonism)?
- Does the person rely on cultural healers (e.g., curandero, shaman, spiritualist, priest, minister, monk)? Who determines when the person is sick and when he or she is healthy? Who determines the type of healer and treatment that should be sought?
- In what types of cultural healing practices does the person engage (use of herbal remedies, potions, massage, wearing of talismans or charms to discourage evil spirits, healing rituals, incantations, prayers)?
- How are biomedical/scientific health care providers perceived? How does the person and his or her family perceive nurses or physicians? What are the expectations of nurses and nursing care?
- What is appropriate "sick role" behavior? Who determines what symptoms constitute disease/illness? Who decides when the person is no longer sick? Who cares for the person at home?
- How does the person's cultural group view mental disorders? Are there differences in acceptable behaviors for physical versus psychological illnesses?

NUTRITION

- What is the meaning of food and eating to the person? With whom does the person usually eat? What types of foods are eaten? What does the person define as food? What does the person believe composes a "healthy" versus an "unhealthy" diet?
- How are foods prepared at home (type of food preparation; cooking oil[s] used; length of time foods are cooked, especially vegetables; amount and type of seasoning added to various foods during preparation)?
- Do religious beliefs and practices influence the person's diet (e.g., amount, type, preparation, or delineation of acceptable food combinations, such as kosher diets)? Does the person abstain from certain foods at regular intervals, on specific dates determined by the religious calendar, or at other times?
- If the person's religion mandates or encourages fasting, what does the term "fast" mean (e.g., refraining from certain types or quantities of foods, eating only during certain times of the day)? For what period of time is the person expected to fast?
- During fasting, does the person refrain from liquids/beverages? Does the religion allow exemption from fasting during illness? If so, does the person believe that an exemption applies to him or her?

SOCIOECONOMIC CONSIDERATIONS

- Who composes the person's social network (family, peers, and cultural healers)? How do they influence the person's health or illness status?

- How do members of the person's social support network define caring (e.g., being continuously present, doing things for the person, looking after the person's family)? What are the roles of various family members during health and illness?
- How does the person's family participate in the nursing care (e.g., bathing, feeding, touching, being present)?
- Does the cultural family structure influence the person's response to health or illness (e.g., beliefs, strengths, weaknesses, and social class)? Is there a key family member whose role is significant in health-related decisions (e.g., grandmother in many black families, eldest adult son in Asian families)?
- Who is the principal wage earner in the person's family? What is the total annual income? (Note: This is a potentially sensitive question that should be asked only if necessary.) Is there more than one wage earner? Are there other sources of financial support (extended family, investments)?
- What impact does economic status have on lifestyle, place of residence, living conditions, ability to obtain health care, discharge planning?

ORGANIZATIONS PROVIDING CULTURAL SUPPORT

- What influence do ethnic/cultural organizations have on the person's receiving health care (e.g., Organization of Migrant Workers, National Association for the Advancement of Colored People [NAACP], Black Political Caucus, churches, schools, Urban League, community-based health care programs and clinics)?

EDUCATIONAL BACKGROUND

- What is the person's highest educational level obtained?
- Can the person read and write English, or is another language preferred? If English is the second language, are materials available in the primary language?
- What learning style is most comfortable/familiar? Does the person prefer to learn through written materials, oral explanation, or demonstration?

RELIGIOUS AFFILIATION

- What is the role of religious beliefs and practices during health and illness?
- Are there healing rituals or practices that the person believes can promote well-being or hasten recovery from illness? If so, who performs these?
- What is the role of significant religious representatives during health and illness? Are there recognized healers (e.g., Islamic imams, Christian Scientist practitioners or nurses, Catholic priests, Mormon elders, Buddhist monks)?

SPIRITUAL CONSIDERATIONS

- Does the person have religious objects in the environment?
- Does the person wear outer- or undergarments having religious significance?
- Are get-well greeting cards religious in nature or from a religious representative?
- Does the person appear to pray at certain times of the day or before meals?
- Does the person make special dietary requests (e.g., kosher diet; vegetarian diet; diet free from caffeine, pork, shellfish, or other specific food items)?
- Does the person read religious magazines or books?
- Does the person mention God (Allah, Buddha, Yahweh, or a synonym), prayer, faith, or other religious topics?
- Is a request made for a visit by a member of the clergy or other religious representative?
- Is there an expression of anxiety or fear about pain, suffering, death?
- Does the person prefer to interact with others or to remain alone?

BIBLIOGRAPHY

Abbott PD et al: Improving your cultural awareness with culture clues, *Nurse Pract* 27(2):44–51, 2002.

American Religious Identification Survey 2001: The City University of New York, NY, 2001. Available at www.gc.cuny.edu/studies/religion ethnicity.htm. (June 5, 2001).

Andrews MM, Boyle JS: Competence in transcultural nursing care, *Am J Nurs* 97(8):16AAA-16DDD, 1997.

Andrews MM, Boyle JS: *Transcultural concepts in nursing care,* ed 4, Philadelphia, 2003, Lippincott Williams & Wilkins.

Andrews MM, Hanson PA: Religion, culture and nursing. In Andrews MM, Boyle JS, editors: *Transcultural concepts in nursing care,* ed 3, Philadelphia, 2003, Lippincott, pp. 432–502.

Broadway B: Faith communities in the United States today. *Washington Post,* March 13, 2001 (Available at washingtonpost/com/we-dyn/articles/A944-2001Mar 13.html).

Campinha-Bacote J: A model and instrument for addressing cultural competence in health care, *J Nurs Educ* 38(5):203–207, 1999.

Campinha-Bacote J, Munoz C: A guiding framework for delivering culturally competent services in case management, *J Case Manag* 12(2):48–52, 2001.

Geisler EM: *Pocket guide to cultural assessment,* ed 2, St Louis, 1998, Mosby.

Kluckhohn FR: Dominant and variant value orientations. In Brink PJ, editor: *Transcultural nursing: a book of readings,* Englewood Cliffs, NJ, 1990, Prentice Hall, pp. 63–81.

Leininger MM: What is transcultural nursing and culturally competent care? *J Transcult Nurs* 10(1):9, 1999.

Leininger MM, McFarland MR: *Transcultural nursing: concepts, theories, research and practices,* New York, 2002, McGraw-Hill.

Lester N: Cultural competence: a nursing dialogue. Part 1, *Am J Nurs* 98(8):26–34, 1998.

Lester N: Cultural competence: a nursing dialogue. Part 2, *Am J Nurs* 98(9):36–43, 1998.

Lipson JG, Steiger NJ: *Self-care nursing in a multicultural context,* Thousand Oaks, Mich, 1996, Sage Publications.

Ludwig-Beymer PA: Transcultural aspects of pain. In Andrews MM, Boyle JS, editors: *Transcultural concepts in nursing care,* ed 4, Philadelphia, 2002, Lippincott, Williams & Wilkins, pp. 405–431.

Meleis AI: Culturally competent care, *J Transcult Nurs* 10(1):12, 1999.

Office of Minority Health: *Assuring cultural competence in health care: recommendations for national standards and an outcomes-focused research agenda.* Washington, DC, 1999, Department of Health and Human Services, U.S. Public Health Service, (Available at www.omhrc.gov/clas/ds.htm).

Pew Research Council: *Americans struggle with religion's role at home and abroad.* The Pew Research Center, March 20, 2002 (Available at www.adherents.com/rel_USA/html).

Smith LS: Concept analysis: cultural competence, *J Cult Divers* 5(1):4–10, 1998.

U.S. Bureau of the Census: *General population characteristics,* 2002 (Available at factfinder.census.gov).

Wenger AF: Cultural context, health, and health care decision making, *J Transcult Nurs* 7(1):3–14, 1995.

Wenger AF: Cultural meaning of symptoms, *Holist Nurs Pract* 7(2):22–35, 1993.

Zatrick DF, Dimsdale JE: Cultural variations in response to painful stimuli, *Psychosom Med* 52:544–557, 1990.

The Interview

*T*he interview is a meeting between you and your patient. The meeting's goal is to record a complete health history. The health history is important in beginning to identify the person's health strengths and problems and as a bridge to the next step in data collection, the physical examination.

The interview is the first and really the most important part of data collection. It collects **subjective data**—what the person says about himself or herself. The interview is the first and the best chance a person has to tell you what *he or she* perceives the health state to be. Once people enter the health care system, they may relinquish some control. At the interview, however, the patient is still in charge. The individual knows everything about his or her own health state, and you know nothing. Your skill in interviewing will glean all the necessary information as well as build rapport for a successful working relationship. When you have a successful interview, you:

1. Gather complete and accurate data about the person's health state, including the description and chronology of any symptoms of illness.
2. Establish rapport and trust so the person feels accepted and thus free to share all relevant data.
3. Teach the person about the health state so that the person can participate in identifying problems.
4. Build rapport for a continuing therapeutic relationship; this rapport facilitates future diagnoses, planning, and treatment.
5. Begin teaching for health promotion and disease prevention.

Consider the interview as being similar to forming a contract between you and your patient. A contract consists of spoken or unspoken rules for behavior. In this case, the contract concerns what the person needs and expects from health care and what you, the health professional, have to offer. Your mutual goal is optimal health for the patient. The contract's terms include:

- Time and place of the interview and succeeding physical examination
- Introduction of yourself and a brief explanation of your role
- The purpose of the interview
- How long it will take
- Expectation of participation for each person
- Presence of any other people (e.g., patient's family, other health professionals, students)
- Confidentiality and to what extent it may be limited
- Any costs that the patient must pay

Although the patient already may know some of this information through telephone contact with receptionists or the admitting office, the remaining points need to be stated clearly at the outset. Any confusion could produce resentment and anger, rather than the openness and trust you need to facilitate the interview.

THE PROCESS OF COMMUNICATION

The vehicle that carries you and your patient through the interview is communication. Communication is exchanging information so that each person clearly understands the other. If you do not understand each other, if you have not *conveyed meaning*, no communication has occurred.

It is challenging to teach the skill of interviewing because initially most students think little needs to be learned. They assume that if they can talk and hear, they can communicate. But much more than talking and hearing is necessary. Communication is all behavior, conscious and unconscious, verbal and nonverbal. *All behavior has meaning.*

SENDING

Likely, you are most aware of *verbal* communication—the words you speak, vocalizations, the tone of voice. *Nonverbal* communication also occurs. This is your body language—posture, gestures, facial expression, eye contact, foot tapping, touch, even where you place your chair. Since nonverbal communication is under less conscious control than verbal communication, nonverbal communication probably is more reflective of your true feelings.

RECEIVING

Being aware of the messages you send is only part of the process. Your words and gestures must be interpreted in a *specific context* to have meaning. You have a specific context in mind when you send your words. The receiver puts his or her own interpretation on them. The receiver attaches meaning determined by his or her past experiences, culture, and self-concept, as well as current physical and emotional state. Sometimes these contexts do not coincide. Remember how frustrating it may have been to try to communicate something to a friend, only to have your message totally misunderstood? Your message can be sabotaged by the listener's bias. It takes mutual understanding by the sender and receiver to have successful communication.

Even greater risk for misunderstanding exists in the health care setting than in a social setting. The patient usually has a health problem, and this factor emotionally charges your professional relationship. It *intensifies* the communication because the person feels dependent on you to get better.

Communication is a *basic skill* that can be learned and polished when you are a beginning practitioner. It is a tool, as basic to quality health care as the tools of inspection or palpation. To maximize your communicating skill, first you need to be aware of internal and external factors and their influence.

INTERNAL FACTORS

Internal factors are those particular to the examiner, what you bring into the interview. Cultivate the three inner factors of liking others, empathy, and the ability to listen.

LIKING OTHERS

One essential factor for an examiner's "goodness of fit" into a helping profession is a genuine liking of other people. This means a generally optimistic view of people: an assumption of their strengths and a tolerance for their weaknesses (Benjamin, 1980). An atmosphere of warmth and caring is necessary. The patient must feel that he or she is accepted unconditionally.

The respect for other people extends to respect for their own control over their health. Your goal is *not* to make your patients dependent on you, but to help them to be increasingly responsible for themselves. You wish to promote their growth. You have the health care resources to offer. Patients must choose how to apply those resources to their own lives.

EMPATHY

Empathy means viewing the world from the other person's inner frame of reference while remaining yourself. Empathy means recognizing and accepting the other person's feelings without criticism. It is described as "feeling *with* the person rather than feeling *like* the person" (Bernstein and Bernstein, 1985). It does not mean you become lost in the other person at the expense of your own self. If this occurred you would cease to be helpful. Rather, it is to *understand with* the person how *he or she* perceives his or her world (Rogers, 1951).

THE ABILITY TO LISTEN

Listening is not a passive role in the communication process; it is active and demanding. Listening requires your complete attention. You cannot be preoccupied with your own needs or the needs of other patients, or you will miss something important with this one. For the time of this interview, no one is more important than this person. This person's needs are your sole concern.

Active listening is the route to understanding. You cannot be thinking of what you are going to say as soon as the person stops for breath. Listen to *what* the person says. The story may not come out in the order you would ask it, or will record it later. Let the person talk from his or her own outline; nearly everything that is said will be relevant. Listen to *the way* a person tells the story, such as difficulty with language, impaired memory, the tone of the person's voice, and even to what the person is leaving out (Clinical Illustration).

Clinical Illustration

Sandra B., 32 years of age, sought care for headaches she had during the last 3 months, which were unresponsive to aspirin and were interfering with her job. She was interviewed for 30 minutes. Through this time she never mentioned her husband, although they had been married only 5 months earlier. Finally, the examiner asked, "I haven't heard you mention your husband. Tell me about him." It unfolded that Sandra's husband lost his job a few months after they were married because of alcohol-related work errors. Although Sandra related extreme personal stress and worry, she never thought that her headaches might be related to the stressful situation.

EXTERNAL FACTORS

Prepare the physical setting. The setting may be in a hospital room, an examination room in an office or clinic, or in the person's home (where you will have less control). In any location, optimal conditions are important to have a smooth interview.

ENSURE PRIVACY

Aim for geographic privacy—a private room in the hospital, clinic, office, or home. This may involve asking an ambulatory roommate to step out for a while or finding an unoccupied room or an empty lounge. If geographic privacy is not available, "psychological privacy" by curtained partitions may suffice as long as the person feels sure no one can overhear the conversation or interrupt.

REFUSE INTERRUPTIONS

Most people resent interruptions except in cases of an emergency. Inform any support staff of your interview, and ask that they not interrupt you during this time. Discourage other health professionals from interrupting you with *their* need for access to the patient. You need to concentrate and to establish rapport. An interruption can destroy in seconds what you have spent many minutes building up.

PHYSICAL ENVIRONMENT

- Set the room temperature at a comfortable level.
- Provide sufficient lighting so that you can see each other clearly. Avoid facing the patient directly toward a strong light where the patient must squint as if on stage.
- Reduce noise. Multiple stimuli are confusing. Turn off the television, radio, and any unnecessary equipment.
- Remove distracting objects or equipment. It is appropriate to leave some professional equipment (oto/ophthalmoscope, blood pressure manometer) in view. However, clutter, stacks of mail, files of other patients, or your lunch should not be seen. The room should advertise the professional nature of the interviewer.
- Place the distance between you and the patient at 4 to 5 feet (twice arm's length). If you place the patient any closer, you may invade his or her private space and you may create anxiety. If you place the patient farther away, you seem distant and aloof. (See the section on Transcultural Considerations for more information.)
- Arrange equal-status seating. Both you and the patient should be comfortably seated, at eye level. Avoid facing a patient across a desk or table because that feels like a barrier. Placing the chairs at 90 degrees is good because it allows the person either to face you or to look straight ahead from time to time (Fig. 4–1). Most important, avoid standing. Standing does two things: (1) it communicates your haste, and (2) it assumes superiority. Standing makes you loom over the patient as an authority figure. When you are sitting, the person feels some control in the setting.
- Arrange a face-to-face position when interviewing the hospitalized bedridden person. The person should not have to stare at the ceiling, because this causes him or her to lose the visual message of your communication.

DRESS

- The patient should remain in street clothes except in the case of an emergency.

4–1 Equal status seating.

- Your appearance and clothing should be appropriate to the setting and should meet conventional professional standards: a uniform or lab coat over conservative clothing, a name tag, and neat hair. Avoid extremes.

NOTE-TAKING

Some use of history forms and note-taking may be unavoidable. When you sit down later to record the interview, you cannot rely completely on memory to furnish details of previous hospitalizations or the review of body systems, for example. But be aware that note-taking during the interview has disadvantages:

- It breaks eye contact too often.
- It shifts your attention away from the person, diminishing his or her sense of importance.
- It can interrupt the patient's narrative flow. You may say "Please slow down; I'm not getting it all." Or, the patient may see you recording furiously, and in an effort to please you, adjust his or her tempo to your writing. Either way, the patient's natural mode of expression is lost.
- It impedes your observation of the patient's nonverbal behavior.
- It is threatening to the patient during the discussion of sensitive issues (e.g., amount of alcohol and drug use, number of sexual partners, or incidence of physical abuse).

So keep note-taking to a minimum, and try to focus your attention on the person. Any recording you do should be secondary to the dialogue and should not interfere with the person's spontaneity. With experience, you will not rely on note-taking as much.

TAPE AND VIDEO RECORDING

An audio tape documents a complete record of what was said during the interview. You cannot refer to it as easily as you can to your notes, but the tape is an excellent teaching tool to study objectively your performance as an interviewer. After listening, other students have commented:

"I never realized how much I talked. I really dominated the patient."

"I have to watch my interrupting. I cut her off that time."

"There. That response really worked. She opened up. I want to be that effective more often."

Tapes demonstrate how you can improve your communication. And, as you gain experience, the tapes also document your advancing skills. This process is very rewarding.

A video recording takes the teaching-learning tool one step further because you can study both verbal and nonverbal communication at the same time. Initial anxiety is common among students who feel self-conscious and fear "making a fool" of themselves on camera, but the video can detect richer detail in nonverbal behavior.

"I must have crossed and uncrossed my legs 20 times! I never realized I did that. My fidgeting sure made Mr. J. look distracted."

"It was good that I leaned toward her when she paused that time. I think it helped her continue."

"I talked for five minutes nonstop about how to perform breast self examination, without ever letting Mrs. S. ask a question!"

If you use any tape recording, some ethical considerations are necessary. Explain to the person the purpose of the recording (whether for teaching, supervision, research), exactly who will hear it (you, your supervisor), and that it will then be destroyed. Obtain consent before you start. Be thoroughly familiar with the equipment; fumbling with the controls is distracting. Arrange the microphone between you and the patient and place the rest of the recording equipment out of sight. It is likely that after a few moments, neither of you will be aware of the recording.

TECHNIQUES OF COMMUNICATION

INTRODUCING THE INTERVIEW

The patient is here and you are ready for the interview. If you are nervous about how to begin, remember to keep the beginning short. Probably, the patient is nervous, too, and is anxious to start. Address the person, using his or her surname, and shake hands if that seems comfortable. Introduce yourself and state your role in the agency (if you are a student, say so). If you are gathering a complete history, give the reason for this interview:

"Mrs. Sanchez, I would like to talk about your illness that caused you to come to the hospital."

"Ms. Taft, I want to ask you some questions about your health so that we can identify what is keeping you healthy and explore any problems."

"Mr. Craig, I want to ask you some questions about your health and your usual daily activities so that we can plan your care here in the hospital."

If the person is in the hospital, more than one health team member may be collecting a history. Patients are apt to feel exasperated because they believe they are repeating the same thing unless you give a reason for this interview.

After this brief introduction, ask an open-ended question (see the following section) and then let the person proceed. You do not need friendly small talk to build rapport. This is not a social visit; the person has some concern to talk about and wants to get on with it. You will build rapport best by letting him or her discuss the concern early.

THE WORKING PHASE

The working phase is the data-gathering phase. Verbal skills for this phase include your questions to the patient and your responses to what the patient has said. Two types of questions exist: open-ended and closed. Each type has a different place and function in the interview.

Open-Ended Questions

The **open-ended** question asks for narrative information. It states the topic to be discussed but only in **general** terms. Use it to begin the interview, to introduce a new section of questions, and whenever the person introduces a new topic.

"Tell me how I can help you."
"What brings you to the hospital?"
"Tell me why you have come here today."
"How have you been getting along?"
"You mentioned shortness of breath. Tell me more about that."
"How have you been feeling since your last appointment?"

The open-ended question is unbiased; it leaves the person free to answer in any way. This question encourages the person to respond in paragraphs and to give a spontaneous account in any order chosen. It lets the person express herself or himself fully.

As the person answers, stop and *listen*. What usually happens is that the patient answers with a short phrase or sentence, pauses, and then looks at you expecting some direction of how to go on. What you do next is the key to the interview. If you pose new questions on other topics, you may lose much of the initial story. Instead, respond to the first statement with "Tell me about it," or "Anything else?" or merely look acutely interested. The person then will tell the story.

Closed or Direct Questions

Closed or **direct** questions ask for specific information. They elicit a short, one- or two-word answer, a yes or no, or a forced choice. Whereas the open-ended question allows the patient to have free rein, the direct question limits his or her answer (Table 4–1).

Use the direct questions after the person's opening narrative to fill in any details he or she left out. Also use direct questions when you need many specific facts, such as when asking about past health problems or during the review of systems. You need direct questions to speed up the interview. Asking all open-ended questions would be unwieldy and may take hours. But be careful not to overuse closed questions. Follow these guidelines:

1. Ask only one direct question at a time. Avoid bombarding the person with long lists: "Have you ever had pain, double vision, watering or redness in the eyes?" Avoid double-barreled questions, such as "Do you exercise and follow a diet for your weight?" The person will not know which question to answer. And if the person answers "yes," you will not know which question the person has answered.
2. Choose language the person understands. You may need to use regional phrases or colloquial expressions. For example, "running off" means running away in standard English, but it means diarrhea to Appalachian mountain people.

Responses—Assisting the Narrative

You have asked the first open-ended question, and the patient answers. As the person talks, your role is to encourage free expression but not let the person wander off course. Your responses help the teller amplify the story.

Some people seek health care for short-term or relatively simple needs. Their history is direct and uncomplicated; for these people, two responses (facilitation and silence) may be all you need to get a complete picture. Other people have a complex story, a long history of a chronic condition, or accompanying emotions. Additional responses help you gather data without cutting them off.

There are nine types of verbal responses in all. The first five responses (facilitation, silence, reflection, empathy, clarification), involve your *reactions* to the facts or feelings the person has communicated. Your response focuses on the patient's frame of reference. Your own frame of reference does not enter into the response. In the last four responses (confrontation, interpretation, explanation, summary), you start to express your *own* thoughts and feelings. The frame of reference shifts from the patient's perspective to yours (Benjamin, 1980). In the first five responses, the patient leads; in the last four responses, you lead.

FACILITATION

These responses encourage the patient to say more, to continue with the story ("mm-hmm, go on, continue, uh-huh"). Also called general leads, these responses show the person you are interested and will listen further. Simply maintaining eye contact, shifting forward in your seat with increased attention, nodding "Yes," or using your hand to gesture, "Yes, go on, I'm with you," encourage the person to continue talking.

SILENCE

Silence is golden after open-ended questions. Your silent attentiveness communicates that the patient has time to think, to organize what he or she wishes to say without interruption from you. This "thinking silence" is the one health

TABLE 4–1: **Comparison of Open-Ended and Closed Questions**	
OPEN-ENDED	**DIRECT, CLOSED**
Use for narrative information	Use for specific information
Calls for long paragraph answers	Calls for short one- to two-word answers
Elicits feelings, opinions, ideas	Elicits cold facts
Builds and enhances rapport	Limits rapport and leaves interaction neutral

professionals interrupt most often. The interruption destroys the person's train of thought. The patient is often interrupted because silence is uncomfortable to beginning examiners. They feel responsible for keeping the dialogue going and feel at fault if it stops. But silence has advantages. One advantage is letting the person collect his or her thoughts. Also, silence gives you a chance to observe the person unobtrusively and to note nonverbal cues. Finally, silence gives you time to plan your next approach.

REFLECTION

This response echoes the patient's words. Reflection is repeating part of what the person has just said. In this example, it focuses further attention on a specific phrase and helps the person continue in his own way:

Patient: I'm here because of my water. It was cutting off.
Response: It was cutting off?
Patient: Yes, yesterday it took me 30 minutes to pass my water. Finally I got a tiny stream, but then it just closed off.

Reflection also can help express feeling behind a person's words. The feeling is already in the statement. You focus on it and encourage the person to elaborate:

Patient: It's so hard having to stay flat on my back in the hospital with this pregnancy. I have two more little ones at home. I'm so worried they are not getting the care they need.
Response: You feel worried and anxious about your children?

Think of yourself as a mirror reflecting the person's words or feelings. This helps the person to elaborate on the problem.

EMPATHY

A physical symptom, condition, or illness often has accompanying emotions. Many people have trouble expressing these feelings, perhaps because of confusion or embarrassment. In the reflecting example above, the person already had stated her feeling and you echoed it. But in the following example, he has not said it yet. An empathic response recognizes a feeling and puts it into words. It names the feeling and allows the expression of it. When the empathic response is used, the patient feels accepted and can deal with the feeling openly.

Patient (sarcastically): This is just great. I have my own business, I direct 20 employees everyday, and now here I am having to call you for every little thing.
Response: It must be hard—one day having so much control, and now feeling dependent on someone else.

Your response does not cut off further communication as would happen by giving false reassurance ("Oh, you'll be back to work in no time"). Also, it does not deny the feeling and indicate that it is not justified ("Now I don't do *everything* for you. Why, you are feeding yourself"). An empathic response recognizes the feeling, accepts it, and allows the person to express it without embarrassment. It strengthens rapport. The patient feels understood, which by itself is therapeutic, because it "bridges the isolation of illness" (Suchman et al., 1997). Other empathic responses are, "This must be very hard for you," "I understand," or just placing your hand on the person's arm (Fig. 4–2).

4–2

CLARIFICATION

Use this when the person's word choice is ambiguous or confusing (e.g., "Tell me what you mean by 'tired blood'"). Clarification also is used to summarize the person's words, simplify the words to make them clearer, then ask if you are on the right track. You are asking for agreement, and the person can then confirm or deny your understanding.

Response: Now as I understand you, this heaviness in your chest comes when you shovel snow or climb stairs, and it goes away when you stop doing those things. Is that correct?
Patient: Yes, that's pretty much it.

CONFRONTATION

Recall that in these last four responses, (confrontation, interpretation, explanation, summary), the frame of reference shifts from the patient's perspective to yours. These responses now include your own thoughts and feelings. Use the last four responses only when merited by the situation. If you use them too often, you take over at the patient's expense. In the case of confrontation, you have observed a certain action, feeling, or statement and you now focus the person's attention on it. You give your honest feedback about what you see or feel. This may focus on a discrepancy: "You say it doesn't hurt, but when I touch you here, you grimace." Or, it may focus on the person's affect: "You look sad" or "You sound angry." Or, you may confront the person when you notice parts of the story are inconsistent: "Earlier you said you were laying off alcohol and just now you said you had a few drinks after work."

INTERPRETATION

This statement is not based on direct observation as is confrontation, but it is based on your inference or conclusion. It links events, makes associations, or implies cause: "It seems that every time you feel the stomach pain, you have had some kind of stress in your life." Interpretation also ascribes feelings and helps the person understand his or her own feelings in relation to the verbal message.

Patient: I have decided I don't want to take any more treatments. But I can't seem to tell my doctor that. Every time she comes in, I tighten up and can't say anything.
Response: Could it be that you're afraid of her reaction?

You do run a risk of making the wrong inference. If this is the case, the person will correct it. But even if the inference is corrected, interpretation helps to prompt further discussion of the topic.

EXPLANATION

With these statements, you inform the person. You share factual and objective information. This may be for orientation to the agency setting: "Your dinner comes at 5:30 PM." Or, it may be to explain cause: "The reason you cannot eat or drink before your blood test is that the food will change the test results."

SUMMARY

This is a final review of what you understand the person has said. It condenses the facts and presents a survey of how you perceive the health problem or need. It is a type of validation in that the person can agree with it or correct it. Both you and the patient should participate. When the summary occurs at the end of the interview, it signals that termination of the interview is imminent.

TEN TRAPS OF INTERVIEWING

The verbal skills discussed above are productive and enhance the interview. Now take time to consider nonproductive, defeating verbal messages, or *traps*. It is easy to fall into these traps because you are anxious to help. The danger is that they restrict the patient's response. The following traps are obstacles to obtaining complete data and to establishing rapport.

1. PROVIDING FALSE ASSURANCE OR REASSURANCE

A woman says, "Oh I just know this lump is going to turn out to be cancer." What happens inside you? The automatic response of many clinicians is to say, "Now don't worry; I'm sure you will be all right." This "courage builder" relieves *your* anxiety and gives you the false sense of having provided comfort. But for the woman it actually closes off communication. It trivializes her anxiety and effectively denies any further talk of it. (Also it promises something that may not happen—that is, she may *not* be all right). Consider instead these responses:

"You are really worried about the lump, aren't you?"
"It must be hard to wait for the biopsy results."

These responses acknowledge the feeling and open the door for more communication.

A genuine, valid form of reassurance does exist. You *can* reassure patients that you are listening to them, that you understand them, that you have hope for them, and that you will take good care of them.

Patient: I feel so lost here since they transferred me to the medical center. No one comes to see me. No one here cares what happens to me.
Response: I care what happens to you. I am here today and I want you to know that I'll be here all week.

This type of reassurance makes a commitment to the patient, and it can have a powerful impact.

2. GIVING UNWANTED ADVICE

Know when to give advice and when to avoid giving it. Often, people seek health care because they want your professional advice and information on the management of a health problem: "My child has chickenpox; how should I take care of him?" This is a straightforward request for information that you have that the parent needs. You respond by giving a health prescription, a therapeutic plan based on your knowledge and experience.

In other situations, advice is different; it is based on a hunch or feeling. It is your personal opinion. Consider the woman who has just left a meeting with her consultant physician: "Dr. Kline just told me my only chance of getting pregnant is to have an operation. I just don't know. What would you do?" Does the woman really want your advice? If you answer, "If I were you, I'd . . . ," then you would be making a mistake. You are not her. If you give your answer, you have shifted the accountability for decision making from her to you. She has not worked out her own solution. She has learned nothing about herself.

Does the woman really want to know what you would do? Probably not. Instead, a better response is reflection:

Response: Have an operation?
Woman: Yes, and I'm terrified of being put to sleep. What if I don't wake up?

Now you know her *real* concern and can help her deal with it. She will have grown in the process and may be better equipped to meet her next decision.

When asked for advice, other preferred responses are,

"What are the pros and cons of _____ [this choice] for you?"
"What concerns do you have?"
"What is holding you back?"

Although it is quicker just to give advice, take the time to involve the patient in a problem-solving process. When a patient participates, he or she is more likely to learn and to change behavior.

3. USING AUTHORITY

"Your doctor/nurse knows best" is a response that promotes dependency and inferiority. The communication pathway looks something like this:

Interviewer:

Patient:

with your talk coming "down" and little from the patient going back "up" (Cornell, 1993). A better approach is to avoid using authority. Although you and the patient cannot have equality of professional skill and experience, you do have equally worthy roles in the health process, each respecting the other.

4. USING AVOIDANCE LANGUAGE

People use euphemisms such as "passed on" to avoid reality or to hide their feelings. They think if they just say the word "death," it might really happen. So to protect themselves, they evade the issue. Although it seems this will make comfortable potentially fearful topics, it does not. Not talking about the fear does not make it go away; it just suppresses the fear and makes it even more frightening. Using direct language is the best way to deal with frightening topics.

5. ENGAGING IN DISTANCING

Distancing is the use of impersonal speech to put space between a threat and the self: "My friend has a problem; she is afraid she . . . " or "There is a lump in the left breast." By using "the" instead of "my," the woman can deny any association with her diseased breast and protect herself from it. Health professionals use distancing, too, to soften reality. This does not work because it communicates to the other person that you also are afraid of the procedure. The use of blunt specific terms actually is preferable to defuse anxiety.

6. USING PROFESSIONAL JARGON

What is called a myocardial infarction in the health profession is called a heart attack by most laypeople. Use of jargon sounds exclusionary and paternalistic. You need to adjust your vocabulary to the person, but avoid sounding condescending.

If a patient uses medical jargon, do not assume he or she always knows the correct meaning. For example, some people think "hypertensive" means that they are very tense. As a result, they take their medication only when feeling stressed and not when they feel relaxed. This misinformation must be corrected. They need to understand that hypertension is a chronic condition that needs consistent medication to avoid side effects. On the other hand, you do not need to feel that it is a moral imperative to correct all misstatements (e.g., when a patient says "prostrate" for prostate gland).

7. USING LEADING OR BIASED QUESTIONS

Asking a man, "You don't smoke, do you?" implies that one answer is "better" than another. If the person wants to please you, either he is forced to answer in a way corresponding to your values or he feels guilty when he must admit the other answer. He risks your disapproval. And if he feels dependent on you for care, the last thing he wants to do is alienate you.

8. TALKING TOO MUCH

Some examiners positively associate helpfulness with verbal productivity. If the air has been thick with their oratory and advice, these examiners leave thinking they have met the patient's needs. Just the opposite is true. Anxious to please the examiner, the patient lets the professional talk at the expense of his or her need to express himself or herself. A good rule for every interviewer is to *listen more than you talk*.

9. INTERRUPTING

Often, when you think you know what the person will say, you interrupt and cut the person off. This does not show that you are clever. Rather, it signals that you are impatient or bored with the interview.

A related trap is preoccupation with yourself by thinking of your next remark while the person is talking. The communication pathway looks like this (Cornell, 1993):

Patient: ⟶   Interviewer: ⟶

As the patient speaks, you are thinking about what to say next. Thus you cannot fully understand what the person says. You are so preoccupied with your own role as the interviewer that you are not really listening. Aim for a second of silence between the person's statement and your next response. Ideally, your communication pathway should look like this:

with two people talking, and two people listening (Cornell, 1993).

10. USING "WHY" QUESTIONS

A young child asks, "Why does the moon look like the end of my fingernail?" The motive behind this question is an innocent search for information. This is quite different from that of an adult's "why" question, such as "*Why* were you so late for your appointment?" The adult's use of why questions usually implies blame and condemnation; it puts the person on the defensive (Benjamin, 1980).

Consider your use of "why" questions in the health care setting. "Why did you take so much medication?" Or, let's say you ask a man who has just come to the emergency department, "Why did you wait so long before coming to the hospital?" The only possible answer to a "why" question is "because . . . " and the man may not know the answer. He may not have worked it out. You sound whining, accusatory, and judgmental. And the man now must produce an excuse to rationalize his own behavior. To avoid this trap, say: "I see you started to have chest pains early in the day. What was happening between the time the pains started and the time you came to the emergency department?"

NONVERBAL SKILLS

Learn to listen with your eyes as well as with your ears. Nonverbal modes of communication include physical appearance, posture, gestures, facial expression, eye contact, voice, and touch. Nonverbal messages are very important in establishing rapport and in conveying information, especially about feelings. Nonverbal messages provide clues to understanding feelings. When nonverbal and verbal messages are congruent, the verbal is reinforced. When they are incongruent, the nonverbal message tends to be the true one, because it is under less conscious control.

PHYSICAL APPEARANCE

In his classic work *The Stress of Life*, Hans Selye (1956) reports his interest in the body's total response to stress began as a student. Unbiased as yet by medical knowledge, he noted that some patients just "looked sick," even though they did not exhibit the specific characteristic signs that would lead to a precise medical diagnosis. Such people simply felt and looked ill or feverish. The same view can work for you. Inattention to dressing or grooming suggests the person is too sick to maintain self-care or has an emotional dysfunction such as depression. Choice of clothing also sends a message, projecting such varied images as role (student, worker, or professional) or attitude (casual, suggestive, or rebellious).

Your own appearance sends a message to the patient. Professional dress varies among agencies and settings. Depending on the setting, the use of a professional uniform may create a positive stereotype (comfort, expertise, or ease of identification) or a negative stereotype (distance, authority, or formality). Whatever your personal choice in clothing or grooming, the aim should be to convey a competent, professional image.

POSTURE

Note the patient's position. An open position with extension of large muscle groups shows relaxation, physical comfort, and a willingness to share information. A closed position with arms and legs crossed looks defensive and anxious. Note any change in posture. If a person in a relaxed position suddenly tenses, it suggests discomfort with the new topic.

Your own calm, relaxed posture creates a feeling of warmth and trust and conveys an interest in the person. Standing and hastily filling out a history form with periodic peeks at your watch communicates that you are busy with many more important things than interviewing this person. Even when your time is limited, appear calm and unhurried. Sit down, even if it is only for a few minutes, and look as if nothing else mattered except this person.

GESTURES

Gestures send messages. For example, nodding or an open turning out of the hand shows acceptance, attention, or agreement. A wringing of the hands often indicates anxiety. Pointing a finger occurs with anger and vehemence. Also, hand gestures can reinforce a person's description of pain. When a crushing substernal chest pain is described, the person often holds the hand twisted into a fist in front of the sternum. Or, pain that is bright and sharply localized may be shown by pointing one finger to the exact spot: "It hurts right here."

FACIAL EXPRESSION

The face reflects a wide variety of relevant emotions and conditions. The expression may look alert, relaxed, and interested or it may look anxious, angry, and suspicious. Physical conditions such as pain or shortness of breath also show in the expression.

Your own expression should reflect a professional who is attentive, sincere, and interested in the patient. Any expression of boredom, distraction, disgust, criticism, or disbelief is picked up by the other person, and rapport will dissolve.

EYE CONTACT

Lack of eye contact suggests that the person is shy, withdrawn, confused, bored, intimidated, apathetic, or depressed. This applies to examiners, too. You should aim to maintain eye contact, but do not "stare down" the person. Do not have a fixed, penetrating look but rather an easy gaze toward the person's eyes, with occasional glances away. One exception to this is when you are interviewing someone from a culture that avoids direct eye contact (see the section on Transcultural Considerations).

VOICE

Beside the spoken words, meaning comes through the tone of voice, the intensity and rate of speech, the pitch, and any pauses. These are just as important as words in conveying meaning. For example, the tone of a person's voice may show sarcasm, disbelief, sympathy, or hostility. An anxious person often speaks in a loud, fast voice. A whining voice is similar; it has a high-pitched wavering quality and long, drawn-out syllables. A soft voice may indicate shyness or fear. A hearing-impaired person may use a loud voice.

Even the use of pauses conveys meaning. When your question is easy and straightforward, a patient's long unexpected pause indicates the person is taking time to think of an answer. This raises some doubt as to the honesty of the answer. Unusually frequent and long pauses, when combined with speech that is slow and monotonous and a weak breathy voice, indicate depression.

TOUCH

The meaning of physical touch is influenced by the person's age, sex, cultural background, past experience, and current setting. The meaning of touch is easily misinterpreted. In most Western cultures, physical touch is reserved for expressions of love and affection or for rigidly defined acts of greeting (see the section on Transcultural Considerations). Do not use touch during the interview unless you know the person well and are sure how it will be interpreted. When appropriate, touch communicates effectively, such as a touch of the hand or arm to signal empathy.

In sum, an examiner's nonverbal messages that are productive and enhancing to the relationship are those that show attentiveness and unconditional acceptance. Defeating, nonproductive nonverbal behaviors are those of inattentiveness, authority, and superiority (Table 4–2).

TABLE 4–2: Nonverbal Behaviors of the Interviewer

POSITIVE	NEGATIVE
Appropriate professional appearance	Appearance objectionable to patient
Equal-status seating	Standing
Close proximity to patient	Sitting behind desk, far away, turned away
Relaxed open posture	Tense posture
Leaning slightly toward person	Slouched back
Occasional facilitating gestures	Critical or distracting gestures: pointing finger, clenched fist, finger-tapping, foot-swinging, looking at watch
Facial animation, interest	Bland expression, yawning, tight mouth
Appropriate smiling	Frowning, lip biting
Appropriate eye contact	Shifty, avoiding eye contact, focusing on notes
Moderate tone of voice	Strident, high-pitched tone
Moderate rate of speech	Rate too slow or too fast
Appropriate touch	Too frequent or inappropriate touch

CLOSING THE INTERVIEW

The session should end gracefully. An abrupt or awkward closing can destroy rapport and leave the person with a negative impression of the whole interview. To ease into the closing, ask the person:

"Is there anything else you would like to mention?"
"Are there any questions you would like to ask?"
"Are there any other areas I should have asked about?"

This gives the person the final opportunity for self-expression. Then, to indicate that closing is imminent, say something like "Our interview is just about over." No new topic should be introduced now. This is a good time to give your summary or a recapitulation of what you have learned during the interview. The summary is a final statement of what you and the patient agree the health state to be. It should include positive health aspects, any health problems that have been identified, any plans for action, or an explanation of the following physical examination. As you part from patients, thank them for the time spent and for their cooperation.

 DEVELOPMENTAL CONSIDERATIONS

INTERVIEWING THE PARENT

When your patient is a child, you must build rapport with two people—the child and the accompanying parent. Greet both by name, but with a younger child (1 to 6 years old), focus more on the parent. By ignoring the child temporarily, you allow the child to size you up from a safe distance. The child can observe your interaction with the parent, see that the parent accepts and likes you, and relax (Fig. 4–3).

Begin by interviewing the parent and child together. If any sensitive topics arise (e.g., the parents' troubled relationship or the child's problems at school or with peers), explore them later when the parent is alone. Provide toys to occupy the child as you and the parent talk. This frees the parent to concentrate on the history. Also, it indicates the child's level of attention span or independent play. Through the interview, be alert to ways the parent and child interact.

For younger children, the parent will provide all or most of the history. Thus you are collecting the child's health data from the parent's frame of reference. Usually, this viewpoint is reliable because most parents have the child's well-being as a priority and see cooperation with you as a way to enhance this well-being. But the possibilities exist for parental bias. Bias can occur when parents are asked to describe the child's achievements, or whenever their own parenting ability seems called into question. For example, if you say "His fever was 103 and you did not bring him in?" you are implying a lack of parenting skill. This puts the parent on the defensive and increases anxiety. Instead, use open-ended questions that increase description and defuse threat, such as "What happened when the fever went up?"

A parent with more than one child has more than one set of data to remember. Be patient as the parent sorts through his or her memory to pull out facts of developmental milestones or past history. A comprehensive history may be lacking if the child is accompanied by a family friend or day care provider instead of the parent.

In collecting developmental data, avoid being judgmental about the age of achievement of certain milestones. Parents are understandably proud of their child's achievements and are sensitive to inferences that these milestones may occur late.

Refer to the child by name—not as "the baby." Refer to the parent by name, and not the demeaning "Mother" or "Dad." Also, be clear when identifying the parents. The mother's present husband may not necessarily be the child's father. Instead of asking about "your husband's" health, ask "Is Joan's father in good health?"

Although most of your communication is with the parent, do not ignore the child completely. You need to make contact to ease into the physical examination later. Begin by asking about the toys the child is playing with or about a special doll or teddy bear brought from home: "Does your doll have a name?" or "What can your truck do?" Stoop down to meet the child at his or her eye level. Adult size can be overwhelming to young children and can emphasize their smallness.

Nonverbal communication is even more important to children than it is to adults. Children are quick to pick up feelings, anxiety, or comfort from nonverbal cues. Keep your physical appearance neat and clean, and avoid formal uniforms that distance you. Keep your gestures slow, deliberate, and close to your body. Children are frightened by quick or grandiose gestures. Do not try to maintain constant eye contact; this feels threatening to a small child. Use a quiet, measured voice, and choose simple words in your speech. Considering the child's level of language development is valuable in planning your communication.

THE INFANT

Nonverbal communication is the primary method. Most infants look calm and relaxed when all their needs are met, and they cry when they are frightened, hungry, tired, or uncom-

4–3

fortable. They respond best to firm, gentle handling and a quiet, calm voice. Your voice is comforting, even though they do not understand the words. Older infants have anxiety toward strangers. They are more cooperative when the parent is kept in view.

THE PRESCHOOLER

A 2- to 6-year-old is egocentric. He or she sees the world mostly from his or her own point of view. Everything revolves around him or her. It may not work to cite the example of another child's behavior to get the child to cooperate. It has no meaning. Only the child's own experience is relevant.

Preschoolers' communication is direct, concrete, literal, and set in the present. Avoid expressions such as "climbing the walls," because they are easily misinterpreted by young children. Use short, simple sentences with a concrete explanation. Take time to give a short simple explanation for any unfamiliar equipment that will be used on the child. Preschoolers can have *animistic* thinking about unfamiliar objects. They may imagine that unfamiliar inanimate objects can come alive and have human characteristics (e.g., that a blood pressure cuff can wake up and bite or pinch).

THE SCHOOL-AGE CHILD

A child 7 to 12 years old can tolerate and understand others' viewpoints. This child is more objective and realistic. He or she wants to know functional aspects—how things work and why things are done.

Children of this age group have the verbal ability to add important data to the history. Interview the parent and child together, but when a presenting symptom or sign exists ask the child about it first, then gather data from the parent. For the well child seeking a checkup, pose questions about school, friends, or activities directly to the child.

THE ADOLESCENT

Adolescents want to be adults, but they do not have the cognitive ability yet to achieve their goal. They are between two stages. Sometimes they are capable of mature actions, and other times they fall back on childhood response patterns, especially in times of stress. You cannot treat adolescents as children, yet you cannot overcompensate and assume that their communication style, learning ability, and motivation are consistently at an adult level.

Adolescents value their peers. They crave acceptance and sameness with their peers. Adolescents think no adult can understand them. Because of this, some act with aloof contempt, answering only in monosyllables. Others make eye contact and tell you what they think you want to hear, but inside they are thinking "You'll never know the full story about me."

This knowledge about adolescents is apt to paralyze you in communicating with them. However, successful communication is possible and rewarding. The guidelines are simple.

The first consideration is your attitude, which must be one of respect. Respect is the most important thing you can com-

municate to the adolescent. The adolescent needs to feel validated as a human being, accepted, and worthy.

Second, your communication must be totally honest. The adolescent's intuition is highly tuned and can detect phoniness or when information is withheld. Always give them the truth. Play it straight or you will lose them. They will cooperate if they understand your rationale.

Stay in character. Avoid using language that is absurd for your age or professional role. It is helpful to understand some of the jargon used by adolescents, but you cannot use those words yourself simply to try to bond with the adolescent. Do not try to be his or her peer. You are not, and they will not accept you as such.

Use icebreakers. Focus first on the adolescent, not on the problem. Although an adult just wants to get on with it and talk about the health concern immediately, the adolescent responds best when the focus is on him or her as a person. Show an interest in the adolescent. Ask open, friendly questions about school, activities, hobbies, friends. Refrain from asking questions about parents and family for now—these issues can be emotionally charged during adolescence.

Do not assume adolescents know *anything* about a health interview or a physical examination. Explain every step and give the rationale. They need direction. They will cooperate when they know the reason for the questions or actions. Encourage their questions. Adolescents are afraid they will sound "dumb" if they ask a question to which they assume everybody else knows the answer.

Keep your questions short and simple. "Why are you here?" sounds brazen to you, but it is effective with the adolescent. Be prepared for the adolescent who does *not* know why he or she is there. Some adolescents are pushed into coming to the examination by a parent.

The communication responses described for the adult need to be reconsidered when talking with the adolescent. Silent periods usually are best avoided. Giving adolescents a little time to collect their thoughts is acceptable, but a silence for other reasons is threatening. Also, avoid reflection. If you use reflection, the adolescent is likely to answer, "What?" They just do not have the cognitive skills to respond to that indirect mode of questioning. Also, adolescents are more sensitive to nonverbal communication than are adults. Be aware of your expressions and gestures. They are also more sensitive to any comment they take to mean criticism from you, and will withdraw.

Later in the interview, after you have developed rapport with the adolescent, you can address the topics that are emotionally charged, including alcohol and drug use, sexual behaviors, suicidal thoughts, and depression. Adolescents will assume that health professionals have similar values and standards of behavior as most of the other authority figures in their lives, and they may be reluctant to share this information. You can assure them that your questions are not intended to be curious or intrusive, but cover topics that are important for most teens and on which you have relevant health information to share.

If confidential material is uncovered during the interview, consider what can remain confidential and what you feel you must share for the well-being of the adolescent. State laws vary about confidentiality with minors, and in some states parents are not notified about, for example, birth control prescriptions or treatment for sexually transmitted diseases (STDs). However, if the adolescent talks about an abusive home situation, state that you must share this information with other health professionals for his or her own protection. Ask the adolescent, "Do you have a problem with that?" and then talk it through. Tell the adolescent, "You will have to trust that I will handle this information professionally and in your best interest."

Finally, take every opportunity for positive reinforcement. Praise every action regarding healthy lifestyle choices: "That's great that you don't smoke. You get lots of gold stars in my book for staying off the cigarettes. It's great for your heart, it will save you lots of money that you can use on other things, and your skin won't be wrinkled when you get older."

THE OLDER ADULT

The aging adult has the developmental task of finding the meaning of life and the purpose of his or her own existence, and adjusting to the inevitability of death. Some people have developed comfortable and satisfying answers and greet you with a calm demeanor and self-assurance. Be alert for the occasional person who sounds hopeless and despairing about life at present and in the future. Symptoms of illness are even more frightening when they mean physical limitation or threaten independence.

Always address the person by the last name (e.g., "Hello, Mr. Choi"; "Good morning, Mrs. Smith"). Some older adults resent being called by their first name by younger persons, and almost all cringe at the ignominious "Grandma" or "Pop."

The interview usually takes longer with older adults because they have a longer story to tell. You may need to break up the interview into more than one visit, collecting the most important historical data first. Or certain portions of the data, such as past history or the review of systems, can be provided on a form that is filled out at home, as long as the person's vision and handwriting are adequate. Take time to review these parts with the person during the interview.

It is important to adjust the pace of the interview to the aging person. The older person has a great amount of background material to sort through, and this takes some time. Also, some aging persons need a greater amount of response time to interpret the question and process their answer. Avoid trying to hurry them along. This approach only affirms their stereotype of younger persons in general and health care providers in particular—that is, people who are merely interested in numbers of patients and filling out forms. Any urge from you to get on with it will surely make them retreat. You will lose valuable data, and their needs will not be met (Fig. 4–4).

Consider physical limitations when planning the interview. An aging person may fatigue earlier and may require that the interview be broken up into shorter segments. For the person with impaired hearing, face directly so that your mouth and face are fully visible. Do not shout; it does not help and actually distorts speech.

4–4

Touch is a nonverbal skill that is very important to older persons. Their other senses may be diminished, and touch grounds you in reality. Also, a hand on the arm or shoulder is an empathic message that communicates you empathize with the person and want to understand his or her problem (see Transcultural Considerations for exceptions).

INTERVIEWING PEOPLE WITH SPECIAL NEEDS

HEARING-IMPAIRED PEOPLE

Although many people will tell you in advance that they have a hearing deficit, others must be recognized by clues, such as staring at your mouth and face, not attending unless looking at you, or speaking in a voice unusually loud or with guttural or garbled sounds. The deaf person may be familiar with some equipment in the hospital or office setting or may have had previous experience with health care settings. But without full communication, the hearing-impaired person is sure to feel isolated and anxious. Ask his or her preferred way to communicate—by signing, lip reading, or writing.

A complete health history requires a sign language interpreter. Since most health care professionals are not proficient in signing, try to find an interpreter through a social service agency or the person's own social network. You may use family members, but be aware that they sometimes edit for the person. Use the same guidelines as for the bilingual interpreter (see the section on Transcultural Considerations).

If the person prefers lip reading, be sure to face him or her squarely and have good lighting on your face. Examiners with a beard, mustache, or foreign accents are less effective. Do not exaggerate your lip movements because this distorts your words. Similarly, shouting distorts the reception of a hearing aid the person may wear. Speak slowly and supplement your voice with appropriate hand gestures or pantomime. Nonverbal cues are important adjuncts because the lip reader understands at best only 50% of your speech when relying solely on vision. Be sure the person understands your questions. Many hearing-impaired people nod "yes" just to be friendly and cooperative but really do not understand.

Written communication is efficient in sections such as past health history or review of systems. For the present history of illness, writing is very time consuming and laborious. The syntax of the person's written words will read normally if the hearing impairment occurred after speech patterns developed. If the deafness occurred before speech patterns developed, the written syntax follows that of signing, which is different from that of English.

ACUTELY ILL PEOPLE

An emergency demands your prompt action. You must combine interviewing with physical examination skills to determine lifesaving actions. Although life support measures may be paramount, still try to interview the person as much as possible. Subjective data are crucial to determine the cause and course of the emergency. Abbreviate your questioning. Identify the main area of distress and question about that. Family or friends often can provide important data.

A hospitalized person with a critical or severe illness is usually too weak, too short of breath, or in too much pain to talk. First attend to the comfort of the person. Then establish a priority; find out immediately what parts of the history are the most relevant. Explore the first concern the person mentions. Begin to use closed, direct questions earlier. Finally, watch that your statements are very clear. When a person is very sick, even the simplest sentence can be misconstrued. The person will react according to preconceived ideas about what a serious illness means, so anything you say should be direct and precise.

PEOPLE UNDER THE INFLUENCE OF STREET DRUGS OR ALCOHOL

It is common for persons under the influence of alcohol or other mood-altering drugs to be admitted to a hospital; all of these drugs affect the central nervous system, increasing the risk for accidents and injuries. Also, chronic use creates complex medical problems that require increasing care.

Many substance abusers are poly-drug abusers. You may be faced with a wide range of patient behaviors due to current influence. Alcohol and the opioids (heroin, meperidine [Demerol], propoxyphene [Darvon]) are central nervous system depressants. Stimulants of the central nervous system (cocaine, amphetamine) can cause an intense high, agitation, and paranoid behavior. Hallucinogens cause bizarre, inappropriate, sometimes even violent behavior accompanied by superhuman strength and insensitivity to pain.

When interviewing a person currently under the influence of alcohol or illicit drugs, ask simple and direct questions. Take care to make your manner and questions nonthreatening. Avoid confrontation at this point. Further, avoid any display of scolding or disgust, because this person may become

belligerent. One priority is to find out the time of the person's last drink and how much he or she drank at this episode as well as the name and amount of other drugs taken. This information will help assess any withdrawal patterns. For your own protection, be aware of hospital security or other personnel who could be called on for assistance.

Once he or she is sober, the hospitalized substance abuser should be assessed for the extent of the problem and the meaning of the problem for the person and family. Initially you will encounter denial and increased defensiveness; special interview techniques are needed.

PERSONAL QUESTIONS

Occasionally, people will ask you questions about *your* personal life or opinions, such as "Are you married?" "Do you have children?" or "Do you smoke?" You do not need to answer every question. You may supply brief information when you feel it is appropriate, but be sensitive to the possibility that there may be a motive behind the personal questions such as loneliness or anxiety. Try directing your response back to the person's frame of reference. You might say something like "No, I don't have children; I wonder if your question is related to how I can help you care for little Jamie?"

SEXUALLY AGGRESSIVE PEOPLE

On some occasions, personal questions extend to flirtatious compliments, seductive innuendo, or advances. Some people experience serious or chronic illness as a threat to their self-esteem and sexual adequacy. This creates anxiety that makes them act out in sexually aggressive ways.

Your response must make it clear that you are a health professional who can best care for the person by maintaining a professional relationship. At the same time, you should communicate that you accept the person and you understand the person's need to be self-assertive but that you cannot tolerate sexual advances. This may be difficult, considering that the person's words or gestures may have left you shocked, embarrassed, or angry. Your feelings are normal. You need to set appropriate verbal boundaries by saying, "I am uncomfortable when you talk to me that way; please don't." A further response that would open communication is: "I wonder if the way you're feeling now relates to your illness or to being in the hospital?"

CRYING

A beginning examiner usually feels horrified when the patient starts crying. But crying actually is a big relief to a person. Health problems come with powerful emotions. Worries about illness, death, or loss take a great amount of energy to keep bottled up inside. When you say something that "makes the person cry," do not think you have hurt the person. You have just hit on a topic that is important. Do not go on to a new topic. Just let the person cry and express his or her feelings fully. You can offer a tissue and wait until the crying subsides to talk. The person will regain control soon.

Clinical Illustration

Alice P., a 49-year-old white divorced female with chronic alcoholism and skin yellow with jaundice has entered treatment for substance abuse. Today, she needs a pelvic examination and Pap smear.

Patient: I haven't had a pelvic exam in 5 years. I had a hysterectomy 18 years ago. They said I had "preinvasive" cancer cells. (At this, Alice's lips fold in, her eyes squeeze shut; she puts hand to mouth, and breathes in audibly in jerks.)

Response: Alice, you look sad. (Puts hand on upper arm.)

Patient: (Crying freely now.) What if you find more cancer now? They can't operate on me with my liver so big. I'd never survive the anesthesia. And my father died of cancer. He had cirrhosis too, and they opened him up and he was full of cancer. He never woke up from surgery and he died 2 weeks later.

Response: I understand how worried you are. I think you have done the right thing to come in for treatment. That took courage. As for today, let's take one step at a time. Today we need to do the pelvic exam and Pap smear. There is no reason today to assume you need an operation. I'll do your exam today and I'll be here all week. We'll work together to help you get through this.

Alice: (Breathing deeply, sitting up straight, arms down and open at sides, making eye contact.) All right. I'm better now. Let's go ahead.

Sometimes your patient looks as if he or she is on the verge of tears but is trying hard to suppress them. Again instead of moving on to something new, acknowledge the expression by saying, "You look sad". Do not worry that you will open an uncontrollable floodgate. The person may cry but will be relieved, and you will have gained insight to a serious concern (Clinical Illustration).

ANGER

Occasionally you will try to interview a person who is already angry. Try not to personalize this anger; usually it does not relate to you. The person is showing aggression as a response to his or her own feelings of anxiety or helplessness. Do ask about the anger and hear the person out. Deal with the angry feelings before you ask anything else. An angry person cannot be an effective participant in a health interview.

Maybe because of an unrelated incident *you* are angry when you come into the interview. When you are angry, say so and tell the patient that you are angry at something or someone else. Otherwise the patient, unusually vulnerable and dependent on you, thinks you are angry at him or her.

THREAT OF VIOLENCE

The health care setting is not immune to violent behavior. An individual may act with such angry gestures that you feel a threat to your personal safety. Other red flag behaviors of a potentially disruptive person include fist clenching, pacing back and forth, a vacant stare, confusion, statements out of touch with reality, statements that do not make sense, a history of recent drug use (alcohol, hallucinogen, cocaine), or perhaps even a recent history of intense bereavement (loss of spouse, loss of job). Trust your instincts. If you sense any suspicious or threatening behavior, act immediately to defuse the situation. Leave the examining room door open and position yourself between the person and the door. Many departments have a prearranged sign or signal so that a co-worker can call 911 and the security department to send help to the setting. Do not raise your own voice or try to argue with the threatening person. Act quite calm and talk to the person in a soft voice. Act interested in what the person is saying, and behave in an unhurried way. Your most important goal is safety; avoid taking any risks.

ANXIETY

Finally, take it for granted that nearly all sick people have some anxiety. This is a normal response to being sick. It makes some people aggressive and others dependent. Remember that the person is not reacting as typically as when he or she is healthy.

TRANSCULTURAL CONSIDERATIONS

CROSS-CULTURAL COMMUNICATION

When two people come from different cultural backgrounds, the probability of miscommunication increases. Verbal and nonverbal communications are influenced by the cultural background of both the health care professional and the patient. *Cross-cultural* or *intercultural communication* refers to the communication process occurring between a health care professional and a patient, each with different cultural backgrounds, in which both attempt to understand the other's point of view from a cultural perspective (Fig. 4–5).

4–5

CULTURAL PERSPECTIVES ON PROFESSIONAL INTERACTIONS

Your professional interaction depends, to a large extent, on the patient's cultural perception of health care providers and the degree of formality/informality that is considered appropriate. For example, some Southeast Asians expect those in authority, such as health care providers, to be authoritarian, directive, and detached. In seeking health care, some Asian Americans may expect the health care provider to intuitively know what is wrong with them, and you may actually lose some credibility by asking a fairly standard interview question such as, "What brings you here?" The Asian person may be thinking, "Don't you know why I'm here? You're supposed to be the one with all the answers."

The emphasis on social harmony among Asians and Native Americans may prevent the full expression of concerns or feelings during the interview. Such reserved behavior may leave you with the impression that the person agrees with or understands your explanation. Nodding or smiling by Asians may only reflect their cultural value for interpersonal harmony, not agreement with you. You may distinguish between socially compliant patient responses aimed at maintaining harmony and genuine concurrence by obtaining validation of your assumptions. You might accomplish this by inviting the person to respond frankly to your suggestions or by giving the person "permission" to disagree.

In contrast, Appalachians traditionally have close family interaction patterns, which often lead them to expect close personal relationships with health care providers. The Appalachian may evaluate your effectiveness on the basis of interpersonal skills rather than professional competencies. Appalachians are likely to be uncomfortable with the impersonal, bureaucratic orientation of most health care institutions. People of Latin American or Mediterranean origins often expect an even higher degree of intimacy and may attempt to involve you in their family system by expecting you to participate in personal activities and social functions. These individuals might come to expect personal favors that extend beyond the scope of your professional practice and may feel it is their privilege to contact you at home during any time of the day or night for care.

ETIQUETTE

Etiquette refers to the conventional code of good manners that governs behavior and varies cross-culturally. Consider the cultural perceptions of some people from Hispanic, Middle Eastern, and African cultures who expect you to engage in conversation of a personal or social nature before they feel comfortable entering into the more personal and intimate aspects of the health history and physical examination. For these people, there is a high value placed on developing interpersonal relationships and getting to know about a person's family, personal concerns, and interests before they allow you to interact therapeutically. Recognizing that time constraints frequently affect the social interchange expected by individuals from some cultures, you should strive to incorporate the person's cultural needs with the health history data categories. For example, using a conversational tone of voice, you might begin the health history by inquiring about the patient's family members and their health.

You should be prepared for the converse; that is, individuals from some cultures may want to interview *you*. They may ask questions about your family, marital status, salary, home address, telephone number, and so forth. Your own cultural beliefs will determine your level of comfort in responding to these questions. Remember that you aren't obligated to answer questions that you deem too personal and always have a right to protect your personal safety. For example, you are discouraged from providing your home telephone number. Rather, you should provide the patient with the hospital, clinic, or agency's business number. If you want the patient to be able to contact you while you're at home, you should ask a secretary or other third party at the health care facility to call your home number. You may want to consider in advance which categories of questions you are willing to discuss and which ones you will politely avoid. If you refuse to answer certain questions about yourself, remember that the person may perceive your behavior as aloof and uncaring. Thus, the manner in which you reply to personal inquiries should be carefully worded, sensitive to the cultural needs of the patient, and congruent with your own cultural beliefs.

When meeting a patient for the first time, it is best to be formal, respectful, and polite. Unless a physical disability or handicap prevents you from doing so, you should be standing when you first greet the person and those accompanying him or her. Another aspect of etiquette concerns the use of *names* and *titles*. In order to ensure that a mutually respectful relationship is established, you should introduce yourself and indicate to the person how you prefer to be called—that is, by first name, last name, and/or title. You should elicit the same information from the patient because this enables you to address the person in a manner that is culturally appropriate and could actually spare you considerable embarrassment. Everyone likes to be called by his or her correct name. You must be certain that you know your patients' names, pronounce them correctly, and follow cultural conventions concerning the use of titles. Avoid being unduly casual or familiar. For example, refrain from routinely using the person's first name before you have been invited to do so. The same guidelines should be followed when addressing the family members and other visitors.

Among Chinese, Vietnamese, and many other Asian groups, the family or surname is written and spoken first, followed by the first or given name. You will notice that this is exactly the opposite of most European-American cultures. Because politeness and formality frequently are valued by those from Asian cultures, you should address the person using the correct title (Mr., Mrs., Ms., Miss, Dr., and so forth) followed by the family or surname. Be aware that some Asians, particularly those who are members of Christian religions, also may have English names. Most Asian women do not use their husband's last name after marriage. You should be especially mindful of this when examining children in the presence of both parents. It is likely that you will need to refer to the husband and wife by different last names (e.g., Mr. Cai and Mrs. Li). In most Asian cultures the child is given the father's last name. Depending on the degree of acculturation, some Asian-Americans switch the order of their names in order to be consistent with the European-American custom. If you are in doubt, be sure to ask the patient or a significant other if the patient is unable to respond.

In traditional Chinese, Japanese, and other Asian cultures, when people are introduced, they show each other respect by bowing. The more profound the bow is, the deeper the respect. For example, it would be appropriate to bow very low to an older adult whose wisdom is highly regarded and less profoundly to an adolescent or a young adult. With Westernization, handshakes are now customary throughout most parts of Asia and among Asian-Americans, but shaking someone's hand too firmly or vigorously is considered rude or intrusive. Most people of Asian descent will expect you to behave in a manner congruent with your cultural heritage. In other words, it is not necessary to bow when greeting Asian-Americans but to greet them as you would other patients.

Because of the importance of family for people from Central and South America, two surnames are used, representing their father's and mother's last names. The paternal name is first, then the maternal name. For example, if the patient's name is Juan Diaz Hernandez, his father's last name is Diaz and his mother's last name is Hernandez. With immigration to the United States or Canada, some people with Spanish surnames drop their mother's name for the sake of brevity. Consider the number of spaces allowed for a person's name on a typical hospital admissions form, and it becomes evident why the name might be shortened. This is unfortunate because people lose part of their name, an important expression of their cultural identity.

Although there are dozens of Arab cultures and subcultures, customs pertaining to names are similar. Both males and females are given a first name as infants. The father's first name is used as the middle name and the last name is the family name. Some may prefer to be addressed as father (*abu*) or mother (*um*) of their oldest son (e.g., abu Walid or father of Walid). Because formality is emphasized in most Arab cultures, you should call patients Mr., Mrs., Ms., Miss, or Dr. followed by their last name unless invited to use more familiar first names or the *abu/um* form of the name. In most Arab cultures, etiquette requires either a gentle kiss on the cheeks or a handshake on arrival and departure for people of the same gender. When an Arab man is introduced to a woman, he usually waits for the woman to extend her hand first. This is done out of respect for the traditional beliefs about modesty in male-female relationships held by some Muslim women. When a handshake is not exchanged, the Muslim woman usually faces the man while bowing her head slightly and crossing her arms across her chest. In lieu of a handshake, this is a widely accepted, culturally appropriate gesture that is used when men and women are introduced in some Arab cultures.

With more than 550 federal and/or state-recognized Native American tribes, there is wide variation in the customs pertaining to names, titles, and etiquette. The majority tend to follow the dominant European-American cultural norms. In the Navajo culture a health care provider may call an older adult "grandfather" or "grandmother" as a sign of respect after getting to know him or her, but should be more formal during the initial introduction. Some Native American and Alaska natives have anglicized traditional names into surnames such as Running Deer, Flying Eagle, or Swift Bear, often reflecting the clan to which the person belongs. You should extend a gentle, nonaggressive handshake when introduced to a Native American patient.

SPACE AND DISTANCE

Both the patient's and your own sense of spatial distance are significant throughout the interview and physical examination, with culturally appropriate distance zones varying widely. For example, you may find yourself backing away from people of Hispanic, East Indian, or Middle Eastern origins who invade your personal space with regularity in an attempt to bring you closer into the space that is comfortable to them. Although you are uncomfortable with their close physical proximity, they are perplexed by your distancing behaviors and may perceive you as aloof and unfriendly. Summarized in Table 4–3 are the four distance zones identified for the functional use of space that are embraced by the dominant cultural group, including that of most health care professionals.

CULTURAL CONSIDERATIONS ON GENDER AND SEXUAL ORIENTATION

Violating cultural norms related to appropriate male-female relationships may jeopardize your professional relationship. Among some Arab-Americans, you may find that an adult male is never alone with a female (except his wife) and is generally accompanied by one or more other males when inter-

TABLE 4–3: **Functional Use of Space**	
ZONE	REMARKS
Intimate zone (0 to 1½ ft)	Visual distortion occurs
	Best for assessing breath and other body odors
Personal distance (1½ to 4 ft)	Perceived as an extension of the self similar to a bubble
	Voice is moderate
	Body odors inapparent
	No visual distortion
	Much of the physical assessment occurs at this distance
Social distance (4 to 12 ft)	Used for impersonal business transactions
	Perceptual information much less detailed
	Much of the interview occurs at this distance
Public distance (12+ ft)	Interaction with others impersonal
	Speaker's voice must be projected
	Subtle facial expressions imperceptible

From Hall E: Proxemics: the study of man's spatial relations. In Galdston I, editor: *Man's image in medicine and anthropology,* New York, 1963, International University Press, pp 109–120.

acting with females. This behavior is culturally very significant; failure to adhere to the *cultural code* (set of rules or norms of behavior used by a cultural group to guide their behavior and interpret situations) is viewed as a serious transgression, often one in which the lone male will be accused of sexual impropriety. The best way to ensure that cultural variables have been considered is to ask the person about culturally relevant aspects of male-female relationships, preferably at the beginning of the interview—before you have an opportunity to violate any culturally based practices. When you have determined that gender differences are important to the patient, you might try strategies such as offering to have a third person present when this is feasible. If a family member or friend has accompanied the patient, you might inquire whether the patient would like that person to be in the examination room during the history and/or physical examination.

The gender issue is further complicated by cultural beliefs about relationships with authority figures and cross-national perspectives on the status of various health care disciplines. For example, in many less developed nations, nursing is a low-status occupation. In some oil-rich Arab countries (e.g., Saudi Arabia, Kuwait), care for the sick is carried out by health care providers who are hired from abroad for the purpose of caring for the bodily needs of the sick, an activity that is considered undignified.

In approaching lesbian, gay, or bisexual individuals, you should be aware of heterosexist biases and the communication of these biases during the interview and physical examination. *Heterosexism* refers to the institutionalized belief that heterosexuality is the only natural choice and assumes it is the norm. For example, most health histories include a question concerning marital status. Although many same-sex couples are in committed, long-term monogamous relationships, seldom is there a category on the standard form that acknowledges this type of relationship. Although technically and legally the person may be single, this trivializes the relationship with his or her significant other. It also may have health-related implications if the person is diagnosed, for example, with a communicable disease, which may range in severity from a minor sore throat to a life-threatening condition such as HIV/AIDS. In extreme cases, lesbians have been subjected to unnecessary diagnostic procedures when the heterosexual assumption was made (Eliason, 1993; MacNeil, 2002).

OVERCOMING COMMUNICATION BARRIERS

Health care providers tend to have stereotypical expectations of the patient's behavior during the interview and physical examination. In general, we expect behavior to consist of undemanding compliance, an attitude of respect for the health care provider, and cooperation with requested behavior throughout the examination. Although patients may ask a few questions for the purpose of clarification, slight deference to recognized authority figures (i.e., health care providers) is expected. Individuals from culturally diverse backgrounds, however, may have significantly different perceptions about the appropriate role of the individual and his or her family when seeking health care. If you find yourself becoming an-noyed that a patient is asking too many questions, assuming a defensive posture, or otherwise feeling uncomfortable, you might pause for a moment to examine the source of the conflict from a cross-cultural perspective.

During illness, culturally acceptable sick role behavior may range from aggressive, demanding behavior to silent passivity. Complaining, demanding behavior during illness is often rewarded with attention among American Jewish and Italian groups, whereas Asians and Native Americans are likely to be quiet and compliant during illness. During the interview, Asians may provide you with the answers they think you want to hear, behavior consistent with the dominant cultural value for harmonious relationships with others. Thus, you should attempt to phrase questions or statements in a neutral manner that avoids foreshadowing an expected response. Appalachian people may reject an interviewer whom they perceive as prying or nosey as a result of a cultural ethic of neutrality that mandates minding one's own business and avoiding assertive or argumentative behavior (Andrews and Boyle, 2002; Leininger and McFarland, 2002; Ludwig-Beymer, 2002; Zatrick and Dimsdale, 1990).

WORKING WITH (AND WITHOUT) AN INTERPRETER

Nearly 45 million people in the United States speak a language other than English at home (U.S. Bureau of the Census, 2000). Many also can read and write other languages. One of the greatest challenges in cross-cultural communication occurs when you and the patient speak different languages (Fig. 4–6). After assessing the language skills of non–English-speaking people, you may find yourself in one of two situations: trying to communicate effectively through an interpreter or trying to communicate effectively when there is no interpreter.

Interviewing the non–English-speaking person requires a bilingual interpreter for full communication. Even the person from another culture or country who has a basic command of English (those for whom English is a second language) may need an interpreter when faced with the anxiety-provoking situation of entering a hospital, describing a

4-6

strange symptom, or discussing sensitive topics such as those related to reproductive or urologic concerns.

It is tempting to ask a relative, friend, or even another patient to interpret because this person is readily available and probably would like to help. This is disadvantageous because it violates confidentiality for the patient, who may not want personal information shared with another. Furthermore, the friend or relative, although fluent in ordinary language usage, is likely to be unfamiliar with medical terminology, hospital or clinic procedures, and medical ethics.

Whenever possible, work with a bilingual team member or a trained medical interpreter. This person knows interpreting techniques, has a health care background, and understands patients' rights. The trained interpreter also is knowledgeable about cultural beliefs and health practices. This person can help you bridge the cultural gap and can advise you concerning the cultural appropriateness of your recommendations.

Although interpreters are trained to remain neutral, they can influence both the content of information exchanged and the nature of the interaction. Many trained medical interpreters are members of the linguistic community they serve. While this is largely beneficial, it has limitations. For example, interpreters often know patients and details of their circumstances before the interview begins. Although acceptance of a code of ethics governing confidentiality and conflicts of interest is part of the training interpreters receive, discord may arise when they relate information that the patient has not volunteered to the examiner.

It should be noted that being bilingual doesn't always mean the interpreter is culturally aware. The Hispanic culture, for example, is so diverse that a Spanish-speaking interpreter from one country, class, race, and gender doesn't necessarily understand the cultural background of a Spanish-speaking person from another country and different circumstances. Even trained interpreters, who are often from urban areas and represent a higher socioeconomic class than the patients for whom they interpret, may be unaware of or embarrassed by rural attitudes and practices.

Although you will be in charge of the focus and flow of the interview, view yourself and the interpreters as a team. Ask the interpreter to meet the patient beforehand to establish rapport and to garner the patient's age, occupation, educational level, and attitude toward health care. This enables the interpreter to communicate on the patient's level.

Allow more time for this interview. With the third person repeating everything, it can take considerably longer than interviewing English-speaking people. You need to focus on priority data.

There are two styles of interpreting—line-by-line and summarizing. Translating line-by-line takes more time, but it ensures accuracy. Use this style for most of the interview. Both you and the patient should speak only a sentence or two, then allow the interpreter some time. Use simple language yourself, not medical jargon that the interpreter must simplify before it can be translated. Summary translation progresses faster and is useful for teaching relatively simple

health techniques with which the interpreter is already familiar. Be alert for nonverbal cues as the patient talks. These cues can give valuable data. A good interpreter also notes nonverbal messages and passes them on to you. Summarized in Table 4–4 are suggestions for the selection and use of an interpreter.

Although use of an interpreter is the ideal, you may find yourself in a situation with a non–English-speaking patient when no interpreter is available. Table 4–5 summarizes some suggestions for overcoming language barriers when no interpreter is present. Communicating with these patients may require that you combine verbal and nonverbal communication.

NONVERBAL CROSS-CULTURAL COMMUNICATION

Basically, there are five types of nonverbal behaviors that convey information about the person: (1) *vocal cues,* such as pitch, tone, and quality of voice, including moaning, crying, and groaning; (2) *action cues,* such as posture, facial expression, and gestures; (3) *object cues,* such as clothes, jewelry, and hair styles: (4) *use of personal and territorial space* in interpersonal transactions and care of belongings; and (5) *touch,* which involves the use of personal space and action (Lapierre and Padgett, 1991).

Unless you make an effort to understand the patient's nonverbal behavior, you may overlook important information such as that conveyed by facial expressions, silence, eye contact, touch, and other body language. Communication patterns vary widely transculturally even for such conventional social behaviors as smiling and handshaking. Among many Hispanic people, for example, smiling and handshaking are considered an integral part of sincere interactions and essential to establishing trust, whereas a Russian person might perceive the same behavior as insolent and frivolous.

Wide cultural variation exists when interpreting **silence.** Some individuals find silence extremely uncomfortable and make every effort to fill conversational lags with words. Conversely, many Native Americans consider silence essential to understanding and respecting the other person. A pause following your question signifies that what has been asked is important enough to be given thoughtful consideration. In traditional Chinese and Japanese cultures, silence may mean that the speaker wishes the listener to consider the content of what has been said before continuing. The English and Arabs may use silence out of respect for another's privacy, whereas the French, Spanish, and Russians may interpret it as a sign of agreement. Asian cultures often use silence to demonstrate respect for elders. Among some black communities, silence is used in response to what they perceive as a ridiculous question.

Eye contact is perhaps among the most culturally variable nonverbal behaviors. Although you probably have been taught to maintain eye contact when speaking with others, individuals from culturally diverse backgrounds may attribute other culturally based meanings to this behavior. Asian, Native American, Indochinese, Arab, and Appalachian people

TABLE 4-4: Use of an Interpreter

Choosing an Interpreter

- Before locating an interpreter, identify the language the person speaks at home. Be aware that it may differ from the language spoken publicly (e.g., French is sometimes spoken by well-educated and upper-class members of certain Asian, African, or Middle Eastern cultures, but it is not the language spoken in the home).
- Whenever possible, use a *trained* interpreter, preferably one who knows medical terminology.
- Avoid interpreters from a rival tribe, state, region, or nation (e.g., a Palestinian who knows Hebrew may not be the best interpreter for a Jewish person).
- Be aware of gender differences between interpreter and patient. In general, the same gender is preferred.
- Be aware of age differences between interpreter and patient. In general, an older, more mature interpreter is preferred to a younger, less experienced one.
- Be aware of socioeconomic differences between interpreter and patient.

Strategies for Effective Use of an Interpreter

- Plan what you want to say ahead of time. Meet privately with the interpreter before the interview. Avoid confusing the interpreter by backing up, hesitating, or inserting a proviso.
- Ask the interpreter to provide a line-by-line verbatim account of the conversation. Ask for a detailed interpretation when provided with brief summaries of longer exchanges between interpreter and patient.
- Be patient. When using an interpreter, interviews often take two to three times longer.
- Longer-than-expected explanatory exchanges are often required to convey the meaning of words such as *stress, depression, allergy, preventive medicine,* and *physical therapy* because there may not be comparable terms in the language the patient understands.
- When discussing diagnostic tests such as mammograms; MRIs (magnetic resonance imaging); CT (computed tomography) scans; or those involving body fluids such as blood, urine, stool, spinal fluid, or saliva, be sure to clarify the nature of the test to the interpreter. Indicate the purpose of the test, exactly what will happen to the patient, approximately how long the test will take, whether the procedure is invasive or noninvasive, and what part(s) of the body will be tested.
- Be aware that the interpreter may modify or edit some aspects of the conversation, especially if he or she thinks you might not understand the cultural context of the patient's response (e.g., traditional or folk beliefs and practices related to healing).
- Avoid ambiguous statements and questions. Refrain from using conditional or indefinite phrasing such as "if," "would," and "could," especially for target languages, such as Khmer (Cambodia), that lack nuances of conditionally or distinctions of time other than simple past and present. Conditional statements may be mistaken for actual agreement or approval of a course of action.
- Avoid abstract expressions, idioms, similes, metaphors, and medical jargon.
- To ensure confidentiality and privacy, avoid using as interpreters children or strangers who may be visiting other patients.
- Be aware that an interpreter who is a nonrelative may seek compensation for services rendered. Be sure to negotiate fees ahead of time.

Recommendations for Institutions

- Maintain a current, computerized list of interpreters who may be contacted as needed.
- Network with area hospitals, colleges, universities, and other organizations that may serve as resources.
- Utilize over-the-telephone interpretation services provided by telephone companies. For example, since 1989, AT&T has operated the Language Line Services, which provides interpretation in more than 140 languages. Services are available around the clock every day of the year. Call (800) 628-8486 for further information on services and charges.

TABLE 4-5: Overcoming Language Barriers: What to Do When No Interpreter is Available

1. Be polite and formal.
2. Pronounce name correctly. Use proper titles of respect, such as "Mr.," "Mrs.," "Ms.," "Dr." Greet the person using the last or complete name.
   Gesture to yourself and say your name.
   Offer a handshake or nod. Smile.
3. Proceed in an unhurried manner. Pay attention to any effort by the patient or family to communicate.
4. Speak in a low, moderate voice. Avoid talking loudly. Remember that there is a tendency to raise the volume and pitch of your voice when the listener appears not to understand. The listener may perceive that you are shouting and/or angry.
5. Use any words that you might know in the person's language. This indicates that you are aware of and respect his or her culture.
6. Use simple words, such as "pain" instead of "discomfort." Avoid medical jargon, idioms, and slang. Avoid using contractions (e.g., don't, can't, won't). Use nouns repeatedly instead of pronouns.
   Example:
   Do not say: "He has been taking his medicine, hasn't he?"
   Do say: "Does Juan take medicine?"
7. Pantomime words and simple actions while you verbalize them.
8. Give instructions in the proper sequence.
   Example:
   Do not say: "Before you rinse the bottle, sterilize it."
   Do say: "First wash the bottle. Second, rinse the bottle."
9. Discuss one topic at a time. Avoid using conjunctions.
   Example:
   Do not say: "Are you cold and in pain?"
   Do say: "Are you cold (while pantomiming)? Are you in pain?"
10. Validate if the person understands by having him or her repeat instructions, demonstrate the procedure, or act out the meaning.
11. Write out several short sentences in English and determine the person's ability to read them.
12. Try a third language. Many Indochinese speak French. Europeans often know two or more languages. Try Latin words or phrases.
13. Ask who among the person's family and friends could serve as an interpreter.
14. Obtain phrase books from a library or bookstore, make or purchase flash cards, contact hospitals for a list of interpreters, and use both a formal and an informal network to locate a suitable interpreter.

may consider direct eye contact impolite or aggressive, and they may avert their eyes when talking with you. Native Americans often stare at the floor during conversations, a culturally appropriate behavior indicating that the listener is paying close attention to the speaker. Some blacks may use *oculistics* (eye-rolling) in response to what is perceived to be a ridiculous question. Among Hispanics, respect dictates appropriate deferential behavior in the form of downcast eyes toward others on the basis of age, sex, social position, economic status, and position of authority. Elders expect respect from younger individuals, adults from children, men from women, teachers from students, and employers from employees. By virtue of your authority status as a health care provider, with Hispanic people, your eye contact is expected but will not necessarily be reciprocated by the person.

In some cultures—including Arab, Hispanic, and black groups—*modesty for both women and men* is interrelated with eye contact. For Muslim-Arab women, modesty is achieved in part by avoiding eye contact with males (except for one's husband in private settings) and keeping the eyes downcast when encountering members of the opposite sex in public situations. In many cultures, the only woman who smiles and establishes eye contact with men in public is likely to be a prostitute. Hasidic Jewish males also have culturally based norms concerning eye contact with females. You may observe the male avoiding direct eye contact and turning his head in the opposite direction when walking past or speaking to a woman. The preceding examples are intended to be illustrative, not exhaustive.

TOUCH

Without doubt, touching the patient is a necessary component of a comprehensive assessment. From a cultural perspective, however, you are urged to give careful consideration to issues concerning **touch**. While recognizing the benefits reported by many in establishing rapport with patients through touch, physical contact with patients conveys various meanings cross-culturally. In many cultures, such as Arab and Hispanic societies, male health care providers may be prohibited from touching or examining either all or certain parts of the female body. In many cultures, adolescent girls may prefer female health care providers or refuse to be examined by a male. You should be aware that the patient's significant others also may exert pressure on nurses by enforcing these culturally meaningful norms in the health care setting.

Touching children also may have associated meaning transculturally. For example, approximately 80% of the world's people believe in *mal ojo*, which literally translated means "evil of the eye." In this culture-bound syndrome, a child's illness may be attributed to excessive admiration by another person. *Mal ojo* is especially prevalent in Hispanic cultures. Many Asians believe that one's strength resides in the head and that touching the head is a sign of disrespect. The clinical significance of this is that you need to be aware that patting the child on the head or examining the fontanel of a Southeast Asian infant, for example, should be avoided or done only with parental permission. Whenever possible, you should explore alternative ways to express affection or to obtain information necessary for assessment of the patient's condition (e.g., hold the child on the lap, observe for other manifestations of increased intracranial pressure or signs of premature fontanel closure, or place one's hand over the mother's while asking for a description of what she feels).

In concluding this section, a brief comment about same-sex relationships is warranted. In some cultures, it is considered an acceptable expression of friendship and affection to openly and publicly hold hands with or embrace members of the same sex without any sexual connotation being associated with the behavior. For example, you may notice that although a Nigerian-American woman may not demonstrate overt affection for her husband or other male family members, she will hold hands with female relatives and friends while walking or talking with them. You may find that a patient displays similar behaviors and should feel free to discuss cultural differences and similarities openly with the person. The discussion should include how each person feels about the cultural practice and exploration of mutually acceptable—and unacceptable—avenues for communicating.

BIBLIOGRAPHY

Andrews MM, Boyle JS: *Transcultural concepts in nursing care,* ed 4, Philadelphia, 2002, Lippincott Williams & Wilkins.

Arnold E, Boggs K: *Interpersonal relationships: professional communication skills for nurses,* ed 3, Philadelphia, 1999, W.B. Saunders.

Benjamin A: *The helping interview,* ed 3, Boston, 1980, Houghton Mifflin.

Bernstein L, Bernstein RS: *Interviewing: a guide for health professionals,* ed 4, E. Norwalk, Conn, 1985, Appleton & Lange.

Cornell D: Saying the words: communication techniques, *Nurs Manage* 24(3):42–44, 1993.

Deering CG, Cody DJ: Communicating with children and adolescents, *Am J Nurs* 102(3):34–42, 2002.

Dernocoeur K, Meade DM: Street smarts: safe and effective use of interpreters, *Emerg Med Serv* 29(4):32, 38, 2000.

Dreher BB: *Communication skills for working with elders,* ed 2, New York, 2001, Springer.

Gulati S: Issues to consider in deaf and hard-of-hearing patients, *Am Fam Physician* 56(8):2057–2064, 1997.

Eliason MJ: Cultural diversity in nursing care: the lesbian, gay or bisexual client, *J Transcult Nurs* 5(1):14–20, 1993.

Enlow AJ, Forde DL, Brummel-Smith K: *Interviewing and patient care,* ed 4, New York, 1996, Oxford University Press.

Heckerson EW, Shepard JM: Creating an effective patient history: mnemonic SAMPLE, *Emerg Med Serv* 28(7):78–81, 1999.

Lapierre ED, Padgett J: How can we become more aware of culturally specific body language and use this awareness therapeutically? *J Psychosoc Nurs Ment Health Serv* 29(11):38–41, 1991.

Leininger MM, McFarland MR: *Transcultural nursing: concepts, theories, research and practices,* New York, 2002, McGraw-Hill.

Ludwig-Beymer PA: Transcultural aspects of pain. In Andrews MM, Boyle JS, editors: *Transcultural concepts in nursing care,* ed 4, Philadelphia, 2003, Lippincott Williams & Wilkins.

Lyles JS et al: Evidence-based patient-centered interviewing, *JCOM* 8(7):28–34, 2001.

MacNeil J: Transcultural nursing care and health perspectives of HIV/AIDS. In Leininger MM, McFarland MR: *Transcultural nursing: concepts, theories, research and practices,* New York, 2002, McGraw-Hill, pp 253–262.

Platt FW et al: "Tell me about yourself": the patient-centered interview, *Ann Intern Med* 134(11):1079–1085, 2001.

Purtilo R, Haddad A: *Health professional and patient interaction,* ed 6, Philadelphia, 2002, W.B. Saunders.

Radziewics R, Baile WF: Communication skills: breaking bad news in the clinical setting, *Oncol Nurs Forum* 28(6):951–953, 2001.

Redelmeier DA et al: "Eliciting an insightful history of present illness, *Can Med Assoc J* 164(55):647–651, 2001.

Redelmeier DA et al: Obtaining a reliable past medical history, *Can Med Assoc J* 164(6):809–813, 2001.

Rogers CR: *Client-centered therapy,* Boston, 1951, Houghton Mifflin.

Sanchez-Gallegos D, Viens DC: When the client is armed or dangerous: management of violent and difficult clients in primary care, *Nurse Pract* 20(6):26–32, 1995.

Selye H: *The stress of life,* New York, 1956, McGraw-Hill.

Suchman AL et al: A model of empathetic communication in the medical interview, *JAMA* 277(8):678–682, 1997.

U.S. Bureau of the Census: *Profile of selected social characteristics: 2000.* Available at factfinder.census.gov/servlet/QTTable?ds_name=D&geo_id=D&qr_name=ACS_C2SS_E ST_G00_QT02&_lang=en (accessed 4/2/2002).

Zatrick DF, Dimsdale JE: Cultural variations in response to painful stimuli, *Psychosom Med* 52:544–557, 1990.

Domestic Violence Assessment

*I*ntimate partner violence and elder abuse are important health problems that health care professionals must recognize and assess. The Joint Commission on the Accreditation of Healthcare Organizations (JCAHO) requires that all health care settings have policies and procedures to assess, document and make referrals for both kinds of family violence along with child abuse, which is outside the scope of this chapter. All of the major nursing and medical organizations such as the American Nurses Association (ANA) and the American Medical Association (AMA) have policy statements recognizing the need for health care professionals to assess family violence.

The Centers for Disease Control and Prevention (CDC) definition for intimate partner violence (IPV) will be used throughout this chapter; the definition identifies two types of IPV:

- Physical and/or sexual violence (use of physical force) or threat of such violence
- Psychological/emotional abuse and/or coercive tactics when there has been prior physical and/or sexual violence between persons who are spouses or nonmarital partners (dating, boyfriend/girlfriend) or former spouses or nonmarital partners (Saltzman et al, 1999).

Although violence by intimates has decreased in the past decade, numbers remaining are substantial. In 1998, approximately 900,000 U.S. women reported physical or sexual assault by intimates, reduced from 1.1 million in 1993 (National Crime Victimization Survey [NCVS], 2000). IPV accounted for 22% of violent crimes against women between 1993 and 1998 (versus 3% for men) (NCVS, 2000). Current rates of IPV (in the past year) range from 1.8% to 14% in population-based studies and up to 44% in health care settings (Jones et al, 1999; Tjaden and Thoennes, 2000). Lifetime estimates vary from 5% to 51% (Tjaden and Thoennes, 2000), with the most usual range between 25% and 35%. Women are significantly more likely to be physically or sexually assaulted by a current or former intimate partner than by an acquaintance, family member, friend, or stranger (Tjaden and Thoennes, 2000). As high as these figures are, it is commonly accepted that they (particularly crime data) represent *under*estimates of the true incidence and prevalence of IPV.

Almost every state has some form of mandatory reporting of abused elderly and other vulnerable patients (the developmentally disabled and the mentally ill). You need to be familiar with specific state reporting requirements in your state of practice. Those who work in communities that border two states will need to be informed about mandatory reporting statutes in both states. In some communities, the reporting mechanism is established county by county, while some states have a statewide hotline. As mandatory reporters of abuse, you need only have suspicion that elder abuse and/or neglect may have occurred in order to generate a call to the authorities. Many nurses, physicians, and social workers are erroneously under the assumption that they must have proof of abuse before calling the hotline. While exact definitions of elder abuse and neglect vary from state to state, the American Medical Association has developed a generic list of definitions that are clinically useful (Table 5–1) (Arvanis et al, 1992).

TABLE 5–1: AMA Definitions for Elder Abuse and Neglect

Physical abuse	Violent acts that result or could result in injury, pain, impairment, and/or disease
Physical neglect	Failure of the family member and/or caregiver to provide basic goods and/or services such as food, shelter, health care, and medications
Psychological abuse	Behaviors that result in mental anguish
Psychological neglect	Failing to provide basic social stimulation
Financial abuse	Intentional misuse of the elderly person's financial/material resources without the informed consent of the person
Financial neglect	Failure to use the assets of the elderly person to provide services needed by the elderly person

Adapted from Arvanis SC et al: *Diagnosis and treatment guidelines on elder abuse and neglect*, Chicago, 1992, American Medical Association.

HEALTH EFFECTS OF VIOLENCE

A persuasive body of knowledge accumulated in the past decade has established that violent experiences have significant effects on women's health. The most obvious health care problem for abused women is injury, with approximately 52% of abused women saying they were injured seriously enough to need medical attention from an abusive incident (Bachman and Saltzman, 1995). Such injuries have particular patterns that can be recognized.

In many controlled investigations of women in a variety of health care settings, abused women also have been found to have significantly more chronic health problems, including significantly more neurologic, gastrointestinal, and gynecologic symptoms and chronic pain (Campbell, 2002; Campbell et al, 2002; Coker et al, 2000; Leserman et al, 1998; Letourneau et al, 1999; McCauley et al, 1995; Plichta, 1996). Abused women have also been shown to visit health care professionals more often than women not battered and to incur more health care costs (Wisner et al, 1999). In terms of mental health, abused women also have significantly more depression, suicidality and PTSD symptoms, as well as problems with substance abuse (Golding, 1999). The forced sex that accompanies physical abuse in 40% to 45% of the cases contributes to a host of reproductive health problems including chronic pelvic pain, unintended pregnancy, STDs (including HIV), and urinary tract infections (Campbell and Soeken, 1999a; Letourneau et al, 1999; Maman et al, 2000). Abuse during pregnancy is also a significant health problem, with serious consequences for both the pregnant mother (e.g., depression, substance abuse) and infant (low birth weight, increased risk of child abuse) (Gazmararian et al, 2000; Murphy et al, 2001).

Although more than half of battered women say they have been injured, only 25% to 30% of abused women say they have actually sought health care for one of the injuries

(Plichta, 1996). Even so, the majority of abused women (80%) say they have been in the health care setting for some reason, either for regular checkups or for one of the long-term health problems described previously. Because many abused women are not yet ready to seek help from a shelter or from the criminal justice system (Landenburger, 1998), the health care system can be an extremely important early point of contact. By uncovering abuse in its early stages, it is hoped that the pattern of violence can be stopped and long-term health problems avoided or minimized.

The health effects of elder abuse are not nearly as well studied. Complications from intentional injury can range from minor pain and discomfort to life-threatening injuries. Bleeding from intentional trauma can cause significant changes in circulatory homeostasis, leading to marked fluctuations in blood pressure and pulse, shock, and then death. Localized infections can progress to generalized sepsis, then death, in aging patients who are immunocompromised. The actual assault or the stress leading up to or following an assault can contribute to cardiac complications. All of the sexually transmitted diseases and sexually related complications that are sequelae of abuse for the younger women are present in the older sexually assaulted women. In addition, postmenopausal women have more friable vaginal mucosal tissue secondary to deestrogenation.

Abuse of the elderly often is coupled with neglect. Neglect can manifest itself with symptoms of dehydration and malnutrition. Neglect can be intentional or nonintentional. Many family members or caretakers working with an aging person consciously, and with malice, withhold food, water, medication, and appropriate necessities, while often concurrently stealing the financial assets of the elderly, dependent person. This type of neglect is often, by definition, criminal in nature.

Other family members or caretakers working with an elderly person struggle with their own severe physical and cognitive health challenges. Their intentions are good; however, the elderly patient may experience profound unintentional neglect. While unintentional neglect is usually not viewed as a crime, it is still reportable to adult protective service agencies. Self-neglect raises often unanswerable questions about one's right to live autonomously versus society's obligation to care for a person who is not able to care for herself or himself. Suspected self-neglect is also a mandatory reportable activity to adult protective services.

SCREENING FOR INTIMATE PARTNER VIOLENCE

Routine, universal screening for intimate partner violence means asking every woman at every health care encounter if she has been abused by a husband, boyfriend or other intimate partner or ex-partner. The majority of both abused and nonabused women say that they are in favor of routine screening and that they believe it would assist women in getting help for the problem (Gielen et al, 2000; Glass, Dearwater and Campbell, 2001). Routine, universal screening for IPV has been called for by most nursing professional organizations (e.g., ANA; American College of Nurse Midwives [ACNM];

Association of Women's Health and Obstetrics and Neonatal Nursing [AWHONN]; Emergency Nurses Association [ENA]; International Association of Forensic Nurses [IAFN]; Nursing Network on Violence Against Women, International [NNVAWI]).

HOW TO SCREEN

The Abuse Assessment Screen (AAS) has been used in many different health care settings, has been translated into at least seven languages, and has strong support for reliability and validity (Soeken et al, 1998). It has never been copyrighted, with the intention that nurses be able to revise and reformat its content to be adaptable to their own health care setting (Fig. 5–1).

Many health care professionals precede the questions with an introduction such as "Because domestic violence is so common in our society, we are asking all women the following questions." Or "Because domestic violence has such serious health care consequences, we are asking all of our female patients the questions that follow." This both alerts the woman that questions about domestic violence are coming and makes sure that the woman knows she is not being singled out for these questions.

The Family Violence Prevention Fund (1999) has developed a protocol for the recommended frequency of screening (Fig. 5–2).

ASSESSMENT

If a woman answers yes to any of the AAS questions, you need to ask questions designed to assess how recent and how serious the abuse was. Asking the woman to "tell me about this abuse in your relationship" is a good way to start. Even if the woman only says yes to the first question and calls the abuse "only emotional" or "not that bad," or says "we just fight a lot" at first, more abuse may be revealed as you gently assess the situation. This type of assessment is often like "peeling layers of an onion," with more violence being uncovered as the assessment continues. This is not "denial" on the woman's part but rather the normal minimization that often accompanies trauma from violence.

It is appropriate for you to show that you are concerned and even distressed about the degree of violence. One message that needs to be conveyed during the assessment is that the abuse is not the woman's fault; this can be said several times. Another important message is that you are concerned and that help is possible. Still another is that several health problems can occur because of domestic violence and that is why it is necessary to conduct a thorough assessment. In fact, in a recent survey of 265 abused women who accepted a referral to a social worker, 59% said it was because the medical provider expressed concern that their presenting health problem was related to IPV (McCaw et al, 2002).

Routine screening for possible elder abuse and neglect can be more complicated than assessments for IPV. The aging can present for health care cognitively and physically intact or with multiple health, physical, and cognitive challenges.

Abuse Assessment Screen
NRCVA, (1988)

Violence is very common in today's world, and it can overlap into our homes. Because violence affects so many people, I now routinely ask all my patients (clients) a few questions about violence in their lives.

All couples argue now and again, even the best of couples.

1. When you and your partner argue, are you ever afraid of him (her)?

2. When you and your partner verbally argue, do you think he (she) tries to emotionally hurt/abuse you?

3. Does your partner try to control you? Where you go? Who you see? How much money you can have?

4. Has your partner (or anyone) ever slapped you, pushed you, hit you, kicked you, or otherwise physically hurt you?

5. Since you have been pregnant (when you were pregnant), has your partner ever bit you, slapped you, pushed you, hit you, kicked you, or otherwise physically hurt you?

6. Has your partner ever forced you into sex when you did not want to participate?

With any yes, say, "Thank you for sharing. Can you tell me more about the last time?"

The Nursing Research Consortium on Violence and Abuse (1988) encourages the reproduction, modification, and/or use of the Abuse Assessment Screen in routine screening for domestic violence.

5–1 Abuse assessment screen (AAS).

Protocol for Screening Summary: Women Over 14 Years of Age

Setting
Frequency of IPV screening

Primary Care
Every first visit for a new chief complaint, every new patient encounter, every new intimate relationship, and all periodic examinations

Emergency Department and Urgent Care
All women, all visits

OB/GYN
Each prenatal and postpartum visit, each new intimate relationship, all routine gynecologic visits (periodic and symptom based), all family planning visits, and all visits in STD and abortion clinics

Mental Health
Every initial assessment, each new intimate relationship, and annually if ongoing or periodic treatment

Inpatient
Part of all admissions and discharge

Source: Family Violence Prevention Fund, 1999. (www.fvpf.org)

5–2 Protocol for screening summary—women over 14 years of age.

Screening for intimate partner violence in the elderly is very similar to screening for IPV among younger women if the patient is cognitively intact. The AAS can be a useful screen for assessing domestic violence among elderly women. You may modify the introductory statement as follows: "Because domestic violence has such serious health care consequences, we are asking women of all ages the following questions."

While some aging women have been in abusive relationships for decades, others are experiencing for the first time physical and sexual violence from normally nonabusive partners who themselves are afflicted with behavior-altering neurological illness (Alzheimer disease, organic brain syndromes). An older battered woman in a long-term abusive relationship may be trying to outlive her abuser, whereas the newly abused older woman may be reluctant to disclose because of embarrassment, shame, and fears that her partner will be institutionalized.

The aging are vulnerable to abuse from other family members and caretakers. The AMA has developed a nine-question clinically effective screen that can be used with elderly persons who are cognitively intact (Table 5–2).

Assessment of physical abuse and/or neglect in the cognitively challenged person is much more complicated. Physical findings that are inconsistent with the history provided by the patient, family member, or caregiver are significant red flags of possible abuse and neglect. Almost all states have some form of mandatory reporting of suspected abuse of patients aged 65 and older. To report abuse, you need not have proof of abuse or neglect, only reasonable cause to suspect that elder abuse or neglect may have occurred.

HISTORY

It is important also to assess and document prior abuse, including prior IPV, childhood physical and sexual abuse, and prior rapes of all kinds (stranger, date, intimate partner). Cumulative trauma has been shown to be associated with more severe mental and physical health problems (Koss et al, 1994; McCauley et al, 1997). Also important to determine is the history of traumatic injuries, since these may have an impact on the current health condition. For instance, a woman may have experienced prior episodes of head trauma and strangulation, both of which may be related to chronic but subtle neurological symptoms and problems (Diaz-Olavarrieta et

al, 1999). Another extremely important area of history and examination in cases of IPV or elder abuse is a mental status examination, both for potential head trauma and neurological symptoms and also for mental health problems. All survivors of violence should be given a mental status examination, with particular attention to the most frequent mental health problems associated with violence: depression, suicidality, PTSD, substance abuse, and anxiety. Chapter 7 gives direction for conducting this part of the history.

PHYSICAL EXAMINATION

Important components of the physical exam of the known survivor of IPV and/or elder abuse include a complete head-to-toe visual examination, especially if the patient is receiving health services secondary to reported abuse. When the examination reveals physical findings, knowledge of basic medical forensic terminology is essential in all documentation. Table 5–3 lists the most common forensic terms with definitions. Please note that the most commonly misused terms are *ecchymosis* and *laceration*. Ecchymoses are not directly related to blunt force trauma that results in bruising, and not all open wounds should be called lacerations (only those related to splitting of tissue from blunt force impact and/or tearing of tissue should be).

Keep in mind the following guidelines when documenting the physical examination:

- *Bruise* can be used interchangeably with *contusion*.
- *Laceration* is related to *avulsion*.
- *Ecchymosis* is related to *(senile) purpura*.
- *Petechia* is related to *purpura*.
- *Rug burn* is more accurately described as a *friction abrasion*.
- *Incision* can be used interchangeably with *cut*.
- *Cut* can be used interchangeably with *sharp injury*.
- *Stab wounds* are penetrating, deep, sharp injuries.
- *Hematoma* is a collection of blood that is often but not always caused by blunt force trauma.

Many practitioners try to date bruises based on the color; however, there is no scientific evidence to support the accurate dating of injuries based on color of the contusion (Langlois and Gresham, 2001). Therefore, trying to accurately date injuries solely by examination is forensically futile. There are, however, some guidelines that can assist in determining if the approximate age of the bruise is consistent with the history being provided by the patient and/or caregiver. A new bruise is usually red and will often develop a purple or purple-blue appearance 12 to 36 hours after blunt-force trauma. The color of bruises (and ecchymoses) generally progresses from purple-blue to bluish-green to greenish-brown to brownish-yellow before fading away.

This process will be the same on all people; however, depending on the color of a person's skin, the process may be more or less visible, and more or less able to be photographed. In general, newer bruises will be mostly reddish-purple, whereas bruises that are beginning to age will be more greenish-brown or brownish-yellow.

There are multiple factors that can contribute to the elderly bruising more readily or more severely than younger

TABLE 5–2: AMA Elder Abuse Screening Questions

1. Has anyone ever touched you inappropriately without your consent?
2. Has anyone ever made you do things you didn't want to do?
3. Has anyone taken things that were yours without first asking?
4. Has anyone ever physically hurt you?
5. Has anyone ever scolded or threatened you?
6. Have you ever signed any documents you did not understand?
7. Are you afraid of anybody at home or who enters your home?
8. Are you alone a lot?
9. Has anyone ever failed to help you take care of yourself when you needed help?

Adapted from Arvanis SC et al: *Diagnosis and treatment guidelines on elder abuse and neglect*, Chicago, 1992, American Medical Association.

people. Medications and abnormal blood values related to medication side effects and underlying hemotologic disorders can affect ease of bruising or the formation of ecchymosis. Common medications that increase risk for bruising or bleeding complications include but are not limited to the following: aspirin, ibuprofen, any of the nonsteroidal anti-inflammatory drugs, warfarin, heparin, valproic acid, prednisone, and clopidogrel. Vitamin nutritional supplements also may contribute to hemotologic complications, especially if the person is already taking a blood-thinning or platelet-altering medication. Bilberry, garlic, ginger, and ginkgo are among the more common supplements linked to increased risk of bruising and/or bleeding complications (Doyle, Harold, and Johnson, 2001).

Any health evaluation for known or suspected elder abuse and neglect should include baseline laboratory tests, including, at a minimum, a complete blood count (CBC) with platelet level, basic blood chemistries (including BUN, creatinine, protein, and albumin), serum liver function tests, a coagulation panel, and a urinalysis (Geroff and Olshaker, 2001).

DOCUMENTATION

Documentation of intimate partner violence and elder abuse must include detailed, nonbiased progress notes, the use of injury maps, and photographic documentation in the health record. Examples of photographic documentation of patients of one of the authors are included in this chapter (Figs. 5–3 through 5–9*).

*Many of these photos were first published in Sheridan, 2001. Reprinted here with the author's permission.

TABLE 5–3: **Forensic Terminology**

Abrasion   A wound caused by rubbing the skin or mucous membrane.

Avulsion   The tearing away of a structure or part.

Bruise   Superficial discoloration due to hemorrhage into the tissues from ruptured blood vessels beneath the skin surface, without the skin itself being broken; also called a contusion.

Contusion   A bruise; injury to tissues without breakage of skin; blood from broken blood vessels accumulates, producing pain, swelling, tenderness.

Cut   See incision.

Ecchymosis   A hemorrhagic spot or blotch, larger than petechia, in the skin or mucous membrane, forming a nonelevated, rounded or regular, blue or purplish patch.

Hematoma   A localized collection of extravasated blood, usually clotted in an organ, space, or tissue.

Hemorrhage   The escape of blood from a ruptured vessel, which can be external, internal, and/or into the skin or other organ.

Incision   A cut or wound made by a sharp instrument; the act of cutting.

Laceration   The act of tearing or splitting; a wound produced by the tearing and/or splitting of body tissue, usually from blunt impact over a bony surface.

Lesion   A broad term referring to any pathologic or traumatic discontinuity of tissue or loss of function of a part.

Patterned injury   An injury caused by an object that leaves a distinct pattern on the skin and/or organ (i.e., being whipped with an extension cord) or an injury caused by a unique mechanism of injury (i.e., immersion burns to the hands [glove burn] or feet [sock burns]).

Pattern of injuries   Injuries, usually bruises and fractures, in various stages of healing.

Petechiae   Minute, pinpoint, nonraised, perfectly round, purplish red spots caused by intradermal or submucous hemorrhage, which later turn blue or yellow.

Puncture   The act of piercing or penetrating with a pointed object or instrument.

Stab wound   A penetrating, sharp, cutting injury that is deeper than it is wide.

Traumatic alopecia   Loss of hair from pulling and yanking or by other traumatic means.

Wound   A general term referring to a bodily injury caused by physical means.

Adapted from Miller BF, Keane CB: *Encyclopedia and dictionary of medicine, nursing, and allied health*, ed 2, Philadelphia, 1978, W.B. Saunders; Sheridan DJ: Treating survivors of intimate partner abuse: Forensic identification and documentation. In Olshaker JS, Jackson ML, Smock WS, editors: *Forensic emergency medicine*, Philadelphia, 2001, W.B. Saunders; *Taber's cyclopedic medical dictionary*, Philadelphia, 1997, F.A. Davis.

5–3 Patterned, fingernail-like scratch abrasions to the left lateral neck from a manual strangulation mechanism of injury.

5–4 Patterned, punchlike abrasion to the mid-forehead from an assailant wearing a ring with a stone; sutured laceration to the left eyebrow; sutured partial-avulsion injury to the nose, punchlike contusion to the left eye involving the sclera, and manual strangulation–related abrasion to the neck.

5–5 Newer, patterned, looped, cordlike contusions to the right upper posterior shoulder and left lower posterior shoulder; patterned, looped, cordlike scar to the right mid-lateral back; scabbed, cordlike abrasions to the mid-back; patterned, kick/stomp heel-like contusion to the left mid-back; and patterned foot/kick/stomplike heel and sole bruise imprint to the upper left posterior, superior shoulder.

5–6 Multiple, patterned-punch–like contusions to the right upper arm.

5–7 Patterned, defensive posture–like bruises to the right forearm.

5–8 Multiple, patterned, "hidden" punch–like contusions to the upper abdomen and lower anterior chest.

5-9 Series of two photographs to illustrate how photographs can be used to demonstrate mechanisms of injuries. **A,** Victim has obvious facial trauma to her left eyelid, left lateral nose, and mouth. The left lateral nose contusion was caused by the nose piece of her glasses being forcefully pushed into her skin from a punch injury to the left eye. The patient's glasses absorbed much of the punch force and were broken (not pictured). A second punch produced the mouth trauma. **B,** The force of the mouth punch caused the upper teeth to leave patterned contusion, abrasion, and minor laceration to the oral mucosa of the upper lip.

Written documentation of histories of IPV and elder abuse need to be verbatim but within reason. It is clinically unrealistic to document verbatim every statement made by an abused patient. However, it is critical to document exceptionally poignant statements made by the victim that identify the reported perpetrator and severe threats of harm made by the reported perpetrator. Other aspects of the abuse history, including reports of past abusive incidents can be paraphrased with the use of partial direct quotations.

When quoting or paraphrasing the history, you should not sanitize the words reportedly heard by the victim. Verbatim documentation of the reported perpetrator's threats interlaced with curses and expletives can be extremely useful in future court proceedings. Also, be careful to use the exact terms an abused patient may use to describe sexual organs or sexually assaultive behaviors.

Photographic documentation in the medical record can be invaluable. Prior written consent to take photographs should be obtained from all cognitively intact, competent adults. Most health facilities have standardized consent to photograph forms. If a patient is unconscious or cognitively impaired, the taking of photographs without consent is generally viewed as ethically sound since it is a noninvasive, painless intervention that has high potential to help a suspected abuse victim. There are advantages and disadvantages to the different photographic systems (Polaroid, 35 mm, and digital) commonly in use (Besant-Matthews and Smock, 2001; Sheridan, 2001). In general, any in-focus picture of injury is better than no picture, regardless of what system is used.

ASSESSING FOR RISK OF HOMICIDE

Women in this country are more often killed by a husband, boyfriend, or ex-husband than by anyone else, and about three fourths of these women have been abused by the man who subsequently killed them (Campbell, Sharps, and Glass, 2001). In a recently completed multicity study of intimate partner homicide of women, 42% of the women killed had been seen somewhere in the health care system (the ED in the majority of cases but also in primary care, prenatal care, and other settings) for something in the year before she was killed (Sharps et al, 2001). These encounters were missed opportunities for health care professionals to identify IPV and intervene to decrease the danger. The same study found reliability and validity support for the Danger Assessment (DA), a 19-item yes/no instrument that has been used extensively by nurses in the health care system as well as advocates in other settings with battered women (Campbell, Sharps, and Glass, 2001) (Fig. 5-10). The instrument starts with a calendar so that women can more accurately see for themselves how frequent and severe the violence has become over the past year. This is also an excellent assessment of frequency and severity for the health care provider. Although there are no predetermined cutoff scores on the DA, the more yes answers there are, the more serious the danger of the woman's situation. In the previously described multicity study, abused women who were the victims of a homicide had an average score of 7.1 on the original 15-item DA. The DA is copyrighted, so users need to use it intact and are asked to communicate with the author if they are planning to use it in research. It can also be downloaded from www.son.jhmi.edu or www.nrcva.com.

DANGER ASSESSMENT
Jacquelyn C. Campbell, Ph.D., R.N.
Copyright 1985, 1988, 2001

Several risk factors have been associated with homicides (murders) of both batterers and battered women in research conducted after the murders have taken place. We cannot predict what will happen in your case, but we would like you to be aware of the danger of homicide in situations of severe battering and for you to see how many of the risk factors apply to your situation.

Using the calendar, please mark the approximate dates during the past year when you were beaten by your husband or partner. Write on that date how bad the incident was according to the following scale:

      1. Slapping, pushing; no injuries and/or lasting pain
      2. Punching, kicking; bruises, cuts, and/or continuing pain
      3. "Beating up"; severe contusions, burns, broken bones
      4. Threat to use weapon; head injury, internal injury, permanent injury
      5. Use of weapon; wounds from weapon

      (If **any** of the descriptions for the higher number apply, use the higher number.)

Mark **Yes** or **No** for each of the following. ("He" refers to your husband, partner, ex-husband, ex-partner, or whoever is currently physically hurting you.)

_____ 1. Has the physical violence increased in severity or frequency over the past year?
_____ 2. Has he ever used a weapon against you or threatened you with a weapon?
_____ 3. Does he ever try to choke you?
_____ 4. Does he own a gun?
_____ 5. Has he ever forced you to have sex when you did not wish to do so?
_____ 6. Does he use drugs? By drugs, I mean "uppers" or amphetamines, speed, angel dust, cocaine, "crack", street drugs or mixtures.
_____ 7. Does he threaten to kill you and/or do you believe he is capable of killing you?
_____ 8. Is he drunk every day or almost every day? (In terms of quantity of alcohol.)
_____ 9. Does he control most or all of your daily activities? For instance: does he tell you who you can be friends with, when you can see your family, how much money you can use, or when you can take the car? (If he tries, but you do not let him, check here: _____)
_____ 10. Have you ever been beaten by him while you were pregnant? (If you have never been pregnant by him, check here: _____)
_____ 11. Is he violently and constantly jealous of you? (For instance, does he say "If I can't have you, no one can."?)
_____ 12. Have you ever threatened or tried to commit suicide?
_____ 13. Has he ever threatened or tried to commit suicide?
_____ 14. Does he threaten to harm your children?
_____ 15. Do you have a child that is not his?
_____ 16. Is he unemployed?
_____ 17. Have you left him during the past year? (If you have *never* lived with him, check here: _____)
_____ 18. Do you currently have another (different) intimate partner?
_____ 19. Does he follow or spy on you, leave threatening notes, destroy your property, or call you when you don't want him to?

_____ Total "Yes" Answers

Thank you. Please talk to your nurse, advocate, or counselor about what the Danger Assessment means in terms of your situation.

5–10 | Danger assessment.

WHEN SHE SAYS NO TO THE AAS BUT THERE ARE OTHER IPV HEALTH INDICATORS

In addition to the AAS, providers need to be alert for the conditions particularly associated with IPV, including gynecological problems (especially STDs, pelvic pain, and complaints of sexual dysfunction), chronic irritable bowel syndrome, back pain, depression, and the presenting symptoms of PTSD (especially problems sleeping and "panic" attacks or problems with "nerves"). When these problems occur, and especially when they persist, a thorough and repeated assessment for domestic violence is needed. In this case, an instrument such as the WEB (Coker et al, 2000) scale might be used in addition to the AAS, or gentle indirect queries (e.g., "I am concerned about your health conditions; is there any chance that stress at home is contributing to these problems?") may be used.

BIBLIOGRAPHY

Arvanis SC et al: *Diagnosis and treatment guidelines on elder abuse and neglect*, Chicago, 1992, American Medical Association.

Bachman R, Saltzman LE: *Violence against women: estimates from the redesigned survey*, Washington, DC, 1995, Bureau of Justice Statistics, National Institute of Justice.

Besant-Matthews PE, Smock WS: Forensic photography in the emergency department. In Olshaker JS, Jackson MC, Smock WS, editors: *Forensic emergency medicine*, Philadelphia, 2001, Lippincott Williams & Wilkins, pp. 257–282.

Campbell J: Nursing assessment for risk of homicide with battered women, *Adv Nurs Sci* 8:36–51, 1986.

Campbell J: *Assessing dangerousness*, Newbury Park, Calif, 1995, Sage.

Campbell J et al: Risk factors for femicide among pregnant and non-pregnant battered women. In Campbell JC, editor: *Empowering survivors of abuse: health care for battered women and their children*, Thousand Oaks, Calif, 1988, Sage.

Campbell J et al: Intimate partner violence and physical health consequences, *Arch Intern Med* 162:1157–1163, 2002.

Campbell J, Soeken K: Forced sex and intimate partner violence: effects on women's health, *Violence Against Women* 5:1017–1035, 1999a.

Campbell J, Soeken KL: Women's responses to battering: a test of the model, *Research in Nursing and Health* 22:49–58, 1999b.

Campbell JC: Health consequences of intimate partner violence, *Lancet* 359(9314):1331–1336, 2002.

Campbell JC, Sharps P, Glass NE: Risk assessment for intimate partner homicide. In Pinard GF, Pagani L, editors: *Clinical assessment of dangerousness: empirical contributions*, New York, 2000, Cambridge University Press.

Coker A et al: Frequency and correlates of intimate partner violence by type: physical, sexual, and psychological battering, *Am J Public Health* 90(4):553–559, 2000.

Diaz-Olavarrieta C et al: Domestic violence against patients with chronic neurologic disorders, *Arch Neurol* 56:681–685, 1999.

Doyle RM, Harold C, Johnson P, editors: *Nursing herbal medicine handbook*, Springhouse, Penn, 2001, Springhouse Corporation.

Family Violence Prevention Fund: *Preventing domestic violence: clinical guidelines on routine screening*, San Francisco, 1999, Family Violence Prevention Fund (www.fvpf.org).

Gazmararian JA et al: Violence and reproductive health: current knowledge and future research directions, *Matern Child Health J* 4(2):79–84, 2000.

Geroff AJ, Olshaker JS: Elder abuse. In Olshaker JS, Jackson MC, Smock WS, editors: *Forensic emergency medicine*, Philadelphia, 2001, Lippincott Williams & Wilkins.

Gielen AC et al: Women's opinions about domestic violence screening and mandatory reporting, *Am J Prev Med* 19(4):279–285, 2000.

Glass NE, Dearwater S, Campbell JC: Intimate partner violence screening and intervention: data from eleven Pennsylvania and California community hospital emergency departments, *J Emerg Nurs* 27(2):141–149, 2001.

Golding JM: Intimate partner violence as a risk factor for mental disorders: a meta-analysis, *J Fam Violence* 14(2):99–132, 1999.

Jones A et al: Annual and lifetime prevalence of partner abuse in a sample of female HMO enrollees, *Womens Health Issues* 9:295–305, 1999.

Koss MP et al: *No safe haven: male violence against women at home, at work, and in the community*, Washington, DC, 1994, APA.

Landenburger K: Exploration of women's identity: clinical approaches with abused women. In Campbell J, editor: *Empowering survivors of abuse: health care for battered women and their children*, Newbury Park, Calif, 1998, Sage.

Langlois NEI, Greshman GA: The aging of bruises: a review and study of the colour changes with time, *Forensic Sci Int* 50:227–238, 2001.

Leserman J et al: Selected symptoms associated with sexual and physical abuse among female patients with gastrointestinal disorders: the impact on subsequent health care visits, *Psychol Med* 28:417–425, 1998.

Letourneau E, Holmes M, Chasedunn-Roark J: Gynecologic health consequences to victims of interpersonal violence, *Womens Health Issues* 9(2):115–120, 1999.

Maman S et al: The intersection of HIV and violence: directions for future research and interventions, *Soc Sci Med* 4:459–478, 2000.

McCauley J et al: The "battering syndrome": prevalence and clinical characteristics of domestic violence in primary care internal medicine practices, *Ann Intern Med* 123(10):737–746, 1995.

McCauley J et al: Clinical characteristics of women with a history of childhood abuse: unhealed wounds, *JAMA* 277(17):1362–1368, 1997.

McCaw B et al: Women referred for on-site domestic violence services in a managed care organization, *Women and Health* 35(2/3):23–40, 2002.

McFarlane J, Parker B, Soeken K: Abuse during pregnancy: associations with maternal health and infant birth weight, *Nurs Res* 45:37–42, 1996.

Miller BF, Keane CB: *Encyclopedia and dictionary of medicine, nursing, and allied health*, ed 2, Philadelphia, 1978, W.B. Saunders.

Murphy CC et al: Abuse: a risk factor for low birth weight? A systematic review and meta-analysis, *Can Med Assoc J* 164(11):1567–1572, 2001.

Plichta SB: Violence and abuse: implications for women's health. In Falik MK, Collins KS, editors: *Women's health, the Commonwealth Fund survey*, Baltimore, 1996, Johns Hopkins University Press.

Rennison C: *Violent victimization and race, 1993-98*, Washington, DC, 2001, Bureau of Justice Statistics, US Department of Justice.

Saltzman LE et al: *Intimate partner violence surveillance: uniform definitions and recommended data elements*, Version 1.0, Atlanta, 1999, National Center for Injury Prevention and Control, Centers for Disease Control and Prevention.

Sharps P et al: Opportunities for prevention of femicide by health care providers, *Prev Med* 33:373–380, 2001.

Sheridan DJ: Treating survivors of intimate partner abuse: forensic identification and documentation. In Olshaker JS, Jackson MC, Smock WS, editors: *Forensic emergency medicine*, Philadelphia, 2001, Lippincott Williams & Wilkins.

Silva C et al: Symptoms of post-traumatic stress disorder in abused women in a primary care setting, *J Womens Health* 6:543–552, 1997.

Soeken K et al: The abuse assessment screen: a clinical instrument to measure frequency, severity, and perpetrator of abuse against women. In Campbell JC, editor: *Empowering survivors of abuse: health care for battered women and their children*, Newbury Park, Calif, 1998, Sage.

Taber's cyclopedic medical dictionary, Philadelphia, 1997, FA Davis.

Tjaden P, Thoennes N: *Full report of the prevalence, incidence, and consequences of violence against women*, Washington, DC, 2000, National Institute of Justice (NCJ-183781).

Wisner CL et al: Intimate partner violence against women: do victims cost health plans more? *J Fam Pract* 48(6):439–443, 1999.

The Complete Health History

The purpose of the health history is to collect **subjective data**—what the person *says* about himself or herself. The history is combined with the **objective data** from the physical examination and laboratory studies to form the data base. The data base is used to make a judgment or a diagnosis about the health status of the individual.

The following health history provides a complete picture of the person's past and present health. It describes the individual as a whole and how the person interacts with the environment. It records health strengths and coping skills. The history should recognize and affirm what the person is doing right: what he or she is doing to help stay well. For the well person, the history is used to assess his or her lifestyle, including such factors as exercise, diet, risk reduction, and health promotion behaviors. For the ill person, it includes a detailed and chronologic record of the health problem. For all, the health history is a screening tool for abnormal symptoms, health problems, and concerns, and it records ways of responding to the health problems.

In many settings the patient fills out a printed history form or checklist. This allows the person ample time to recall and consider such items as dates of health landmarks and relevant family history. The interview is then used to validate the written data and to collect more data on lifestyle management and current health problems.

Although history forms vary, most contain information in this sequence of categories:

1. Biographical data
2. Reason for seeking care
3. Present health or history of present illness
4. Past history
5. Family history
6. Review of systems
7. Functional assessment or activities of daily living (ADLs)

The health history discussed in the following section follows this format and presents a generic data base for all practitioners. Those in primary care settings may use all of it, whereas those in a hospital may focus primarily on the history of present illness and the functional, or patterns of living, data.

THE HEALTH HISTORY—THE ADULT

BIOGRAPHICAL DATA

Name, address and phone number, age and birthdate, birthplace, gender, marital status, race, ethnic origin, occupation, usual and present (an illness or disability may have prompted change in occupation).

SOURCE OF HISTORY

1. Record who furnishes the information—usually the person herself or himself, although the source may be a relative or friend.
2. Judge how reliable the informant seems and how willing he or she is to communicate. A reliable person always gives the same answers, even when questions are rephrased or are repeated later in the interview.
3. Note any special circumstances, such as the use of an interpreter. Sample statements include:

Patient herself, who seems reliable.
Patient's son, John Ramirez, who seems reliable.
Mrs. R. Fuentes, interpreter for Theresa Castillo who does not speak English.

REASON FOR SEEKING CARE*

This is a brief spontaneous statement in the person's own words that describes the reason for the visit. Think of it as the "title" for the story to follow. It states one (possibly two) symptoms or signs and their duration. A **symptom** is a subjective sensation that the person

---

*In the past, this statement was called the "Chief Complaint" (CC). This title is avoided now because it labels the person a "complainer," and more importantly, does not include wellness needs.

feels from the disorder. A **sign** is an objective abnormality that you as the examiner could detect on physical examination or in laboratory reports. Whatever the person says is the reason for seeking care is recorded, enclosed in quotation marks to indicate the person's exact words.

"Chest pain" for 2 hours.
"Earache and fussy all night."
"Need yearly physical for work."
"Want to start jogging and need checkup."

The reason for seeking care is not a diagnostic statement. Avoid translating it into the terms of a medical diagnosis. For example, Mr. J. Schmidt enters with shortness of breath, and you ponder writing "emphysema." Even if he is known to have emphysema from previous visits, it is not the chronic emphysema that prompted *this visit,* but rather the "increasing shortness of breath" for 4 hours.

Some people try to self-diagnose based on similar signs and symptoms in their relatives or friends, or based on conditions they know they have. Rather than record a woman's statement that she has "strep throat," ask her what symptoms she has that make her think this is true and record those symptoms.

Occasionally a person may list *many* reasons for seeking care. The most important reason to the person may not necessarily be the one stated first. Try to focus on which is the most pressing concern by asking the person which one prompted him or her to seek help *now.*

PRESENT HEALTH OR HISTORY OF PRESENT ILLNESS

For the well person, this is a short statement about the general state of health.

For the ill person, this section is a chronologic record of the reason for seeking care, from the time the symptom first started until now. Isolate each reason for care identified by the person and say, for example, "Please tell me all about your headache, from the time it started until the time you came to the hospital." If the concern started months or years ago, record what occurred during that time and find out why the person is seeking care *now.*

As the person talks, do not jump to conclusions and bias the story by adding your opinion. Collect *all* the data first. Although you want the person to respond in a narrative format without interruption from you, your final summary of any symptom the person has should include these *eight critical characteristics:*

1. **Location.** Be specific; ask the person to point to the location. If the problem is pain, note the precise site. "Head pain" is vague, whereas descriptions such as "pain behind the eyes," "jaw pain," and "occipital pain" are more precise and are diagnostically significant. Is the pain localized to this site or radiating? Is the pain superficial or deep?
2. **Character** or **Quality.** This calls for specific descriptive terms such as burning, sharp, dull, aching, gnawing, throbbing, shooting, viselike. Use similes—does blood in the stool look like sticky tar? Does blood in vomitus look like coffee grounds?
3. **Quantity** or **Severity.** Attempt to quantify the sign or symptom such as "profuse menstrual flow soaking five pads per hour." The symptom of pain is difficult to quantify because of individual interpretation. What one person may identify as "terrible pain," another may describe as "not too bad." With pain, avoid adjectives and ask how it affects daily activities. Then the person might say, "I was so sick I was doubled up and couldn't move," or "I was able to go to work, but then I came home and went to bed."
4. **Timing** (Onset, Duration, Frequency). When did the symptom first appear? Give the specific date and time, or state specifically how long ago the symptom started prior to arrival (PTA). "The pain started yesterday" will not mean much when you return to read the record in the future. The report must include questions such as: How long did the symptom last (duration)? Was it steady (constant) or did it come and go during that time (intermittent)? Did it resolve completely and reappear days or weeks later (cycle of remission and exacerbation)?

5. **Setting.** Where was the person or what was the person doing when the symptom started? What brings it on? For example, "Did you notice the chest pain after shoveling snow, or did the pain start by itself?"

6. **Aggravating** or **Relieving Factors.** What makes the pain worse? Is it aggravated by weather, activity, food, medication, standing bent over, fatigue, time of day, season, and so on? What relieves it (e.g., rest, medication, or ice pack)? What is the effect of any treatment? Ask, "What have you tried?" or "What seems to help?"

7. **Associated Factors.** Is this primary symptom associated with any others (e.g., urinary frequency and burning associated with fever and chills)? Review the body system related to this symptom now rather than wait for the review of systems.

8. **Patient's Perception.** Find out the meaning of the symptom by asking how it affects daily activities. Also ask directly, "What do you think it means?" This is crucial because it alerts you to potential anxiety if the person thinks the symptom may be ominous.

You may find it helpful to organize this same question sequence into the mnemonic PQRSTU to help remember all the points. Note that you still need to address the patient's perception of the problem.

P: **Provocative** or **Palliative.** What brings it on? What were you doing when you first noticed it? What makes it better? Worse?

Q: **Quality** or **Quantity.** How does it look, feel, sound? How intense/severe is it?

R: **Region** or **Radiation.** Where is it? Does it spread anywhere?

S: **Severity Scale.** How bad is it (on a scale of 1 to 10)? Is it getting better, worse, staying the same?

T: **Timing.** Onset—Exactly when did it first occur? Duration—How long did it last? Frequency—How often does it occur?

U: **Understand Patient's Perception** of the problem. What do you think it means?

PAST HEALTH

Past health events may have residual effects on the current health state. Also, the previous experience with illness may give clues as to how the person responds to illness and to the significance of illness for him or her.

CHILDHOOD ILLNESSES. Measles, mumps, rubella, chicken pox, pertussis, and strep throat. Avoid recording "usual childhood illnesses," because an illness common in the person's childhood (e.g., measles) may be unusual today. Ask about serious illnesses that may have sequelae for the person in later years (e.g., rheumatic fever, scarlet fever, and poliomyelitis).

ACCIDENTS OR INJURIES. Auto accidents, fractures, penetrating wounds, head injuries (especially if associated with unconsciousness), and burns.

SERIOUS OR CHRONIC ILLNESSES. Diabetes, hypertension, heart disease, sickle-cell anemia, cancer, and seizure disorder.

HOSPITALIZATIONS. Cause, name of hospital, how the condition was treated, how long the person was hospitalized, and name of the physician.

OPERATIONS. Type of surgery, date, name of the surgeon, name of hospital, and how the person recovered.

OBSTETRIC HISTORY. Number of pregnancies (gravidity), number of deliveries in which the fetus reached full term (term), number of preterm pregnancies (preterm), number of incomplete pregnancies (abortions), and number of children living (living). This is recorded: Grav _____ Term _____ Preterm _____ Ab _____ Living _____. For each complete pregnancy, note the course of pregnancy; labor and delivery; sex, weight, and condition of each infant; and postpartum course. For any incomplete pregnancies, record the duration and whether the pregnancy resulted in spontaneous (S) or induced (I) abortion.

IMMUNIZATIONS. Measles-mumps-rubella, polio, diphtheria-pertussis-tetanus, hepatitis B, *Haemophilus influenzae* type b, pneumococcal vaccine. Note the date of the last tetanus immunization, last tuberculosis skin test, and last flu shot.

LAST EXAMINATION DATE. Physical, dental, vision, hearing, electrocardiogram, chest x-ray examinations.

ALLERGIES. Note both the allergen (medication, food, or contact agent, such as fabric or environmental agent) and the reaction (rash, itching, runny nose, watery eyes, difficulty breathing). With a drug, this symptom should not be a side effect but a true allergic reaction.

CURRENT MEDICATIONS. Note all prescription and over-the-counter medications. Ask specifically about vitamins, birth control pills, aspirin, and antacids, because many people do not consider these to be medications. For each medication, note the name, dose, and schedule, and ask "How often do you take it each day?" "What is it for?" and "How long have you been taking it?"

FAMILY HISTORY

Ask about the age and health or the age and cause of death of blood relatives, such as parents, grandparents, and siblings. These data may have genetic significance for the patient. Also ask about close family members, such as spouse and children. You need to know about the person's prolonged contact with any communicable disease or the effect of a family member's illness on this person.

Specifically ask for any family history of heart disease, high blood pressure, stroke, diabetes, blood disorders, cancer, sickle-cell anemia, arthritis, allergies, obesity, alcoholism, mental illness, seizure disorder, kidney disease, and tuberculosis. Construct a family tree, or genogram, to show this information clearly and concisely (Fig. 6–1).

REVIEW OF SYSTEMS

The purposes of this section are (1) to evaluate the past and present health state of each body system, (2) to double-check in case any significant data were omitted in the present illness section, and (3) to evaluate health promotion practices. The order of the examination of body systems is roughly head-to-toe. The items within each system are not inclu-

FAMILY TREE, or GENOGRAM

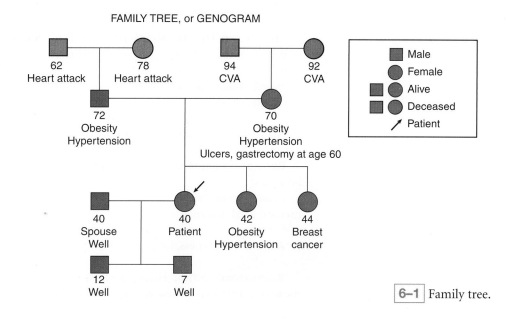

6–1 Family tree.

sive, and only the most common symptoms are listed. If the present illness section covered one body system, you do not need to repeat all the data here. For example, if the reason for seeking care is earache, the present illness section describes most of the symptoms listed for the auditory system. Just ask now what was not asked in the present illness section. Medical terms are listed here, but they need to be translated for the patient. (Note that symptoms and health promotion activities are only listed here. These terms are repeated and expanded in each related physical examination chapter, along with suggested ways to pose questions and a rationale for each question.)

When recording information, avoid writing "negative" after the system heading. You need to record the *presence* or *absence* of all symptoms, otherwise the reader does not know about which factors you asked.

A common mistake made by beginning practitioners is to record some physical finding or objective data here, such as "skin warm and dry." Remember that the history should be limited to patient statements, or subjective data—factors that the person *says* were or were not present.

GENERAL OVERALL HEALTH STATE. Present weight (gain or loss, period of time, by diet or other factors), fatigue, weakness or malaise, fever, chills, sweats or night sweats.

SKIN. History of skin disease (eczema, psoriasis, hives), pigment or color change, change in mole, excessive dryness or moisture, pruritus, excessive bruising, rash or lesion.

HAIR. Recent loss, change in texture. Nails: change in shape, color, or brittleness.
Health Promotion. Amount of sun exposure; method of self-care for skin and hair.

HEAD. Any unusually frequent or severe headache, any head injury, dizziness (syncope) or vertigo.

EYES. Difficulty with vision (decreased acuity, blurring, blind spots), eye pain, diplopia (double vision), redness or swelling, watering or discharge, glaucoma or cataracts.
Health Promotion. Wears glasses or contacts; last vision check or glaucoma test; and how coping with loss of vision if any.

EARS. Earaches, infections, discharge and its characteristics, tinnitus or vertigo.
Health Promotion. Hearing loss, hearing aid use, how loss affects the daily life, any exposure to environmental noise, and method of cleaning ears.

NOSE AND SINUSES. Discharge and its characteristics, any unusually frequent or severe colds, sinus pain, nasal obstruction, nosebleeds, allergies or hay fever, or change in sense of smell.

MOUTH AND THROAT. Mouth pain, frequent sore throat, bleeding gums, toothache, lesion in mouth or tongue, dysphagia, hoarseness or voice change, tonsillectomy, altered taste.
Health Promotion. Pattern of daily dental care, use of prostheses (dentures, bridge), and last dental checkup.

NECK. Pain, limitation of motion, lumps or swelling, enlarged or tender nodes, goiter.

BREAST. Pain, lump, nipple discharge, rash, history of breast disease, any surgery on the breasts.
Health Promotion. Performs breast self-examination, including its frequency and method used, last mammogram.

AXILLA. Tenderness, lump or swelling, rash.

RESPIRATORY SYSTEM. History of lung diseases (asthma, emphysema, bronchitis, pneumonia, tuberculosis), chest pain with breathing, wheezing or noisy breathing, shortness of breath, how much activity produces shortness of breath, cough, sputum (color, amount), hemoptysis, toxin or pollution exposure.

Health Promotion. Last chest x-ray study.

CARDIOVASCULAR. Precordial or retrosternal pain, palpitation, cyanosis, dyspnea on exertion (specify amount of exertion, e.g., walking one flight of stairs, walking from chair to bath, or just talking), orthopnea, paroxysmal nocturnal dyspnea, nocturia, edema, history of heart murmur, hypertension, coronary artery disease, anemia.

Health Promotion. Date of last ECG or other heart tests.

PERIPHERAL VASCULAR. Coldness, numbness and tingling, swelling of legs (time of day, activity), discoloration in hands or feet (bluish red, pallor, mottling, associated with position, especially around feet and ankles), varicose veins or complications, intermittent claudication, thrombophlebitis, ulcers.

Health Promotion. Does the work involve long-term sitting or standing? Avoid crossing legs at the knees. Wear support hose.

GASTROINTESTINAL. Appetite, food intolerance, dysphagia, heartburn, indigestion, pain (associated with eating), other abdominal pain, pyrosis (esophageal and stomach burning sensation with sour eructation), nausea and vomiting (character), vomiting blood, history of abdominal disease (ulcer, liver or gallbladder, jaundice, appendicitis, colitis), flatulence, frequency of bowel movement, any recent change, stool characteristics, constipation or diarrhea, black stools, rectal bleeding, rectal conditions (hemorrhoids, fistula).

Health Promotion. Use of antacids or laxatives. (Alternatively, diet history and substance habits can be placed here.)

URINARY SYSTEM. Frequency, urgency, nocturia (the number of times the person awakens at night to urinate, recent change), dysuria, polyuria or oliguria, hesitancy or straining, narrowed stream, urine color (cloudy or presence of hematuria), incontinence, history of urinary disease (kidney disease, kidney stones, urinary tract infections, prostate), pain in flank, groin, suprapubic region, or low back.

Health Promotion. Measures to avoid or treat urinary tract infections, use of Kegel exercises after childbirth.

MALE GENITAL SYSTEM. Penis or testicular pain, sores or lesions, penile discharge, lumps, hernia.

Health Promotion. Perform testicular self-examination? How frequently?

FEMALE GENITAL SYSTEM. Menstrual history (age at menarche, last menstrual period, cycle and duration, any amenorrhea or menorrhagia, premenstrual pain or dysmenorrhea, intermenstrual spotting), vaginal itching, discharge and its characteristics, age at menopause, menopausal signs or symptoms, postmenopausal bleeding.

Health Promotion. Last gynecologic checkup and last Papanicolaou test.

SEXUAL HEALTH. Presently in a relationship involving intercourse? Are the aspects of sex satisfactory to the patient and partner? Any dyspareunia (for female), any changes in erection or ejaculation (for male), and use of contraceptive? Is the contraceptive method satisfactory? Aware of contact with a partner who has any sexually transmitted disease (gonorrhea, herpes, chlamydia, venereal warts, HIV/AIDS, or syphilis)?

MUSCULOSKELETAL SYSTEM. History of arthritis or gout. In the joints: pain, stiffness, swelling (location, migratory nature), deformity, limitation of motion, noise with joint motion? In the muscles: any pain, cramps, weakness, gait problems or problems with coordinated activities? In the back: any pain (location and radiation to extremities), stiffness, limitation of motion, or history of back pain or disk disease?

Health Promotion. How much walking per day? What is the effect of limited range of motion on daily activities, such as on grooming, feeding, toileting, dressing? Are any mobility aids used?

NEUROLOGIC SYSTEM. History of seizure disorder, stroke, fainting, blackouts. In motor function: weakness, tic or tremor, paralysis, or coordination problems. In sensory function: numbness and tingling (paresthesia). In cognitive function: memory disorder (recent or distant, disorientation). In mental status: any nervousness, mood change, depression, or any history of mental health dysfunction or hallucinations.

Health Promotion. Alternatively, data about interpersonal relationships, coping patterns placed here.

HEMATOLOGIC SYSTEM. Bleeding tendency of skin or mucous membranes, excessive bruising, lymph node swelling, exposure to toxic agents or radiation, blood transfusion and reactions.

ENDOCRINE SYSTEM. History of diabetes or diabetic symptoms (polyuria, polydipsia, polyphagia), history of thyroid disease, intolerance to heat and cold, change in skin pigmentation or texture, excessive sweating, relationship between appetite and weight, abnormal hair distribution, nervousness, tremors, and need for hormone therapy.

FUNCTIONAL ASSESSMENT (INCLUDING ACTIVITIES OF DAILY LIVING)

Functional assessment measures a person's self-care ability in the areas of general physical health or absence of illness; ADLs, such as bathing, dressing, toileting, eating, walking; instrumental activities of daily living (IADLs), or those needed for independent living, such as housekeeping, shopping, cooking, doing laundry, using the telephone, managing finances; nutrition; social relationships and resources; self-concept and coping; and home environment.

Functional assessment may mean organizing the entire assessment around functional "pattern areas" (Gordon, 2000). Instruments that emphasize functional categories may help in leading to a nursing diagnosis.

Functional assessment may also mean that the health history may be supplemented by a standardized instrument on functional assessment. These instruments objectively measure a person's present functional status and monitor any changes over time (Granger et al., 1979; Katz et al., 1963; Linn and Linn, 1982; Mahoney and Barthel, 1965; Pearlman, 1987).

Whether or not you use any of these formalized instruments, functional assessment questions such as those listed in the following section should be included in the standard health history. These questions provide data on the lifestyle and type of living environment to which the person is accustomed. Since some of the data may be judged private by the individual, the questions are best asked at this later point in the interview after you have had time to establish rapport.

SELF-ESTEEM, SELF-CONCEPT. Education (last grade completed, other significant training), financial status (income adequate for lifestyle and/or health concerns), value-belief system (religious practices and perception of personal strengths).

ACTIVITY/EXERCISE. A daily profile reflecting usual daily activities: ask "Tell me how you spend a typical day." Note ability to perform ADLs: independent or needs assistance with feeding, bathing, hygiene, dressing, toileting, bed to chair transfer, walking, standing, or climbing stairs. Any use of wheelchair, prostheses, or mobility aids?

Record leisure activities enjoyed and exercise pattern (type, amount per day or week, method of warm-up session, method of monitoring the body's response to exercise).

SLEEP/REST. Sleep patterns, daytime naps, any sleep aids used.

NUTRITION/ELIMINATION. Record the diet by a recall of all food and beverages taken over the last 24 hours (see Chapter 8 for suggested method of inquiry). "Is that menu typical of most days?" Describe eating habits and current appetite. Ask "Who buys food and prepares food?" "Are your finances adequate for food?" "Who is present at mealtimes?" Indicate any food allergy or intolerance. Record daily intake of caffeine (coffee, tea, cola drinks).

Ask about usual pattern of bowel elimination and urinating including problems with mobility or transfer in toileting, continence, use of laxatives.

INTERPERSONAL RELATIONSHIPS/RESOURCES. Social roles: "How would you describe your role in the family?" "How would you say you get along with family, friends, and co-workers?" Ask about support systems composed of family and significant others: "To whom could you go for support with a problem at work, with your health, or a personal problem?" Include contact with spouse, siblings, parents, children, friends, organizations, workplace: "Is time spent alone pleasurable and relaxing, or isolating?"

SPIRITUAL RESOURCES. Many people believe in a relationship between spirituality and health, and they may wish to have spiritual matters addressed in the traditional health care setting. Use the faith, influence, community, and address (FICA) questions to incorporate the person's spiritual values into the health history (Post et al., 2000). *Faith:* "Does religious faith or spirituality play an important part in your life? Do you consider yourself to be a religious or spiritual person?" *Influence:* "How does your religious faith or spirituality influence the way you think about your health or the way you care for yourself?" *Community:* "Are you a part of any religious or spiritual community or congregation?" *Address:* "Would you like me to address any religious or spiritual issues or concerns with you?"

COPING AND STRESS MANAGEMENT. Kinds of stresses in life, especially in the last year, any change in lifestyle or any current stress, methods tried to relieve stress, and if these have been helpful.

PERSONAL HABITS. Tobacco, alcohol, street drugs: "Do you smoke cigarettes (pipe, use chewing tobacco)?" "At what age did you start?" "How many packs do you smoke per day?" "How many years have you smoked?" Record the number of packs smoked per day (PPD) and duration, e.g., 1 PPD × 5 years. Then ask, "Have you ever tried to quit?" and "How did it go?" to introduce plans about smoking cessation.

ALCOHOL. Health care professionals often fail to question about alcohol unless problems are obvious. However, alcohol interacts adversely with all medications; is a factor in many social problems such as assaults, rapes, high-risk sexual behavior, and child abuse; contributes to half of all fatal traffic accidents; and accounts for 5% of all deaths in the United States. The latter figure is actually an underestimate because alcohol-related conditions are underreported on death certificates (U.S. Department of Health and Human Services, 1997).

Be alert, then, to early signs of hazardous alcohol use. Ask whether the person drinks alcohol. If yes, ask specific questions about the amount and frequency of alcohol use: "When was your last drink of alcohol?" "How much did you drink that time?" "Out of the last 30 days, about how many days would you say that you drank alcohol?" "Have you ever had a drinking problem?"

You may wish to use a screening questionnaire to identify excessive or uncontrolled drinking, such as the Alcohol Use Disorder Identification Test (AUDIT) (Volk et al., 1997), or the Cut down, Annoyed, Guilty, and Eye-opener (**CAGE**) test (Ewing, 1984):

- Have you ever thought you should Cut down your drinking?
- Have you ever been Annoyed by criticism of your drinking?
- Have you ever felt Guilty about your drinking?
- Do you drink in the morning? (i.e., an Eye opener?)

If the person answers "yes" to two or more CAGE questions, you should suspect alcohol abuse and continue with a more complete substance abuse assessment. If the person answers "no" to drinking alcohol, ask the reason for this decision (psychosocial, legal, health). Any history of alcohol treatment? Involvement in recovery activities? History of family member with problem drinking?

STREET DRUGS. Ask specifically about marijuana, cocaine, crack cocaine, amphetamines, and barbiturates. Indicate frequency of use and how has usage affected work or family.

ENVIRONMENT/HAZARDS. Housing and neighborhood (living alone, knowledge of neighbors), safety of area, adequate heat and utilities, access to transportation, and involvement in community services. Note environmental health, including hazards in workplace, hazards at home, use of seat belts, geographic or occupational exposures, and travel or residence in other countries, including time spent abroad during military service.

INTIMATE PARTNER VIOLENCE. Begin with open-ended questions: "How are things at home?" and "Do you feel safe?" These are valuable initial screening questions, because some people may not recognize that they are in abusive situations or may be reluctant to admit it due to guilt, fear, shame, or denial (Asher et al., 2001). If the person responds to feeling unsafe, follow up with closed-ended questions: "Have you ever been emotionally or physically abused by your partner or someone important to you?" "Within the last year, have you been hit, slapped, kicked, pushed or shoved, or otherwise physically hurt by your partner or ex-partner?" "If yes, by whom?" "Number of times?" "Does your partner ever force you into having sex?" "Are you afraid of your partner or expartner?"

OCCUPATIONAL HEALTH. Ask the person to describe his or her job. Ever worked with any health hazard, such as asbestos, inhalants, chemicals, repetitive motion? Wear any protective equipment? Any work programs in place that monitor exposure? Aware of any health problems now that may be related to work exposure?

Note the timing of the reason for seeking care, and whether it may be related to work or home activities, job titles, or exposure history. Take a careful smoking history, which may contribute to occupational hazards. Finally, ask the person what he or she likes or dislikes about the job.

PERCEPTION OF HEALTH

Ask the person questions such as: "How do you define health?" "How do you view your situation now?" "What are your concerns?" "What do you think will happen in the future?" "What are your health goals?" "What do you expect from us as nurses, physicians, (or other health care providers)?"

 DEVELOPMENTAL CONSIDERATIONS

CHILDREN AND ADOLESCENTS

The health history is adapted to include information specific for the age and developmental stage of the child (e.g., the mother's health during pregnancy, labor and delivery, and the perinatal period). Note that the developmental history and nutritional data are listed as separate sections because of their importance for current health.

Biographic Data
Include the child's name, nickname, address and phone number, parents' names and work numbers, child's age and birthdate, birthplace, sex, race, ethnic origin, and information on other children and family members at home.

Source of History
1. Person providing information and relation to child
2. Your impression of reliability of information
3. Any special circumstances, e.g., the use of an interpreter

Reason for Seeking Care
Record the parent's spontaneous statement. Because of the frequency of well child visits for routine health care, there will be more reasons such as "time for the child's checkup" or "she needs the next baby shot." Reasons for health problems may be initiated by the child, parent, or by a third party such as the classroom teacher.

Sometimes the reason stated may not be the real reason for the visit. A parent may have a "hidden agenda," such as the mother who brought her 4-year-old child in because "she looked pale." Further questioning revealed that the mother had heard recently from a former college friend whose own 4-year-old child had just been diagnosed with leukemia.

Present Health or History of Present Illness

If the parent or child seeks routine health care, include a statement about the usual health of the child and any common health problems or major health concerns.

Describe any presenting symptom or sign, using the same format as for the adult. Some additional considerations include:

- Severity of pain: "How do you know the child is in pain" (e.g., pulling at ears alerts parent to ear pain)? Note effect of pain on usual behavior (e.g., does it stop child from playing?).
- Associated factors, such as relation to activity, eating, and body position.
- The parent's intuitive sense of a problem. As the constant caregiver, this intuitive sense is often very accurate. Even if proved otherwise, this factor gives you an idea of parent's area of concern.
- Parent's coping ability and reaction of other family members to child's symptoms or illness.

Past Health

PRENATAL STATUS. How was this pregnancy spaced? Was it planned? What was the mother's attitude toward the pregnancy? What was the father's attitude? Was there medical supervision for the mother? At what month was the supervision started? What was the mother's health during pregnancy? Were there any complications (bleeding, excessive nausea and vomiting, unusual weight gain, high blood pressure, swelling of hands and feet, infections—rubella or sexually transmitted diseases, falls)? During what month were diet and medications prescribed and/or taken during pregnancy (dose and duration)? Record the mother's use of alcohol, street drugs, or cigarettes and any x-ray studies taken during pregnancy.

Start with an open-ended question: "Tell me about your pregnancy." If she questions the relevancy of the statement, mention that these questions are important to gain a complete picture of the child's health.

LABOR AND DELIVERY. Parity of the mother, duration of the pregnancy, name of the hospital, course and duration of labor, use of anesthesia, type of delivery (vertex, breech, cesarean section), birth weight, Apgar scores, onset of breathing, any cyanosis, need for resuscitation, and use of special equipment or procedures.

POSTNATAL STATUS. Any problems in the nursery, length of hospital stay, neonatal jaundice, whether the baby was discharged with the mother, whether the baby was breast or bottle fed, weight gain, any feeding problems, "blue spells," colic, diarrhea, patterns of crying and sleeping, the mother's health postpartum, and the mother's reaction to the baby.

CHILDHOOD ILLNESSES. Age and any complications of measles, mumps, rubella, chickenpox, whooping cough, strep throat, and frequent ear infections. Also, any recent exposure to illness.

SERIOUS ACCIDENTS OR INJURIES. Age of occurrence, extent of injury, how the child was treated, and complications of auto accidents, falls, head injuries, fractures, burns, and poisonings.

SERIOUS OR CHRONIC ILLNESSES. Age of onset, how the child was treated, and complications of meningitis or encephalitis; seizure disorders; asthma, pneumonia, and other chronic lung conditions; rheumatic fever; scarlet fever; diabetes; kidney problems; sickle-cell anemia; high blood pressure; and allergies.

OPERATIONS OR HOSPITALIZATIONS. Reason for care, age at admission, name of surgeon or primary care providers, name of hospital, duration of stay, how child reacted to hospitalization, and any complications. (If child reacted poorly, he or she may be afraid now and will need special preparation for the examination that is to follow.)

IMMUNIZATIONS. Age when administered, date administered, and any reactions following immunizations. Appendix A lists suggested immunization schedules. Because of recent outbreaks of measles across the United States, the American Academy of Pediatrics now is recommending two doses of the measles-mumps-rubella vaccine, one at 12 to 15 months and one at age 4 to 6 years (American Academy of Pediatrics, 2002).

ALLERGIES. Any drugs, foods, contact agents, and environmental agents to which the child is allergic, and reaction to allergen. Note allergic reactions particularly common in childhood, such as allergic rhinitis, insect hypersensitivity, eczema, and urticaria.

MEDICATIONS. Any prescription and over-the-counter medications (or vitamins) the child takes, including the dose, daily schedule, why the medication is given, and any problems.

Developmental History
GROWTH. Height and weight at birth and at 1, 2, 5, and 10 years, any periods of rapid gain or loss, and process of dentition (age of tooth eruption and pattern of loss).

MILESTONES. Age when child first held head erect, rolled over, sat alone, walked alone, cut his or her first tooth, said his or her first words with meaning, spoke in sentences, was toilet trained, tied shoes, dressed without help. Does the parent believe this development has been normal? How does this child's development compare with siblings or peers?

CURRENT DEVELOPMENT (CHILDREN 1 MONTH THROUGH PRESCHOOL). Gross motor skills (rolls over, sits alone, walks alone, skips, climbs), fine motor skills (inspects hands, brings hands to mouth, pincer grasp, stacks blocks, feeds self, uses crayon to draw, uses scissors), language skills (vocalizes, first words with meaning, sentences, persistence of baby talk, speech problems), and personal-social skills (smiles, tracks movement with eyes to midline, past midline, attends to sound by turning head, recognizes own name). If the child is undergoing toilet training, indicate the method used, age of bladder/bowel control, parents' attitude toward toilet training, and terms used for toileting.

SCHOOL-AGE CHILD. Gross motor skills (runs, jumps, climbs, rides bicycle, general coordination), fine motor skills (ties shoelace, uses scissors, writes name and numbers, draws pictures), and language skills (vocabulary, verbal ability, able to tell time, reading level).

Nutritional History
The amount of nutritional information needed depends on the child's age; the younger the child is, the more detailed and specific the data should be. For the infant, record whether breastfeeding or bottle-feeding is used. If the child is breastfed, record nursing frequency and duration, any supplements (vitamin, iron, fluoride, bottles), family support for nursing, and age and method of weaning. If the child is bottle-fed, record type of formula used, frequency and amount, any problems with feeding (spitting up, colic, diarrhea), supplements used, and any bottle propping. Record introduction of solid foods (age when the child began eating solids, which foods, whether foods are home or commercially made, amount given, child's reaction to new food, parent's reaction to feeding).

For preschool- and school-age children and adolescents, record the child's appetite, 24-hour diet recall (meals, snacks, amounts), vitamins taken, how much junk food is eaten, who eats with the child, food likes and dislikes, and parent's perception of child's nutrition.

A week-long diary of food intake may be more accurate than a spot 24-hour recall. Also, consider cultural practices in assessing child's diet (see Transcultural Considerations).

Family History
As with the adult, diagram a family tree for the child, including siblings, parents, and grandparents. Give the age, health, or age and cause of death of each. Ask specifically for the family history of heart disease, high blood pressure, diabetes, blood disorders, cancer, sickle-cell anemia, arthritis, allergies, obesity, cystic fibrosis, alcoholism, mental illness,

seizure disorder, kidney disease, mental retardation, learning disabilities, birth defects, and sudden infant death. (When interviewing the mother, ask about the "child's father," not "your husband," in case of the separation of the child's biologic parents.)

Review of Systems

GENERAL. Significant gain or loss of weight, failure to gain weight appropriate for age, frequent colds, ear infections, illnesses, energy level, fatigue, overactivity, and behavior change (irritability, increased crying, nervousness).

SKIN. Birthmarks, skin disease, pigment or color change, mottling, change in mole, pruritus, rash, lesion, acne, easy bruising or petechiae, easy bleeding, and changes in hair or nails.

HEAD. Headache, head injury, dizziness.

EYES. Strabismus, diplopia, pain, redness, discharge, cataracts, vision changes, reading problems. Is the child able to see the board at school? Does the child sit too close to the television?
Health Promotion. Use of eyeglasses, date of last vision screening.

EARS. Earaches, frequency of ear infections, myringotomy tubes in ears, discharge (characteristics), cerumen, ringing or crackling, and whether parent perceives any hearing problems.
Health Promotion. How does the child clean his or her ears?

NOSE AND SINUSES. Discharge and its characteristics, frequency of colds, nasal stuffiness, nosebleeds, and allergies.

MOUTH AND THROAT. History of cleft lip or palate, frequency of sore throats, toothache, caries, sores in mouth or tongue, tonsils present, mouth breathing, difficulty chewing, difficulty swallowing, and hoarseness or voice change.
Health Promotion. Child's pattern of brushing teeth and last dental checkup.

NECK. Swollen or tender glands, limitation of movement, or stiffness.

BREAST. For preadolescent and adolescent girls, when did they notice that their breasts were changing? What is the girl's self-perception of development? For older adolescents, does the girl perform breast self-examination? (See Chapter 17 for suggested phrasing of questions.)

RESPIRATORY SYSTEM. Croup or asthma, wheezing or noisy breathing, shortness of breath, chronic cough.

CARDIOVASCULAR SYSTEM. Congenital heart problems, history of murmur, and cyanosis (what prompts this condition). Is there any limitation of activity, or can the child keep up with peers? Is there any dyspnea on exertion, palpitations, high blood pressure, or coldness in the extremities?

GASTROINTESTINAL SYSTEM. Abdominal pain, nausea and vomiting, history of ulcer, frequency of bowel movements, stool color and characteristics, diarrhea, constipation or stool-holding, rectal bleeding, anal itching, history of pinworms, and use of laxatives.

URINARY SYSTEM. Painful urination, polyuria/oliguria, narrowed stream, urine color (cloudy, dark), history of urinary tract infection, whether toilet trained, when toilet training was planned, any problems, bedwetting (when the child started, frequency, associated with stress, how child feels about it).

MALE GENITAL SYSTEM. Penis or testicular pain, whether told if testes are descended, any sores or lesions, discharge, hernia or hydrocele, or swelling in scrotum during crying. For the preadolescent and adolescent boy, has he noticed any change in the penis and scrotum?

Is the boy familiar with normal growth patterns, nocturnal emissions, and sex education? Screen for sexual abuse. (See Chapter 24 for suggested phrasing of questions.)

FEMALE GENITAL SYSTEM. Has the girl noted any genital itching, rash, vaginal discharge? For the preadolescent and adolescent girl, when did menstruation start? Was she prepared? Screen for sexual abuse. (See Chapter 26 for suggested phrasing of questions.)

SEXUAL HEALTH. What is the child's attitude toward the opposite sex? Who provides sex education? How does the family deal with sex education, masturbation, dating patterns? Is the adolescent in a relationship involving intercourse? Does he or she have information on birth control and sexually transmitted diseases? (See Chapters 24 and 26 for suggested phrasing of questions.)

MUSCULOSKELETAL SYSTEM. In bones and joints: arthritis, joint pain, stiffness, swelling, limitation of movement, gait strength and coordination. In muscles: pain, cramps, and weakness. In the back: pain, posture, spinal curvature, and any treatment.

NEUROLOGIC SYSTEM. Numbness and tingling. (Behavior and cognitive issues are covered in the sections on development and interpersonal relationships.)

HEMATOLOGIC SYSTEMS. Excessive bruising, lymph node swelling, and exposure to toxic agents or radiation.

ENDOCRINE SYSTEM. History of diabetes or thyroid disease; excessive hunger, thirst, or urinating; abnormal hair distribution; and precocious or delayed puberty.

Functional Assessment (Including Activities of Daily Living)

INTERPERSONAL RELATIONSHIPS. Within the family constellation, record the child's position in family; whether the child is adopted; who lives with the child; who is the primary caretaker; who is the caretaker if both parents work outside of the home; any support from relatives, neighbors, or friends; and the ethnic or cultural milieu.

Indicate family cohesion. Does the family enjoy activities as a unit? Has there been a recent family change or crisis (death, divorce, move)? Record information on child's self-image and level of independence. Does the child use a security blanket or toy? Is there any repetitive behavior (bed-rocking, head-banging), pica, thumb-sucking, or nail-biting? Note method of discipline used. Indicate type used at home. How effective is it? Who disciplines the child? Is there any occurrence of negativism, temper tantrums, withdrawal, or aggressive behavior?

Provide information on the child's friends: whether the child makes friends easily. How does the child get along with friends? Does he or she play with same-age or older or younger children?

ACTIVITY AND REST. Record the child's play activities. Indicate amount of active and quiet play, outdoor play, time watching television, and special hobbies or activities. Record sleep and rest. Indicate pattern and number of hours at night and during the day and the child's routine at bedtime. Is the child a sound sleeper, or is he or she wakeful? Does the child have nightmares, night terrors, or somnambulation? How does the parent respond? Does the child have naps during the day?

Record school attendance. Has the child had any experience with day care or nursery school? In what grade is the child in school? Has the child ever skipped a grade or been held back? Does the child seem to like school? What is his or her school performance? Are the parent and child satisfied with the performance? Were days missed in school? Provide a reason for the absence. (These questions give an important index to child's functioning outside the home.)

ECONOMIC STATUS. Ask about the mother's occupation and father's occupation. Indicate the number of hours each parent is away from home. Do parents perceive their income as adequate? What is the effect of illness on financial status?

HOME ENVIRONMENT. Where does family live (house, apartment)? Is the size of the home adequate? Is there access to an outdoor play area? Does the child share a room, have his or her own bed, and have toys appropriate for his or her age?

ENVIRONMENTAL HAZARDS. Inquire about home safety (precautions for poisons, medications, household products, presence of gates for stairways, and safe yard equipment). Provide information on the child's residence (adequate heating, ventilation, bathroom facilities), neighborhood (residential or industrial, age of neighbors, safe play areas, playmates available, distance to school, amount of traffic, is area remote or congested and overcrowded, is crime a problem, presence of air or water pollution), and automobile (child safety seat, seat belts).

COPING/STRESS MANAGEMENT. Does the child have the ability to adapt to new situations? Record recent stressful experiences (death, divorce, move, loss of special friend). How does the child cope with stress? Has there been any recent change in behavior or mood? Has counseling ever been sought?

HABITS. Has the child ever tried cigarette smoking? How much did he or she smoke? Has the child ever tried alcohol? How much alcohol did he or she drink weekly or daily? Has the child ever tried other drugs (marijuana, cocaine, amphetamines, barbiturates)?

HEALTH PROMOTION. Who is the primary health care provider? When was the child's last checkup? Who is the dental care provider, and when was the last dental checkup? Provide date and result of screening for vision, hearing, urinalysis, phenylketonuria, hematocrit, tuberculosis skin test, sickle-cell trait, blood lead, and other tests specific for high-risk populations.

THE OLDER ADULT

This health history includes the same format as that described for the younger adult, as well as some additional questions. These questions address ways in which the ADLs may have been affected by normal aging processes or by the effects of chronic illness or disability. There is no specific age at which to ask these additional questions. Use them when it seems appropriate.

It is important for you to recognize positive health measures: what the person has been doing to help himself or herself stay well and to live to an older age. Older people have spent a lifetime with a traditional health care system that searches only for pathology and what is wrong with their health. It may be a pleasant surprise to have a health professional affirm the things that they are "doing right" and to note health strengths.

As you study the following, keep in mind the format for the "younger" adult. Only *additional* questions or a varying focus are addressed here.

Reason for Seeking Care

It may take time to figure out the reason that the older person has come in for an examination. An aging person may shrug off a symptom as evidence of growing old and may be unsure whether it is "worth mentioning." Also, some older people have a conservative philosophy toward their health status: "If it isn't broken, don't fix it." These people come for care only when something is blatantly wrong.

Another older person may have many chronic problems, such as diabetes, hypertension, or constipation. It is challenging to filter out what brought the person in this time. The final statement should be the *person's* reason for seeking care, not your assumption of what the problem is.

Past Health

GENERAL HEALTH. Health state in the last 5 years.

ACCIDENTS OR INJURIES, SERIOUS OR CHRONIC ILLNESSES, HOSPITALIZATIONS, OPERATIONS. These areas may produce lengthy responses, and the person probably will not relate them in chronologic order. Let the person talk freely; you can reorder the events later when you do the write-up. The amount of data included here can indicate the amount of stress the person has faced during his or her lifetime. This section of the history can be filled out at home or before the interview if the person's vision and writing ability are adequate. Then you can concentrate remaining time of the interview on reviewing pertinent data and on the present health of the person.

LAST EXAMINATION. Most recent mammography, proctoscopy, and tonometry.

OBSTETRIC STATUS. It is *not* necessary to collect a detailed account of each pregnancy and delivery if the woman has passed menopause and has no gynecologic symptoms. Merely record the number of pregnancies and the health of each newborn.

CURRENT MEDICATIONS. For each medication, record the name, purpose, and daily schedule. Does the person have a system to remember to take the medicine? Does medicine seem to work? Are there any side effects? If so, does the person feel like skipping medicine because of them? Also consider the following issues:

- Some older persons take a large number of drugs, prescribed by different physicians.
- The person may not know drug name or purpose. When this occurs, ask the person to bring in the drug to be identified.
- Is cost a problem? When the person is unable to afford a drug, he or she may decrease the dosage, take one pill instead of two, or not refill the empty bottle immediately.
- Is traveling to the pharmacy to refill a prescription a problem?
- Is the person taking any over-the-counter medications? Some people use a local pharmacist for self-treatment.
- Has the person ever shared medications with neighbors or friends? Some establish "lay referral" networks by comparing symptoms and thus medications.

Family History

This is not as useful in predicting which familial diseases the person may contract, because most of those will have occurred at an earlier age. But these data are useful to assess which diseases or causes of death of relatives the person has experienced. Also it describes the person's existing social network.

Review of Systems

Remember that these are *additional* items to question for the older adult. Refer to the history for the younger adult for the basic list.

GENERAL. Present weight and what the person would like to weigh (gives idea of body image).

SKIN. Change in sensation to pain, heat, or cold.

EYES. Use of bifocal glasses, any trouble adjusting to far vision (problems with stairs).

EARS. Increased sensitivity to background noise and whether conversation sounds garbled or distorted.

MOUTH. Use of dentures, when the person wears them (always, all day, only at meals, only at social occasions, or never), method of cleaning, any difficulty wearing the dentures (loose, pain, makes whistling or clicking noise), cracks at corners of the mouth.

RESPIRATORY SYSTEM. Shortness of breath and level of activity that produces it. Shortness of breath often is an early sign of cardiac dysfunction, but many older people dismiss it as "a cold" or getting "winded" because of old age.

CARDIOVASCULAR SYSTEM. If chest pain occurs, the person may not feel it as intensely as a younger person. Instead, the older adult may feel dyspnea on exertion.

PERIPHERAL VASCULAR SYSTEM. Wears constrictive clothing, garters, or rolls stockings at knees. Any color change at feet or ankles.

URINARY SYSTEM. Urinary retention, incomplete emptying, straining to urinate, change in force of stream. If a weakened stream occurs, men may note the need to stand closer to the toilet. Women may note incontinence when coughing, laughing, or sneezing.

SEXUAL HEALTH. Ask about any changes in sexual relationship the person has experienced. Note for men it is normal for an erection to develop slowly. (See Chapter 24.) Note for women any vaginal dryness or pain with intercourse. Note for all whether aspects of sex are satisfactory and whether adequate privacy exists for sexual relationship.

MUSCULOSKELETAL SYSTEM. Gait change (balance, weakness, difficulty with steps, fear of falling), use of any assistive device (cane, walker). Any joint stiffness? During what part of the day does the stiffness occur? Does pain or stiffness occur with activity or rest?

NEUROLOGIC SYSTEM. Any problem with memory (recent or remote) or disorientation (time of day, in what settings)?

Functional Assessment (Including Activities of Daily Living)

Functional assessment measures how a person manages day-to-day activities. For older people, the meaning of health becomes those activities that they can or cannot do. The *impact* of a disease on their daily activities and overall quality of life (called the *disease burden*) is more important to older people than the actual disease diagnosis or pathology. Thus the functional assessment—because it emphasizes function—is very important in assessing older people.

Many functional assessment instruments are available that objectively measure a person's present functional status and monitor any changes over time. Most instruments measure the performance of specific tasks such as the ADLs and IADLs. The Comprehensive Older Person's Evaluation (Table 6–1) is particularly useful because it contains the basic ADL/IADL functional assessment as well as physical, social, psychologic, demographic, financial, and legal issues.

Whether or not a standardized instrument is used, the following functional assessment questions are important additions to the older adult's health history.

SELF-CONCEPT, SELF-ESTEEM. When the aging person was an adolescent, educational opportunities were not as available as they are today, nor were they equally available for women. The aging person may be sensitive about having achieved only the level of elementary school education or less.

OCCUPATION. Past positions, volunteer activities, and community activities. Many people continue to work past the age of 65; they grew up with a strong work ethic and are proud to continue. If the person is retired, how has he or she adjusted to the change in role? It may mean loss of social role or social status, loss of personal relationships formed at work, and reduced income.

ACTIVITY AND EXERCISE. How does the person spend a typical day in work, hobbies, and leisure activities? Is there any day this routine changes (e.g., Sunday visits from family)? Note that the person suffering from chronic illness or disability may have a self-care deficit, musculoskeletal changes such as arthritis, and mental confusion.

List significant leisure activities, hobbies, sports, and community activities. Is there a community senior citizen center available for nutrition, social network, and screening of health status?

What is the type, amount, and frequency of the exercise? Is a warm-up included? How does the body respond?

SLEEP AND REST. Usual sleep pattern: feel rested during the day? Is energy sufficient to carry out daily activities? Need naps? Is there a problem with night wakenings (nocturia, shortness of breath, light sleep, insomnia [difficulty falling asleep, awakening during night,

TABLE 6–1: Comprehensive Older Person's Evaluation

Name (print): _____   Date of Visit: _____

Chief complaint: _____

Today I will ask you about your overall health and function and will be using a questionnaire to help me obtain this information. The first few questions are to check your memory.

Preliminary Cognition Questionnaire: *Record if answer is correct with (+); if answer is incorrect, with (−). Record total number of errors.*

	(+, −)
1) What is the date today?	_____
2) What day of the week is it?	_____
3) What is the name of this place?	_____
4) What is your telephone number or room number?	
(record answer: _____)	_____
If subject does not have phone, ask:	
What is your street address?	
5) How old are you? *(record answer: _____)*	_____
6) When were you born? *(record answer from records if patient cannot answer: _____)*	_____
7) Who is the president of the United States now?	_____
8) Who was the president just before him?	_____
9) What was your mother's maiden name?	_____
10) Subtract 3 from 20 and keep subtracting from each new number you get, all the way down.	_____
Total errors	_____

If more than 4 errors, ask #11. If more than 6 errors, complete questionnaire from informant.

11) Do you think you would benefit from a legal guardian, someone who would be responsible for your legal and financial matters?
Do you have a living will? Would you like one?
   a) No
   b) Has functioning legal guardian for sole purpose of managing money
   (describe:_____)
   c) Has legal guardian
   d) Yes

Demographic Section

1) Patient's race or ethnic background *(record: _____)*
2) Patient's gender *(circle)*   Male   Female
3) How far did you go in school?
   a) Postgraduate education
   b) Four-year degree
   c) College or technical school
   d) High school complete
   e) High school incomplete
   f) 0–8 years

Social Support Section: Now there are a few questions about your family and friends.

4) Are you married, widowed, separated, divorced, or have you never been married?
   a) Now married
   b) Widowed
   c) Separated
   d) Divorced
   e) Never married
5) Who lives with you? *(circle all responses)*
   a) Spouse
   b) Other relative or friend *(specify: _____)*
   c) Group living situation (non-health)
   d) Lives alone
   e) Nursing home, number of years _____

6) Have you talked to any friends or relatives by phone during the last week?
   a) Yes
   b) No
7) Are you satisfied by seeing your relatives and friends as often as you want to, or are you somewhat dissatisfied about how little you see them?
   a) Satisfied *(skip to #8)*
   b) No *(ask A)*
      A) Do you feel you would like to be involved in a Senior Citizens Center for social events, or perhaps meals?
         1) No
         2) Is involved *(describe: _____)*
         3) Yes
8) Is there someone who would take care of you for as long as you needed if you were sick or disabled?
   a) Yes *(skip to C)*
   b) No *(ask A)*
      A) Is there someone who would take care of you for a short time?
         1) Yes *(skip to C)*
         2) No *(ask B)*
      B) Is there someone who could help you now and then?
         1) Yes *(ask C)*
         2) No *(ask C)*
      C) Whom would we call in case of an emergency?
         (record name and telephone: _____
         _____ *)*

Financial Section

9) Do you own, or are you buying, your own home?
   a) Yes *(skip to #10)*
   b) No *(ask A)*
      A) Do you feel you need assistance with housing?
         1) No
         2) Has subsidized or other housing assistance
         3) Yes *(describe: _____)*
      B) What type of housing did you have prior to coming here?
10) Are you covered by private medical insurance, Medicare, Medicaid, or some disability plan? *(circle all that apply)*
   a) Private insurance *(specify and skip to #11):* _____
   b) Medicare
   c) Medicaid
   d) Disability *(specify and ask A: _____)*
   e) None
   f) Other *(specify: _____)*
      A) Do you feel you need additional assistance with your medical bills?
         1) No
         2) Yes
11) Which of these statements best describes your financial situation?
   a) My bills are no problem to me *(skip to #12)*
   b) My expenses make it difficult to meet my bills *(ask A)*
   c) My expenses are so heavy that I cannot meet my bills *(ask A)*
      A) Do you feel that you need financial assistance such as: *(circle all that apply)*
         1) Food stamps
         2) Social Security or disability payments
         3) Assistance in paying your heating or electrical bills
         4) Other financial assistance *(describe: _____)*

Reprinted with permission from Pearlman R: Development of a functional assessment questionnaire for geriatric patients: COPE, *J Chronic Dis* 40:85S–94S, 1987. With permission from Elsevier Science.

TABLE 6–1: Comprehensive Older Person's Evaluation—cont'd

Psychological Health Section: The next few questions are about how you feel about your life in general. There are no right or wrong answers, only what best applies to you. Please answer yes or no to each question.

	Yes	No
12) Is your daily life full of things that keep you interested?	___	___
13) Have you, at times, very much wanted to leave home?	___	___
14) Does it seem that no one understands you?	___	___
15) Are you happy most of the time?	___	___
16) Do you feel weak all over much of the time?	___	___
17) Is your sleep fitful and disturbed?	___	___

18) Taking everything into consideration, how would you describe your satisfaction with your life in general at the present time—good, fair, or poor?
   a) Good
   b) Fair
   c) Poor

19) Do you feel you now need help with your mental health; for example, a counselor or psychiatrist?
   a) No
   b) Has (*specify:* _____)
   c) Yes

Physical Health Section: The next few questions are about your health.

20) During the past month (30 days), how many days were you so sick that you couldn't do your usual activities, such as working around the house or visiting with friends? _____

21) Relative to other people your age, how would you rate your overall health at the present time: excellent, good, fair, poor, or very poor?
   a) Excellent (*skip to* #22)
   b) Very good (*skip to* #22)
   c) Good (*ask* A)
   d) Fair (*ask* A)
   e) Poor (*ask* A)
      A) Do you feel you need additional medical services such as a doctor, nurse, visiting nurse, or physical therapist? (*circle all that apply*)
         1) Doctor
         2) Nurse
         3) Visiting nurse
         4) Physical therapist
         5) None

22) Do you use an aid for walking, such as a wheelchair, walker, cane, or anything else? (*circle aid usually used*)
   a) Wheelchair
   b) Other (*specify:* _____)
   c) Visiting nurse
   d) Walker
   e) None

23) How much do your health troubles stand in the way of your doing things you want to do: not at all, a little, or a great deal?
   a) Not at all (*skip to* #24)
   b) A little (*ask* A)
   c) A great deal (*ask* A)
      A) Do you think you need assistance to do your daily activities; for example, do you need a live-in aide or choreworker?
         1) LIve-in aide
         2) Choreworker
         3) Has aide, choreworker, or other assistance (*describe:* _____)
         4) None needed

24) Have you had, or do you currently have, any of the following health problems? *If yes, place an "X" in appropriate box and describe; medical record information may be used to help complete this section.*)

	HX	CURRENT	DESCRIBE
a) Arthritis or rheumatism?			
b) Lung or breathing problem?			
c) Hypertension?			
d) Heart trouble?			
e) Phlebitis or poor circulation problems in arms or legs?			
f) Diabetes or low blood sugar?			
g) Digestive ulcers?			
h) Other digestive problem?			
i) Cancer?			
j) Anemia?			
k) Effects of stroke?			
l) Other neurological problem? (specify: _____)			
m) Thyroid or other glandular problem? (specify: _____)			
n) Skin disorders such as pressure sores, leg ulcers, burns?			
o) Speech problem?			
p) Hearing problem?			
q) Vision or eye problem?			
r) Kidney or bladder problems, or incontinence?			
s) A problem of falls?			
t) Problem with eating or your weight? (specify: _____)			
u) Problem with depression or your nerves? (specify: _____)			
v) Problem with your behavior (specify: _____)			
w) Problem with your sexual activity?			
x) Problem with alcohol?			
y) Problem with pain?			
z) Other health problems? (specify: _____)			

Immunizations: _____
_____

Continued

TABLE 6–1: Comprehensive Older Person's Evaluation—cont'd

25) What medications are you currently taking, or have been taking, in the last month? (May I see your medication bottles?) *(If patient cannot list, ask categories a–r and note dosage and schedule, or obtain information from medical or pharmacy records and verify accuracy with the patient.)*

Allergies:

	Rx (DOSAGE AND SCHEDULE)
a) Arthritis medication	
b) Pain medication	
c) Blood pressure medication	
d) Water pills or pills for fluid	
e) Medication for your heart	
f) Medication for your lungs	
g) Blood thinners	
h) Medication for your circulation	
i) Insulin or diabetes medication	
j) Seizure medication	
k) Thyroid pills	
l) Steroids	
m) Hormones	
n) Antibiotics	
o) Medicine for nerves or depression	
p) Prescription sleeping pills	
q) Other prescription drugs	
r) Other nonprescription drugs	

26) Many people have problems remembering to take their medications, especially ones they need to take on a regular basis. How often do you forget to take your medications? Would you say you forget often, sometimes, rarely, or never?
a) Never
b) Rarely
c) Sometimes
d) Often

Activities of Daily Living: The next set of questions asks whether you need help with any of the following activities of daily living.

27) I would like to know whether you can do these activities without any help at all, or if you need assistance to do them. Do you need help to: *(If yes, describe, including patient needs.)*

	YES	NO	DESCRIBE (INCLUDE NEEDS)
a) Use the telephone?			
b) Get to places out of walking distance (using transportation)?			
c) Shop for clothes and food?			
d) Do your housework?			
e) Handle your money?			
f) Feed yourself?			
g) Dress and undress yourself?			
h) Take care of your appearance?			
i) Get in and out of bed?			
j) Take a bath or shower?			
k) Prepare your meals?			
l) Do you have any problem getting to the bathroom on time?			

28) During the past 6 months, have you had any help with such things as shopping, housework, bathing, dressing, and getting around?
a) Yes *(specify: _____)*
b) No

Signature of person completing the form:

_____

early morning wakening])? If no routine, do you tend to nap all afternoon? Does insomnia worsen with lack of a daily schedule?

NUTRITION/ELIMINATION. Record a 24-hour recall. Is this typical of most days? (Nutrition may vary greatly. Ask the person to keep a weekly log to bring in.) What are the meal patterns? Are there three full meals or five to six smaller meals per day? How many convenience foods and soft foods are used? Who prepares meals? Eat alone? Who shops for food? How are groceries transported home? Is the income adequate for groceries? Is there a problem preparing meals (adequate vision, motor deficit, adequate energy)? Are the appliances and water and utilities adequate for meal preparation? Is there any difficulty chewing or swallowing? What are the food preferences (aging persons often eat high amounts of carbohydrates because these foods are cheaper, easier to make, and easier to chew)?

INTERPERSONAL RELATIONSHIPS/RESOURCES. Who else is at home with you? Live alone? Is this satisfactory? Have a pet? How close are family or friends? How often do you see family or friends? If infrequent, do you experience this as a loss?

Do you live with family, such as a spouse, children, or a sibling? Is this a satisfactory arrangement? What is the role in family for preparation of meals, housework, and other activities? Are there any conflicts?

On whom do you depend for emotional support? For help with problems? Who meets affection needs?

COPING AND STRESS MANAGEMENT. Has there been a recent change in lifestyle, such as loss of occupation, spouse, friends, move from home, illness of self or family member, or has income been decreased? How dealing with stress? If a loved one has died, how responding to the loss? "How do you feel about being 'alone' and having to take on unfamiliar responsibilities now?"

ENVIRONMENTAL/HAZARDS. Home safety: one floor or are there stairs, state of repair, is money adequate to maintain home, exits for fire, heating and utilities adequate, how long in the present home? Transportation: own automobile, last driver's test, consider self a safe driver, income adequate for maintenance, public transportation access, receive drives from community resources, friends? Neighborhood: secure in personal safety at day or night; danger of loss of possessions; amount of noise and pollution; access to family and friends, grocery store, drug store, laundry, church, temple, mosque, health care facilities?

BIBLIOGRAPHY

American Academy of Pediatrics: *Recommended childhood and adolescent immunization schedule United States, 2003.* Available at www.cispimmunize.org (December 2002).

Andrews MM, Boyle JS, editors: *Transcultural concepts in nursing care,* ed 3, Philadelphia, 1999, Lippincott Williams & Wilkins.

Asher J, Crespo E, Sugg NK: Domestic violence: detection and treatment, *Patient Care* 35(7):68–87, 2001.

Campbell LA, Thompson BL: Evaluating elderly patients: a critique of comprehensive functional assessment tools, *Nurse Pract* 15(8):11–18, 1990.

Cole-Kelly K, Seaburn D: Five areas of questioning to promote a family oriented approach in primary care, *Fam Syst Health* 17(3):341–348, 1999.

Ewing JA: Detecting alcoholism: the CAGE questionnaire, *JAMA* 252:1905–1907, 1984.

Fleming KC et al: Practical functional assessment of elderly persons: a primary care approach, *Mayo Clin Proc* 70:890–910, 1995.

Gordon M: *Manual of nursing diagnosis,* ed 9, St Louis, 2000, Mosby.

Granger CV, Albrecht GL, Hamilton BB: Outcome of comprehensive medical rehabilitation: measures of PULSES profile and the Barthel index, *Arch Phys Med Rehabil* 60:145–154, 1979.

Granger CV et al: Reliability of a brief outpatient functional outcome assessment measure, *Am J Phys Med Rehabil* 74(6):469–475, 1995.

Katz S et al: Studies of illness in the aged. The Index of ADL: a standardized measure of biological and psychosocial function, *JAMA* 185:94–98, 1963.

Kempen GIJ et al: The assessment of ADL among frail elderly in an interview survey: self-report versus performance-based tests and determinants of discrepancies, *J Gerontol* 51B(5):254–260, 1996.

Leininger M: *Culture care diversity and universality: a theory of nursing,* New York, 1991, National League for Nursing.

Lekan-Rutledge D: Functional assessment. In Matteson M, McConnell ES, Linton AD: *Gerontological nursing,* ed 2, Philadelphia, 1997, W.B. Saunders.

Linn MW, Linn BS: The rapid disability rating scale—2, *J Am Geriatr Soc* 30(6):378–382, 1982.

Maddox M: Spiritual assessments in primary care, *Nurse Pract* 27(2):12–14, 2002.

Mahoney FI, Barthel DW: Functional evaluation: the Barthel Index, *Md State Med J* 14:61–65, 1965.

Pearlman R: Development of a functional assessment questionnaire for geriatric patients: the comprehensive older person's evaluation (COPE), *J Chronic Dis* 40:85S–94S, 1987.

Porter SC et al: Parents as direct contributors to the medical record: validation of their electronic input, *Ann Emerg Med* 35(4):346–352, 2000.

Post SG, Puchalski CM, Larson DB: Physician and patient spirituality: professional boundaries, competency, and ethics, *Ann Intern Med* 132:578–583, 2000.

Schoultz J, Tanner B, Harrigan R: Culturally appropriate guidelines for alcohol and drug abuse prevention, *Nurse Pract* 25(11):50–56, 2000.

Staab AM: Adult immunization: recommendations for optimal protection, *Clin Rev* 8(10):55–77, 1998.

Stone AT, Wyman JF, Salisbury SS, editors: *Clinical gerontological nursing: a guide to advanced practice,* ed 2, Philadelphia, 1998, W.B. Saunders.

U.S. Department of Health and Human Services: *Alcohol and health* (Publication No. 97-4017), Alexandria, Va, 1997, National Institutes of Health, National Institute on Alcohol Abuse and Alcoholism.

Volk RJ et al: The Alcohol Use Disorders Identification Test (AUDIT) as a screen for at-risk drinking in primary care patients of different racial/ethnic backgrounds, *Addiction* 92(2):197–206, 1997.

Mental Status Assessment

Structure and Function

DEFINING MENTAL STATUS

Mental status is a person's emotional and cognitive functioning. Optimal functioning aims toward simultaneous life satisfaction in work, in caring relationships, and within the self. Mental health is relative and ongoing. Everyone has "good" and "bad" days. Usually, mental status strikes a balance, allowing the person to function socially and occupationally.

The stress surrounding a traumatic life event (death of a loved one, serious illness) tips the balance, causing transient dysfunction. This is an expected response to a trauma. Mental status assessment at this time can identify remaining strengths and can help the individual mobilize resources and use coping skills.

A **mental disorder** is apparent when a person's response is much greater than the expected reaction to a traumatic life event. A mental disorder is defined as a significant behavioral or psychological *pattern* that is associated with distress (a painful symptom) or disability (impaired functioning) and has a significant risk of pain, disability, or death, or a loss of freedom (American Psychiatric Association, 1994). Mental disorders include **organic disorders** (due to brain disease of *known* specific organic cause, e.g., delirium, dementia, intoxication, and withdrawal) and **psychiatric mental illness** (in which organic etiology has not yet been established, e.g., anxiety disorder or schizophrenia). Mental status assessment documents a dysfunction and determines how that dysfunction affects self-care in everyday life.

Mental status cannot be scrutinized directly like the characteristics of skin or heart sounds. Its functioning is *inferred* through assessment of an individual's behaviors:

Consciousness: being aware of one's own existence, feelings, and thoughts and aware of the environment. This is the most elementary of mental status functions.

Language: using the voice to communicate one's thoughts and feelings. This is a basic tool of humans, and its loss has a heavy social impact on the individual.

Mood and affect: both of these elements deal with the prevailing feelings; **affect** is a temporary expression of feelings or state of mind, and **mood** is more durable, a prolonged display of feelings that color the whole emotional life.

Orientation: the awareness of the objective world in relation to the self.

Attention: the power of concentration, the ability to focus on one specific thing without being distracted by many environmental stimuli.

Memory: the ability to lay down and store experiences and perceptions for later recall. *Recent* memory evokes day-to-day events; *remote* memory brings up years' worth of experiences.

Abstract reasoning: pondering a deeper meaning beyond the concrete and literal.

Thought process: the *way* a person thinks, the logical train of thought.

Thought content: *what* the person thinks—specific ideas, beliefs, the use of words.

Perceptions: an awareness of objects through the five senses.

DEVELOPMENTAL CONSIDERATIONS

INFANTS AND CHILDREN

The maturation of emotional and cognitive functioning is described in detail in Chapter 2. It is difficult to separate and trace the development of just one aspect of mental status. All aspects are interdependent. For example, consciousness is rudimentary at birth because the cerebral cortex is not yet developed; the infant cannot distinguish the self from the mother's body. Consciousness gradually develops along with language, so that by 18 to 24 months the child learns that he or she is separate from objects in the environment and has words to express this. We also can trace language development: from the differentiated crying at 4 weeks, the cooing at 6 weeks, through one-word sentences at 1 year to multiword sentences at 2 years. Yet the concept of language as a social tool of communication occurs around 4 to 5 years of age, coincident with the child's readiness to cooperatively play with other children.

Attention gradually increases in span through preschool years so that, by school age, most children are able to sit and concentrate on their work for a period of time. Some children are late in developing concentration. School readiness coincides with the development of the thought process; around age 7, thinking becomes more logical and systematic, and the child is able to reason and understand. Abstract thinking, the ability to consider a hypothetical situation, usually develops between ages 12 and 15, although a few adolescents never achieve it.

THE AGING ADULT

The aging process leaves the parameters of mental status mostly intact. There is no decrease in general knowledge and little or no loss in vocabulary. Response time is slower than in youth; it takes a bit longer for the brain to process information and react to it. Thus performance on timed intelligence tests may be lower for the aging person—not because intelligence has declined, but because it takes longer to respond to the questions. The slower response time affects new learning; if a new presentation is rapidly paced, the older person does not have time to respond to it (Birren and Schaie, 2001).

Recent memory, which requires some processing (e.g., medication instructions, 24-hour diet recall, names of new acquaintances), is somewhat decreased with aging. Remote memory is not affected.

Age-related changes in sensory perception can affect mental status. For example, vision loss (as detailed in Chapter 14) may result in apathy, social isolation, and depression. Hearing changes are common in older adults (see the discussion of presbycusis in Chapter 15). Age-related hearing loss involves high sound frequencies. Consonants are high-frequency sounds, so older people who have difficulty hearing them have problems with normal conversation. This problem produces frustration, suspicion, and social isolation, and also makes the person look confused.

The era of older adulthood contains more potential for loss than do earlier eras, such as loss of loved ones, loss of job status and prestige, loss of income, and the loss of an energetic and resilient body. The grief and despair surrounding these losses can affect mental status. These losses can result in disorientation, disability, or depression.

COMPONENTS OF THE MENTAL STATUS EXAMINATION

The full mental status examination is a systematic check of emotional and cognitive functioning. The steps described here, though, rarely need to be taken in their entirety. Usually, you can assess mental status through the context of the health history interview. During that time, keep in mind the four main headings of mental status assessment:

Appearance, Behavior, Cognition,
and Thought processes, or
A, B, C, T

Integrating the mental status examination into the health history interview is sufficient for most people. You will collect ample data to be able to assess mental health strengths and coping skills, and to screen for any dysfunction.

It is necessary to perform a full mental status examination when you discover any abnormality in affect or behavior, and in the following situations:

• Family members concerned about a person's behavioral changes, such as memory loss, inappropriate social interaction.
• Brain lesions (trauma, tumor, brain attack [formerly known as cerebrovascular accident or stroke]). A mental status assessment documents any emotional or cognitive change associated with the lesion. Not recognizing these changes hinders care planning and creates problems with social readjustment.
• Aphasia (the impairment of language secondary to brain damage). A mental status examination assesses language dysfunction as well as any emotional problems associated with it, such as depression or agitation.
• Symptoms of psychiatric mental illness, especially with acute onset.

In every mental status examination, note these factors from the health history that could affect your interpretation of the findings:

• Any known illnesses or health problems, such as alcoholism or chronic renal disease.
• Current medications whose side effects may cause confusion or depression.
• The usual educational and behavioral level—note that factor as the normal baseline, and do not expect performance on the mental status examination to exceed it.
• Responses to personal history questions, indicating current stress, social interaction patterns, sleep habits, drug and alcohol use.

In the following examination, the sequence of steps forms a *hierarchy* in which the most basic functions (consciousness, language) are assessed first. The first steps must be accurately assessed to ensure validity for the steps to follow. That is, if consciousness is clouded, then the person cannot be expected to have full attention and to cooperate with new learning. Or, if language is impaired, subsequent assessment of new learning or abstract reasoning (anything that requires language functioning) can give erroneous conclusions.

 Objective Data

EQUIPMENT NEEDED

(Occasionally)
Pencil, paper, reading material

NORMAL RANGE OF FINDINGS	ABNORMAL FINDINGS
APPEARANCE	
POSTURE. *Posture* is erect and *position* is relaxed.	Sitting on edge of chair or curled in bed, tense muscles, frowning, darting watchful eyes, restless pacing occur with anxiety and with hyperthyroidism. Sitting slumped in chair, slow walk, dragging feet occur with depression and some organic brain diseases.

NORMAL RANGE OF FINDINGS	ABNORMAL FINDINGS
BODY MOVEMENTS. *Body movements* are voluntary, deliberate, coordinated, and smooth and even.	Restless, fidgety movements, or hyperkinetic appearance occur with anxiety. Apathy and psychomotor slowing occur with depression and organic brain disease. Abnormal posturing and bizarre gestures occur with schizophrenia. Facial grimaces.
DRESS. *Dress* is appropriate for setting, season, age, gender, and social group. Clothing fits and is put on appropriately.	Inappropriate dress can occur with organic brain syndrome. Eccentric dress combination and bizarre make-up occur with schizophrenia or manic syndrome.
GROOMING AND HYGIENE. The person is clean and well groomed; hair is neat and clean; women have moderate or no make-up; men are shaved or beard or mustache are well groomed. Nails are clean (though some jobs leave nails chronically dirty). Note: A disheveled appearance in a previously well-groomed person is significant. Use care in interpreting clothing that is disheveled, bizarre, or in poor repair, because these sometimes reflect the person's economic status or a deliberate fashion trend.	Unilateral neglect (total inattention to one side of body) occurs following some cerebrovascular accidents. Inappropriate dress, poor hygiene, and lack of concern with appearance occur with depression and severe Alzheimer's disease. Meticulously dressed and groomed appearance and fastidious manner may occur with obsessive-compulsive disorders.

BEHAVIOR

LEVEL OF CONSCIOUSNESS. The person is awake, alert, aware of stimuli from the environment and within the self, and responds appropriately to stimuli.	Lethargic, obtunded. See Table 7–3, Levels of Consciousness.
FACIAL EXPRESSION. The look is appropriate to the situation and changes appropriately with the topic. There is comfortable eye contact unless precluded by cultural norm, e.g., Native American.	Flat, masklike expression occurs with parkinsonism and depression.
SPEECH. Judge the quality of speech by noting that the person makes laryngeal sounds effortlessly and shares conversation appropriately.	Dysphonia is abnormal volume, pitch, see Table 7–4. Monopolizes interview. Silent, secretive, or uncommunicative.
The pace of the conversation is moderate, and stream of talking is fluent.	Slow, monotonous speech with parkinsonism, depression. Rapid-fire, pressured, and loud talking occur with manic syndrome.
Articulation (ability to form words) is clear and understandable.	Dysarthria is distorted speech, see Table 7–4. Misuse of words; omits letters, syllables, or words; transposes words; occurs with aphasia. Circumlocution, or repetitious abnormal patterns: neologism, echolalia, see Table 7–6.
Word choice is effortless and appropriate to educational level. The person completes sentences, occasionally pausing to think.	Unduly long word-finding or failure in word search occurs with aphasia.
MOOD AND AFFECT. Judge this by body language and facial expression, and by asking directly, "How do you feel today," or "How do you usually feel?" The mood should be appropriate to the person's place and condition and change appropriately with topics. The person is willing to cooperate with you.	See Table 7–5, Abnormalities of Mood and Affect. Wide mood swings occur with manic syndrome. Bizarre mood is apparent in schizophrenia.

NORMAL RANGE OF FINDINGS	ABNORMAL FINDINGS

COGNITIVE FUNCTIONS

ORIENTATION. You can discern orientation through the course of the interview, or ask for it directly, using tact. "Some people have trouble keeping up with the dates while in the hospital. Do you know today's date?" Assess:

Time: day of week, date, year, season
Place: where person lives, present location, type of building, name of city and state
Person: own name, age, who examiner is, type of worker

Many hospitalized people normally have trouble with the exact date but are fully oriented on the remaining items.

Disorientation occurs with organic brain disorders, such as delirium and dementia. Orientation is usually lost in this order—first to time, then to place, and rarely to person.

ATTENTION SPAN. Check the person's ability to concentrate by noting whether he or she completes a thought without wandering. Note any distractibility or difficulty attending to you. Or, give a series of directions to follow and note the correct sequence of behaviors, such as "Please take this glass of water with your left hand, drink from it, shift it to your right hand, and set it on the table." Note that attention span commonly is impaired in people who are anxious, fatigued, or drug intoxicated.

Digression from initial thought. Irrelevant replies to questions. Easily distracted; "stimulus bound," i.e., any new stimulus quickly draws attention. Confusion, negativism.

RECENT MEMORY. Assess recent memory in the context of the interview by the 24-hour diet recall or by asking the time the person arrived at the agency. Ask questions you can corroborate. This screens for the occasional person who confabulates or makes up answers to fill in the gaps of memory loss.

Recent memory deficit occurs with organic disorders, e.g., delirium, dementia, amnestic syndrome, or Korsakoff's syndrome in chronic alcoholism.

REMOTE MEMORY. In the context of the interview, ask the person verifiable past events; for example, ask to describe past health, the first job, birthday and anniversary dates, and historical events that are relevant for that person.

Remote memory is lost when cortical storage area for that memory is damaged, such as in Alzheimer's dementia or any disease that damages the cerebral cortex.

NEW LEARNING—THE FOUR UNRELATED WORDS TEST. This tests the person's ability to lay down new memories. It is a highly sensitive and valid memory test. It requires more effort than does the recall of personal or historic events. It also avoids the danger of unverifiable material.

To the person, say, "I am going to say four words. I want you to remember them. In a few minutes I will ask you to recall them." To be sure the person has understood, have the words repeated. Pick four words with semantic and phonetic diversity:

1. brown	1. fun
2. honesty	2. carrot
3. tulip	3. ankle
4. eyedropper	4. loyalty

After 5 minutes, ask for the recall of the four words. To test the duration of memory, ask for a recall at 10 minutes and at 30 minutes. The normal response for persons under 60 years is an accurate three- or four-word recall after a 5-, 10-, and 30-minute delay (Strub and Black, 1999).

People with Alzheimer's dementia score a zero- or one-word recall. Impaired new learning ability also occurs with anxiety (due to inattention and distractibility) and depression (due to lack of effort mobilized to remember).

Additional Testing for Persons with Aphasia

WORD COMPREHENSION. Point to articles in the room, parts of the body, articles from pockets, and ask the person to name them.

READING. Ask the person to read available print. Be aware that reading is related to educational level. Use caution that you are not just testing literacy.

Aphasia is the loss of the ability to speak or write coherently, or to understand speech or writing, due to a brain attack (cerebral vascular accident or CVA). See Table 7–4, Speech Disorders.

NORMAL RANGE OF FINDINGS	ABNORMAL FINDINGS
WRITING. Ask the person to make up and write a sentence. Note coherence, spelling, and parts of speech (the sentence should have a subject and verb).	Reading and writing are important in planning health teaching and rehabilitation.

Higher Intellectual Function

These tests measure problem-solving and reasoning abilities. Results are closely related to the person's general intelligence and must be assessed considering educational and cultural background. Tests of higher intellectual functioning have been used to discriminate between organic brain disease and psychiatric disorders; errors on the tests indicate organic dysfunction.

Although they have been widely used, there is little evidence that most of these tests are valid in detecting organic brain disease (Keller and Manschreck, 1981). Furthermore, most of these tests have little relevance for daily clinical care. Thus, many time-honored, standard tests of higher intellectual function are not discussed here, such as fund of general knowledge, digit span repetition, calculation, proverb interpretation and similarities to test abstract reasoning, or hypothetical situations to test judgment.

Judgment

A person exercises judgment when he or she can compare and evaluate the alternatives in a situation and reach an appropriate course of action. Rather than testing the person's response to a hypothetical situation (e.g., "What would you do if you found a stamped, addressed envelope lying on the sidewalk?"), you should be more interested in the person's judgment about daily or long-term life goals, the likelihood of acting in response to delusions or hallucinations, and the capacity for violent or suicidal behavior.

To assess judgment in the context of the interview, note what the person says about job plans, social or family obligations, and plans for the future. Job and future plans should be realistic, considering the person's health situation. Also, ask the person to describe the rationale for personal health care, and how he or she decided about whether or not to comply with prescribed health regimens. The person's actions and decisions should be realistic.

Impaired judgment (unrealistic or impulsive decisions, wish fulfillment) occurs with mental retardation, emotional dysfunction, schizophrenia, and organic brain disease.

THOUGHT PROCESSES AND PERCEPTIONS

THOUGHT PROCESSES. Ask yourself, "Does this person make sense? Can I follow what the person is saying?" The *way* a person thinks should be logical, goal directed, coherent, and relevant. The person should complete a thought.

Illogical, unrealistic thought processes. Digression from initial thought. Ideas run together. Evidence of blocking (person stops in middle of thought). See Table 7–6, Abnormalities of Thought Process.

THOUGHT CONTENT. *What* the person says should be consistent and logical.

Obsessions, compulsions. See Table 7–7, Abnormalities of Thought Content.

PERCEPTIONS. The person should be consistently aware of reality. The perceptions should be congruent with yours. Ask the following questions:

- How do people treat you?
- Do other people talk about you?
- Do you feel like you are being watched, followed, or controlled?
- Is your imagination very active?
- Have you heard your name when alone?

Illusions, hallucinations. See Table 7–8, Abnormalities of Perception. Auditory and visual hallucinations occur with psychiatric and organic brain disease and with psychedelic drugs. Tactile hallucinations occur with alcohol withdrawal.

SCREEN FOR SUICIDAL THOUGHTS. When the person expresses feelings of sadness, hopelessness, despair or grief, it is important to assess any possible risk of

NORMAL RANGE OF FINDINGS	ABNORMAL FINDINGS

physical harm to himself or herself. Begin with more general questions. If you hear affirmative answers, continue with more specific questions:

- Have you ever felt so blue you thought of hurting yourself?
- Do you feel like hurting yourself now?
- Do you have a plan to hurt yourself?
- What would happen if you were dead?
- How would other people react if you were dead?

It is very difficult to question people about possible suicidal wishes, especially for beginning examiners. Examiners fear invading privacy and may have their own normal denial of death and suicide. However, the risk is far greater if you skip these questions when you have the slightest clue that they are appropriate. You may be the only health professional to pick up clues of suicide risk. You are responsible for encouraging the person to talk about suicidal thoughts. Sometimes you cannot prevent a suicide when someone really wishes to kill himself or herself. However, for the people who are ambivalent, and they are the majority, you can buy time so the person can be helped to find an alternate route to the situation. Share any concerns you have about a person's suicide ideation with a mental health professional.

> A precise suicide plan to take place in the next 24 to 48 hours using a lethal method constitutes high risk. Important clues and warning signs of suicide:
>   Prior suicide attempts
>   Depression, hopelessness
>   Social withdrawal, running away
>   Self-mutilation
>   Hypersomnia or insomnia
>   Slowed psychomotor activity
>   Anorexia
>   Verbal suicide messages (defeat, failure, worthlessness, loss, giving up, desire to kill self)
>   Death themes in art, jokes, writing, behaviors
>   Saying goodbye (giving away prized possessions)
>   Additional content on mental disorders is listed in Table 7–9, Delirium, Dementia, and Amnestic Disorders; Table 7–10, Substance Use Disorders; Table 7–11, Schizophrenia; Table 7–12, Mood Disorders; and Table 7–13, Anxiety Disorders.

SUPPLEMENTAL MENTAL STATUS EXAMINATION

The MiniMental State is a simplified scored form of the cognitive functions of the mental status examination (Folstein et al., 1975; replicated by Depaulo and Folstein, 1978; Table 7–1). It is quick and easy, includes a standard set of only 11 questions, and requires only 5 to 10 minutes to administer. It is useful for both initial and serial measurement, so you can demonstrate worsening or improvement of cognition over time and with treatment. It concentrates only on cognitive functioning, not on mood or thought processes. It is a valid detector of organic disease; thus it is a good screening tool to detect dementia and delirium and to differentiate these from psychiatric mental illness.

The maximum score on the test is 30; people with normal mental status average 27. Scores between 24 and 30 indicate no cognitive impairment.

> Scores that occur with dementia and delirium are classified as follows: 18–23 = mild cognitive impairment; 0–7 = severe cognitive impairment.

DEVELOPMENTAL CONSIDERATIONS
Infants and Children

The mental status assessment of infants and children covers behavioral, cognitive, and psychosocial development, and examines how the child is coping with his or her environment. Essentially, you will follow the same A-B-C-T guidelines as for the adult, with special consideration for developmental milestones. Your best examination "technique" arises from thorough knowledge of developmental milestones as described in Chapter 2. Abnormalities are often problems of *omission;* the child does not achieve a milestone you would expect.

The parent's health history, especially the sections on the developmental history and personal history, yields most of the mental status data.

TABLE 7–1: MiniMental State Examination

NAME OF SUBJECT _____   Age _____

NAME OF EXAMINER _____   Years of School Completed _____

Approach the patient with respect and encouragement.

Ask: Do you have any trouble with your memory?   ☐ Yes ☐ No   Date of Examination _____

May I ask you some questions about your memory?   ☐ Yes ☐ No

SCORE ITEM

5 ( )   **TIME ORIENTATION**
Ask: What is the year _____ (1), season _____ (1),
month of the year _____ (1), date _____ (1),
day of the week _____ (1)?

5 ( )   **PLACE ORIENTATION**
Ask: Where are we now? What is the state _____ (1), city _____ (1),
part of the city _____ (1), building _____ (1),
floor of the building _____ (1)?

3 ( )   **REGISTRATION OF THREE WORDS**
Say: Listen carefully. I am going to say three words. You say them back after I stop.
Ready? Here they are . . . PONY (wait 1 second), QUARTER (wait 1 second), ORANGE (wait one second).
What were those words?
_____ (1)
_____ (1)
_____ (1)
Give 1 point for each correct answer, then repeat them until the patient learns all three.

5 ( )   **SERIAL 7s AS A TEST OF ATTENTION AND CALCULATION**
Ask: Subtract 7 from 100 and continue to subtract 7 from each subsequent remainder until I tell you to stop.
What is 100 take away 7? _____ (1)
Say: Keep Going. _____ (1), _____ (1),
_____ (1), _____ (1),

3 ( )   **RECALL OF THREE WORDS**
Ask: What were those three words I asked you to remember? Give one point for each correct answer.
_____ (1),
_____ (1),
_____ (1),

2 ( )   **NAMING**
Ask: What is this? (show pencil) _____ (1). What is this? (show watch) _____ (1).

1 ( )   **REPETITION**
Say: Now I am going to ask you to repeat what I say. Ready? No ifs, ands, or buts.
Now you say that. _____ (1)

3 ( )   **COMPREHENSION**
Say: Listen carefully because I am going to ask you to do something:
Take this paper in your left hand (1), fold it in half (1), and put it on the floor. (1)

1 ( )   **READING**
Say: Please read the following and do what it says, but do not say it aloud. (1)

Close your eyes

1 ( )   **WRITING**
Say: Please write a sentence. If patient does not respond, say: Write about the weather. (1)

_____

1 ( )   **DRAWING**
Say: Please copy this design.

TOTAL SCORE _____   Assess level of consciousness along a continuum

		Alert	Drowsy		Stupor		Coma

	YES	NO		YES	NO	FUNCTION BY PROXY
Cooperative:	☐	☐	Deterioration from previous			Please record date when patient was last able to perform the following tasks.
Depressed:	☐	☐	level of functioning:	☐	☐	
Anxious:	☐	☐	Family History of Dementia:	☐	☐	Ask caregiver if patient independently handles:
Poor Vision:	☐	☐	Head Trauma:	☐	☐	
Poor Hearing:	☐	☐	Stroke:	☐	☐	
Native Language:			Alcohol Abuse:	☐	☐	
			Thyroid Disease:	☐	☐	

	YES	NO	DATE
Money/Bills:	☐	☐	____
Medication:	☐	☐	____
Transportation:	☐	☐	____
Telephone:	☐	☐	____

From Folstein MF, Folstein SE, McHugh PR: Mini-mental state, *J Psychiatr Res* 12:189–198, 1975. Reprinted with permission. © 1975, 1998 Mini-Mental LLC.

TABLE 7–2: Behavioral Checklist

1. Prefers to play alone	15. Seems afraid of someone or something
2. Gets hurt in major accidents	16. Is nervous and jumpy
3. Does he/she ever play with fire?	17. Has a nervous habit
4. Has difficulties with teachers	18. Does not show feelings
5. Gets poor grades in school	19. Fights with other children
6. Is absent from school	20. Is understanding of other people's feelings
7. Becomes angry easily	21. Refuses to share
8. Daydreams	22. Shows jealousy
9. Feels unhappy	23. Takes things that are not his/hers
10. Acts younger than other children his/her age	24. Blames others for his/her troubles
11. Does not listen to parents	25. Prefers to play with children not his/her age
12. Does not tell the truth	26. Gets along well with grownups
13. Unsure of himself/herself	27. Teases others
14. Has trouble sleeping	

Scoring is a point system: 0—never; 1—sometimes; 2—often. Scoring is reversed for items 20 and 26. Scores between 15 and 22 indicate closer following; scores above 22 warrant psychiatric evaluation.

From Jellinek M, Evans N, Knight R: Use of a behavior checklist on a pediatric inpatient unit, *J Pediatr* 94:156–158, 1979.

NORMAL RANGE OF FINDINGS

ABNORMAL FINDINGS

In addition, the Denver II screening test (see Chapter 2) gives you a chance to interact directly with the young child to assess mental status. For the child from birth to 6 years of age, the Denver II helps identify those who may be slow in development in behavioral, language, cognitive, and psychosocial areas. An additional language test is the Denver Articulation Screening Exam.

For school-age children, ages 7 to 11, who have grown beyond the age when developmental milestones are very useful, the "Behavioral Checklist" (Table 7–2) is an additional tool that can be given to the parent along with the history. It covers five major areas: mood, play, school, friends, and family relations. It is easy to administer and lasts about 5 minutes.

For the adolescent, follow the same A-B-C-T guidelines as described for the adult.

The Aging Adult

It is important to conduct even a brief examination of all older people admitted to the hospital. Confusion is common in aging people and is easily misdiagnosed. Between one third and one half of older adults admitted to acute-care medical and surgical services show varying degress of confusion. In the community, about 5% of adults over 65 and almost 20% of those over 75 have some degree of clinically detectable impaired cognitive function (Kane et al, 1999).

Check sensory status before assessing any aspect of mental status. Vision and hearing changes due to aging may alter alertness and leave the person looking confused. When older people cannot hear your questions, they may test worse than they actually are. One group of 21 older people with psychiatric mental illness tested significantly better when they wore hearing aids (Kreeger et al, 1995).

Follow the same A-B-C-T guidelines as described for the younger adult with these *additional* considerations:

BEHAVIOR

LEVEL OF CONSCIOUSNESS. In a hospital or extended care setting, the Glasgow Coma Scale (see Chapter 23) is a quantitative tool that is useful in testing consciousness in aging persons in whom confusion is common. It gives a numerical value to the person's response in eye-opening, best verbal response, and best motor response. This system avoids ambiguity when numerous examiners care for the same person.

NORMAL RANGE OF FINDINGS	ABNORMAL FINDINGS

COGNITIVE FUNCTIONS

ORIENTATION. Many aging persons experience social isolation, loss of structure without a job, a change in residence, or some short-term memory loss. These factors affect orientation, and this person may not provide the precise date or complete name of agency. You may consider aging persons oriented if they know *generally* where they are and the present period. That is, consider them oriented to time if the year and month are correctly stated. Orientation to place is accepted with the correct identification of the type of setting (e.g., the hospital) and the name of the town.

NEW LEARNING. In people of normal cognitive function, an age-related decline occurs in performance in the Four Unrelated Words Test described on p. 109 (Strub and Black, 1993). Persons in the eighth decade average two of four words recalled over 5 minutes. They will improve their performance at 10 and 30 minutes after being reminded by verbal cues (e.g., "one word was a color; a common flower in Holland is _____").

> People with Alzheimer's dementia do not improve their performance on subsequent trials.

SUPPLEMENTAL MENTAL STATUS EXAMINATION

SET TEST. The Set Test was developed specifically for use with an aging population. The original study tested people 65 to 85 years of age. It is a quantifiable test, designed to screen for dementia (Isaacs and Kennie, 1973). The test is easy to administer and takes less than 5 minutes. Ask the person to name 10 items in each of four categories or sets: fruits, animals, colors, and towns (FACT). Do not coach, prompt, or hurry the person. Each correct answer is one point. The maximum total score is 40. No one with a score over 25 has been found to have dementia. (Note: Since this is a verbal test, do not use it with persons with hearing impairments or aphasia.)

> Set Test scores of less than 15 indicate dementia. Scores between 15 and 24 show less association with dementia and should be evaluated carefully.

The Set Test is a more holistic approach to testing cognitive function. It assesses mental function as a whole instead of examining individual parts of cognitive function. That is, by asking the person to categorize, name, remember, and count the items in the test, you are really assessing this person's alertness, motivation, concentration, short-term memory, and problem-solving ability.

SUMMARY CHECKLIST: Mental Status Assessment

1. Appearance
- Posture
- Body movements
- Dress
- Grooming and hygiene

2. Behavior
- Level of consciousness
- Facial expression
- Speech (quality, pace, articulation, word choice)
- Mood and affect

3. Cognitive functions
- Orientation
- Attention span
- Recent and remote memory
- New learning—the Four Unrelated Words test
- Judgment

4. Thought processes
- Thought processes
- Thought content
- Perceptions
- Screen for suicidal thoughts (when indicated)

5. Perform the MiniMental State Examination

See Health Promotion Guide on CD

Application and Critical Thinking

SAMPLE CHARTING

Appearance: Person's posture is erect, with no involuntary body movements. Dress and grooming are appropriate for season and setting.

Behavior: Person is alert, with appropriate facial expression and fluent, understandable speech. Affect and verbal responses are appropriate.

Cognitive functions: Oriented to time, person, place. Able to attend cooperatively with examiner. Recent and remote memory intact. Can recall four unrelated words at 5-, 10-, and 30-minute testing intervals. Future plans include returning to home and to local university once individual therapy is established and medication is adjusted.

Thought processes: Perceptions and thought processes are logical and coherent. No suicide ideation.
   Score on MiniMental State Examination is 28.

FOCUSED ASSESSMENT: CLINICAL CASE STUDY

Lola P. is a 79-year-old white married woman, with a recent hospitalization for evaluation of increasing memory loss, confusion, and socially inappropriate behavior. Her family reports that Mrs. P's hygiene and grooming have decreased; she eats very little and has lost weight, does not sleep through the night, has angry emotional outbursts that are unlike her former demeanor, and does not recognize her younger grandchildren. Her husband reports that she has drifted away from the stove while cooking, allowing food to burn on the stovetop. He has found her wandering through the house in the middle of the night, unsure of where she was. She used to "talk on the phone for hours" but now he has to push her into conversations. During this hospitalization, Mrs. P. has undergone a series of medical tests, including a negative lumbar puncture test, normal electroencephalogram (EEG), and a benign head computed tomography (CT) scan. Her physician now suggests a diagnosis of senile dementia of the Alzheimer's type (SDAT).

Appearance: Sitting quietly, somewhat slumped, picking on loose threads on her dress. Hooded, zippered sweatshirt top worn over dress. Hair is gathered in loose ponytail with stray wisps. No make-up.

Behavior: Awake and gazing at hands and lap. Expression is flat and vacant. Will make eye contact when called by name, although gaze quickly shifts back to lap. Speech is a bit slow but articulate; some trouble with word choice.

Cognitive functions: Oriented to person and place. Can state the season, but not the day of the week or the year. Is not able to repeat the correct sequence of complex directions involving lifting and shifting glass of water to the other hand. Scores a one-word recall on the Four Unrelated Words test. Cannot tell examiner how she would plan a grocery shopping trip.

Thought processes: Experiences blocking in train of thought. Thought content is logical. Acts cranky and suspicious with family members. No suicide ideation.
   MiniMental State Examination score is 17, and shows poor recall ability and marked difficulty with serial 7s.

ASSESSMENT

Chronic confusion
Impaired social interaction
Impaired memory
Wandering

NURSING DIAGNOSES COMMONLY ASSOCIATED WITH MENTAL HEALTH DISORDERS

RELATED FACTORS (Etiology)	DEFINING CHARACTERISTICS (Symptoms and Signs)
DIAGNOSIS: Powerlessness	
Immobility	Anger
Difficulty in performing self-care	Violent behavior
Low self-esteem	Anxiety
Cultural role	Resentment
Communication barriers	Guilt
Loss of financial independence	Apathy
Lifestyle of helplessness	Devalues own feelings or opinions

RELATED FACTORS (Etiology)	DEFINING CHARACTERISTICS (Symptoms and Signs)

DIAGNOSIS: Powerlessness—cont'd

Lack of knowledge or skills	Reluctance to express true feelings, fearing alienation from
Health care environment	caregiver
Illness-related regimen	Verbal expressions of having no control over situation,
	outcome, or self-care
	Expressions of doubt about self-worth role performance

DIAGNOSIS: Spiritual Distress

Loss of significant others	Feeling separated or alienated from deity
Challenged belief and value system	Feelings of helplessness or hopelessness
Beliefs opposed by family, peers, or health care providers	Expresses concerns about meaning of life and death and/or
Disruption in usual religious activity	belief system
Effects of personal and family disasters or major life changes	Verbalizes inner conflict about beliefs
	Inability to participate in usual religious practices
	Regards illness as punishment

DIAGNOSIS: Disturbed Thought Processes

Psychological conflicts	Agitation or depressed behavior
Social isolation	Altered sleep patterns
Side effects of sedatives, narcotics, or anesthetics	Inappropriate affect or social behavior
Sleep deprivation	Cognitive dissonance
Sensory overload or deprivation	Confabulations
Stress	Delusions or hallucinations
Anxiety	Disorientation to time, place, person
Depression	Distractibility
Effects of aging	Egocentricity
Emotional trauma	Fabrication
Exposure to unfamiliar environment	Hyper/hypovigilance
Fear of the unknown	Impaired ability to make decisions, solve problems, reason,
Impaired judgment	abstract, conceptualize, calculate
Limited attention span	Inaccurate interpretation of environment
Loss of memory	Inability to perceive and/or repeat message clearly
Negative reactions from others	Memory deficits
Actual loss of:	Non–reality-based thinking
• Control	Nonsensical speech
• Familiar objects	Obsessions
• Routine surroundings	
• Significant other	

DIAGNOSIS: Risk for Violence (Self-Directed or Other-Directed)

Substance abuse or withdrawal	Rage
Toxic reaction to medication	Overt and aggressive acts
Explosive, impulsive, immature personality	Self-destructive behavior
Paranoia	Aggression
Panic state	Increased motor activity
Rage reaction	Hostile, threatening verbalizations
Manic excitement	Body language: clenched fists, facial expressions, rigid
Loneliness	posture, tautness
Perceived threat to self-esteem	Provocative behavior
Response to catastrophic event	Increasing anxiety level
Suicidal behavior	Depression
Change in mental or physical health status	Paranoid ideation
Feelings of alienation	Expresses intent to harm self or others
Physical, sexual, or psychologic abuse	Possession of destructive means: gun, knife, or other
Manipulative behavior	weapon

RELATED FACTORS (Etiology)

DEFINING CHARACTERISTICS (Symptoms and Signs)

DIAGNOSIS: Risk for Violence (Self-Directed or Other-Directed)

Developmental crisis
Lack of support systems
Actual or potential loss of significant other
Significant change in lifestyle

Hallucinations, delusions

ADDITIONAL RELATED NURSING DIAGNOSES

ACTUAL	RISK/WELLNESS
Impaired Adjustment	**Risk**
Anxiety (see Chapter 18)	Risk for Caregiver role strain
Acute Confusion	Risk for Powerlessness
Chronic Confusion	Risk for Suicide
Ineffective Coping	**Wellness**
Dysfunctional Family processes: Alcoholism	Readiness for enhanced Coping
Impaired Memory	Readiness for enhanced Family processes
Disturbed Personal identity	Readiness for enhanced Spiritual well-being
Chronic low Self-esteem	
Situational low Self-esteem	
Self-mutilation	
Impaired Social interaction	
Social isolation	
Wandering	

ABNORMAL FINDINGS

Abnormal Findings

TABLE 7–3: Levels of Consciousness

These terms are commonly used in clinical practice. They spread over a continuum from full alertness to deep coma. The terms are qualitative and therefore are not always reliable. (A *quantitative* tool that serves the same purpose and eliminates ambiguity is the Glasgow Coma Scale in Chapter 23.) These terms are widely accepted, however, and are useful as long as all co-workers agree on definitions and are consistent in their application. To increase clarity when using these terms, record also:

1. The level of stimulus used, ranging progressively from
   a. Name called in normal tone of voice
   b. Name called in loud voice
   c. Light touch on person's arm
   d. Vigorous shake of shoulder
   e. Pain applied

2. The person's response
   a. Amount and quality of movement
   b. Presence and coherence of speech
   c. Opening of eyes and making of eye contact
3. What the person does on cessation of your stimulus

(1) Alert
Awake or readily aroused, oriented, fully aware of external and internal stimuli and responds appropriately, conducts meaningful interpersonal interactions.

(2) Lethargic (or Somnolent)
Not fully alert, drifts off to sleep when not stimulated, can be aroused to name when called in normal voice but looks drowsy, responds appropriately to questions or commands but thinking seems slow and fuzzy, inattentive, loses train of thought, spontaneous movements are decreased.

(3) Obtunded
(Transitional state between lethargy and stupor; some sources omit this level.)
Sleeps most of time, difficult to arouse—needs loud shout or vigorous shake, acts confused when is aroused, converses in monosyllables, speech may be mumbled and incoherent, requires constant stimulation for even marginal cooperation.

(4) Stupor or Semi-Coma
Spontaneously unconscious, responds only to persistent and vigorous shake or pain; has appropriate motor response (i.e., withdraws hand to avoid pain); otherwise can only groan, mumble, or move restlessly; reflex activity persists.

(5) Coma
Completely unconscious, no response to pain or to any external or internal stimuli (e.g., when suctioned, does not try to push the catheter away), light coma has some reflex activity but no purposeful movement, deep coma has no motor response.

Acute Confusional State (Delirium)
Clouding of consciousness (dulled cognition, impaired alertness); inattentive; incoherent conversation; impaired recent memory and confabulatory for recent events; often agitated and having visual hallucinations; disoriented, with confusion worse at night when environmental stimuli are decreased.

Adapted from Strub RL, Black FW: *The mental status examination in neurology,* ed 3, Philadelphia, 1993, F.A. Davis, with permission.

TABLE 7–4: **Speech Disorders**

CONDITION	DISORDER OF	DESCRIPTION
Dysphonia	Voice	Difficulty or discomfort in talking, with abnormal pitch or volume, due to laryngeal disease. Voice sounds hoarse or whispered, but articulation and language are intact.
Dysarthria	Articulation	Distorted speech sounds; speech may sound unintelligible; basic language (word choice, grammar, comprehension) intact.
Aphasia	Language comprehension and production secondary to brain damage	True language disturbance, defect in word choice and grammar or defect in comprehension; defect is in *higher* integrative language processing.

TYPES OF APHASIA

An earlier dichotomy classified aphasias as expressive (difficulty producing language) or receptive (difficulty understanding language). Since all people with aphasia have some difficulty with expression, beginning examiners tend to classify them all as expressive. The following system is more descriptive.

CONDITION	DESCRIPTION
Global aphasia	The most common and severe form. Spontaneous speech is absent or reduced to a few stereotyped words or sounds. Comprehension is absent or reduced to only the person's own name and a few select words. Repetition, reading, and writing are severely impaired. Prognosis for language recovery is poor. Caused by a large lesion that damages most of combined anterior and posterior language areas.
Broca's aphasia	Expressive aphasia. The person can understand language but cannot express him- or herself using language. This is characterized by nonfluent, dysarthric, and effortful speech. The speech is mostly nouns and verbs (high-content words) with few grammatic fillers, termed "agrammatic" or "telegraphic" speech. Repetition and reading aloud are severely impaired. Auditory and reading comprehensions are surprisingly intact. Lesion is in anterior language area called the *motor speech cortex* or *Broca's area.*
Wernicke's aphasia	Receptive aphasia. The linguistic opposite of Broca's aphasia. The person can hear sounds and words but cannot relate them to previous experiences. Speech is fluent, effortless, and well articulated but has many paraphasias (word substitutions that are malformed or wrong) and neologisms (made-up words) and often lacks substantive words. Speech can be totally incomprehensible. Often, there is a great urge to speak. Repetition, reading, and writing also are impaired. Lesion is in posterior language area called the *Association auditory cortext* or *Wernicke's area.*

(For a discussion of other types of aphasia [e.g., conduction, anomic, transcortical, and so on], please consult a neurology text.)

ABNORMAL FINDINGS

TABLE 7–5: Abnormalities of Mood and Affect

TYPE OF MOOD OR AFFECT	DEFINITION	CLINICAL EXAMPLE
Flat affect (blunted affect)	Lack of emotional response; no expression of feelings; voice monotonous and face immobile	Topic varies, expression does not
Depression	Sad, gloomy, dejected; symptoms may occur with rainy weather, after a holiday, or with an illness; if the situation is temporary, symptoms fade quickly	"I've got the blues."
Depersonalization (lack of ego boundaries)	Loss of identity, feels estranged, perplexed about own identity and meaning of existence	"I don't feel real." "I feel like I'm not really here."
Elation	Joy and optimism, overconfidence, increased motor activity, not necessarily pathologic	"I'm feeling very happy."
Euphoria	Excessive well-being, unusually cheerful or elated, which is inappropriate considering physical and mental condition, implies a pathologic mood	"I am high." "I feel like I'm flying." "I feel on top of the world."
Anxiety	Worried, uneasy, apprehensive from the anticipation of a danger whose source is unknown	"I feel nervous and high strung." "I worry all the time." "I can't seem to make up my mind."
Fear	Worried, uneasy, apprehensive; external danger is known and identified	Fear of flying in airplanes
Irritability	Annoyed, easily provoked, impatient	Person internalizes a feeling of tension, and a seemingly mild stimulus "sets him (or her) off"
Rage	Furious, loss of control	Person has expressed violent behavior toward self or others
Ambivalence	The existence of opposing emotions toward an idea, object, person	A person feels love and hate toward another at the same time
Lability	Rapid shift of emotions	Person expresses euphoric, tearful, angry feelings in rapid succession
Inappropriate affect	Affect clearly discordant with the content of the person's speech	Laughs while discussing admission for liver biopsy

TABLE 7–6: **Abnormalities of Thought Process**

Type of Process	Definition	Clinical Example
Blocking	Sudden interruption in train of thought, unable to complete sentence, seems related to strong emotion	"Forgot what I was going to say."
Confabulation	Fabricates events to fill in memory gaps	Gives detailed description of his long walk around the hospital although you know Mr. J remained in his room all afternoon.
Neologism	Coining a new word; invented word has no real meaning except for the person; may condense several words	"I'll have to turn on my thinkilator."
Circumlocution	Round-about expression, substituting a phrase when cannot think of name of object	Says "the thing you open the door with" instead of "key."
Circumstantiality	Talks with excessive and unnecessary detail, delays reaching point; sentences have a meaningful connection but are irrelevant (this occurs normally in some people)	"When was my surgery? Well I was 28, I was living with my aunt, she's the one with psoriasis, she had it bad that year because of the heat, the heat was worse then than it was the summer of '82, . . . "
Loosening associations	Shifting from one topic to an unrelated topic; person seems unaware that topics are unconnected	"My boss is angry with me and it wasn't even my fault. *(pause)* I saw that movie too, Lassie. I felt really bad about it. But she kept trying to land the airplane and she never knew what was going on."
Flight of ideas	Abrupt change, rapid skipping from topic to topic, practically continuous flow of accelerated speech; topics usually have recognizable associations or are plays on words	"Take this pill? The pill is blue. I feel blue. *(sings)* She wore blue velvet."
Word salad	Incoherent mixture of words, phrases, and sentences; illogical, disconnected, includes neologisms	"Beauty, red based five, pigeon, the street corner, sort-of."
Perseveration	Persistent repeating of verbal or motor response, even with varied stimuli	"I'm going to lock the door, lock the door. I walk every day and I lock the door. I usually take the dog and I lock the door."
Echolalia	Imitation, repeats others' words or phrases, often with a mumbling, mocking, or mechanical tone	Nurse: "I want you to take your pill." Patient *(mocking):* "Take your pill. Take your pill."
Clanging	Word choice based on sound, not meaning, includes nonsense rhymes and puns	"My feet are cold. Cold, bold, told. The bell tolled for me."

TABLE 7–7: **Abnormalities of Thought Content**

TYPE OF CONTENT	DEFINITION	CLINICAL EXAMPLE
Phobia	Strong, persistent, irrational fear of an object or situation; feels driven to avoid it	Cats, dogs, heights, enclosed spaces
Hypochondriasis	Morbid worrying about his or her own health, feels sick with no actual basis for that assumption	Preoccupied with the fear of having cancer; any symptom or physical sign means cancer
Obsession	Unwanted, persistent thoughts or impulses; logic will not purge them from consciousness; experienced as intrusive and senseless	Violence (parent having repeated impulse to kill a loved child); contamination (becoming infected by shaking hands)
Compulsion	Unwanted repetitive, purposeful act; driven to do it; behavior thought to neutralize or prevent discomfort or some dreaded event	Hand-washing, counting, checking and rechecking, touching
Delusions	Firm, fixed, false beliefs; irrational; person clings to delusion despite objective evidence to contrary	Grandiose—person believes he or she is God; famous, historical, or sports figure; or other well-known person Persecution—"They are out to get me."

TABLE 7–8: **Abnormalities of Perception**

TYPE OF PERCEPTION	DEFINITION	CLINICAL EXAMPLE
Hallucination	Sensory perceptions for which there are no external stimuli; may strike any sense: visual, auditory, tactile, olfactory, gustatory	Visual: seeing an image (ghost) of a person who is not there; auditory: hearing voices or music
Illusion	*Mis*perception of an actual existing stimulus, by any sense	Folds of bedsheets appear to be animated

TABLE 7–9: Delirium, Dementia, and Amnestic Disorders*

Delirium

A. **Disturbance of consciousness** (i.e., reduced clarity of awareness of the environment) with reduced ability to focus, sustain, or shift attention

B. A **change in cognition** (such as memory deficit, disorientation, language disturbance) or the development of a perceptual disturbance

C. The disturbance **develops over a short period of time** (usually hours to days) and tends to fluctuate during the course of the day

Delirium may be due to a **general medical condition:** systemic infections, metabolic disorders (e.g., hypoxia, hypercarbia, hypoglycemia), fluid or electrolyte imbalances, liver or kidney disease, thiamine deficiency, postoperative states, hypertensive encephalopathy, or following seizures or head trauma.
Delirium also may be **substance-induced** (i.e., due to a drug of abuse, a medication, or toxin exposure).

Dementia

A. The development of multiple cognitive deficits manifested by both
  1. **Memory impairment** (impaired ability to learn new information or to recall previously learned information), and
  2. One (or more) of the following **cognitive disturbances:**
    a. Aphasia (language disturbance)
    b. Apraxia (impaired ability to carry out motor activities despite intact motor function)
    c. Agnosia (failure to recognize or identify objects despite intact sensory function)
    d. Disturbance in executive functioning (i.e., planning, organizing, sequencing, abstracting)

B. The cognitive deficits must be sufficiently severe to cause **impairment in occupational or social functioning** and must represent a decline from a previously higher level of functioning

Dementias have a common symptom presentation but are differentiated based on etiology, which include senile dementia of the Alzheimer's type or SDAT (course is characterized by gradual onset and continuing cognitive decline); dementia due to cerebrovascular disease (characterized by focal neurologic signs and symptoms, e.g., exaggeration of deep tendon reflexes, extensor plantar response, gait abnormalities, weakness of an extremity); human immunodeficiency virus disease; head trauma; Parkinson's disease, and others.

Amnestic Disorder

A. The development of **memory impairment** (inability to learn new information or to recall previously learned information) in the absence of other significant cognitive impairments

B. The memory disturbance causes significant **impairment in social or occupational functioning** and represents a significant decline from a previous level of functioning

This may be due to pathology (closed head trauma, penetrating missile wounds, surgical intervention, hypoxia, infarction of the posterior cerebral artery, herpes simplex encephalitis), or it may be substance induced (e.g., alcohol-induced amnestic disorder due to thiamine deficiency associated with prolonged, heavy ingestion of alcohol).

*The terms *organic mental disorder* and *organic brain syndrome* are no longer used for these disorders. These diagnostic categories are meant to be illustrative, not inclusive. Please refer to the original source for additional details and for further categories.
  Adapted from the American Psychiatric Association: *Diagnostic and statistical manual of mental disorders,* ed 4, Washington, DC, 1994, American Psychiatric Association. Reprinted with permission from the *Diagnostic and Statistical Manual of Mental Disorders,* ed 4. © 1994 American Psychiatric Association.

ABNORMAL FINDINGS

TABLE 7-10: Substance Use Disorders

"Substances" refer to those agents taken nonmedically to alter mood or behavior

Intoxication: ingestion of substance produces maladaptive behavior changes due to effects on the central nervous system

Abuse: daily use needed to function, inability to stop, impaired social and occupational functioning, recurrent use when it is physically hazardous, substance-related legal problems

Dependence: physiologic dependence on substance

Tolerance: requires increased amount of substance to produce same effect

Withdrawal: cessation of substance produces a syndrome of physiologic symptoms

SUBSTANCE	INTOXICATION	WITHDRAWAL
Alcohol	**Appearance.** Unsteady gait, incoordination, nystagmus, flushed face **Behavior.** Sedation, relief of anxiety, dulled concentration, impaired judgment, expansive, uninhibited behavior, talkativeness, slurred speech, impaired memory, irritability, depression, emotional lability	**Uncomplicated.** (Shortly after cessation of drinking, lasts 5 to 7 days.) Coarse tremor of hands, tongue, eyelids; anorexia; nausea and vomiting; malaise; autonomic hyperactivity (tachycardia, sweating, elevated blood pressure); headache; insomnia; anxiety; depression or irritability; transient hallucinations or illusions **Withdrawal delirium, "delirium tremens."** (Much less common than uncomplicated, occurs within 1 week of cessation.) Coarse, irregular tremor; marked autonomic hyperactivity (tachycardia, sweating); vivid hallucinations; delusions; agitated behavior; fever
Sedatives, hypnotics	Similar to alcohol **Appearance.** Unsteady gait, incoordination **Behavior.** Talkativeness, slurred speech, inattention, impaired memory, irritability, emotional lability, sexual aggressiveness, impaired judgment, impaired social or occupational functioning	Anxiety or irritability; nausea or vomiting; malaise; autonomic hyperactivity (tachycardia, sweating); orthostatic hypotension; coarse tremor of hands, tongue, and eyelids; marked insomnia; grand mal seizures
Nicotine	**Appearance.** Alerting, increased systolic blood pressure, increased heart rate, vasoconstriction **Behavior.** Nausea, vomiting, indigestion (first use); loss of appetite, head rush, dizziness, jittery feeling, mild stimulant	Vasodilation, headaches; anger, irritability, frustration, anxiety, nervousness, awakening at night, difficulty concentrating, depression, hunger, impatience or restlessness, desire to smoke
Cannabis (marijuana)	**Appearance.** Injected (reddened) conjunctivae, tachycardia, dry mouth, increased appetite, especially for "junk" food **Behavior.** Euphoria, anxiety, slowed time perception, increased perceptions, impaired judgment, social withdrawal, suspiciousness or paranoid ideation	
Cocaine	**Appearance.** Pupillary dilation, tachycardia or bradycardia, elevated or lowered blood pressure, sweating, chills, nausea, vomiting, weight loss **Behavior.** Euphoria, talkativeness, hypervigilance, pacing, psychomotor agitation, impaired social or occupational functioning, fighting, grandiosity, visual or tactile hallucinations	Dysphoric mood (anxiety, depression, irritability), fatigue, insomnia or hypersomnia, psychomotor agitation

Continued

TABLE 7–10: Substance Use Disorders—cont'd

SUBSTANCE	INTOXICATION	WITHDRAWAL
Amphetamines	Similar to cocaine **Appearance.** Pupillary dilation, tachycardia, or bradycardia, elevated or lowered blood pressure, sweating or chills, nausea and vomiting, weight loss **Behavior.** Elation, talkativeness, hypervigilance, psychomotor agitation, fighting, grandiosity, impaired judgment, impaired social and occupational functioning	Dysphoric mood (anxiety, depression, irritability), fatigue, insomnia or hypersomnia, psychomotor agitation
Opiates (morphine, heroin, meperidine)	**Appearance.** Pinpoint pupils, decreased blood pressure, pulse, respirations, and temperature **Behavior.** Lethargy; somnolence; slurred speech; initial euphoria followed by apathy, dysphoria, and psychomotor retardation; inattention; impaired memory; impaired judgment; impaired social or occupational functioning	Dilated pupils, lacrimation, runny nose, tachycardia, fever, elevated blood pressure, piloerection, sweating, diarrhea, yawning, insomnia, restlessness, irritability, depression, nausea, vomiting, malaise, tremor, muscle and joint pains; symptoms are remarkably similar to clinical picture of influenza

TABLE 7–11: Schizophrenia*

A. Characteristic Symptoms

Two (or more) of the following, each present for a significant part of a 1-month period:

1. Delusions, i.e., involving a phenomenon that the person's culture would regard as totally implausible, such as thought broadcasting, being controlled by a dead person
2. Hallucinations (auditory are more common), e.g., voices speaking directly to the person or commenting on his or her ongoing behavior
3. Disorganized speech, e.g., frequent derailment or incoherence
4. Grossly disorganized or catatonic behavior
5. Negative symptoms, i.e., affective flattening, alogia (inability to speak), or avolition

B. Social/Occupational Dysfunction

One or more major areas of functioning such as work, interpersonal relations, or self-care are markedly below the level achieved prior to onset of the disturbance

C. Duration

Continuous signs persist for at least 6 months, including at least 1 month of symptoms from criterion A (i.e., active phase) and may include periods of prodromal or residual symptoms

*These diagnostic categories are meant to be illustrative, not inclusive. The reader is referred to the original source or a psychiatry textbook for further categories and schizophrenia subtypes, such as Paranoid Type, Catatonic Type, Disorganized Type.

Adapted from American Psychiatric Association: *Diagnostic and statistical manual of mental disorders,* ed 4, Washington, DC, 1994, American Psychiatric Association. Reprinted with permission from the *Diagnostic and Statistical Manual of Mental Disorders,* ed 4, © 1994 American Psychiatric Association.

TABLE 7–12: Mood Disorders*

Major Depressive Episode
Characteristics

A. Five (or more) of the following symptoms present during the same 2-week period and represent a change from previous functioning; at least one of the symptoms is either (1) depressed mood, or (2) loss of interest or pleasure.

Note: Do not include symptoms that are clearly caused by a general medical condition, or delusions, or hallucinations.

1. **Depressed mood** most of the day nearly every day, as indicated by either subjective report (e.g., feels sad or empty) or by observation by others (e.g., appears tearful).
   Note: In children and adolescents, can be irritable mood
2. Markedly **diminished interest or pleasure** in all, or almost all, activities most of the day nearly every day
3. Significant **weight loss** when not dieting, weight gain (e.g., a change of >5% body weight in a month), or decrease or increase in appetite nearly every day.
   Note: In children, consider failure to make expected weight gains
4. **Insomnia** or hypersomnia nearly every day
5. **Psychomotor agitation** or retardation nearly every day
6. **Fatigue** or loss of energy nearly every day
7. Feelings of **worthlessness** or excessive or inappropriate guilt nearly every day
8. **Diminished ability to think** or concentrate, or indecisiveness, nearly every day
9. Recurrent **thoughts of death** (not just fear of dying), recurrent suicidal ideation without a specific plan, or a suicide attempt or a specific plan for committing suicide

B. The symptoms cause clinically significant distress or impairment in social, occupational, or other important areas of functioning.

C. The symptoms are not due to the direct physiologic effects of a substance (e.g., drug of abuse, a medication) or a general medical condition (e.g., hypothyroidism) and are not better accounted for by bereavement, as with loss of a loved one (unless persist for longer than 2 months or are characterized by functional impairment, morbid preoccupation with worthlessness, suicidal ideation, psychotic symptoms, or psychomotor retardation).

Manic Episode
Characteristics

A. A distinct period of abnormally and **persistently elevated, expansive, or irritable mood,** lasting at least 1 week (or any duration if hospitalization is necessary).

B. During this period of mood disturbance, three (or more) of the following symptoms have persisted (four if the mood is only irritable):

1. Inflated self-esteem or grandiosity
2. Decreased need for sleep (e.g., feels rested after only 3 hours of sleep)
3. More talkative than usual or pressure to keep talking
4. Flight of ideas or subjective experience that thoughts are racing
5. Distractibility (i.e., attention too easily drawn to unimportant or irrelevant external stimuli)
6. Increase in goal-directed activity (either socially, at work or school, or sexually) or psychomotor agitation
7. Excessive involvement in pleasurable activities that have a high potential for painful consequences (e.g., engaging in unrestrained buying sprees, sexual indiscretions, or foolish business investments)

C. The mood disturbance is sufficiently severe to cause marked impairment in occupational functioning or in usual social activities or relationships with others, or to necessitate hospitalization to prevent harm to self or others, or there are psychotic features.

D. The symptoms are not due to the direct physiologic effects of a substance (e.g., a drug of abuse, a medication) or a general medical condition (e.g., hyperthyroidism).

Major depressive disorder is characterized by one or more major depressive episodes (i.e., at least 2 weeks of depressed mood or loss of interest accompanied by at least four additional symptoms of depression); **dysthymic disorder** is characterized by at least 2 years of depressed mood for more days than not, accompanied by additional depressive symptoms; **bipolar disorder** is characterized by one or more manic episodes usually accompanied by major depressive episodes.

*These diagnostic categories are meant to be illustrative, not inclusive. The reader is referred to the original source or a psychiatry textbook for further categories, such as personality disorders or somatiform disorders.
  Adapted from American Psychiatric Association: *Diagnostic and statistical manual of mental disorders,* ed 4, Washington, DC, 1994, American Psychiatric Association. Reprinted with permission from the *Diagnostic and Statistical Manual of Mental Disorders,* ed 4. © 1994 American Psychiatric Association.

TABLE 7–13: Anxiety Disorders*

Panic Attack

A discrete period of **intense fear or discomfort,** in which four (or more) of the following symptoms developed abruptly and reached a peak within 10 minutes:

1. Palpitations, pounding heart, or accelerated heart rate
2. Sweating
3. Trembling or shaking
4. Sensations of shortness of breath or smothering
5. Feeling of choking
6. Chest pain or discomfort
7. Nausea or abdominal distress
8. Feeling dizzy, unsteady, lightheaded, or faint
9. Derealization (feelings of unreality) or depersonalization (being detached from oneself)
10. Fear of losing control or going crazy
11. Fear of dying
12. Paresthesias (numbness or tingling sensations)
13. Chills or hot flashes

Agoraphobia

A. Anxiety about being in places or situations from which escape might be difficult (or embarrassing) or in which help may not be available in the event of having a panic attack or paniclike symptoms—agoraphobic fears typically involve being outside the home alone; being in a crowd or standing in a line; being on a bridge; and traveling in a bus, train, or automobile.

B. The situations are avoided (e.g., travel is restricted), are endured with marked distress or with anxiety about having a panic attack or paniclike symptoms, or require the presence of a companion.

Panic Disorder

A. Both 1. and 2. occur:

1. Recurrent unexpected panic attacks (see above)
2. At least one of the attacks has been followed by 1 month (or more) of one (or more) of the following:
   a. Persistent concern about having additional attacks
   b. Worry about the implications of the attack or its consequences (e.g., losing control, having a heart attack, "going crazy")
   c. A significant change in behavior related to the attacks

B. Agoraphobia may be present or absent.

Specific Phobia

A. Marked and persistent fear that is excessive or unreasonable, cued by a specific object or situation (e.g., flying, heights, animals, receiving an injection, seeing blood).

B. Exposure to the phobic stimulus almost invariably provokes an immediate anxiety response, which may be a panic attack. Note: In children, the anxiety may be expressed by crying, tantrums, freezing, or clinging.

C. The person recognizes that the fear is excessive or unreasonable.

D. The phobic situation is avoided or is endured with intense anxiety or distress.

E. This interferes significantly with the person's normal routine, occupational (or academic) functioning, or social activities or relationships.

*These diagnostic categories are meant to be illustrative, not inclusive. The reader is referred to the original source or a psychiatry textbook for further details and categories of anxiety disorders.

Adapted from American Psychiatric Association: *Diagnostic and statistical manual of mental disorders,* ed 4, Washington, DC, 1994, American Psychiatric Association. Reprinted with permission from the *Diagnostic and Statistical Manual of Mental Disorders,* ed 4. © 1994 American Psychiatric Association.

TABLE 7–13: Anxiety Disorders—cont'd

Social Phobia

A. A marked and persistent fear of one or more social or performance situations in which the person is exposed to unfamiliar people or to possible scrutiny by others; the individual fears that he or she will act in a way (or show anxiety symptoms) that will be humiliating or embarrassing.

B.–E.: The same as in specific phobia.

Obsessive-Compulsive Disorder

A. Person has either obsessions:

1. Recurrent and persistent thoughts, impulses, or images that are experienced as intrusive and inappropriate and that cause marked anxiety or distress
2. The thoughts, impulses, or images are not simply excessive worries about real-life problems
3. The person attempts to ignore or suppress such thoughts, impulses, or images, or to neutralize them with some other thought or action
4. The person recognizes that the obsessional thoughts are a product of his or her own mind (not imposed from without)

or compulsions:

1. Repetitive behaviors (e.g., hand-washing, ordering, checking) or mental acts (e.g., praying, counting, repeating words silently) that the person feels driven to perform in response to an obsession, or according to rules that must be applied rigidly
2. The behaviors or mental acts are aimed at preventing or reducing distress or at preventing some dreaded event or situation

B. At some point, the person has recognized that the obsessions or compulsions are excessive or unreasonable.

C. The obsessions or compulsions cause marked distress; are time consuming; or significantly interfere with the person's normal routine, occupational (or academic) functioning, or usual social activities or relationships.

Posttraumatic Stress Disorder

A. The person has been exposed to a traumatic event in which
1. The person experienced, witnessed, or was confronted with the actual or threatened death or serious injury of self or others
2. The person's response involved intense fear, helplessness, or horror

B. The traumatic event is persistently reexperienced by:
1. Recurrent and intrusive distressing recollections of the event, including images, thoughts, or perceptions
2. Recurrent distressing dreams of the event
3. Acting or feeling as if the traumatic event were recurring

C. Persistent avoidance of stimuli associated with the trauma and numbing of general responsiveness (e.g., feeling of detachment or estrangement from others, unable to have loving feelings, sense of a foreshortened future).

D. Persistent symptoms of increased arousal:
1. Difficulty falling or staying asleep
2. Irritability or outbursts of anger
3. Difficulty concentrating
4. Hypervigilance
5. Exaggerated startle response

Generalized Anxiety Disorder

A. Excessive anxiety and worry occurring more days than not for at least 6 months about a number of events or activities (such as work or school performance).

B. The person finds it difficult to control the worry.

C. The anxiety and worry are associated with three (or more) of the following:
1. Restlessness or feeling keyed up or on edge
2. Being easily fatigued
3. Difficulty concentrating or mind going blank
4. Irritability
5. Muscle tension
6. Sleep disturbance

BIBLIOGRAPHY

American Psychiatric Association: *Diagnostic and statistical manual of mental disorders,* ed 4, Washington, DC, 1994, American Psychiatric Association.

Birren JE, Schaie KW, editors: *Handbook of the psychology of aging,* ed 5, San Diego, 2001, Academic Press.

Brackley MH: Mental health assessment/mental status examination, *Nurse Practitioner Forum* 8(3):105–113, Sept 1997.

Clark CC: Posttraumatic stress disorder: how to support healing, *Am J Nurs* 97(8):27–32, 1997.

Depaulo JR Jr, Folstein MF: Psychiatric disturbances in neurological patients: detection, recognition and hospital course, *Ann Neurol* 4:225–228, Aug 1978.

Dubin S: The mini-mental state exam, *Am J Nurs* 98(11):16D, Nov 1998.

Folstein MF, Folstein SE, McHugh PR: "Mini-mental state": a practical method for grading the cognitive state of patients for the clinician, *J Psychiatr Res* 12:189–198, 1975.

Inouye SK et al: Importance of functional measures in predicting mortality among older hospitalized patients, *JAMA* 279(15): 1187–1193, April 15 1998.

Isaacs B, Kennie A: The set test as an aid to the detection of dementia in old people, *Br J Psychiatry* 123:467–470, 1973.

Kane RL, Ouslander JG, Abrass IB: *Essentials of clinical geriatrics,* ed 4, New York, 1999, McGraw-Hill.

Keller MB, Manschreck TC: The bedside mental status examination-reliability and validity, *Compr Psychiatry* 22(5):500–511, 1981.

Kreeger JL et al: Effect of hearing enhancement on mental status ratings in geriatric psychiatric patients, *Am J Psychiatry* 152(4): 629–631, Apr 1995.

Lang MM: Screening for cognitive impairment in the older adult, *Nurse Pract* 26(11):26–43, Nov 2001.

Lucas BD: Coping with psychiatric emergencies in the office, *Patient Care for the Nurse Practitioner* 2(2):25–42, Feb 1999.

Mangino M, Middlemiss C: Alzheimer's disease: preventing and recognizing a misdiagnosis, *Nurs Pract* 22(10):58–75, 1997.

McCrea M: Standardized mental status assessment of sports concussion, *Clin J Sport Med* 11(3):176–181, July 2001.

Norton JW: Personality disorders in the primary care setting, *Nurse Pract* 25(12):40–63, 2000.

O'Keefe KP, Sanson TG: Elderly patients with altered mental status, *Emerg Med Clin North Am* 16(4):701–715, Nov 1998.

Rapp CG et al: Acute confusion assessment instruments: clinical versus research usability, *Appl Nurs Res* 13(1):37–45, Feb 2000.

Reeves RR, Pendarvis EJ, Kimble R: Unrecognized medical emergencies admitted to psychiatric units, *Am J Emerg Med* 18(4):390–393, Jul 2000.

Solnek BL, Seiter T: How to diagnose and treat depression, *Nurse Pract* 27(10):12–23, Oct 2002.

Souder E, O'Sullivan PS: Nursing documentation versus standardized assessment of cognitive status in hospitalized medical patients, *Appl Nurs Res* 13(1):29–36, Feb 2000.

Strub RL, Black FW: *The mental status examination in neurology,* ed 4, Philadelphia, 1999, F.A. Davis.

Sulkowski JA, Judy KD: Acute mental status changes, *AACN Clin Issues* 8(3):319–334, Aug 1997.

Sullivan-Marx EM: Delirium and physical restraint in the hospitalized elderly, *Image* 26(4):295–300, 1994.

Tocchi C: Altered mental status—understanding a comprehensive differential, *Clinical Letter for Nurse Practitioners* 4(3):1–6, May-June 2000.

Tully MW et al: The Eating Behavior Scale: a simple method of assessing functional ability in patients with Alzheimer's disease, *J Gerontol Nurs* 23(7):9–15, July 1997.

Nutritional Assessment

Structure and Function

DEFINING NUTRITIONAL STATUS

Nutritional status refers to the degree of balance between nutrient intake and nutrient requirements. This balance is affected by many factors, including physiologic, psychosocial, developmental, cultural, and economic.

Optimal nutritional status is achieved when sufficient nutrients are consumed to support day-to-day body needs and any increased metabolic demands due to growth, pregnancy, or illness. Persons having optimal nutritional status are more active, have fewer physical illnesses, and live longer than persons who are malnourished.

Undernutrition occurs when nutritional reserves are depleted and/or when nutrient intake is inadequate to meet day-to-day needs or added metabolic demands. Vulnerable groups—infants, children, pregnant women, recent immigrants, persons with low incomes, hospitalized people, and aging adults—are at risk for impaired growth and development, lowered resistance to infection and disease, delayed wound healing, longer hospital stays, and higher health care costs.

Overnutrition is caused by the consumption of nutrients—especially calories, sodium, and fat—in excess of body needs. A major nutritional problem today, overnutrition can lead to obesity and related diseases (e.g., type 2 diabetes, heart disease). An estimated 13% of children (ages 6 to 11), 14% of adolescents (ages 12 to 19), and 61% of adults in the United States are overweight or obese (NCHS, 1999). These data are of considerable concern because they represent notable increases in prevalence from previous surveys (NHANES III, 1988–1994). Being overweight during childhood and adolescence is associated with increased risk for becoming overweight during adulthood (NCHS, 1999).

 DEVELOPMENTAL CONSIDERATIONS

INFANTS AND CHILDREN

The time from birth to 4 months of age is the most rapid period of growth in the life cycle. Although infants lose weight during the first few days of life, birth weight is usually regained by the 7th to 10th day after birth. Thereafter, infants double their birth weight by 4 months and triple it by 1 year of age. Breastfeeding is recommended for full-term infants for the 1st year of life because breast milk is ideally formulated to promote normal infant growth and development and natural immunity. Although relatively few contraindications to breastfeeding exist, women who are human immunodeficiency virus (HIV) positive should not breastfeed, since HIV can be transmitted through breast milk. The number of pounds gained during the second year approximates the birth weight.

Infants increase their length by 50% during the first year of life and double it by 4 years of age. Brain size also increases very rapidly during infancy and childhood. By age 2 years, the brain has reached 50% of its adult size; by age 4, 75%; and by age 8, 100%. For this reason, infants and children younger than 2 should not drink skim or low-fat milk or be placed on low-fat diets—fat (calories and essential fatty acids) is required for proper growth and central nervous system development.

The Recommended Dietary Intakes for infants and children are illustrated in Appendix C.

ADOLESCENCE

Following a period of slow growth in late childhood, adolescence is characterized by rapid physical growth and endocrine and hormonal changes. Caloric and protein requirements increase to meet this demand, and because of bone growth and increasing muscle mass (and, in girls, the onset of menarche), calcium and iron requirements also increase. Typically, these increased requirements cannot be met by three meals per day; therefore, nutritious snacks play an important role in achieving adequate nutrient intake. The recommended ranges of caloric and protein intakes for adolescents are shown in Appendix C.

In general, boys grow taller and have less body fat than girls. The percent of body fat increases in females to about 25% and decreases in males (replaced by muscle mass) to about 12%. Typically, girls double their body weight between the ages of 8 and 14; boys double their body weight between the ages of 10 and 17 years.

PREGNANCY AND LACTATION

To support the synthesis of maternal and fetal tissues, sufficient calories, protein, vitamins, and minerals must be consumed. The National Academy of Sciences (NAS) recommends a weight gain of 25 to 35 lb for women of normal weight, 28 to 40 lb for underweight women, and 15 to 25 lb for overweight women. See Appendix C for increased requirements of pregnancy and lactation. Appendix D gives recommended weight gain guidelines based on body mass index, and illustrates curves of desirable weight gain during pregnancy, as recommended by the Subcommittee on Nutritional Status and Weight Gain During Pregnancy (National Academy of Sciences, 1990).

ADULTHOOD

During adulthood, growth and nutrient needs stabilize. Most adults are in relatively good health. However, unhealthy habits such as cigarette smoking, stressful lifestyles, lack of exercise, excessive alcohol intake, and diets high in saturated fat, cholesterol, salt, and sugar and low in fiber can be factors in the development of hypertension, obesity, atherosclerosis, cancer, osteoporosis, and diabetes mellitus. The adult years, therefore, are an important time for education, to preserve health and to prevent or delay the onset of chronic disease.

The RDAs for this group (persons aged 23 to 50 years) for protein, energy, vitamin, and mineral intakes are shown in Appendix C.

THE AGING ADULT

As people age, a number of changes occur that make them prone to undernutrition or overnutrition. Poor physical or mental health, social isolation, alcoholism, limited functional ability, poverty, and polypharmacy are the major risk factors for malnutrition in older adults (Drewnowski & Shultz, 2001). Normal physiological changes in aging adults that directly affect nutritional status include poor dentition, decreased visual acuity, decreased saliva production, slowed gastrointestinal motility, decreased gastrointestinal absorption, and diminished olfactory and taste sensitivity.

Socioeconomic conditions frequently have a significant effect on the nutritional status of the aging adult. Decline of extended families and increased mobility of families reduce available support systems. Facilities for meal preparation and eating, transportation to grocery stores, physical limitations, income, and social isolation are frequent problems and can obviously interfere with the acquisition of a balanced diet. Medications must also be considered, because aging adults frequently take multiple medications that have a potential for interaction with nutrients and with one another.

Important nutritional features of the older years are a decrease in energy requirements due to loss of lean body mass, the most metabolically active tissue, and an increase in fat mass. Between the ages of 51 and 75, energy needs decrease by approximately 200 kcal/day in both men and women. After age 75, energy needs decrease by 500 kcal and 400 kcal/day in males and females, respectively. The protein requirement of 0.8 g/kg/day for younger adults is appropriate for the healthy older person.

TRANSCULTURAL CONSIDERATIONS

Because foods and eating customs are culturally distinct, each person has a unique cultural heritage that may affect nutritional status. Immigrants commonly maintain traditional eating customs long after the language and manner of dress of an adopted country become routine (especially for holidays and observance of religious customs). Occupation, class, religion, gender, and health awareness also have a great bearing on eating customs. Within the last decade, hundreds of thousands of Southeast Asians, Mexicans, and Cubans have immigrated to the United States. Not only do their food habits change to accommodate their new cultures, but their food habits have influence on their adoptive country. The popularity of tofu, stir-fried vegetables, tortillas, and rice and beans is just one example of these influences on American eating habits (Fig. 8–1).

Newly arriving immigrants may be at nutritional risk for a variety of reasons. They frequently come from countries with limited food supplies caused by poverty, poor sanitation, war, or political strife. General undernutrition, hypertension, diarrhea, lactose intolerance, osteomalacia (soft bones), scurvy, and dental caries are among the more common nutrition-related problems of new immigrants from developing countries.

When immigrants arrive in the United States, other factors contribute to their nutritional problems: They are in a new country with a completely new language, culture, and society. They are faced with unfamiliar foods, food storage, food preparation, and food-buying habits. Many familiar foods are difficult or impossible to obtain. Low income may also limit their access to familiar foods. When traditional food habits are disrupted by a new culture, borderline deficiencies or adverse nutritional consequences may result. As an example, Japanese immigrants to the United States have increased risk of colon and breast cancer as they adapt to a diet in the United States that is higher in saturated fats and cholesterol (Ishida, 2001).

Cultural heritage also plays a role in nutrient needs. For example, studies have shown that black women have lower hemoglobin levels than white women independent of iron intake, and that their risk for osteoporosis is significantly less despite lower overall calcium intake. Or, cultural values may conflict with optimum nutrition (e.g., many cultures worldwide consider obesity an indication of beauty, affluence, and well-being).

Because rapid changes in eating patterns and customs are occurring in all countries, what are considered customs today may not be considered traditional in a few years. The best way to learn about the eating patterns of a people is to talk with them, eat with them, and ask about their dietary customs. It is important to keep in mind that recent immigrant groups, such as the Southeast Asians, are often shorter and weigh less than their Western counterparts, so American standard tables of weight for age, height for age, and weight for height may not be appropriate to evaluate growth and development of immigrant children. At present no reliable standards to evaluate every immigrant group exist.

The cultural factors that must be considered are the cultural definition of food, frequency and number of meals eaten away from home, form and content of ceremonial meals, amount and types of foods eaten, and regularity of food consumption. Because inaccuracies may occur, the 24-hour dietary recalls or 3-day food records used traditionally

8–1

for assessment may be inadequate when dealing with people from culturally diverse backgrounds. Standard dietary handbooks may fail to provide culture-specific diet information because nutritional content and exchange tables are generally based on Western diets (Pennington, 1998). Another source of error may originate from cultural patterns of eating. For example, many low-income ethnic groups eat sparingly or moderately during the week (i.e., simple rice or bean dishes), whereas weekend meals are markedly more elaborate (i.e., meats, fruits, vegetables, and sweets are added).

Although you may assume that the term "food" is a universal concept, you should have the person clarify what is meant by the term. For example, certain Latin American groups do not consider chili peppers—an important source of vitamins A and C—to be food and thus fail to list them as vegetables on daily food records. Among Vietnamese refugees, the dietary intake of calcium may appear inadequate, particularly with the low consumption of dairy products common among members of this group. Daily soups prepared by soaking bones in acidified broth or pickled or sweet and sour meats such as pork ribs (vinegar leaches calcium from the bones and makes it available to the body) are, however, commonly consumed, thus providing adequate quantities of calcium to meet daily requirements. Tofu is also a good source of calcium if calcium salts are used to precipitate the curd. For Mexican Americans, tortillas prepared from corn treated with lime water significantly increase dietary calcium. In Middle Eastern countries, yogurt and feta cheese are the major dietary sources of calcium since milk is not commonly consumed by adults.

Food itself is only one part of eating. In some cultures, social contacts during meals are restricted to members of the immediate or extended family. For example, in some Middle Eastern cultures, men and women eat meals separately, or women may be permitted to eat with their husbands, but not with other males. Among some Hispanic groups, the male breadwinner is served first, then women and children. Etiquette during meals, the use of hands, type of eating utensils (e.g., chopsticks, special flatware), and protocols governing the order in which foods is consumed during a meal all vary cross-culturally.

DIETARY PRACTICES OF SELECTED CULTURAL GROUPS

It is necessary to avoid *cultural stereotyping*, the tendency to view individuals of common cultural backgrounds similarly and according to a preconceived notion of how they "ought"

TABLE 8–1: Religious Dietary Practices

RELIGIOUS GROUP	FOOD RESTRICTIONS
Church of Jesus Christ of Latter-Day Saints (Mormons)	No alcoholic beverages No stimulants (caffeinated beverages such as coffee, tea, sodas) Avoid medicines containing caffeine and/or alcohol such as the following: analgesics (e.g., Anacin, Bromo-Seltzer, Empirin, Excedrin), stimulants (e.g., No-Doz, Vivarin, Caffedrine), weight-loss aids (e.g., Dexatrim and related products), and cold medicines (e.g., Nyquil). Observant Mormons fast (refrain from food and liquids) on the first Sunday of each month.

Judaism
  Orthodox—strict observance
  Conservative—nominal observance
  Reform—less ceremonial emphasis and minimum observance of dietary laws
	The *laws of kashrut* dictate which foods are permissible under religious law:
	1. Only meat from cloven-hoofed animals that chew cud (cattle, sheep, goat, ox, or deer) is allowed. These animals must be slaughtered ritually in a manner that results in minimal pain to the animal and maximal blood drainage. There are two methods used to prepare *kosher* (meaning "properly preserved" or "fit for eating") meats: (a) The meat is soaked in cold water for 30 minutes, salted, and drained to deplete blood content. It is then washed under cold water and drained again before cooking, *or* (b) the meat is first prepared by quickly searing or cooking over an open flame, which permits liver to be eaten.
	2. Meat and dairy products cannot be served at the same meal, nor can they be cooked or served in the same set of dishes or eaten with the same utensils. Fish, eggs, vegetables, and fruits are considered *parve* or neutral and may be eaten with dairy products or meat meals.
	3. Fish with fins and scales are allowed. No shellfish (crab, lobster, shrimp, clam, oyster) or scavenger fish (catfish, shark, porpoise) may be eaten. Crocodile, frog, snail, snake, and tortoise also are prohibited.
	Additional dietary laws are followed during the week of Passover. No bread or product with yeast may be eaten; instead *matzah* or unleavened bread is eaten. Products that are fermented or can cause fermenting or souring may not be eaten.

Islam	Pork, pork products, animal shortening, and alcohol are strictly prohibited. The slaughter of poultry, beef, and lamb must be done ritually by a Muslim to ensure that it is *halal.* Fasting is common. During the month of Ramadan, no foods or beverages are consumed until after sunset.
Roman Catholicism	Abstinence from meat and meat products (gravy, soups) and fasting on Ash Wednesday and the Fridays during a 40-day period of religious observance called *Lent.* Rules of fasting apply to those between the ages of 12 and 65.
Seventh-Day Adventism	Fermented or alcoholic beverages are prohibited. Optional vegetarianism may take three forms: (a) strict vegetarians (syn. *vegans*)—people who include no animal-derived products in their diet; (b) ovolactovegetarians—people who use milk, milk products, and eggs but no meats in their diet; and (c) semivegetarians—Adventists who refrain from pork or pork products, shellfish, and blood. Snacking between meals is discouraged.

to behave. For example, despite widely held stereotypes, we know that there are Chinese who do not like rice, Italians who despise spaghetti, Irish who dislike corned beef and cabbage, and so forth. Aggregate dietary preferences among people from certain cultural groups, however, can be described (e.g., characteristic ethnic dishes, methods of food preparation). Refer to nutrition texts on the topic for detailed information about culture-specific diets and the nutritional value of ethnic foods.

Cultural food preferences are often interrelated with religious dietary beliefs and practices. Many religions use foods as symbols in celebrations and rituals. Knowing the person's religious practices related to food enables you to suggest improvements or modifications that do not conflict with dietary laws. Table 8–1 summarizes dietary practices for selected religious groups.

Other issues are fasting and other religious observations that may limit a person's food or liquid intake during specified times (e.g., many Catholics fast and abstain from meat on Ash Wednesday and the Fridays of Lent. Muslims fast from dawn to sunset during the month of Ramadan in the Islamic calendar and eat only twice a day—before dawn and after sunset; Jews observe a 24-hour fast on Yom Kippur).

PURPOSES AND COMPONENTS OF NUTRITIONAL ASSESSMENT

Nutritional status can be determined by the application of nutritional assessment techniques. In general, these techniques are noninvasive, inexpensive, and easy to perform.

The purposes of nutritional assessment are to (1) identify individuals who are malnourished or are at risk of developing malnutrition, (2) provide data for designing a nutrition plan of care that will prevent or minimize the development of malnutrition, and (3) establish baseline data for evaluating the efficacy of nutritional care.

Nutrition screening, the first step in assessing nutritional status, may be completed in any setting (e.g., clinic, home, hospital, long-term care). Based on easily obtained data, nutrition screening is a quick and easy way to identify individuals at nutrition risk, such as those with weight loss, inadequate food intake, or recent illness. Parameters used for nutrition screening typically include weight and weight history, conditions associated with increased nutritional risk, diet information, and routine laboratory data. A variety of valid tools are available for screening different populations. For example, the Admission Nutrition Screening Tool (Kovacevich et al., 1997) was validated for use by nurses in hospitalized patients (Table 8–2), and the Nutrition Screening Initiative form (see Fig. 8–2) was designed and validated in the outpatient, geriatric population (Dwyer, 1991).

Individuals identified at nutritional risk during screening should undergo a **comprehensive nutritional assessment,** which includes dietary history and intake information, physical examination for clinical signs, anthropometric measures, and laboratory tests. The skills needed to collect the dietary history and to perform the physical examination are described in the Subjective Data and Objective Data sections

TABLE 8–2: Admission Nutrition Screening Tool

A. DIAGNOSIS

If the patient has at least ONE of the following diagnoses, circle and proceed to section E to consider the patient AT NUTRITIONAL RISK and stop here.

- Anorexia nervosa/bulimia nervosa
- Malabsorption (celiac sprue, ulcerative colitis, Crohn's disease, short bowel syndrome)
- Multiple trauma (closed head injury, penetrating trauma, multiple fractures)
- Decubitus ulcers
- Major gastrointestinal surgery within the past year
- Cachexia (temporal wasting, muscle wasting, cancer, cardiac)
- Coma
- Diabetes
- End-stage liver disease
- End-stage renal disease
- Nonhealing wounds

B. NUTRITION INTAKE HISTORY

If the patient has at least ONE of the following symptoms, circle and proceed to section E to consider the patient AT NUTRITIONAL RISK and stop here.

- Diarrhea (>500 ml × 2 days)
- Vomiting (>5 days)
- Reduced intake (<$\frac{1}{2}$ normal intake for >5 days)

C. IDEAL BODY WEIGHT STANDARDS

Compare the patients' current weight for height to the ideal body weight chart.

If at <80% of ideal body weight, proceed to section E to consider the patient AT NUTRITIONAL RISK and stop here.

D. WEIGHT HISTORY

Any recent unplanned weight loss? No ___ Yes ___ Amount (lbs or kg) _____

    If yes, within the past _____ weeks or _____ months

    Current weight (lbs or kg) _____

    Usual weight (lbs or kg) _____

    Height (ft, in, or cm) _____

Find percentage of weight loss:

$$\frac{\text{Usual wt} - \text{current wt}}{\text{Usual wt}} \times 100 = \underline{\quad}\% \text{ wt loss}$$

Compare the % wt loss with the chart values and circle appropriate value

Length of Time	Significant (%)	Severe (%)
1 week	1–2	>2
2–3 weeks	2–3	>3
1 month	4–5	>5
3 months	7–8	>8
5+ months	10	>10

If the patient has experienced a significant or severe weight loss, proceed to section E and consider the patient AT NUTRITIONAL RISK

E. NURSE ASSESSMENT

Using the above criteria, what is this patient's nutritional risk? (circle one)

    LOW NUTRITIONAL RISK   AT NUTRITIONAL RISK

Adapted from Kovacevich DS et al: Nutrition risk classification: a valid and reproducible tool for nurses. *Nutr Clin Practice* 12:20–25, 1997. Used with permission.

The warning signs of poor nutritional health are often overlooked. Use this checklist to find out if you or someone you know is at nutritional risk.

DETERMINE YOUR NUTRITIONAL HEALTH

Read the statements below. Circle the number in the yes column for those that apply to you or someone you know. For each yes answer, score the number in the box. Total your nutritional score.

	YES
I have an illness or condition that made me change the kind and/or amount of food I eat.	2
I eat fewer than 2 meals per day.	3
I eat few fruits or vegetables, or milk products.	2
I have 3 or more drinks of beer, liquor or wine almost every day.	2
I have tooth or mouth problems that make it hard for me to eat.	2
I don't always have enough money to buy the food I need.	4
I eat alone most of the time.	1
I take 3 or more different prescribed or over-the-counter drugs a day.	1
Without wanting to, I have lost or gained 10 pounds in the last 6 months.	2
I am not always physically able to shop, cook, and/or feed myself.	2
TOTAL	

Total Your Nutritional Score. If it's —

0-2   Good! Recheck your nutritional score in 6 months.

3-5   You are at moderate nutritional risk. See what can be done to improve your eating habits and lifestyle. Your office on aging, senior nutrition program, senior citizens center, or health department can help. Recheck your nutritional score in 3 months.

6 or more   You are at high nutritional risk. Bring this checklist the next time you see your doctor, dietitian or other qualified health or social service professional. Talk with them about any problems you may have. Ask for help to improve your nutritional health.

These materials developed and distributed by the Nutrition Screening Initiative, a project of:

 AMERICAN ACADEMY OF FAMILY PHYSICIANS

 THE AMERICAN DIETETIC ASSOCIATION

 NATIONAL COUNCIL ON THE AGING, INC.

Remember that warning signs suggest risk, but do not represent diagnosis of any condition.

8–2

---

that follow. Table 8–3 is an example of a form for compiling comprehensive nutritional assessment data.

Various methods for collecting current dietary intake information are available—24-hour recall, food frequency questionnaire, and food diary. During hospitalization, documentation of nutritional intake can best be achieved through calorie counts of nutrients consumed and/or infused.

The easiest and most popular method for obtaining information about dietary intake is the **24-hour recall**. The individual or family member completes a questionnaire or is interviewed and asked to recall everything eaten within the last 24 hours. However, several significant sources of error may occur when this method is used: (1) the individual or family member may not be able to recall the type or amount of food eaten; (2) intake within the last 24 hours may be atypical of usual intake; (3) the individual or family member may alter the truth for a variety of reasons; and (4) snack items and use of gravies, sauces, and condiments may be underreported.

To counter some of the difficulties inherent in the 24-hour recall method, a **food frequency questionnaire** may also be completed. With this tool, information is collected on how many times per day, week, or month the individual eats particular foods. Drawbacks to the use of the food frequency questionnaire are (1) it does not quantify amount of intake, and (2) like the 24-hour recall, it relies on the individual's or family member's memory for how often a food was eaten.

Food diaries or records require asking the individual or family member to write down everything consumed for a certain period of time. Three days—two weekdays and one weekend day—are customarily used. A food diary is most complete and accurate if the individual is instructed to record information immediately after eating. Potential problems with the food diary include (1) noncompliance, (2) inaccurate recording, (3) atypical intake on the recording days, and (4) conscious alteration of diet during the recording period.

Direct observation of the feeding and eating process can lead to detection of problems not readily identified through standard nutrition interviews. For example, observing the typical feeding techniques used by a parent or caregiver and the interaction between the individual and caregiver can be of value when assessing failure to thrive in children or unintentional weight loss in older adults.

TABLE 8–3: Comprehensive Nutritional Assessment Form

Scored
PG-SGA

Institutional Code: _____ Patient Code: _____
Setting: Input   Output Clinic/Office   Homecare   Hospice
Patient Name: _____
Medical Record # (optional): _____
Sex: Male   Female   Age: _____

History

---

1. Weight   *See Table A*

In summary of my current and recent weight:
I currently weigh about _____ pounds
I am about _____ feet _____ inches tall
Six months ago I weighed about _____ pounds
One month ago I weighed about _____ pounds
During the past two weeks, my weight has
☐ decreased (1)   ☐ not changed (0)   ☐ increased (0)

---

2. Food Intake

As compared to my normal, I would rate my food intake
during the past month as either:
☐ unchanged (0)
☐ more than usual (1)
☐ less than usual (1)
    I am now taking: ☐ little solid food (2)
                              ☐ only liquids (3)
                              ☐ only nutritional supplements (3)
                              ☐ very little of anything (4)

---

3. Symptoms

During the past two weeks, I have had the following problems that kept me from eating enough (check all that apply):
☐ no problems eating (0)
☐ no appetite, just did not feel like eating (3)
☐ nausea (1)   ☐ vomiting (3)
☐ constipation (1)   ☐ diarrhea (3)
☐ mouth sores (2)   ☐ dry mouth (1)
☐ pain: (where?) (3) _____
☐ things taste funny or have no taste (1)
☐ smells bother me (1)
☐ other* (1) _____

---

4. Functional Capacity

Over the past month, I would rate my activity as generally:
☐ normal with no limitations (0)
☐ not my normal self, but able to be up and about with fairly
    normal activities (1)
☐ not feeling up to most things, but in bed less than half the
    day (2)
☐ able to do little activity and spend most of the day in bed
    or chair (3)
☐ pretty much bedridden, rarely out of bed (3)

Patient Signature _____

---

*Depression, money, dental problems, etc.

The Remainder of this Form will be Completed by Your Doctor, Nurse, or Therapist. Thank You.

5. Disease and Its Relationship to Nutritional Requirements   *See Table B*
Primary diagnoses (specify) _____
Stage, if known _____
Metabolic demand: *See Table C* ☐ no stress   ☐ low stress   ☐ moderate stress   ☐ high stress

Physical
For each trait specify: 0 = normal   1 = mild   2 = moderate   3 = severe   *See Table D*
____ loss of subcutaneous   ____ muscle wasting   ____ ankle edema   ____ sacral edema   ____ ascites
    fat (triceps, chest)   (quadriceps, deltoids)

SGA Rating
Select One   *See Table E*
☐ A: well nourished   ☐ B: moderately (or suspected) malnourished   ☐ C: severely malnourished
Clinician Signature _____   RD RN PA MD DO Other: _____   Date _____

Table A. Criteria for Scoring Weight Loss

Weight loss in 6 months	Points	Weight loss in 1 month	Points
20% or greater	4	10% or greater	4
10–19.9%	3	5–9.9%	3
6–9.9%	2	3–4.9%	2
2–5.9%	1	2–2.9%	1
0–1.9%	0	0–1.9%	0

Table continued on following page

TABLE 8–3: Comprehensive Nutritional Assessment Form—cont'd

Table B. Scoring Criteria for Diseases or Conditions

Category	Points
Cancer	1
AIDS	1
Pulmonary or cardiac cachexia	1
Presence of decubitus, open wound, or fistula	1
Presence of trauma	1
Age greater than 65 years	1

Table C. Scoring of Metabolic Stressors

Stressor	None (0)	Low (1)	Moderate (2)	High (3)
Fever (° F)*	No fever	>99 and <101	≥101 and <102	≥102
Fever duration	No fever	<72 hr		Lasting >72 hr
Steroids	No steroids	Low-dose steroids (<10 mg prednisone equivalents/day)	Moderate steroids (≥10, <30 mg prednisone equivalents/day)	High-dose steroids (≥30 mg prednisone equivalents/day)

Table D. Components of Quick Physical Examination (none to +++)

Fat status	Muscle status	Fluid status
Eyes	Temples	Skin and skin turgor
Triceps fat pinch	Shoulders	Eyes
Anterior lower ribs	Clavicle	Ankles
	Scapula	Sacrum
	Thumb/index press	Abdomen for ascites
	Thigh and calf	

Table E. PG-SGA Staging Guide

Variable	Stage A: Well Nourished	Stage B: Moderately Malnourished or Suspected of Being Malnourished	Stage C: Severely Malnourished
Weight	No weight loss or recent nonfluid weight gain	a. Approximately 5% weight loss within 1 month (or 10% in 6 months) b. No weight stabilization or weight (i.e., continued loss)	a. >5% loss in one month (or >10% loss in 6 months) b. No weight stabilization or weight gain
Intake	No deficit or significant recent improvement	Definite decrease in intake	Severe deficit in intake
Nutrition impact symptoms	None or significant recent improvement allowing adequate intake	Presence of nutrition impact symptoms (Box 3 of PG-SGA)	Presence of nutrition impact symptoms (Box 3 of PG-SGA)
Functionality	No deficit or significant recent improvement	Moderate functional deficit or recent functional deterioration	Severe functional deficit or recent significant functional deterioration
Physical exam	No deficit or chronic deficit in the face of recent improvement in all history categories listed above	Evidence of mild to moderate loss of • Subcutaneous fat and/or • Muscle mass and/or • Muscle tone on palpation	Obvious signs of malnutrition (e.g., severe loss of subcutaneous tissues, possible edema)

The PG-SGA scoring is based on the points found in parentheses on the PG-SGA form. Where a point score is not included on the form, Tables A through E are used for scoring.

Table F. Triaging Nutritional Intervention

Additive scores are used to define specific nutritional intervention pathways including education and/or symptom management, aggressive oral nutrition, enteral/parenteral triage.

An additive score of 0 to 1 indicates that no intervention is required at this time. Although these examples include only the patient section of the form, the total additive scores include addition of both the patient and clinician scores.

An additive score of 2 to 3 is an indication for patient education by a dietitian or nurse, with pharmacologic triage by the nurse or physician as indicated by the symptom survey.

An additive score of 4 to 8 requires the intervention of the dietitian, working in conjunction with the nurse or physician as indicated by the symptom check-off for pharmacologic management.

An additive score of ≥9 indicates a critical need for symptom management and/or nutritional intervention. These patients require an interdisciplinary discussion to address all the aspects that have an impact on the nutritional status as well as to address the potential need for nonoral nutritional options, including enteral or parenteral. This decision should be dictated by the presence or absence GI function.

© Ottery 1997

*PG-SGA = Patient-Generated Subjective Global Assessment. © Ottery 1997.
For additional information concerning the PG-SGA, contact F. Ottery, MD, PhD, at (215)351-4050 or noatpres@mem.po.com.

The Food Guide Pyramid (Fig. 8–3), dietary guidelines (Table 8–4), and the RDAs (Appendix C) are most often used as a basis for determining nutritional adequacy of diet. The Food Guide Pyramid has been modified for use with various personal preferences (e.g., vegetarian, athletes), as well as with cultural (e.g., Native American, African-American) and age-related (e.g., children, older adults) groups. Refer to nutrition texts for examples of these specific Food Guide Pyramids. One shortcoming of the RDAs is that they are not meant to be applied to sick individuals, whose nutrient requirements may be very different from those of healthy individuals. Specific nutrient values of foods can be obtained from several publications (e.g., *Bowes and Church's Food Values of Portions Commonly Used,* Pennington, 1998) and from nutrition labels and food manufacturers' information.

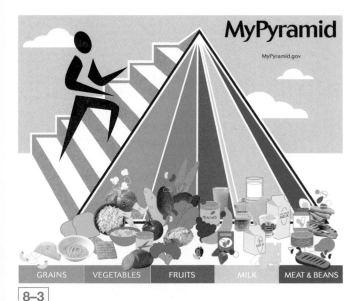

8–3

TABLE 8–4: Summary of Major Dietary Guidelines

1. Reduce overall fat consumption to about 30% of total calorie intake
2. Increase complex carbohydrate intake (fruits, vegetables, grains) to about 60% of total calorie intake; reduce intake of refined and processed sugars to about 10% of total calorie intake
3. Limit protein consumption to about 10% of total calorie intake
4. Reduce cholesterol consumption to about 300 mg/d
5. Limit intake of sodium to about 3–5 g/d
6. Increase fiber intake to 25–35 g/d
7. Eat a variety of foods in each of the major food groups and maintain a healthy weight

Subjective Data

1. Eating patterns
2. Usual weight
3. Changes in appetite, taste, smell, chewing, swallowing
4. Recent surgery, trauma, burns, infection
5. Chronic illnesses
6. Vomiting, diarrhea, constipation
7. Food allergies or intolerances
8. Medications and/or nutritional supplements
9. Self-care behaviors
10. Alcohol or illegal drug use
11. Exercise and activity patterns
12. Family history

EXAMINER ASKS

1. Eating patterns.
- Number of meals/snacks per day?
- Kind and amount of food eaten?
- Fad or special diets?
- Where is food eaten?
- Food preferences and dislikes?
- Religious or cultural restrictions?
- Able to feed self?

RATIONALE

Most individuals are knowledgeable about, or interested in, the foods they consume. If misconceptions are present, begin gradual instruction to correct them. Ethnic/religious beliefs or feeding difficulties may affect intake of certain foods.

EXAMINER ASKS	RATIONALE
2. Usual weight. What is your usual weight? • 20% below or above desirable weight? • Recent weight change? • How much lost or gained? • Over what time period? • Reason for loss or gain?	Persons who have had a recent, unintentional weight loss or who are obese are at nutritional risk. Underweight individuals are vulnerable because their fuel reserves may be depleted. Excess weight is associated with a number of health problems, ranging from hypertension to cancer. Protein and calorie needs are often overlooked in acutely ill obese persons.
3. Changes in appetite, taste, smell, chewing, swallowing. • Type of change? • When did change occur?	Poor appetite, taste and smell alterations, as well as chewing and swallowing difficulties interfere with adequate nutrient intake and increase the likelihood of nutritional risk.
4. Recent surgery, trauma, burns, infection. • When? • Type? • How treated? • Conditions that increase nutrient loss (e.g., draining wounds, effusions, blood loss, dialysis)?	Persons who have had recent surgery, trauma, sepsis, or conditions causing nutrient losses may have caloric and nutrient needs that are two or three times greater than normal.
5. Chronic illnesses. • Type? • When diagnosed? • How treated? • Dietary modifications? • Recent cancer chemotherapy or radiation therapy?	Individuals with chronic illnesses that affect nutrient use (e.g., diabetes mellitus, pancreatitis, or malabsorption) or those receiving cancer treatment are twice as likely to have nutritional deficits.
6. Vomiting, diarrhea, constipation. Any problems? • Due to? • How long?	Gastrointestinal symptoms such as vomiting, diarrhea, or constipation may interfere with nutrient intake or absorption.
7. Food allergies or intolerances. • Any problematic foods? • Type of reaction? • How long?	Food allergies, especially peanut allergies, are on the rise and a major health concern. Refer to published guidelines for more information on the management of food allergies. Intolerances may result in nutrient deficiencies (e.g., diarrhea after milk ingestion).
8. Medications and/or nutritional supplements. • Prescription medications? • Nonprescription? • Use over a 24-hour period? • Type of vitamin/mineral, herbal, or alternative supplement? • Amount? • Duration of use?	Analgesics, antacids, anticonvulsants, antibiotics, diuretics, laxatives, antineoplastic drugs, steroids, and oral contraceptives are among the drugs that can interact with nutrients, impairing their digestion, absorption, metabolism, or utilization. Vitamin/mineral supplements may cause harmful side effects if taken in large amounts.

EXAMINER ASKS	RATIONALE
	Use of herbal/alternative supplements is commonly not reported, so be sure to ask about intake and to discuss proper use and potential adverse effects. Refer to National Center for Complementary and Alternative Medicine website in reference list and other reliable alternative therapy resources.
9. Self-care behaviors. • Meal preparation facilities? • Transportation for travel to market? • Adequate income for food purchase? • Who prepares meals and does shopping? • Environment during mealtimes?	Socioeconomic factors may interfere with ingestion of adequate amounts of food or usual diet.
10. Alcohol or illegal drug use. • When was last drink of alcohol? • Amount taken that episode? • Amount alcohol each day? Each week? • Duration of use? • (Repeat questions for each drug used.)	These agents are often substituted for nutritious foods and may increase requirements for some nutrients. Also, pregnant women who smoke, drink alcohol, or use illegal drugs give birth to a disproportionate number of infants with low birth weights, failure to thrive, and other complications.
11. Exercise and activity patterns. • Amount? • Type?	Caloric and nutrient needs increase with increased activity and exercise, especially competitive sports and manual labor. Inactive or sedentary lifestyles often lead to excess weight gain.
12. Family history. Family or personal history of heart disease, osteoporosis, cancer, gout, GI disorders, obesity, or diabetes? • Effect of each on eating patterns? • Effect on activity patterns?	Long-term nutritional deficiencies or excesses may first become manifest as disease, such as these common examples during the adult years. Early identification of nutritional alterations permits dietary and activity modifications to occur promptly—at a time when the body can recover more fully.

Additional History for Infants and Children

Dietary histories of infants and children are generally obtained from the child's parents, guardian, baby sitter, or day care center. Usually, the person responsible for food preparation is able to provide a fairly accurate dietary history. Having the caregivers keep a thorough daily food diary and occasionally requesting 24-hour recalls during clinic visits are the most commonly employed techniques for this population group.

1. Gestational nutrition. • Maternal history of alcohol or illegal drug use? • Any diet-related complications during gestation? • Infant's birth weight? • Any evidence of delayed physical or mental growth?	Low birth weight (<2500 g) is a major factor in infant morbidity and mortality. Poor gestational nutrition, low maternal weight gain, and maternal alcohol and drug use—all factors in low birth weight—can lead to birth defects and delayed growth and development.

EXAMINER ASKS	RATIONALE
2. Infant breastfed or bottle fed. • Type, frequency, amount, and duration of feeding? • Any difficulties encountered? • Timing and method of weaning?	Well-nourished infants experience appropriate physical and social growth and development. Inexperienced mothers may encounter problems with either breastfeeding or bottle-feeding or have questions about whether the infant is receiving adequate amounts of food.
3. Child's willingness to eat what you prepare. • Any special likes or dislikes? • How much will child eat? • How do you control non-nutritious snack foods? • How do you avoid food aspiration?	The preschool period is one of increasing growth for the child. Lifelong food habits are forming. Use of small portions, finger foods, simple meals, and nutritious snacks are strategies to improve dietary intake. Foods likely to be aspirated should be avoided (e.g., hot dogs, nuts, grapes, round candies, popcorn).

Additional History for the Adolescent

EXAMINER ASKS	RATIONALE
1. Your present weight. • What would you like to weigh? • How do you feel about your present weight? • On any special diet to lose weight? • On other diets to lose weight? If so, were they successful? • Constantly think about "feeling fat?" • Intentionally vomit or use laxatives or diuretics after eating?	Obesity, particularly in girls, may precipitate fad dieting and malnutrition. Also, because of adolescents' increased body awareness and self-consciousness, they are prone to develop eating disorders such as anorexia nervosa or bulimia, conditions in which the real or perceived body image does not compare favorably to an ideal image—that found in advertisements or pictures of fashion models.
2. Use of anabolic steroids or other agents to increase muscle size and physical performance? • When? • How much? • Any problems?	Once confined to male professional athletes, the use of anabolic steroids and other performance-enhancing agents now extends to junior high, high school, and college males and females. Adverse effects include personality disorders, aggressiveness, and liver and other organ damage.
3. What snacks or fast foods do you like to eat? • When? • How much?	An accurate dietary history may be difficult to obtain from the adolescent because of the frequency of between-meal snacks and meals eaten on the run. These often are omitted or forgotten during the interview or in a food diary.
4. Age first started menstruating. • What is your menstrual flow like?	Menarche is usually delayed if malnutrition is present. Likewise, amenorrhea or scant menstrual flow is associated with nutritional deficiency.

EXAMINER ASKS	RATIONALE

Additional History for the Pregnant Female

1. How many times have you been pregnant?
  • When?
  • Any problems encountered during previous pregnancies?
  • Problems this pregnancy?

If the mother is multiparous, with pregnancies occurring less than 1 year apart, there is a greatly increased chance that her nutritional reserves are depleted. Note previous complications of pregnancy such as excessive vomiting, anemia, or gestational diabetes. Slower gastrointestinal motility and pressure from the fetus may cause constipation, hemorrhoids, and indigestion. A past history of giving birth to a low-birth-weight infant suggests past nutritional problems. Giving birth to an infant with a birth weight of 4.5 kg (10 lbs) or more may signal the presence of *latent* diabetes in the mother.

2. What foods do you prefer when pregnant?
  • What foods do you avoid?
  • Crave any particular foods?

The expectant mother may be extremely vulnerable to familial, cultural, and traditional influences for food choices. Cravings for or aversions to particular foods are common, and should be evaluated for their potential contribution to, or interference with, dietary intake.

Additional History for the Aging Adult

1. How does your diet differ from when you were in your 40s and 50s?
  • Why?
  • What factors affect the way you eat?

Note any physiologic or psychologic changes of aging or socioeconomic changes that affect nutritional status.

2. Review the "Determine Your Nutritional Health" checklist (see Fig. 8–2).

The Nutritional Screening Initiative (White et al., 1991) is a three-step approach for nutrition screening of the elderly. The nutrition checklist in Figure 8–2 is completed by the older person or caregiver and identifies major risk factors and indicators of poor nutritional status. Persons identified at risk should undergo level 1 and/or level 2 screening depending on whether they are at moderate or high risk of poor nutritional status. (See sample forms in Jarvis C: *Laboratory Manual for Physical Examination and Health Assessment.*)

Objective Data

CLINICAL SIGNS

Observation of an individual's general appearance—obese, cachectic (fat and muscle wasting), or edematous—can provide clues to overall nutritional status. More specific clinical signs and symptoms suggestive of nutritional deficiencies can be detected through a physical examination. Because clinical signs are late manifestations of malnutrition, only in areas in which rapid turnover of epithelial tissue occurs—skin, hair, mouth, lips, and eyes—are the nutritional deficiencies readily detectable. These signs may also be nonnutritional in origin. Therefore, laboratory testing is required to make an accurate diagnosis. Laboratory tests for assessment of nutritional status are reviewed later in this chapter. Clinical signs of various nutritional deficiencies are summarized in Table 8–5 and are depicted in the section on abnormalities at the end of this chapter (see Table 8–7).

EQUIPMENT NEEDED

Lange or Harpenden skinfold calipers
Ross insertion tape or other measurement tape
Anthropometer
Pen or pencil
Nutritional assessment data form

TABLE 8–5: Clinical Signs of Malnutrition

AREA OF EXAMINATION	NORMAL APPEARANCE	SIGNS ASSOCIATED WITH MALNUTRITION	NUTRIENT DEFICIENCY
Skin	Smooth, no signs of rashes, bruises, flaking	Dry, flaking, scaly	Vitamin A, vitamin B-complex, linoleic acid
		Petechiae/ecchymoses	Vitamins C and K
		Follicular hyperkeratosis (dry, bumpy skin)	Vitamin A, linoleic acid
		Cracks in skin, lesions on the hands, legs, face, or neck	Niacin, tryptophan
		Pellagrous dermatosis (hyperpigmentation of skin exposed to sunlight)	Niacin
		Nasolabial seborrhea	Riboflavin, vitamin B_6
		Acneiform forehead rash	Vitamin B_6
		Eczema	Linoleic acid
		Xanthomas (excessive deposits of cholesterol)	Excessive serum levels of LDLs or VLDLs
Hair	Shiny, firm, does not fall out easily, healthy scalp	Dull, dry, sparse	Protein, zinc, linoleic acid
		Color changes	Copper or protein
		Corkscrew hair	Copper
Eyes	Corneas are clear, shiny; membranes are pink and moist; no sores at corners of eyelids	Foamy plaques (Bitot's spots)	Vitamin A
		Dryness (xerophthalmia)	Vitamin A
		Softening (keratomalacia)	Vitamin A
		Pale conjunctivae	Iron, vitamins B_6, B_{12}
		Red conjunctivae	Riboflavin
		Blepharitis	B-complex, biotin
Lips	Smooth, not chapped or swollen	Cheilosis (vertical cracks in lips)	Riboflavin, niacin
		Angular stomatitis (red cracks at sides of mouth)	Riboflavin, niacin, iron, vitamin B_6
Tongue	Red in appearance; not swollen or smooth, no lesions	Glossitis (beefy red)	Vitamin B-complex
		Pale	Iron
		Papillary atrophy	Niacin
		Papillary hypertrophy	Multiple nutrients
		Magenta/purplish colored	Riboflavin
Gums	Reddish-pink, firm, no swelling or bleeding	Bleeding	Vitamin C
Nails	Smooth, pink	Brittle, ridged, or spoon shaped (koilonychia)	Iron
		Splinter hemorrhages	Vitamin C
Musculoskeletal	Erect posture, no malformations, good muscle tone, can walk or run without pain	Pain in calves, thighs	Thiamine
		Osteomalacia	Vitamin D, calcium
		Rickets	Vitamin D, calcium
		Joint pain	Vitamin C
		Muscle wasting	Protein, carbohydrate, fat
Neurologic	Normal reflexes, appropriate affect	Peripheral neuropathy	Thiamine, vitamin B_6
		Hyporeflexia	Thiamine
		Disorientation or irritability	Vitamin B_{12}

NORMAL RANGE OF FINDINGS	ABNORMAL FINDINGS

ANTHROPOMETRIC MEASURES

Anthropometry is the measurement and evaluation of growth, development, and body composition. The most commonly used anthropometric measures are height, weight, triceps skinfold thickness, elbow breadth, and arm and head circumferences. Measurement of height, weight, and head circumference is described in Chapter 10.

Derived Weight Measures

Three derived weight measures are used to depict changes in body weight.

Body weight as a percentage of ideal body weight is calculated using the following formula:

$$\text{Percent ideal body weight} = \frac{\text{Current weight}}{\text{Ideal weight}} \times 100$$

(Ideal weight is based on the Metropolitan Life Insurance Tables, 1983; cited in Chapter 10.)

The **percent usual body weight** is calculated as follows:

$$\text{Percent usual body weight} = \frac{\text{Current weight}}{\text{Usual weight}} \times 100$$

Recent weight change is calculated using the following formula:

$$\frac{\text{Usual weight} - \text{Current weight}}{\text{Usual weight}} \times 100$$

A current weight of 80 to 90 percent of ideal weight is suggestive of mild malnutrition; 70 to 80 percent, of moderate malnutrition; and less than 70 percent, of severe malnutrition.
Obesity is defined as >120 percent ideal body weight.

A current weight of 85 to 95 percent of usual body weight is an indication of mild malnutrition; 75 to 84 percent, of moderate malnutrition; and less than 75 percent, of severe malnutrition.

An unintentional loss of >5 percent of body weight over 1 month, >7.5 percent of body weight over 3 months, or >10 percent of body weight over 6 months is considered clinically significant.

Body Mass Index

Body mass index is a practical marker of optimal weight for height and an indicator of obesity or protein-calorie malnutrition (see Appendix E). It is calculated by:

$$\text{Body mass index} = \frac{\text{Weight (in kilograms)}}{\text{Height (in meters)}^2}$$

$$\text{or} \quad \frac{\text{Weight (in pounds)}}{\text{Height (in inches)}^2} \times 703$$

BMI interpretation (NIH, 2000):
<18.5	Underweight
18.5–24.9	Normal weight
25.0–29.9	Overweight
30.0–39.9	Obesity
≥40	Extreme obesity

Waist-to-Hip Ratio

The waist-to-hip ratio assesses body fat distribution as an indicator of health risk (Folsom et al., 1993). Obese persons with a greater proportion of fat in the upper body, especially in the abdomen, have android obesity; obese persons with most of their fat in the hips and thighs have gynoid obesity. The equation is:

$$\text{Waist-to-hip ratio} = \frac{\text{Waist circumference}}{\text{Hip circumference}}$$

where waist circumference is measured in inches at the smallest circumference below the rib cage and above the umbilicus, and hip circumference is measured in inches at the largest circumference of the buttocks.

A waist-to-hip ratio of 1.0 or greater in men or 0.8 or greater in women is indicative of android (upper body obesity) and increasing risk for obesity-related diseases and early mortality.

NORMAL RANGE OF FINDINGS

Skinfold Thickness

Skinfold thickness measurements provide an estimate of body fat stores or the extent of obesity or undernutrition. Although other sites can be used (biceps, subcapsular, or suprailiac skinfolds), the triceps skinfold (TSF) is most commonly selected because of its easy accessibility and because standards and techniques are most developed for this site. To measure TSF thickness:

1. Have the ambulatory person stand with arms hanging freely at the sides and back to the examiner. (Nonambulatory persons should lie on one side. The uppermost arm should be fully extended, with the palm of the hand resting on the thigh.)
2. Using the thumb and forefinger of your left hand, gently grasp a fold of skin and fat on the posterior aspect of the person's left upper arm, midway between the acromion process of the scapula and the olecranon process (the tip of the elbow). Gently pull the skinfold away from the underlying muscle (Fig. 8–4).

8–4

3. While grasping the skinfold, pick up the calipers with your right hand and depress the spring-loaded lever. Apply caliper jaws horizontally to the fat fold. Release the lever of the calipers while holding the skinfold. Wait 3 seconds, then take a reading. Repeat three times and average the three skinfold measurements (Fig. 8–5).

TSF values that are 10% below or above standard are suggestive of undernutrition and overnutrition, respectively.

8–5

NORMAL RANGE OF FINDINGS	ABNORMAL FINDINGS

4. Record measurements to the nearest 5 mm (0.5 cm) on the nutritional assessment data form. Compare the person's measurements with standards by age, sex, and body frame size (see Appendixes F and G).

Conditions such as edema or subcutaneous emphysema may produce falsely high readings. Nonreproducible readings may be due to instrument malfunctions, use of plastic calipers (which are less accurate), or examiner error.

Mid-Upper Arm Circumference

Mid-upper arm circumference (MAC) estimates skeletal muscle mass and fat stores.

1. Have the person stand or sit with arm hanging fully extended and relaxed by the side of the body.
2. Loop the insertion tape or measuring tape around the arm at the midpoint of the upper arm (midway between the acromion and olecranon processes).
3. Position the tape horizontally at the midpoint, then tighten it firmly around the arm, but not so tightly as to cause skin contour indentation or pinching (Fig. 8–6).

8–6

4. Note and record the measurement (in centimeters) on the appropriate form. Compare with norms (Appendix H).

For example, a normal mid-upper arm circumference for a 20-year-old female ranges from 23 to 34.5 cm; for a 20-year-old male, the normal range is 27.2 to 37.2 cm. Remember that accurate MAC and TSF measurements are difficult to obtain and interpret in older adults because of sagging skin, changes in fat distribution, and declining muscle mass.

Individuals whose measurements fall below the 10th percentile or above the 95th percentile warrant further medical and nutritional evaluation. Very high or very low readings may be due to examiner error.

Derived Anthropometric Measures

Although the MAC is of little value in and of itself, when combined with the TSF measurement, it is possible to indirectly determine the arm muscle *circumference* and arm muscle *area*.

NORMAL RANGE OF FINDINGS	ABNORMAL FINDINGS

NORMAL RANGE OF FINDINGS

Mid-upper arm muscle circumference (MAMC) estimates skeletal muscle reserves or the amount of lean body mass and is derived from the TSF and MAC measures using the following formula:

$$MAMC = MAC - (\pi \times TSF)$$

where

$$\pi = 3.14$$
$$MAC = \text{Mid-upper arm circumference (in cm)}$$
$$TSF = \text{Triceps skinfold (in mm)}$$
$$MAMC = \text{Mid-upper arm muscle circumference (in cm)}$$

Record calculation on data forms. Compare with norms (Appendix H).

Mid-arm muscle area (MAMA) is a good indicator of lean body mass and thus skeletal protein reserves. These reserves are important in growing children and are especially valuable in evaluating persons who may be malnourished because of chronic illness, multiple surgeries, or inadequate dietary intake.

The equation for calculating MAMA is

$$MAMA = \frac{(MAC - MAMC)^2}{4\,\pi}$$

where

$$MAMA = \text{mid-arm muscle area (in cm}^2\text{)}$$
$$MAC = \text{mid-upper arm circumference (in cm)}$$
$$MAMC = \text{mid-upper arm muscle circumference (in cm)}$$
$$4\,\pi = 4 \times 3.14 = 12.56$$

Record calculation on data forms. Compare with norms (Appendices F and G).

Two newer techniques to measure body composition are **bioelectrical impedance analysis (BIA)** and **dual-energy x-ray absorptiometry (DEXA)**. Both BIA and DEXA measure fat and lean body mass; in addition, DEXA measures bone mineral density (Bolanowski and Nilsson, 2001).

Arm Span or Total Arm Length

Measurement of arm span is useful for those situations in which height is difficult to measure, such as in children with cerebral palsy or scoliosis or in aging persons with spinal curvature. Arm span, which is nearly equivalent to height, is sometimes used clinically instead of height (Gabriella and Sinclair, 1997; Rueben et al., 1995). Ask the person to hold the arms straight out from the sides of the body. Measure the distance from the tip of the middle finger on one hand to that on the other hand.

Frame Size

Frame size is calculated to determine appropriate range of ideal body weight. Most weight standards, such as the Metropolitan Life Insurance Tables of ideal weight for height, contain classifications of weight by frame size. Elbow breadth, a measure of skeletal breadth, is the most accurate method to determine frame size (Frisancho and Flegel, 1983). To measure it, you must be familiar with the use of flat-blade sliding calipers or a broad-blade anthropometer.

1. Instruct the person to extend the right arm forward, perpendicular to the body. Bend the elbow to a 90-degree angle, with the palm of the hand turned laterally (Fig. 8–7).
2. Facing the person, place the calipers on the condyles of the humerus (a broad-blade anthropometer may be needed if the calipers do not extend to the breadth of the elbow).
3. Read the distance between the condyles; record measurement (in centimeters) on the appropriate form. Using the norms (Appendix I), assess whether the person has small, medium, or large frame size.

ABNORMAL FINDINGS

MAMC is dependent on accurate measurement of the MAC and TSF. In general, a MAMC that is 90% of standard is suggestive of mild malnutrition, 60% to 90% suggests moderate malnutrition, and less than 60% is indicative of severe malnutrition.

MAMA is considered to be a more sensitive measure of long-standing malnutrition than MAMC. A MAMA of 90% of standard reflects mild malnutrition; 60% to 90% moderate malnutrition; and less than 60% severe malnutrition.

8–7

NORMAL RANGE OF FINDINGS	ABNORMAL FINDINGS

 DEVELOPMENTAL CONSIDERATIONS

Infants, Children, and Adolescents

WEIGHT. During infancy, childhood, and adolescence, height and weight should be measured at regular intervals, because longitudinal growth is one of the best indices of nutritional status over time. See Chapter 10 for techniques.

SKINFOLD THICKNESS. Determination of skinfold thickness and/or body mass index may be useful in evaluating childhood and teenage overnutrition.

An estimated 15% of children and teenagers in the United States are obese.

The Pregnant Female

WEIGHT. Measure weight monthly up to 30 weeks' gestation, then every 2 weeks until the last month of pregnancy, when weight should be measured weekly. Appendix D illustrates approximate weight gain considered normal for each week of pregnancy.

The expectant mother should be considered at nutritional risk if her weight is 10% or more below ideal or 20% or more above the norm for her height and age group.

The Aging Adult

HEIGHT. With age, height declines in both men and women very slowly from the early 30s, leading to an average 2.9-cm loss in men and 4.9-cm loss in women (Gabriella and Sinclair, 1997; Rueben et al., 1995). Height measures may not be accurate in individuals confined to a bed or wheelchair or those over 60 years of age (because of osteoporotic changes). Therefore, arm span, which is correlated with height, may be a better measure for the elderly.

OTHER MEASUREMENTS. MAC and TSF measures may not be accurate and are difficult to obtain in older adults (because of sagging skin, changes in fat distribution, and declining muscle mass). (See Frisancho [1984] for data on weight and TSF thickness by height in U.S. men and women age 55 to 74 years.) Body mass index and waist-to-hip ratio are better indicators of obesity in this age group.

LABORATORY STUDIES

Routine laboratory tests are of particular value in nutritional assessment because they are objective, can detect preclinical nutritional deficiencies, and can be used to confirm subjective findings. Use caution, however, when interpreting test results that may be outside normal ranges, because they do not always reflect a nutritional problem and because standards for aging adults have not yet been firmly established.

The best routinely performed laboratory indicators of nutritional status are hemoglobin, hematocrit, cholesterol, triglycerides, total lymphocyte count, and serum albumin. Glucose, low- and high-density lipoproteins, prealbumin, transferrin, and total protein levels also provide meaningful information.

HEMOGLOBIN. The hemoglobin determination is used to detect iron deficiency anemia. Normal values are as follows: **infants,** 1 to 3 days—14.5 to 22.5 g/dl, 2 months—9.0 to 14.0 g/dl; **children,** 6 to 12 years—11.5 to 15.5 g/dl; **adults,** males—14 to 18 g/dl, females—12 to 16 g/dl.

Increased hemoglobin levels are suggestive of hemoconcentration due to polycythemia vera or dehydration.
Decreased hemoglobin levels may indicate anemia, recent hemorrhage, or hemodilution caused by fluid retention.

HEMATOCRIT. Hematocrit, a measure of cell volume, is also an indicator of iron status. Normal values are as follows: **infants,** 1 to 3 days—44 to 72%, 2 months—28 to 42%; **children,** 6 to 12 years—35 to 45%; **adults,** males—37 to 49%, females—36 to 46%.

A low value indicates insufficient hemoglobin formation, and for this reason, hematocrit and hemoglobin values should be interpreted together.

NORMAL RANGE OF FINDINGS

ABNORMAL FINDINGS

CHOLESTEROL. Total cholesterol is measured to evaluate fat metabolism and to assess the risk of cardiovascular disease. Normal cholesterol concentrations vary with age and gender and may range from 120 mg/dl to 200 mg/dl.

Coronary artery disease risk steadily increases as serum cholesterol rises. Serum cholesterol levels of 200 to 239 mg/dl (borderline high) are associated with moderate risk and 240 mg/dl or more (high) with high risk of coronary artery disease, myocardial infarction, stroke, and peripheral vascular disease.

TRIGLYCERIDES. Serum triglycerides are used to screen for hyperlipidemia and to determine the risk of coronary artery disease. Triglyceride values are age related. Some controversy exists over the most appropriate normal ranges, but the following are fairly widely accepted: **ages 0 to 19,** 10 to 100 mg/dl; **ages 20 to 65,** 40 to 200 mg/dl.

Serum triglyceride levels are also associated with coronary artery disease. Serum triglycerides are categorized as: *borderline,* 250 to 500 mg/dl, or *high,* more than 500 mg/dl.

TOTAL LYMPHOCYTE COUNT. The most commonly used tests of immune function are total lymphocyte count (TLC) and skin testing, also called delayed cutaneous hypersensitivity testing. TLC is an important indicator of visceral protein status and therefore of cellular immune function.

The TLC is derived from the white blood cell count (WBC) and the differential count:

$$TLC = WBC \times \frac{\text{Number of lymphocytes in differential}}{100 \text{ cells}}$$

where TLC is calculated in cells per cubic millimeter.

Normal values for all age categories are between 1800 and 3000 cells/mm^3.

Nonnutritional factors that affect TLC include hypoalbuminemia, metabolic stress (e.g., major surgery, trauma, sepsis), infection, cancer, and chronic diseases.

Total lymphocyte counts of 1500 to 1800 indicate mild lymphocyte depletion; 900 to 1500, moderate depletion; and less than 900, severe depletion.

SKIN TESTING. Adequate immunity can also be demonstrated by a positive reaction to multiple skin test antigens. In these tests of immune function, at least six antigens are injected intradermally in the forearm area, and the response (redness and/or induration) is noted at 24 and 48 hours. A 5-mm or greater response to more than one antigen is generally considered to be a positive reaction (i.e., indicative of adequate immunity).

Commonly used antigens include *Candida,* tetanus toxoid, diphtheria toxoid, streptococcus, old tuberculin, proteus, and trichophyton.

A response of less than 5 mm indicates anergy or immunoincompetence. Anergy occurs with malnutrition, hepatic failure, infection, and immunosuppressive drugs (e.g., chemotherapy agents, steroids).

Lymphopenia and the lack of a positive response to skin test antigens place the person at increased risk of infection, sepsis, and other complications.

SERUM PROTEINS. **Serum albumin** is another common measurement of visceral protein status. Because of its relatively long half-life (17 to 20 days) and large body pool (4.0 to 5.0 g/kg), albumin is not an early indicator of protein malnutrition.

Normal serum albumin concentration in infants and children older than 6 months and adults ranges from 3.5 to 5.5 g/dl.

Low serum albumin levels may be caused by reasons other than protein-calorie malnutrition—for example, altered hydration status and decreased liver function.

In general, a serum albumin level of 2.8 to 3.5 g/dl represents moderate visceral protein depletion, and less than 2.8 g/dl denotes severe depletion (Wallach, 1996).

NORMAL RANGE OF FINDINGS

Levels of **serum transferrin**, an iron-transport protein, can be measured directly or by an indirect measurement of total iron-binding capacity. Serum transferrin, with a half-life of 8 to 10 days, may be a more sensitive indicator of visceral protein status than albumin.

The most widely used formula for computing serum transferrin is

$$\text{Serum Transferrin} = (0.8 \times \text{Total Iron-Binding Capacity}) - 43$$

The normal values for serum transferrin are 170 to 250 mg/dl.

Prealbumin, or thyroxine-binding prealbumin, serves as a transport protein for thyroxine (T_4) and retinol-binding protein. With a shorter half-life (48 hours) than either albumin or transferrin, prealbumin is sensitive to acute changes in protein status and sudden demands on protein synthesis. Normal prealbumin levels range from 15 to 25 mg/dl.

NITROGEN BALANCE. Nitrogen balance is also used as an index of protein nutritional status. Nitrogen is released with the catabolism of amino acids and is excreted in the urine as urea. Nitrogen balance therefore indicates whether the person is anabolic (positive nitrogen balance) or catabolic (negative nitrogen balance).

Nitrogen balance is estimated by a formula based on urine urea nitrogen (UUN) excreted during the previous 24 hours:

$$\text{Nitrogen} = \text{Nitrogen intake} - \text{Nitrogen excretion}$$
$$= \text{Protein intake}/6.25 - (\text{24-hour UUN} + 4)$$

where

Nitrogen balance is determined in grams
24-hour UNN = Urinary urea nitrogen, measured in grams
4 = Nonurea nitrogen losses via feces, skin, sweat, and lungs, measured in grams

CREATININE-HEIGHT INDEX. The creatinine-height index (CHI) is a method of estimating the amount of skeletal muscle mass. Creatinine is derived from the breakdown of creatine, an energy-containing complex found in muscle. Creatinine is excreted unchanged in the urine at a constant rate in proportion to the amount of body muscle.

Creatinine height index is calculated by first measuring urinary creatinine using a carefully collected 24-hour urine specimen. This value is then compared with ideal urinary creatinine levels from a creatinine-for-height-standard table, by means of the following equation:

$$\text{CHI} = \frac{\text{Actual 24-hour urine creatinine}}{\text{Ideal 24-hour urine creatinine for height}} \times 100$$

The person's CHI is then compared with a CHI standard table to determine the degree of skeletal muscle depletion.

ABNORMAL FINDINGS

Levels of 150 to 170 mg/dl are considered evidence of mild deficiency; 100 to 150 mg/dl, moderate deficiency; and levels less than 100 mg/dl, severe deficiency (Lee and Nieman, 2003). Because a variety of clinical conditions can alter serum albumin and transferrin levels, consider the person's history in conjunction with these values for accurate interpretation.

Prealbumin levels are elevated in renal disease and reduced by surgery, trauma, burns, and infection. Prealbumin levels of 10 to 15 mg/dl indicate mild depletion; 5 to 10 mg/dl, moderate depletion; and less than 5 mg/dl, severe depletion.

In response to stress and increased protein demand, the body rapidly mobilizes its protein compartments, which results in increased production of urea and excretion of urea in the urine. With infection, an estimated loss of 9 to 11 g/day of UUN can be expected. In patients with major burns, 12 to 18 g/day of urea nitrogen may be expected in the urine (Blackburn et al., 1977).

The validities of CHI and nitrogen balance studies are dependent on the accuracy of the 24-hour urine collection. Failure to obtain an accurate sample, abnormal renal function, and certain other conditions can result in underestimation of creatinine and nitrogen losses.

Assuming an accurate 24-hour urine specimen has been collected, a CHI of 60% to 80% of standard indicates a moderate deficit in body mass. A value of less than 60% indicates a severe deficit of body muscle mass (Blackburn et al., 1977). Stress, fever, and trauma can increase urinary creatinine excretion.

DEVELOPMENTAL CONSIDERATIONS

In infancy and childhood, laboratory tests are performed only when undernutrition is suspected or if the child has acute or chronic illnesses that affect nutritional status.

During adolescence, unless overt disease is suspected, laboratory evaluation of hemoglobin and hematocrit levels and urinalysis for glucose and protein levels are adequate.

In pregnancy, hemoglobin and hematocrit values can be used to detect deficiencies of protein, folacin, vitamin B_{12}, and iron. Urine is frequently tested for glucose and protein (albumin), which can signal diabetes, preeclampsia, and renal disease.

In older adulthood, all serum and urine data must be interpreted with an understanding of declining renal efficiency and a tendency for aging adults to be overhydrated or underhydrated.

 TRANSCULTURAL CONSIDERATIONS

Biocultural Variations in Laboratory Studies

Biocultural variations occur with some laboratory tests, such as *hemoglobin/hematocrit, serum cholesterol,* and *serum transferrin.* The normal *hemoglobin level* for blacks is 1 g lower than levels for other groups, a factor that should be considered in the treatment of anemia. Data indicate that Native Americans, Hispanics, Asian Americans, and whites do not differ in this factor.

The difference between blacks and whites with respect to *serum cholesterol* is quite interesting. At birth, blacks and whites have similar serum cholesterol levels, but during childhood blacks have higher serum cholesterol levels than whites (5 mg/100 ml). These differences reverse during adulthood, when black adults have lower serum cholesterol levels than white adults. The Pima Indians have considerably lower serum cholesterol levels than whites, both during childhood (20 to 30 mg/100 ml lower) and adulthood (50 to 60 mg/100 ml lower).

In a study of children 1 to $3^1/_2$ years of age, *serum transferrin* levels were found to differ between white and black children. The mean value for white children was 200 to 400 mg/100 ml, whereas the mean for black children was 341.4. The higher serum transferrin levels in black children may be due to their lowered hemoglobin/hematocrit levels. Transferrin levels increase in the presence of anemia. If the hemoglobin and hematocrit levels are normally lower in blacks, then higher transferrin levels should be considered normal (Jackson, 1990).

SERIAL ASSESSMENT

To monitor nutritional status in malnourished individuals or in individuals at risk for malnutrition, serial measurements of nutritional assessment parameters are made at routine intervals. At a minimum, weight and dietary intake should be evaluated weekly. Because the other nutritional assessment parameters change more slowly, data on these indicators may be collected biweekly or monthly.

Based on the findings of the nutritional assessment, the type of malnutrition can be diagnosed. The four major types of malnutrition are obesity, marasmus, kwashiorkor, and marasmus-kwashiorkor mix (Table 8–6). Each type of malnutrition has characteristic clinical and laboratory findings and a distinct cause.

SUMMARY CHECKLIST: Nutritional Assessment

1. Obtain a health history relevant to nutritional status
2. Elicit dietary history, if indicated
3. Inspect skin, hair, eyes, oral cavity, nails, and musculoskeletal and neurologic systems for clinical signs and symptoms suggestive of nutritional deficiencies
4. Measure height, weight, and other anthropometric parameters, as indicated
5. Review relevant laboratory tests

Application and Critical Thinking

SAMPLE CHARTING

SUBJECTIVE

No history of diseases or surgery that would alter intake/requirements; no recent weight changes; no appetite changes. Socioeconomic history is noncontributory. Does not smoke; drink alcohol; or use illegal, prescription, or over-the-counter drugs. No food allergies. Sedentary lifestyle; plays golf once per week.

OBJECTIVE

Dietary intake is adequate to meet protein and energy needs. No clinical signs of nutrient deficiencies. Height, weight, and screening laboratory tests within normal ranges.

FOCUSED ASSESSMENT: CLINICAL CASE STUDY 1

R.G. is a 33-year-old gay male diagnosed as HIV seropositive 5 years ago.

SUBJECTIVE

He presents to the Infectious Disease Clinic with a 2-week history of diarrhea and anorexia, and a weight loss of 17 kg. Daily caloric intake averages 1000 kcal (usual intake is 2000 kcal). Describes diarrhea as "runny" and occurring 4 to 6 times a day.

OBJECTIVE

Inspection. Slightly raised patches resembling milk curds present in mouth and throat. General appearance is pale and cachectic.
Anthropometric. Height is 166.4 cm (65.5 inches). Current weight is 50.9 kg (112 lb); usual and ideal body weight is 68 kg (150 lb). TSF measures 8.5 mm (normal value is 12.5).
Laboratory. Serum albumin (1.86 g/dl) and total lymphocyte count (1000/mm³) are well below normal ranges. Stool is of watery consistency; stool analysis reveals *Cryptosporidium* infection.

ASSESSMENT

- Imbalanced nutrition: less than body requirements R/T anorexia, fever, diarrhea, and oral *Candida albicans*
- Protein-calorie malnutrition (marasmus)

FOCUSED ASSESSMENT: CLINICAL CASE STUDY 2

E.F. is an 87-year-old widow who lives alone in her own home. She has enjoyed good health all of her life.

SUBJECTIVE

During the past year, she has experienced declining memory and no longer cooks or drives. Relies on children to take her grocery shopping and prepare occasional meals. Income adequate. Describes her appetite as excellent. Spends her days watching television and reading. Experiences occasional constipation. Eats a well-balanced diet and enjoys high-carbohydrate foods such as cookies, candy, and doughnuts because they are easy to chew. Caloric intake is 1800 kcal/day.

OBJECTIVE

Inspection. No clinical signs of nutrient deficiencies.
Anthropometric. Height is 160 cm (63 inches). Current weight is 56.8 kg (125 lb); usual weight is 56.8 kg (125 lb), and ideal weight is 56.4 kg (124 lb).
Laboratory. Hemoglobin, hematocrit, and albumin values within normal limits.

ASSESSMENT

- Normal nutriture
- Constipation related to inactivity and diet high in refined carbohydrates

NURSING DIAGNOSES COMMONLY ASSOCIATED WITH NUTRITIONAL DISORDERS

RELATED FACTORS (Etiology)	DEFINING CHARACTERISTICS (Symptoms and Signs)

DIAGNOSIS: Imbalanced Nutrition: Less than Body Requirements

Increased energy and nutrient needs:	Loss of body weight with adequate food intake
Periods of rapid growth and development	Body weight 20% or more under ideal weight for height
Pregnancy	Aversion to eating
Draining wounds	Diarrhea and/or steatorrhea
Infection	Inadequate food intake
Surgery	Triceps skinfold (TSF) <60% of standard measurement
Inadequate nutrient intake:	Midarm circumference (MAC <60% of standard
Anorexia	measurement)
Nausea and vomiting	Abdominal pain or cramping
Fatigue	Sore, inflamed buccal cavity
Socioeconomic factors	Pale conjunctival and mucous membranes
Substance abuse	Poor muscle tone or skin turgor
Maldigestion or malabsorption (short bowel syndrome,	Loss of hair
pancreatitis)	Decreased serum albumin or total protein
Drug-nutrient interactions	Decreased serum transferrin or iron binding capacity
Alteration in taste or smell	Metabolic demands in excess of intake
Dysphagia	Anemia
Inability to chew	Lack of interest in food
Decreased level of consciousness	Reported or evidence of lack of food
Stress	
Decreased salivation	
Effects of hypercatabolic states (cancer, burns, infection)	
Effects of aging—decreased sense of taste	

DIAGNOSIS: Imbalanced Nutrition: More than Body Requirements

Lack of physical exercise/decreased activity pattern	Weight 10%–20% over ideal for height and frame
Eating in response to stress or emotional trauma	Reported and observed dysfunctional eating patterns:
Eating as a comfort measure/substitute gratification	Pairing food with other activities
Learned eating behaviors	Concentrating food intake at end of day
Decreased metabolic need	Eating in response to external cues such as time of day
Lack of knowledge regarding nutritional needs	Eating in response to internal cues other than hunger, e.g.,
Perceived lack of control	anxiety
Ethnic and cultural values	Sedentary activity level
Lack of social support for weight loss	Body mass index >27
Decreased self-esteem	TSF >15 mm for men and >25 mm for women
Negative body image	Serum cholesterol ≥200 mg/dl
	Serum triglycerides >250 mg/dl

OTHER RELATED NURSING DIAGNOSES

ACTUAL	RISK/WELLNESS
Disturbed Body image (see Chapter 13)	**Risk**
Ineffective Breastfeeding	Risk for constipation
Constipation	Risk for deficient fluid volume
Diarrhea	Risk for imbalanced fluid volume
Deficient Fluid volume (see Chapter 12)	**Wellness**
Excess Fluid volume (see Chapter 18)	Compliance with prescribed diet
Deficient Knowledge: nutrition	Increasing knowledge about adequate nutrition
Impaired Oral mucous membrane (see Chapter 16)	Improving nutritional intake
Feeding Self-care deficit	
Impaired Skin integrity (see Chapter 12)	
Impaired Swallowing	

Abnormal Findings

TABLE 8–6: Classification of Malnutrition

TYPE/ETIOLOGY	CLINICAL FEATURES	ANTHROPOMETRIC MEASURES	LABORATORY FINDINGS
Obesity due to caloric excess, refers to weights more than 20% above ideal body weight. Persons who are 100% or more above ideal body weight are categorized as morbidly obese. The causes of overweight and obese conditions are complex and multifaceted; genetic, social, cultural, pathologic, psychologic, and physiologic factors have all been implicated. Regardless of its cause, the underlying problem is usually an imbalance of caloric intake and caloric expenditure. In most cases, a small caloric surplus over a long period of time results in the extra pounds. Although visceral protein levels and immunocompetence are generally normal in the obese individual, anthropometric measures are above normal.	Obese appearance	Weight >120% standard for height Body mass index >27 Triceps skinfold (TSF) >10% standard Waist-to-hip ratio >1.0 (men) or >0.8 (women)	Serum cholesterol ≥200 mg/dl Serum triglycerides >250 mg/dl
Marasmus (protein-calorie malnutrition) is due to inadequate intake of protein and calories or prolonged starvation. Anorexia, bowel obstruction, cancer cachexia, and chronic illness are among the clinical conditions leading to marasmus. Marasmus is characterized by decreased anthropometric measures—weight loss and subcutaneous fat and muscle wasting. Visceral protein levels may remain within normal ranges.	Starved appearance 	Weight ≤80% standard for height TSF <90% standard Midarm muscle circumference (MAMC) ≤90% standard	Creatinine-height index <80% standard

Table continued on following page

TABLE 8–6: Classification of Malnutrition—cont'd

TYPE/ETIOLOGY	CLINICAL FEATURES	ANTHROPOMETRIC MEASURES	LABORATORY FINDINGS
Kwashiorkor (protein malnutrition) is due to diets that may be high in calories but that contain little or no protein, e.g., low-protein liquid diets, fad diets, and long-term use of dextrose-containing intravenous fluids. Individuals with kwashiorkor, in contrast to those with marasmus, have decreased visceral protein levels and depressed immune function, but generally they have adequate anthropometric measures. These individuals may therefore appear well nourished or even obese.	Well-nourished appearance Edematous	Weight $\geq$100% standard for height TSF $\geq$100% standard	Serum albumin <3.5 g/dl Serum transferinn <150 mg/dl Lymphocytes <1,500 mm^3 Anergy
Marasmus/kwashiorkor mix is due to prolonged inadequate intake of protein and calories (e.g., severe starvation, severe catabolic states). This mix combines elements of both marasmus and kwashiorkor. Nutritional assessment findings include muscle, fat, and visceral protein wasting, along with immune incompetence. Individuals with marasmus-kwashiorkor mix are usually those who have undergone acute catabolic stress, such as major surgery, trauma, or burns in combination with prolonged starvation. Without nutritional support, this type of malnutrition is associated with the highest risk of morbidity and mortality.	Emaciated appearance	Weight $\leq$70% standard TSF $\leq$80% standard MAMC $\leq$60% standard	Serum albumin <2.8 g/dl Serum transferrin <100 mg/dl Lymphocytes <900 mm^3 Anergy Creatinine-height index $\leq$60% standard

TABLE 8–7: Abnormalities Due to Nutritional Deficiencies

Pellagra

Pigmented keratotic scaling lesions resulting from a deficiency of niacin. These lesions are especially prominent in areas exposed to the sun, such as hands, forearms, neck, and legs.

Kwashiorkor

Occurs in children and adults whose diets contain mostly carbohydrate and little or no protein and are under stress (growth, parasitic or viral infections, major surgery, trauma, or burns). Accompanying signs include generalized edema, scaling areas of decreased pigmentation, and decreased hair pigmentation.

Follicular Hyperkeratosis

Dry, bumpy skin associated with vitamin A and/or linoleic acid (essential fatty acid) deficiency. Linoleic acid deficiency may also result in eczematous skin, especially in infants.

Scorbutic Gums

Deficiency of vitamin C. Gums are swollen, ulcerated, and bleeding due to vitamin C–induced defects in oral epithelial basement membrane and periodontal collagen fiber synthesis.

Bitot's Spots

Foamy plaques of the cornea that are a sign of vitamin A deficiency. Severe depletion may result in conjunctival xerosis (drying) and progress to corneal ulceration, and finally destruction of the eye (keratomalacia).

Table continued on following page

TABLE 8–7: Abnormalities due to Nutritional Deficiencies—cont'd

Magenta Tongue

"Magenta tongue" is a sign of riboflavin deficiency. In contrast, a pale tongue is probably attributable to iron deficiency; a beefy red–colored tongue is caused by vitamin B-complex deficiency.

Rickets

Sign of vitamin D and calcium deficiencies in children (disorders of cartilage cell growth, enlargement of epiphyseal growth plates) and adults (osteomalacia).

HIV Infection Discordant Twins   ▶

An HIV-infected 4¹⁄₂-year-old girl with her uninfected twin brother. The girl has been sickly since shortly after birth and suffers from HIV-associated malnutrition.

BIBLIOGRAPHY

Adult Treatment Panel III (ATP III): Executive summary of the third report of the National Cholesterol Education Program (NCEP) Expert Panel on Detection, Evaluation, and Treatment of High Blood Cholesterol in Adults, *JAMA* 285:2486–2497, 2001.

Anonymous: Position of the American Dietetic Association: child and adolescent food and nutrition programs, *J Am Diet Assoc* 96(9):913–917, 1996.

Arrowsmith H: A critical evaluation of the use of nutrition screening tools by nurses, *Br J Nurs* 22(8):1483–1490, 1999.

Battaglia FC, Thureen PJ: Nutrition of the fetus and premature infant, *Nutrition* 13(10):903–906, 1997.

Blackburn GL et al: Nutritional and metabolic assessment of the hospitalized patient, *J Parenter Enteral Nutr* 1(1):11–22, 1977.

Bolanowski M, Nilsson BE: Assessment of human body composition using dual-energy x-ray absorptiometry and bioelectrical impedance analysis, *Med Sci Monit* 7(5):1029–1033, 2001.

Drewnowski A, Shultz JM: Impact of aging on eating behaviors, food choices, nutrition, and health status, *J Nutr Health Aging* 5(2):75–79, 2001.

Dwyer JT: *Screening older Americans' nutritional health: current practices and future possibilities* [monograph], Washington, DC, 1991, Nutrition Screening Initiative.

Fischback F: *A manual of laboratory and diagnostic tests,* ed 6, Philadelphia, 2000, Lippincott, Williams and Wilkins.

Frisancho AR: New standards of weight and body composition by frame size and height for assessment of nutritional status of adults and the elderly, *Am J Clin Nutr* 40:808–819, 1984.

Frisancho AR: *Anthropometric standards for the assessment of growth and nutritional status,* Ann Arbor, Mich, 1990, University of Michigan Press.

Frisancho AR, Flegel PN: Elbow breadth as a measure of frame size for U.S. males and females, *Am J Clin Nutr* 31:311–314, 1983.

Gabriella SE, Sinclair AJ: Diagnosing undernutrition in elderly people, *Rev Clin Gerontol* 7:367–371, 1997.

Gentleman B: Malnutrition in the older adult, *Nurse Pract* 25(11):73–76, 2001.

Giotta MP: Nutrition during pregnancy: reducing obstetric risk, *J Perinat Neonatal Nurs* 6(4):1–12, 1993.

Graves DE, Suitor CW: *Celebrating diversity: approaching families through their food,* Arlington, Va, 1998, National Center for Education in Maternal and Child Health.

Ishida DN: Making inroads on cancer prevention and control with Asian Americans, *Semin Oncol Nurs* 17(3):220–228, 2001.

Jackson RT: Separate hemoglobin standards for blacks and whites: a critical review of the case for separate and unequal hemoglobin standards, *Med Hypotheses* 32:181–189, 1990.

Keithley JK, Keller A, Vazquez J: Promoting good nutrition: using the food guide pyramid in clinical practice, *MedSurg Nurs* 5(6):397–403, 1996.

Kolasa KM, Weismiller DG: Nutrition during pregnancy, *Am Fam Physician* 56(1):205–212, 1997.

Kovacevich DS et al: Nutrition risk classification: a valid and reproducible tool for nurses, *Nutr Clin Pract* 12:20–25, 1997.

Lee RD, Nieman DC: *Nutritional assessment,* ed 3, New York, 2003, McGraw-Hill.

Mahan KL, Escott-Stump S: *Krauses's food, nutrition, and diet therapy,* ed 10, Philadelphia, 2000, W.B. Saunders.

Muscari ME: Screening for anorexia and bulimia, *Am J Nurs* 98(11):22–24, 1998.

National Academy of Sciences: *Nutrition during pregnancy,* Washington, DC, 1990, National Academy Press.

National Academy of Sciences: *Nutrition during lactation,* Washington, DC, 1991, National Academy Press.

National Center for Complementary and Alternative Medicine (NCCAM) website: http://nccam.nih.gov [accessed May 1, 2002].

National Center for Health Statistics (NCHS): *Overweight prevalence,* U.S. Department of Health and Human Services, Centers for Disease Control and Prevention, 1999. [Retrieved April 18, 2002, from http://www.cdc.gov/nchs/fastats/overwt.htm.

National Health and Nutrition Examination Survey (NHANES): *NHANES Data,* U.S. Department of Health and Human Services, Centers for Disease Control and Prevention, 2002. [Retrieved April 18, 2002, from http://www.cdc.gov/nchs/nhanes.htm.

National Institutes of Health: *The practical guide: identification, evaluation, and treatment of overweight and obesity in adults* [monograph], Washington, DC, 2000, NHLBI Obesity Education Initiative.

North American Nursing Diagnosis Association: *Nursing Diagnosis: Definitions and Classification 2001–2002,* Philadelphia, 2001, Nursecom.

Nutrition Interventions Manual for Professionals Caring for Older Americans: *Project of the American Academy of Family Physicians, The American Dietetic Association, and National Council on Aging,* Washington, DC, 1994, Nutrition Screening Initiative.

Ottery FD: Definition of standardized nutritional assessment and interventional pathways in oncology, *Nutrition* 12(suppl 1):S15–S19, 1996.

Pennington JAT: *Bowes and Church's food values of portions commonly used,* ed 17, Philadelphia, 1998, J.B. Lippincott.

Recommended Dietary Allowances (RDA). National Academy of Sciences, Food and Nutrition Board (n.d.). [Retrieved April 18, 2002, from http://www.nal.usda.gov/fnic/dga/rda.pdf.]

Rueben DB, Greendale GA, Harrison GG: Nutrition screening in older person, *J Am Geriatr Soc* 43(4):415–425, 1995.

Sampson HA: Peanut allergy, *N Engl J Med* 346(17):1294–1299, 2002.

Sermet-Gaudelus I et al: Simple pediatric nutritional risk score to identify at risk of malnutrition, *Am J Clin Nutr* 72(1):64–70, 2000.

Shopbell JM, Hopkins B, Shronts EP: Nutrition screening and assessment. In Gotschlich M: *The science and practice of nutrition support: a case-based core curriculum,* Dubuque, Iowa, 2001, Kendall/Hunt.

Spector RE: *Cultural diversity in health and illness,* ed 5, Upper Saddle River, NJ, 2000, Prentice Hall.

Subcommittee on Nutritional Status and Weight Gain During Pregnancy, Food and Nutrition Board, National Academy of Sciences: *Nutrition during pregnancy.* Parts I and II, Washington, DC, 1990, National Academy Press.

Sucher KP, Kittler PG: *Food and culture in America: a nutrition handbook,* ed 3, Australia, 2001, Wadsworth/Thomson.

White JV et al: Nutrition screening initiative: development and implementation of the public awareness checklist and screening tools, *J Am Diet Assoc* 92:163–167, 1992.

White JV, Ham RJ, Lipschitz DA: *Nutrition screening initiative: toward a common view* [Monograph], Washington, DC, 1991, Nutrition Screening Initiative.

Nutrition-Related Internet Sites

American Dietetic Association: http://www.eatright.org

Consumer Information Center—the Food Guide Pyramid: http://www.pueblo.gsa.gov/cic_text/food/food-pyramid/main.htm

FDA Food Safety: www.foodsafety.gov

International Food Information Council: http://www.ific.org/food

Mayo Clinic Food and Nutrition Center: http://mayohealth.org

National Eating Disorders Organization: http://www.nationaleating disorders.org

National Institutes of Health—Guidelines for Obesity: http://www.nhlbi.nih.gov/guidelines/obesity/ob_home.htm

U.S. Food and Nutrition Information Center: http://www.nal.usda.gov/fnic/etext/fnic.html

CHAPTER 9

Assessment Techniques and the Clinical Setting

The health history described in the preceding chapters provides **subjective** data for health assessment, the individual's *own* perception of the health state. Unit 3 presents **objective** data, the signs perceived by the examiner through the physical examination.

The physical examination requires that the examiner develop technical skills and a knowledge base. The technical skills are the tools to gather data. You will relate those data to your knowledge base and to your previous experience. A sturdy knowledge base enables you to look *for,* rather than merely look *at.* Consider a statement by the eighteenth century German poet Goethe: "We see only what we know." To recognize a significant finding, you need to know what to look for.

CULTIVATING YOUR SENSES

You will use your senses—sight, smell, touch, and hearing—to gather data during the physical examination. You always have perceived the world through your senses, but now they will be focused in a new way. Applying your senses to assess each individual's health state may seem awkward at first, but this will be polished with repetition and tutored practice. The skills requisite for the physical examination are **inspection, palpation, percussion,** and **auscultation.** The skills are performed one at a time and in this order.

INSPECTION

Inspection is concentrated watching. It is close, careful scrutiny, first of the individual as a whole and then of each body system. Inspection begins the moment you first meet the individual and develop a "general survey." (Specific data to consider for the general survey are presented in the following chapter.) Then as you proceed through the examination, start the assessment of each body system with inspection.

Inspection always comes first. Initially you may feel embarrassed "staring" at the person without also "doing something." But do not be too eager to touch the person. A focused inspection takes time and yields a surprising amount of data. Train yourself not to rush through inspection by placing your hands in your pockets or holding them behind your back.

Learn to use each person as his or her own control and compare the right and left sides of the body. The two sides are nearly symmetric. Inspection requires good lighting, adequate exposure, and occasional use of certain instruments (otoscope, ophthalmoscope, penlight, nasal and vaginal specula) to enlarge your view.

PALPATION

Palpation follows and often confirms points you noted during inspection. Palpation applies your sense of touch to assess these factors: texture, temperature, moisture, organ location and size, as well as any swelling, vibration or pulsation, rigidity or spasticity, crepitation, presence of lumps or masses, and presence of tenderness or pain. Different parts of the hands are best suited for assessing different factors:

- Fingertips—best for fine tactile discrimination, as of skin texture, swelling, pulsation, and determining presence of lumps
- A grasping action of the fingers and thumb—to detect the position, shape, and consistency of an organ or mass
- The dorsa (backs) of hands and fingers—best for determining temperature because the skin here is thinner than on the palms
- Base of fingers (metacarpophalangeal joints) or ulnar surface of the hand—best for vibration.

Your palpation technique should be slow and systematic. A person stiffens when touched suddenly, making it difficult for you to feel very much. Use a calm, gentle approach. Warm your hands by kneading them together or holding them under warm water. Identify any tender areas, and palpate them last.

Start with light palpation to detect surface characteristics and to accustom the person to being touched. Then perform deeper palpation, perhaps by helping the person use relaxation techniques such as imagery or deep breathing. Your sense of touch becomes blunted with heavy or continuous pressure. When deep palpation is needed (as for abdominal contents), intermittent pressure is better than one long continuous palpation. Avoid any situation in which deep palpation could cause internal injury or pain.

Bimanual palpation requires the use of both of your hands to envelop or capture certain body parts or organs—such as the kidneys, uterus, or adnexa—for more precise delimitation (see Chapters 21 and 26).

PERCUSSION

Percussion is tapping the person's skin with short, sharp strokes to assess underlying structures. The strokes yield a palpable vibration and a characteristic sound that depicts the location, size, and density of the underlying organ. Why learn percussion when an x-ray study is so much more accurate? Because your percussing hands are always available, are easily portable, give instant feedback, and have no radiactive side effects. Percussion has the following uses:

- Mapping out the *location* and *size* of an organ by exploring where the percussion note changes between the borders of an organ and its neighbors.
- Signaling the *density* (air, fluid, or solid) of a structure by a characteristic note.
- Detecting an abnormal mass if it is fairly superficial; the percussion vibrations penetrate about 5 cm deep—a deeper mass would give no change in percussion.
- Eliciting pain if the underlying structure is inflamed, as with sinus areas or over the kidney.
- Eliciting a deep tendon reflex using the percussion hammer.

Two methods of percussion can be used—*direct* (sometimes called immediate) and *indirect* (or mediate). In direct percussion the striking hand directly contacts the body wall. This produces a sound and is used in percussing the infant's thorax or the adult's sinus areas. *Indirect* percussion is used more often and involves both hands. The striking hand contacts the stationary hand fixed on the person's skin. This yields a sound and a subtle vibration. The procedure is as follows.

The Stationary Hand

Hyperextend the middle finger (sometimes called the pleximeter) and place its distal portion, the phalanx and distal interphalangeal joint, *firmly* against the person's skin. Avoid the person's ribs and scapulae. Percussing over a bone yields no data because it always sounds "dull." Lift the rest of the stationary hand up off the person's skin (Fig. 9–1). Otherwise the resting hand will dampen off the produced vibrations, just as a drummer uses the hand to halt a drum roll.

The Striking Hand

Use the middle finger of your dominant hand as the *striking finger* (sometimes called the plexor) (Fig. 9–2). Hold your forearm close to the skin surface, with your upper arm and shoulder steady. Scan your muscles to make sure they are steady but not rigid. The action is all in the wrist, and it *must* be relaxed. Spread your fingers, swish your wrist, and bounce your middle finger off the stationary one. Aim for just behind the nail bed or at the distal interphalangeal joint; the goal is to hit the portion of the finger that is pushing the hardest into the skin surface. Flex the striking finger so that its tip, not the finger pad, makes contact. It hits directly at right angles to the stationary finger.

Percuss two times in this location using even, staccato blows. Lift the striking finger off quickly; a resting finger damps off vibrations. Then move to a new body location and repeat, keeping your technique even. The force of the blow determines the loudness of the note. You do not need a very loud sound; use just enough force to achieve a clear note. The thickness of the person's body wall will be a factor. You will need a stronger percussion stroke for persons with obese or very muscular body walls.

Percussion can be an awkward technique for beginning examiners. You may feel surprised and embarrassed if your striking finger misses your stationary hand completely. You may wince if the fingernail of your striking finger is too long and painfully gouges your stationary finger. As with all new skills, refinement follows practice. After a few weeks your hand placement becomes precise and feels natural, and your ears learn to perceive the subtle difference in percussion notes.

9–1

9–2

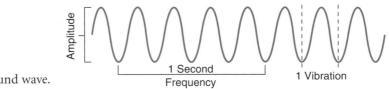

9–3 Sound wave.

Amplitude

1 Second
Frequency

1 Vibration

Production of Sound

All sound results from vibration of some structure (Fig. 9–3). Percussing over a body structure causes vibrations that produce characteristic waves and are heard as "notes" (Table 9–1). Each of the five percussion notes is differentiated by the following components:

1. **Amplitude** (or intensity), a loud or soft sound. The louder the sound, the greater the amplitude. Loudness depends on the force of the blow and the structure's ability to vibrate.
2. **Pitch** (or frequency), the number of vibrations per second, written as "cps," or cycles per second. More rapid vibrations produce a high-pitched tone; slower vibrations yield a low-pitched tone.
3. **Quality** (timbre), a subjective difference due to a sound's distinctive overtones. A pure tone is a sound of one frequency. Variations within a sound wave produce overtones. Overtones allow you to distinguish a C on a piano from a C on a violin.
4. **Duration,** the length of time the note lingers.

A basic principle is that a structure with relatively more air (such as the lungs) produces a louder, deeper, and longer sound because it vibrates freely, whereas a denser, more solid structure (such as the liver) gives a softer, higher, shorter sound because it does not vibrate as easily. Although Table 9–1 describes five "normal" percussion notes, varia-

tions occur in clinical practice. The "note" you hear depends on the nature of the underlying structure, as well as the thickness of the body wall and your correct technique. Do not learn these various notes just from written description. Practice on a willing partner.

AUSCULTATION

Auscultation is listening to sounds produced by the body, such as the heart and blood vessels and the lungs and abdomen. Likely you already have heard certain body sounds with your ear alone—for example, the harsh gurgling of very congested breathing. However, most body sounds are very soft and must be channeled through a **stethoscope** for you to evaluate them. The stethoscope does not magnify sound but does block out extraneous room sounds. Of all the equipment you will use, the stethoscope quickly becomes a very personal instrument. Take time to learn its features and to fit one individually to yourself.

The fit and quality of the stethoscope are important. You cannot assess what you cannot hear through a poor instrument. The slope of the earpiece should point forward toward your nose. This matches the natural slope of your ear canal and efficiently blocks out environmental sound. If necessary, twist the earpieces to parallel the slope of your ear canals. The earpieces should fit snugly, but if they hurt, they are inserted

TABLE 9–1: Characteristics of Percussion Notes

	AMPLITUDE	PITCH	QUALITY	DURATION	SAMPLE LOCATION
Resonant	Medium-loud	Low	Clear, hollow	Moderate	Over normal lung tissue
Hyperresonant	Louder	Lower	Booming	Longer	Normal over child's lung Abnormal in the adult, over lungs with increased amount of air, as in emphysema
Tympany	Loud	High	Musical and drumlike (like the kettle drum)	Sustained longest	Over air-filled viscus, e.g., the stomach, the intestine
Dull	Soft	High	Muffled thud	Short	Relatively dense organ, as liver or spleen
Flat	Very soft	High	A dead stop of sound, absolute dullness	Very short	When no air is present, over thigh muscles, bone, or over tumor

9-4 Stethoscope diaphragm *(left)* and bell *(right)*.

too far. Adjust the tension and experiment with different rubber or plastic earplugs to achieve the most comfort. The tubing should be of thick material, with an internal diameter of 4 mm ($^1/_8$ in), and about 30 to 36 cm (12 to 14 in) long. Longer tubing may distort the sound.

Choose a stethoscope with two endpieces—a diaphragm and a bell (Fig. 9–4). You will use the **diaphragm** most often because its flat edge is best for high-pitched sounds—breath, bowel, and normal heart sounds. (Since your stethoscope touches many people, clean the endpieces with an alcohol swab to eliminate a possible vector of infection.) Hold the diaphragm firmly against the person's skin—firm enough to leave a slight ring afterward. The **bell** endpiece has a deep, hollow cuplike shape. It is best for soft, low-pitched sounds such as extra heart sounds or murmurs. Hold it lightly against the person's skin—just enough that it forms a perfect seal. Any harder causes the person's skin to act as a diaphragm, obliterating the low-pitched sounds.

Before you can evaluate body sounds, you must eliminate any confusing artifacts:

- Any extra room noise can produce a "roaring" in your stethoscope, so the room must be quiet.
- Keep the examination room warm. If the person starts shivering, the involuntary muscle contractions could drown out other sounds.
- Warm the stethoscope endpiece by rubbing it in your palm. This avoids the "chandelier sign" elicited when placing a cold endpiece on a warm chest!
- The friction on the endpiece from a male's hairy chest causes a crackling sound that mimics an abnormal breath sound called *crackles* or *rales.* To minimize this problem, wet the hair before auscultating the area.

- Never listen through a gown. Reach under a gown to listen, but take care that no clothing rubs on the stethoscope.
- Finally, avoid your own "artifact," such as breathing on the tubing, or the "thump" from bumping the tubing together.

Auscultation is a skill that beginning examiners are eager to learn, but one that is difficult to master. First you must learn the wide range of normal sounds. Once you can recognize normal sounds, you can distinguish the abnormal sounds and "extra" sounds. Be aware that in some body locations you may hear more than one sound; this can be confusing. You will need to listen selectively, to only one thing at a time. As you listen, ask yourself: What am I *actually hearing?* . . . What *should* I be hearing at this spot?

SETTING

The examination room should be warm and comfortable, quiet, private, and well lit. When possible, stop any distracting noises—such as humming machinery, radio or television, or people talking—that could make it difficult to hear body sounds. Your time with the individual should be secure from interruptions from other health care personnel. Lighting with natural daylight is best, although it is often not available; artificial light from two sources will suffice and will prevent shadows. A wall-mounted or gooseneck stand lamp is needed for high-intensity lighting.

Position the examination table so that both sides of the person are easily accessible (Fig. 9–5). The table should be at a height at which you can stand without stooping and should be equipped to raise the person's head up to 45 degrees. A roll-up stool is used for the sections of the examination for which you must be sitting. A bedside stand or table is needed to lay out all your equipment.

9-5

EQUIPMENT

During the examination, you do not want to be searching for equipment or to have to leave the room to find an item. Have all your equipment at easy reach and laid out in an organized fashion (Fig. 9–6). The following items are usually needed for a screening physical examination:

- Platform scale with height attachment
- Skinfold calipers
- Sphygmomanometer
- Stethoscope with bell and diaphragm endpieces
- Thermometer
- Flashlight or penlight
- Otoscope/ophthalmoscope
- Tuning fork
- Nasal speculum (if a short, broad speculum is not included with the otoscope)
- Tongue depressor
- Pocket vision screener
- Skin-marking pen
- Flexible tape measure and ruler marked in centimeters
- Reflex hammer

- Sharp object (split tongue blade)
- Cotton balls
- Bivalve vaginal speculum
- Clean gloves
- Materials for cytologic study
- Lubricant
- Fecal occult blood test materials

Most of the equipment is described as it comes into use throughout the text. However, consider these introductory comments on the otoscope and ophthalmoscope.

The **otoscope** funnels light into the ear canal and onto the tympanic membrane. The base serves both as the power source by holding a battery and as the handle. To attach the head, press it down onto the male adaptor end of the base and turn clockwise until you feel a stop. To turn the light on, press the red button rheostat down and clockwise. (Always turn it off after use to increase the life of the bulb and battery.) Five specula, each a different size, are available to attach to the head (Fig. 9–7). (The short, broad speculum is for viewing the nares.) Choose the largest one that will fit comfortably into the person's ear canal. See Chapter 15 for technique on use of the otoscope.

9–6

9–7   Otoscope.

9–8   Ophthalmoscope.

The **ophthalmoscope** illuminates the internal eye structures. Its system of lenses and mirrors enables you to look through the pupil at the fundus (background) of the eye, much like looking through a keyhole at a room beyond. The ophthalmoscope head attaches to the base male adaptor just as the otoscope head does (Fig. 9–8). The head has five different parts:

1. Viewing aperture, with five different apertures
2. Aperture selector dial on the front
3. Mirror window on the front
4. Lens selector dial
5. Lens indicator

Select the aperture to be used (Fig. 9–9).

◯   Large (full spot) for dilated pupils

◦   Small for undilated pupils

◉   Red-free filter — a green beam, used to examine the optic disc for hemorrhage (which looks black) and melanin deposits (which look gray)

⊕   Grid — to determine fixation pattern and to assess size and location of lesions on the fundus

▯   Slit — to examine the anterior portion of the eye and to assess elevation or depression of lesions on the fundus

9–9

Rotating the lens selector dial brings the object into focus. The lens indicator shows a number, or *diopter*, that indicates the value of the lens in position. The black numbers indicate a positive lens, from 0 to +40. The red numbers indicate a negative lens, from 0 to −20. The ophthalmoscope can compensate for myopia (nearsightedness) or hyperopia (farsightedness) but will not correct for astigmatism. See Chapter 14 for details on how to hold the instrument and what to inspect.

The following equipment occasionally will be used, depending on the individual's needs: goniometer to measure joint range of motion, Doppler sonometer to augment pulse or blood pressure measurement, fetoscope for auscultating fetal heart tones, and pelvimeter to measure pelvic width.

For a child you also will need appropriate pediatric-sized endpieces for stethoscope and otoscope specula, materials for developmental assessment, age-appropriate toys, and a nipple or pacifier for an infant.

A CLEAN FIELD

Do not let your stethoscope become a *staph*-oscope! Stethoscopes and other equipment that are frequently used on many patients can become a common vehicle for transmission of infection. Cleaning with an alcohol swab between patients is an effective control.

Designate a "clean" versus a "used" area for handling of your equipment. In a hospital setting, you may use the bedside stand for your clean surface and the overbed table for the used equipment surface. Or in a clinic setting, use two separate areas of the pull-up table. Distinguish the clean area by one or two disposable paper towels. On the towels, place all the new, newly cleaned, or newly alcohol-swabbed equipment that you will use on this patient. Use alcohol swabs to clean all equipment that you carry from patient to patient (e.g., your stethoscope endpieces, the reflex hammer, ruler). As you proceed through the examination, pick up each piece of equipment from the clean area, and after use on the patient, relegate it to the used area or (as in the case of tongue blades, gloves) throw it directly in the trash.

A SAFER ENVIRONMENT

In addition to monitoring the cleanliness of your equipment, take all steps to avoid any possible transmission of infection between patients or between patient and examiner. A *nosocomial* infection (an infection acquired during hospitalization) is a hazard because hospitals have sites that are possible reservoirs for virulent microorganisms. Some of these microorganisms have become resistant to antibiotics, such as methicillin-resistant *Staphylococcus aureus* (MRSA), vancomycin-resistant *Enterococcus* (VRE), or multidrug-resistant tuberculosis. Other microorganisms include those for which there is currently no known cure, such as HIV.

The single most important step to decrease risk of microorganism transmission is to wash your hands promptly and thoroughly for 10 to 15 seconds (or longer if hands appear visibly soiled). Wash hands (1) before and after physical contact with each patient; (2) after inadvertent contact with blood, body fluids, secretions, and excretions; (3) after contact with any equipment contaminated with body fluids; and (4) after removing gloves.

Wear gloves when the potential exists for contact with any body fluids (e.g., blood, mucous membranes, body fluids, drainage, open skin lesions). Wearing gloves is *not* a protective substitute to washing hands, however, because gloves may have undetectable holes or may become torn during use, or hands may become contaminated as gloves are removed. Wear a gown, mask, and protective eyewear when the potential exists for any blood or body fluid spattering (e.g., suctioning, arterial puncture).

The Centers for Disease Control and Prevention (CDC) guidelines include the latest epidemiologic information for decreasing transmission of bloodborne and other infections in hospitals (Garner, 1996). The guidelines include two tiers of precautions. **Standard Precautions** (Table 9–2) are intended for use with *all* patients regardless of their risk or presumed infection status. Standard precautions are designed to reduce the risk of transmission of microorganisms from both recognized and unrecognized sources, and they apply to (1) blood; (2) all body fluids, secretions, and excretions *except sweat*, whether or not they contain visible blood; (3) nonintact skin; and (4) mucous membranes (Garner, 1996).

The second tier is **Transmission-Based Precautions,** intended for use with patients with documented or suspected transmissible infections. They are designed *in addition to* Standard Precautions to interrupt transmission in hospitals.

TABLE 9–2: Standard Precautions for Use With All Patients

A. **Wash hands** after touching blood, body fluids, secretions, excretions, and contaminated items, whether or not wearing gloves. Wash hands immediately after gloves are removed and between patient contacts. May need to wash hands between procedures on the same patient to prevent cross-contamination of different body sites.

B. **Wear clean gloves** when touching blood, body fluids, secretions, excretions, items contaminated with these, mucous membranes, and nonintact skin. Change gloves between tasks and procedures on the same patient after contact with material that may contain a high concentration of microorganisms. Remove gloves promptly after use, before touching noncontaminated items, and before going to another patient, and wash hands immediately.

C. **Wear a mask and eye protection** to protect mucous membranes during procedures and patient care activities that are likely to generate splashes of blood, body fluids, secretions, and excretions.

D. **Wear a gown** (clean, nonsterile, appropriate to activity) to protect skin and prevent soiling of clothing during procedures and patient care activities that are likely to generate splashes of blood, body fluids, secretions, or excretions. Remove a soiled gown promptly and wash hands.

E. **Take care with used patient care equipment,** soiled with blood, body fluids, secretions, and excretions; handle it in a manner that prevents skin and mucous membrane exposure, contamination of clothing, and transfer of microorganisms to other patients and environments. Do not use the reusable equipment on another patient until it has been cleaned and reprocessed appropriately. Discard single-use items appropriately.

F. **Design and follow adequate hospital or clinic procedures** for the routine care, cleaning, and disinfection of environmental surfaces, beds, bed rails, bedside equipment, and other frequently touched surfaces.

G. **Take care with used linen** soiled with blood, body fluids, secretions, and excretions; handle, transport, and process this linen in a manner that prevents skin and mucous membrane exposure and contamination of clothing, and that avoids transfer of microorganisms to other patients and environments.

H. **Prevent injuries due to bloodborne pathogens** when using or handling needles, scalpels, and other sharp instruments. Never recap used needles, manipulate them using both hands, or direct the point of a needle toward any part of the body; rather, use either a one-handed "scoop" technique or an appropriate mechanical device. Do not remove used needles from disposable syringes by hand or otherwise bend, break, or manipulate used needles by hand. Place used disposable syringes, needles, scalpel blades, and other sharp items in appropriate puncture-resistant containers.

Use mouthpieces, resuscitation bags, or other ventilation devices instead of mouth-to-mouth resuscitation methods in areas where the need for resuscitation is predictable.

I. **Place in a private room** any patient who contaminates the environment or who does not or cannot assist in appropriate hygiene or environmental control.

Adapted from Garner JS: *Guidelines for isolation precautions in hospitals,* Atlanta, GA, 1996, Public Health Service, U.S. Department of Health and Human Services, Centers for Disease Control and Prevention.

There are three types of transmission-based precautions: airborne, droplet, and contact. They may be combined for diseases that have multiple routes of transmission, such as varicella (chickenpox) (Appendices B and J).

THE CLINICAL SETTING

GENERAL APPROACH

Consider your emotional state and that of the person being examined. The patient is usually anxious due to the anticipation of being examined by a stranger and the unknown outcome of the examination. If anxiety can be reduced, the person will feel more comfortable and the data gathered will more closely describe the person's natural state. Anxiety can be reduced by an examiner who is confident and self-assured, as well as considerate and unhurried.

Usually, a beginning examiner feels anything *but* self-assured! Most worry about their technical skill, about missing something significant, or about forgetting a step. Many are embarrassed themselves about encountering a partially dressed individual. All these fears are natural and common. The best way to minimize them is with a lot of tutored practice on a healthy willing subject, usually a fellow student. You have to feel comfortable with your motor skills before you can absorb what you are actually seeing or hearing in a "real" patient. This comes with practice under the guidance of an experienced tutor, in an atmosphere in which it is acceptable to make mistakes and to ask questions. Your subject should "act like a patient" so that you can deal with the "real" situation while still in a safe setting. After you feel comfortable with the laboratory setting, accompany your tutor as he or she examines an actual patient so that you can observe an experienced examiner.

HANDS ON

With this preparation, it is possible to interact with your own patient in a confident manner. Begin by measuring the person's height, weight, blood pressure, temperature, pulse, and respirations (see Chapter 10). If needed, measure visual acuity at this time using the Snellen eye chart. All of these are familiar, relatively nonthreatening actions; they will gradually accustom the person to the examination. Then ask the person to change into an examining gown, leaving his or her underpants on. This will feel more comfortable, and the underpants can easily be removed just before the genital examination. Unless your assistance is needed, leave the room as the person undresses.

As you reenter the room, wash your hands in the person's presence. This indicates you are protective of this person and are starting fresh for him or her. Explain each step in the examination and how the person can cooperate. Encourage the person to ask questions. Keep your own movements slow, methodical, and deliberate.

Begin by touching the person's hands, checking skin color, nail beds, and metacarpophalangeal joints (Fig. 9–10; see Chapters 12 and 22). Again, this is a less threatening way to ease a person into being touched. Most people are used to having relative strangers touch their hands.

As you proceed through the examination, avoid distractions and concentrate on one step at a time. The sequence of the steps may differ depending on the age of the person and your own preference. However, you should establish a system that works for you and stick to it to avoid omissions. Organize the steps so the person does not change positions too often. Although proper exposure is necessary, use additional drapes to maintain the person's privacy and to prevent chilling.

Do not hesitate to write out the examination sequence and refer to it as you proceed. The patient will accept this as quite natural if you explain you are making brief notations to ensure accuracy. Many agencies use a printed form. You will find that you will glance at the form less and less as you gain experience. Even with a form, you sometimes may forget a step in the examination. When you realize this, perform the maneuver in the next logical place in the sequence. (See Chapter 28 for the sequence of steps in the complete physical examination.)

As you proceed through the examination, occasionally offer some brief teaching about the person's body. For example, you might say, "This tapping on your back (percussion) is a little like playing different drums. The different notes I hear tell me where each organ starts and stops. You probably can hear the difference yourself from within your body." Or, "Everyone has two sounds for each heartbeat, something like this—lub-dup. Your own beats sound normal." Do not do this with every single step, or you will be hard pressed to make a comment when you do come across an abnormality. But some sharing of information builds rapport and increases the person's confidence in you as an examiner. It also gives the person a little more control in a situation in which it is easy to feel completely helpless.

At some point, you will want to linger in one location to concentrate on some complicated findings. To avoid anxiety, tell the person, "I always listen to heart sounds on a number of places on the chest. Just because I am listening a long time does not necessarily mean anything is wrong with you." And it follows that sometimes you *will* discover a finding that may be abnormal and you want another examiner to double-check. You need to give the person some information, yet you

9–10

should not alarm the person unnecessarily. Say something like, "I do not have a complete assessment of your heart sounds. I want Ms. Wright to listen to you too."

At the end of the examination, summarize your findings and share the necessary information with the person. Thank the person for the time spent. In a hospital setting, apprise the person of what is scheduled next. Before you leave a hospitalized person, lower the bed; make the person comfortable and safe; and return the bedside table, television, or any equipment to the way it was originally.

 DEVELOPMENTAL CONSIDERATIONS

Children are different from adults. Their difference in size is obvious. Their bodies grow in a predictable pattern that is assessed during the physical examination. However, their behavior is also different. Behavior grows and develops through predictable stages, just as the body does. Each examiner needs to know the expected emotional and cognitive features of these stages and to perform the physical examination based on developmental principles (Berk, 2001; Hockenberry, 2003).

With all children, the goal is to increase their comfort in the setting. This approach reveals their natural state as much as possible and will give them a more positive memory of health care providers. Remember that a "routine" examination is anything but routine to the child. You can increase their comfort by attending to the following developmental principles and approaches. The *order* of the developmental stages is more meaningful than the exact chronological age. Each child is an individual and will not fit exactly into one category. For example, if your efforts to "play games" with the preschooler are rebuffed, modify your approach to the security measures used with the toddler.

The Infant

Erikson defines the major task of infancy as establishing trust. An infant is completely dependent on the parent for his or her basic needs. If these needs are met promptly and consistently, the infant feels secure and learns to trust others.

Position
- The parent always should be present to understand normal growth and development and for the child's feeling of security.
- Place the neonate or young infant flat on a padded examination table (Fig. 9–11). The infant also may be held against the parent's chest for some steps.
- Once the baby can sit without support (around 6 months), as much of the examination as possible should be performed while the infant is in the parent's lap.
- By 9 to 12 months, the infant is acutely aware of the surroundings. Anything outside the infant's range of vision is "lost," so the parent must be in full view.

Preparation
- Timing should be 1 to 2 hours after feeding, when the baby is not too drowsy or too hungry.

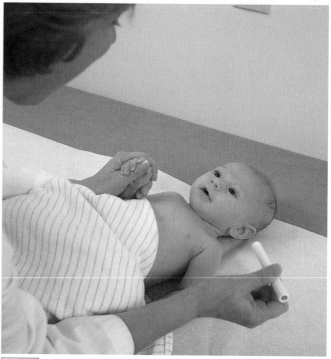

9–11

- Maintain a warm environment. A neonate may require an overhead radiant heater.
- An infant will not object to being nude. Have the parent remove outer clothing, but leave a diaper on a boy.
- An infant does not mind being touched, but make sure your hands and stethoscope endpiece are warm.
- Use a soft, crooning voice during the examination; the baby responds more to the feeling in the tone of the voice than to what is actually said.
- An infant likes eye contact; lock eyes from time to time.
- Smile; a baby prefers a smiling face to a frowning one. (Often beginning examiners are so absorbed in their technique that they look serious or stern.) Take time to play.
- Keep movements smooth and deliberate, not jerky.
- Use a pacifier for crying or during invasive steps.
- Offer brightly colored toys for a distraction when the infant is fussy.
- Let an older baby touch the stethoscope or tongue blade.

Sequence
- Seize the opportunity with a sleeping baby to listen to heart, lung, and abdomen sounds first.
- Perform least distressing steps first. (See the sequence in Chapter 28.) Save the invasive steps of examination of the eye, ear, nose, and throat until last.
- Elicit the Moro or "startle" reflex at the end of the examination because it may cause the baby to cry.

The Toddler

This is Erikson's stage of developing autonomy. However, the need to explore the world and be independent is in conflict with the basic dependency on the parent. This often results in frustration and negativism. The toddler may be difficult to

9–12

examine; do not take this personally. Since he or she is acutely aware of the new environment, the toddler may be frightened and cling to the parent. Also, the toddler has fear of invasive procedures and dislikes being restrained (Fig. 9–12).

Position

- The toddler should be sitting up on the parent's lap for all of the examination. When the toddler must be supine (as in the abdominal examination), move chairs to sit knee-to-knee with parent. Have the toddler lie in the parent's lap with the toddler's legs in your lap.
- Enlist the aid of a cooperative parent to help position the toddler during invasive procedures. The child's legs can be captured between the parent's. An arm of the parent can encircle the child's head, holding it against the chest, and the other arm can hold the child's arms. (See Fig. 16–22.)

Preparation

- Children 1 or 2 years of age can understand symbols, so a security object, such as a special blanket or teddy bear, is helpful.
- Begin by greeting the child and the accompanying parent by name, but with a child 1 to 6 years old, focus more on the parent. By essentially "ignoring" the child at first, you allow the child to adjust gradually and to size you up from a safe distance. Then turn your attention gradually to the child, at first to a toy or object the child is holding, or perhaps to compliment a dress, the hair, or what a big girl or boy the child is. If the child is ready, you will note these signals: eye contact with you, smiling, talking with you, or accepting a toy or a piece of equipment.
- A 2-year-old child does not like to take off his or her clothes; have the parent undress the child one part at a time.
- Children 1 or 2 years of age like to say "No." Do not offer a choice when there really is none. Avoid saying, "May I listen to your heart now?" When the 1- or 2-year-old child says "No," and you go ahead and do it anyway, you lose trust. Instead, use clear firm instructions, in a tone that expects cooperation, "Now it is time for you to lie down so I can check your tummy."

- Also, 1- or 2-year-old children like to make choices. When possible, enhance autonomy by offering the *limited option:* "Shall I listen to your heart next, or your tummy?"
- Demonstrate the procedures on the parent (see Fig. 15–14).
- Praise the child when he or she is cooperative.

Sequence

- Collect some objective data during the history, which is a less stressful time. While you are focusing on the parent, note the child's gross motor and fine motor skills and gait.
- Begin with "games," such as the Denver II test or cranial nerve testing.
- Start with nonthreatening areas. Save distressing procedures—such as examination of the head, ear, nose, or throat—for last.

THE PRESCHOOL CHILD

The child at this stage displays developing initiative. The preschooler takes on tasks independently and plans the task and sees it through. A child of this age is often cooperative, helpful, and easy to involve. However, children of this age have fantasies and may see illness as punishment for being "bad." The concept of body image is limited. The child fears any body injury or mutilation, so he or she will recoil from invasive procedures (e.g., tongue blade, rectal temperature, injection, and venipuncture).

Position

- With a 3-year-old child, the parent should be present and may hold the child on his or her lap (Fig. 9–13).
- A 4- or 5-year-old child usually feels comfortable on the examining table, with the parent present.

Preparation

- A preschooler can talk. Verbal communication becomes helpful now, but remember that the child's understanding is still limited. Use short, simple explanations.
- The preschooler is usually willing to undress. Leave underpants on until the genital examination.

9–13

9-14

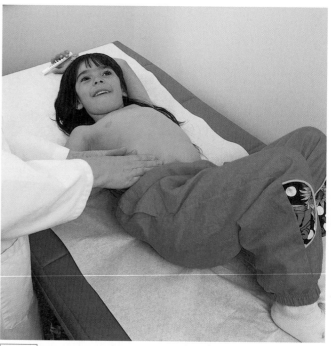

9-15

- Talk to the child and explain the steps in the examination exactly.
- Do not allow a choice when there is none.
- As with the toddler, enhance the autonomy of the preschooler by offering choice when possible.
- Allow the child to play with equipment to reduce fears (Fig. 9–14).
- A preschooler likes to help; have the child hold the stethoscope for you.
- Use games. Have the child "blow out" the light on the penlight as you listen to the breath sounds. Or, pretend to listen to the heart sounds of the child's teddy bear first. One technique that is absorbing to a preschooler is to trace their shape on the examining table paper (Hockenberry et al., 2003). You can comment on how big the child is, then fill in the outline with a heart or stomach and listen to the paper doll first. After the examination, the child can take the paper doll home as a souvenir.
- Use a slow, patient, deliberate approach. Do not rush.
- During the examination give the preschooler needed feedback and reassurance: "Your tummy feels just fine."
- Compliment the child on his or her cooperation.

Sequence
- Examine the thorax, abdomen, extremities, and genitalia first. Although the preschooler is usually cooperative, continue to assess head, eye, ear, nose, and throat last.

THE SCHOOL-AGE CHILD

During the school-age period, the major task of the child is developing industry. The child is developing basic competency in school and in social networks and desires the approval of parents and teachers. When successful, the child has a feeling of accomplishment. During the examination, the child is cooperative and is interested in learning about the body. Language is more sophisticated now, but do not overestimate and treat the school-age child as a small adult. The child's level of understanding does not match that of his or her speech.

Position
- The school-age child should be sitting on the examination table.
- A 5-year-old child has a sense of modesty. To maintain privacy, let the older child (an 11- or 12-year-old child) decide whether parents or siblings should be present.

Preparation
- Break the ice with small talk about family, school, friends, music, or sports.
- The child should undress himself or herself, leave underpants on, and use a gown and drape.
- Demonstrate equipment—a school-age child is curious to know how equipment works.
- Comment on the body and how it works (Fig. 9–15). An 8- or 9-year-old child has some understanding of the body and is interested to learn more. It is rewarding to see the child's eyes light up when he or she hears the heart sounds.

Sequence
- As with the adult, progress from head to toes.

THE ADOLESCENT

The major task of adolescence is developing a self-identity. This takes shape from various sets of values and different social roles (son or daughter, sibling, and student). In the end, each person needs to feel satisfied and comfortable with who he or she is. In the process, the adolescent is increasingly self-conscious and introspective. Peer group values and acceptance are important.

Position
- The adolescent should be sitting on the examination table.
- Examine the adolescent alone, without parent or sibling present.

Preparation
- The body is changing rapidly. During the examination, the adolescent needs feedback that his or her own body is healthy and developing normally.
- The adolescent has keen awareness of body image, often comparing himself or herself to peers. Apprise the adolescent of the wide variation among teenagers on the rate of growth and development (see Sex Maturity Rating, Chapters 17, 24, and 26).
- Communicate with some care. Do not treat the teenager like a child, but do not overestimate and treat him or her like an adult either.
- Since the person is idealistic at this age, the adolescent is ripe for health teaching. Positive attitudes developed now may last through adult life. Focus your teaching on ways the adolescent can promote wellness.

Sequence
- As with the adult, a head-to-toe approach is appropriate. Examine genitalia last, and do it quickly.

THE AGING ADULT

During later years, the tasks are developing the meaning of life and one's own existence and adjusting to changes in physical strength and health.

Position
- The older adult should be sitting on the examination table; a frail older adult may need to be supine.
- Arrange the sequence to allow as few position changes as possible.
- Allow rest periods when needed.

Preparation
- Adjust examination pace to meet possible slowed pace of the aging person. It is better to break the complete examination into a few visits than to rush through the examination and turn off the person.
- Use physical touch (unless there is a cultural contraindication). This is especially important with the aging person because other senses, such as vision and hearing, may be diminished.

- Do not mistake diminished vision or hearing for confusion. Confusion of sudden onset may signify a disease state. It is noted by short-term memory loss, diminished thought process, diminished attention span, and labile emotions (see Mental Status Assessment, Chapter 7).
- Be aware that aging years contain more of life's stress. Loss is inevitable, including changes in physical appearance of the face and body, declining energy level, loss of job through retirement, loss of financial security, loss of long-time home, and death of friends or spouse. How the person adapts to these losses significantly affects health assessment.

Sequence
- Use the head-to-toe approach as in the younger adult.

THE ILL PERSON

For the person in some distress, alter the position during the examination. For example, a person with shortness of breath or ear pain may want to sit up, whereas a person with faintness or overwhelming fatigue may want to be supine. Initially it may be necessary just to examine the body areas appropriate to the problem, collecting a *mini–data base*. You may return to finish a complete assessment after the initial distress is resolved.

BIBLIOGRAPHY

Berk LE: *Development through the lifespan,* ed 2, Boston, 2001, Allyn and Bacon.

Garner JS, Hospital Infection Control Practices Advisory Committee: *Guideline for isolation precautions in hospitals,* Atlanta, Ga, 1996, Public Health Service, U.S. Department of Health and Human Services, Centers for Disease Control and Prevention.

Goldberg EA: Physical assessment of children ages 1 to 10 years, *ANNA J* 24(2):209–217, 1997.

Grenier M et al: Clinical comparison of acoustic and electronic stethoscopes and design of a new electronic stethoscope, *Am J Cardiol* 81(5):653–656, Mar 1, 1998.

Hockenberry M et al: *Wong's nursing care of infants and children,* ed 7, St Louis, 2003, Mosby.

O'Keefe M: Revitalizing the art of auscultation, *JEMS* 26(5):79–80, May 2001.

Perkin RM, Van Stralen D: 20 things you may not know about pediatrics, *JEMS* 25(3):38–49, Mar 2000.

Ricchini W: Sound advice about stethoscopes, *Adv Nurse Pract* 6(5):65–66, May 1998.

Romig LE: PREP for peds: size-up & approach tips for pediatric calls, *JEMS* 26(5):24–33, May 2001.

Stone JT, Wyman JF, Salisbury SA: *Clinical gerontological nursing: a guide to advance practice,* ed 2, Philadelphia, 1998, W.B. Saunders.

Thofern UAR: Bacterial contamination of hospital physicians' stethoscopes, *Infect Control Hosp Epidemiol* 21(9):558–559, Sep 2000.

Thomas DO: Assessing children—it's different, *RN* 19:38–45, Apr 1996.

CHAPTER 10

General Survey, Measurement, Vital Signs

Objective Data

The general survey is a study of the whole person, covering the general health state and any obvious physical characteristics. It is an introduction for the physical examination that will follow; it should give an overall impression, a "gestalt," of the person (see Sample Charting). Objective parameters are used to form the general survey, but these apply to the whole person, not just to one body system.

Launch a general survey at the moment you first encounter the person. What leaves an immediate impression? Does the person stand promptly as his or her name is called and walk easily to meet you? Or does the person look sick, rising slowly or with effort, with shoulders slumped and eyes without luster or downcast? Is the hospitalized person conversing with visitors, involved in reading or television, or lying perfectly still? Even as you introduce yourself and shake hands, you collect data. Does the person fully extend the arm, shake your hand firmly, make eye contact, or smile? Are the palms dry or wet and clammy? As you proceed through the health history, the measurements, and the vital signs, note the following points that will add up to the general survey. Consider these four areas: **physical appearance**, **body structure**, **mobility**, and **behavior**.

NORMAL RANGE OF FINDINGS	ABNORMAL FINDINGS

THE GENERAL SURVEY

Physical Appearance

Age—The person appears his or her stated age.

Appears older than stated age, as with chronic illness, chronic alcoholism.
Delayed or precocious puberty.

Sex—Sexual development is appropriate for gender and age.

Level of consciousness—The person is alert and oriented, attends to your questions and responds appropriately.

Confused, drowsy, lethargic (see Table 7–3, Levels of Consciousness).

Skin color—Color tone is even, pigmentation varying with genetic background, skin is intact with no obvious lesions.

Pallor, cyanosis, jaundice, erythema, any lesions (see Chapter 12).

Facial features—Facial features are symmetric with movement.

Immobile, masklike, asymmetric, drooping (see Table 13–5, Abnormal Facial Appearances with Chronic Illness).

No signs of acute distress are present.

Respiratory signs—shortness of breath, wheezing.
Pain, indicated by facial grimace, holding body part.

Body Structure

Stature—The height appears within normal range for age, genetic heritage (see Measurement, p. 178).

Excessively short or tall (see Table 10–6, Abnormalities in Body Height and Proportion).

Nutrition—The weight appears within normal range for height and body build; body fat distribution is even.

Cachectic, emaciated.
Simple obesity, with even fat distribution.
Centripetal (truncal) obesity—fat concentrated in face, neck, trunk, with thin extremities, as in Cushing's syndrome (hyperadrenalism) (see Table 10–6).

Symmetry—Body parts look equal bilaterally and are in relative proportion to each other.

Unilateral atrophy or hypertrophy.
Asymmetric location of a body part.

NORMAL RANGE OF FINDINGS	ABNORMAL FINDINGS
Posture—The person stands comfortably erect as appropriate for age. Note the normal "plumb line" through anterior ear, shoulder, hip, patella, ankle. Exceptions are the standing toddler who has a normally protuberant abdomen ("toddler lordosis") and the aging person who may be stooped with kyphosis.	Rigid spine and neck; moves as one unit, e.g., arthritis. Stiff and tense, ready to spring from chair, fidgety movements. Shoulders slumped; looks deflated, e.g., depression.
Position—The person sits comfortably in a chair or on the bed or examination table, arms relaxed at sides, head turned to examiner.	Tripod—leaning forward with arms braced on chair arms, occurs with chronic pulmonary disease. Sitting straight up and resists lying down, e.g., congestive heart failure. Curled up in fetal position, e.g., acute abdominal pain.
Body build, contour—proportions are 1. Arm span (fingertip to fingertip) equals height. 2. Body length from crown to pubis roughly equal to length from pubis to sole. Obvious physical deformities—note any congenital or acquired defects.	Elongated arm span, arm span greater than height, e.g., Marfan's syndrome hypogonadism (see Table 10–6). Missing extremities or digits; webbed digits; shortened limb.
Mobility **Gait**—Normally, the base is as wide as the shoulder width; foot placement is accurate; the walk is smooth, even, and well-balanced; and associated movements, such as symmetric arm swing, are present.	Exceptionally wide base. Staggered, stumbling. Shuffling, dragging, nonfunctional leg. Limping with injury. Propulsion—difficulty stopping (see Table 23–6, Abnormal Gaits).
Range of motion—Note full mobility for each joint, and that movement is deliberate, accurate, smooth, and coordinated. (See Chapter 22 for information on more detailed testing of joint range of motion.) No involuntary movement.	Limited joint range of motion. Paralysis—absent movement. Movement jerky, uncoordinated. Tics, tremors, seizures (see Table 23–5, Abnormalities in Muscle Movement).
Behavior **Facial expression**—The person maintains eye contact (unless a cultural taboo exists), expressions are appropriate to the situation, e.g., thoughtful, serious, or smiling. (Note expressions both while the face is at rest and while the person is talking.)	Flat, depressed, angry, sad, anxious. However, note that anxiety is common in ill people. Also, some people smile when they are anxious.
Mood and affect—The person is comfortable and cooperative with the examiner and interacts pleasantly.	Hostile, distrustful, suspicious, crying.
Speech—Articulation (the ability to form words) is clear and understandable.	Dysarthria and dysphagia (see Table 7–4, Speech Disorders). Speech defect, monotone, garbled speech.
The stream of talking is fluent, with an even pace. The person conveys ideas clearly. Word choice is appropriate to culture and education. The person communicates in prevailing language easily by himself or herself or with an interpreter.	Extremes of few words or of constant talking.

NORMAL RANGE OF FINDINGS	ABNORMAL FINDINGS

Dress—Clothing is appropriate to the climate, looks clean and fits the body, and is appropriate to the person's culture and age group; for example, normally, Amish women wear clothing from the nineteenth century, Indian women may wear saris. Culturally determined dress should not be labeled as bizarre by Western standards.

Trousers too large and held up by belt suggest weight loss, as does the addition of new holes in belt. If the belt is moved to a looser fit, it may indicate obesity or ascites.

Consistent wear of certain clothing may provide clues: long sleeves may conceal needle marks of drug abuse; broad-brimmed hats may reveal sun intolerance; Velcro fasteners instead of buttons may indicate chronic motor dysfunction.

Personal hygiene—The person appears clean and groomed appropriately for his or her age, occupation, and socioeconomic group. (Note that a wide variation of dress and hygiene is "normal." Many cultures do not include use of deodorant or women shaving legs.)

Hair is groomed, brushed. Women's make-up is appropriate for age and culture.

In a previously carefully groomed woman, unkempt hair and absent make-up may indicate malaise or illness.

MEASUREMENT

Weight

Use a standardized *balance* or electronic standing scale. Instruct the person to remove his or her shoes and heavy outer clothing before standing on the scale. When a sequence of repeated weights is necessary, aim for approximately the same time of day and the same type of clothing worn each time. Record the weight in kilograms and in pounds.

Show the person how his or her own weight matches up to the recommended range for height (Table 10–1). Compare the person's current weight with that from the previous health visit. A recent weight loss may be explained by successful dieting. A weight gain usually reflects overabundant caloric intake, unhealthy eating habits, and sedentary lifestyle.

An unexplained weight loss may be a sign of a short-term illness (e.g., fever, infection, disease of the mouth or throat) or a chronic illness (endocrine disease, malignancy, mental health dysfunction).

Obesity is >120% ideal body weight and occasionally may be due to endocrine disorders, drug therapy (e.g., corticosteroids), or mental depression.

TABLE 10–1: Height and Weight Tables for Men and Women According to Frame, Ages 25–59

HEIGHT*		WEIGHT†			HEIGHT*		WEIGHT†		
FEET	INCHES	SMALL FRAME	MEDIUM FRAME	LARGE FRAME	FEET	INCHES	SMALL FRAME	MEDIUM FRAME	LARGE FRAME
MEN					**WOMEN**				
5	2	128-134	131-134	138-150	4	10	102-111	109-121	118-131
5	3	130-136	133-143	140-153	4	11	103-113	111-123	120-134
5	4	132-138	135-145	142-156	5	0	104-115	113-126	122-137
5	5	134-140	137-148	144-160	5	1	106-118	115-129	125-140
5	6	136-142	139-151	146-164	5	2	108-121	118-132	128-143
5	7	138-145	142-154	149-168	5	3	111-124	121-135	131-147
5	8	140-148	145-157	152-172	5	4	114-127	124-138	134-151
5	9	142-151	148-160	155-176	5	5	117-130	127-141	137-155
5	10	144-154	151-163	158-180	5	6	120-133	130-144	140-159
5	11	146-157	154-166	161-184	5	7	123-136	133-147	143-163
6	0	149-160	157-170	164-188	5	8	126-139	136-150	146-167
6	1	152-164	160-174	168-192	5	9	129-142	139-153	149-170
6	2	155-168	164-178	172-197	5	10	132-145	142-156	152-173
6	3	158-172	167-182	176-202	5	11	135-148	145-159	155-176
6	4	162-176	171-187	181-207	6	0	138-151	148-162	158-179

*Shoes with 1-inch heels.
†Weight in pounds. Men: allow 5 lb of clothing. Women: allow 3 lb of clothing.
Courtesy of Metropolitan Life Insurance Company, 1983.

NORMAL RANGE OF FINDINGS	ABNORMAL FINDINGS

NORMAL RANGE OF FINDINGS

Height

Use the measuring pole on the balance scale. Align the extended headpiece with the top of the head. The person should be shoeless, standing straight, and looking straight ahead.

Note that measurement of skinfold thickness is described in Chapter 8.

VITAL SIGNS

Temperature

Cellular metabolism requires a stable core, or "deep body," temperature of a mean of 37.2° C (99° F). The body maintains a steady temperature through a thermostat, or feedback mechanism, regulated in the hypothalamus of the brain. The thermostat balances heat production (from metabolism, exercise, food digestion, external factors) with heat loss (through radiation, evaporation of sweat, convection, conduction).

The various routes of temperature measurement reflect the body's core temperature. The normal oral temperature in a resting person is 37° C (98.6° F), with a range of 35.8° C to 37.3° C (96.4° F to 99.1° F). The rectal temperature measures 0.4° C to 0.5° C (0.7° F to 1° F) higher. The normal temperature is influenced by

- A diurnal cycle of 1° F to 1.5° F, with the trough occurring in the early morning hours and the peak occurring in late afternoon to early evening.
- The menstruation cycle in women. Progesterone secretion, occurring with ovulation at midcycle, causes a 0.5° F to 1.0° F rise in temperature that continues until menses.
- Exercise. Moderate to hard exercise increases body temperature.
- Age. Wider normal variations occur in the infant and young child due to less effective heat control mechanisms. In older adults, temperature is usually lower than in other age groups, with a mean of 36.2° C (97.2° F).

The **oral** temperature is accurate and convenient. The oral sublingual site has a rich blood supply from the carotid arteries that quickly responds to changes in inner core temperature.

Due to environmental concerns of mercury pollution from medical waste incinerators, most medical settings are replacing mercury-containing oral thermometers and sphygmomanometers with electronic equipment (Goldman and Shannon, 2001). When the *mercury-in-glass* thermometer is the only equipment available, shake it down to 35.5° C (96° F) and place it at the base of the tongue in either of the posterior sublingual pockets—*not* in front of the tongue. Instruct the person to keep his or her lips closed. Leave in place 3 to 4 minutes if the person is afebrile, and up to 8 minutes if febrile. (Take other vital signs during this time.) Wait 15 minutes if the person has just taken hot or iced liquids and 2 minutes if he or she has just smoked.

The **electronic thermometer** has the advantages of swift and accurate measurement (usually in 20 to 30 seconds) as well as safe, unbreakable, disposable probe covers. The instrument must be fully charged and correctly calibrated. Most children enjoy watching their temperature numbers advance on the box.

The **axillary** temperature is safe and accurate for infants and young children when the environment is reasonably controlled (see Developmental Considerations, p. 189).

Take a **rectal** temperature only when the other routes are not practical—for example, for comatose or confused persons; for persons in shock; or for those who cannot close the mouth because of breathing or oxygen tubes, wired mandible, or other facial dysfunction or if no tympanic membrane thermometer equipment is available. Wear gloves and insert a lubricated rectal probe cover on an electronic thermometer only 2 to 3 cm (1 in) into the adult rectum, directed toward the umbilicus. (For a glass thermometer, leave in place for 2½ minutes.) Disadvantages to the rectal route are patient discomfort and the time-consuming and disruptive nature of the activity.

ABNORMAL FINDINGS

The thermostatic function of the hypothalamus may become scrambled during illness or central nervous system disorders.

Hyperthermia, or fever, is caused by pyrogens secreted by toxic bacteria during infections or from tissue breakdown such as that following myocardial infarction, trauma, surgery, or malignancy. Neurologic disorders (e.g., a cerebral vascular accident, cerebral edema, brain trauma, tumor, or surgery) also can reset the brain's thermostat at a higher level, resulting in heat production and conservation.

Hypothermia is usually due to accidental, prolonged exposure to cold. It also may be purposefully induced to lower the body's oxygen requirements during heart or peripheral vascular surgery, neurosurgery, amputation, or gastrointestinal hemorrhage.

NORMAL RANGE OF FINDINGS

The **tympanic membrane thermometer** (TMT) senses the infrared emissions of the tympanic membrane (eardrum). The tympanic membrane shares the same vascular supply that perfuses the hypothalamus (the internal carotid artery); thus it is an accurate measurement of core temperature (Gilbert et al, 2002).

The tympanic membrane thermometer is a noninvasive, nontraumatic device that is extremely quick and efficient. The probe tip has the shape of an otoscope, the instrument used to inspect the ear. Gently place the covered probe tip in the person's ear canal (see Fig. 10–14 on p. 194). Do not force it and do not occlude the canal. Activate the device and you can read the temperature in 2 to 3 seconds.

There is minimal chance of cross-contamination using the tympanic thermometer because the ear canal is lined with skin and not mucous membrane. This thermometer is successful in use with unconscious patients or with those who are unable or unwilling to cooperate with traditional techniques (i.e., those in critical care units, emergency departments, recovery areas, labor and delivery units). Some clinicians favor the use of the tympanic thermometer over the usual rectal and oral thermometers because of its speed, convenience, safety, reduced risk of injury and infection, and noninvasiveness.

Report the temperature in degrees Celsius unless your agency uses the Fahrenheit scale. Use this conversion:

$$\text{Degrees C} = \tfrac{5}{9}\,(F - 32)$$
$$\text{Degrees F} = (\tfrac{9}{5} \cdot C) + 32$$

Familiarize yourself with both scales. Note that it is far easier to learn to *think* in the centigrade scale than to take the time for paper-and-pencil conversions. Begin by memorizing these convenient equivalents:

$$104.0° \text{ F} = 40.0° \text{ C}; \quad 98.6° \text{ F} = 37.0° \text{ C}; \quad 95.0° \text{ F} = 35.0° \text{ C}.$$

Pulse

With every beat, the heart pumps an amount of blood—the **stroke volume**—into the aorta. This is about 70 ml in the adult. The force flares the arterial walls and generates a pressure wave, which is felt in the periphery as the **pulse**. Palpating the peripheral pulse gives the rate and rhythm of the heartbeat, as well as local data on the condition of the artery. The *radial* pulse is usually palpated while vital signs are measured.

Using the pads of your first three fingers, palpate the radial pulse at the flexor aspect of the wrist laterally along the radius bone (Fig. 10–1). Push until you feel the strongest pulsation. If the rhythm is regular, count the number of beats in 30 seconds and multiply by 2. Although the 15-second interval is frequently practiced, any one-beat error in counting results in a recorded error of four beats per minute. The 30-second interval is the most accurate and efficient when heart rates are normal or rapid and when rhythms are regular. However, if the rhythm is irregular, count for a full minute (Sneed and Hollerbach, 1992). As you begin the counting interval, start your count with "zero" for the first pulse felt. The second pulse felt is "one," and so on. Assess the pulse, including (1) rate, (2) rhythm, (3) force, and (4) elasticity.

10–1

NORMAL RANGE OF FINDINGS

RATE. In the resting adult, the normal heart rate range is 60 to 100 beats per minute (bpm). The rate normally varies with age, being more rapid in infancy and childhood and more moderate during adult and older years. The rate also varies with gender; after puberty, females have a slightly faster rate than males (Table 10–2).

TABLE 10–2: Normal Resting Pulse Rates Across Age Groups

AGE	AVERAGE (BEATS PER MINUTE)	NORMAL LIMITS
Newborn	120	70-190
1 yr	120	80-160
2 yr	110	80-130
4 yr	100	80-120
6 yr	100	75-115
8 yr	90	70-110
10 yr	90	70-110
12 yr		
Female	90	70-110
Male	85	65-105
14 yr		
Female	85	65-105
Male	80	60-100
16 yr		
Female	80	60-100
Male	75	55-95
18 yr		
Female	75	55-95
Male	70	50-90
Well-conditioned athlete	May be 50-60	50-100
Adult	74-76	60-100
Aging	74-76	60-100

In the adult, a heart rate less than 60 bpm is **bradycardia**. This occurs normally in the well-trained athlete whose heart muscle develops along with the skeletal muscles. The stronger, more efficient heart muscle pushes out a larger stroke volume with each beat, thus requiring fewer beats per minute to maintain a stable cardiac output. (Review the equation CO = SV × R, or Cardiac Output = Stroke Volume × Rate, in Chapter 19.) A more rapid heart rate, over 100 bpm, is **tachycardia**. It occurs normally with anxiety or with increased exercise to match the body's demand for increased metabolism.

Some researchers propose that the range of normal resting heart rate for adults should be shifted down to new limits of 50 to 90 bpm, rather than the traditional 60 to 100 bpm (Spodick, 1993). Revising the limits down would account for the physically fit individuals who have resting heart rates well below 60 and often 50 bpm. Also, lowering the tachycardia threshold would agree with studies that show heart rates over 90 bpm do occur with conditions of sepsis and following myocardial infarction.

RHYTHM. The rhythm of the pulse normally has an even tempo. However, one irregularity that is commonly found in children and young adults is **sinus arrhythmia.** Here the heart rate varies with the respiratory cycle, speeding up at the peak of inspiration and slowing to normal with expiration. Inspiration momentarily causes a decreased stroke volume from the left side of the heart; to compensate, the heart rate increases. (See Chapter 19 for a full discussion on sinus arrhythmia.) If any other irregularities are felt, auscultate heart sounds for a more complete assessment (see Chapter 19).

For descriptions of abnormal rates and rhythms, see Table 20–1, Variations in Arterial Pulse.

NORMAL RANGE OF FINDINGS	ABNORMAL FINDINGS

FORCE. The force of the pulse shows the strength of the heart's stroke volume. A "weak, thready" pulse reflects a decreased stroke volume (e.g., as occurs with hemorrhagic shock). A "full, bounding" pulse denotes an increased stroke volume, as with anxiety, exercise, and some abnormal conditions. The pulse force is recorded using a three-point scale:

3+—Full, bounding
2+—Normal
1+—Weak, thready
0—Absent

Some agencies use a four-point scale; make sure your system is consistent with that used by the rest of your staff. Either scale is somewhat subjective. Experience will increase your clinical judgment.

ELASTICITY. With normal elasticity, the artery feels springy, straight, resilient.
Chapter 19 presents assessment of the precordium, including listening to the heart rate and rhythm as well as the quality of heart sounds. Chapter 20, on peripheral vascular assessment, presents further data on other pulse sites.

Respirations

Normally, a person's breathing is relaxed, regular, automatic, and silent. Since most people are unaware of their breathing, do not mention that you will be counting the respirations, because sudden awareness may alter the normal pattern. Instead, maintain your position of counting the radial pulse and unobtrusively count the respirations. Count for 30 seconds or for a full minute if you suspect an abnormality. Avoid the 15-second interval. The result can vary by a factor of $+$ or $-$ 4, which is significant with such a small number.

Note that respiratory rates presented in Table 10–3 normally are more rapid in infants and children. Also, a fairly constant ratio of pulse rate to respiratory rate exists, which is about 4:1. Normally, both pulse and respiratory rates rise as a response to exercise or anxiety. More detailed assessment on respiratory status is presented in Chapter 18.

TABLE 10–3: Normal Respiratory Rates	
AGE	BREATHS PER MINUTE
Neonate	30-40
1 yr	20-40
2 yr	25-32
4 yr	23-30
6 yr	21-26
8 yr	20-26
10 yr	20-26
12 yr	18-22
14 yr	18-22
16 yr	16-20
18 yr	12-20
Adult	10-20

Blood Pressure

Blood pressure (BP) is the force of the blood pushing against the side of its container, the vessel wall. The strength of the push changes with the event in the cardiac cycle. The **systolic** pressure is the maximum pressure felt on the artery dur-

NORMAL RANGE OF FINDINGS	ABNORMAL FINDINGS

ing left ventricular contraction, or systole. The **diastolic** pressure is the elastic recoil, or resting, pressure that the blood exerts constantly between each contraction. The **pulse pressure** is the difference between the systolic and diastolic and reflects the stroke volume (Fig. 10–2). The **mean arterial pressure (MAP)** is the pressure forcing blood into the tissues, averaged over the cardiac cycle. This is not an arithmetic average of systolic and diastolic pressures because diastole lasts longer. Rather, it is a value closer to diastolic pressure plus one third the pulse pressure.

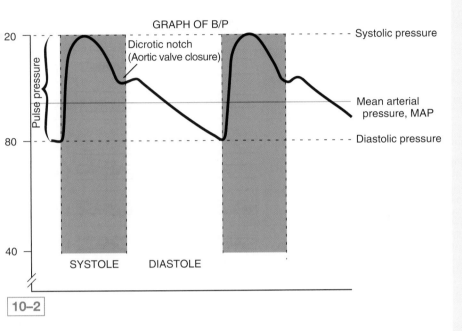

GRAPH OF B/P

Systolic pressure

Dicrotic notch
(Aortic valve closure)

Mean arterial
pressure, MAP

Diastolic pressure

Pulse pressure

SYSTOLE   DIASTOLE

10–2

The average BP in the young adult is 120/80 mm Hg, although this varies normally with many factors, such as:

- **Age.** Normally, a gradual rise occurs through childhood and into the adult years (see Fig. 10–17).
- **Sex.** Before puberty, no difference exists between males and females. After puberty, females usually show a lower BP reading than male counterparts. After menopause, BP in females is higher than in male counterparts.
- **Race.** In the United States, a black adult's BP is usually higher than that of a white person of the same age. The incidence of hypertension is twice as high in blacks as in whites. The reasons for this difference are not understood fully but appear to be due to genetic heritage and environmental factors.
- **Diurnal rhythm.** A daily cycle of a peak and a trough occurs: the BP climbs to a high in late afternoon or early evening and then declines to an early morning low.
- **Weight.** BP is higher in obese persons than in persons of normal weight of the same age (including adolescents).
- **Exercise.** Increasing activity yields a proportionate increase in BP. Within 5 minutes of terminating the exercise, the BP normally returns to baseline.
- **Emotions.** The BP momentarily rises with fear, anger, and pain as a result of stimulation of the sympathetic nervous system.
- **Stress.** The BP is elevated in persons experiencing continual tension because of their lifestyle, occupational stress, or life problems.

FACTORS CONTROLLING BLOOD PRESSURE

FACTOR	CONDITION	RESULT
Cardiac output	↑ with heavy exercise to meet body demand for increased metabolism	↑ BP
	↓ with pump failure (weak pumping action after myocardial infarction, or in shock)	↓ BP
Vascular resistance	↑ resistance (vasoconstriction)	↑ BP
	↓ resistance (vasodilatation)	↓ BP
Volume	↓ volume (hemorrhage)	↓ BP
	↑ volume (increased sodium and water retention, intravenous fluid overload)	↑ BP
Viscosity	↑ viscosity (increased hematocrit in polycythemia)	↑ BP
Elasticity of arterial walls	↑ rigidity, hardening as in arteriosclerosis (heart pumping against greater resistance)	↑ BP

10–3

The level of **BP** is determined by five factors:

1. **Cardiac output.** If the heart pumps more blood into the container (i.e., the blood vessels), the pressure on the container walls increases (Fig. 10–3).
2. **Peripheral vascular resistance.** This is the opposition to blood flow through the arteries. When the container becomes smaller (e.g., such as with constricted vessels), the pressure needed to push the contents becomes greater.
3. **Volume of circulating blood.** This is how tightly the blood is packed into the arteries. Increasing the contents in the container increases the pressure.
4. **Viscosity.** The "thickness" of blood is determined by its formed elements, the blood cells. When the contents are thicker, the pressure increases.
5. **Elasticity of vessel walls.** When the container walls are stiff and rigid, the pressure needed to push the contents increases.

Blood pressure is measured using a stethoscope and a *sphygmomanometer* of either the aneroid or mercury type. As mentioned, the mercury sphygmomanometer is being replaced in medical settings. The aneroid gauge is subject to drift; it must be recalibrated at least once each year and it must rest at zero.

The cuff consists of an inflatable rubber bladder inside a cloth cover. The width of the rubber bladder should equal 40% of the circumference of the person's arm. The length of the bladder should equal 80% of this circumference.

Available cuffs include six sizes that fit newborns to the extra-large adult, as well as tapered cuffs for the cone-shaped obese arm, and thigh cuffs. Match the appropriate size cuff to the person's arm size and shape and not to the person's age (Fig. 10–4).

The cuff size is important; using a cuff that is too narrow yields a falsely high BP because it takes extra pressure to compress the artery.

NORMAL RANGE OF FINDINGS	ABNORMAL FINDINGS

Thigh cuff or large arm cuff

Standard adult arm cuff

10–4

ARM PRESSURE. A comfortable, relaxed person yields a valid blood pressure. Many people are anxious at the beginning of an examination; allow at least a 5-minute rest before measuring the BP. Then take two or more BP measurements separated by two minutes.

For each person, verify BP in both arms once, either on admission or for the first complete physical examination. It is not necessary to continue to check both arms for screening or monitoring. Occasionally a 5- to 10-mm Hg difference may occur in BP in the two arms (if values are different, use the higher value).

A difference in the two arms of more than 10 to 15 mm Hg may indicate arterial obstruction on the side with the lower reading.

The person may be sitting or lying, with the bare arm supported at heart level. (If used, place the mercury manometer so that it is vertical and at your eye level.) When sitting, the patient's feet should be flat on the floor, because BP has a false high measurement when legs are crossed versus uncrossed (Keele-Smith and Price-Daniel, 2001).

Palpate the brachial artery, which is located just above the antecubital fossa, medial to the biceps tendon. With the cuff deflated, center it about 2.5 cm (1 in) above the brachial artery and wrap it evenly.

Now palpate the brachial or the radial artery (Fig. 10–5). Inflate the cuff until the artery pulsation is obliterated and then 20 to 30 mm Hg beyond. This will avoid missing an **auscultatory gap,** which is a period when Korotkoff's sounds disappear during auscultation (Table 10–4).

An auscultatory gap occurs in about 5% of people, most often in hypertension due to a noncompliant arterial system.

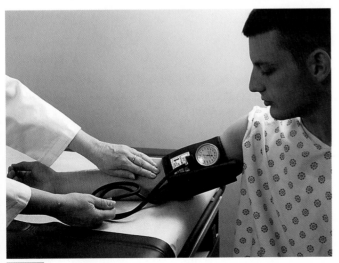

10–5

TABLE 10–4: Korotkoff Sounds

PHASE	QUALITY	DESCRIPTION	RATIONALE
Cuff correctly inflated	No sound		Cuff inflation compresses brachial artery. Cuff pressure exceeds heart's systolic pressure, occluding brachial artery blood flow.
I	Tapping	Soft, clear tapping, increasing in intensity	The SYSTOLIC pressure. As the cuff pressure lowers to reach intraluminal systolic pressure, the artery opens, and blood first spurts into the brachial artery. Blood is at very high velocity because of small opening of artery and large pressure difference across opening. This creates turbulent flow, which is audible.
Auscultatory gap*	No sound	Silence for 30–40 mm Hg	Sounds temporarily disappear during end of phase I, then reappear in phase II. Common with hypertension. If undetected, results in falsely low systolic or falsely high diastolic reading.
II	Swooshing	Softer murmur follows tapping	Turbulent blood flow through still partially occluded artery.
III	Knocking	Crisp, high-pitched sounds	Longer duration of blood flow through artery. Artery closes just briefly during late diastole.
IV	Abrupt muffling	Sound mutes to a low-pitched, cushioned murmur; blowing quality	Artery no longer closes in any part of cardiac cycle. Change in quality, not intensity.
V	Silence		Decreased velocity of blood flow. Streamlined blood flow is silent. The last audible sound (marking the disappearance of sounds) is DIASTOLIC pressure. The fifth Korotkoff sound is now used to define diastolic pressure in all age groups (JNC-VI, 1997).

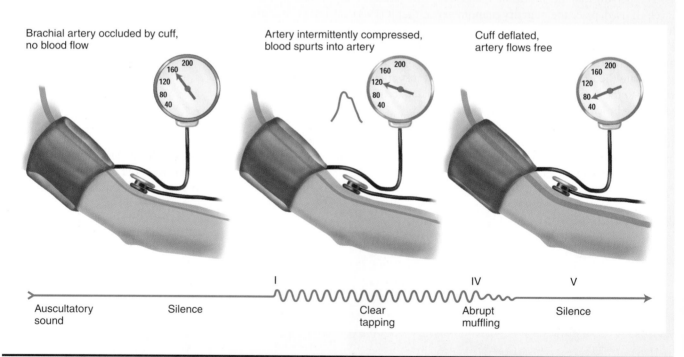

*This is an abnormal finding.

NORMAL RANGE OF FINDINGS

Deflate the cuff quickly and completely; then wait 15 to 30 seconds before re-inflating so that the blood trapped in the veins can dissipate. Place the bell of the stethoscope over the site of the brachial artery, making a light but airtight seal (Fig. 10–6). The diaphragm endpiece is usually adequate, but the bell is designed to pick up low-pitched sounds such as the sounds of a blood pressure reading. So if you have a bell, use it.

Rapidly inflate the cuff to the maximal inflation level you determined. Then deflate the cuff slowly and evenly, about 2 mm Hg per heartbeat. Note the points at which you hear the first appearance of sound, the muffling of sound, and the final disappearance of sound. These are phases I, IV, and V of **Korotkoff's sounds,** which are the components of a BP reading first described by a Russian surgeon in 1905 (see Table 10–4).

10–6

For all age groups, the fifth Korotkoff phase is now used to define diastolic pressure (Joint National Committee–VII[JNC-VII], 2003). However, when a variance greater than 10 to 12 mm Hg exists between phases IV and V, record *both* phases along with the systolic reading (e.g., 142/98/80). Clear communication is important because the results significantly affect diagnosis and planning of care. See Table 10–5 for a list of common errors in blood pressure measurement.

ORTHOSTATIC (OR POSTURAL) VITAL SIGNS. Take serial measurements of pulse and blood pressure when: you suspect volume depletion; when the person is known to have hypertension or is taking antihypertensive medications; or when the person reports fainting or syncope. Have the person rest supine for 2 or 3 minutes, take baseline readings of pulse and BP, and then repeat the measurements with the person sitting and then standing. For the person who is too weak or dizzy to stand, assess supine and then sitting with legs dangling. When the position is changed from supine to standing, normally a slight decrease (less than 10 mm Hg) in systolic pressure may occur.

Hypotension, abnormally low BP; **hypertension,** abnormally high BP (see parameters in Table 10–7, Abnormalities in Blood Pressure).

Orthostatic hypotension, a drop in systolic pressure of more than 20 mm Hg, and/or orthostatic pulse increases of 20 bpm or more, occurs with a quick change to a standing position. These changes are due to abrupt peripheral vasodilatation without a compensatory increase in cardiac output. Orthostatic changes also occur with prolonged bedrest, older age, hypovolemia, and some drugs.

TABLE 10–5: Common Errors in Blood Pressure Measurement

FACTOR	RESULT	RATIONALE
Taking blood pressure reading when person is anxious or angry or has just been active	Falsely high	Sympathetic nervous system stimulation
Faulty arm position		
Above level of heart	Falsely low	Eliminates effect of hydrostatic pressure
Below level of heart	Falsely high	Additional force of gravity added to brachial artery pressure
Person supports own arm	Falsely high diastolic	Sustained isometric muscular contraction
Faulty leg position (e.g., person's legs are crossed)	Falsely high systolic and diastolic	Translocation of blood volume from dependent legs to thoracic area
Examiner's eyes are not level with meniscus of mercury column		
Looking up at meniscus	Falsely high	Parallax
Looking down on meniscus	Falsely low	
Inaccurate cuff size*		
Cuff too narrow for extremity	Falsely high	Needs excessive pressure to occlude brachial artery
Cuff wrap is too loose or uneven, or bladder balloons out of wrap	Falsely high	Needs excessive pressure to occlude brachial artery
Failure to palpate radial artery while inflating		
Inflating not high enough	Falsely low systolic	Miss initial systolic tapping or may tune in during *auscultatory gap* (tapping sounds disappear for 10 to 40 mm Hg and then return; common with hypertension)
Inflating cuff too high	Pain	
Pushing stethoscope too hard on brachial artery	Falsely low diastolic	Excessive pressure distorts artery and the sounds continue
Deflating cuff		
Too quickly	Falsely low systolic and/or, falsely high diastolic	Insufficient time to hear tapping
Too slowly	Falsely high diastolic	Venous congestion in forearm makes sounds less audible
Halting during descent and reinflating cuff to recheck systolic	Falsely high diastolic	Venous congestion in forearm
Failure to wait 1–2 min before repeating entire reading	Falsely high diastolic	Venous congestion in forearm
Any observer error		
Examiner's "subconscious bias"; a preconceived idea of what blood pressure reading *should* be due to person's age, race, sex, weight, history, or condition	Error anywhere	
Examiner's haste	Error anywhere	
Faulty technique		
Examiner's digit preference, "hears" more results that end in zero than would occur by chance alone (e.g., 130/80)		
Diminished hearing acuity		
Defective or inaccurately calibrated equipment		

*This is the most common error.

Record the BP using even numbers. Also record the person's position, arm used, and cuff size if different from the standard adult cuff. Record the pulse rate and rhythm, noting whether the pulse is regular.

NORMAL RANGE OF FINDINGS

THIGH PRESSURE. When BP measured at the arm is excessively high, particularly in adolescents and young adults, compare it with the thigh pressure to check for **coarctation** of the aorta (a congenital form of narrowing). Normally, the *thigh pressure is higher* than that in the arm. If possible, turn the person into the prone position on the abdomen. (If the person must remain in the supine position, bend the knee slightly.) Wrap a large cuff, 18 to 20 cm, around the lower third of the thigh, centered over the popliteal artery on the back of the knee. Auscultate the popliteal artery for the reading (Fig. 10–7). Normally, the systolic value is 10 to 40 mm Hg higher in the thigh than in the arm, and the diastolic pressure is the same.

ABNORMAL FINDINGS

With **coarctation of the aorta,** arm pressures are high. Thigh pressure is *lower* because the blood supply to the thigh is below the constriction.

10–7

 DEVELOPMENTAL CONSIDERATIONS

Infants and Children

GENERAL SURVEY

Physical appearance, body structure, mobility—note the same basic elements as with the adult, with consideration to age and development.

Behavior—note the response to stimuli and level of alertness appropriate for age.

Parental bonding—note the child's interactions with parents, that parent and child show a mutual response and are warm and affectionate, appropriate to the child's condition. The parent provides appropriate physical care of child and promotes new learning.

Some signs of child abuse are that the child avoids eye contact; the child exhibits no separation anxiety when you would expect it for age; the parent is disgusted by child's odor, sounds, drooling, or stools.

Deprivation of physical or emotional care.

Signs of physical abuse (see Chapter 12).

MEASUREMENT

WEIGHT. Weigh an infant on a platform-type balance scale (Fig. 10–8). To check calibration, set the weight at zero and observe the beam balance. Guard the baby so that he or she does not fall. Weigh to the nearest 10 g ($^{1}/_{2}$ oz) for infants and 100 g ($^{1}/_{4}$ lb) for toddlers.

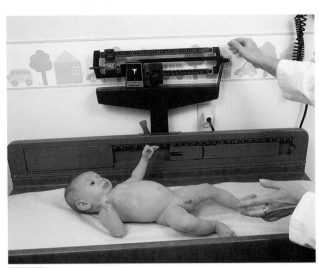

10–8

By age 2 or 3 years, use the upright scale. Leave underpants on the child. Some young children are fearful of the rickety standing platform and may prefer sitting on the infant scale. Use the upright scale with preschoolers and school-age children, maintaining modesty with light clothing (Fig. 10–9).

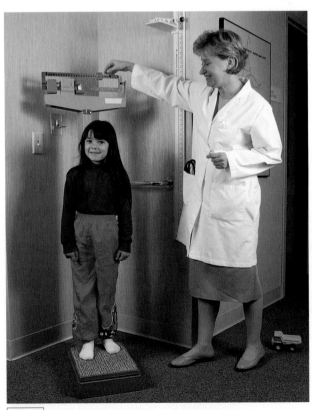

10–9

NORMAL RANGE OF FINDINGS	ABNORMAL FINDINGS

LENGTH. Until age 2 years, measure the infant's body length supine using a horizontal measuring board (Fig. 10–10). Hold the head in the midline. Because the infant normally has flexed legs, extend them momentarily by holding the knees together and pushing them down until the legs are flat on the table. Avoid using a tape measure along the infant's length because this is inaccurate.

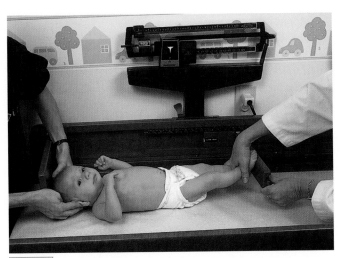

10–10

By age 2 or 3 years, measure the child's height by standing the child against the pole on the platform scale or back against a flat ruler taped to the wall (Fig. 10–11). (Sometimes a child will stand more erect against the solid wall than against the narrow measuring pole on the scale.) Encourage the child to stand straight and tall and to look straight ahead without tilting the head. The shoulders, buttocks, and heels should touch the wall. Hold a book or flat board on the child's head at a right angle to the wall. Mark just under the book, noting the measure to the nearest 1 mm ($^1/_8$ in).

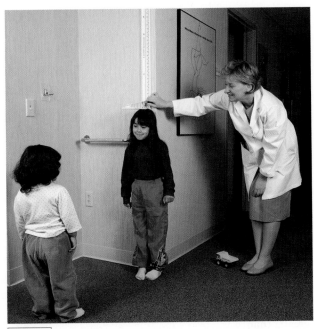

10–11

NORMAL RANGE OF FINDINGS

Physical growth is perhaps the best index of a child's general health. The child's height and weight are recorded at every health care visit to determine normal growth patterns. The results are plotted on growth charts based on data from the National Center for Health Statistics (NCHS). (See Appendix K for samples of the two groups of charts: one group for weight and height charts from birth to 36 months for girls and boys, and the second group from 2 to 18 years for males and females.)

Healthy childhood growth is continuous but uneven, with rapid growth spurts occurring during infancy and adolescence. Results are more reliable when comparing numerous growth measures over a long time. These charts also compare the individual child's measurements against the general population. Normal limits range from the 5th to the 95th percentile on the standardized charts.

Use your judgment and consider the genetic background of the small-for-age child. Explore the growth patterns of the parents and siblings. Be aware that the statistical averages for the United States charts are based on norms for white children and may not necessarily generalize to other ethnic groups. Studies indicate that black children weigh less than white children during the first 2 years of life, but afterward black children tend to be taller and heavier than white children of the same age. Asian children (particularly girls) are found to be shorter and lighter than white counterparts (Barr et al, 1972; Robson et al, 1975). Race-specific standards are needed before making judgments on growth of infants and children. Otherwise an excessive number of black infants or Asian children may be judged to be below normal when they actually may be normal for their own population group (see Transcultural Considerations, p. 199).

HEAD CIRCUMFERENCE. Measure the infant's head circumference at birth and at each well child visit up to age 2 years, then yearly up to 6 years (Fig. 10–12). Circle the tape around the head at the prominent frontal and occipital bones; the widest span is correct. Plot the measurement on standardized growth charts. Compare the infant's head size with that expected for age. A series of measurements is more valuable than a single figure to show the *rate* of head growth.

10–12

The newborn's head measures about 32 to 38 cm (average around 34 cm) and is about 2 cm larger than the chest circumference. The chest grows at a faster rate than the cranium; at some time between 6 months and 2 years, both measurements are about the same, and after age 2, the chest circumference is greater than the head circumference.

ABNORMAL FINDINGS

Further explore any growth measure that

- Falls below the 5th or above the 95th percentile with no genetic explanation
- Shows a wide percentile difference between height and weight—for example, a 10th percentile height with a 95th percentile weight
- Shows that growth has suddenly stopped when it had been steady
- Fails to show normal growth spurts during infancy and adolescence

Enlarged head circumference occurs with increased intracranial pressure (see Chapter 13, Head and Neck).

NORMAL RANGE OF FINDINGS	ABNORMAL FINDINGS

Measurement of the chest circumference is valuable in a comparison with the head circumference but not necessarily by itself. Encircle the tape around the chest at the nipple line. It should be snug, but not so tight that it leaves a mark (Fig. 10–13).

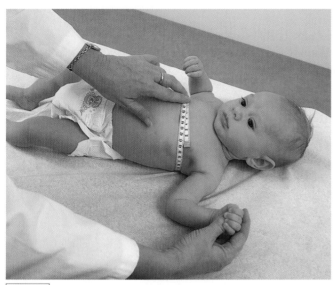

10–13

ASSESSMENT OF GESTATIONAL AGE. Occasionally, you will need to compare birth weight with a newborn's gestational age (GA) to assess maturity. Fetal maturity is the ability of the infant's organ systems to adapt to extrauterine life and is closely related to GA. GA is the number of weeks from the first day of the mother's last menstrual period (LMP) to the newborn's date of birth. Normal GA for a full-term newborn is 38 to 42 weeks.

The most commonly used method of assessing GA is the New Ballard Score (Ballard et al, 1991). Examine the newborn regarding the six neuromuscular maturity signs and the six physical maturity signs described on the form, and record the scores in each adjacent box (Appendix L). Scores range from 0 to 4 or 5, with the new addition of −1 scores that reflect signs of extreme prematurity. Add the two maturity scores to determine the maturity rating, and compare this maturity rating with the corresponding week of GA. Then enter the newborn's weight, length, and head circumference on the three grids at the vertical axis for the newborn's GA (Appendix L). Plotted scores that fall within the 10th to the 90th percentile show that a newborn is AGA, or appropriate for gestational age. That indicates this newborn grew at a normal rate during fetal life, regardless of being born at term, preterm, or postterm.

At the 50th percentile, a baby of average GA (40 weeks) measures an average weight of 3200 g (7 lb, 1 oz), an average length of 49 cm (19.3 in), and an average head circumference of 34 cm (13.5 in).

VITAL SIGNS

Measure vital signs with the same purpose and frequency as you would in an adult. With an *infant,* reverse the order of vital sign measurement to respiration, pulse, and temperature. Taking a rectal temperature may cause the infant to cry, which will increase the respiratory and pulse rate, thus masking the normal resting values. A *preschooler's* normal fear of body mutilation is increased with any invasive procedure. Whenever possible, avoid the rectal route and take a tympanic, inguinal, or axillary temperature. When this is not feasible, use the reverse

Preterm—less than 38 weeks
Postterm—more than 42 weeks

SGA, or small for gestational age, occurs with scores below the 10th percentile, indicating the infant grew at a retarded rate during fetal life. LGA, or large for gestational age, occurs with scores above the 90th percentile, indicating this infant grew at an accelerated rate during fetal life.

order and measure the rectal temperature last. Promote the cooperation of the *school-age child* by explaining the procedure completely and encouraging the child to handle the equipment. Your approach to measuring vital signs with the *adolescent* is much the same as with the adult.

TEMPERATURE

TYMPANIC. The TMT is useful with toddlers who squirm at the restraint needed for the rectal route, and it is useful with preschoolers who are not yet able to cooperate for an oral temperature yet fear the disrobing and invasion of a rectal temperature. The TMT measurement is so rapid that it is usually over before the child realizes it (Fig. 10–14).

10–14

The TMT use with newborns has remained questionable. Cusson, Madonia, and Taekman (1997) found that the temperature of the environment has a significant effect on temperature measurements. The superheated environment of the radiant warmer and particularly the incubator resulted in a significant elevation of tympanic membrane temperature over rectal, inguinal, or axillary measurement—a difference that could influence clinical management. They recommended the inguinal route. However, for infants in room-air bassinets, the TMT thermometers were recommended because the differences between tympanic and rectal or axillary measurements were much less (Cusson et al, 1997). Lanham et al (1999) found the results of tympanic temperature measurement in children under 6 years to be unacceptably low, and that some children with fever would be missed by this method. Their study did not support the use of TMT to detect fever in children under 6 years of age. Similarly, in a study of healthy newborns, Sganga et al (2000) found that tympanic thermometers had a lack of correlation with other methods, making them a poor choice for healthy newborns.

INGUINAL. The inguinal route is safer than the rectal site. Its results may be closer to core temperature than the axillary site because the inguinal area has a rich supply of blood vessels, it lacks the brown fat tissue that interferes with axillary temperatures, and you can form a tight skin-to-skin seal (Cusson et al, 1997). Abduct the infant's leg and locate the femoral pulse. Place the bulb of the thermometer lateral to the pulse site, and adduct the leg to create a seal. (In a glass thermometer, a stable temperature will register in 3 to 5 minutes.)

NORMAL RANGE OF FINDINGS

ABNORMAL FINDINGS

AXILLARY. The axillary route is safer and more accessible than the rectal route; however, its accuracy and reliability have been questioned (Cusson et al, 1997). When cold receptors are stimulated, brown fat tissue in the area releases heat through chemical energy, which artificially raises skin temperature. Studies on preterm infants show only small differences between axillary and rectal temperature measurement, which may be because brown fat is not present until 34 weeks' gestation (Bliss-Holtz, 1995). When the axillary route is used, place the tip well into the axilla, and hold the child's arm close to the body. (In a glass thermometer, a stable axillary temperature will register by $5^1/_2$ minutes.)

ORAL. Use the oral route when the child is old enough to keep the mouth closed. This is usually at age 5 or 6, although some 4-year-old children can cooperate. When available, use an electronic thermometer because it is unbreakable and it registers quickly.

RECTAL. Use this route with infants or with other age groups when other routes are not feasible, such as with the child who is unable to cooperate, agitated, unconscious, critically ill, or prone to seizure. An infant may be supine or side lying, with the examiner's hand flexing the knees up onto the abdomen. (When supine, cover the boy's penis with a diaper.) An infant also may lie prone across the adult's lap. Separate the buttocks with one hand, and insert the lubricated electronic rectal probe *no farther than* 2.5 cm (1 in). Any deeper insertion risks rectal perforation because the colon curves posteriorly at 3 cm ($1^1/_4$ in). (In a glass thermometer, a temperature will register by 3 minutes.)

Normally, rectal temperatures measure higher in infants and young children than in adults, with an average of 37.8° C (100° F) at 18 months. Also, the temperature normally may be elevated in the late afternoon, after vigorous playing or after eating.

Up to ages 6 to 8, children have higher fevers with illness than adults do. Even with minor infections, fevers may elevate to 39.5° C to 40.5° C (103° to 105° F).

PULSE

Palpate or auscultate an apical rate with infants and toddlers. (See Chapter 19 for location of apex and technique.) In children older than 2 years, use the radial site. Count the pulse for a full minute to take into account normal irregularities, such as sinus arrhythmia. The heart rate normally fluctuates more with infants and children than with adults in response to exercise, emotion, and illness.

RESPIRATIONS

Watch the infant's abdomen for movement, because the infant's respirations are normally more diaphragmatic than thoracic (Fig. 10–15). Count a full minute, because the pattern varies significantly from rapid breaths to short periods of apnea. Note the normal rate in Table 10–4.

10–15

NORMAL RANGE OF FINDINGS	ABNORMAL FINDINGS

BLOOD PRESSURE

In children age 3 and older, and in younger children at risk, measure a routine BP at least annually. For accurate measurement in children, make some adjustment in the choice of equipment and technique. The most common error is to use the incorrect size cuff. The cuff width must cover two thirds of the upper arm, and the cuff bladder must completely encircle it.

Use a pediatric-sized endpiece on the stethoscope to locate the sounds. If possible, allow a crying infant to become quiet for 5 to 10 minutes before measuring the BP; crying may elevate the systolic pressure by 30 to 50 mm Hg. New guidelines state that the disappearance of sound (phase V Korotkoff) can now be used for the diastolic reading in children as well as adults (JNC-VI, 1997; NHBPEP, 1996). Note the new guidelines for normal BP values by age groups *based on the child's height* (Appendix M). In children, height is more strongly correlated with BP than is age. The new charts avoid the misclassification as normotensive or hypertensive of children who are at the extremes of normal growth (NHBPEP, 1996). That is, for children of the same age, BP classified as 90th and 95th percentiles are lower for very short children, while tall children are given a higher normal range.

Children under 3 years of age have such small arm vessels that it is difficult to hear Korotkoff's sounds using a stethoscope. Instead, use an electronic BP device that uses *oscillometry,* such as Dinamap, and gives a digital readout for systolic, diastolic, and MAP and pulse. Or use a *Doppler* ultrasound device to amplify the sounds. This instrument is easy to use and can be used by one examiner. (Note the technique for using the Doppler on p. 198).

Further explore any blood pressure that is greater than the 95th percentile and refer for diagnostic evaluation. For the child whose BP falls in the 90 to 95th percentile and whose high BP cannot be explained by height or weight, monitor the BP every 6 months.

The Aging Adult

GENERAL SURVEY

Physical appearance—By the eighth and ninth decades, body contour is sharper, with more angular facial features, and body proportions are redistributed. (See measuring weight and height, p. 178.)

Posture—A general flexion occurs by the eight or ninth decade.

Gait—Older adults often use a wider base to compensate for diminished balance, arms may be held out to help balance, and steps may be shorter or uneven.

MEASUREMENT

WEIGHT. The aging person appears sharper in contour with more prominent bony landmarks than the younger adult. Body weight decreases during the 80s and 90s. This factor is more evident in males, perhaps because of greater muscle shrinkage. The distribution of fat also changes during the 80s and 90s. Even with good nutrition, subcutaneous fat is lost from the face and periphery

10–16

NORMAL RANGE OF FINDINGS	ABNORMAL FINDINGS

(especially the forearms), whereas additional fat is deposited on the abdomen and hips (Fig. 10–16).

HEIGHT. By the 80s and 90s, many people are shorter than they were in their 70s. This results from shortening in the spinal column due to thinning of the vertebral disks and shortening of the individual vertebrae as well as the postural changes of kyphosis and slight flexion in the knees and hips. Since long bones do not shorten with age, the overall body proportion looks different—a shorter trunk with relatively long extremities (see Fig. 10–16).

VITAL SIGNS

TEMPERATURE. Changes in the body's temperature regulatory mechanism leave the aging person less likely to develop fever but at a greater risk of developing hypothermia. Thus the temperature is a less reliable index of the older person's true health state. Sweat gland activity is also diminished.

PULSE. The normal range of heart rate is 60 to 100 bpm, but the rhythm may be slightly irregular. The radial artery may feel stiff, rigid, and tortuous in an older person, although this condition does not necessarily imply vascular disease in the heart or brain. The increasingly rigid arterial wall needs a faster upstroke of blood, so the pulse is actually easier to palpate.

RESPIRATIONS. Aging causes a decrease in vital capacity and a decreased inspiratory reserve volume. You may note a shallower inspiratory phase and an increased respiratory rate.

BLOOD PRESSURE. The aorta and major arteries tend to harden with age. As the heart pumps against a stiffer aorta, the systolic pressure increases, leading to a widened pulse pressure (see Fig. 10–17 for mean BP readings in apparently healthy persons from birth to old age). With many older people, both the systolic and diastolic pressures increase, making it difficult to distinguish normal aging values from abnormal hypertension.

10–17 Mean blood pressure readings in apparently healthy people, birth to old age.

ADDITIONAL TECHNIQUES

The Doppler Technique

In many situations, pulse and BP measurement are enhanced using an electronic device, the *Doppler ultrasonic flowmeter.* The Doppler technique works by a principle discovered in the nineteenth century by an Austrian physicist, Johannes Doppler. Sound varies in pitch in relation to the distance between the sound source and the listener; the pitch is higher when the distance is small, and the pitch lowers as the distance increases. Think of a railroad train speeding toward you; its train whistle sounds higher the closer it gets, and the pitch of the whistle lowers as the train fades away.

In this case, the sound source is the blood pumping through the artery in a rhythmic manner. A handheld transducer picks up changes in sound frequency as the blood flows and ebbs and it amplifies them. The listener hears a whooshing pulsatile beat.

The Doppler technique is used to locate the peripheral pulse sites (see Chapter 20 for further discussion of this technique). For BP measurement, the Doppler technique will augment Korotkoff's sounds (Fig. 10–18). Through this technique, you can evaluate sounds that are hard to hear with a stethoscope, such as those in critically ill individuals with a low BP, in infants with small arms, and in obese persons in whom the sounds are muffled by layers of fat. Also, proper cuff placement is difficult on the obese person's cone-shaped upper arm. In this situation, you can place the cuff on the more even forearm and hold the Doppler probe over the radial artery. For either location, use the following procedure:

10–18

- Apply coupling gel to the transducer probe.
- Turn Doppler flowmeter on.
- Touch the probe to the skin, holding the probe perpendicular to the artery.
- A pulsatile whooshing sound indicates location of the artery. You may need to rotate the probe, but maintain contact with the skin. Do not push the probe too hard or you will wipe out the pulse.
- Inflate the cuff until the sounds disappear; then proceed another 20 to 30 mm Hg beyond that point.
- Slowly deflate the cuff, noting the point at which the first whooshing sounds appear. This is the systolic pressure.
- It is difficult to hear the muffling of sounds or a reliable disappearance of sounds indicating the diastolic pressure (phases IV and V of Korotkoff's sounds). However, the systolic pressure alone gives valuable data on the level of tissue perfusion and on blood flow through patent vessels.

NORMAL RANGE OF FINDINGS	ABNORMAL FINDINGS

PROMOTING HEALTH AND SELF-CARE

As you measure height and weight and collect vital signs, it is a good time to begin a teaching plan to help the individual keep these physical signs within normal limits. The 2003 Joint National Committee on Detection, Evaluation, and Treatment of High Blood Pressure considers the following **lifestyle modifications** to be the foundation of hypertension control. Even if your patient is normotensive and has body weight in normal limits, the following lifestyle modifications will help keep blood pressure under control (JNC-VII, 2003).

- Lose weight, if you are more than 10% above ideal weight.
- Limit alcohol intake to no more than 1 oz of ethanol (i.e., 24 oz [720 ml] of beer, 10 oz [300 ml] of wine, or 2 oz [60 ml] of 100-proof whiskey) per day or 0.5 oz (15 ml) of ethanol per day for women and lighter-weight people.
- Get regular aerobic exercise (e.g., a 30- to 45-minute brisk walk) most days of the week.
- Cut sodium intake from the average 150 mmol/L (150 mEq/L) to less than 100 mmol/L (100 mEq/L) per day (less than 2.3 g of sodium or 6 g of sodium chloride).
- Include the recommended daily allowances of potassium, calcium, and magnesium in your diet.
- Stop smoking.
- Reduce dietary saturated fat and cholesterol.

 See Health Promotion Guide on CD

TRANSCULTURAL CONSIDERATIONS

General Appearance

Cultural differences are found in the body proportions of individuals. In general, white males are 1.27 cm (0.5 in) taller than black males, whereas white and black women are, on the average, the same height. Sitting-to-standing height ratios reveal that blacks of both sexes have longer legs and shorter trunks than whites. Because proportionately most of the weight is in the trunk, white men appear more obese than black men. Asians are markedly shorter, weigh less, and have smaller body frames.

Despite their longer legs, black women are consistently heavier than white women at every age, with black women carrying an average of 9.1 kg (20 lb) more than white women between the ages of 35 and 64 years (Overfield, 1995).

Bone length, as revealed by stature, shows definite biocultural differences, with blacks having longer legs and arms than whites. Asians and Native Americans have, on the average, proportionately longer trunks and shorter limbs than whites. Blacks tend to be wide shouldered and narrow hipped, whereas Asians tend to be wide hipped and narrow shouldered. Shoulder width is largely produced by the clavicle. Because the clavicle is a long bone, this explains why taller people have wide shoulders, whereas shorter people have narrower shoulders.

Although not all groups have been studied, research on selected populations reveals that children of some immigrant groups to the United States are taller than their peers in the country of origin. For example, Japanese Americans residing in Hawaii are taller than those Japanese living in Japan. Although the sitting-to-standing height ratio is the same, Italians in California are 3.8 cm (1.5 in) taller than those of the same age living in Italy (Hulse, 1968; Overfield, 1995). This indicates that the increase in height occurs in both the long bones and the spine (Brues, 1977).

The height increase in migrants is theorized to be the result of two factors: (1) better nutrition provided in the United States and (2) decreased interference with growth from infectious diseases during the formative years. Furthermore, the overall height of Americans increased 1.8 cm (0.7 in) for men and 1.3 cm (0.5 in) for women during the 10-year period studied (Abraham et al, 1976).

Biocultural differences also exist in the amount of body fat and the distribution of fat throughout the body. In general, individuals from lower socioeconomic groups are more obese than those from middle socioeconomic groups, who are more obese than members from upper socioeconomic groups. In addition to socioeconomic considerations, blacks tend to have smaller (1 mm) skinfold thicknesses in their arms than whites, but the distribution of fat on the trunk is similar.

Application and Critical Thinking

SAMPLE CHARTING

A.J. is a 47-year-old black female high school principal, well nourished, well developed, appears stated age. She is alert, oriented, cooperative, with no signs of acute distress. Ht 163 cm (5'4"), Wt 57 kg (126 lbs), TPR 37° C—76—14, B/P 146/84 right arm, sitting.

FOCUSED ASSESSMENT: CLINICAL CASE STUDY*

Mrs. Grazia Sanchez is a 76-year-old Hispanic female, retired secretary, in previous good health, who is brought to the emergency department by her 83-year-old husband. They have both been ill during the night with nausea, vomiting, abdominal pain, and diarrhea, which they attribute to eating "bad food" at a buffet-style restaurant the night before. Mr. Sanchez's condition has improved during the next day, but Mrs. Sanchez is worse, with severe vomiting, diarrhea, weakness, dizziness, and abdominal pain.

SUBJECTIVE

Extreme fatigue. Weakness and dizziness occur whenever patient tries to sit or stand up: "Feels like I'm going to black out." Severe nausea and vomiting, thirsty but cannot keep anything down; even sips of water result in "dry heaves." Abdominal pain is moderate aching, intermittent. Diarrhea is watery brown stool, profuse during the night, somewhat diminished now.

OBJECTIVE

Vital signs: temp 99° F, BP (supine) 102/64, pulse (supine) 70, regular rhythm, respirations 18.

Helped to seated, leg dangling position, vitals: BP 74/52, pulse 138, regular rhythm, respirations 20. Skin pale and moist (diaphoretic).

Reports lightheaded and dizzy in seated position. Returned to supine.

Respiratory: breath sounds clear in all fields, no adventitious sounds.

Cardiovascular: regular rate (70 bpm) and rhythm when supine, S_1 and S_2 are not accentuated or diminished, no extra sounds. All pulses present, 2+ and equal bilaterally. Carotids 2+ with no carotid bruit.

Abdomen: bowel sounds hyperactive, skin pale and moist, abdomen soft and mildly tender to palpation. No enlargement of liver or spleen.

Neuro: level of consciousness alert and oriented; pupils equal, round, react to light and accommodation. Sensory status normal. Mild weakness in arms and legs. Gait and standing leg strength not tested due to inability to stand. Deep tendon reflexes 2+ and equal bilaterally. Babinski reflex → down-going toes.

ASSESSMENT

Orthostatic hypotension, orthostatic pulse increase, and syncopal symptoms, R/T hypovolemia
Diarrhea, possibly R/T ingestion of contaminated food
Risk for hyperthermia, R/T dehydration and aging
Deficient fluid volume

NURSING DIAGNOSES COMMONLY ASSOCIATED WITH MEASUREMENT OR VITAL SIGN DISORDERS

RELATED FACTORS (Etiology)	DEFINING CHARACTERISTICS (Symptoms and Signs)
DIAGNOSIS: Hyperthermia	
Dehydration	Increase in body temperature above normal range
Effects of	Skin flushed or warm to the touch
Illness or trauma involving temperature regulation	Increased respiratory rate
Medications/anesthesia	Tachycardia
Aging	Seizures/convulsions

*Please note that space does not allow a detailed plan for each clinical case study in this text. Please consult the appropriate text for current treatment plan.

RELATED FACTORS (Etiology)	DEFINING CHARACTERISTICS (Symptoms and Signs)
DIAGNOSIS: Hyperthermia—cont'd	
Exposure to hot environment	Shivering
Inability to perspire	Weakness, faintness
Inability to regulate environmental temperature	Perspiration
No air conditioning	Verbal reports of feeling hot
Isolette temperature for infants	
Increased metabolic rate	
Vigorous activity	

OTHER RELATED NURSING DIAGNOSES

ACTUAL	RISK/WELLNESS
Hypothermia	**Risk**
Imbalanced Nutrition: less than body requirements	Risk for imbalanced Body temperature
Imbalanced Nutrition: more than body requirements	Risk for deficient Fluid volume
Bathing/hygiene Self-care deficit	**Wellness**
Dressing/grooming Self-care deficit	Enhanced Health-seeking behavior R/T request for hyper-
Ineffective Thermoregulation	tension management by diet and exercise

Abnormal Findings

TABLE 10–6: Abnormalities in Body Height and Proportion

Hypopituitary Dwarfism

Deficiency in growth hormone in childhood results in retardation of growth and delayed puberty. The 9-year-old girl at left appears much younger than her chronological age, with infantile facial features and chubbiness. The age-matched girl at right shows increased height, more mature facies, and loss of infantile fat.

Gigantism

Excessive secretion of growth hormone by the anterior pituitary. When this occurs during childhood, before closure of bone epiphyses in puberty, it causes increased height (here 2.09 m, or 6 ft 9 in), and weight and delayed sexual development.

Acromegaly (Hyperpituitarism)

Excessive secretion of growth hormone in adulthood, after normal completion of body growth, causes over-growth of bone in the face, head, hands, and feet, but no change in height. Internal organs also enlarge (e.g., cardiomegaly).*

*Reprinted from the Clinical Slide Collection on the Rheumatic Diseases. © 1991, 1995, 1997. Used by permission of the American College of Rheumatology.

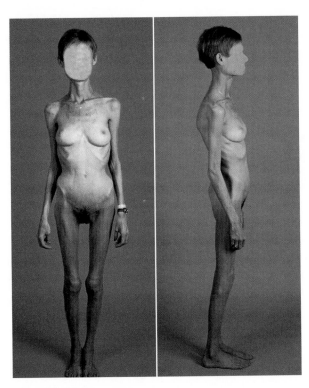

Anorexia Nervosa

A serious psychological disorder characterized by severe and debilitating weight loss and amenorrhea in an otherwise healthy adolescent or young woman. Behavior is characterized by fanatic concern about weight, distorted body image (perceives self as fat despite skeletal appearance), starvation diets, frenetic exercise patterns, and striving for perfection.

Marfan's Syndrome

Abraham Lincoln, Paganini, and Rachmaninoff are thought to have had this inherited connective tissue disorder, characterized by tall, thin stature (greater than 95th percentile), arachnodactyly (long, thin fingers), hyperextensible joints, arm span greater than height, pubis-to-sole measurement exceeding crown-to-pubis measurement, sternal deformity, high-arched narrow palate, and pes planus. Early morbidity and mortality occur due to cardiovascular complications such as mitral regurgitation and aortic dissection.

◀ Achondroplastic Dwarfism

Congenital skeletal malformation due to genetic disorder characterized by relatively large head, short stature, and short limbs, and often thoracic kyphosis, prominent lumbar lordosis, and abdominal protrusion. The mean adult height in men is about 131.5 cm (51.8 in) and in women about 125 cm (49.2 in).

Endogenous Obesity—Cushing's Syndrome

Either administration of adrenocorticotropic hormone (ACTH) or excessive production of ACTH by the pituitary will stimulate the adrenal cortex to secrete excess cortisol. This causes Cushing's syndrome, characterized by weight gain and edema with central trunk and cervical obesity (buffalo hump) and round plethoric face (moon face). Excessive catabolism causes muscle wasting; weakness; thin arms and legs; reduced height; and thin, fragile skin with purple abdominal striae, bruising, and acne. Note the obesity here is markedly different from *exogenous obesity* due to excessive caloric intake, in which body fat is evenly distributed and muscle strength is intact.

TABLE 10–7: Abnormalities in Blood Pressure

Hypotension

In normotensive adults: <95/60
In hypertensive adults: <the person's average reading, but >95/60
In children: <expected value for age

Occurs with	Rationale
Acute myocardial infarction	Decreased cardiac output
Shock	Decreased cardiac output
Hemorrhage	Decrease in total blood volume
Vasodilatation	Decrease in peripheral vascular resistance
Addison's disease (hypofunction of adrenal glands)	

Associated Symptoms and Signs

In conditions of decreased cardiac output, a low BP is accompanied by an increased pulse, dizziness, diaphoresis, confusion, and blurred vision. The skin feels cool and clammy because the superficial blood vessels constrict to shunt blood to the vital organs. An individual having an acute MI (myocardial infarction) may also complain of crushing substernal chest pain, high epigastric pain, and shoulder or jaw pain.

Hypertension

Essential or Primary Hypertension
This occurs from no known cause but is responsible for about 95% of cases of hypertension in adults.

Classification and Follow-Up of Blood Pressure for Adults Age 18 and Older*

BP CLASSIFICATION	SBP* mmHg	DBP* mHg	LIFESTYLE MODIFICATION	INITIAL DRUG THERAPY	
				WITHOUT COMPELLING INDICATION	WITH COMPELLING INDICATIONS
Normal	<120	and <80	Encourage		
Prehypertension	120–139	or 80–89	Yes	No antihypertensive drug indicated.	Drug(s) for compelling indications.***
Stage 1 Hypertension	140–159	or 90–99	Yes	Thiazide-type diuretics for most. May consider ACEI, ARB, BB, CCB, or combination.	Drug(s) for the compelling indications.*** Other antihypertensive drugs (diuretics, ACEI, ARB, BB, CCB) as needed.
Stage 2 Hypertension	≤160	or ≥100	Yes	Two-drug combination for most** usually Thiazide-type diuretic and ACEI, or ARB or BB or CCB).	Drug(s) for the compelling indications.*** Other antihypertensive drugs (diuretics, ACEI, ARB, BB, CCB) as needed.

DBP, diastolic blood pressure; SBP, systolic blood pressure.
Drug abbreviations: ACEI, angiotensin converting enzyme inhibitor; ARB, angiotensin receptor blocker; BB, beta-blocker; CCB, calcium channel blocker.
*Treatment determined by highest BP category.
**Initial combined therapy should be used cautiously in those at risk for orthostatic hypotension.
***Treat patients with chronic kidney disease or diabetes to BP goal of <130/80 mmHg.
   Data on classification of hypertension in adults adapted from the Joint National Committee VII: The Seventh Report of the Joint National Committee on Prevention, Detection, Evaluation and Treatment of High Blood Pressure, *JAMA* 289:2560–2572, May 21, 2003, and http://www.nhlbi.nih.gov/guidelines/hypertension.

Cardiovascular Risk Stratification in Patients With Hypertension

Major Risk Factors

Smoking

Dyslipidemia

Diabetes mellitus

Age >60 y

Sex (men and postmenopausal women)

Family history of cardiovascular disease: women <65 y
    or men <55 y

Target Organ Damage/Clinical Cardiovascular Disease

Heart diseases
    Left ventricular hypertrophy
    Angina or prior myocardial infarction
    Prior coronary revascularization
    Heart failure

Stroke or transient ischemic attack

Nephropathy

Peripheral arterial disease

Retinopathy

Lifestyle Modifications for Hypertension Prevention and Management

- Lose weight if overweight
- Limit alcohol intake to no more than 1 oz (30 ml) of ethanol (e.g., 24 oz [720 ml] of beer, 10 oz [300 ml] of wine, or 2 oz [60 ml] of 100-proof whiskey) per day or 0.5 oz (15 ml) of ethanol per day for women and lighter-weight people
- Increase aerobic physical activity (30–45 min most days of the week)
- Reduce sodium intake to no more than 100 mmol/d (2.4 g of sodium or 6 g of sodium chloride)
- Maintain adequate intake of dietary potassium (approximately 90 mmol/d)
- Maintain adequate intake of dietary calcium and magnesium for general health
- Stop smoking and reduce intake of dietary saturated fat and cholesterol for overall cardiovascular health

BIBLIOGRAPHY

Abraham SJ, Clifford L, Najjar MF: Height and weight of adults 18–74 years of age in the United States, *Advancedata* 3:1–8, 1976.

Bailey J, Rose P: Temperature measurement in the preterm infant: a literature review, *J Neonat Nurs* 6(1):28–32, Jan 2000.

Ballard JL et al: New Ballard score, expanded to extremely premature infants, *J Pediatr* 119:417–423, 1991.

Barr GD, Allen CM, Shinefield HR: Height and weight of 7,500 children of three skin colors, *Am J Dis Child* 124:866–872, 1972.

Beevers G, Lip GYH, O'Brien E: ADB of hypertension: blood pressure measurement: part II—conventional sphygmomanometry: technique of auscultatory blood pressure measurement, *BMJ* 322(7293):1043–1047, Apr 2001.

Blacher J et al: Pulse pressure not mean pressure determines cardiovascular risk in older hypertensive patients, *Arch Intern Med* 160(8):1085–1089, Apr 2000.

Blazys D: Orthostatic blood pressure, *J Emerg Nurs* 26(5):479–480, Oct 2000.

Bliss-Holtz J: Methods of newborn infant temperature monitoring: a research review, *Issues Compr Pediatr Nurs* 18(4):287–298, Oct-Dec 1995.

Brues AM: *People and races,* New York, 1977, Macmillan.

Canzanello VJ, Jensen PL, Schwartz GL: Are aneroid sphygmomanometers accurate in hospital and clinic settings? *Arch Intern Med* 161(5):729–731, Mar 2001.

Cunha BA: Relative bradycardia as a diagnostic clue, *Patient Care* 34(3):223–227, Feb 2000.

Cusson RM, Madonia JA, Taekmen JB: The effect of environment on body site temperatures in full-term neonates, *Nurs Res* 46(4):202–207, Jul-Aug 1997.

Elliott WJ: Which blood pressure measurement is more important in the elderly? *Arch Intern Med* 159(11):1165–1166, Jun 1999.

Faria SH: Assessment of peripheral arterial pulses, *Home Care Provid* 4(4):140–141, Aug 1999.

Foster-Fitzpatrick L et al: The effects of crossed leg on blood pressure measurement, *Nurs Res* 48(2):105–108, Mar-Apr 1999.

Gilbert M, Barton AJ, Counsell CM: Comparison of oral and tympanic temperatures in adult surgical patients, *Appl Nurs Res* 15(1):42–47, Feb 2002.

Goldberg EA: Physical assessment of children ages 1 to 10 years, *ANNA J* 24(2):209–217, Apr 1997.

Goldman LR, Shannon MW: Technical report: mercury in the environment: implications for pediatricians, *Pediatrics* 108(1):197–205, Jul 2001.

Giuliano KK et al: Temperature measurement in critically ill adults: a comparison of tympanic and oral methods, *Am J Crit Care* 9(4):254–261, Jul 2000.

Hines SE: Performing a focused physical examination, *Patient Care* 34(23):76–106, Dec 2000.

Hockenberry MJ et al: *Wong's nursing care of infants and children,* ed 7, St Louis, 2003, Mosby.

Hulse FS: *The breakdown of isolates and hybrid vigor among the Italian Swiss,* Proceedings of the 12th International Congress on Genetics 2:177, 1968.

Hwu Y, Coates VE, Lin F: A study of the effectiveness of different measuring times and counting methods of human radial pulse rates, *J Clin Nurs* 9(1):146–152, Jan 2000.

Joint National Committee VII: The seventh report of the Joint National Committee on the Prevention, Detection, Evaluation, and Treatment of High Blood Pressure, *JAMA* 289:2560–2572, May 21, 2003, and http://www.nhlbi.nih.gov/guidelines/hypertension.

Karch AM, Karch FE: When a blood pressure isn't routine, *Am J Nurs* 100(3):23, Mar 2000.

Keele-Smith R, Price-Daniel C: Effects of crossing legs on blood pressure measurement, *Clin Nurs Res* 10(2):202–213, May 2001.

Lanham DM et al: Accuracy of tympanic temperature readings in children under 6 years of age, *Pediatr Nurs* 25(1):39–42, Jan-Feb 1999.

LoBuono C, Pinkowish MD: Pulse pressure as a predictor of coronary heart disease, *Patient Care Nurse Pract* 2(10):56, Oct 1999.

Moody LY: Pediatric cardiovascular assessment and referral in the primary care setting, *Nurse Pract* 22(1):120–134, Jan 1997.

National High Blood Pressure Education Program (NHBPEP): Update on the 1987 task force report on high blood pressure in children and adolescents, *Pediatrics* 98(4):649–667, 1996.

O'Brien E: Replacing the mercury sphygmomanometer: requires clinicians to demand better automated devices, *BMJ* 320(7238):815–816, Mar 2000.

Overfield T: *Biologic variation in health and illness: race, age and sex differences,* Menlo Park, Calif, 1995, Addison Wesley.

Pesola GR et al: The normal difference in bilateral indirect blood pressure recordings in normotensive individuals, *Am J Emerg Med* 19(1):43–45, Jan 2001.

Rice KL: Measuring thigh BP, *Nursing* 29(8):58–59, Aug 1999.

Robson JR et al: Growth standards for infants and children: a cross-sectional study, *Pediatrics* 56:1014–1020, 1975.

Ryan-Krause P: Identify and manage Marfan syndrome in children, *Nurse Pract* 27(10):26-36, Oct 2002.

Sachse D: Acromegaly, *Am J Nurs* 101(11):69–77, Nov 2001.

Sganga A et al: A comparison of four methods of normal newborn temperature measurement, *MCN* 25(2):66–79, Mar-Apr 2000.

Sneed NV, Hollerbach AD: Accuracy of heart rate assessment in atrial fibrillation, *Heart Lung* 21(5):427–433, Sep-Oct 1992.

Spodick DH: Redefinition of normal sinus heart rate, *Chest* 104(3):939–941, 1993.

Tobin LJ: Evaluating mild to moderate hypertension, *Nurse Pract* 24(5):22-41, May 1999.

Yarows SA, Qian K: Accuracy of aneroid sphygmomanometers in clinical usage, *Blood Press Monit* 6(2):101–106, Apr 2001.

CHAPTER 11

Pain Assessment: The Fifth Vital Sign

Structure and Function

NEUROANATOMIC PATHWAY

Pain is a highly complex and subjective experience that originates from the central (CNS) or peripheral nervous system (PNS) or both. Specialized nerve endings called **nociceptors** are designed to detect painful sensations from the periphery and transmit them to the central nervous system. Nociceptors are located within the skin; connective tissue; muscle; and the thoracic, abdominal, and pelvic viscera. These nociceptors can be stimulated directly by trauma or injury or secondarily by chemical mediators that are released from the site of tissue damage.

Nociceptors carry the pain signal to the central nervous system by two primary sensory (or afferent) fibers: **Aδ and C fibers** (Fig. 11-1). Aδ fibers are myelinated and larger in diameter, and they transmit the pain signal rapidly to the CNS.

Very localized, short-term, and sharp sensations result from Aδ fiber stimulation. In contrast, C fibers are unmyelinated and smaller, and they transmit the signal more slowly. Sensations are diffuse and aching, and they persist after the initial injury.

Peripheral sensory Aδ and C fibers enter the spinal cord by posterior nerve roots within the dorsal horn by the tract of Lissauer. The fibers synapse with **interneurons** located within a specified area of the cord called the **substantia gelatinosa**. A cross section shows that the gray matter of the spinal cord is divided into a series of consecutively numbered laminae (layers of nerve cells) (see Fig. 11-1). The substantia gelatinosa is lamina II, which receives sensory input from various areas of the body. The pain signals then cross over to the other side of the spinal cord and ascend to the brain by the **anterolateral spinothalamic tract**.

11–1

② TRANSMISSION

The pain impulse moves from the spinal cord to the brain.

Spinothalamic tract neuron

Opioid receptors

Nociceptor

③ PERCEPTION OF PAIN

④ MODULATION

Neurons from brain stem release neurotransmitters that block the pain impulse.

Spinothalamic tract neuron

Neuron from brain stem

Nociceptor

Opioid receptors

Noxious stimuli

① TRANSDUCTION

• Injured tissue releases chemicals that propagate pain message.
• Action potential moves along an afferent fiber to the spinal cord.

Na^+ K^+
Na^+ K^+
Na^+ Na^+
          Na^+
          Na^+

Nociceptor

PAT THOMAS

11–2

NOCICEPTION

It is important to understand that pain occurs on a cellular level. Only then can you appreciate a patient's report of painful sensations that may develop after the initial site of injury heals. **Nociception** is the term used to describe how noxious stimuli are typically perceived as pain. Nociception can be divided into four phases: (1) transduction, (2) transmission, (3) perception, and (4) modulation (Fig. 11-2).

Initially, the first phase of **transduction** occurs when a noxious stimulus in the form of traumatic or chemical injury, burn, incision, or tumor takes place in the periphery. The periphery includes the skin, as well as somatic and visceral structures. These injured tissues then release a variety of chemicals, including substance P, histamine, prostaglandins, serotonin, and bradykinin. These chemicals are neurotransmitters that propagate a pain message, or action potential, along afferent nerve fibers to the spinal cord. These nerve fibers terminate in the dorsal horn of the spinal cord. Because the initial afferent fibers stop in the dorsal horn, a second set of neurotransmitters carry the pain impulse across the synaptic cleft to the dorsal horn neurons. These neurotransmitters include substance P, glutamate, and adenosine triphosphate (ATP).

In the second phase, known as **transmission**, the pain impulse moves from the level of the spinal cord to the brain. Within the spinal cord, at the site of the synaptic cleft are opioid receptors that can block this pain signaling with endogenous or exogenous opioids. However, if left uninterrupted, the pain impulse moves to the brain via various ascending fibers within the spinothalamic tract that terminate in the brain stem and thalamus. Once the pain impulse moves through the thalamus, the message is dispersed to higher cortical areas via mechanisms that are not clearly understood at this time.

The third phase, **perception**, indicates the conscious awareness of a painful sensation. Cortical structures such as the limbic system account for the emotional response to pain, and somatosensory areas can characterize the sensation. Only when the noxious stimuli are interpreted in these higher cortical structures can this sensation be identified as pain.

Lastly, the pain message is inhibited through the phase of **modulation**. Descending pathways from the brain stem to the spinal cord produce a third set of neurotransmitters that slow down or impede the pain impulse, producing an analgesic effect. These neurotransmitters include serotonin; norepinephrine; neurotensin; γ-aminobutyric acid (GABA); and our own endogenous opioids, β-endorphins, enkephalins, and dynorphins.

NEUROPATHIC PAIN

Neuropathic pain indicates a type of pain that does not adhere to the typical and rather predictable phases inherent in nociceptive pain. Neuropathic pain implies an abnormal processing of the pain message. It is this type of pain that is most difficult to assess and treat. Pain is often perceived long after the site of injury heals. Pain is sustained on a neurochemical level that cannot be identified by x-ray, computerized axial tomography (CAT scan), or magnetic resonance imaging (MRI). The abnormal processing of the pain impulse can be continued by the peripheral or central nervous system. Exact mechanisms are unclear to date. A proposed mechanism is that injury to peripheral neurons can result in spontaneous and repetitive firing of nerve fibers, almost seizurelike in activity (Fig. 11-3). Neuropathic pain may be sustained centrally in a phenomenon known as neuronal "wind-up." Within the dorsal horn of the spinal cord, neurons are thought to be transformed into a hyperexcitable state and a minimal stimulus can ultimately spiral into a much larger painful effect.

SOURCES OF PAIN

Pain sources are based upon their origin. **Visceral** pain originates from the larger interior organs (i.e., kidney, stomach, intestine, gallbladder, pancreas). The pain can stem from direct injury to the organ, or from stretching of the organ from tumor, ischemia, distention, or severe contraction. Examples of visceral pain include ureteral colic, acute appendicitis, ulcer pain, and cholecystitis. The pain impulse is transmitted by ascending nerve fibers along with nerve fibers of the autonomic nervous system. That is why visceral pain often presents along with autonomic responses such as vomiting, nausea, pallor, and diaphoresis. **Deep somatic pain** comes from sources such as the blood vessels, joints, tendons, muscles, and bone. Injury may result from pressure, trauma, or ischemia. **Cutaneous pain** is derived from skin surface and subcutaneous tissues. The injury is superficial, with a sharp, burning sensation.

In past literature, you may have come across the term "psychogenic" pain. This term was attributed to pain with no known physical cause and assumed to have a psychiatric or emotional cause. It often was used as a derogatory label. Psychogenic is an obsolete term and is not accepted by the International Association for the Study of Pain. Linking pain to a mental disorder negates the person's pain report. A clinician's lack of awareness and understanding of neuropathic pain may contribute to this mislabeling.

Pain that is felt at a particular site but originates from another location is termed **referred pain**. Both sites are innervated by the same spinal nerve, and it is difficult for the brain to differentiate the point of origin. Referred pain may originate from visceral or somatic structures. Various structures maintain their same embryonic innervation. For example, an inflamed appendix in the right lower quadrant of the abdomen may have referred pain in the periumbilical area. It is useful to have knowledge of areas of referred pain for diag-

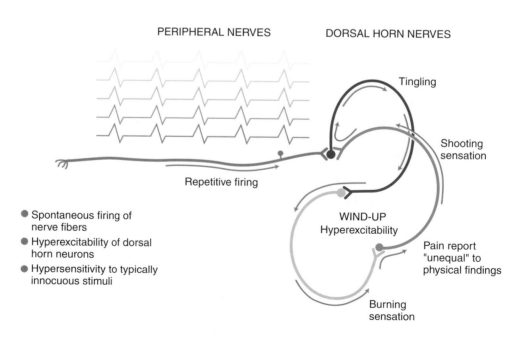

PERIPHERAL NERVES   DORSAL HORN NERVES

Tingling

Shooting
sensation

Repetitive firing

WIND-UP
Hyperexcitability

Pain report
"unequal" to
physical findings

Burning
sensation

● Spontaneous firing of
  nerve fibers
● Hyperexcitability of dorsal
  horn neurons
● Hypersensitivity to typically
  innocuous stimuli

NEUROPATHIC MECHANISMS

11–3

nostic purposes (see Table 21-2, Common Sites of Referred Abdominal Pain, p. 593).

TYPES OF PAIN (by duration)

Pain can be classified by its duration. The duration can provide information on possible underlying mechanisms and treatment decisions. Pain is divided into acute or chronic categories. **Acute pain** is short term and self-limiting, often follows a predictable trajectory, and dissipates after an injury heals. Examples of acute pain include surgery, trauma, and kidney stones. Acute pain serves a self-protective purpose; acute pain warns the individual of actual or potential tissue damage.

In contrast, **chronic pain** is diagnosed when the pain continues for 6 months or longer. It can last 5, 15, or 20 years and beyond. Chronic pain can be further divided into malignant (cancer related) and nonmalignant. Malignant pain often parallels the pathology created by the tumor cells. The pain is induced by tissue necrosis or stretching of an organ by the growing tumor. The pain fluctuates within the course of the disease. Chronic nonmalignant pain is often associated with musculoskeletal conditions, such as arthritis, low back pain, or fibromyalgia. Chronic pain does not stop when the injury heals. It persists after the predicted trajectory. Chronic pain outlasts its protective purpose, and the level of pain intensity does not correspond with the physical findings. Unfortunately, many patients with chronic pain are not believed and often are labeled as malingers, attention seekers, drug seekers, and so forth. Chronic pain originates from abnormal processing of pain fibers from peripheral or central sites. Because the pain is transmitted on a cellular level, our current technology—including x-rays, CAT scans, and MRIs—is unable to detect this process. Therefore the most important and reliable indicator for pain is the patient's self-report.

 DEVELOPMENTAL CONSIDERATIONS

INFANTS

Infants have the same capacity for pain as adults. By 20 weeks' gestation, ascending fibers, neurotransmitters, and the cerebral cortex are developed and functioning to the extent that the fetus is capable of feeling pain (Anand, 1993). However, inhibitory neurotransmitters are in insufficient supply until birth at full term. Therefore the preterm infant is rendered more sensitive to painful stimuli.

Preverbal infants are at high risk for undertreatment of pain because of persistent myths and beliefs that infants do not remember pain. In fact, new research indicates that repetitive and poorly controlled pain in infants (daily heal sticks, venipunctures) can result in lifelong adverse consequences such as neurodevelopmental problems, poor weight gain, learning disabilities, psychiatric disorders, and alcoholism (Anand, 2000).

THE AGING ADULT

No evidence exists to suggest that older individuals perceive pain to a lesser degree or that sensitivity is diminished. Although pain is a common experience among individuals 65 years of age and older, it is *not* a normal process of aging. Pain indicates pathology or injury. Pain should never be considered something to tolerate or accept in one's later years. Unfortunately, many clinicians and older adults wrongfully assume that pain should be expected in aging, which leads to less aggressive treatment. Older adults have additional fears about becoming dependent, undergoing invasive procedures, taking pain medications, and having a financial burden. The most common pain-producing conditions for aging adults include pathologies such as arthritis, osteoarthritis, osteoporosis, peripheral vascular disease, cancer, peripheral neuropathies, angina, and chronic constipation.

The somatosensory cortex is generally unaffected by dementia of the Alzheimer's type. Sensory discrimination is preserved in cognitively intact and impaired adults (Vreeling et al, 1995). Because the limbic system is affected by Alzheimer's disease, current research focuses on how the person interprets and reports these pain messages (Buffum et al, 2001; Scherder et al, 1999).

GENDER DIFFERENCES

Gender differences are influenced by societal expectations, hormones, and genetic makeup. Traditionally, men have been raised to be more stoic about pain, and more affective or emotional displays of pain are accepted for women. Hormonal changes are found to have strong influences on pain sensitivity for women. Women are two to three times more likely to experience migraines during childbearing years (Fillingim, 2000); are more sensitive to pain during the premenstrual period (Fillingim, 2000); and are six times more likely to have fibromyalgia (Fillingim, 2000). With recent findings from the Human Genome Project, genetic differences between both sexes may account for the differences in pain perception (Mogil, 2002). A pain gene exists, which helps to explain why some people feel more/less pain even with the same stimulus. Efforts are being made to tailor pharmacological agents to improve pain treatment based upon genetic sequencing.

 TRANSCULTURAL CONSIDERATIONS

Please review the cultural variations in Chapter 3. As clinicians, adopt the habit of asking each patient how he or she typically behaves when in pain.

Most of the research conducted on racial differences and pain has focused on the disparity in management of pain for various races—comparing pain treatment for individuals of color (e.g., blacks, Hispanics) with the standard treatment for individuals with similar injuries or diseases. Various studies describe how black and Hispanic patients are often prescribed and administered less analgesic therapy than white patients who present with similar symptoms (Edwards, Fillingim, and Keefe, 2001).

Subjective Data

Pain is defined as an "unpleasant sensory and emotional experience associated with actual or potential tissue damage or described in terms of such damage. Pain is always subjective" (American Pain Society, 1992, p. 250). "Pain is whatever the experiencing person says it is, existing whenever he says it does," (McCaffery, 1968, p. 95).

The subjective report is the most reliable indicator of pain. With knowledge that pain occurs on a neurochemical level, the clinician cannot base the diagnosis of pain exclusively on physical examination findings, although these findings can lend support. At this time, x-rays, CAT scans, and MRIs are not sensitive enough to identify minute damage to nerve fibers.

EXAMINER ASKS	RATIONALE
Initial Pain Assessment	
1. Where is your pain?	Pain may be localized or occurring in multiple sites.
2. When did your pain start?	Identifies onset and duration. Chronic pain is defined as pain that persists after injury heals; pain that occurs for 6 months or longer.
3. What does your pain feel like? • Burning, stabbing, aching • Throbbing, firelike, squeezing • Cramping, sharp, itching, tingling • Shooting, crushing, sharp, dull	Identifies quality of pain and helps differentiate between nociceptive and neuropathic pain mechanisms. Neuropathic pain is described as burning, shooting, and tingling. Nociceptive pain originating from visceral sites is described as aching if localized and cramping if poorly localized, and from somatic sites it is described as throbbing/aching.
4. How much pain do you have now?	Identifies intensity (refer to various intensity scales).
5. What makes your pain better or worse? (Include behavioral, pharmacologic, nonpharmacologic interventions)	Identifies alleviating and aggravating factors. Evaluates effectiveness of current treatment.
6. How does pain limit your function or activities?	Identifies degree of impairment and quality of life.
7. How do you usually behave when you are in pain? How would others know you are in pain?	Nonverbal behaviors are extremely variable, especially for chronic pain syndromes. Will aid in detection and assessment.
8. What does this pain mean to you? Why do you think you are having pain?	Can identify myths, misconceptions, beliefs, such as "I'm getting old"; "It's a punishment from God."

Pain Assessment Tools

Pain is multidimensional in scope, encompassing physical, affective, and functional domains. Various tools have been developed to capture unidimensional aspects (i.e., intensity) or multidimensional components. Select the pain assessment tool based upon its purpose, time involved in administration, and the patient's ability to comprehend and complete the tool. First, teach patients how to use each tool, with practice sessions to strengthen the validity and reliability of the response. Enlarge the print when appropriate for individuals with impaired vision. The printed language should be translated to the native language of the patient.

Standardized **overall pain assessment tools** are more useful for chronic pain conditions or particularly problematic acute pain problems. A few examples include the Initial Pain Assessment, The Brief Pain Inventory, and the McGill Questionnaire.

In the **Initial Pain Assessment** (McCaffery and Pasero, 1999), the clinician asks the patient to answer eight questions concerning location, duration, quality, intensity, and aggravating/relieving factors. Further, the clinician adds questions about manner of expressing pain and the effects of pain that impairs one's quality of life (Fig. 11-4).

Initial Pain Assessment Tool

Patient's Name _____ Age _____ Date _____
Diagnosis _____ Physician _____ Room _____
                                        Nurse _____

1. LOCATION: Patient or nurse mark drawing.

2. INTENSITY: Patient rates the pain. Scale used _____
   Present: _____
   Worst pain gets: _____
   Best pain gets: _____
   Acceptable level of pain: _____

3. QUALITY: (Use patient's own words, e.g., prick, ache, burn, throb, pull, sharp) _____

4. ONSET, DURATION, VARIATION, RHYTHMS: _____

5. MANNER OF EXPRESSING PAIN: _____

6. WHAT RELIEVES THE PAIN? _____

7. WHAT CAUSES OR INCREASES THE PAIN? _____

8. EFFECTS OF PAIN: (Note decreased function, decreased quality of life.)
   Accompanying symptoms (e.g., nausea) _____
   Sleep _____
   Appetite _____
   Physical activity _____
   Relationship with others (e.g., irritability) _____
   Emotions (e.g., anger, suicidal, crying) _____
   Concentration _____
   Other _____

9. OTHER COMMENTS: _____

10. PLAN: _____

11-4

The Brief Pain Inventory (Daut and Cleeland, 1982) asks the patient to rate the pain within the past 24 hours using graduated scales (0-10) with respect to its impact on areas such as mood, walking ability, and sleep (Fig. 11-5). **The Short-Form McGill Pain Questionnaire** (Melzack, 1987, not pictured) asks the patient to rank a list of descriptors in terms of their intensity and to give an overall intensity rating to his or her pain.

Pain rating scales are unidimensional and are intended to reflect pain intensity. They come in various forms. Pain rating

---

Brief Pain Inventory

Date ____/____/____   Time: _____

Name: _____
          Last   First   Middle initial

1. Throughout our lives, most of us have had pain from time to time (such as minor headaches, sprains, and toothaches). Have you had pain other than these everyday kinds of pain today?
   1. Yes   2. No

2. On the diagram, shade in the areas where you feel pain. Put an X on the area that hurts the most.

Right   Left   Left   Right

3. Please rate your pain by circling the one number that best describes your pain at its **worst** in the past 24 hours.

   0   1   2   3   4   5   6   7   8   9   10
   No   Pain as bad as
   pain   you can imagine

4. Please rate your pain by circling the one number that best describes your pain at its **least** in the past 24 hours.

   0   1   2   3   4   5   6   7   8   9   10
   No   Pain as bad as
   pain   you can imagine

5. Please rate your pain by circling the one number that best describes your pain on the **average**.

   0   1   2   3   4   5   6   7   8   9   10
   No   Pain as bad as
   pain   you can imagine

6. Please rate your pain by circling the one number that tells how much pain you have **right now**.

   0   1   2   3   4   5   6   7   8   9   10
   No   Pain as bad as
   pain   you can imagine

7. What treatments or medications are you receiving for your pain?

   _____

   _____

8. In the past 24 hours, how much **relief** have pain treatments or medications provided? Please circle the one percentage that most shows how much relief you have received.

   0% 10 20 30 40 50 60 70 80 90 100%
   No   Complete
   relief   relief

9. Circle the one number that describes how, during the past 24 hours, pain has **interfered** with your:
   A: General activity

   0   1   2   3   4   5   6   7   8   9   10
   Does not   Completely
   interfere   interferes

   B: Mood

   0   1   2   3   4   5   6   7   8   9   10
   Does not   Completely
   interfere   interferes

   C: Walking ability

   0   1   2   3   4   5   6   7   8   9   10
   Does not   Completely
   interfere   interferes

   D: Normal work (includes both work outside the home and housework)

   0   1   2   3   4   5   6   7   8   9   10
   Does not   Completely
   interfere   interferes

   E: Relations with other people

   0   1   2   3   4   5   6   7   8   9   10
   Does not   Completely
   interfere   interferes

   F: Sleep

   0   1   2   3   4   5   6   7   8   9   10
   Does not   Completely
   interfere   interferes

   G: Enjoyment of life

   0   1   2   3   4   5   6   7   8   9   10
   Does not   Completely
   interfere   interferes

11-5

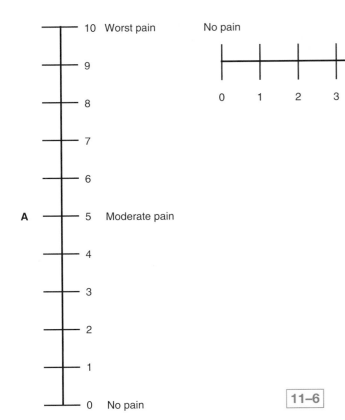

11-6

scales can indicate a baseline intensity, track changes, and give some degree of evaluation to a treatment modality. **Numeric rating scales** ask the patient to choose a number that rates the level of pain, with 0 being no pain and the highest anchor 10 indicating the worst pain. It can be administered verbally or visually along a vertical or horizontal line (Fig. 11-6).

In general, older adults find the numeric rating scale abstract and have difficulty responding, especially with a fluctuating chronic pain experience. An alternative is the simple

Descriptor Scale that lists words that describe different levels of pain intensity, such as *no pain, mild pain, moderate pain,* and *severe pain*. Older adults will often respond to scales in which words are selected. Again, it is essential to teach the person how to use the scale to enhance accuracy.

Infants and Children

Because infants are "preverbal and incapable of self report," pain assessment is dependent upon behavioral and physiologic cues. Refer to the Objective Data section. It is important to underscore the understanding that infants do feel pain.

Children 2 years of age can report pain and point to its location. They cannot rate pain intensity at this developmental level. It is helpful to ask the parent or caregiver what words their child uses to report pain (e.g., boo–boo, owie). Be aware that some children will try to be "grown up and brave" and often deny having pain in the presence of a stranger or if they are fearful of receiving a "shot." Rating scales can be introduced at 4 or 5 years of age. The Wong-Baker Scale is one example; the child is asked to choose a face that shows, "how much hurt you have now" (Fig. 11-7). Similarly, the Oucher Scale (Beyer, 1983) has six photographs of young boys' faces with different expressions of pain, ranked on a 0-5 scale of increasing intensity. The child is asked to point at the face that best matches his or her hurt/pain.

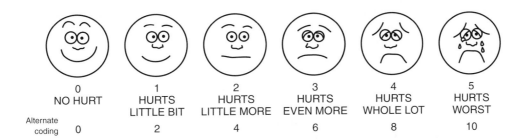

Original instructions:
Explain to the person that each face is for a person who feels happy because he has no pain (hurt) or sad because he has some or a lot of pain. **Face 0** is very happy because he doesn't hurt at all. **Face 1** hurts just a little bit. **Face 2** hurts a little more. **Face 3** hurts even more. **Face 4** hurts a whole lot. **Face 5** hurts as much as you can imagine, although you don't have to be crying to feel this bad. Ask the person to choose the face that best describes how he is feeling. Rating scale is recommended for persons age 3 years and older.

Brief word instructions:
Point to each face using the words to describe the pain intensity. Ask the child to choose face that best describes own pain and record the appropriate number.

11-7 | Wong-Baker FACES Pain Rating Scale. (From Wong DL, Hockenberry-Eaton M, Wilson D, Winkelstein ML, Schwartz P: *Wong's essentials of pediatric nursing,* ed 6, St Louis, 2001, Mosby, p. 1301. Copyright by Mosby, Inc. Reprinted by permission.)

Objective Data

PREPARATION

The physical exam process can help you understand the nature of the pain. Consider whether this is an acute or chronic condition. Recall that physical findings may not always support the patient's pain complaints, particularly for chronic pain syndromes. Pain should not be discounted when objective, physical evidence is not found. Based on the patient's pain report, make every effort to reduce or eliminate the pain with appropriate analgesic and nonpharmacologic intervention. According to the American Pain Society (1992), "In cases in which the cause of acute pain is uncertain, establishing a diagnosis is a priority, but symptomatic treatment of pain should be given while the investigation is proceeding. With occasional exceptions, (e.g., the *initial* examination of the patient with an acute condition of the abdomen), it is rarely justified to defer analgesia until a diagnosis is made. In fact, a comfortable patient is better able to cooperate with diagnostic procedures" (p. 3).

EQUIPMENT NEEDED

Tape measure to measure circumference of swollen joints or extremities
Tongue blade

NORMAL RANGE OF FINDINGS	ABNORMAL FINDINGS

THE JOINTS

Note the size and contour of the joint. Measure circumference of the involved joint for comparison with baseline. Check active or passive range of motion (see complete technique, Chapter 22). Joint motion normally causes no tenderness, pain, or crepitation.

Swelling, inflammation, injury, deformity, diminished range of motion, increased pain on palpation.
Crepitation is an audible and palpable crunching that accompanies movement.

THE MUSCLES AND SKIN

Inspect the skin and tissues for color, swelling, and any masses or deformity.

Bruising, lesions, open wounds, tissue damage, atrophy, bulging, change in hair distribution.

To assess for changes in sensation, ask the person to close his or her eyes. Test the person's ability to perceive sensation by breaking a tongue blade in two lengthwise. Lightly press the sharp and blunted ends on the skin in a random fashion and ask to identify it as sharp or dull (see Fig. 23-23). This test will help you identify location and extent of altered sensation.

Absent pain sensation (analgesia); increased pain sensation (hyperalgesia); or if a severe pain sensation is evoked with a stimulus that does not normally induce pain (e.g., the blunt end of the tongue blade; cotton ball; clothing) (allodynia).

THE ABDOMEN

Observe for contour and symmetry. Palpate for muscle guarding and organ size (see complete technique in Chapter 21). Note any areas of referred pain (see Table 21-2).

Swelling, bulging, herniation, inflammation, organ enlargement.

Table 11-1 lists physiologic changes resulting from poorly controlled pain.

NONVERBAL BEHAVIORS OF PAIN

When the individual cannot verbally communicate the pain, you can (to a limited extent) identify pain using behavioral cues. Recall that individuals react to painful stimuli with a wide variety of behaviors. Behaviors are influenced by a wide variety of factors, including the nature of the pain (acute versus chronic), age, and cultural and gender expectations.

Acute Pain Behaviors

Because acute pain involves autonomic responses and has a protective purpose, individuals experiencing moderate to intense levels of pain *may* exhibit the following behaviors:

guarding, grimacing, vocalizations such as moaning, agitation, restlessness, stillness, diaphoresis, or change in vital signs. This list of behaviors is not exhaustive because they should not be used exclusively to deny or confirm the presence of pain. For example, in a postoperative patient, pulse and blood pressure can be altered by a fluid volume, medications, and blood loss.

Chronic Pain Behaviors

Persons with chronic pain often live with the experience for months and years. One cannot function physiologically and go on with life in a repetitive state of grimacing, diaphoresis, guarding, etc. The person adapts over time, and clinicians cannot look for or anticipate the same acute pain behaviors to exist in order to confirm a pain diagnosis. Chronic pain behaviors have even more variability. Persons with chronic pain typically try to give little indication that they are in pain and therefore are at higher risk for underdetection (Fig. 11-8). Behaviors that have been associated with chronic pain include bracing, rubbing, diminished activity, sighing, and change in appetite. Whenever possible it is best to ask the person how he or she acts or behaves when in pain. Chronic pain behaviors, such as being with other people, movement, exercise, prayer, sleeping, or inactivity, underscore the more subtle, less antici-

11–8

pated ways in which persons behave when they are experiencing chronic pain. Sleeping is one way persons behave in response to chronic pain in order to self distract. Unfortunately, clinical staff may inadvertently interpret this behavior as "comfort" and do not follow up with an appropriate pharmacologic intervention.

 DEVELOPMENTAL CONSIDERATIONS

Infants

Most pain research on infants has focused on acute, procedural pain. We have a limited understanding of how to assess chronic pain in the infant. At this time, there is no one assessment tool that adequately identifies pain in the infant. Using a multidimensional approach for the whole infant is encouraged. Changes in facial activity and body movements may help assess pain. Much effort and time is spent on decoding facial expressions (e.g., taut tongue, bulging brow, closing of eye fissures), which may be difficult for the general practitioner to carry out in a busy clinical setting.

One tool that has been developed for postoperative pain in preterm and term neonates is the CRIES developed by Krechel and Bildner (1995). It measures physiologic and behavioral indicators on a 3-point scale (Fig. 11-9).

Because the sympathetic nervous system is engaged particularly in acute episodes of pain, physiologic changes take place that may indicate the presence of pain. These include sweating, increases in blood pressure and heart rate, vomiting, nausea, and changes in oxygen saturation. However, like the adult, these physiologic changes cannot be used exclu-

TABLE 11-1: Physiologic Changes from Poorly Controlled Pain

Pain is not a benign symptom. Poorly controlled acute and chronic pain have a negative impact on physiologic systems.

PHYSIOLOGIC SYSTEM	ACUTE PAIN RESPONSES
Cardiac	Tachycardia
	Elevated blood pressure
	Increased myocardial oxygen demand
	Increased cardiac output
Pulmonary	Hypoventilation
	Hypoxia
	Decreased cough
	Atelectasis
Gastrointestinal	Nausea
	Vomiting
	Ileus
Renal	Oliguria
	Urinary retention
Musculoskeletal	Spasm
	Joint stiffness
Endocrine	Increased adrenergic activity
Central nervous system	Fear
	Anxiety
	Fatigue
Immune	Impaired cellular immunity
	Impaired wound healing
Poorly controlled chronic pain	Depression
	Isolation
	Limited mobility and function
	Confusion
	Family distress
	Diminished quality of life

CRIES Neonatal Postoperative Pain Measurement Score

		0	1	2
	Crying	No	High pitched	Inconsolable
	Requires O_2 for sat >95%	No	<30%	>30%
	Increased vital signs	HR and BP = or < preop	HR or BP ↑ <20% of preop	HR or BP ↑ >20% of preop
	Expression	None	Grimace	Grimace/grunt
	Sleepless	No	Wakes at frequent intervals	Constantly awake

Neonatal pain assessment tool developed at the University of Missouri-Columbia. Copyright S. Krechel, MD, and J. Bildner, RNC, CNS.

CODING TIPS FOR USING CRIES

Crying

The characteristic cry of pain is *high pitched*.
If no cry or cry that is not high pitched, score 0.
If cry is high pitched but baby is easily consoled, score 1.
If cry is high pitched and baby is inconsolable, score 2.

Requires O_2 for sat >95%

Look for *changes* in oxygenation. Babies experiencing pain manifest decreases in oxygenation as measured by Tco_2 or oxygen saturation.
If no oxygen is required, score 0.   (Consider other causes of changes in oxygenation,
If >30% O_2 is required, score 1.   such as atelectasis, pneumothorax, over-sedation)
If <30% O_2 is required, score 2.

Increased vital signs

NOTE: Take blood presssure last as this may wake child, causing difficulty with other assessments.
Use baseline preoperative parameters from a nonstressed period.
Multiply baseline HR × 0.2 and then add this to baseline HR to determine the HR, which is 20% over baseline.
Do likewise for BP. Use mean BP.
If HR and BP are both unchanged or less than baseline, score 0.
If HR or BP is increased but increase is <20% of baseline, score 1.
If either one is increased >20% over baseline, score 2.

Expression

The facial expression most often associated with pain is a grimace. This may be characterized by brow lowering, eyes squeezed shut, deepening of the nasolabial furrow, open lips and mouth.
If no grimace is present, score 0.
If grimace alone is present, score 1.
If grimace and noncry vocalization grunt are present, score 2.

Sleepless

This parameter is scored based on the infant's state during the hour preceding this recorded score.
If the child has been continuously asleep, score 0.
If he or she has awakened at frequent intervals, score 1.
If he or she has been awake constantly, score 2.

11–9

sively to confirm or deny pain because of other factors such as stress, medications, and fluid changes.

Note that these measures target acute pain. No biological markers have been identified for long-term chronic pain in infants or children. Therefore evaluate the whole individual. Look for changes in temperament, expression, and activity. If a procedure or disease process is known to induce pain in adults (e.g., circumcision, surgery, sickle cell disease, cancer), it *will* induce pain in the infant or child.

The Aging Adult

Although pain should not be considered a "normal" part of aging, it is prevalent. When the patient reports a history of conditions such as osteoarthritis, peripheral vascular disease, cancer, osteoporosis, angina, or chronic constipation, be alert and anticipate a pain problem. Older adults will often deny having pain for fear of dependency, further testing or invasive procedures, cost, and fear of taking pain killers or becoming a drug addict. During the interview you must establish an empathic and caring rapport to gain trust.

When you look for behavioral cues, look at changes in functional status. Observe for changes in dressing, walking, toileting, or involvement in activities. A slowness and rigidity may develop, and fatigue may occur. Look for a sudden onset of acute confusion, which may indicate poorly controlled pain. However, you will need to rule out other competing explanations such as infection or adverse reaction from medications.

Application and Critical Thinking

SAMPLE CHARTING

SUBJECTIVE

Starting within the past 2 weeks, states having severe epigastric pain within a half hour of eating greasy fatty foods. Pain is stabbing and squeezing in nature with radiation to right shoulder blade. Rates pain as a 10 on a 0-10 scale. Nausea accompanies pain. Takes antacids with minimal relief. Pain diminishes after bringing knees to chest and "not moving" for a 1-hour period.

OBJECTIVE

Patient diaphoretic, grimacing, and having difficulty concentrating. Breathless during history. Arms guarding upper abdominal area. Abdomen distended. Severe tenderness noted upon light left upper quadrant and epigastric palpation. Bowel sounds hyperactive in all four quadrants.

FOCUSED ASSESSMENT: CLINICAL CASE STUDY 1

R.M. is a 20-year-old African American male diagnosed with sickle cell crisis. Admitted to the emergency department.

SUBJECTIVE

Within the past 48 hours, R.M. reports increasing pain in upper and lower extremity joints and swelling of right knee. States having "stomach flu" 1 week before with periods of vomiting and diarrhea. Pain is aching and constant in nature. Rates pain as 10+ on a 0-10 scale. Reports difficulty walking and climbing stairs. Taking ibuprofen, two tablets every 4 hours, and using ice packs with no relief.

OBJECTIVE

Requiring assistance to sit on exam table. Unable to bear weight on right leg. Affect flat, clenches jaw during position changes. Tenderness localized in elbow, wrist, finger, and knee joints. Diminished range of motion in wrists and knees (right knee 36 centimeters, left knee 30 centimeters diameter). Right knee warm and boggy to touch.

ASSESSMENT

Acute pain

FOCUSED ASSESSMENT: CLINICAL CASE STUDY 2

A.G. is an 85-year-old Irish-American female with a 20-year history of osteoarthritis.

SUBJECTIVE

A.G. reports increased pain and stiffness in her neck, arms, and lower back for the past month. Denies radiation of pain. Denies tingling or numbness in upper or lower extremities.

Having difficulty getting in and out of bathtub and dressing herself. Describes pain as aching, with good and bad days. Becomes frustrated when asked to rate her pain intensity. Replies "I don't know what number to give; it hurts a lot, on and off." Takes acetaminophen extra strength, two tablets, when the pain "really gets the best of me," with some degree of relief. Does not take part in "field trips" offered by assisted living facility because she "hurts too much."

OBJECTIVE

Localized tenderness noted upon palpation to C3 and C4; unable to flex neck to chest. Crepitus noted in both shoulder joints. No swelling noted. Muscle strength 1+ and equal for upper extremities. Lumbar area tender to moderate palpation. Rubs lower back frequently; limited flexion at the waist. Gait slow and unsteady. Facial expression stoic.

ASSESSMENT

Chronic pain

ABNORMAL FINDINGS

Abnormal Findings

Complex Regional Pain—Type I (Reflexive Sympathetic Dystrophy)

This pain syndrome has more overt physical changes than most pain problems. Injury can occur months before the pain syndrome develops. A key feature is that a typically innocuous stimulus (e.g., a light brush of a cotton ball or clothing) can create a severe, intense painful response. Complex regional pain—type I is found in upper or lower extremities. It is neuropathic in nature with an underlying "wind-up" mechanism suspected. On examination the affected extremity becomes less functional and develops changes such as widespread "burning" pain, atrophy of muscle, edema, cool shiny skin, diminished hair and nail growth, and decreased range of motion.

BIBLIOGRAPHY

American Pain Society (APS): *Principles of analgesic use in the treatment of acute and cancer pain,* ed 3, Glenview, Ill, 1992, Author.

Anand KJS: Effects of perinatal pain and stress, *Prog Brain Res* 122:117-119, 2000.

Anand KJS: The applied physiology of pain. In Anand KJS, McGrath RJ, editors: *Pain in neonates,* Amsterdam, 1993, Elsevier.

Banasik JL: Pain. In Copstead LE, Banasik, JL, editors: *Pathophysiology: biological and behavioral perspectives,* ed 2, Philadelphia, 2000, W.B. Saunders.

Beyer JE: *The oucher: a user's manual and technical report,* Evanston, Ill, 1983, Judson.

Buffum MD, Miaskowski C, Sands L, Brod M: A pilot study of the relationship between discomfort and agitation in patients with dementia, *Geriatr Nurs* 22(2):80-85, 2001.

Curtis S, Kolytolo C, Broome ME: Somatosensory function and pain. In Mattson Porth C, editor: *Pathophysiology: concepts in altered health states,* ed 5, Philadelphia, 2002, Lippincott.

Daut RL, Cleeland CS: The prevalence and severity of pain in cancer, *Cancer* 50:1913-1918, 1982.

Dellasega C, Keiser CL: Pharmacologic approaches to chronic pain in the older adult, *Nurse Pract* 22(5):20-37, 1997.

Edwards CL, Fillingim RB, Keefe F: Race, ethnicity and pain, *Pain* 94(2):133-137, 2001.

Fillingim RB: *Sex, gender and pain,* Seattle, 2000, IASP Press.

Hummel P, Puchalski M: Assessment and management of pain in infancy, *Newborn and Infant Nursing Reviews* 1(2):114-121, 2001.

International Association for the Study of Pain: Assess the person, not just the pain, *Pain Clinical Updates* 1(3):1-4, 1993.

International Association for the Study of Pain: Pain measurement in children, *Pain Clinical Updates* 1(3):2, 1995.

Krechel SW, Bildner J: CRIES: a new neonatal postoperative pain measurement score. Initial testing of validity and reliability, *Paediatr Anaesth* 5(1):53-61, 1995.

Mayer DD, Torma L, Byock I, Norris K: Speaking the language of pain, *Am J Nurs* 101(2):44-50, 2001.

McCaffery M: *Nursing practice theories related to cognition, bodily pain, and man-environment interactions,* Los Angeles, 1968, UCLA, Students' Store.

McCaffery M, Pasero C: *Pain: clinical manual,* ed 2, St Louis, 1999, Mosby.

Melzack R: The short-form McGill Pain Questionnaire, *Pain* 30:191-197, 1987.

Mogil JS: Pain genetics: pre- and post-genomic findings. *International Association for the Study of Pain Technical Corner Newsletter,* (2):3-6, 2002.

Turk DC, Melzack R, editors: *Handbook of pain assessment,* New York, 1992, The Guilford Press.

Vreeling FW, Houx PJ, Jolles J, Verhey FR: Primitive reflexes in Alzheimer's disease and vascular dementia, *J Geriatr Psychiatry Neurol* 8(2):111-117, 1995.

Weisse CS, Sorum PC, Sanders KN, Syat BS: Do gender and race affect decisions about pain management? *J Gen Intern Med* 16(4):211-217, 2001.

Wong D, Baker C: *Reference manual for the Wong-Baker FACES pain rating scale,* Tulsa, 1995, Wong and Baker.

Skin, Hair, and Nails

http://evolve.elsevier.com/Jarvis/

Structure and Function

Think of the skin as the body's largest organ system—it covers 20 square feet of surface area in the average adult. The skin is the sentry that guards the body from environmental stresses (e.g., trauma, pathogens, dirt) and adapts it to other environmental influences (e.g., heat, cold).

SKIN

The skin has two layers—the outer highly differentiated *epidermis* and the inner supportive *dermis* (Fig. 12–1). Beneath these layers is a third layer, the *subcutaneous* layer of adipose tissue.

Epidermis

The *epidermis* is thin but tough. Its cells are bound tightly together into sheets that form a rugged protective barrier. It is stratified into several zones. The inner **stratum germinativum,** or basal cell layer, forms new skin cells. Their major ingredient is the tough, fibrous protein *keratin.* The melanocytes interspersed along this layer produce the pigment *melanin,* which gives brown tones to the skin and hair. All people have the same number of melanocytes; however,

the amount of melanin they produce varies with genetic, hormonal, and environmental influences.

From the basal layer the new cells migrate up and flatten into the **stratum corneum.** This outer horny cell layer consists of dead keratinized cells that are interwoven and closely packed. The cells are constantly being shed, or desquamated, and are replaced with new cells from below. The epidermis is completely replaced every 4 weeks. In fact, each person sheds about 1 lb of skin each year.

The epidermis is uniformly thin except on the surfaces that are exposed to friction, such as the palms and the soles. On these surfaces, skin is thicker because of work and weight bearing. The epidermis is avascular; it is nourished by blood vessels in the dermis below.

Skin color is derived from three sources: (1) mainly from the brown pigment melanin, (2) also from the yellow-orange tones of the pigment carotene, and (3) from the red-purple tones in the underlying vascular bed. All people have skin of varying shades of brown, yellow, and red; the relative proportion of these shades affects the prevailing color. Skin color is further modified by the thickness of the skin and by the presence of edema.

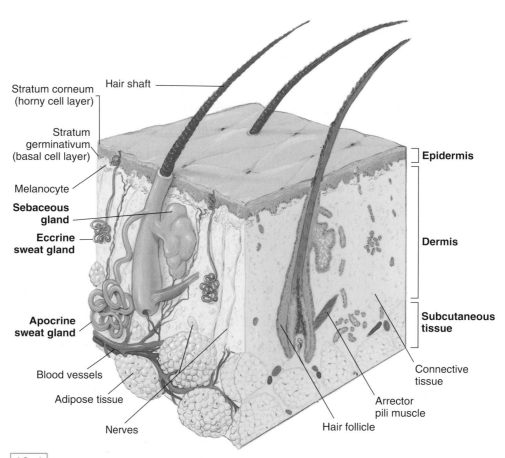

Stratum corneum (horny cell layer)
Hair shaft
Stratum germinativum (basal cell layer)
Epidermis
Melanocyte
Sebaceous gland
Dermis
Eccrine sweat gland
Apocrine sweat gland
Subcutaneous tissue
Blood vessels
Connective tissue
Adipose tissue
Arrector pili muscle
Nerves
Hair follicle

12–1

Dermis

The *dermis* is the inner supportive layer consisting mostly of connective tissue, or *collagen.* This is the tough, fibrous protein that enables the skin to resist tearing. The dermis also has resilient elastic tissue that allows the skin to stretch with body movements. The nerves, sensory receptors, blood vessels, and lymphatics lie in the dermis. Also, appendages from the epidermis—such as the hair follicles, sebaceous glands, and sweat glands—are embedded in the dermis.

Subcutaneous Layer

The *subcutaneous layer* is adipose tissue, which is made up of lobules of fat cells. The subcutaneous tissue stores fat for energy, provides insulation for temperature control, and aids in protection by its soft cushioning effect. Also, the loose subcutaneous layer gives skin its increased mobility over structures underneath.

EPIDERMAL APPENDAGES

These structures are formed by a tubular invagination of the epidermis down into the underlying dermis.

Hair

Hair is *vestigial* for humans; it no longer is needed for protection from cold or trauma. However, hair is highly significant in most cultures for its cosmetic and psychological meaning (see Transcultural Considerations).

Hairs are threads of keratin. The hair *shaft* is the visible projecting part, and the *root* is below the surface embedded in the follicle. At the root the *bulb matrix* is the expanded area where new cells are produced at a high rate. Hair growth is cyclical, with active and resting phases. Each follicle functions independently so that while some hairs are resting, others are growing. Around the hair follicle are the muscular *arrector pili,* which contract and elevate the hair so that it resembles "goose flesh" when the skin is exposed to cold or in emotional states.

People have two types of hair. Fine, faint **vellus hair** covers most of the body (except the palms and soles, the dorsa of the distal parts of the fingers, the umbilicus, the glans penis, and inside the labia). The other type is **terminal hair,** the darker thicker hair that grows on the scalp and eyebrows and, after puberty, on the axillae, pubic area, and the face and chest in the male.

Sebaceous Glands

These glands produce a protective lipid substance, *sebum,* which is secreted through the hair follicles. Sebum oils and lubricates the skin and hair and forms an emulsion with water that retards water loss from the skin. (Dry skin results from loss of water, not directly from loss of oil.) Sebaceous glands are everywhere except on the palms and soles. They are most abundant in the scalp, forehead, face, and chin.

Sweat Glands

There are two types. The **eccrine** glands are coiled tubules that open directly onto the skin surface and produce a dilute saline solution called *sweat.* The evaporation of sweat reduces body temperature. Eccrine glands are widely distributed through the body and are mature in the 2-month-old infant.

The **apocrine** glands produce a thick, milky secretion and open into the hair follicles. They are located mainly in the axillae, anogenital area, nipples, and navel and are vestigial in humans. They become active during puberty, and secretion occurs with emotional and sexual stimulation. Bacterial flora residing on the skin surface react with apocrine sweat to produce characteristic musky body odor. The functioning of apocrine glands decreases in the aging adult.

Nails

The nails are hard plates of keratin on the dorsal edges of the fingers and toes (Fig. 12–2). The nail plate is clear, with fine longitudinal ridges that become prominent in aging. Nails take their pink color from the underlying nail bed of highly vascular epithelial cells. The lunula is the white opaque semilunar area at the proximal end of the nail. It lies over the nail matrix where new keratinized cells are formed. The nail folds overlap the posterior and lateral borders. The cuticle works like a gasket to cover and protect the nail matrix.

Posterior nail fold

Cuticle

Lunula

Lateral nail fold

Nail plate

Nail matrix

Nail bed

12–2

FUNCTION OF THE SKIN

The skin is a waterproof, almost indestructible covering that has protective and adaptive properties:

- **Protection.** Skin minimizes injury from physical, chemical, thermal, and light wave sources.
- **Prevents penetration.** Skin is a barrier that stops invasion of microorganisms and loss of water and electrolytes from within the body.
- **Perception.** Skin is a vast sensory surface holding the neurosensory end-organs for touch, pain, temperature, and pressure.
- **Temperature regulation.** Skin allows heat dissipation through sweat glands and heat storage through subcutaneous insulation.

- **Identification.** People identify one another by unique combinations of facial characteristics, hair, skin color, and even fingerprints. Self-image is often enhanced or deterred by the way society's standards of beauty measure up to each person's perceived characteristics.
- **Communication.** Emotions are expressed in the sign language of the face and in the body posture. Vascular mechanisms such as blushing or blanching also signal emotional states.
- **Wound repair.** Skin allows cell replacement of surface wounds.
- **Absorption and excretion.** Skin allows limited excretion of some metabolic wastes, by-products of cellular decomposition such as minerals, sugars, amino acids, cholesterol, uric acid, and urea.
- **Production of vitamin D.** The skin is the surface on which ultraviolet light converts cholesterol into vitamin D.

 DEVELOPMENTAL CONSIDERATIONS

INFANTS AND CHILDREN

The hair follicles develop in the fetus at 3 months' gestation; by midgestation most of the skin is covered with **lanugo,** the fine downy hair of the newborn. In the first few months after birth, this is replaced by fine vellus hair. Terminal hair on the scalp, if present at birth, tends to be soft and to suffer a patchy loss, especially at the temples and occiput. Also present at birth is **vernix caseosa,** the thick, cheesy substance made up of sebum and shed epithelial cells.

The newborn's skin is similar in structure to the adult's, but many of its functions are not fully developed. The newborn's skin is thin, smooth, and elastic and is relatively more permeable than that of the adult, so the infant is at greater risk for fluid loss. Sebum, which holds water in the skin, is present for the first few weeks of life, producing milia and cradle cap in some babies. Then sebaceous glands decrease in size and production and do not resume functioning until puberty. Temperature regulation is ineffective. Eccrine sweat glands do not secrete in response to heat until the first few months of life and then only minimally throughout childhood. The skin cannot protect much against cold because it cannot contract and shiver and because the subcutaneous layer is inefficient. Also, the pigment system is inefficient at birth.

As the child grows, the epidermis thickens, toughens, and darkens and the skin becomes better lubricated. Hair growth accelerates. At puberty, secretion from apocrine sweat glands increases in response to heat and emotional stimuli, producing body odor. Sebaceous glands become more active—the skin looks oily, and acne develops. Subcutaneous fat deposits increase, especially in females.

Secondary sex characteristics that appear during adolescence are evident in the integument (i.e., skin). In the female the diameter of the areola enlarges and darkens, and breast tissue develops. Coarse pubic hair develops in males and females, then axillary hair, and then coarse facial hair in males.

THE PREGNANT FEMALE

The change in hormone levels results in increased pigment in the areolae and nipples, vulva, and sometimes in the midline of the abdomen (**linea nigra**) or in the face (**chloasma**). Hyperestrogenemia probably also causes the common vascular spiders and palmar erythema. Connective tissue develops increased fragility, resulting in **striae gravidarum,** which may develop in the skin of the abdomen, breasts, or thighs. Metabolism is increased in pregnancy; as a way to dissipate heat, the peripheral vasculature dilates, and the sweat and sebaceous glands increase secretion. Fat deposits are laid down, particularly in the buttocks and hips, as maternal reserves for the nursing baby.

THE AGING ADULT

The skin is a mirror that reflects aging changes that proceed in *all* our organ systems; it just happens to be the one organ we can view directly. The aging process carries a slow atrophy of skin structures. The aging skin loses its elasticity; it folds and sags. By the 70s to 80s, it looks parchment thin, lax, dry, and wrinkled.

The epidermis's outer layer, *stratum corneum,* thins and flattens. This allows chemicals easier access into the body. Wrinkling occurs because the underlying dermis thins and flattens. A loss of elastin, collagen, and subcutaneous fat occurs as well as a reduction in muscle tone. The loss of collagen increases the risk for shearing, tearing injuries.

Sweat glands and sebaceous glands decrease in number and function, leaving dry skin. Decreased response of the sweat glands to thermoregulatory demand also puts the aging person at greater risk for heat stroke. The vascularity of the skin diminishes, while the vascular fragility increases; a minor trauma may produce dark red discolored areas, or **senile purpura.**

Sun exposure and, to a somewhat lesser extent, cigarette smoking further accentuate aging changes in the skin. Coarse wrinkling, decreased elasticity, atrophy, speckled and uneven coloring, more pigment changes, and a yellowed leathery texture occur. Chronic sun damage is even more prominent in pale or light-skinned persons.

An accumulation of factors place the aging person at risk for skin disease and breakdown: the thinning of the skin, the decrease in vascularity and nutrients, the loss of protective cushioning of the subcutaneous layer, a lifetime of environmental trauma to skin, the social changes of aging (e.g., less nutrition, limited financial resources), the increasingly sedentary lifestyle, and the chance of immobility. When skin breakdown does occur, subsequent cell replacement is slower, and wound healing is delayed.

In the aging hair matrix, the number of functioning melanocytes decreases so the hair looks gray or white and feels thin and fine. A person's genetic script determines the onset of graying and the number of gray hairs. Hair distribution changes. Males may have a symmetrical W-shaped balding in the frontal areas. Some testosterone is present in both males and females; as it decreases with age, axillary and pubic hair decrease. As the female's estrogen also decreases, testosterone is unopposed and the female may develop some bristly facial hairs. Nails grow more slowly. Their surface is lusterless and is characterized by longitudinal ridges due to local trauma at the nail matrix.

Because the aging changes in the skin and hair can be viewed directly, they carry profound psychological impact. For many people, self-esteem is linked to a youthful appearance. This view is compounded by media advertising in Western society. Although sagging and wrinkling skin and graying and thinning hair are normal processes of aging, they prompt a loss of self-esteem for many adults.

TRANSCULTURAL CONSIDERATIONS

Awareness of normal biocultural differences and the ability to recognize the unique clinical manifestations of disease are especially important for darkly pigmented people. As described earlier, melanin is responsible for the various colors and tones of skin observed among people from culturally diverse backgrounds. Melanin protects the skin against harmful ultraviolet rays, a genetic advantage accounting for the lower incidence of skin cancer among darkly pigmented blacks and Native Americans. Areas of the skin affected by hormones and, in some cases, differing for culturally diverse people, are the sexual skin areas, such as the nipples, areola, scrotum, and labia majora. In general, these areas are darker than other parts of the skin in both adults and children, especially among blacks and Asians.

The apocrine and eccrine sweat glands are important for fluid balance and for thermoregulation. When apocrine gland secretions are contaminated by normal skin flora, odor results. Most Asians and Native Americans have a mild body odor or none at all, whereas whites and blacks tend to have strong body odor. The amount of chloride excreted by sweat glands varies widely, and blacks have lower salt concentrations in their sweat than whites do.

Inuits have made an interesting environmental adaptation, whereby they sweat less than whites on their trunks and extremities but more on their faces. This adaptation allows for temperature regulation without causing perspiration and dampness of their clothes, which would decrease their ability to insulate against severe cold weather and would pose a serious threat to their survival.

Perhaps one of the most obvious and widely variable racial differences occurs with the hair. The hair of blacks varies widely in texture. It is very fragile and ranges from long and straight to short, spiraled, thick, and kinky. The hair and scalp have a natural tendency to be dry and require daily combing, gentle brushing, and the application of oil. In comparison, people of Asian backgrounds generally have straight, silky hair.

Hair condition is significant in diagnosing and treating certain disease states. For example, hair texture becomes dry, brittle, and lusterless with inadequate nutrition. The hair of black children with severe malnutrition (e.g., marasmus) frequently changes not only in texture but in color. The child's hair often becomes less kinky and assumes a copper-red color.

Subjective Data

1. Previous history of skin disease (allergies, hives, psoriasis, eczema)	**4.** Excessive dryness or moisture	**9.** Hair loss
	5. Pruritus	**10.** Change in nails
2. Change in pigmentation	**6.** Excessive bruising	**11.** Environmental or occupational hazards
3. Change in mole (size or color)	**7.** Rash or lesion	**12.** Self-care behaviors
	8. Medications	

EXAMINER ASKS	RATIONALE
1. Previous history of skin disease. Any **previous skin disease** or problem?	
• How was this treated?	Significant familial predisposition: allergies, hay fever, psoriasis, atopic dermatitis (eczema), acne.
• Any family history of allergies or allergic skin problem?	
• Any known allergies to drugs, plants, animals?	Identify offending allergen.
• Any birthmarks, tattoos?	Use of nonsterile equipment to apply tattoos increases risk of hepatitis C.
2. Change in pigmentation. Any **change in skin color** or **pigmentation?**	Localized change: hypopigmentation—loss of pigmentation; hyperpigmentation—increase in color.
• A generalized color change (all over), or localized?	Generalized change suggests systemic illness: pallor, jaundice, cyanosis.

EXAMINER ASKS	RATIONALE
3. Change in mole. Any **change in a mole:** color, size, shape, sudden appearance of tenderness, bleeding, itching? • Any "sores" that do not heal?	Signs suggest neoplasm in pigmented nevus. Person may be unaware of change in nevus on back or buttocks that he or she cannot see.
4. Excessive dryness or moisture. Any change in the feel of your skin: temperature, **moisture,** texture? • Any excess **dryness**? Is this seasonal or constant?	Seborrhea—oily. Xerosis—dry.
5. Pruritus. Any skin itching? Is this mild (prickling, tingling) or intense (intolerable)? • Does it awaken you from sleep? • Where is the itching? When did it start? • Any other skin pain or soreness? Where?	Pruritus is the most common of skin symptoms; occurs with dry skin, aging, drug reactions, allergy, obstructive jaundice, uremia, lice. Presence or absence of pruritus may be significant for diagnosis. Scratching may cause excoriation of primary lesion.
6. Excessive bruising. Any excess **bruising?** Where on the body? • How did this happen? • How long have you had it?	Multiple cuts and bruises, bruises in various stages of healing, bruises above knees and elbows, and illogical explanation—consider the possibility of abuse. Frequent falls may be due to dizziness of neurologic or cardiovascular origin. Also, frequent minor trauma may be a side effect of alcoholism or other drug abuse.
7. Rash or lesion. Any skin **rash or lesion?** • Onset. When did you first notice it? • Location. Where did it start? • Where did it spread? • Character or quality. Describe the color. • Is it raised or flat? Any crust, odor? Does it feel tender, warm? • Duration. How long have you had it? • Setting. Anyone at home or work with a similar rash? Have you been camping, acquired a new pet, tried a new food, drug? Does the rash seem to come with stress? • Alleviating and aggravating factors. What home care have you tried? Bath, lotions, heat? Do they help, or make it worse? • Associated symptoms. Any itching, fever? • What do you think rash/lesion means? • Coping strategies. How has rash/lesion affected your self-care, hygiene, ability to function at work/home/socially?	Rashes are a common cause of seeking health care. A careful history is important; it may be an accurate predictor of the type of lesion you will see in the examination and its cause. Identify the primary site—it may give clue to cause. Migration pattern, evolution. Identify new or relevant exposure. Identify any household or social contacts with similar symptoms. Myriad over-the-counter remedies are available. Many people try them and seek professional help only when they do not see improvement. Assess person's perception of cause. May need to deal with fear of cancer, tick-borne illnesses, or sexually transmitted diseases. Assess effectiveness of coping strategies. Chronic skin diseases may increase risk of loss of self-esteem, social isolation, and anxiety.

EXAMINER ASKS	RATIONALE
• Any new or increased stress in your life?	Stress can exacerbate chronic skin illness.
8. Medications. What **medications** do you take? • Prescription and over-the-counter? • Recent change?	Drugs may produce allergic skin eruption: aspirin, antibiotics, barbiturates, some tonics. Drugs may increase sunlight sensitivity and give burn response: sulfonamides, thiazide diuretics, oral hypoglycemic agents, and tetracycline. Drugs can cause hyperpigmentation: antimalarials, antineoplastic agents, hormones, metals, tetracycline.
• How long on medication?	Even after a long time on medication, a person may develop sensitivity.
9. Hair loss. Any recent **hair loss?** • A gradual or sudden onset? Symmetrical? Associated with fever, illness, increased stress?	Alopecia is a significant loss. A full head of hair equates with vitality in many cultures. If this is treated as a trivial problem, the person may seek alternative, unproven methods of treatment.
• Any unusual hair growth? • Any recent change in texture, appearance?	Hirsutism.
10. Change in nails. Any **change in nails:** shape, color, brittleness? Do you tend to bite or chew nails?	
11. Environmental or occupational hazards. Any **environmental** or **occupational hazards?** • Any hazard-related problems with your occupation, such as dyes, toxic chemicals, radiation? • How about hobbies? Do you perform any household or furniture repair work? • How much sun exposure do you get from outdoor work, leisure activities, sunbathing, tanning salons?	Majority of skin neoplasms result from occupational or environmental agents. People at risk include coal workers; farmers exposed to the sun, sailors, outdoor workers; also creosote workers, roofers. Unprotected sun exposure accelerates aging and produces lesions. At more risk: light-skinned people, those over 40, and those regularly in sun.
• Recently been bitten by insect: bee, tick, mosquito?	Identify contactants that produce lesions or contact dermatitis.
• Any recent exposure to plants, animals in yard work, camping?	For people with chronic recurrent urticaria (hives), tell them to keep diary of meals and environment to identify precipitating factors.
12. Self-care behaviors. What do you do to care for your skin, hair, nails? What cosmetics, soaps, chemicals do you use? • Clip cuticles on nails, use adhesive for false fingernails?	Assess **self-care** and influence on self-concept—may be important with this society's media stress on high norms of beauty. Many over-the-counter remedies are costly and exacerbate skin problems.
• If you have allergies, how do you control your environment to minimize exposure? • Do you perform a skin self-examination?	

EXAMINER ASKS	RATIONALE

Additional History for Infants and Children

1. Does the child have any birthmarks?

2. Was there any change in skin color as a newborn?
  • Any jaundice? Which day after birth?
  • Any cyanosis? What were the circumstances?

3. Have you noted any rash or sores? What seems to bring it on?
  • Have you introduced a new food or formula? When? Does your child eat chocolate, cow's milk, eggs?

Generalized rash—consider allergic reaction to new food.
Irritability and general fussiness may indicate the presence of pruritus.

4. Does the child have any diaper rash? How do you care for this? How do you wash diapers? How often do you change diapers? How do you clean skin?

Occlusive diapers or infrequent changing may cause rash. Infant may be allergic to certain detergent or to disposable wipes.

5. Does the child have any burns or bruises?
  • Where?
  • How did it happen?

A careful history is important to distinguish expected childhood bumps and bruises from any lesion that may indicate child abuse or neglect: cigarette burns; excessive bruising, especially above knees or elbows; linear whip marks. With abuse the history often will not coincide with the physical appearance and location of lesion.

6. Has the child had any exposure to contagious skin conditions: scabies, impetigo, lice? Or to communicable diseases: measles, chickenpox, scarlet fever? Or to toxic plants: poison ivy?
  • Are the child's vaccinations up to date?

7. Does the child have any habits or habitual movements, such as nailbiting, twisting hair, rubbing head on mattress?

8. What steps are taken to protect the child from sun exposure? What about sunscreens and sunblocks? How do you treat a sunburn?

Between 60% and 80% of a person's lifetime sun exposure occurs before 18 years of age. One or more severe sunburns during childhood double the risk of malignant melanoma in later life (Heffernan and O'Sullivan, 1998).

Additional History for the Adolescent

1. Have you noticed any skin problems such as pimples, blackheads?
  • How long have you had them?
  • How do you treat this?
  • How do you feel about it?

About 70% of teens will have acne, and the psychological effect often is more significant than the physical effect. Self-treatment is common. Many myths surround the cause of acne. Cause is unknown; acne is not caused by poor diet, oily complexion, or contagion, and has no relation to sexual practices.

EXAMINER ASK	RATIONALE

Additional History for the Aging Adult

1. What changes have you noticed in your skin in the last few years?

Assess impact of aging on self-concept. Normal aging changes may cause distress. Note that many changes attributed to aging are due to chronic sun damage. Most skin cancers appear in aging people, although sun damage often begins decades earlier.

2. Any delay in wound healing?
   • Any skin itching?

Pruritus is very common with aging. Consider side effects of medicine or systemic disease (e.g., liver or kidney disease, cancer, lymphoma), but senile pruritus is usually due to dry skin (xerosis). Exacerbated by too-frequent bathing or use of soap. Scratching with dirty, jagged fingernails produces excoriations.

3. Any other skin pain?

Some diseases, such as herpes zoster (shingles), produce more intense sensations of pain, itching in aging people. Other diseases (e.g., diabetes) may reduce pain sensation in extremities. Also, some aging people tolerate chronic pain as "part of growing old," and hesitate to "complain."

4. Any change in feet, toenails? Any bunions? Is it possible to wear shoes?

Some aging people cannot reach down to their feet to give self-care.

5. Do you experience frequent falls?

Multiple bruises, trauma from falls.

6. Any history of diabetes, peripheral vascular disease?

Risk for skin lesions in feet or ankles.

7. What do you do to care for your skin?

Application of bland lotions is important to retain moisture in aging skin. Dermatitis may ensue from certain cosmetics, creams, ointments, and dyes applied to achieve a youthful appearance.
Aging skin has a delayed inflammatory response when exposed to irritants. If the person is not alerted by warning signs (e.g., pruritus, redness), exposure may continue and dermatitis may ensue.

Objective Data

PREPARATION

Try to control external variables that may influence skin color and confuse your findings, both in light-skinned and in dark-skinned persons (Table 12–1).

Learn to consciously attend to skin characteristics. The danger is one of omission. You grow so accustomed to seeing the skin that you are likely to ignore it as you assess the organ systems underneath. Yet the skin holds information about the body's circulation, nutritional status, and signs of systemic diseases as well as topical data on the integument itself.

Know the person's normal skin coloring. Baseline knowledge is important to assess color or pigment changes. If this is the first time you are examining the person, ask about his or her usual skin color and about any self-monitoring practices.

THE COMPLETE PHYSICAL EXAMINATION. Although it is presented alone in this chapter, skin assessment is *integrated* throughout the complete examination; it is not a separate step. At the beginning of the examination, assessing the person's hands and fingernails is a nonthreatening way to accustom him or her to your touch. Most people are used to having relative strangers shake their hand or touch their arm. As you move through the examination, scrutinize the outer skin surface first before you concentrate on the underlying structures. Separate intertriginous areas (areas with skinfolds) such as under large breasts, obese abdomen, and the groin and inspect them thoroughly. These areas are dark, warm, and moist and provide the perfect conditions for irritation or infection. Last, always remove the person's socks and inspect the feet, toenails, and the area between the toes.

THE REGIONAL EXAMINATION. At times, an individual seeks health care because of a skin change and your assessment will be focused on the skin alone. Ask the person to remove his or her clothing and assess the skin as one entity. Stand back at first to get an overall impression; this helps reveal distribution patterns. Then inspect lesions carefully. With a skin rash, check all areas of the body because there are some locations the person cannot see. You cannot rely on the history alone that the rash is limited to one location. Inspect mucous membranes, too, because some disorders have characteristic lesions here.

The skills used are inspection and palpation because some skin changes have accompanying signs that can be felt.

EQUIPMENT NEEDED

Strong direct lighting (natural daylight is ideal to evaluate skin characteristics but is usually not available in the clinical area)
Small centimeter ruler
Penlight
Gloves
Needed for special procedures:
  Wood's light (filtered ultraviolet light)
  Magnifying glass, for minute lesions
  Materials for laboratory tests: potassium hydroxide (KOH), glass slide

TABLE 12–1: External Variables Influencing Skin Color

VARIABLE	CAUSES	MISLEADING OUTCOME
Emotions		
Fear, anger	⟶ Peripheral vasoconstriction	⟶ False pallor
Embarrassment	⟶ Flushing in face and neck	⟶ False erythema
Environment		
Hot room	⟶ Vasodilatation	⟶ False erythema
Chilly or air-conditioned room, mist tents	⟶ Vasoconstriction	⟶ False pallor, coolness
Cigarette smoking	⟶ Vasoconstriction	⟶ False pallor
Physical		
Prolonged elevation	⟶ Decreased arterial perfusion	⟶ Pallor, coolness
Dependent position	⟶ Venous pooling	⟶ Redness, warmth, distended veins
Immobilization, prolonged inactivity	⟶ Slowed circulation	⟶ Pallor, coolness, nail beds pale, prolonged capillary filling time

Data from Roach L. Dark skins: recognizing and interpreting color changes. *Crit Care Update* 5–15, 1977.

NORMAL RANGE OF FINDINGS	ABNORMAL FINDINGS

INSPECT AND PALPATE THE SKIN

Color

GENERAL PIGMENTATION. Observe the skin tone. Normally it is consistent with genetic background and varies from pinkish tan to ruddy dark tan or from light to dark brown and may have yellow or olive overtones. Dark-skinned people normally have areas of lighter pigmentation on the palms, nail beds, and lips (Fig. 12–3, *A*).

An acquired condition is **vitiligo,** the complete absence of melanin pigment in patchy areas of white or light skin on the face, neck, hands, feet, body folds, and around orifices (Fig. 12–3, *B*). Vitiligo can occur in all races, although dark-skinned people are more severely affected and potentially suffer a greater threat to their body image.

12–3 A

12–3 **B**, Vitiligo.

General pigmentation is darker in sun-exposed areas. Common (benign) pigmented areas also occur:

- **Freckles** (ephelides)—small, flat macules of brown melanin pigment that occur on sun-exposed skin (Fig. 12–4, *A*).
- **Mole** (nevus)—a proliferation of melanocytes, tan to brown color, flat or raised. Acquired nevi are characterized by their symmetry, small size (6 mm or less), smooth borders, and single uniform pigmentation. The **junctional nevus** (Fig. 12–4, *B*) is macular only and occurs in children and adolescents. It progresses to the **compound nevi** in young adults (Fig. 12–4, *C*) that are macular and papular. The intradermal nevus (mainly in older age) has nevus cells in only the dermis.
- **Birthmarks**—may be tan to brown in color.

Danger signs: abnormal characteristics of pigmented lesions are summarized in the mnemonic **ABCDE:**

Asymmetry of a pigmented lesion (one that is *not* regularly round or oval)

Border irregularity (notching, scalloping, ragged edges or poorly defined margins)

Color variation (areas of brown, tan, black, blue, red, white, or combination thereof)

Diameter greater than 6 mm (i.e., the size of a pencil eraser), although early melanomas may be diagnosed at a smaller size (Oliviero, 2002).

Elevation and **E**nlargement

Additionally, individuals may report change in mole's size, a new pigmented lesion, and development of itching, burning, or bleeding in a mole. Any of these signs should raise suspicion of malignant melanoma and warrant referral.

A	B	C

12–4 **A**, Freckles. **B**, Junctional nevus. **C**, Compound nevus.

WIDESPREAD COLOR CHANGE. Note any color change over the entire body skin, such as pallor (white), erythema (red), cyanosis (blue), and jaundice (yellow). Note whether the color change is transient and expected or if it is due to pathology.

In dark-skinned people the amount of normal pigment may mask color changes. Lips and nail beds show some color change, but they vary with the person's skin color and may not always be accurate signs. The more reliable sites are those with the least pigmentation, such as under the tongue, the buccal mucosa, the palpebral conjunctiva, and the sclera. See Table 12–2 on p. 249 for specific clues to assessment.

PALLOR. When the red-pink tones from the oxygenated hemoglobin in the blood are lost, the skin takes on the color of connective tissue (collagen), which is mostly white. Pallor is common in acute high-stress states, such as anxiety or fear, due to the powerful peripheral vasoconstriction from sympathetic nervous system stimulation. The skin also looks pale with vasoconstriction from exposure to cold and cigarette smoking and in the presence of edema.

Look for pallor in dark-skinned people by the absence of the underlying red tones that normally give brown or black skin its luster. The brown-skinned individual demonstrates pallor with a more yellowish-brown color, and the black-skinned person will appear ashen or gray. Generalized pallor can be observed in the mucous membranes, lips, and nail beds. The palpebral conjunctiva and nail beds are preferred sites for assessing the pallor of anemia. When inspecting the conjunctiva, lower the lid sufficiently to visualize the conjunctiva near the *outer* canthus as well as the inner canthus. The coloration is often lighter near the inner canthus.

Ashen gray color in dark skin or marked pallor in whites occurs with anemia, shock, arterial insufficiency (see Table 12–2).

The pallor of impending shock is accompanied by other subtle manifestations, such as increasing pulse rate, oliguria, apprehension, and restlessness.

Anemias, particularly chronic iron deficiency anemia, may show "spoon" nails, with a concave shape. A lemon yellow tint of the face and slightly yellow sclera accompany pernicious anemia, also indicated by neurologic deficits and a red, painful tongue. Fatigue, exertional dyspnea, rapid pulse, dizziness, and impaired mental function accompany most severe anemias.

Erythema occurs with polycythemia, venous stasis, carbon monoxide poisoning, and the extravascular presence of red blood cells (petechiae, ecchymosis, hematoma) (see Tables 12–2 and 12–7).

ERYTHEMA. This is an intense redness of the skin due to excess blood (hyperemia) in the dilated superficial capillaries. This sign is *expected* with fever, local inflammation, or with emotional reactions such as blushing in vascular flush areas (cheeks, neck, and upper chest).

When erythema is associated with fever or localized inflammation, it is characterized by increased skin temperature due to the increased rate of blood flow through the blood vessels. Since you cannot see inflammation in dark-skinned persons, it is often necessary to palpate the skin for increased warmth, taut or tightly pulled surfaces that may be indicative of edema, and hardening of deep tissues or blood vessels.

CYANOSIS. This is a bluish mottled color that signifies decreased perfusion; the tissues are not adequately perfused with oxygenated blood. Be aware that cyanosis can be a nonspecific sign. A person who is anemic could have hypoxemia without ever looking blue because not enough hemoglobin is present (either oxygenated or reduced) to color the skin. On the other hand, a person with polycythemia (an increase in the number of red blood cells) looks ruddy blue at all times and may not necessarily be hypoxemic. This person just is unable to fully oxygenate the massive numbers of red blood cells. Lastly, do not confuse cyanosis with the common and normal bluish tone on the lips of dark-skinned persons of Mediterranean origin.

Cyanosis is difficult to observe in darkly pigmented persons (see Table 12–2). Given that most conditions causing cyanosis also cause decreased oxygenation of the brain, other clinical signs—such as changes in level of consciousness and signs of respiratory distress—will be evident.

Cyanosis indicates hypoxemia and occurs with shock, heart failure, chronic bronchitis, and congenital heart disease.

NORMAL RANGE OF FINDINGS

ABNORMAL FINDINGS

JAUNDICE. Jaundice is exhibited by a yellow color, indicating rising amounts of bilirubin in the blood. Except for physiological jaundice in the newborn (p. 241), jaundice does not occur normally. Jaundice is *first* noted in the junction of the hard and soft palate in the mouth and in the sclera. But do not confuse scleral jaundice with the normal yellow subconjunctival fatty deposits that are common in the outer sclera of dark-skinned persons. The scleral yellow of jaundice extends up to the edge of the iris.

Jaundice occurs with hepatitis, cirrhosis, sickle-cell disease, transfusion reaction, and hemolytic disease of the newborn.

As levels of serum bilirubin rise, jaundice is evident in the skin over the rest of the body. This is best assessed in direct natural daylight. Common calluses on palms and soles often look yellow—do not interpret these as jaundice.

Light or clay-colored stools and dark golden urine often accompany jaundice in both light- and dark-skinned people.

Temperature

Note the temperature of your own hands. Then use the backs (dorsa) of your hands to palpate the person and check bilaterally. The skin should be warm, and the temperature should be equal bilaterally; warmth suggests normal circulatory status. Hands and feet may be slightly cooler in a cool environment.

HYPOTHERMIA. Generalized coolness may be induced, such as in hypothermia used for surgery or high fever. Localized coolness is expected with an immobilized extremity, as when a limb is in a cast or with an intravenous infusion.

General hypothermia accompanies central circulatory disturbance, such as in shock.
Localized hypothermia occurs in peripheral arterial insufficiency and Raynaud's disease.

HYPERTHERMIA. Generalized hyperthermia occurs with an increased metabolic rate, such as in fever, or after heavy exercise. A localized area feels hyperthermic with trauma, infection, or sunburn.

Hyperthyroidism has an increased metabolic rate, causing warm, moist skin.

Moisture

Perspiration appears normally on the face, hands, axilla, and skinfolds in response to activity, a warm environment, or anxiety. **Diaphoresis,** or profuse perspiration, accompanies an increased metabolic rate, such as occurs in heavy activity or fever.

Diaphoresis occurs with thyrotoxicosis and with stimulation of the nervous system with anxiety or pain.

Look for **dehydration** in the oral mucous membranes. Normally there is none, and the mucous membranes look smooth and moist. Be aware that dark skin may normally look dry and flaky, but this does not necessarily indicate systemic dehydration.

With dehydration, mucous membranes look dry and the lips look parched and cracked. With extreme dryness the skin is fissured, resembling cracks in a dry lake bed.

Texture

Normal skin feels smooth and firm, with an even surface.

Hyperthyroidism—skin feels smoother and softer, like velvet.
Hypothyroidism—skin feels rough, dry, and flaky.

Thickness

The epidermis is uniformly thin over most of the body, although thickened callus areas are normal on palms and soles. A callus is a circumscribed overgrowth of epidermis and is an adaptation to excessive pressure from the friction of work and weight bearing.

Very thin, shiny skin (atrophic) occurs with arterial insufficiency.

NORMAL RANGE OF FINDINGS	ABNORMAL FINDINGS

Edema

Edema is fluid accumulating in the intercellular spaces; it is not present normally. To check for edema, imprint your thumbs firmly against the ankle malleolus or the tibia. Normally the skin surface stays smooth. If your pressure leaves a dent in the skin, "pitting" edema is present. Its presence is graded on a four-point scale:

1 + Mild pitting, slight indentation, no perceptible swelling of the leg
2 + Moderate pitting, indentation subsides rapidly
3 + Deep pitting, indentation remains for a short time, leg looks swollen
4 + Very deep pitting, indentation lasts a long time, leg is very swollen

This scale is somewhat subjective; outcomes vary among examiners (see further content on grading scale in Chapter 20).

Edema masks normal skin color as well as obscures pathological conditions such as jaundice or cyanosis because the fluid lies between the surface and the pigmented and vascular layers. It makes dark skin look lighter.

Edema is most evident in dependent parts of the body (feet, ankles, and sacral areas), where the skin looks puffy and tight. Edema makes the hair follicles more prominent, so you note a pig-skin or orange-peel look (called *peau d'orange*).

Unilateral edema—consider a local or peripheral cause.

Bilateral edema or edema that is generalized over the whole body *(anasarca)*—consider a central problem such as heart failure, kidney failure.

Mobility and Turgor

Pinch up a large fold of skin on the anterior chest under the clavicle (Fig. 12–5). Mobility is the skin's ease of rising, and turgor is its ability to return to place promptly when released. This reflects the elasticity of the skin.

Mobility is decreased when edema is present.

Poor turgor is evident in severe dehydration or extreme weight loss; the pinched skin recedes slowly or "tents" and stands by itself.

Scleroderma, literally "hard skin," is a chronic connective tissue disorder associated with decreased mobility (see Table 13–5).

12–5

Vascularity or Bruising

Cherry (senile) angiomas are small (1 to 5 mm), smooth, slightly raised bright red dots that commonly appear on the trunk in all adults over 30 (Fig. 12–6). They normally increase in size and number with aging and are not significant.

Any bruising (ecchymosis) should be consistent with the expected trauma of life. There are normally no venous dilatations or varicosities.

Multiple bruises at different stages of healing and excessive bruises above knees or elbows should raise concern about physical abuse (see Table 12–6).

12–6 Cherry angioma.

NORMAL RANGE OF FINDINGS

Document the presence of any tattoos (a permanent skin design from indelible pigment) on the person's chart. Advise the person that the use of tattoo needles and tattoo parlor equipment of doubtful sterility increases the risk of hepatitis C.

Lesions

If any lesions are present, note the:
1. Color.
2. Elevation: flat, raised, or pedunculated.
3. Pattern or shape: the grouping or distinctness of each lesion, for example, annular, grouped, confluent, linear. The pattern may be characteristic of a certain disease.
4. Size, in centimeters: Use a ruler to measure. Avoid household descriptions such as "quarter size" or "pea size."
5. Location and distribution on body: Is it generalized or localized to area of a specific irritant; around jewelry, watchband, around eyes?
6. Any exudate. Note its color and/or odor.

Palpate lesions. Wear a glove if you anticipate contact with blood, mucosa, any body fluid, or skin lesion. Roll a nodule between the thumb and index finger to assess depth. Gently scrape a scale to see if it comes off. Note the nature of its base or if it bleeds when the scale comes off. Note the surrounding skin temperature. However, the erythema associated with rashes is not always accompanied by noticeable increases in skin temperature.

Does the lesion blanch with pressure or stretch? Stretching the area of skin between your thumb and index finger decreases (blanches) the normal underlying red tones, thus providing more contrast and brightening the macules. Red macules from dilated blood vessels *will* blanch momentarily, whereas those from extravasated blood (petechiae) do not. Blanching also helps identify a macular rash in dark-skinned people.

Use a magnifier and light for closer inspection of the lesion (Fig. 12–7). Use a Wood's light (i.e., an ultraviolet light filtered through a special glass) to detect fluorescing lesions. With the room darkened, shine the Wood's light on the area.

12–7

POTASSIUM HYDROXIDE (KOH) PREPARATION. Microscopic examination of skin scrapings helps diagnose superficial fungal infections. Use a sharp sterile blade and lightly scrape the scale from the edge of a scaling lesion. Place on a clean slide. Add a drop of 10% to 20% potassium hydroxide (KOH) to dissolve nonfungal skin debris and send to the lab.

ABNORMAL FINDINGS

Needle marks or tracks from intravenous injection of street drugs may be visible on the antecubital fossae, forearms, or on any available vein.

Lesions are traumatic or pathological changes in previously normal structures. When a lesion develops on previously unaltered skin, it is **primary.** However, when a lesion changes over time or changes because of a factor such as scratching or infection, it is **secondary.** Study Table 12–3 for the shapes and Tables 12–4 and 12–5 for the characteristics of primary and secondary skin lesions. The terms used (*macule, papule,* etc.) are helpful to describe any lesion you encounter.

Note the pattern and characteristics of common skin lesions (see Table 12–8) and malignant skin lesions (Table 12–9), and lesions associated with AIDS (Table 12–10).

Lesions with blue-green fluorescence indicate fungal infection, such as tinea capitis (scalp ringworm).

NORMAL RANGE OF FINDINGS	ABNORMAL FINDINGS

INSPECT AND PALPATE THE HAIR

Color

Hair color comes from melanin production and may vary from pale blonde to total black. Graying begins as early as the third decade of life because of reduced melanin production in the follicles. Genetic factors affect the age of onset of graying.

Texture

Scalp hair may be fine or thick and may look straight, curly, or kinky. It should look shiny, although this characteristic may be lost with the use of some beauty products such as dyes, rinses, or permanents.

Note dull, coarse, or brittle scalp hair.

Gray, scaly, well-defined areas with broken hairs accompany tinea capitis, a ringworm infection found mostly in school-age children (see Table 12–11).

Distribution

Fine vellus hair coats the body, whereas coarser terminal hairs grow at the eyebrows, eyelashes, and scalp. During puberty, distribution conforms to normal male and female patterns. At first, coarse curly hairs develop in the pubic area, then in the axillae, and last in the facial area in boys. In the genital area the female pattern is an inverted triangle; the male pattern is an upright triangle with pubic hair extending up to the umbilicus. In Asians, body hair may be diminished.

Genital hair absent or with abnormal configuration suggests endocrine abnormalities.

Hirsutism—excess body hair. In females, this forms a male pattern of hair distribution on the face and chest and indicates endocrine abnormalities (see Table 12–11).

Lesions

Separate the hair into sections and lift it, observing the scalp. With a history of itching, inspect the hair behind the ears and in the occipital area as well. All areas should be clean and free of any lesions or pest inhabitants. Many people normally have seborrhea (dandruff), which is indicated by loose white flakes.

Head or pubic lice. Distinguish dandruff from nits (eggs) of lice, which are oval, adherent to hair shaft, and cause intense itching (see Table 12–11).

INSPECT AND PALPATE THE NAILS

Shape and Contour

The nail surface is normally slightly curved or flat, and the posterior and lateral nail folds are smooth and rounded. Nail edges are smooth, rounded, and clean, suggesting adequate self-care.

Jagged nails, bitten to the quick, or traumatized nail folds from chronic nervous picking suggest nervous habits.

Chronically dirty nails suggest poor self-care or some occupations in which it is impossible to keep them clean.

THE PROFILE SIGN. View the index finger at its profile and note the angle of the nail base; it should be about 160 degrees (Fig. 12–8). The nail base is firm to palpation. Curved nails are a variation of normal with a convex profile. They may look like clubbed nails, but notice that the angle between nail base and nail is normal, i.e., 160 degrees or less.

Clubbing of nails occurs with congenital chronic cyanotic heart disease and with emphysema and chronic bronchitis.

In early clubbing, the angle straightens out to 180 degrees and the nail base feels spongy to palpation.

Normal 160°

Curved nail 160° or less

Early clubbing 180°

12–8

NORMAL RANGE OF FINDINGS	ABNORMAL FINDINGS

Consistency

The surface is smooth and regular, not brittle or splitting.

Pits, transverse grooves, or lines may indicate a nutrient deficiency or may accompany acute illness in which nail growth is disturbed (see Table 12–12).

Nail thickness is uniform.

Nails are thickened and ridged with arterial insufficiency.

The nail is firmly adherent to the nail bed, and the nail base is firm to palpation.

A spongy nail base accompanies clubbing.

Color

The translucent nail plate is a window to the even, pink nail bed underneath.

Dark-skinned people may have brown-black pigmented areas or linear bands or streaks along the nail edge (Fig. 12–9). All people normally may have white hairline linear markings from trauma or picking at the cuticle (Fig. 12–10). Note any abnormal marking in the nail beds.

Cyanosis or marked pallor.

Brown linear streaks (especially sudden appearance) are abnormal in light-skinned people and may indicate melanoma.

Splinter hemorrhages, transverse ridges, or Beau's lines (see Table 12–12).

12–9 Linear pigmentation.

12–10 Leukonychia striata.

CAPILLARY REFILL. Depress the nail edge to blanch and then release, noting the return of color. Normally, color return is instant, or at least within a few seconds in a cold environment. This indicates the status of the peripheral circulation. A sluggish color return takes longer than 1 or 2 seconds.

Inspect the toenails. Separate the toes and note the smooth skin in between.

Cyanotic nail beds or sluggish color return: consider cardiovascular or respiratory dysfunction.

PROMOTING HEALTH AND SELF-CARE

Teach Skin Self-Examination

Teach all adults to examine their skin once a month, using the ABCDE rule (see p. 231) to raise warning signals of any suspicious lesions. Use a well-lighted room that has a full-length mirror. It helps to have a small handheld mirror. Ask a relative to search skin areas difficult to see (e.g., behind ears, back of neck, back). Follow the sequence outlined in Figure 12–11 and report any suspicious lesions promptly to a physician or nurse.

1. Undress completely. Check forearms, palms, space between fingers. Turn over hands and study the backs.

2. Face mirror; bend arms at elbow. Study arms in mirror.

3. Face mirror and study entire front of body. Start at face, neck, torso, working down to lower legs.

4. Pivot to right side facing mirror. Study sides of upper arms, working down to ankles. Repeat with left side.

5. With back to mirror, study buttocks, thighs, lower legs.

6. Use the hand-held mirror to study upper back.

7. Use the hand-held mirror to study scalp, lifting the hair. A blow-dryer on a cool setting helps to lift hair.

8. Sit on chair or bed. Study insides of each leg and soles of feet. Use the small mirror to help.

12–11 Skin self-examination.

 DEVELOPMENTAL CONSIDERATIONS

Infants

SKIN COLOR—GENERAL PIGMENTATION. Black newborns initially have lighter-toned skin than their parents because of a pigment function that is not yet in full production. Their full melanotic color is evident in the nail beds and scrotal folds. The **mongolian spot** is a common variation of hyperpigmentation in

NORMAL RANGE OF FINDINGS	ABNORMAL FINDINGS

12–12 Mongolian spot.

black, Asian, Native American, and Hispanic newborns (Fig. 12–12). It is a blue-black to purple macular area at the sacrum or buttocks, but sometimes it occurs on the abdomen, thighs, shoulders, or arms. It is due to deep dermal melanocytes. It gradually fades during the first year. By adulthood these spots are lighter but are frequently still visible. Mongolian spots are present in 90% of blacks, 80% of Asians and Native Americans, and 9% of whites. If you are unfamiliar with mongolian spots, be careful not to confuse them with bruises. Recognition of this normal variation is particularly important when dealing with children who might be erroneously identified as victims of child abuse.

Bruising is a common soft tissue injury that follows a rapid, traumatic, or breech birth.

Multiple bruises in various stages of healing, or pattern injury, suggest child abuse (see Table 12–6).

The **café au lait spot** is a large round or oval patch of light-brown pigmentation (hence, the name "coffee with milk"), which is usually present at birth (Fig. 12–13). Most often these patches are normal.

Six or more café au lait macules, each more than 1.5 cm in diameter, are diagnostic of neurofibromatosis, an inherited neurocutaneous disease.

12–13 Café au lait spot.

NORMAL RANGE OF FINDINGS   **ABNORMAL FINDINGS**

SKIN COLOR CHANGE. Three erythematous states are common variations in the neonate:

1. The newborn's skin has a beefy red flush for the first 24 hours because of vasomotor instability; then the color fades to its normal color.
2. Another finding, the **Harlequin color change,** occurs when the baby is in a side-lying position. The lower half of the body turns red and the upper half blanches with a distinct demarcation line down the midline. The cause is unknown, and its occurrence is transient.
3. Finally, **erythema toxicum** is a common rash that appears in the first 3 to 4 days of life. Sometimes called the "flea bite" rash or newborn rash, it consists of tiny, punctate, red macules and papules on the cheeks, trunk, chest, back, and buttocks (Fig. 12–14). The cause is unknown; no treatment is needed.

12–14 Erythema toxicum.

Two temporary cyanotic conditions may occur:

1. A newborn may have **acrocyanosis,** a bluish color around the lips, hands and fingernails, and feet and toenails. This may last for a few hours and disappear with warming.
2. **Cutis marmorata** is a transient mottling in the trunk and extremities in response to cooler room temperatures (Fig. 12–15). It forms a reticulated red or blue pattern over the skin.

Persistent generalized cyanosis indicates distress, such as cyanotic congenital heart disease.

Persistent or pronounced cutis marmorata occurs with Down syndrome or prematurity.

Green-brown discoloration of the skin, nails, and cord occurs with passing of meconium in utero, indicating fetal distress.

12–15 Cutis marmorata.

NORMAL RANGE OF FINDINGS

Physiological jaundice is a common variation in about half of all newborns. A yellowing of the skin, sclera, and mucous membranes develops after the 3rd or 4th day of life because of the increased numbers of red blood cells that hemolyze following birth. The hemoglobin in the red blood cells is metabolized by the liver and spleen; its pigment is converted into bilirubin.

Carotenemia also produces a yellow-orange color in light-skinned persons but no yellowing in the sclera or mucous membranes. It comes from ingesting large amounts of foods containing carotene, a vitamin A precursor. Carotene-rich foods are popular as prepared infant foods, and the absorption of carotene is enhanced by mashing, pureeing, and cooking. The color is best seen on the palms and soles, the forehead, tip of the nose and nasolabial folds, the chin, behind the ears, and over the knuckles; it fades to normal color within 2 to 6 weeks of withdrawing carotene-rich foods from the diet.

MOISTURE. The vernix caseosa is the moist, white, cream-cheese–like substance that covers part of the skin in all newborns. Perspiration is present after 1 month of age.

TEXTURE. A common variation occurring in the infant is **milia** (Fig. 12–16). Milia are tiny while papules on the cheeks, forehead, and across the nose and chin due to sebum that occludes the opening of the follicles. Tell parents not to squeeze the lesions; milia resolve spontaneously within a few weeks.

12–16 Milia.

THICKNESS. In the neonate, the epidermis is normally thin but you will also note well-defined areas of subcutaneous fat. The baby's skin dimples over joints, but there is no break in the skin. Check for any defect or break in the skin, especially over the length of the spine.

MOBILITY AND TURGOR. Test mobility and turgor over the abdomen in an infant.

ABNORMAL FINDINGS

Jaundice on the first day of life may indicate hemolytic disease. Jaundice after 2 weeks of age may indicate biliary tract obstruction.

Green-tinged vernix occurs with meconium staining.

In children, excessive sweating may accompany hypoglycemia, heart disease, or hyperthyroidism.

Lack of subcutaneous fat occurs in prematurity and malnutrition.

A red sacrococcygeal dimple occurs with a pilonidal cyst or sinus (see Table 25–1).

Poor turgor, or "tenting," indicates dehydration or malnutrition.

NORMAL RANGE OF FINDINGS

ABNORMAL FINDINGS

VASCULARITY OR BRUISING.   Some vascular markings are common birthmarks in the newborn. A **storkbite** (salmon patch) is a flat, irregularly shaped red or pink patch found on the forehead, eyelid, or upper lip, but most commonly at the back of the neck (nuchal area) (Fig. 12–17). It is present at birth and usually fades during the first year.

Port-wine stain, strawberry mark (immature hemangioma), cavernous hemangioma (see Table 12–6).

Bruising may suggest abuse (see Table 12–7).

12-17 Storkbite.

HAIR.   A newborn's skin is covered with fine downy lanugo (Fig. 12–18), especially in a preterm infant. Dark-skinned newborns have more lanugo than lighter-skinned newborns. Scalp hair may be lost in the few weeks following birth, especially at the temples and occiput. It grows back slowly.

Scaly crusted scalp occurs with seborrheic dermatitis (cradle cap [see Table 12–10]).

NAILS.   A newborn's nail beds may be blue (cyanotic) for the first few hours of life; then they turn pink.

12-18 Lanugo.

Adolescents

The increase in sebaceous gland activity creates increased oiliness and **acne.** Acne is the most common skin problem of adolescence. Almost all teens have some acne, even if it is the milder form of open comedones (blackheads) (Fig. 12–19, *A*) and closed comedones (whiteheads). Severe acne includes papules, pustules, and nodules (Fig. 12–19, *B*). Acne lesions usually appear on the face and sometimes on

NORMAL RANGE OF FINDINGS	ABNORMAL FINDINGS

the chest, back, and shoulders. Acne may appear in children as early as 7 to 8 years of age; then the lesions increase in number and severity and peak at 14 to 16 years in girls and at 16 to 19 years in boys.

12-19 **A,** Open comedones. **B,** Acne.

The Pregnant Female

Striae are jagged linear "stretch marks" of silver to pink color that appear during the second trimester on the abdomen, breasts, and sometimes thighs. They occur in one half of all pregnancies. They fade after delivery but do not disappear. Another skin change on the abdomen is the **linea nigra,** a brownish black line down the midline (see Fig. 27–3). **Chloasma** is an irregular brown patch of hyperpigmentation on the face. It may occur with pregnancy or in women taking oral contraceptive pills. Chloasma disappears after delivery or stopping the pills. **Vascular spiders** occur in two thirds of pregnancies in white women and less often in blacks. These lesions have tiny red centers with radiating branches and occur on the face, neck, upper chest, and arms.

NORMAL RANGE OF FINDINGS	ABNORMAL FINDINGS

The Aging Adult

SKIN COLOR AND PIGMENTATION. Common variations of hyperpigmentation are:

SENILE LENTIGINES. These are commonly called liver spots and are small, flat, brown macules (Fig. 12–20). These circumscribed areas are clusters of melanocytes that appear following extensive sun exposure. They appear on the forearms and dorsa of the hands. They are not malignant and require no treatment.

12–20 Lentigines.

12–21 Seborrheic keratosis.

KERATOSES. These lesions are raised, thickened areas of pigmentation that look crusted, scaly, and warty. One type, **seborrheic keratosis,** looks dark, greasy, and "stuck on" (Fig. 12–21). They develop mostly on the trunk but also on the face and hands and on unexposed as well as on sun-exposed areas. They do not become cancerous.

Another type, **actinic (senile** or **solar) keratosis,** is less common (Fig. 12–22). These lesions are red-tan scaly plaques that increase over the years to become raised and roughened. They may have a silvery-white scale adherent to the plaque. They occur on sun-exposed surfaces and are directly related to sun exposure. They are premalignant and may develop into squamous cell carcinoma.

MOISTURE. Dry skin (xerosis) is common in the aging person because of a decline in the size, number, and output of the sweat glands and sebaceous glands. The skin itches and looks flaky and loose.

TEXTURE. Common variations occurring in the aging adult are **acrochordons,** or "skin tags," which are overgrowths of normal skin that form a stalk and are polyplike (Fig. 12–23). They occur frequently on eyelids, cheeks and neck, and axillae and trunk.

12–23 Skin tags.

12–22 Actinic keratosis.

NORMAL RANGE OF FINDINGS

ABNORMAL FINDINGS

Sebaceous hyperplasia consists of raised yellow papules with a central depression. They are more common in men, occurring over the forehead, nose, or cheeks. They have a pebbly look (Fig. 12–24).

12–24 | Sebaceous hyperplasia.

THICKNESS. With aging, the skin looks as thin as parchment and the subcutaneous fat diminishes. Thinner skin is evident over the dorsa of the hands, forearms, lower legs, dorsa of feet, and over bony prominences. The skin may feel thicker over the abdomen and chest.

MOBILITY AND TURGOR. The turgor is decreased (less elasticity), and the skin recedes slowly or "tents" and stands by itself (Fig. 12–25).

12–25

HAIR. With aging, the hair growth decreases, and the amount decreases in the axillae and pubic areas. After menopause, white women may develop bristly hairs on the chin or upper lip resulting from unopposed androgens. In men, coarse terminal hairs develop in the ears, nose, and eyebrows, although the beard is unchanged. Male-pattern balding, or alopecia, is a genetic trait. It is usually a gradual receding of the anterior hairline in a symmetric W shape. In men and women, scalp hair gradually turns gray because of the decrease in melanocyte function.

NAILS. With aging, the nail growth rate decreases, and local injuries in the nail matrix may produce longitudinal ridges. The surface may be brittle or peeling and sometimes yellowed. Toenails also are thickened and may grow misshapen, almost grotesque. The thickening may be a process of aging or it may be due to chronic peripheral vascular disease.

Fungal infections are common in aging, with thickened crumbling toenails and erythematous scaling on contiguous skin surfaces.

1. **Inspect the skin:**
   Color
   General pigmentation
   Areas of hypopigmentation or
     hyperpigmentation
   Abnormal color changes
2. **Palpate the skin:**
   Temperature
   Moisture
   Texture
   Thickness
   Edema
   Mobility and turgor
   Hygiene
   Vascularity or bruising

3. **Note any lesions:**
   Color
   Shape and configuration
   Size
   Location and distribution on body
4. **Inspect and palpate the hair:**
   Texture
   Distribution
   Any scalp lesions

5. **Inspect and palpate the nails:**
   Shape and contour
   Consistency
   Color
6. **Teach skin self-examination**

See Health Promotion Guide on CD

Application and Critical Thinking

SAMPLE CHARTING

SUBJECTIVE

No history of skin disease; no present change in pigmentation or in nevi; no pruritus, bruising, rash, or lesions. On no medications. No work-related skin hazards. Uses sun block cream when outdoors.

OBJECTIVE

Skin: color tan-pink, even pigmentation, with no nevi. Warm to touch, dry, smooth, and even. Turgor good, no lesions.
   Hair: even distribution, thick texture, no lesions or pest inhabitants.
   Nails: no clubbing or deformities. Nail beds pink with prompt capillary refill.

FOCUSED ASSESSMENT: CLINICAL CASE STUDY 1*

Ethan E. is a 3-year-old white male presenting with his mother, who seeks health care because of Ethan's fever, fatigue, and rash of 3 days' duration.

SUBJECTIVE

2 weeks PTA (prior to arrival)—Ethan was playing with child who was subsequently diagnosed as having chickenpox.

   3 days PTA—mother reports fever 100° to 101° F and fatigue, irritability. That evening noted "tiny blisters" on chest and back.

   1 day PTA—blisters on chest changed to white with scab on top. New eruption of blisters on shoulders, thighs, face. Intense itching and scratching.

OBJECTIVE

Temp 38.0° C (100.4° F), P 110, R 24
   Skin: generalized vesiculopustular rash covering face, trunk, upper arms, and thighs. Small vesicles on face, pustules and red-honey–colored crusts on trunk. Otherwise skin is warm and dry, turgor good.
   Ears: tympanic membranes pearl-gray with landmarks intact. No discharge.
   Mouth and throat: mucosa dark pink, no lesions. Tonsils 1 +, no exudate. No lymphadenopathy.
   Heart: S₁, S₂ normal, not accentuated or diminished, no murmurs or extra sounds.
   Lungs: hyperresonant to percussion. Breath sounds clear, no adventitious sounds.

*Please note that space does not allow a detailed plan for each sample clinical problem in the text. Please consult the appropriate text for current treatment plans.

ASSESSMENT

Varicella
Impaired skin integrity R/T infection and scratching

FOCUSED ASSESSMENT: CLINICAL CASE STUDY 2

Myra G. is a 79-year-old white, widowed, retired college professor, in good health up until recent hospitalization following a fall.
    Problem List   1   Fractured right hip—hip pinning   11/24   11/27

SUBJECTIVE

Aching pain in left hip (nonoperative side).

OBJECTIVE

Erosion 2 × 2 cm with surrounding erythema covering L ischium. Erosion is moist, no active bleeding. Area very warm and tender to touch.

ASSESSMENT

Pressure sore, L hip
Impaired skin integrity R/T immobility and pressure
Acute pain

NURSING DIAGNOSES COMMONLY ASSOCIATED WITH SKIN, HAIR, AND NAIL DISORDERS

RELATED FACTORS (Etiology)	DEFINING CHARACTERISTICS (Symptoms and Signs)
DIAGNOSIS: Impaired Skin Integrity	
Altered	Blisters
Nutritional state	Bruising
Oxygen transport	Callus
Sensation	Chafing
Autoimmune dysfunction	Cyanosis
Decreased circulation	Disruption of
Edema	Skin surface
Effects of aging, medication	Skin layers
Infection	Dryness
Skeletal prominence	Erythema
Excretions/secretions	Induration
Allergy (drugs, foods)	Lesions
Chemical substances on skin	Necrosis
Immobility	Pallor
Insect/animal bites	Pruritus
Pressure	
Radiation	
Restraint	
Stress	
Surgery	

Continued

NURSING DIAGNOSES COMMONLY ASSOCIATED WITH SKIN, HAIR, AND NAIL DISORDERS—cont'd

RELATED FACTORS (Etiology)	DEFINING CHARACTERISTICS (Symptoms and Signs)

DIAGNOSIS: Self-Care Deficit: Bathing Hygiene

Effects of
  Aging
  Trauma
  Surgery
  Chronic illness
Muscular weakness
Fatigue
Pain
Immobility
Presence of external devices—intravenous lines, casts, traction
Visual impairment
Stiffness
Depression
Knowledge deficit
Lack of motivation
Perceptual or cognitive impairment
Confusion
Grieving
	Dirt or stains on body
	Requests help in bathing
	Body odor
	Halitosis
	Inability to wash body or body parts

DIAGNOSIS: Deficient Fluid Volume

Loss of body fluids or electrolytes
Diaphoresis
Diarrhea
Increased insensible water loss
Nausea and/or vomiting
Excessive drainage through artificial orifices or lumens, wounds, or drainage tubes
Diuretic therapy
Exposure to extreme heat
Excessive use of alcohol, enemas, or laxatives
	Concentrated urine, blood
	Decreased
	  Blood pressure
	  Skin turgor
	  Urine output
	Dry skin
	Dry mucous membranes
	Increased
	  Body temperature
	  Pulse rate
	Thirst
	Sudden weight loss

OTHER RELATED NURSING DIAGNOSES

ACTUAL	RISK/WELLNESS
Disturbed **B**ody image Deficient **K**nowledge **P**ain Chronic or situational low **S**elf-esteem Ineffective **T**hermoregulation	**Risk** Risk for Infection Risk for impaired Skin integrity Risk for Trauma **Wellness** Enhanced Health-seeking behavior R/T request for information on skin self-exam

Abnormal Findings

TABLE 12–2: Detecting Color Changes in Light and Dark Skin

ETIOLOGY	NOTE APPEARANCE	
	LIGHT SKIN	DARK SKIN
Pallor		
Anemia—decreased hematocrit Shock—decreased perfusion, vasoconstriction	Generalized pallor	Brown skin appears yellow-brown, dull; black skin appears ashen gray, dull; skin loses its healthy glow—check areas with least pigmentation, such as conjunctivae, mucous membranes
Local arterial insufficiency	Marked localized pallor, e.g., lower extremities, especially when elevated	Ashen gray, dull; cool to palpitation
Albinism—total absence of pigment melanin throughout the integument	Whitish pink	Tan, cream, white
Vitiligo—patchy depigmentation from destruction of melanocytes	Patchy milky white spots, often symmetrical bilaterally	Same
Cyanosis		
Increased amount of unoxygenated hemoglobin Central—chronic heart and lung disease cause arterial desaturation Peripheral—exposure to cold, anxiety	Dusky blue Nail beds dusky	Dark but dull, lifeless; only severe cyanosis is apparent in skin—check conjunctivae, oral mucosa, nail beds
Erythema		
Hyperemia—increased blood flow through engorged arterioles, such as in inflammation, fever, alcohol intake, blushing	Red, bright pink	Purplish tinge, but difficult to see; palpate for increased warmth with inflammation, taut skin, and hardening of deep tissues
Polycythemia—increased red blood cells, capillary stasis	Ruddy blue in face, oral mucosa, conjunctiva, hands and feet	Well concealed by pigment—check for redness in lips
Carbon monoxide poisoning	Bright cherry red in face and upper torso	Cherry red color in nail beds, lips, and oral mucosa
Venous stasis—decreased blood flow from area, engorged venules	Dusky rubor of dependent extremities; a prelude to necrosis with pressure sore	Easily masked; use palpation for warmth or edema
Jaundice		
Increased serum bilirubin, over 2 to 3 mg/100 ml due to liver inflammation or hemolytic disease, such as after severe burns, some infections	Yellow in sclera, hard palate, mucous membranes, then over skin	Check sclera for yellow near limbus; do not mistake normal yellowish fatty deposits in the periphery under the eyelids for jaundice—jaundice best noted in junction of hard and soft palate and also palms
Carotenemia—increased serum carotene from ingestion of large amounts of carotene-rich foods	Yellow-orange in forehead, palms and soles, nasolabial folds, but no yellowing in sclera or mucous membranes	Yellow-orange tinge in palms and soles
Uremia—renal failure causes retained uro-chrome pigments in the blood	Orange-green or gray overlying pallor of anemia; may also have ecchymoses and purpura	Easily masked; rely on laboratory and clinical findings

Continued

TABLE 12–2: Detecting Color Changes in Light and Dark Skin—cont'd

ETIOLOGY	NOTE APPEARANCE	
	LIGHT SKIN	DARK SKIN

Brown-Tan

Addison's disease—cortisol deficiency stimulates increased melanin production	Bronzed appearance, an "eternal tan," most apparent around nipples, perineum, genitalia, and pressure points (inner thighs, buttocks, elbow, axillae)	Easily masked; rely on lab and clinical findings
Café au lait spots—due to increased melanin pigment in basal cell layer	Tan to light brown, irregularly shaped, oval patch with well-defined borders	

TABLE 12–3: Common Shapes and Configurations of Lesions

ANNULAR, or circular, begins in center and spreads to periphery, e.g., tinea corporis or ringworm, tinea versicolor, pityriasis rosea.

CONFLUENT, lesions run together, e.g, urticaria (hives).

◀ **DISCRETE,** distinct, individual lesions that remain separate, e.g., molluscum.

TABLE 12–3: Common Shapes and Configurations of Lesions—cont'd

GROUPED, clusters of lesions, e.g., vesicles of contact dermatitis

GYRATE, twisted, coiled spiral, snakelike.

TARGET, or iris, resembles iris of eye, concentric rings of color in the lesions, e.g., erythema multiforme.

LINEAR, a scratch, streak, line, or stripe.

POLYCYCLIC, annular lesions grow together, e.g., lichen planus, psoriasis.

ZOSTERIFORM, linear arrangement along a nerve route, e.g., herpes zoster.

TABLE 12–4: Primary Skin Lesions*

Macule

Solely a color change, flat and circumscribed, of less than 1 cm. Examples: freckles, flat nevi, hypopigmentation, petechiae, measles, scarlet fever.

Patch

Macules that are larger than 1 cm. Examples: mongolian spot, vitiligo, café au lait spot, chloasma, measles rash.

Papule

Something you can feel, i.e., solid, elevated, circumscribed, less than 1 cm diameter, due to superficial thickening in the epidermis. Examples: elevated nevus (mole), lichen planus, molluscum, wart (verruca).

Plaque

Papules coalesce to form surface elevation wider than 1 cm. A plateaulike, disk-shaped lesion. Examples: psoriasis, lichen planus.

Nodule

Solid, elevated, hard or soft, larger than 1 cm. May extend deeper into dermis than papule. Examples: xanthoma, fibroma, intradermal nevi.

Tumor

Larger than a few centimeters in diameter, firm or soft, deeper into dermis; may be benign or malignant, although "tumor" implies "cancer" to most people. Examples: lipoma, hemangioma.

Wheal

Superficial, raised, transient, and erythematous; slightly irregular shape due to edema (fluid held diffusely in the tissues). Examples: mosquito bite, allergic reaction, dermographism.

*The immediate result of a specific causative factor; primary lesions develop on previously unaltered skin.

TABLE 12–4: Primary Skin Lesions—cont'd

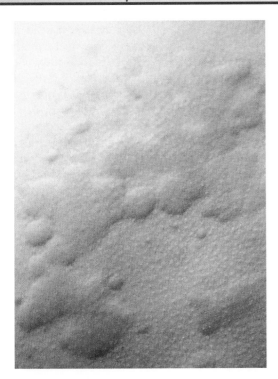

Urticaria (Hives)

Wheals coalesce to form extensive reaction, intensely pruritic.

Reprinted from Atlas of Allergies, 2nd edition, Fireman, 1995, by permission of the publisher Mosby.

Vesicle

Elevated cavity containing free fluid, up to 1 cm. Clear serum flows if wall is ruptured. Examples: herpes simplex, early varicella (chickenpox), herpes zoster (shingles), contact dermatitis.

Bulla

Larger than 1 cm diameter; usually single chambered (unilocular); superficial in epidermis; it is thin walled, so it ruptures easily. Examples: friction blister, pemphigus, burns, contact dermatitis.

Cyst

Encapsulated fluid-filled cavity in dermis or subcutaneous layer, tensely elevating skin. Examples: sebaceous cyst, wen.

Pustule

Turbid fluid (pus) in the cavity. Circumscribed and elevated. Examples: impetigo, acne.

TABLE 12–5: Secondary Skin Lesions*

DEBRIS ON SKIN SURFACE

Crust

The thickened, dried-out exudate left when vesicles/pustules burst or dry up. Color can be red-brown, honey, or yellow, depending on the fluid's ingredients (blood, serum, pus). Examples: impetigo (dry, honey-colored), weeping eczematous dermatitis, scab following abrasion.

Scale

Compact, desiccated flakes of skin, dry or greasy, silvery or white, from shedding of dead excess keratin cells. Examples: following scarlet fever or drug reaction (laminated sheets), psoriasis (silver, micalike), seborrheic dermatitis (yellow, greasy), eczema, ichthyosis (large, adherent, laminated), dry skin.

BREAK IN CONTINUITY OF SURFACE

Fissure

Linear crack with abrupt edges, extends into dermis, dry or moist. Examples: cheilosis—at corners of mouth due to excess moisture; athlete's foot.

Erosion

Scooped out but shallow depression. Superficial; epidermis lost; moist but no bleeding; heals without scar because erosion does not extend into dermis.

*Resulting from a change in a primary lesion due to the passage of time; an evolutionary change.
Note: Combinations of primary and secondary lesions may coexist in the same person. Such combined designations may be termed papulosquamous, maculopapular, vesiculopustular, or papulovesicular.

TABLE 12–5: Secondary Skin Lesions—cont'd

Ulcer

Deeper depression extending into dermis, irregular shape; may bleed; leaves scar when heals. Examples: stasis ulcer, pressure sore, chancre.

Excoriation

Self-inflicted abrasion; superficial; sometimes crusted; scratches from intense itching. Examples: insect bites, scabies, dermatitis, varicella.

Scar

After a skin lesion is repaired, normal tissue is lost and replaced with connective tissue (collagen). This is a permanent fibrotic change. Examples: healed area of surgery or injury, acne.

Atrophic Scar

Resulting skin level depressed with loss of tissue; a thinning of the epidermis. Example: striae.

Lichenification

Prolonged intense scratching eventually thickens the skin and produces tightly packed sets of papules; looks like surface of moss (or lichen).

Keloid

A hypertrophic scar. The resulting skin level is elevated by excess scar tissue, which is invasive beyond the site of original injury. May increase long after healing occurs. Looks smooth, rubbery, "clawlike," and has a higher incidence among blacks.

ABNORMAL FINDINGS

TABLE 12–6: Vascular Lesions

HEMANGIOMAS

Due to a benign proliferation of blood vessels in the dermis.

Strawberry Mark (Immature Hemangioma)

A raised bright red area with well-defined borders about 2 to 3 cm in diameter. It does not blanch with pressure. It consists of immature capillaries, is present at birth or develops in the first few months, and usually disappears by age 5 to 7. Requires no treatment, although parental and peer pressure may prompt treatment.

◄ Port-Wine Stain (Nevus Flammeus)

A large, flat macular patch covering the scalp or face, frequently along the distribution of cranial nerve V. The color is dark red, bluish, or purplish and intensifies with crying, exertion, or exposure to heat or cold. The marking consists of mature capillaries. It is present at birth and usually does not fade. The use of yellow light lasers now makes photoablation of the lesion possible, with minimal adverse effects.

Cavernous Hemangioma (Mature)

A reddish-blue, irregularly shaped, solid and spongy mass of blood vessels. It may be present at birth, may enlarge during the first 10 to 15 months, and will not involute spontaneously.

TELANGIECTASES

Due to vascular dilatation; permanently enlarged and dilated blood vessels that are visible on the skin surface. Examples are as follows.

◄ Spider or Star Angioma

A fiery red, star-shaped marking with a solid circular center. Capillary radiations extend from the central arterial body. With pressure, note a central pulsating body and blanching of extended legs. Develops on face, neck, or chest; may be associated with pregnancy, chronic liver disease, or estrogen therapy, or may be normal.

TABLE 12–6: Vascular Lesions—cont'd

◀ Venous Lake

A blue-purple dilatation of venules and capillaries in a star-shaped, linear, or flaring pattern. Pressure causes them to empty or disappear. Located on the legs near varicose veins and also on the face, lips, ears, and chest.

PURPURIC LESIONS

Due to blood flowing out of breaks in the vessels. Red blood cells and blood pigments are deposited in the tissues (extravascular). Difficult to see in dark-skinned people.

◀ Petechiae

Tiny punctate hemorrhages, less than 2 mm, round and discrete, dark red, purple, or brown in color. Due to bleeding from superficial capillaries; will not blanch. May indicate abnormal clotting factors. In dark-skinned people, petechiae are best visualized in the areas of lighter melanization, such as the abdomen, buttocks, and volar surface of the forearm. When the skin is black or very dark brown, petechiae cannot be seen in the skin. Most of the diseases that cause bleeding and microembolism formation—such as thrombocytopenia, subacute bacterial endocarditis, and other septicemias—are characterized by the presence of petechiae in the mucous membranes as well as on the skin. Thus you should inspect for petechiae in the mouth, particularly the buccal mucosa, and in the conjunctivae.

Purpura ▶

Confluent and extensive patch of petechiae and ecchymoses, flat macular hemorrhage. Seen in generalized disorders such as thrombocytopenia and scurvy. Also occurs in old age as blood leaks from capillaries in response to minor trauma and diffuses through dermis.

Table continued on following page

TABLE 12–6: Vascular Lesions—cont'd

LESIONS DUE TO TRAUMA OR ABUSE

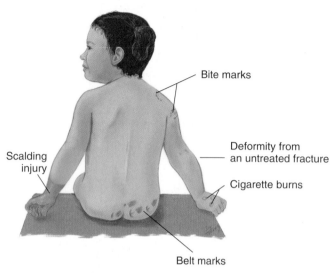

Bite marks

Deformity from an untreated fracture

Cigarette burns

Scalding injury

Belt marks

◀ Pattern Injury

Pattern injury is a bruise or wound whose shape suggests the instrument or weapon that caused it, e.g., belt buckle, broomstick, burning cigarette, pinch marks, bite marks, or scalding hot liquid. Inflicted scalding-water immersion burns usually have a clear border, like a glove or sock, indicating body part was held under water intentionally. Deformity results from an untreated fracture because the bone heals out of alignment.

These physical signs suggest child abuse, together with a history that does not match the severity or type of injury, and indicates impaired or dysfunctional parent-child relationship.

Scalp petechiae

Hematoma

Hematoma

A hematoma is a bruise you can feel. It elevates the skin and is seen as swelling. Multiple petechiae and purpura may occur on the face when prolonged vigorous crying or coughing raises venous pressure.

1
2
3
4
5

Ecchymosis (Bruise)

A large patch of capillary bleeding into tissues. Color in light-skinned person is first 1—red-blue or purple immediately after or within 24 hours of trauma and generally progresses to 2—blue to purple; 3—blue-green; 4—yellow; 5—brown to disappearing. A recent bruise in dark-skinned person is deep, dark purple. Pressure on a bruise will *not* cause it to blanch. A bruise usually occurs from trauma; also from bleeding disorders and liver dysfunction.

TABLE 12–7: Common Skin Lesions in Children

Diaper Dermatitis

Red, moist maculopapular patch with poorly defined borders in diaper area, extending along inguinal and gluteal folds. History of infrequent diaper changes or occlusive coverings. Inflammatory disease due to skin irritation from ammonia, heat, moisture, occlusive diapers.

Intertrigo (Candidiasis)

Scalding red, moist patches with sharply demarcated borders, some loose scales. Usually in genital area extending along inguinal and gluteal folds. Aggravated by urine, feces, heat, and moisture, the *Candida* fungus infects the superficial skin layers.

Impetigo

Moist, thin-roofed vesicles with thin, erythematous base. Rupture to form thick, honey-colored crusts. Contagious bacterial infection of skin; most common in infants and children.

Atopic Dermatitis (Eczema)

Erythematous papules and vesicles, with weeping, oozing, and crusts. Lesions usually on scalp, forehead, cheeks, forearms and wrists, elbows, backs of knees. Paroxysmal and severe pruritus. Family history of allergies.

Table continued on following page

TABLE 12–7: Common Skin Lesions in Children–cont'd

Measles (Rubeola) in Dark Skin

Measles (Rubeola) in Light Skin

Red-purple maculopapular blotchy rash in dark skin (on left) and in light skin (on right) appears on 3rd or 4th day of illness. Rash appears first behind ears and spreads over face, then over neck, trunk, arms, and legs; looks "coppery" and dose not blanch. Also characterized by Koplik's spots in mouth—bluish white, red-based elevations of 1 to 3 mm.

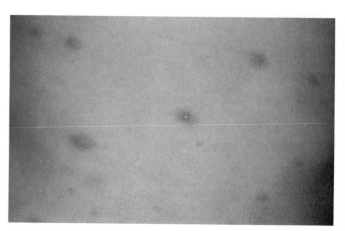

German Measles (Rubella)

Pink papular rash (similar to measles but paler) first appears on face, then spreads. Distinguished from measles by presence of neck lymphadenopathy and absence of Koplik's spots.

Chickenpox (Varicella)

Small tight vesicles first appear on trunk, then spread to face, arms, and legs (not palms or soles). Shiny vesicles on an erythematous base are commonly described as the "dewdrop on a rose petal." Vesicles erupt in succeeding crops over several days, then become pustules, and then crusts. Intensely pruritic.

TABLE 12–8: Common Skin Lesions—cont'd

Primary Contact Dermatitis

Local inflammatory reaction to an irritant in the environment or an allergy. Characteristic location of lesions often
gives clue. Often erythema shows first, followed by
swelling, wheals (or urticaria), or maculopapular vesicles,
scales. Frequently accompanied by intense pruritus.
Example here: poison ivy.

Allergic Drug Reaction

Erythematous and symmetric rash, usually generalized.
  Some drugs produce urticarial rash or vesicles and bullae.
  History of drug ingestion.

Tinea Corporis (Ringworm of the Body)

Scales—hyperpigmented in whites, depigmented in dark-
skinned persons—on chest, abdomen, back of arms
forming multiple circular lesions with clear centers.

Tinea Pedis (Ringworm of the Foot)

"Athlete's foot," a fungal infection, first appears as small vesicles between toes, sides of feet, soles. Then grows scaly and
hard. Found in chronically warm moist feet: children after
gymnasium activities, athletes, aging adults who cannot
dry their feet well.

Table continued on following page

TABLE 12–8: Common Skin Lesions—cont'd

Psoriasis

Scaly erythematous patch, with silvery scales on top. Usually on scalp, outside of elbows and knees, low back, and anogenital area.

Labial Herpes Simplex (Cold Sores)

Herpes simplex virus (HSV) infection has a prodrome of skin tingling and sensitivity. Lesion then erupts with tight vesicles followed by pustules, and then produces acute gingivostomatitis with many shallow, painful ulcers. Common location is upper lip, also in oral mucosa and tongue.

Herpes Zoster (Shingles)

Small grouped vesicles emerge along route of cutaneous sensory nerve, then pustules, then crusts. Caused by the varicella zoster virus (VZV), a reactivation of the dormant virus of chickenpox. Acute appearance, practically always unilateral, does not cross midline. Commonly on trunk, can be anywhere. If on ophthalmic branch of cranial nerve V, it poses risk to eye. Most common in adults over 50. Pain is often severe and long lasting in aging adults, called *postherpetic neuralgia.*

Tinea Versicolor

Fine, scaling, round patches of pink, tan, or white that (hence the name) do not tan in sunlight, due to a superficial fungal infection. Usual distribution is on neck, trunk, and upper arms—a short-sleeved turtleneck sweater area. Most common in otherwise healthy young adults.

Erythema Migrans of Lyme Disease

Lyme disease is not fatal, but may have serious arthritic, cardiac, or neurological sequelae. It is caused by a spirochete bacterium carried by the black or dark brown deer tick. Deer ticks are common in the Northeast, upper Midwest, and California (with cases occurring in people who spend time outdoors) in May through September. The first stage (early localized LD) has the distinctive bull's eye, red macular or papular rash (shown above) in 50% of cases. The rash radiates from the site of the tick bite (5 cm or larger), with some central clearing, and is usually located in axilla, midriff, inquina, or behind knee, with regional lymphadenopathy. Rash fades in 4 weeks; untreated individual then may have disseminated disease with fatigue, anorexia, fever, chills, joint or muscle aches. Antibiotic treatment shortens symptoms and decreases risk of sequelae.

TABLE 12–9: Malignant Skin Lesions

Basal Cell Carcinoma

Usually starts as a skin-colored papule (may be deeply pigmented) with a translucent top and overlying telangiectasia. Then develops rounded pearly borders with central red ulcer, or looks like large open pore with central yellowing. Most common form of skin cancer; slow but inexorable growth.

Squamous Cell Carcinoma

Erythematous scaly patch with sharp margins, 1 cm or more. Develops central ulcer and surrounding erythema. Usually on hands or head, areas exposed to solar radiation. Less common than basal cell carcinoma but grows rapidly.

Malignant Melanoma

Half of these lesions arise from preexisting nevi. Usually brown; can be tan, black, pink-red, purple, or mixed pigmentation. Often irregular or notched borders. May have scaling, flaking, oozing texture. Common locations are on the trunk and back in men and women, on the legs in women, and on the palms, soles of feet, and the nails in blacks.

TABLE 12–10: Skin Lesions Associated with AIDS

Epidemic Kaposi's Sarcoma: Patch Stage

An aggressive form of Kaposi's sarcoma is one of the diseases that characterize the epidemic AIDS. Here, multiple patch-stage early lesions are faint pink on the temple and beard area. They easily could be mistaken for bruises or nevi and be ignored.

Epidemic Kaposi's Sarcoma: Advanced Disease

Advanced stage, widely disseminated lesions involving skin, mucous membranes, and visceral organs. Here, violet-colored tumors over the nose and face, and a tiny cherry-red tumor nodule is on the inner canthus of the right eye.

◀ Epidemic Kaposi's Sarcoma: Plaque Stage

Evolving lesions develop into raised papules or thickened plaques. These are oval in shape and vary in color from red to brown.

TABLE 12–11: Infectious Disease as a Biological Weapon

Anthrax

Cutaneous anthrax is caused by *Bacillus anthracis* (an encapsulated, spore-forming bacteria) when it contracts a preexisting lesion or broken skin, usually on the head, neck, or extremities. After 3 days, a red, raised, pruritic papule appears, followed by a round ulcer with surrounding vesicles a few days later (forearm lesion on left). Area edema and tender lymphadenopathy are common. A tough, painless, black scab or *eschar,* forms in a few weeks (neck lesion on right), which loosens and falls off in another few weeks. Antibiotics decrease the risk of systemic disease.

◀ Smallpox (Variola Major)

Smallpox is a viral infection with no known treatment, which was declared eradicated worldwide in 1980 by the World Health Organization, and routine vaccination stopped. Disease is spread by direct contact or inhalation of respiratory droplets. After exposure and an incubation period of 10–12 days, the person develops flu-like symptoms of malaise, fever, myalgia, headache, vomiting; then a maculopapular rash appears, first on the oral mucosa, face and arms, later on the trunk. Lesions are uniform in appearance and become vesicular, then pustular and umbilicated (as opposed to chickenpox lesions that are in various stages, more superficial, and are more numerous on the trunk). In a few weeks, the lesions form crusts and drop away leaving pitted scars. The present treatment is supportive only, and mortality rate is 30–40%.

TABLE 12–12: Abnormal Conditions of Hair

Seborrheic Dermatitis (Cradle Cap)

Thick, yellow to white, greasy, adherent scales with mild erythema on scalp and forehead; very common in early infancy. Resembles eczema lesions except cradle cap is distinguished by absence of pruritus, "greasy" yellow-pink lesions, and negative family history of allergy.

Tinea Capitis (Scalp Ringworm)

Rounded patchy hair loss on scalp, leaving broken-off hairs, pustules, and scales on skin. Due to fungal infection; lesions may fluoresce blue-green under Wood's light. Usually seen in children and farmers; highly contagious, may be transmitted by another person, by domestic animals, or from soil.

Toxic Alopecia

Patchy, asymmetric balding that accompanies severe illness or use of chemotherapy where growing hairs are lost and resting hairs are spared. Regrowth occurs after illness or discontinuation of toxin.

Alopecia Areata

Sudden appearance of a sharply circumscribed, round or oval balding patch, usually with smooth, soft, hairless skin underneath. Unknown cause; when limited to a few patches, person usually has complete regrowth.

TABLE 12–12: Abnormal Conditions of Hair—cont'd

Traumatic Alopecia: Traction Alopecia

Linear or oval patch of hair loss along hair line, a part, or scattered distribution; due to trauma from hair rollers, tight braiding, tight ponytail, barrettes.

Trichotillomania

Traumatic self-induced hair loss usually due to compulsive twisting or plucking. Forms irregularly shaped patch, with broken-off, stublike hairs of varying lengths; person is never completely bald. Occurs as child rubs or twists area absently while falling asleep, reading, or watching television. In adults it can be a serious problem and is usually a sign of a personality disorder.

Pediculosis Capitis (Head Lice)

History includes intense itching of the scalp, especially the occiput. The nits (eggs) of lice are easier to see in the occipital area and around the ears, appearing as 2- to 3-mm oval translucent bodies, adherent to the hair shafts. Common among school-age children. Over-the-counter pediculicide shampoos are available; however, nit removal by daily combing of wet hair with a fine-tooth metal comb is especially important.

Folliculitis

Superficial infection of hair follicles. Multiple pustules, "whiteheads," with hair visible at center and erythematous base. Usually on arms, legs, face, and buttocks.

Table continued on following page

TABLE 12–12: Abnormal Conditions of Hair—cont'd

Hirsutism

Excess body hair in females forming a male sexual pattern (upper lip, face, chest, abdomen, arms, legs); due to endocrine or metabolic dysfunction or occasionally idiopathic.

Furuncle and Abscess

Red, swollen, hard, tender, pus-filled lesion due to acute localized bacterial (usually staphylococcal) infection; usually on back of neck, buttocks, occasionally on wrists or ankles. Furuncles are due to infected hair follicles, whereas abscesses are due to traumatic introduction of bacteria into the skin. Abscesses are usually larger and deeper than furuncles.

TABLE 12–13: Abnormal Conditions of the Nails

Paronychia

Red, swollen, tender inflammation of the nail folds. Acute paronychia is usually a bacterial infection; chronic paronychia is most often a fungal infection from a break in the cuticle in those who perform "wet" work.

Koilonychia (Spoon Nails)

Thin, depressed nails with lateral edges tilted up, forming a concave profile. May be congenital or a hereditary trait; if all nails are involved, may be due to iron deficiency anemia.

Beau's Line

Transverse furrow or groove. A depression across the nail that extends down to the nail bed. Occurs with any trauma that temporarily impairs nail formation, such as acute illness, toxic reaction, or local trauma. Dent appears first at the cuticle and moves forward as nail grows.

TABLE 12–13: Abnormal Conditions of the Nails—cont'd

Splinter Hemorrhages

Red-brown linear streaks, embolic lesions, occur with subacute bacterial endocarditis; also may occur with minor trauma.

Late Clubbing

Proximal edge of nail elevates; angle is greater than 180 degrees. Distal phalanx looks rounder and wider. Seen with chronic obstructive pulmonary disease and congenital heart disease with cyanosis. Occurs first in thumb and index finger.

Reprinted from the Clinical Slide Collection on the Rheumatic Diseases. © 1991, 1995, 1997. Used by permission of the American College of Rheumatology.

Onycholysis

This is a slow, persistent fungal infection of fingernails and, more often, toenails, common in older adults. Fungus causes change in color (green where nail plate separated from bed), texture, thickness, with nail crumbling or breaking, and loosening of the nail plate, usually beginning at the distal edge and progressing proximally.

Pitting

Sharply defined pitting and crumbling of the nails with distal detachment often occurs with psoriasis.

Habit-Tic Dystrophy

Depression down middle of nail or multiple horizontal ridges, due to continuous picking of cuticle by another finger of same hand, which causes injury to nail base and nail matrix.

BIBLIOGRAPHY

Bjorgen S: Herpes zoster, *Am J Nurs* 98(2):46–47, Feb 1998.

Bower MG: Managing dog, cat, and human bite wounds, *Nurse Pract* 26(4):36–47, Apr 2001.

Cuevas T: Identifying and treating rosacea, *Nurse Pract* 26(6)13–25, Jun 2001.

Dixon TC, Guillemin J: Anthrax, *N Engl J Med* 341(11):815–825, Sep 9, 1999.

Edmond RT, Bowl HAK, Welsby P: *Color atlas of infectious diseases,* ed 3, St Louis, 1996, Mosby.

Fell E: Update on Lyme disease and other tick-borne illnesses, *Nurse Pract* 25(10):38–57, Oct 2000.

Friedman-Kien AE: *Color atlas of AIDS,* ed 2, Philadelphia, 1996, W.B. Saunders.

Habif TP et al: *Skin disease: diagnosis and treatment,* St Louis, 2001, Mosby.

Heffernan AE, O'Sullivan A: Pediatric sun exposure, *Nurse Pract* 23(7):67–86, Jul 1998.

Henderson DA et al: Smallpox as a biological weapon, *JAMA* 281(22):2127–2137, Jun 9, 1999.

Ingelsby TV et al: Anthrax as a biological weapon, *JAMA* 281(18):1735–1745, May 12, 1999.

Leffell DJ, Brash DE: Sunlight and skin cancer, *Sci Amer* 275(1):54–59, Jul 1996.

Levin S: Effect of age, ethnic background and disease on sweat chloride, *Isr J Med Sci* 2(3):333–337, 1966.

Lindow KB: Understanding rosacea, *Am J Nurs* 101(10):44–52, Oct 2001.

Lookingbill DP, Marks JG: *Principles of dermatology,* ed 3, Philadelphia, 2000, W.B. Saunders.

Mayer BW, Burns P: Differential diagnosis of abuse injuries in infants and young children, *Nurse Pract* 25(10):15–37, Oct 2000.

Milles CL, Riley PA, Kessenich CR: Onychomycosis: diagnosis and systemic treatment, *Nurse Pract* 23(12):40–51, Dec 1998.

Nicol NH: Managing atopic dermatitis in children and adults, *Nurse Pract* 25(4):58–81, Apr 2000.

Oliviero MC: How to diagnose malignant melanoma, *Nurse Pract* 27(2):26–37, Feb 2002.

Persell DJ et al: Preparing for bioterrorism: category A agents, *Nurse Pract* 26(12):12–29, Dec 2001.

Phillips LP, Caruso ES, Paine LL: Primary care for women: comprehensive dermatologic assessment, *J Nurse Midwifery* 40(2):172–186, Mar-Apr 1995.

Polednak A: Connective tissue responses in negroes in relation to disease, *Am J Physical Anthropol* 41:49–55, 1974.

Reifsnider E: Common adult infectious skin conditions, *Nurs Pract* 22(11):17–33, Nov 1997.

Reilly CM, Deason D: Smallpox, *Am J Nurs* 102(2):51–55, Feb 2002.

Resnick B: Dermatologic problems in the elderly, *Primary Care Pract* 1(1):14–31, Mar-Apr 1997.

Santangelo J: Acute seroconversion of HIV infection in the ambulatory care setting, *Nurse Pract* 26(4):48–56, Apr 2001.

Schaefer O: Regional sweating in Eskimos compared with Caucasians, *Can J Physiol Pharmacol* 52(5):960–965, 1974.

Simmerman JM: Advances in DNA vaccines, *Nurse Pract* 27(1):53–61, Jan 2002.

Sinni-McKeehen B: Scaling skin disorders, *Primary Care Pract* 1(1):3–13, Mar-Apr 1997.

Starr C: Anthrax: know the guidelines for management, *Am J Nurs* 101(12):48–51, Dec 2001.

Sugar NF, Taylor JA, Feldman KW: Bruises in infants and toddlers, *Arch Pediatr Adolesc Med* 153:399–403, Apr 1999.

Sullivan JR, Shear NH: Drug eruptions and other adverse drug effects in aged skin, *Clin Geriatr Med* 18(1):21–42, Feb 2002.

Taffe AM: Acne treatment: a comprehensive review of pharmacotherapy, *Lippincotts Primary Care Pract* 1(1):70–87, Mar-Apr 1997.

Talbot L, Curtis L: The challenges of assessing skin indicators in people of color, *Home Healthc Nurse* 14(3):167–171, 1996.

Turnbull R: Skin assessment in children: a methodical approach, *Nurs Times* 96(41):33–34, 2000.

U.S. Preventive Services Task Force: Screening for skin cancer: recommendations and rationale, *Am J Nurs* 102(5):97–101, 2002.

Head and Neck, Including Regional Lymphatics

http://evolve.elsevier.com/Jarvis/

Structure and Function

THE HEAD

The **skull** is a rigid bony box that protects the brain and special sense organs, and it includes the bones of the cranium and the face (Fig. 13–1). Note the location of these **cranial bones:** frontal, parietal, occipital, and temporal. Use these names to describe any of your findings in the corresponding areas.

The adjacent cranial bones unite at meshed immovable joints called the **sutures.** The bones are not firmly joined at birth; this allows for the mobility and change in shape needed for the birth process. The sutures gradually ossify during early childhood. The **coronal** suture *crowns* the head from ear to ear at the union of the frontal and parietal bones. The **sagittal** suture *separates* the head lengthwise between the two parietal bones. The **lambdoid** suture separates the parietal bones crosswise from the occipital bone.

The 14 **facial bones** also articulate at sutures (note the nasal bone, zygomatic bone, and maxilla), except for the mandible (the lower jaw). It moves up, down, and sideways from the temporomandibular joint, which is anterior to each ear.

The cranium is supported by the cervical vertebra: C1, the "atlas"; C2, the "axis"; and down to C7. The C7 vertebra has a long spinous process that is palpable when the head is flexed. Feel this useful landmark, the **vertebra prominens,** on your own neck.

The human **face** has myriad appearances and a large array of facial expressions that reflect mood. The expressions are formed by the facial muscles (Fig. 13–2), which are mediated by cranial nerve VII, the facial nerve. Facial muscle function is symmetric bilaterally, except for an occasional quirk or wry expression.

Facial structures also are symmetric; the eyebrows, eyes, ears, nose, and mouth appear about the same on both sides. The palpebral fissures—the openings between the eyelids—are equal bilaterally. Also, the nasolabial folds, the creases extending from the nose to each corner of the mouth, should look symmetric. Facial sensations of pain or touch are mediated by the three sensory branches of cranial nerve V, the trigeminal nerve. (Testing for sensory function is described in Chapter 23, Neurological System.)

Two pairs of **salivary glands** are accessible to examination on the face (Fig. 13–3). The **parotid** glands are in the cheeks over the mandible, anterior to and below the ear. They are the largest of the salivary glands but are not normally palpable. The **submandibular** glands are beneath the mandible at the angle of the jaw. A third pair, the **sublingual** glands, lie in the floor of the mouth. (Salivary gland function follows in Chapter 16.) The **temporal artery** lies superior to the temporalis muscle, and its pulsation is palpable anterior to the ear.

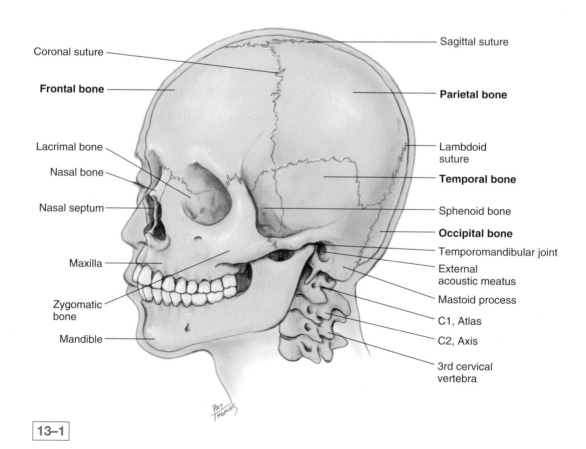

Coronal suture

Frontal bone

Lacrimal bone

Nasal bone

Nasal septum

Maxilla

Zygomatic bone

Mandible

Sagittal suture

Parietal bone

Lambdoid suture

Temporal bone

Sphenoid bone

Occipital bone

Temporomandibular joint

External acoustic meatus

Mastoid process

C1, Atlas

C2, Axis

3rd cervical vertebra

13–1

Frontalis

Orbicularis oculi

Palpebral fissure

Nasolabial fold

Orbicularis oris

Galea aponeurotica

Temporalis

Zygomaticus

Masseter

Buccinator

Sternocleidomastoid

Trapezius

13–2 Facial muscles.

Sternomastoid muscle

Internal jugular vein

External jugular vein

Clavicle

Temporal artery

Parotid gland

Submandibular gland

Sublingual gland

External carotid artery

Internal carotid artery

Common carotid artery

13-3

Sternomastoid muscle
Trapezius muscle
Omohyoid muscle
Clavicle
Anterior triangle
Posterior triangle

13–4

THE NECK

The **neck** is delimited by the base of the skull and inferior border of the mandible above, and by the manubrium sterni, the clavicle, the first rib, and the first thoracic vertebra below. Think of the neck as a *conduit* for the passage of many structures, which are lying in close proximity: vessels, muscles, nerves, lymphatics, and viscera of the respiratory and digestive systems. Blood vessels include the common and internal carotid arteries and their associated veins. The internal carotid branches off the common carotid and runs inward and upward to supply the brain; the external carotid supplies the face, salivary glands, and superficial temporal area. The carotid artery and internal jugular vein lie beneath the sternomastoid muscle. The external

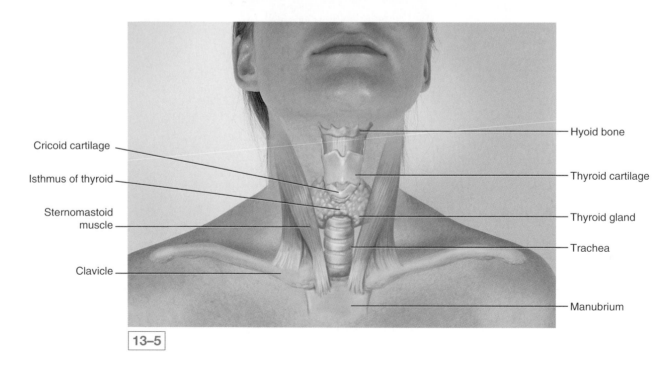

Cricoid cartilage
Isthmus of thyroid
Sternomastoid muscle
Clavicle
Hyoid bone
Thyroid cartilage
Thyroid gland
Trachea
Manubrium

13–5

jugular vein runs diagonally across the sternomastoid muscle. (Assessment of the neck vessels is discussed in Chapter 19.)

The major **neck muscles** are the **sternomastoid** and the **trapezius** (Fig. 13–4); they are innervated by cranial nerve XI, the spinal accessory. The sternomastoid muscle arises from the sternum and the medial part of the clavicle and extends diagonally across the neck to the mastoid process behind the ear. It accomplishes head rotation and head flexion. The two trapezius muscles form a trapezoid shape on the upper back. Each arises from the occipital bone and the vertebrae and extends fanning out to the scapula and clavicle. The trapezius muscles move the shoulders and extend and turn the head.

The sternomastoid muscle divides each side of the neck into two triangles. The **anterior triangle** lies in front, between the sternomastoid and the midline of the body, with its base up along the lower border of the mandible and its apex down at the suprasternal notch. The **posterior triangle** is behind the sternomastoid muscle, with the trapezius muscle on the other side and with its base along the clavicle below. It contains the posterior belly of the omohyoid muscle. These triangles are helpful guidelines when describing findings in the neck.

The **thyroid gland** is an important endocrine gland with a rich blood supply. It straddles the trachea in the middle of the neck (Fig. 13–5). This highly vascular endocrine gland synthesizes and secretes thyroxine (T_4) and triiodothyronine (T_3), hormones that stimulate the rate of cellular metabolism. The gland has two lobes, both conical in shape, each curving posteriorly between the trachea and the sternomastoid muscle. The lobes are connected in the middle by a thin isthmus lying over the second and third tracheal rings. (Sometimes a third lobe, the pyramidal lobe, is present. It is cone shaped, usually on the left, and extends up toward the hyoid bone from the isthmus or from the neighboring lobe.)

Just above the thyroid isthmus, within about 1 cm, is the **cricoid** cartilage or upper tracheal ring. The **thyroid** cartilage is above that, with a small palpable notch in its upper edge. This is the prominent "Adam's apple" in males. The highest is the **hyoid** bone, palpated high in the neck at the level of the floor of the mouth.

LYMPHATICS

The head and neck have a rich supply of **lymph nodes** (Fig. 13–6). Although sources differ as to their nomenclature, one commonly used system is given here. Note that their labels correspond to adjacent structures.

- *Preauricular,* in front of the ear
- *Posterior auricular* (mastoid), superficial to the mastoid process
- *Occipital,* at the base of the skull
- *Submental,* midline, behind the tip of the mandible
- *Submandibular,* halfway between the angle and the tip of the mandible
- *Jugulodigastric,* under the angle of the mandible
- *Superficial cervical,* overlying the sternomastoid muscle
- *Deep cervical,* deep under the sternomastoid muscle
- *Posterior cervical,* in the posterior triangle along the edge of the trapezius muscle
- *Supraclavicular,* just above and behind the clavicle, at the sternomastoid muscle

Posterior auricular
Occipital
Jugulodigastric
Superficial cervical
Posterior cervical
Supraclavicular
Preauricular
Submandibular
Submental
Deep cervical chain

13–6

13-7

You also should be familiar with the direction of the drainage patterns of the lymph nodes (Fig. 13–7). When nodes are abnormal, check the area they drain for the source of the problem. Explore the area proximal (upstream) to the location of the abnormal node.

The lymphatic system is an extensive vessel system, which is separate from the cardiovascular system and is phylogenetically older. It is described in full in Chapter 20. The lymphatics are a major part of the immune system, whose job it is to detect and eliminate foreign substances from the body. The vessels allow the flow of clear, watery fluid (lymph) from the tissue spaces into the circulation. Lymph nodes are small, oval clusters of lymphatic tissue that are set at intervals along the lymph vessels like beads on a string. The nodes filter the

lymph and engulf pathogens, preventing potentially harmful substances from entering the circulation. Nodes are located throughout the body but are accessible to examination only in four areas: head and neck, arms, axillae, and inguinal region. The greatest supply is in the head and neck.

DEVELOPMENTAL CONSIDERATIONS

INFANTS AND CHILDREN

The bones of the neonatal skull are separated by sutures and by **fontanels,** the spaces where the sutures intersect (Fig. 13–8). These membrane-covered "soft spots" allow for growth of the brain during the 1st year. They gradually ossify; the triangle-

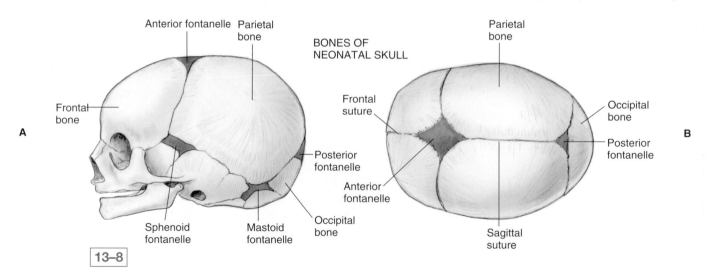

BONES OF NEONATAL SKULL

Anterior fontanelle Parietal bone Frontal bone Sphenoid fontanelle Mastoid fontanelle Posterior fontanelle Occipital bone

Parietal bone Frontal suture Anterior fontanelle Occipital bone Posterior fontanelle Sagittal suture

A B

13-8

shaped posterior fontanel is closed by 1 to 2 months, and the diamond-shaped anterior fontanel closes between 9 months and 2 years.

During the fetal period, head growth predominates. Head size is greater than chest circumference at birth. The head size grows during childhood, reaching 90% of its final size when the child is 6 years old. But during infancy, trunk growth predominates so that head size changes in proportion to body height. Facial bones grow at varying rates, especially nasal and jaw bones. In the toddler the mandible and maxilla are small and the nasal bridge is low, so that the whole face seems small compared with the skull.

Lymphoid tissue is well developed at birth and grows to adult size when the child is 6 years old. The child's lymphatic tissue continues to grow rapidly until age 10 or 11, actually exceeding its adult size before puberty. Then the lymphatic tissue slowly atrophies.

The appearance of acne in adolescence was discussed in the previous chapter. Facial hair also appears on boys at this time—first on the upper lip, then on cheeks and lower lip, and last on the chin. A noticeable enlargement of the thyroid cartilage occurs, and with it, the voice deepens.

THE PREGNANT FEMALE

The thyroid gland enlarges slightly during pregnancy due to hyperplasia of the tissue and increased vascularity.

THE AGING ADULT

The facial bones and orbits appear more prominent, and the facial skin sags due to decreased elasticity, decreased subcutaneous fat, and decreased moisture in the skin. The lower face may look smaller if teeth have been lost.

Subjective Data

1. Headache	3. Dizziness	5. Lumps or swelling
2. Head injury	4. Neck pain, limitation of motion	6. History of head or neck surgery

EXAMINER ASKS	RATIONALE
1. Headache. Any *unusually frequent* or *unusually severe* **headaches?** • Onset. When did *this kind* of headache start? • Gradual, over hours, or a day? • Or, suddenly, over minutes, or less than 1 hour? • Ever had *this kind* of headache before? • Location. Where do you feel it: frontal, temporal, behind your eyes, like a band around the head, in the sinus area, or in the occipital area? • Is pain localized on one side, or all over? • Character. Throbbing (pounding, shooting) or aching (viselike, constant pressure, dull)? • Is it mild, moderate, or severe? • Course and duration. What time of day do the headaches occur: morning, evening, awaken you from sleep? How long do they last? Hours, days? Have you noted any daily headaches, or several within a time period?	This is a more meaningful question than "Do you ever have headaches?" because most people have had at least one headache. Since many conditions have a headache as a symptom, a detailed history is important. A red flag is a severe headache in an adult or child who has never had it before. Tension headaches tend to be occipital or frontal or with bandlike tightness; migraines (vascular) tend to be supraorbital, retroorbital, or frontotemporal; cluster headaches (vascular) produce pain around the eye, temple, forehead, and cheek. Unilateral or bilateral, e.g., with cluster headaches pain is always unilateral and always on the same side of the head. Character is typically viselike with tension headache, throbbing with migraine or temporal arteritis. Quantity is often severe with migraine, or excruciating with cluster headache. Migraines occur about two per month, each lasting 1 to 3 days; one to two cluster headaches occur per day, each lasting $1/2$ to 2 hours for 1 or 2 months; then complete remission may last for months or years.

EXAMINER ASKS	RATIONALE

EXAMINER ASKS

- Precipitating factors. What brings it on: activity or exercise, work environment, emotional upset, anxiety, alcohol? (Also note signs of depression.)

- Associated factors. Any relation to other symptoms: any nausea and vomiting? (Note which came first, headache or nausea.) Any vision changes, pain with bright lights, neck pain or stiffness, fever, weakness, moodiness, stomach problems?

- Do you have any other illness?

- Do you take any medications?

- What makes it worse: movement, coughing, straining, exercise?
- Pattern. Any family history of headache?
  What is the frequency of your headaches: once a week? Are your headaches occurring closer together?
  Are they getting worse? Or are they getting better?
  (For females) When do they occur in relation to your menstrual periods?
- Effort to treat. What seems to help: going to sleep, medications, positions, rubbing the area?

- Coping strategies. How have these headaches affected your self-care, or your ability to function at work, home, and socially?

2. Head injury. Any **head injury** or blow to your head?
- Onset. When? Please describe exactly what happened.
- Setting: any hazardous conditions? Were you wearing a helmet or hard hat?
- How about yourself just before injury: dizzy, lightheaded, had a blackout, had a seizure?
  Lose consciousness and then fall? (Note which came first.)
  Knocked unconscious? Or did you fall and lose consciousness a few minutes later?
- Any history of illness, e.g., heart trouble, diabetes, epilepsy?
- Location. Exactly where did you hit your head?
- Duration. How long were you unconscious?
  Any symptoms afterward—headache, vomiting, projectile vomiting?
  Any change in level of consciousness since injury: dazed or sleepy?

- Associated symptoms. Any pain in the head or the neck, vision change, discharge from ear or nose—is it bloody or watery? Are you able to move all extremities? Any tremors, staggered walk, numbness and tingling?
- Pattern. Symptoms become worse, better, unchanged since injury?
- Effort to treat. Emergency department or hospitalized? Any medications?

RATIONALE

Alcohol ingestion and daytime napping typically precipitate cluster headaches, whereas alcohol, letdown after stress, menstruation, and eating chocolate or cheese precipitate migraines.

Nausea, vomiting, and visual disturbances are associated with migraines; eye reddening and tearing, eyelid drooping, rhinorrhea, and nasal congestion are associated with cluster headaches; anxiety and stress are associated with tension headaches; nuchal rigidity and fever are associated with the headache of meningitis or encephalitis.

Hypertension, fever, hypothyroidism, and vasculitis produce headaches.

Oral contraceptives, bronchodilators, alcohol, nitrates, as well as carbon monoxide inhalation, produce headaches.

Migraines are associated with family history of migraine.

With migraines, people lie down to feel better, whereas with cluster headaches they need to move—even to pace the floor—to feel better.

Loss of consciousness *before* a fall may have a cardiovascular cause, e.g., heart block.

A change in level of consciousness is of prime importance in evaluating a neurologic deficit.

EXAMINER ASKS	RATIONALE
3. Dizziness. Experienced any **dizziness?** (Determine exactly what the person means by dizziness.) Was it a feeling of lightheadedness or of falling? Or was it a spinning sensation?	Dizziness is a lightheaded, swimming sensation or a feeling of falling. True *vertigo* is true rotational spinning due to neurologic dysfunction (labyrinthine-vestibular apparatus, vestibular nuclei in brain stem). When vertigo is *objective*, the perception is that the room spins. When vertigo is *subjective*, the perception is that the person spins.
• Onset. Abrupt or gradual? After a change in position, such as sudden standing? • Associated factors. Any nausea and vomiting, pallor, immobility, decreased hearing acuity, or tinnitus along with the dizziness?	
4. Neck Pain. Any **neck pain?** • Onset. How did the pain start: injury, automobile accident, after lifting, from a fall? Or with fever? Or did it have a gradual onset?	Acute onset of stiffness along with headache and fever occurs with meningeal inflammation.
• Location. Does pain radiate? To the shoulders, arms? • Associated symptoms. Any **limitations to range of motion,** numbness or tingling in shoulders, arms, or hands? • Precipitating factors. What movements cause pain? Do you need to lift or bend at work or home? Does stress seem to bring it on?	Pain creates a vicious circle. Tension increases pain and disability, which produces more anxiety.
• Coping strategies. Able to do your work, to sleep?	
5. Lumps or swelling. Any **lumps or swelling** in the neck? Any recent infection? Any tenderness? For a lump that persists, how long have you had it? Has it changed in size?	Tenderness suggests acute infection. A persistent lump arouses suspicion of malignancy. For those over 40 years, suspect malignancy until proven otherwise.
• Any history of prior irradiation of head, neck, upper chest?	Increased risk for salivary and thyroid tumors.

• Any difficulty swallowing?
• Do you smoke? For how long? How many packs a day? Do you chew tobacco?
• When was your last alcohol drink? How much alcohol do you drink a day?
	Dysphagia.
	    Smoking and chewing tobacco increase risk of oral and respiratory cancer.
	    Smoking and large alcohol consumption together increase the risk of cancer.

• Ever had a thyroid problem? Overfunctioning or underfunctioning? How was it treated: surgery, irradiation, any medication?	
6. History of head or neck surgery. Ever had surgery of the head or neck? For what condition? When did the surgery occur? How do you feel about results?	Surgery for head and neck cancer often is disfiguring and increases risk of body image disturbance.

Additional History for Infants and Children

1. Did the mother use alcohol or street drugs during pregnancy? How often? How much was used per episode?	Alcohol increases the risk of fetal alcohol syndrome, which has distinctive facial features (see Table 13–3). Cocaine use causes neurological, developmental, and emotional problems.

EXAMINER ASKS	RATIONALE
2. Was delivery vaginal or by cesarean section? Any difficulty? Use of forceps?	Forceps may increase the risk of caput succedaneum, cephalhematoma, and Bell's palsy.
3. What were you told about the baby's growth? Was it on schedule? Did the head seem to grow and fontanels close on schedule? At what age (in months) did the baby achieve head control?	

Additional History for the Aging Adult

1. If dizziness is a problem, how does this affect your daily activities? Are you able to drive safely, maneuver about the house safely?

Assess self-care. Assess potential for injury.

2. If neck pain is a problem, how does this affect your daily activities? Are you able to drive, perform at work, do housework, sleep, look down when using stairs?

Objective Data

NORMAL RANGE OF FINDINGS	ABNORMAL FINDINGS

THE HEAD

INSPECT AND PALPATE THE SKULL

Size and Shape

Note the general size and shape. *Normocephalic* is the term that denotes a round symmetric skull that is appropriately related to body size. Be aware that "normal" includes a wide range of sizes.

Deformities: microcephaly, abnormally small head; macrocephaly, abnormally large head (hydrocephaly, acromegaly, Paget's disease), see Table 13–1, p. 291.

To assess shape, place your fingers in the person's hair and palpate the scalp. The skull normally feels symmetric and smooth. The cranial bones that have normal protrusions are the forehead, the lateral edge of each parietal bone, the occipital bone, and the mastoid process behind each ear. There is no tenderness to palpation.

Note lumps, depressions, or abnormal protrusions.

Temporal Area

Palpate the temporal artery above the zygomatic (cheek) bone between the eye and top of the ear.

The artery looks more tortuous and feels hardened and tender with temporal arteritis.

The temporomandibular joint is just below the temporal artery and anterior to the tragus. Palpate the joint as the person opens the mouth, and note normally smooth movement with no limitation or tenderness.

Crepitation, limited range of motion, or tenderness.

INSPECT THE FACE

Facial Structures

Inspect the face, noting the facial expression and its appropriateness to behavior or reported mood. Anxiety is common in the hospitalized or ill person.

Hostility or embarrassment.
Tense, rigid muscles may indicate anxiety or pain; a flat affect may indicate depression; excessive smiling may be inappropriate.

Although the shape of facial structures may vary somewhat among races, they always should be symmetric. Note symmetry of eyebrows, palpebral fissures, nasolabial folds, and sides of the mouth.

Marked asymmetry with central brain lesion (e.g., brain attack) or with peripheral cranial nerve VII damage (Bell's palsy). See Table 13–5.

NORMAL RANGE OF FINDINGS	ABNORMAL FINDINGS

Note any abnormal facial structures (coarse facial features, exophthalmos, changes in skin color or pigmentation), or any abnormal swelling. Also note any involuntary movements (tics) in the facial muscles. Normally none occur.

Edema in the face occurs first around the eyes (periorbital) and the cheeks where the subcutaneous tissue is relatively loose.

Note grinding of jaws, tics, fasciculations, or excessive blinking.

THE NECK

INSPECT AND PALPATE THE NECK

Symmetry

Head position is centered in the midline, and the accessory neck muscles should be symmetrical. The head should be held erect and still.

Head tilt occurs with muscle spasm. Rigid head and neck occur with arthritis.

Range of Motion (ROM)

Note any limitation of movement during active motion. Ask the person to touch the chin to the chest, turn the head to the right and left, try to touch each ear to the shoulder (without elevating shoulders), and to extend the head backward. When the neck is supple, motion is smooth and controlled.

Note pain at any particular movement.

Note ratchety or limited movement due to cervical arthritis or inflammation of neck muscles. With arthritis, the neck is rigid and the person turns at the shoulders rather than the neck.

Test muscle strength and the status of cranial nerve XI by trying to resist the person's movements with your hands as the person shrugs the shoulders and turns the head to each side.

As the person moves the head, note enlargement of the salivary glands and lymph glands. Normally no enlargement is present. Note a swollen parotid gland when the head is extended; look for swelling below the angle of the jaw. Also, note thyroid gland enlargement. Normally none is present.

Thyroid enlargement may be a unilateral lump, or it may be diffuse and look like a doughnut lying across the lower neck (see Table 13–2).

Also note any obvious pulsations. The carotid artery runs medial to the sternomastoid muscle, and it creates a brisk localized pulsation just below the angle of the jaw. Normally, there are no other pulsations while the person is in the sitting position (see Chapter 19, Heart and Neck Vessels).

Lymph Nodes

Using a gentle circular motion of your fingerpads, palpate the lymph nodes (Fig. 13–9). (Normally, the salivary glands are not palpable. When symptoms warrant, check for parotid tenderness by palpating in a line from the outer corner of the eye to the lobule of the ear.) Beginning with the preauricular lymph nodes in front of the ear, palpate the 10 groups of lymph nodes in a routine order. Many nodes are closely packed, so you must be systematic and thorough in your examination. Once you establish your sequence, do not vary or you may miss some small nodes.

The parotid is swollen with mumps (see Table 13–2).

Parotid enlargement has been found with AIDS.

13–9

NORMAL RANGE OF FINDINGS

Use gentle pressure because strong pressure could push the nodes into the neck muscles. It is usually most efficient to palpate with both hands, comparing the two sides symmetrically. However, the submental gland under the tip of the chin is easier to explore with one hand. When you palpate with one hand, use your other hand to position the person's head. For the deep cervical chain, tip the person's head toward the side being examined to relax the ipsilateral muscle (Fig. 13–10). Then you can press your fingers under the muscle. Search for the supraclavicular node by having the person hunch the shoulders and elbows forward (Fig. 13–11); this relaxes the skin. The inferior belly of the omohyoid muscle crosses the posterior triangle here; do not mistake it for a lymph node.

13–10

13–11

If any nodes are palpable, note their location, size, shape, delimitation (discrete or matted together), mobility, consistency, and tenderness. Cervical nodes often are palpable in healthy persons, although this palpability decreases with age (Fig. 13–12). Normal nodes feel movable, discrete, soft, and nontender.

Lymphadenopathy is enlargement of the lymph nodes (>1 cm) due to infection, allergy, or neoplasm.

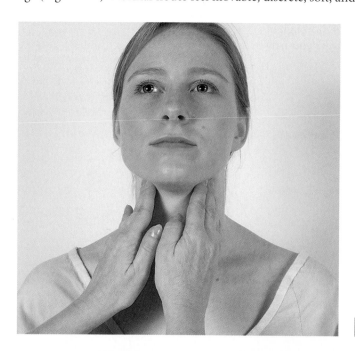

13–12

NORMAL RANGE OF FINDINGS

If nodes are enlarged or tender, check the area they drain for the source of the problem. For example, those in the upper cervical or submandibular area often relate to inflammation or a neoplasm in the head and neck. Follow up on or refer your findings. An enlarged lymph node, particularly when you cannot find the source of the problem, deserves prompt attention.

Trachea

Normally, the trachea is midline; palpate for any tracheal shift. Place your index finger on the trachea in the sternal notch, and slip it off to each side (Fig. 13–13). The space should be symmetric on both sides. Note any deviation from the midline.

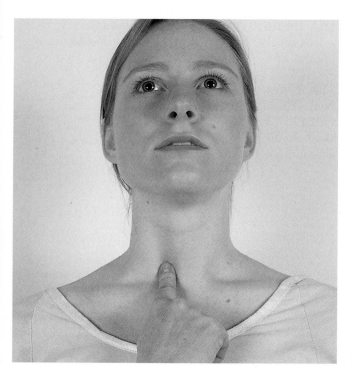

13–13

Thyroid Gland

The thyroid gland is difficult to palpate; arrange your setting to maximize your likelihood of success. Position a standing lamp to shine tangentially across the neck to highlight any possible swelling. Supply the person with a glass of water, and first inspect the neck as the person takes a sip and swallows. Thyroid tissue moves up with a swallow.

ABNORMAL FINDINGS

The following criteria are common clues but are not definitive in all circumstances.

- Acute infection—nodes are bilateral, enlarged, warm, tender, and firm but freely movable.
- Chronic inflammation; e.g., in tuberculosis the nodes are clumped.
- Cancerous nodes are hard, unilateral, nontender, and fixed.
- Nodes with HIV infection are enlarged, firm, nontender, and mobile. Occipital node enlargement is common with HIV infection.
- A single, enlarged, nontender, hard, left supraclavicular node (Virchow's node) may indicate neoplasm in thorax or abdomen.
- Painless, rubbery, discrete nodes that gradually appear occur with Hodgkin's lymphoma.

Conditions of tracheal shift:
- The trachea is *pushed to the unaffected* (or healthy) side with an aortic aneurysm, a tumor, unilateral thyroid lobe enlargement, and pneumothorax.
- The trachea is *pulled toward the affected* (diseased) side with large atelectasis, pleural adhesions, or fibrosis.
- Tracheal tug is a rhythmic downward pull that is synchronous with systole and that occurs with aortic arch aneurysm.

Look for diffuse enlargement or a nodular lump.

NORMAL RANGE OF FINDINGS	ABNORMAL FINDINGS

POSTERIOR APPROACH. To palpate, move behind the person (Fig. 13–14). Ask the person to sit up very straight and then to bend the head slightly forward and to the right. This will relax the neck muscles. Use the fingers of your left hand to push the trachea slightly to the right.

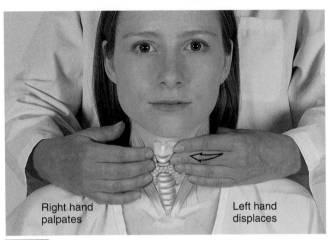

Right hand palpates

Left hand displaces

13–14

Then curve your right fingers between the trachea and the sternomastoid muscle, retracting it slightly, and ask the person to take a sip of water. The thyroid moves up under your fingers with the trachea and larynx as the person swallows. Reverse the procedure for the left side.

Usually you cannot palpate the normal adult thyroid. If the person has a long, thin neck, you sometimes will feel the isthmus over the tracheal rings. The lateral lobes usually are not palpable; check them for enlargement, consistency, symmetry, and the presence of nodules.

Abnormalities: enlarged lobes that are easily palpated before swallowing, or are tender to palpation; or the presence of nodules or lumps. See Table 13–2.

ANTERIOR APPROACH. This is an alternate method of palpating the thyroid, but it is more awkward to perform, especially for a beginning examiner. Stand facing the person. Ask him or her to tip the head forward and to the right. Use your right thumb to displace the trachea slightly to the person's right. Hook your left thumb and fingers around the sternomastoid muscle. Feel for lobe enlargement as the person swallows (Fig. 13–15).

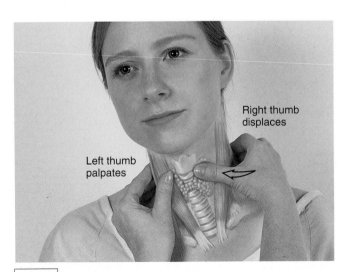

Right thumb displaces

Left thumb palpates

13–15

NORMAL RANGE OF FINDINGS	ABNORMAL FINDINGS

NORMAL RANGE OF FINDINGS

Auscultate the Thyroid

If the thyroid gland is enlarged, auscultate it for the presence of a **bruit.** This is a soft, pulsatile, whooshing, blowing sound heard best with the bell of the stethoscope. The bruit is not present normally.

 DEVELOPMENTAL CONSIDERATIONS

Infants and Children

SKULL

Measure an infant's **head size** with measuring tape at each visit up to age 2, then yearly up to age 6. (Measurement of head circumference is presented in detail in Chapter 10.)

The newborn's head measures about 32 to 38 cm (average around 34 cm), and is 2 cm larger than chest circumference. At age 2, both measurements are the same. During childhood the chest circumference grows to exceed head circumference by 5 to 7 cm.

Observe the infant's head from all angles, not just the front. The contour should be symmetric. Some racial variation occurs in normal head shapes; Nordic children tend to have long heads, and Asian children have broad heads.

Two common variations in the newborn cause the shape of the skull to look markedly asymmetric: A **caput succedaneum** is edematous swelling and ecchymosis of the presenting part of the head due to birth trauma (Fig. 13–16). It feels soft, and it may extend across suture lines. It gradually resolves during the first few days of life and needs no treatment.

ABNORMAL FINDINGS

A bruit occurs with accelerated or turbulent blood flow, indicating hyperplasia of the thyroid, e.g., hyperthyroidism.

Note an abnormal increase in head size or failure to grow.

Microcephalic—head circumference below norms for age.

Macrocephalic—an enlarged head for age, or rapidly increasing in size e.g., hydrocephalus (increased cerebrospinal fluid).

Frontal bulges, or "bossing," occur with prematurity, rickets.

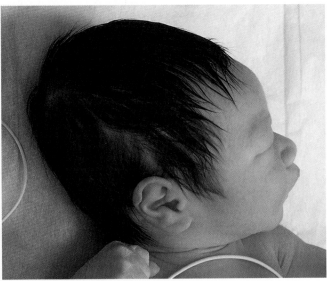

| 13–16 | Caput succedaneum.

NORMAL RANGE OF FINDINGS

ABNORMAL FINDINGS

A **cephalhematoma** is a subperiosteal hemorrhage, which is also a result of birth trauma (Fig. 13–17). It is soft, fluctuant, and well defined over one cranial bone because the periosteum (i.e., the covering over each bone) holds the bleeding in place. It appears several hours after birth and gradually increases in size. No discoloration is present, but it looks bizarre, so parents need reassurance that it will be reabsorbed during the first few weeks of life without treatment. Rarely, a large hematoma may persist to 3 months.

An infant with cephalhematoma is at greater risk for jaundice as the red blood cells within the hematoma are broken down and reabsorbed.

A

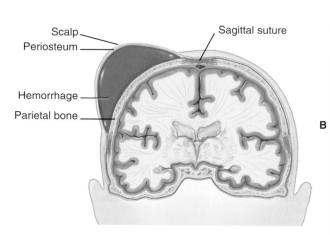

B

Scalp
Periosteum
Hemorrhage
Parietal bone
Sagittal suture

13–17 A, Cephalhematoma.

As you palpate the newborn's head, the suture lines feel like ridges. By 5 to 6 months, they are smooth and not palpable.

A newborn's head may feel asymmetric and the involved ridges more prominent due to *molding* of the cranial bones during engagement and passage through the birth canal. Molding is overriding of the cranial bones; usually, the parietal bone overrides the frontal or occipital bone. Reassure parents that this lasts only a few days or a week. Babies delivered by cesarean section are noted for their evenly round heads. Also, some asymmetry may occur if an infant continually sleeps in one position; this is a flattening of the dependent cranial bone, usually the occiput.

Gently palpate the skull and **fontanels** while the infant is calm and somewhat in a sitting position (crying, lying down, or vomiting may cause the anterior fontanel to look full and bulging). The skull should feel smooth and fused except at the fontanels. The fontanels feel firm, slightly concave, and well defined against the edges of the cranial bones. You may see slight arterial pulsations in the anterior fontanel.

The posterior fontanel may not be palpable at birth. If it is, it measures 1 cm and closes by 1 to 2 months. The anterior fontanel may be small at birth and enlarge to 2.5 cm by 2.5 cm. A large diameter of 4 to 5 cm occasionally may be normal under 6 months. A small fontanel usually is normal. The anterior fontanel closes between 9 months and 2 years. Early closure may be insignificant if head growth proceeds normally.

Sutures palpable when the child is older than 6 months.

Marked asymmetry, as in *craniosynostosis,* a severe deformity due to premature closure of the sutures. Premature closing of the sagittal suture results in a long, narrow head.

Flattening also occurs with rickets or mental retardation.

A true tense or bulging fontanel occurs with acute increased intracranial pressure.
Depressed and sunken fontanels occur with dehydration or malnutrition.
Marked pulsations occur with increased intracranial pressure.

Delayed closure or larger-than-normal fontanel size occurs with hydrocephalus, Down syndrome, hypothyroidism, or rickets.
A small fontanel is a sign of microcephaly, as is early closure.

NORMAL RANGE OF FINDINGS

Note the infant's **head posture** and **head control.** The infant can turn the head side to side by 2 weeks and shows the **tonic neck reflex** when supine and the head is turned to one side (extension of same arm and leg, flexion of opposite arm and leg). The tonic neck reflex disappears between 3 and 4 months, and then the head is maintained in the midline. Head control is achieved by 4 months, when the baby can hold the head erect and steady when pulled to a vertical position. (See Chapter 22, Musculoskeletal System, and Chapter 23, Neurological System, for further details.)

FACE

Check **facial features** for symmetry, appearance, and presence of swelling. Note symmetry of wrinkling when the infant cries or smiles, e.g., both sides of the lips rise and both sides of forehead wrinkle. Children love to comply when you ask them to "make a face." Normally, no swelling is evident. Parotid gland enlargement is seen best when the child sits and looks up at the ceiling; the swelling appears below the angle of the jaw.

NECK

An infant's neck looks short; it lengthens during the first 3 to 4 years. You can see the neck better by supporting the infant's shoulders and tilting the head back a little. This positioning also enhances palpation of the trachea, which is buried deep in the neck. Feel for the row of cartilaginous rings in the midline or just slightly to the right of midline.

Assess muscle development with gentle passive ROM. Cradle the infant's head with your hands and turn it side to side and test forward flexion, extension, and rotation. Note any resistance to movement, especially flexion. Ask a child to actively move through the ROM, as you would an adult.

During infancy, cervical lymph nodes are not palpable normally. But a child's lymph nodes are—they feel more prominent than an adult's until after puberty, when lymphoid tissue begins to atrophy. Palpable nodes less than 3 mm are normal. They may be up to 1 cm in size in the cervical and inguinal areas but are discrete, move easily, and are nontender. Children have a higher incidence of infection, so you will expect a greater incidence of inflammatory adenopathy. No other mass should occur in the neck.

The thyroid gland is difficult to palpate in an infant due to the short, thick neck. The child's thyroid may be palpable normally.

SPECIAL PROCEDURES

PALPATION. *Craniotabes* is a softening of the skull's outer layer. With a newborn, pressure along the suture of the parietal and occipital bones above the ear produces a snapping sensation due to the pliable skull bone. It is like indenting a Ping-Pong ball and feeling it snap back. Do not attempt this unless craniotabes is suspected because of other abnormal findings, and even then avoid excessive pressure. Craniotabes may be normal, especially with premature infants.

PERCUSSION. With an infant, you may directly percuss with your plexor finger against the head surface. This yields a resonant or "cracked pot" sound, which is normal before closure of the fontanels.

AUSCULTATION. Bruits are common in the skull in children under 4 or 5 years of age or in children with anemia. They are systolic or continuous and are heard over the temporal area.

ABNORMAL FINDINGS

Tonic neck reflex beyond 5 months may indicate brain damage.

In children, head tilt occurs with habit spasm, poor vision, and brain tumor.

Head lag after 4 months may indicate mental or motor retardation.

Unilateral immobility indicates nerve damage (central or peripheral), e.g., note angle of mouth droop on paralyzed side.

Some facies are characteristic of congenital abnormalities or chronic allergy. See Tables 13–3 and 13–4.

A short neck or webbing (loose fanlike folds) may indicate congenital abnormality, e.g., Down or Turner syndrome, or it may occur alone.

Head tilt and limited ROM occur with torticollis (wryneck), or from sternomastoid muscle injury during birth or a congenital defect.

Resistance to flexion (nuchal rigidity) and pain on flexion indicate meningeal irritation or meningitis.

Cervical nodes >1 cm are considered enlarged.

Thyroglossal duct cyst—cystic lump high up in midline, freely movable, and rises up when swallowing.

Supraclavicular nodes enlarge with Hodgkin's disease.

Craniotabes may occur with rickets, hydrocephaly, or congenital syphilis.

The sound occurs with hydrocephalus due to separation of cranial sutures (Macewen's sign).

After 5 years of age, bruits indicate increased intracranial pressure, aneurysm, or arteriovenous shunt.

NORMAL RANGE OF FINDINGS

ABNORMAL FINDINGS

TRANSILLUMINATION. Use this procedure if you suspect an abnormal head size or an intracranial lesion. In a completely darkened room, hold a rubber-collared flashlight firmly against the infant's skull. You need a tight fit against the head. Explore all regions of the head: frontal, both sides, occiput (Fig. 13–18). A small ring of light around the flashlight is normal (less than 2 cm in the frontal area, less than 1 cm in the occipital area). But you should not see a larger halo around the rubber collar.

Presence of a halo of light through the skull indicates a loss or thinning of cerebral cortex. If the cortex is absent, the entire cranium lights up (Fig. 13–19).

13–18

13–19 Hydranencephaly.

The Pregnant Female

During the second trimester, chloasma may show on the face. This is a blotchy, hyperpigmented area over the cheeks and forehead that fades after delivery. The thyroid gland may be palpable normally during pregnancy.

The Aging Adult

The temporal arteries may look twisted and prominent. In some aging adults, a mild rhythmic tremor of the head may be normal. *Senile tremors* are benign and include head nodding (as if saying yes or no) and tongue protrusion. If some teeth have been lost, the lower face looks unusually small, with the mouth sunken in.

The neck may show an increased cervical concave curve when the head and jaw are extended forward to compensate for kyphosis of the spine. During the examination, direct the aging person to perform ROM slowly; he or she may experience dizziness with side movements. An aging person may have prolapse of the submandibular glands, which could be mistaken for a tumor. But drooping submandibular glands will feel soft and be present bilaterally.

SUMMARY CHECKLIST: Head and Neck, Including Regional Lymphatics Exam

1. Inspect and palpate the skull
General size and contour
Note any deformities, lumps, tenderness
Palpate temporal artery, temporomandibular joint

2. Inspect the face
Facial expression
Symmetry of movement (cranial nerve VII)
Any involuntary movements, edema, lesions

3. Inspect and palpate the neck
Active ROM
Enlargement of salivary glands, lymph nodes, thyroid gland
Position of the trachea

4. Auscultate the thyroid (if enlarged) for bruit

SAMPLE CHARTING

SUBJECTIVE

Denies any unusually frequent or severe headache; no history of head injury, dizziness, or syncope; no neck pain, limitation of motion, lumps, or swelling.

OBJECTIVE

Head. Normocephalic, no lumps, no lesions, no tenderness.
Face. Symmetric, no weakness or drooping, no involuntary movements.
Neck. Supple with full ROM, no pain. Symmetric, no lymphadenopathy or masses. Trachea midline, thyroid not palpable. No bruits.

FOCUSED ASSESSMENT: CLINICAL CASE STUDY 1

Frank V. is a 57-year-old insurance executive who is in his fourth postoperative day after a transurethral resection of the prostate gland. He also has chronic hypertension, managed by oral hydrochlorothiazide, exercise, and a low-salt diet.

SUBJECTIVE

Complaining of dizziness, a lightheaded feeling that occurred on standing and cleared on sitting. No previous episodes of dizziness. Denies palpitations, nausea, or vomiting. States urine pink tinged as it was yesterday with no red blood. No pain meds today. On second day of same antihypertensive medication he took before surgery.

OBJECTIVE

BP 142/88 RA sitting, 94/58 RA standing. Pulse 94 sitting and standing, regular rhythm, no skipped beats. Temp 37° C. Color tannish-pink, no pallor, skin warm and dry. Neuro: alert and oriented to person, place, and time. Speech clear and fluent. Moving all extremities, no weakness. No nystagmus, no ataxia, past pointing normal. Romberg's sign negative (normal). Intake/output in balance. Urine faint pink tinged, no clots.
    Lab: Hct 45, serum chemistries normal.

ASSESSMENT

Orthostatic hypotension
Risk for injury R/T orthostatic hypotension

FOCUSED ASSESSMENT: CLINICAL CASE STUDY 2

Mara is a 19-year-old single white female college student with a past history of good health and no chronic illnesses; she enters the outpatient clinic today stating, "I think I've had a stroke!"

SUBJECTIVE

One day PTA: first noticed at dinner at college cafeteria when joking with friends, started to stick out tongue and roll tongue and could not do it, right side of tongue was not working. Mara left room to look in mirror and became scared; when smiled, noticed right side was not working. Tried to pucker lips, could not. Could not whistle, could not raise eyebrow, "I looked like a Vulcan." No other movement disorder below neck. Mild pain behind right ear with buzzing in ear. Able to sleep last night, but roommate said Mara's right eyelid did not close completely during sleep.

    Today: still no movement on complete right side of face. Feeling self-conscious in class and during conversations with friends. Now has taste aversion, fluids with high water content taste especially bitter. No hearing loss.

OBJECTIVE

T 37° C, P 64, R 14, B/P 108/78.
    Forehead appears smooth and immobile on right, unable to wrinkle right side. Unable to close right eye, Bell's phenomenon present when attempts to close (right eyeball rolls upward), right palpebral fissure

Continued

appears wider. No corneal reflex on right. Unable to whistle or puff right cheek. Absent nasolabial fold on right. Mouth droops on right, sags on right when tries to smile. Slight drooling. Left side of face responds appropriately to all these movements. Superficial sensation intact.

Rest of musculoskeletal system intact: able to hold balance while standing, able to walk, walk heel-to-toe, do knee bend on each knee. Arm strength and range of motion intact.

ASSESSMENT

Right-sided facial paralysis, consistent with Bell's palsy
Disturbed body image R/T effects of loss of facial function
Risk for deficient fluid volume R/T taste aversion and dietary alteration
Risk for sensory deficit, visual impairment, R/T effects of neurological impairment

NURSING DIAGNOSES COMMONLY ASSOCIATED WITH HEAD AND NECK DISORDERS

RELATED FACTORS (Etiology)	DEFINING CHARACTERISTICS (Symptoms and Signs)
DIAGNOSIS: Disturbed Body image	

Effects of loss of body part(s)
Effects of loss of body function
	Verbal or nonverbal response to actual or perceived change in structure and/or function
	Verbalization of
	    Fear of rejection or of reaction by others
	    Negative feelings about body
	Not looking at and/or touching body part
	Preoccupation with loss or change
	Refusal to verify actual change or loss
	Hiding or overexposing body part
	Change in social involvement
	Depersonalization of part or loss by use of impersonal pronouns

DIAGNOSIS: Impaired Swallowing	

Neuromuscular impairment
    Decreased/absent gag reflex
    Facial paralysis
    Decreased strength or excursion of muscles of mastication
Mechanical obstruction
    Edema
    Tracheostomy tube
    Tumor
Limited awareness
Excessive/inadequate salivation
Fatigue
Reddened, irritated oropharyngeal cavity
	Observed evidence of difficulty swallowing
	Evidence of aspiration
	Reported pain on swallowing
	Dehydration
	Weight loss

OTHER RELATED NURSING DIAGNOSES

ACTUAL	RISK
Pain (see Chapter 14) Disturbed Sensory perception	Risk for ineffective Airway clearance Risk for deficient Fluid volume Risk for Infection

ASSESSMENT VIDEO CRITICAL THINKING QUESTIONS

The Saunders *Physical Examination and Health Assessment* videos "Head, Eyes, and Ears" and "Nose, Mouth, Throat, and Neck" will direct you to consider the following:

1. How do examination techniques and findings differ when palpating the head of an adult and the head of an infant?

2. Describe characteristics of normal and abnormal cervical lymph nodes.

Abnormal Findings

TABLE 13-1: Abnormalities in Head Size and Contour

Hydrocephalus

Obstruction of drainage of cerebrospinal fluid results in excessive accumulation, increasing intracranial pressure, and enlargement of the head. The face looks small compared with the enlarged cranium. The increasing pressure also produces dilated scalp veins, frontal bossing, and downcast or "setting sun" eyes (sclera visible above iris). The cranial bones thin, sutures separate, and percussion yields a "cracked pot" sound (Macewen's sign).

Paget's Disease of Bone (Osteitis Deformans)

A localized bone disease of unknown etiology that softens, thickens, and deforms bone. It affects 3% of adults over age 40 and 10% over age 80 and occurs more often in males. The disease is characterized by bowed long bones, sudden fractures, frontal bossing, and enlarging skull bones which form an acorn-shaped cranium. Enlarging skull bones press on cranial nerves, causing symptoms of headache, vertigo, tinnitus, progressive deafness, as well as optic atrophy and compression of the spinal cord.

Reprinted from the Clinical Slide Collection on the Rheumatic Diseases. © 1991, 1995, 1997. Used by permission of the American College of Rheumatology.

Acromegaly

Excessive secretion of growth hormone from the pituitary, after puberty, creates an enlarged skull and thickened cranial bones. Note the elongated head, massive face, prominent nose and lower jaw, heavy eyebrow ridge, and coarse facial features, especially when compared with the same woman's face on the left pictured several years before she had a pituitary tumor.

TABLE 13–2: Swellings on the Head or Neck

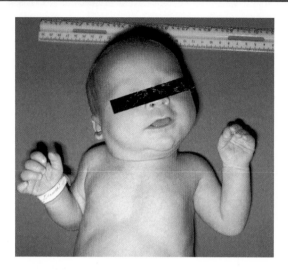

Torticollis (Wryneck)

A hematoma in one sternomastoid muscle, probably injured by intrauterine malposition, results in head tilt to one side and limited neck ROM to the opposite side. You will feel a firm, discrete, nontender mass in mid-muscle on the involved side. This requires treatment, or the muscle becomes fibrotic and permanently shortened with permanent limitation of ROM, asymmetry of head and face, and visual problems from a nonhorizontal position of the eyes.

Thyroid—Multiple Nodules

Multiple nodules usually indicate inflammation or a multinodular goiter rather than a neoplasm. However, suspect any rapidly enlarging or firm nodule.

Thyroid—Single Nodule (not illustrated)

Most solitary nodules are benign, although a solitary nodule poses a greater risk of malignancy than do multiple nodules and poses a greater risk in a young person. Suspect any painless, rapidly growing nodule, especially the appearance of a single nodule in a young person. Cancerous nodules tend to be hard and are fixed to surrounding structures.

Pilar Cyst (Wen)

Smooth, firm, fluctuant swelling on the scalp. Tense pressure of the contents causes overlying skin to be shiny and taut. It is a benign growth.

Parotid Gland Enlargement

Rapid painful inflammation of the parotid occurs with mumps. Parotid swelling also occurs with blockage of a duct, abscess, or tumor. Note swelling anterior to lower ear lobe.

TABLE 13–3: Pediatric Facial Abnormalities

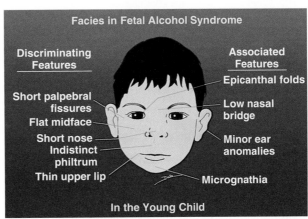

Fetal Alcohol Syndrome

A pregnant woman who abuses alcohol is at great risk of producing a baby with a wide range of growth and developmental abnormalities. Facial malformations may be recognizable at birth. Characteristic facies include narrow palpebral fissures, epicanthal folds, and midfacial hypoplasia.

Congenital Hypothyroidism

Thyroid deficiency at an early age produces impaired growth and neurological deficit. Without neonatal screening, characteristic facies develop by 3 to 6 months of age: low hairline, hirsute forehead, swollen eyelids, narrow palpebral fissures, widely spaced eyes, depressed nasal bridge, puffy face, thick tongue protruding through an open mouth, and a dull expression. Head size is normal, but the anterior and posterior fontanels are wide open.

Down Syndrome

Chromosomal aberration (trisomy 21). Head and face characteristics may include upslanting eyes with inner epicanthal folds, flat nasal bridge, small broad flat nose, protruding thick tongue, ear dysplasia, short broad neck with webbing, and small hands with single palmar crease.

Table continued on following page

ABNORMAL FINDINGS

TABLE 13–3: Pediatric Facial Abnormalities—cont'd

Atopic (Allergic) Facies

Children with chronic allergies such as atopic dermatitis often develop characteristic facial features. These include exhausted face, blue shadows below the eyes ("allergic shiners") from sluggish venous return, a double or single crease on the lower eyelids (Morgan's lines), central facial pallor, and open-mouth breathing (allergic gaping). The open mouth breathing can lead to malocclusion of the teeth and malformed jaw because the child's bones are still forming.

Allergic Salute and Crease

The transverse line on the nose is also a feature of chronic allergies. It is formed when the child chronically uses the hand to push the nose up and back (the "allergic salute") to relieve itching and to free swollen turbinates, which allows air passage.

TABLE 13–4: Abnormal Facial Appearances With Chronic Illnesses

Parkinson's Syndrome

A deficiency of the neurotransmitter dopamine and degeneration of the basal ganglia in the brain. The immobility of features produces a face that is flat and expressionless, "mastlike," with elevated eyebrows, staring gaze, oily skin, and drooling.

Cushing's Syndrome

With excessive secretion of corticotropin hormone (ACTH) and chronic steroid use, the person develops a plethoric, rounded, "moonlike" face, prominent jowls, red cheeks, hirsutism on the upper lip, lower cheeks, and chin, and acneiform rash on the chest.

TABLE 13-4: Abnormal Facial Appearances With Chronic Illnesses—cont'd

Hyperthyroidism

Goiter is an increase in the size of the thyroid gland and occurs with hyperthyroidism, Hashimoto's thyroiditis, and hypothyroidism. Graves' disease (shown here) is the most common cause of hyperthyroidism, manifested by goiter and exophthalmos (bulging eyeballs). Symptoms include nervousness, fatigue, weight loss, muscle cramps, and heat intolerance; signs include tachycardia, shortness of breath, excessive sweating, fine muscle tremor, thin silky hair and skin, infrequent blinking, and a staring appearance.

Myxedema (Hypothyroidism)

A deficiency of thyroid hormone, when severe, causes a nonpitting edema or myxedema. Note puffy edematous face, especially around eyes (periorbital edema), coarse facial features, dry skin, and dry coarse hair and eyebrows.

Bell's Palsy (Right Side)

A **lower motor neuron** lesion (**peripheral**), producing cranial nerve VII paralysis, which is almost always unilateral. It has a rapid onset, and its cause is currently thought to be herpes simplex virus (HSV). Note complete paralysis of one half of the face; person cannot wrinkle forehead, raise eyebrow, close eye, whistle, or show teeth on the right side. Usually presents with smooth forehead, wide palpebral fissure, flat nasolabial fold, drooling, and pain behind the ear.

Brain Attack or Cerebrovascular Accident

An **upper motor neuron** lesion (**central**). A "stroke" is an acute neurologic deficit due to an obstruction of a cerebral vessel, as in atherosclerosis, or a rupture in a cerebral vessel. Note paralysis of lower facial muscles, but also note that the upper half of face is not affected due to the intact nerve from the unaffected hemisphere. The person is still able to wrinkle the forehead and to close the eyes.

Table continued on following page

TABLE 13–4: Abnormal Facial Appearances With Chronic Illnesses—cont'd

Cachectic Appearance

Accompanies chronic wasting diseases such as cancer, dehydration, and starvation. Features include sunken eyes; hollow cheeks; and exhausted, defeated expression.

Scleroderma

Literally, "hard skin," this collagen disease is characterized by chronic hardening and shrinking of connective tissue. This can occur in any body organ (skin, heart, esophagus, kidney, lung). Characteristic facies: hard, shiny skin on forehead and cheeks; thin, pursed lips with radial furrowing; absent skinfolds; muscle atrophy on face and neck; absence of expression.

Reprinted from the Clinical Slide Collection on the Rheumatic Diseases, © 1991, 1995, 1997. Used by permission of the American College of Rheumatology.

BIBLIOGRAPHY

Billue JS: Bell's palsy: an update on idiopathic facial paralysis, *Nurse Pract* 22(8):88–107, Aug 1997.

Burke M: Dizziness in the elderly: etiology and treatment, *Nurse Pract* 20(12):28–35, Dec 1995.

Chabon SL: Identification and evaluation of thyroid nodules, *Lippincotts Prim Care Pract* 1(5):499–506, Nov–Dec 1997.

Costa M: Trigeminal neuralgia, *Am J Nurs* 98(6):42–43, Jun 1998.

Diamond S et al: Migraine: new perspectives on diagnosis and therapy, *Consultant* 40(11):S7–S32, Sep 2000.

Dowd TR: Primary care approach to lymphadenopathy, *Nurs Pract* 19(12):36–43, Dec 1994.

Gilkison CR: Thyrotoxicosis: recognition and management, *Lippincotts Prim Care Pract* 1(5):485–498, Nov–Dec 1997.

Karmel-Ross K, Lepp M: Assessment and treatment of children with congenital muscular torticollis, *Phys Occup Ther Pediatr* 17(2):21–67, 1997.

Kingston L, Reynolds D, Phillips LP: Primary care for women: comprehensive assessment of the head and neck, *J Nurse Midwifery* 40(2):187–201, Mar–Apr 1995.

Malchiodi L: Thyroid storm, *Am J Nurs* 102(5):33–35, May 2002.

Moloney MF et al: Caring for the woman with migraine headaches, *Nurse Pract* 25(2):17–41, Feb 2000.

Prisco MK: Evaluating neck masses, *Nurse Pract* 25(4):30–51, Apr 2000.

Schilling JS: Hyperthyroidism: diagnosis and management of Graves' disease, *Nurse Pract* 22(6):72–97, Jun 1997.

Scripture DL: Hyperthyroidism: an unusual case presentation, *Nurse Pract* 23(2):50–55, Feb 1998.

Weiss J: Assessing and managing the patient with headaches, *Nurse Pract* (24)7:18–37, Jul 1999.

Eyes

http://evolve.elsevier.com/Jarvis/

Structure and Function

EXTERNAL ANATOMY

The eye is the sensory organ of vision. Humans are very visual beings. Over half of the neocortex is involved with processing visual information (Wehenmeyer and Gallman, 2002).

Because this sense is so important to humans, the eye is well protected by the bony orbital cavity, which is surrounded with a cushion of fat. The **eyelids** are like two movable shades that further protect the eye from injury, strong light, and dust. The upper eyelid is the larger and more mobile one. The eyelashes are short hairs in double or triple rows that curve outward from the lid margins, filtering out dust and dirt.

The **palpebral fissure** is the elliptical open space between the eyelids (Fig. 14–1). When closed, the lid margins approximate completely. When open, the upper lid covers part of the iris. The lower lid margin is just at the **limbus,** the border between the cornea and sclera. The **canthus** is the corner of the eye, the angle where the lids meet. At the inner canthus the **caruncle** is a small fleshy mass containing sebaceous glands.

Within the upper lid, **tarsal plates** are strips of connective tissue that give it shape (Fig. 14–2). The tarsal plates contain the **meibomian glands,** modified sebaceous glands that secrete an oily lubricating material onto the lids. This stops the tears from overflowing and helps to form an airtight seal when the lids are closed.

The exposed part of the eye has a transparent protective covering, the **conjunctiva.** The conjunctiva is a thin mucous membrane folded like an envelope between the eyelids and the eyeball. The *palpebral* conjunctiva lines the lids and is clear, with many small blood vessels. It forms a deep recess and then folds back over the eye. The *bulbar* conjunctiva overlays the eyeball, with the white sclera showing through.

At the limbus the conjunctiva merges with the cornea. The cornea covers and protects the iris and pupil.

The **lacrimal apparatus** provides constant irrigation to keep the conjunctiva and cornea moist and lubricated (Fig. 14–3). The lacrimal gland, in the upper outer corner over the eye, secretes tears. The tears wash across the eye and are drawn up evenly as the lid blinks. The tears drain into the **puncta,** visible on the upper and lower lids at the inner canthus. The tears then drain into the nasolacrimal sac, through the one-half-inch-long nasolacrimal duct, and empty into the inferior meatus inside the nose. A tiny fold of mucous membrane prevents air from being forced up the nasolacrimal duct when the nose is blown.

EXTRAOCULAR MUSCLES

Six muscles attach the eyeball to its orbit (Fig. 14–4) and serve to direct the eye to points of interest. These extraocular muscles give the eye both straight and rotary movement. The four straight, or *rectus,* muscles are the superior, inferior, lateral, and medial rectus muscles. The two slanting, or *oblique,* muscles are the superior and inferior muscles.

Each muscle is coordinated, or yoked, with one in the other eye. This ensures that when the two eyes move, their axes always remain parallel (called *conjugate movement*). Parallel axes are important because the human brain can tolerate seeing only one image. Although some animals can perceive two different pictures through each eye, human beings have a binocular, single-image visual system. This occurs because our eyes move as a pair. For example, the two yoked muscles that allow looking to the far right are the right lateral rectus and the left medial rectus.

14–1

14–2 Anterior eye structures.

Labels (top to bottom):
Bony orbit
Orbicularis oculi m.
Palpebral conjunctiva
Bulbar conjunctiva
Posterior chamber
Anterior chamber
Cornea
Tarsal plate
Meibomian glands
Sclera

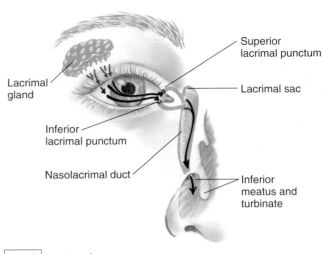

14–3 Lacrimal apparatus.

Labels:
Lacrimal gland
Superior lacrimal punctum
Lacrimal sac
Inferior lacrimal punctum
Nasolacrimal duct
Inferior meatus and turbine

Movement of the **extraocular muscles** (below) is stimulated by three **cranial nerves.** Cranial nerve VI, the abducens nerve, innervates the lateral rectus muscle (which abducts the eye); cranial nerve IV, the trochlear nerve, innervates the superior oblique muscle; and cranial nerve III, the oculomotor nerve, innervates all the rest—the superior, inferior, and medial rectus and the inferior oblique muscles.

A
Medial rectus m.
Superior oblique m. (passing through trochlea)
Superior rectus m.
Optic nerve
Lateral rectus m.
Inferior rectus m.
Inferior oblique m.

14–4 A, Muscle attachments; B, direction of movement.

B
Superior rectus c.n. III
Inferior oblique c.n. III
Inferior oblique c.n. III
Superior rectus c.n. III
Lateral rectus c.n. VI
Medial rectus c.n. III
Lateral rectus c.n. VI
Inferior rectus c.n. III
Superior oblique c.n. IV
Superior oblique c.n. IV
Inferior rectus c.n. III

INTERNAL ANATOMY

The eye is a sphere composed of three concentric coats: (1) the outer fibrous **sclera,** (2) the middle vascular **choroid,** and (3) the inner nervous **retina** (Fig. 14–5). Inside the retina is the transparent vitreous body. The only parts accessible to examination are the sclera anteriorly and the retina through the ophthalmoscope.

THE OUTER LAYER

The **sclera** is a tough, protective, white covering. It is continuous anteriorly with the smooth, transparent cornea, which covers the iris and pupil. The cornea is part of the refracting media of the eye, bending incoming light rays so they will be focused on the inner retina.

The **cornea** is very sensitive to touch; contact with a wisp of cotton stimulates a blink in both eyes, called the *corneal reflex.* The trigeminal nerve (cranial nerve V) carries the afferent sensation into the brain, and the facial nerve (cranial nerve VII) carries the efferent message that stimulates the blink.

THE MIDDLE LAYER

The **choroid** has dark pigmentation to prevent light from reflecting internally and is heavily vascularized to deliver blood to the retina. Anteriorly, the choroid is continuous with the ciliary body and the iris. The muscles of the ciliary body control the thickness of the lens. The iris functions as a diaphragm, varying the opening at its center, the pupil. This controls the amount of light admitted into the retina. The muscle fibers of the iris contract the pupil in bright light and to accommodate for near vision, and dilate the pupil when the light is dim and for far vision. The color of the iris varies from person to person.

The **pupil** is round and regular. Its size is determined by a balance between the parasympathetic and sympathetic chains of the autonomic nervous system. Stimulation of the parasympathetic branch, through cranial nerve III, causes constriction of the pupil. Stimulation of the sympathetic branch dilates the pupil and elevates the eyelid. As mentioned earlier, the pupil size also reacts to the amount of ambient light and to accommodation, or focusing an object on the retina.

The **lens** is a biconvex disc located just posterior to the pupil. The transparent lens serves as a refracting medium, keeping a viewed object in continual focus on the retina. Its thickness is controlled by the ciliary body; the lens bulges for focusing on near objects, and flattens for far objects.

The **anterior chamber** is posterior to the cornea and in front of the iris and lens. It contains the aqueous humor that is produced continually by the ciliary body. The continuous flow of fluid serves to deliver nutrients to the surrounding tissues and to drain metabolic wastes. Intraocular pressure is determined by a balance between the amount of aqueous produced and resistance to its outflow at the angle of the anterior chamber.

THE INNER LAYER

The **retina** is the visual receptive layer of the eye in which light waves are changed into nerve impulses. The retinal

14–5

14-6

structures viewed through the ophthalmoscope are the optic disc, the retinal vessels, the general background, and the macula (Fig. 14–6).

The **optic disc** (or optic papilla) is the area in which fibers from the retina converge to form the optic nerve. Located toward the nasal side of the retina, it has these characteristics: a color that varies from creamy yellow-orange to pink; a round or oval shape; margins that are distinct and sharply demarcated, especially on the temporal side; and a physiologic cup, the smaller circular area inside the disc where the blood vessels exit and enter.

The **retinal vessels** normally include a paired artery and vein extending to each quadrant, growing progressively smaller in caliber as they reach the periphery. The arteries appear brighter red and narrower than the veins, and the arteries have a thin sliver of light on them (the arterial light reflex). The general background of the fundus varies in color, depending on the person's skin color. The **macula** is located on the temporal side of the fundus. It is a slightly darker pigmented region surrounding the **fovea centralis,** the area of sharpest and keenest vision. The macula receives and transduces light from the center of the visual field.

VISUAL PATHWAYS AND VISUAL FIELDS

Objects reflect light. The light rays are refracted through the transparent media (cornea, aqueous humor, lens, and vitreous body) and strike the retina. The retina transforms the light stimulus into nerve impulses that are conducted through the optic nerve and the optic tract to the visual cortex of the occipital lobe.

The image formed on the retina is upside down and reversed from its actual appearance in the outside world (Fig. 14–7). That is, an object in the upper temporal visual

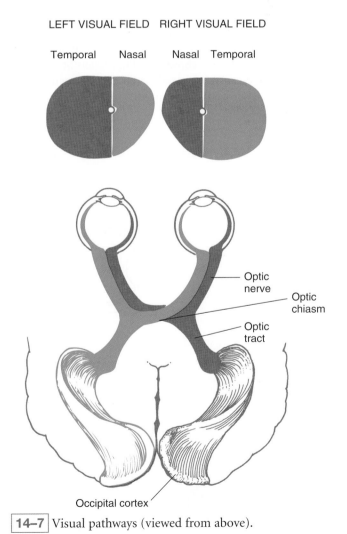

14-7 Visual pathways (viewed from above).

field of the right eye reflects its image onto the lower nasal area of the retina. All retinal fibers collect to form the optic nerve, but they maintain this same spatial arrangement, with nasal fibers running medially and temporal fibers running laterally.

At the optic chiasm, nasal fibers (from both temporal visual fields) cross over. The left optic tract now has fibers from the left half of each retina, and the right optic tract contains fibers only from the right. Thus the right side of the brain looks at the left side of the world.

VISUAL REFLEXES

PUPILLARY LIGHT REFLEX

The pupillary light reflex is the normal constriction of the pupils when bright light shines on the retina (Fig. 14–8). It is a subcortical reflex arc (i.e., a person has no conscious control over it); the afferent link is cranial nerve II, the optic nerve, and the efferent path is cranial III, the oculomotor nerve. When one eye is exposed to bright light, a *direct light reflex* occurs (constriction of that pupil) as well as a *consensual light reflex* (simultaneous constriction of the other pupil). This happens because the optic nerve carries the sensory afferent message in and then synapses with both sides of the brain. For example, consider the light reflex in a person who is blind in one eye. Stimulation of the normal eye produces both a direct and a consensual light reflex. Stimulation of the blind eye causes no response because the sensory afferent in cranial nerve II is destroyed.

FIXATION

This is a reflex direction of the eye toward an object attracting a person's attention. The image is fixed in the center of the visual field, the fovea centralis. This consists of very rapid ocular movements to put the target back on the fovea, and somewhat slower (smooth pursuit) movements to track the target and keep its image on the fovea. These ocular movements are impaired by drugs, alcohol, fatigue, and inattention.

ACCOMMODATION

This is adaptation of the eye for near vision. It is accomplished by increasing the curvature of the lens through movement of the ciliary muscles. Although the lens cannot be observed directly, the components of accommodation that can be observed are convergence (motion toward) of the axes of the eyeballs and pupillary constriction.

 DEVELOPMENTAL CONSIDERATIONS

INFANTS AND CHILDREN

At birth, eye function is limited but it matures fully during the early years. Peripheral vision is intact in the newborn. The macula, the area of keenest vision, is absent at birth but is developing by 4 months and is mature by 8 months. Eye movements may be poorly coordinated at birth. By 3 to 4 months of age, the infant establishes binocularity and can fixate on a single image with both eyes simultaneously. Most neonates (80%) are born farsighted; this gradually decreases after 7 to 8 years of age.

14–8

In structure, the eyeball reaches adult size by 8 years. At birth, the iris shows little pigment, and the pupils are small. The lens is nearly spherical at birth, growing flatter throughout life. Its consistency changes from that of soft plastic at birth to rigid glass in old age.

THE AGING ADULT

Changes in eye structure contribute greatly to the distinct facial changes of the aging person. The skin loses its elasticity, causing wrinkling and drooping; fat tissues and muscles atrophy; and the external eye structures appear as on p. 324. Lacrimal glands involute, causing decreased tear production and a feeling of dryness and burning.

On the globe itself, the cornea may show an infiltration of degenerative lipid material around the limbus (see discussion of *arcus senilis,* p. 325). Pupil size decreases. The lens loses elasticity, becoming hard and glasslike. This glasslike quality decreases the lens's ability to change shape in order to accommodate for near vision; this condition is termed **presbyopia.** The average age at which people experience presbyopia is 40 years (Friedman, Pineda, and Kaiser, 1998). By 70 years of age, the normally transparent fibers of the lens begin to thicken and yellow. This is nuclear sclerosis, or the beginning of a senile cataract.

Inside the globe, floaters appear in the vitreous due to debris that can accumulate because the vitreous is not continuously renewed as the aqueous humor is. Visual acuity may diminish gradually after 50 years of age, and even more so after 70 years. Near vision is commonly affected due to the decreased power of accommodation in the lens (presbyopia). As early as the fourth decade, a person may have blurred vision and difficulty reading. Also, the aging person needs more light to see because of a decreased adaptation to darkness, and this condition may affect the function of night driving.

In the aging population the most common causes of decreased visual functioning are:

1. Cataract formation, or lens opacity. Some cataract formation should be expected by age 70. Studies indicate that 46% of people age 75 to 85 have developed cataracts (Kane, Ouslander, and Abrass, 2003).
2. Glaucoma, or increased ocular pressure. The incidence increases with age to 7.2% at ages 75 to 85, affecting men at higher rates than women (Kane et al., 2003). Chronic, open-angle glaucoma is the most common type and involves a gradual loss of peripheral vision.
3. Macular degeneration. Loss of central vision, the area of clearest vision, is the most common cause of blindness. It affects 28% of those age 75 to 85, with women affected more often than men (Kane et al., 2003). With this, the person is unable to read fine print, sew, or do fine work and may have difficulty distinguishing faces. Depending on how much the lifestyle is oriented around activities requiring close work, loss of central vision may cause great distress. Peripheral vision is not affected, so the person can mange self-care and will not become completely disabled.

TRANSCULTURAL CONSIDERATIONS

Racial differences are evident in the palpebral fissures. Persons of Asian origins are often identified by their characteristic eyes, whereas the presence of narrowed palpebral fissures in non-Asian individuals may be diagnostic of a serious congenital anomaly, *Down syndrome.*

Culturally based variability exists in the color of the iris and in retinal pigmentation, with darker irides having darker retinas behind them. Individuals with light retinas generally have better night vision but can suffer pain in an environment that has too much light.

RACIAL VARIATIONS IN DISEASE

Primary open-angle glaucoma affects blacks three to six times more often than whites and is six times more likely to cause blindness in blacks than in whites (Friedman et al., 1998). Reasons for this are not known. What is even more surprising is that the efficacy of treatment approach to glaucoma may be different for blacks and whites (Gaasterland et al., 1998). For blacks, the best outcomes were when the regimen started with argon laser treatments and then was followed, if necessary, by a trabeculectomy (surgery to create a tunnel between the anterior chamber in the eye and the subconjunctival space, thereby helping the drainage of aqueous humor). For whites, outcomes were better when the regimen started with the trabeculectomy, and then later included the laser treatments if needed. It is not known why racial groups respond differently to treatment.

Subjective Data

1. Vision difficulty (decreased acuity, blurring, blind spots)	4. Redness, swelling	8. Use of glasses or contact lenses
2. Pain	5. Watering, discharge	9. Self-care behaviors
3. Strabismus, diplopia	6. Past history of ocular problems	
	7. Glaucoma	

EXAMINER ASKS	RATIONALE
1. Vision difficulty (decreased acuity, blurring, blind spots). Any difficulty seeing or any blurring? Come on suddenly, or progress slowly? In one eye or both?	

EXAMINER ASKS	RATIONALE

- Constant, or does it come and go?
- Do objects appear out of focus, or does it feel like a clouding over objects? Does it feel like "grayness" of vision?
- Do spots move in front of your eyes? One or many? In one or both eyes?

Floaters are common with myopia or after middle age due to condensed vitreous fibers. Usually not significant, but acute onset of floaters ("shade" or "cobwebs") may occur with retinal detachment.

- Any halos/rainbows around objects? Or rings around lights?

Halos around lights occur with acute narrow-angle glaucoma.

- Any blind spot? Does it move as you shift your gaze? Any loss of peripheral vision?

Scotoma, a blind spot in the visual field surrounded by an area of normal or decreased vision, occurs with glaucoma, with optic nerve and visual pathway disorders.

- Any night blindness?

Night blindness occurs with optic atrophy, glaucoma, or vitamin A deficiency.

2. Pain. Any **eye pain?** Please describe.
- Come on suddenly?

Consider *sudden onset* of eye symptoms or vision change (pain, floaters, blind spot, loss of peripheral vision) as a possible emergency. Refer immediately.

- Quality—a burning or itching?
- Or sharp, stabbing pain or pain with bright light?
- A foreign body sensation? Or deep aching? Or headache in brow area?

Quality is valuable diagnostic indicator. *Photophobia* is inability to tolerate light. (Note: some common eye diseases cause no pain, e.g., refractive errors, cataract, glaucoma.)

3. Strabismus, diplopia. Any history of crossed eyes? Now or in the past? Does this occur with eye fatigue?
- Ever see double? Constant, or does it come and go? In one eye or both?

Strabismus is a deviation in the anteroposterior axis of the eye.
Diplopia is the perception of two images of a single object.

4. Redness, swelling. Any **redness** or **swelling** in the eyes?
- Any infections? Now or in the past?
- When do these occur? In a particular time of year? Are they seasonal?

5. Watering, discharge. Any **watering** or excessive tearing?

Lacrimation (tearing) and epiphora (excessive tearing) are due to irritants or obstruction in drainage of tears.

- Any **discharge?** Any matter in the eyes? Is it hard to open your eyes in the morning? What color is the discharge?
- How do you remove matter from eyes?

Purulent discharge is thick and yellow. Crusts form at night. Assess hygiene practices and knowledge of cross-contamination.

6. Past history of ocular problems. Any **past history** of injury or surgery to eye? Or any history of allergies?

Allergens may cause irritation of conjunctiva or cornea, e.g., make-up, contact lens solution.

7. Glaucoma. Ever been tested for **glaucoma?** Results?
- Any family history of glaucoma?

Glaucoma is an eye disease characterized by increased intraocular pressure.

8. Use of glasses or contact lenses. Do you wear **glasses** or **contact lenses?** How do they work for you?
- Last time your prescription was checked? Was it changed?

EXAMINER ASKS	RATIONALE
• If you wear contact lenses, are there any problems such as pain, photophobia, watering, or swelling?	
• How do you care for contacts? How long do you wear them? How do you clean them? Do you remove them for certain activities?	Assess self-care behaviors.
9. Self-care behaviors. Last vision test? Who tested it?	**Self-care** behaviors for eyes and vision.
• Ever tested for color vision?	
• Any environmental conditions at home or at work that may affect your eyes? For example, flying sparks, metal bits, smoke, dust, chemical fumes? If so, do you wear goggles to protect your eyes?	Ocular diseases or injuries may be work related—e.g., an auto mechanic with a foreign body from metal working.
10. What medications are you taking? Systemic or topical? Do you take any medication specifically for the eyes?	Some medications have ocular side effects; e.g., prednisone may cause cataracts or increased intraocular pressure.
11. If you have experienced a vision loss, how do you cope? Do you have books with large print, books on audio tape, Braille?	
• Do you maintain living environment the same?	A constant spatial layout eases navigation through the home.
• Do you sometimes fear complete loss of vision?	

Additional History for Infants and Children

1. Any vaginal infections in the mother at time of delivery?	Genital herpes and gonorrhea vaginitis have ocular sequelae for the newborn.
2. Considering age of child, which developmental milestones of vision have you (parent) noted?	The parent is most often the one to detect vision problems.
3. Does the child have routine vision testing at school?	
4. Are you (parent) aware of safety measures to protect child's eyes from trauma? Do you inspect toys?	
• Have you taught the child safe care of sharp objects, and how to carry and how to use them?	

Additional History for the Aging Adult

1. Have you noticed any visual difficulty with climbing stairs or driving? Any problem with night vision?	Any loss of depth perception or central vision.
2. When was the last time you were tested for glaucoma?	
• Any aching pain around eyes? Any loss of peripheral vision?	
• If you have glaucoma, how do you manage your eyedrops?	Compliance may be a problem if symptoms are absent. Assess ability to administer eyedrops.
3. Is there a history of cataracts? Any loss or progressive blurring of vision?	
4. Do your eyes ever feel dry? burning? What do you do for this?	Decreased tear production may occur with aging.
5. Any decrease in usual activities, such as reading or sewing?	Macular degeneration causes a loss in central vision acuity.

Objective Data

PREPARATION

Position the person sitting up with the head at your eye level.

EQUIPMENT NEEDED

Snellen eye chart
Handheld visual screener
Opaque card or occluder
Penlight
Applicator stick
Ophthalmoscope

NORMAL RANGE OF FINDINGS

ABNORMAL FINDINGS

TEST CENTRAL VISUAL ACUITY

Snellen Eye Chart

The Snellen alphabet chart is the most commonly used and accurate measure of visual acuity. It has lines of letters arranged in decreasing size.

Place the Snellen alphabet chart in a well-lit spot at eye level. Position the person on a mark exactly 20 feet from the chart. Hand the person an opaque card with which to shield one eye at a time during the test; inadvertent peeking may result when shielding the eye with the person's own fingers (Fig. 14–9). If the person wears glasses or contact lenses, leave them on. Remove only reading glasses because they will blur distance vision. Ask the person to read through the chart to the smallest line of letters possible. Encourage the person to try the next smallest line also. (Note: Use a Snellen "E" chart for people who cannot read letters. See p. 321.)

Hesitancy, squinting, leaning forward, misreading letters.

14–9

Record the result using the numeric fraction at the end of the last successful line read. Indicate whether or not the person missed any letters or if corrective lenses were worn—for example, "O.D.* 20/30—1, with glasses."

---

*O.D., oculus dexter, or right eye.

NORMAL RANGE OF FINDINGS	ABNORMAL FINDINGS

Normal visual acuity is 20/20. Contrary to some people's impression, the numeric fraction is *not* a percentage of normal vision. Instead, the top number (numerator) indicates the distance the person is standing from the chart, while the denominator gives the distance at which a normal eye could have read that particular line. Thus "20/20" means, "You can read at 20 feet what the normal eye could have read at 20 feet."

The larger the denominator, the poorer the vision. If vision is poorer than 20/30, refer to an ophthalmologist or optometrist. Impaired vision may be due to refractive error, opacity in the media (cornea, lens, vitreous), or disorder in the retina or optic pathway.

If the person is unable to see even the largest letters, shorten the distance to the chart until it is seen and record that distance (e.g., "10/200"). If visual acuity is even lower, assess whether the person can count your fingers when they are spread in front of the eyes or distinguish light perception using your penlight.

Near Vision

For people over 40 years of age or for those who report increasing difficulty reading, test near vision using a handheld vision screener with various sizes of print (e.g., a Jaeger card) (Fig. 14–10). Hold the card in good light about 35 cm (14 inches) from the eye—this distance equals the print size on the 20-ft chart. Test each eye separately, with glasses on. A normal result is "14/14" in each eye, read without hesitancy and without moving the card closer or farther away. When no vision screening card is available, ask the person to read from a magazine or newspaper.

Presbyopia, the decrease in power of accommodation with aging, is suggested when the person moves the card farther away.

14-10

NORMAL RANGE OF FINDINGS   **ABNORMAL FINDINGS**

TEST VISUAL FIELDS

Confrontation Test

This is a gross measure of peripheral vision. It compares the person's peripheral vision with your own, assuming yours is normal (Fig. 14–11). Position yourself at eye level with the person, about 2 ft away. Direct the person to cover one eye with an opaque card, and with the other eye to look straight at you. Cover your own eye opposite to the person's covered one. Hold a pencil or your flicking finger as a target midline between you and the other person, and slowly advance it in from the periphery in several directions.

14-11

Ask the person to say "now" as the target is first seen; this should be just as you see the object also. (This works with all but the temporal visual field, with which you would need a 6-ft arm to avoid being seen initially! With the temporal direction, start the object somewhat behind the person.) Estimate the angle between the anteroposterior axis of the eye and the peripheral axis where the object is first seen. Normal results are about 50 degrees upward, 90 degrees temporal, 70 degrees down, and 60 degrees nasal (Fig. 14–12).

If the person is unable to see the object as examiner does, the test suggests peripheral field loss. Refer to an optometrist for more precise testing using a tangent screen (see Table 14–1 on p. 330).

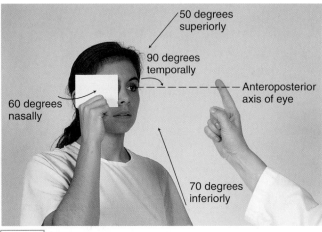

50 degrees superiorly

90 degrees temporally

Anteroposterior axis of eye

60 degrees nasally

70 degrees inferiorly

14–12 Range of peripheral vision.

NORMAL RANGE OF FINDINGS	ABNORMAL FINDINGS

INSPECT EXTRAOCULAR MUSCLE FUNCTION

Corneal Light Reflex (The Hirschberg Test)

Assess the parallel alignment of the eye axes by shining a light toward the person's eyes. Direct the person to stare straight ahead as you hold the light about 30 cm (12 inches) away. Note the reflection of the light on the corneas; it should be in exactly the same spot on each eye. See Figure 14–33 for symmetry of the corneal light reflex.

Asymmetry of the light reflex indicates deviation in alignment due to eye muscle weakness or paralysis. If you see this, perform the cover test.

Cover Test

This test detects small degrees of deviated alignment by interrupting the fusion reflex that normally keeps the two eyes parallel. Ask the person to stare straight ahead at your nose even though the gaze may be interrupted. With an opaque card, cover one eye. As it is covered, note the uncovered eye. A normal response is a steady fixed gaze (Fig. 14–13, *A*).

Meanwhile, the macular image has been suppressed on the covered eye. If muscle weakness exists, the covered eye will drift into a relaxed position. Now uncover the eye and observe it for movement. It should stare straight ahead (Fig. 14–13, *B*). If it jumps to reestablish fixation, eye muscle weakness exists. Repeat with the other eye.

If the eye jumps to fixate on the designated point, it was out of alignment before.

A **phoria** is a mild weakness noted only when fusion is blocked. **Tropia** is more severe—a constant malalignment of the eyes (see Table 14–2).

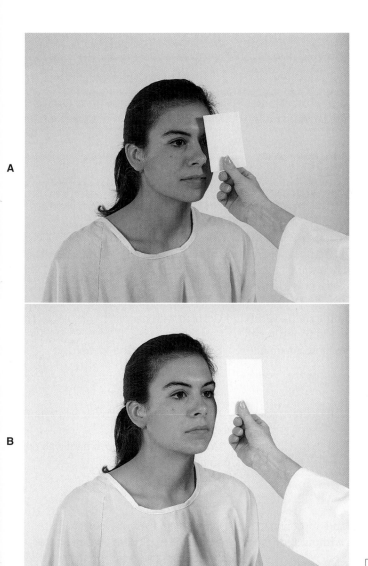

A

B

14–13

NORMAL RANGE OF FINDINGS	ABNORMAL FINDINGS

Diagnostic Positions Test

Leading the eyes through the six cardinal positions of gaze will elicit any muscle weakness during movement (Fig. 14–14). Ask the person to hold the head steady and to follow the movement of your finger, pen, or penlight only with the eyes. Hold the target back about 12 inches so the person can focus on it comfortably, and move it to each of the six positions, hold it momentarily, then back to center. Progress clockwise. A normal response is parallel tracking of the object with both eyes.

Eye movement is not parallel. Failure to follow in a certain direction indicates weakness of an extraocular muscle (EOM) or dysfunction of cranial nerve innervating it.

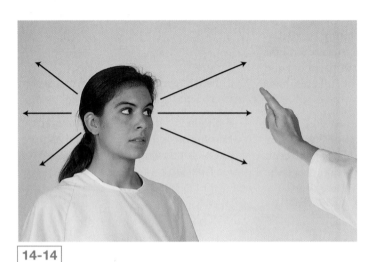

14-14

In addition to parallel movement, note any **nystagmus,** a fine oscillating movement best seen around the iris. Mild nystagmus at extreme lateral gaze is normal; nystagmus at any other position is not.

Nystagmus occurs with disease of the semicircular canals in the ears, a paretic eye muscle, multiple sclerosis, or brain lesions.

Finally, note that the upper eyelid continues to overlap the superior part of the iris, even during downward movement. You should not see a white rim of sclera between the lid and the iris. If noted, this is termed "lid lag."

Lid lag occurs with hyperthyroidism.

INSPECT EXTERNAL OCULAR STRUCTURES

Begin with the most external points, and logically work your way inward.

General

Already you will have noted the person's ability to move around the room, with vision functioning well enough to avoid obstacles, and to respond to your directions. Also note the facial expression; a relaxed expression accompanies adequate vision.

Groping with hands.

Squinting or craning forward.

Eyebrows

Normally the eyebrows are present bilaterally, move symmetrically as the facial expression changes, and have no scaling or lesions.

Absent lateral third of brow with hypothyroidism.
Unequal or absent movement with nerve damage.
Scaling with seborrhea.

Eyelids and Lashes

The upper lids normally overlap the superior part of the iris, and approximate completely with the lower lids when closed. The skin is intact without redness, swelling, discharge, or lesions.

Lid lag with hyperthyroidism.
Incomplete closure creates risk for corneal damage.

NORMAL RANGE OF FINDINGS

The palpebral fissures are horizontal in non-Asians, whereas Asians normally have an upward slant.

Note that the eyelashes are evenly distributed along the lid margins and curve outward.

Eyeballs
The eyeballs are aligned normally in their sockets with no protrusion or sunken appearance. Blacks normally may have a slight protrusion of the eyeball beyond the supraorbital ridge.

Conjunctiva and Sclera
Ask the person to look up. Using your thumbs, slide the lower lids down along the bony orbital rim. Take care not to push against the eyeball. Inspect the exposed area (Fig. 14–15). The eyeball looks moist and glossy. Numerous small

14-15

blood vessels normally show through the transparent conjunctiva. Otherwise, the conjunctivae are clear and show the normal color of the structure below—pink over the lower lids and white over the sclera. Note any color change, swelling, or lesions.

The sclera is china white, although blacks occasionally have a gray-blue or "muddy" color to the sclera. Also in dark-skinned people, you normally may see small brown macules (like freckles) on the sclera, which should not be confused with foreign bodies or petechiae. Lastly, blacks may have yellowish fatty deposits beneath the lids away from the cornea. Do not confuse these yellow spots with the overall scleral, yellowing that accompanies jaundice.

ABNORMAL FINDINGS

Ptosis, drooping of upper lid.
Periorbital edema, lesions (see Tables 14–3 and 14–4 on pp. 332 and 334).

Ectropion and entropion (see Table 14–3).

Exophthalmos (protruding eyes) and enophthalmos (sunken eyes) (see Table 14–3).

General reddening (see Table 14–5).
Cyanosis of the lower lids.
Pallor near the outer canthus of the lower lid may indicate anemia (the inner canthus normally contains less pigment).

Scleral icterus is an even yellowing of the sclera extending up to the cornea, indicating jaundice.
Tenderness, foreign body, discharge, or lesions.

Eversion of the Upper Lid

This maneuver is not part of the normal examination, but it is useful when you must inspect the conjunctiva of the upper lid, as with eye pain or suspicion of a foreign body. Most people are apprehensive of any eye manipulation. Enhance their cooperation by using a calm and gentle, yet deliberate, approach.

1. Ask the person to keep both eyes open and look down. This relaxes the eyelid, whereas closing it would tense the orbicularis muscle.
2. Slide the upper lid up along the bony orbit to lift up the eyelashes.
3. Grasp the lashes between your thumb and forefinger and gently pull down and outward.
4. With your other hand, place the tip of an applicator stick on the upper lid above the level of the internal tarsal plates (Fig. 14–16).

14-16

5. Gently push down with the stick as you lift the lashes up. This uses the edge of the tarsal plate as a fulcrum and flips the lid inside out. Take special care not to push in on the eyeball.
6. Secure the everted position by holding the lashes against the bony orbital rim (Fig. 14–17).

14-17

NORMAL RANGE OF FINDINGS

7. Inspect for any color change, swelling, lesion, or foreign body.
8. To return to normal position, gently pull the lashes outward as the person looks up.

Lacrimal Apparatus

Ask the person to look down. With your thumbs, slide the outer part of the upper lid up along the bony orbit. Inspect for any redness or swelling.

Normally the puncta drain the tears into the lacrimal sac. Presence of excessive tearing may indicate blockage of the nasolacrimal duct. Check this by pressing the index finger against the sac, just inside the lower orbital rim, not against the side of the nose (Fig. 14–18). Pressure will slightly evert the lower lid, but there should be no other response to pressure.

14-18

INSPECT ANTERIOR EYEBALL STRUCTURES

Cornea and Lens

Shine a light from the side across the cornea, and check for smoothness and clarity. This oblique view highlights any abnormal irregularities in the corneal surface. There should be no opacities (cloudiness) in the cornea, the anterior chamber, or the lens behind the pupil. Do not confuse an **arcus senilis** with an opacity. The arcus senilis is a normal finding in aging persons and is illustrated on p. 325.

Iris and Pupil

The iris normally appears flat, with a round regular shape and even coloration. Note the size, shape, and equality of the pupils. Normally the pupils appear round, regular, and of equal size in both eyes. In the adult, resting size is from 3 to 5 mm. A small number of people (5%) normally have pupils of two different sizes, which is termed **anisocoria.**

ABNORMAL FINDINGS

Swelling of the lacrimal gland may show as a visible bulge in the outer part of the upper lid.

Puncta red, swollen, tender to pressure. Watch for any regurgitation of fluid out of the puncta, which confirms duct blockage.

A corneal abrasion causes irregular ridges in reflected light, producing a shattered look to light rays (see Table 14–6).

Irregular shape.

Although they may be normal, all unequally sized pupils call for a consideration of central nervous system injury.

NORMAL RANGE OF FINDINGS	ABNORMAL FINDINGS

NORMAL RANGE OF FINDINGS

To test the **pupillary light reflex,** darken the room and ask the person to gaze into the distance. (This dilates the pupils.) Advance a light in from the side* and note the response. Normally you will see (1) constriction of the same-sided pupil (a *direct light reflex*), and (2) simultaneous constriction of the other pupil (a *consensual light reflex*).

In the acute care setting, gauge the pupil size in millimeters, both before and after the light reflex. Recording the pupil size in millimeters is more accurate when many nurses and physicians care for the same person, or when small changes may be significant signs of increasing intracranial pressure. Normally, the resting size is 3, 4, or 5 mm and decreases equally in response to light. A normal response is designated by:

$$R\frac{3}{1} = \frac{3}{1}L$$

This indicates that both pupils measure 3 mm in the resting state and that both constrict to 1 mm in response to light. A graduated scale printed on a handheld vision screener or taped onto a tongue blade facilitates your measurement (see Fig. 23–57 in Chapter 23).

Test for **accommodation** by asking the person to focus on a distant object (Fig. 14–19). This process dilates the pupils. Then have the person shift the gaze to a near object, such as your finger held about 7 to 8 cm (3 inches) from the nose. A normal response includes (1) pupillary constriction and (2) convergence of the axes of the eyes.

14–19 Far vision—pupils dilate.   Near vision—pupils constrict.

Record the normal response to all these maneuvers as PERRLA, or Pupils Equal, Round, React to Light and Accommodation.

INSPECT THE OCULAR FUNDUS

The ophthalmoscope enlarges your view of the eye so that you can inspect the **media** (anterior chamber, lens, vitreous) and the **ocular fundus** (the internal surface of the retina). It accomplishes this by directing a beam of light through the pupil to illuminate the inner structures. Thus, using the ophthalmoscope is like peering through a keyhole (the pupil) into an interesting room beyond.

*Always advance the light in from the *side* to test the light reflex. If you advance from the front, the pupils will constrict to accommodate for near vision. Thus you do not know what the pure response to the light would have been.

ABNORMAL FINDINGS

Dilated pupils.
Dilated and fixed pupils.
Constricted pupils.

Unequal or no response to light (see Table 14–7).

Absence of constriction or convergence.
Asymmetric response.

The ophthalmoscope should function as an appendage of your own eye. This takes some practice. Practice holding the instrument and focusing at objects around the room before you approach a "real" person. Hold the ophthalmoscope right up to your eye, braced firmly against the cheek and brow. Extend your index finger onto the lens selector dial so that you can refocus as needed during the procedure without taking your head away from the ophthalmoscope to look. Now look about the room, moving your head and the instrument together as one unit. Keep both your eyes open; just view the field through the ophthalmoscope.

Recall that the ophthalmoscope contains a set of lenses that control the focus (Fig. 14–20). The unit of strength of each lens is the *diopter*. The black numbers indicate a positive diopter; they focus on objects nearer in space to the ophthalmoscope. The red numbers show a negative diopter and are for focusing on objects farther away.

14–20

To examine a person, darken the room to help dilate the pupils. (Dilating eyedrops are not needed during a screening examination. When indicated, they dilate the pupils for a wider look at the fundus background and macular area. Eyedrops are used only when glaucoma can be completely ruled out, because dilating the pupils in the presence of glaucoma can precipitate an acute episode.) Remove eyeglasses from yourself or the other person; they obstruct close movement and you can compensate for their correction by using the diopter setting. Contact lenses may be left in; they pose no problem as long as they are clean.

Select the large round aperture with the white light for the routine examination. If the pupils are small, use the smaller white light. (Although the instrument has other shape and colored apertures, these are rarely used in a screening examination.) The light must have maximum brightness; replace old or dim batteries.

NORMAL RANGE OF FINDINGS	ABNORMAL FINDINGS

Tell the person, "Please keep looking at that light switch (or mark) on the wall across the room, even though my head will get in the way." Staring at a distant fixed object helps to dilate the pupils and to hold the retinal structures still.

Match sides with the person. That is, hold the ophthalmoscope in your *right* hand up to your *right* eye to view the person's *right* eye. You must do this to avoid bumping noses during the procedure. Place your free hand on the person's shoulder or forehead (Fig. 14–21, *A*). This helps orient you in space, because once you have the ophthalmoscope in position, you only have a very narrow range of vision. Also, your thumb can anchor the upper lid and help prevent blinking.

14–21

A

Begin about 25 cm (10 inches) away from the person at an angle about 15 degrees lateral to the person's line of vision. Note the red glow filling the person's pupil. This the **red reflex,** caused by the reflection of your ophthalmoscope light off the inner retina. Keep sight of the red reflex, and steadily move closer to the eye. If you lose the red reflex, the light has wandered off the pupil and onto the iris or sclera. Adjust your angle to find it again.

As you advance, adjust the lens to +6 and note any opacities in the media. These appear as dark shadows or black dots interrupting the red reflex. Normally, none are present.

Cataracts appear as opaque black areas against the red reflex (see Table 14–8).

14–21

B

NORMAL RANGE OF FINDINGS	ABNORMAL FINDINGS

Progress toward the person until your foreheads almost touch (Fig. 14–21, *B*). Adjust the diopter setting to bring the ocular fundus into sharp focus. If you and the person have normal vision, this should be at 0. Moving the diopters compensates for nearsightedness or farsightedness. Use the red lenses for nearsighted eyes and the black for farsighted eyes (Fig. 14–22).

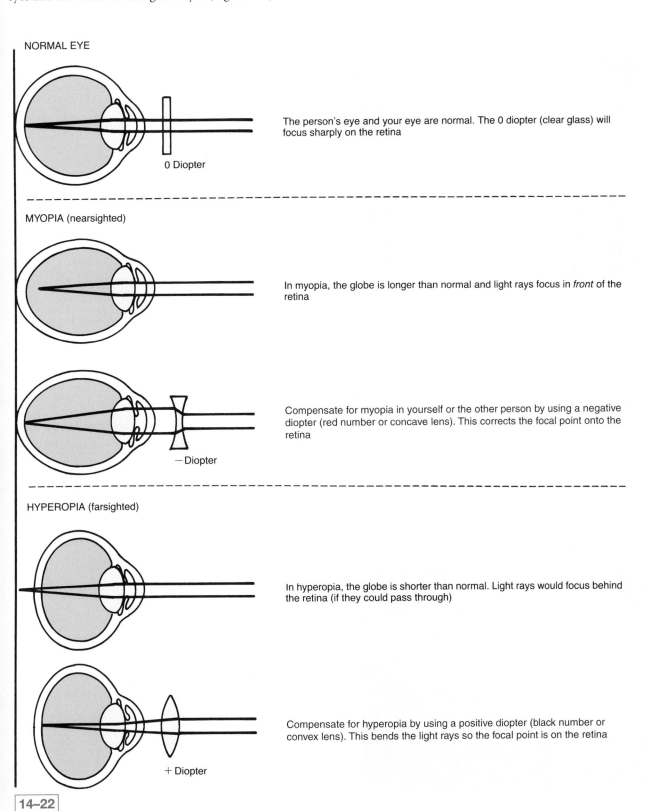

NORMAL EYE

0 Diopter

The person's eye and your eye are normal. The 0 diopter (clear glass) will focus sharply on the retina

MYOPIA (nearsighted)

In myopia, the globe is longer than normal and light rays focus in *front* of the retina

— Diopter

Compensate for myopia in yourself or the other person by using a negative diopter (red number or concave lens). This corrects the focal point onto the retina

HYPEROPIA (farsighted)

In hyperopia, the globe is shorter than normal. Light rays would focus behind the retina (if they could pass through)

+ Diopter

Compensate for hyperopia by using a positive diopter (black number or convex lens). This bends the light rays so the focal point is on the retina

14–22

NORMAL RANGE OF FINDINGS

ABNORMAL FINDINGS

Moving in on the 15-degree lateral line should bring your view just to the optic disc. If the disc is not in sight, track a blood vessel as it grows larger and it will lead you to the disc. Systematically inspect the structures in the ocular fundus: (1) optic disc, (2) retinal vessels, (3) general background, and (4) macula (Fig. 14–23). (Note the illustration here shows a large area of the fundus. Your actual view through the ophthalmoscope is much smaller—slightly larger than 1 disc diameter.)

14–23 Normal ocular fundus.

Optic Disc

The most prominent landmark is the optic disc, located on the nasal side of the retina. Explore these characteristics:

1. **Color**	Creamy yellow-orange to pink.
2. **Shape**	Round or oval.
3. **Margins**	Distinct and sharply demarcated, although the nasal edge may be slightly fuzzy.
4. **Cup-disc ratio**	Distinctness varies. When visible, physiologic cup is a brighter yellow-white than rest of the disc. Its width is not more than one half the disc diameter.

Two normal variations may occur around the disc margins. A **scleral crescent** is a gray-white new moon shape (Fig. 14–24). It occurs when pigment is absent in the choroid layer and you are looking directly at the sclera. A **pigment crescent** is black; it is due to accumulation of pigment in the choroid.

14–24 Scleral crescent.

Pallor. Hyperemia.
Irregular.
Blurred margins.

Cup extending to the disc border (see Table 14–9).

NORMAL RANGE OF FINDINGS

The diameter of the disc, or DD, is a standard of measure for other fundus structures (Fig. 14–25). To describe a finding, note its clock-face position as well as its relationship to the disc in size and distance (e.g., "...at 5:00, 3 DD from the disc").

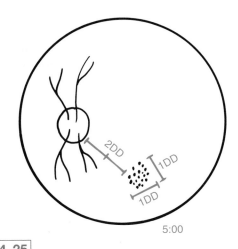

5:00

14–25

Retinal Vessels

This is the only place in the body where you can view blood vessels directly. Many systemic diseases that affect the vascular system show signs in the retinal vessels. Follow a paired artery and vein out to the periphery in the four quadrants (see Fig. 14–23), noting these points:

1. **Number**	A paired artery and vein pass to each quadrant. Vessels look straighter at the nasal side.
2. **Color**	Arteries are brighter red than veins. Also, they have the arterial light reflex, with a thin stripe of light down the middle.
3. **A:V ratio**	The ratio comparing the artery-to-vein width is 2:3 or 4:5.
4. **Caliber**	Arteries and veins show a regular decrease in caliber as they extend to periphery.
5. **A-V (arteriovenous) crossing**	An artery and vein may cross paths. This is not significant if within 2 DD of disc and if no sign of interruption in blood flow is seen. There should be no indenting or displacing of vessel.
6. **Tortuosity**	Mild vessel twisting when present in both eyes is usually congenital and not significant.
7. **Pulsations**	Present in veins near disc as their drainage meets the intermittent pressure of arterial systole. (Often hard to see.)

General Background of the Fundus

The color normally varies from light red to dark brown-red, generally corresponding with the person's skin color. Your view of the fundus should be clear; no lesions should obstruct the retinal structures.

ABNORMAL FINDINGS

Absence of major vessels.

Arteries too constricted.
Veins dilated.

Focal constriction.
Neovascularization.

Crossings more than 2 DD away from disc.
Nicking or pinching of underlying vessel.
Vessel engorged peripheral to crossing (see Table 14–10).

Extreme tortuosity or marked asymmetry in two eyes.

Absent pulsations.

Abnormal lesions: hemorrhages, exudates, microaneurysms.

NORMAL RANGE OF FINDINGS	ABNORMAL FINDINGS

Macula

The macula is 1 DD in size and located 2 DD temporal to the disc. Inspect this area last in the funduscopic examination. A bright light on this area of central vision causes some watering and discomfort and pupillary constriction. Note that the normal color of the area is somewhat darker than the rest of the fundus but is even and homogeneous. Clumped pigment may occur with aging.

Clumped pigment occurs with trauma or retinal detachment.

Within the macula, you may note the foveal light reflex. This is a tiny white glistening dot reflecting your ophthalmoscope light.

Hemorrhage or exudate in the macula occurs with senile macular degeneration.

 DEVELOPMENTAL CONSIDERATIONS

Infants and Children

The eye examination is often deferred at birth because of transient edema of the lids from birth trauma or from the instillation of silver nitrate at birth. The eyes should be examined within a few days and at every well child visit thereafter.

VISUAL ACUITY. The child's age determines the screening measures used. With a newborn, test visual reflexes and attending behaviors. Test **light perception** using the blink reflex; the neonate blinks in response to bright light (Fig. 14–26). Also, the pupillary light reflex shows that the pupils constrict in response to light. These reflexes indicate that the lower portion of the visual apparatus is intact. But you cannot infer that the infant can *see;* that requires later observation to show that the brain has received images and can interpret them.

Absent blinking.
Absent pupillary light reflex, especially after 3 weeks, indicates blindness.

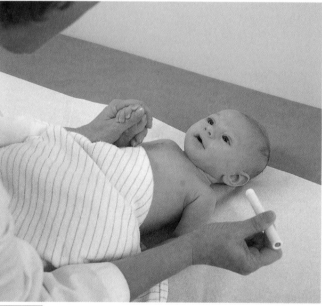

14–26

As you introduce an object to the infant's line of vision, note these attending behaviors:

Birth to 2 weeks—Refusal to reopen eyes after exposure to bright light; increasing alertness to object; infant may fixate on an object.
By 2 to 4 weeks—Infant can fixate on an object.
By 1 month—Infant can fixate and follow a light or bright toy.
By 3 to 4 months—Infant can fixate, follow, and reach for the toy.
By 6 to 10 months—Infant can fixate and follow the toy in all directions.

NORMAL RANGE OF FINDINGS

The Allen test (picture cards) screens children from $2\frac{1}{2}$ years to 2 years and 11 months of age and is even reliable with cooperative toddlers as young as 2 years of age. The test contains seven cards of familiar objects (birthday cake, teddy bear, tree, house, car, telephone, and horse and rider). First, show the pictures up close to the child to make sure the child can identify them. Then, present each picture at a distance of 15 ft. Results are normal if the child can name three out of seven cards within three to five trials.

Use a picture chart or the Snellen E chart for the preschooler from 3 to 6 years of age. The E chart shows the capital letter E in varying sizes pointing in different directions. The child points his or her fingers in the direction the "table legs" are pointing. By 7 to 8 years of age when the child is familiar with reading letters, begin to use the standard Snellen alphabet chart. Normally a child achieves 20/20 acuity by 6 to 7 years of age (Fig. 14–27).

ABNORMAL FINDINGS

The National Society for Prevention of Blindness states these criteria for referral:

1. Age 3—vision 20/50 or less in either eye.
2. Age 4 and over—20/40 or less in either eye.
3. Difference between two eyes is one line or more.
4. Child shows other signs of vision impairment, regardless of acuity.

Screen two separate times before referral.

14–27

NORMAL RANGE OF FINDINGS

ABNORMAL FINDINGS

VISUAL FIELDS. Assess peripheral vision with the confrontation test in children older than 3 years when the preschooler is able to stay in position. As with the adult, the child should see the moving target at the same time your normal eyes do. Often a young child forgets to say "now" or "stop" as the moving object is seen. Rather, note the instant the child's eyes deviate or head shifts position to gaze at the moving object. Match this nearly automatic response with your own sighting.

COLOR VISION. Color blindness is an inherited recessive X-linked trait affecting about 8% of white males and 4% of black males. It is rare in females (0.4%). "Color deficient" is a more accurate term, because the condition is relative and not disabling. Often, it is just a social inconvenience, although it may affect the person's ability to discern traffic lights, or it may affect school performance in which color is a learning tool.

Test only boys for color vision, once between the ages of 4 and 8. Use Ishihara's test, a series of polychromatic cards. Each card has a pattern of dots printed against a background of many colored dots. Ask the child to identify each pattern. A boy with normal color vision can see each pattern. A color blind person cannot see the letter against the field color.

EXTRAOCULAR MUSCLE FUNCTION. Testing for **strabismus** (squint, crossed eye) is an important screening measure during early childhood. Strabismus causes disconjugate vision because one eye deviates off the fixation point. To avoid diplopia or unclear images, the brain begins to suppress data from the weak eye (a suppression scotoma). Then visual acuity in this otherwise normal eye begins to deteriorate from disuse. Early recognition and treatment are essential to restore binocular vision. Diagnosis after 6 years of age has a poor prognosis. Test malalignment by the corneal light reflex and the cover test.

Check the **corneal light reflex** by shining a light toward the child's eyes. The light should be reflected at exactly the same spot in the two corneas (see Fig. 14–29 on p. 323). Some asymmetry (where one light falls off center) under 6 months of age is normal.

Perform the **cover test** on all children as described on p. 309. Some examiners omit the opaque card and place their hand on the child's head. The examiner's thumb extends down and blocks vision over the eye without actually touching the eye. One can use a familiar character puppet to attract the child's attention. The normal results are the same as those listed in the adult section.

Function of the extraocular muscles during movement can be assessed during the early weeks by the child's following a brightly colored toy as a target. An older infant can sit on the parent's lap as you move the toy in all directions. After 2 years of age, direct the child's gaze through the six cardinal positions of gaze. You may stabilize the child's chin with your hand to prevent him or her from moving the entire head.

EXTERNAL EYE STRUCTURES. Inspect the ocular structures as described in the earlier section. A neonate usually holds the eyes tightly shut. Do not attempt to pry them open; that just increases contraction of the orbicularis oculi muscle. Hold the newborn supine and gently lower the head; the eyes will open. Also, the eyes will open when you hold the infant at arm's length and slowly turn the infant in one direction (Fig. 14–28). In addition to inspecting the ocular structures, this also tests the vestibular function reflex. That is, the baby's eyes will look in the same direction as the body is being turned. When the turning stops, the eyes will shift to the opposite direction after a few quick beats of nystagmus. Also termed "doll's eyes," this reflex disappears by 2 months of age.

Untreated strabismus can lead to permanent visual damage. The resulting loss of vision due to disuse is **amblyopia ex anopsia.**

Asymmetry in the corneal light reflex after 6 months is abnormal and must be referred.

NORMAL RANGE OF FINDINGS	ABNORMAL FINDINGS

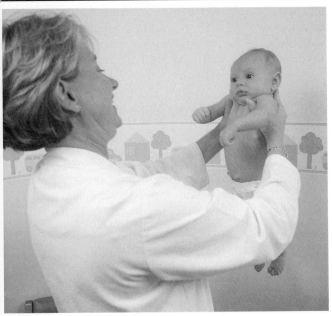

14–28

EYELIDS AND LASHES. Normally the upper lids overlie the superior part of the iris. In newborns the *setting-sun sign* is common. The eyes appear to deviate down, and you see a white rim of sclera over the iris. It may show as you rapidly change the neonate from a sitting to a supine position.

Many infants have an *epicanthal fold,* an excess skinfold extending over the inner corner of the eye, partly or totally overlapping the inner canthus. It occurs frequently in Asian children and in 20% of whites. In non-Asians it disappears as the child grows, usually by 10 years of age. While they are present, epicanthal folds give a false appearance of malalignment, termed **pseudostrabismus** (Fig. 14–29). Yet the corneal light reflex is normal.

14–29 Pseudostrabismus.

Asian infants normally have an upward slant of the palpebral fissures. Entropion, a turning inward of the eyelid, is found normally in some Asian children. If the lashes do not abrade the corneas, it is not significant.

The setting-sun sign also occurs with hydrocephalus as the globes protrude.

Blank sunken eyes accompany malnutrition, dehydration, and a severe illness.

An upward lateral slope together with epicanthal folds and hypertelorism (large spacing between eyes) occurs with Down syndrome.

NORMAL RANGE OF FINDINGS

ABNORMAL FINDINGS

CONJUNCTIVA AND SCLERA. A newborn may have a transient chemical conjunctivitis due to the instillation of silver nitrate. This appears within 1 hour and lasts not more than 24 hours after birth. The sclera should be white and clear, although it may have a blue tint due to thinness at birth. The lacrimal glands are not functional at birth.

Ophthalmia neonatorum (conjunctivitis of the newborn) is a purulent discharge due to a chemical irritant or a bacterial or viral agent from the birth canal.

IRIS AND PUPILS. The iris normally is blue or slate gray in light-skinned newborns and brown in dark-skinned infants. By 6 to 9 months, the permanent color is differentiated. Brushfield's spots, or white specks around the edge of the iris, occasionally may be normal.

Absence of iris color occurs with albinism.
Brushfield's spots usually suggest Down syndrome.

A searching nystagmus is common just after birth. The pupils are small but constrict to light.

Constant nystagmus, prolonged setting-sun sign, marked strabismus, and slow lateral movements suggest vision loss.

THE OCULAR FUNDUS. The amount of data gathered during the funduscopic examination depends on the child's ability to hold the eyes still and on your ability to glean as much data as possible in a brief period of time.

A complete funduscopic examination is difficult to perform on an infant, but at least check the red reflex when the infant fixates at the bright light for a few seconds. Note any interruption.

An interruption in the red reflex indicates an opacity in the cornea or lens. An absent red reflex occurs with congenital cataracts or retinal disorders.

Perform a funduscopic examination on an infant between 2 and 6 months of age. Position the infant (up to 18 months) lying on the table. The fundus appears pale, and the vessels are not fully developed. There is no foveal light reflection because the macula area will not be mature until 1 year.

Papilledema is rare in the infant because the fontanels and open sutures will absorb any increased intracranial pressure if it occurs.

Inspect the fundus of the young child and school-age child as described in the preceding section on the adult. Allow the child to handle the equipment. Explain why you are darkening the room and that you will leave a small light on. Assure the child that the procedure will not hurt. Direct the young child to look at an appealing picture, perhaps a toy or an animal, during the examination.

The Aging Adult

VISUAL ACUITY. Perform the same examination as described in the adult section. Central acuity may decrease, particularly after 70 years of age. Peripheral vision may be diminished.

OCULAR STRUCTURES. The eyebrows may show a loss of the outer one third to one half of hair due to a decrease in hair follicles. The remaining brow hair is coarse (Fig. 14–30). As a result of atrophy of elastic tissues, the skin around the eyes may show wrinkles or crow's feet. The upper lid may be so elongated as to rest on the lashes, resulting in a pseudoptosis.

14–30

NORMAL RANGE OF FINDINGS

The eyes may appear sunken due to atrophy of the orbital fat. Also, the orbital fat may herniate, causing bulging at the lower lids and inner third of the upper lids.

The lacrimal apparatus may decrease tear production, causing the eyes to look dry and lusterless and the person to report a burning sensation. **Pingueculae** commonly show on the sclera (Fig. 14–31). These yellowish elevated nodules are due to a thickening of the bulbar conjunctiva from prolonged exposure to sun, wind, and dust. Pingueculae appear at the 3 and 9 o'clock positions—first on the nasal side, then on the temporal side.

14–31 Pinguecula.

The cornea may look cloudy with age. An **arcus senilis** is commonly seen around the cornea (Fig. 14–32). This is a gray-white arc or circle around the limbus; it is due to deposition of lipid material. As more lipid accumulates, the cornea may look thickened and raised, but the arcus has no effect on vision.

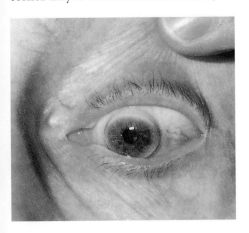

14–32 Arcus senilis.

Xanthelasma are soft, raised yellow plaques occurring on the lids at the inner canthus (Fig. 14–33). They commonly occur around the fifth decade of life and more frequently in women. They occur with both high and normal blood levels of cholesterol and have no pathologic significance.

14–33 Xanthelasma.

Pupils are small in old age, and the pupillary light reflex may be slowed. The lens loses transparency and looks opaque.

ABNORMAL FINDINGS

Ectropion (lower lid dropping away) and entropion (lower lid turning in) (see Table 14–3).

Distinguish from the abnormal **pterygium**, also an opacity on the bulbar conjunctiva, but one that grows over the cornea (see Table 14–6).

NORMAL RANGE OF FINDINGS

THE OCULAR FUNDUS. Retinal structures generally have less shine. The blood vessels look paler, narrower, and attenuated. Arterioles appear paler and straighter, with a narrower light reflex. More arteriovenous crossing defects occur.

A normal development on the retinal surface is **drusen,** or benign degenerative hyaline deposits (Fig. 14–34). They are small, round, yellow dots that are scattered haphazardly on the retina. Although they do not occur in a pattern, they are usually symmetrically placed in the two eyes. They have no effect on vision.

14–34 Drusen.

ABNORMAL FINDINGS

Drusen are easily confused with the abnormal finding *hard exudates,* which occur with a more circular or linear pattern (see Table 14–11).

SUMMARY CHECKLIST: Eye Exam

1. Test visual acuity
Snellen eye chart
Near vision (those older than 40 years or those having difficulty reading)

2. Test visual fields—confrontation test

3. Inspect extraocular muscle function
Corneal light reflex (Hirschberg test)
Cover test
Diagnostic positions test

4. Inspect external eye structures
General
Eyebrows
Eyelids and lashes
Eyeball alignment
Conjunctiva and sclera
Lacrimal apparatus

5. Inspect anterior eyeball structures
Cornea and lens
Iris and pupil
Size, shape, and equality
Pupillary light reflex
Accommodation

6. Inspect the ocular fundus
Optic disc (color, shape, margins, cup-disc ratio)
Retinal vessels (number, color, artery-vein [A : V] ratio, caliber, arteriovenous crossings, tortuosity, pulsations)
General background (color, integrity)
Macula

 See Health Promotion Guide on CD

Application and Critical Thinking

SAMPLE CHARTING

SUBJECTIVE

Vision reported good with no recent change. No eye pain, no inflammation, no discharge, no lesions. Wears no corrective lenses, vision last tested 1 year PTA, test for glaucoma at that time was normal.

OBJECTIVE

Snellen chart—O.D. 20/20, O.S. 20/20 −1. Fields normal by confrontation. Corneal light reflex symmetric bilaterally. Diagnostic positions test shows EOMs intact. Brows and lashes present. No ptosis. Conjunctiva clear. Sclera white. No lesions. PERRLA.

Fundi: Red reflex present bilaterally. Discs flat with sharp margins. Vessels present in all quadrants without crossing defects. Retinal background has even color with no hemorrhages or exudates. Macula has even color.

FOCUSED ASSESSMENT: CLINICAL CASE STUDY 1

Emma K. is a 34-year-old married, white, female homemaker, brought to the Emergency Department by police following a reported domestic quarrel.

SUBJECTIVE

States husband struck her about the face and eyes with his fists about 1 hour PTA. "I ruined the dinner again. I can't do anything right." Pain in left cheek and both eyes felt immediately and continues. Alarmed at "bright red blood on eyeball." No bleeding from eye area or cheek. Vision intact just after trauma. Now reports difficulty opening lids.

OBJECTIVE

Sitting quietly and hunched over, hands over eyes. Voice tired and flat. L cheek swollen and discolored, no laceration. Lids edematous and discolored both eyes. No skin laceration. L lid swollen almost shut. L eye—round 1-mm bright red patch over lateral aspect of globe. No active bleeding out of eye, iris intact, anterior chamber clear. R eye—conjunctiva clear, sclera white, cornea and iris intact, anterior chamber clear. PERRLA. Pupils R 4/1 = 4/1 L. Vision 14/14 both eyes by Jaeger card.

ASSESSMENT

Ecchymoses L cheek and both eyes
Subconjunctival hemorrhage L eye
Pain R/T inflammation
Chronic low self-esteem R/T effects of domestic violence

FOCUSED ASSESSMENT: CLINICAL CASE STUDY 2

Sam T. is a 63-year-old married, white, male postal carrier admitted to the Medical Center for surgery for suspected brain tumor. Following postanesthesia recovery, Sam T. is admitted to the Neurology ICU, awake, lethargic with slowed but correct verbal responses, oriented × 3, moving all four extremities, vital signs stable. Pupils R 4/2 = 4/2 L with sluggish response. Assessments are made q 15 minutes.

SUBJECTIVE

No response now to verbal stimuli.

OBJECTIVE

Semicomatose—no response to verbal stimuli, does withdraw R arm and leg purposefully to painful stimuli. No movement L arm or leg. Pupils R 5/5 ≠ L 4/2. Vitals remain stable as noted on graphic sheet.

ASSESSMENT

Unilateral dilated and fixed R pupil
Clouding of consciousness
Focal motor deficit—no movement L side
Ineffective tissue perfusion R/T interruption of cerebral flow

Continued

FOCUSED ASSESSMENT: CLINICAL CASE STUDY 3

Trung Q. is a 4-year-old male born in Southeast Asia who arrived in this country 1 month PTA. Lives with parents, 2 siblings. Speaks only native language; here with uncle, who acts as interpreter.

SUBJECTIVE

Seeks care because RN in church sponsoring family noted "crossed eyes." Uncle states vision seemed normal to parents. Plays with toys and manipulates small objects without difficulty. Identifies objects in picture books; does not read.

OBJECTIVE

With uncle interpreting directions for test to Trung, vision by Snellen **E** chart—O.D. 20/30, O.S. 20/50 −1. Fields seem intact by confrontation—jerks head to gaze at object entering field.

EOMs—asymmetric corneal light reflex with outward deviation L eye. Cover test—as R eye covered, L eye jerks to fixate, R eye steady when uncovered. As L eye covered, R eye holds steady gaze, L eye jerks to fixate as uncovered. Diagnostic positions—able to gaze in six positions, although L eye obviously malaligned at extreme medial gaze.

Eye structures—brows and lashes present and normal bilaterally. Upward palpebral slant, epicanthal folds bilaterally—consistent with racial heritage. Conjunctiva clear, sclera white, iris intact, PERRLA.

Fundi—discs flat with sharp margins. Observed vessels normal. Unable to see in all four quadrants, unable to see macular area.

ASSESSMENT

L exotropia
Abnormal vision in L eye
Disturbed visual sensory perception R/T effects of neurologic impairment

FOCUSED ASSESSMENT: CLINICAL CASE STUDY 4

Vera K. is an 87-year-old widowed, black, female homemaker, living independently, who is admitted to hospital for observation and adjustment of digitalis medication. Cardiac status has been stable during hospital stay.

SUBJECTIVE

Reports desire to monitor own medication at home but fears problems due to blurred vision. First noted distant vision blurred 5 years ago but near vision seemed to improve at that time, "I started to read better without my glasses!" Since then, blurring at distant vision has increased, near vision now blurred also.

Able to navigate home environment without difficulty. Fixes simple meals with cold foods. Receives hot meal from "Meals on Wheels" at lunch. Enjoys television, though it looks somewhat blurred. Unable to write letters, sew, or read paper, which she regrets.

OBJECTIVE

Vision by Jaeger card O.D. 20/200, O.S. 20/400 −1, with glasses on. Fields intact by confrontation. EOMS intact. Brow hair absent lateral third. Upper lids have folds of redundant skin but lids do not droop. Lower lids and lashes intact. Xanthelasma present both inner canthi. Conjunctiva clear, sclera white, iris intact, L pupil looks cloudy, PERRLA, pupils R 3/2 = 3/2 L.

Fundi: Red reflex has central dark spot both eyes. Discs flat, with sharp margins. Observed vessels normal. Unable to see in all four quadrants or macular area due to small pupils.

ASSESSMENT

Central opacity, both eyes
Central visual acuity deficit, both eyes
Deficient diversional activity R/T poor vision

NURSING DIAGNOSES COMMONLY ASSOCIATED WITH THE EYES AND VISUAL DISORDERS

RELATED FACTORS (Etiology)	DEFINING CHARACTERISTICS (Symptoms and Signs)
DIAGNOSIS: Disturbed **V**isual sensory perception	
Restriction of head/neck motion	Headache
Effects of	Blurring
Aging	Spots
Stress	Double vision
Neurologic impairment	Excessive tearing
Failure to use protective eye devices	Inflammation
Improper use of contact lens	Lack of blink or corneal reflex
Difficulty in adjusting to corrective lens	Squinting
Persistent visual stimulation	Holding objects too close or at a distance for viewing
	Colliding with objects
	Abnormal results of vision testing
DIAGNOSIS: Deficient **D**iversional activity	
Effects of chronic illness	Restlessness
Physical limitations	Napping during day
Poor vision	Apathy or hostility
Social isolation	Complaints of boredom
Decreased economic resources	Verbalizes desire for activity
Confined to bed rest	Inability to participate in usual activities or hobbies because
Preoccupation with job	of physical limitations
	Depression
	Preoccupation with self
	Weight loss or gain
DIAGNOSIS: Impaired **H**ome maintenance	
Impaired mental status	Offensive odors
Effects of chronic debilitating disease (loss of vision)	Presence of rodents or vermin
Inadequate support system	Accumulation of dirt, food, dirty laundry, or hygienic wastes
Substance abuse	Reports by patient or family of difficulty maintaining home
Depression	in comfortable fashion
Lack of knowledge	Inappropriate room temperature
Lack of motivation	Lack of necessary equipment
Decreased financial resources	

OTHER RELATED NURSING DIAGNOSES

ACTUAL	RISK/WELLNESS
Anxiety	**Risk**
Pain	Risk for Injury
Self-care deficit	**Wellness**
Social isolation	Progressive adjustment to vision changes
	Participating in satisfying activities

ASSESSMENT VIDEO CRITICAL THINKING QUESTIONS

The Saunders *Physical Examination and Health Assessment* video "Head, Eyes, and Ears" will direct you to consider the following:

1. In addition to the screening vision test using the Snellen eye chart, what other vision tests could you use and why would you use them?

2. Describe the following abnormal findings, which may be found during inspection of the eyelids: exophthalmos, ptosis, ectropion, hordeolum, chalazion, and carcinoma.

Abnormal Findings

TABLE 14–1: Visual Field Loss

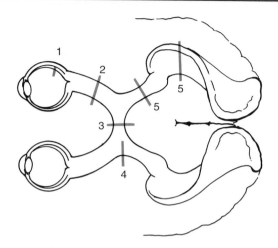

1. Retinal damage
   - Macula—central blind area, e.g., diabetes:

   - Localized damage—blind spot (scotoma) corresponding to particular area:

   - Increasing intraocular pressure—decrease in peripheral vision, e.g., glaucoma. Starts with paracentral scotoma in early stage:

   - Retinal detachment. Person has shadow or diminished vision in one quadrant or one half visual field:

2. Lesion in globe or optic nerve.
   Injury here yields one blind eye, or unilateral blindness:

3. Lesion at optic chiasm (e.g., pituitary tumor)—Injury to crossing fibers only yields a loss of nasal part of each retina and a loss of both temporal visual fields. Bitemporal (heteronymous) hemianopsia:

4. Lesion of outer uncrossed fibers at optic chiasm, e.g., aneurysm of left internal carotid artery exerts pressure on uncrossed fibers. Injury yields left nasal hemianopsia:

5. Lesion R optic tract or R optic radiation.
   Visual field loss in R nasal and L temporal fields.
   Loss of same half visual field in both eyes is homonymous hemianopsia:

TABLE 14–2: Extraocular Muscle Dysfunction

CORNEAL LIGHT REFLEX

A, Pseudostrabismus.

◀ **Symmetric Corneal Light Reflex**

A. **Pseudostrabismus** has the appearance of strabismus due to epicanthic fold but is normal for a young child.

B, Left esotropia.

C, Exotropia

Asymmetric Corneal Light Reflex

Strabismus is true disparity of the eye axes. This constant malalignment is also termed *tropia* and is likely to cause amblyopia.
B. Esotropia—inward turn of the eye.
C. Exotropia—outward turning of the eyes.

COVER TEST

D, Right, or uncovered eye, is weaker

E, Left, or covered eye, is weaker.

D. Uncovered eye—If it jumps to fixate on designated point, it was out of alignment before (i.e., when you cover the stronger eye, the weaker eye now tries to fixate).
Phoria—mild weakness, apparent only with the cover test and less likely to cause amblyopia than a tropia but still possible.

E. Covered eye—If this is the weaker eye, once macular image is suppressed it will drift to relaxed position.
    As eye is uncovered—If it jumps to reestablish fixation, weakness exists.
    Esophoria—nasal (inward) drift.
    Exophoria—temporal (outward) drift.

Table continued on following page

TABLE 14–2: Extraocular Muscle Dysfunction—cont'd

DIAGNOSTIC POSITIONS TEST

(Paralysis apparent during movement through six cardinal positions of gaze.)

If eye will not turn:	Indicates paralysis in:	or cranial nerve
Straight nasal	Medial rectus	III
Up and nasal	Inferior oblique	III
Up and temporal	Superior rectus	III
Straight temporal	Lateral rectus	VI
Down and temporal	Inferior rectus	III
Down and nasal	Superior oblique	IV

TABLE 14–3: Abnormalities in the Eyelids

Periorbital Edema

Lids are swollen and puffy. Lid tissues are loosely connected so excess fluid is easily apparent. This occurs with local infections; crying; and systemic conditions such as congestive heart failure, renal failure, allergy, hypothyroidism (myxedema).

Exophthalmos (Protruding Eyes)

Exophthalmos is a forward displacement of the eyeballs and widened palpebral fissures. Note "lid lag," the upper lid rests well above the limbus and white sclera is visible. Acquired bilateral exophthalmos is associated with thyrotoxicosis.

Table continued on following page

ABNORMAL FINDINGS

TABLE 14–3: Abnormalities in the Eyelids—cont'd

Enophthalmos (Sunken Eyes) (not illustrated)

A look of narrowed palpebral fissures shows with enophthalmos, in which the eyeballs are recessed. Bilateral enophthalmos is caused by loss of fat in the orbits and occurs with dehydration and chronic wasting illnesses. For illustration, see Cachexia in Table 11–5.

Ptosis (Drooping Upper Lid)

Ptosis occurs from neuromuscular weakness (e.g., myasthenia gravis with bilateral fatigue as the day progresses), oculomotor cranial nerve III damage, or sympathetic nerve damage (e.g., Horner's syndrome). It is a positional defect that gives the person a sleepy appearance and impairs vision.

Upward Palpebral Slant

Although normal in many children, when combined with epicanthal folds, hypertelorism (large spacing between the eyes), and Brushfield spots (light-colored areas in outer iris), indicates Down syndrome.

Ectropion

The lower lid is loose and rolling out, does not approximate to eyeball. Puncta cannot siphon tears effectively, so excess tearing results. The eyes feel dry and itchy because the tears do not drain correctly over the corner and toward the medial canthus. Exposed palpebral conjunctiva increases risk for inflammation. Occurs in aging due to atrophy of elastic and fibrous tissues, but may result from trauma.

Entropion

The lower lid rolls in due to spasm of lids or scar tissue contracting. Constant rubbing of lashes may irritate cornea. The person feels a "foreign body" sensation.

TABLE 14–4: Lesions on the Eyelids

Blepharitis (Inflammation of the Eyelids)

Red, scaly, greasy flakes and thickened, crusted lid margins occur with staphylococcal infection or seborrheic dermatitis of the lid edge. Symptoms include burning, itching, tearing, foreign body sensation, and some pain.

Chalazion

A beady nodule protruding on the lid, chalazion is an infection or retention cyst of a meibomian gland. It is a nontender, firm, discrete swelling with freely movable skin overlying the nodule. If it becomes inflamed, it points inside and not on lid margin (in contrast with stye).

Hordeolum (Stye)

Hordeolum is a localized staphylococcal infection of the hair follicles at the lid margin. It is painful, red, and swollen—a pustule at the lid margin. Rubbing the eyes can cause cross-contamination and development of another stye.

Dacryocystitis (Inflammation of the Lacrimal Sac)

Dacryocystitis is infection and blockage of sac and duct. Pain, warmth, redness, and swelling occur below the inner canthus toward nose. Tearing is present. Pressure on sac yields purulent discharge from puncta.

◀ ### Basal Cell Carcinoma

Carcinoma is rare, but it occurs most often on the lower lid and medial canthus. It looks like a papule with an ulcerated center. Note the rolled-out pearly edges. Metastasis is rare but should be referred for removal.

Dacryoadenitis (Inflammation of the Lacrimal Gland) (not illustrated)

Dacryoadenitis is an infection of the lacrimal gland. Pain, swelling, and redness occur in the outer third of upper lid. It occurs with mumps, measles, and infectious mononucleosis, or from trauma.

TABLE 14–5: Vascular Disorders of the External Eye

Conjunctivitis

Infection of the conjunctiva, "pink eye," has red beefy-looking vessels at periphery but usually clearer around iris (although here it is severe). This is common due to bacterial or viral infection, allergy, or chemical irritation. Purulent discharge accompanies bacterial infection. Preauricular lymph node is often swollen and painful, with a history of upper respiratory infection. Symptoms include itching, burning, foreign body sensation, and eyelids stuck together on awakening.

Subconjunctival Hemorrhage

A red patch on the sclera, subconjunctival hemorrhage looks alarming but is usually not serious. The red patch has sharp edges like a spot of paint, although here it is extensive. It occurs from increased intraocular pressure from coughing, sneezing, weight lifting, labor during childbirth, straining at stool, or trauma.

Iritis (Circumcorneal Redness)

Deep dull red halo around the iris and cornea. Note red is around iris, in contrast with conjunctivitis, in which redness is more prominent at the periphery. Pupil shape may be irregular from swelling of iris. Person also has marked photophobia, constricted pupil, blurred vision, and throbbing pain. Warrants immediate referral.

Acute Glaucoma

Acute, narrow-angle glaucoma shows a circumcorneal redness around the iris, with a dilated pupil. Pupil is oval, dilated; cornea looks "steamy"; and anterior chamber is shallow. Acute glaucoma occurs with sudden increase in intraocular pressure due to blocked outflow from anterior chamber. The person experiences a sudden clouding of vision, sudden eye pain, and halos around lights. This requires emergency treatment to avoid permanent vision loss.

TABLE 14–6: Abnormalities on the Cornea and Iris

Pterygium

A triangular opaque wing of bulbar conjunctiva grows toward the center of the cornea. It usually invades from nasal side, and it may obstruct vision as it covers pupil. Occurs usually from chronic exposure to hot, dry, sandy climate, which stimulates the growth of a pinguecula into a pterygium.

Corneal Abrasion

Irregular ridges usually visible only when fluorescein stain reveals yellow-green branching. Top layer of corneal epithelium removed, from scratches or poorly fitting or overworn contact lenses. Because the area is rich in nerve endings, the person feels intense pain, a foreign body sensation, and lacrimation, redness, and photophobia.

Normal Anterior Chamber (for Contrast)

A light directed across the eye from the temporal side illuminates the entire iris evenly because the normal iris is flat and creates no shadow.

Shallow Anterior Chamber

The iris is pushed anteriorly because of increased intraocular pressure. Because direct light is received from the temporal side, only the temporal part of iris is illuminated; the nasal side is shadowed, the "shadow sign." This may be a sign of acute angle-closure glaucoma.

Hyphema

Blood in anterior chamber is a serious result of trauma or spontaneous hemorrhage. Suspect scleral rupture or major intraocular trauma. Note that gravity settles blood.

Hypopyon

Purulent matter in anterior chamber occurs with iritis and with inflammation in the anterior chamber.

TABLE 14–7: Abnormalities in the Pupil

A. Unequal Pupil Size—Anisocoria

Although this exists normally in 5% of the population, consider central nervous system disease.

C. Constricted and Fixed Pupils—Miosis

Miosis occurs with the use of pilocarpine drops for glaucoma treatment, the use of narcotics, with iritis, and with brain damage of pons.

E. Argyll Robertson Pupil

No reaction to light, pupil does constrict with accommodation. Small and irregular bilaterally. Argyll Robertson pupil occurs with central nervous system syphilis, brain tumor, meningitis, and chronic alcoholism.

G. Cranial Nerve III Damage

Unilateral dilated pupil with no reaction to light or accommodation, occurs with oculomotor nerve damage. May also have ptosis with eye deviating down and laterally.

B. Monocular Blindness

When light is directed to the blind eye, no response occurs in either eye. When light is directed to normal eye, both pupils constrict (direct and consensual response to light) as long as the oculomotor nerve is intact.

D. Dilated and Fixed Pupils—Mydriasis

Enlarged pupils occur with stimulation of the sympathetic nervous system, reaction to sympathomimetic drugs, use of dilating drops, acute glaucoma, past or recent trauma. Also, they herald central nervous system injury, circulatory arrest, or deep anesthesia.

F. Tonic Pupil (Adie's Pupil)

Sluggish reaction to light and accommodation. Tonic pupil is usually unilateral, a large regular pupil that does react, but sluggishly after long latent time. No pathologic significance.

H. Horner's Syndrome

Unilateral, small, regular pupil does react to light and accommodation. Occurs with Horner's syndrome, a lesion of the sympathetic nerve. Also, note ptosis and absence of sweat (anhidrosis) on same side.

TABLE 14–8: Opacities in the Lens

Senile Cataracts

Central Gray Opacity—Nuclear Cataract

Nuclear cataract shows as an opaque gray surrounded by black background as it forms in the center of lens nucleus. Through the ophthalmoscope, it looks like a black center against the red reflex. It begins after age 40 and develops slowly, gradually obstructing vision.

Star-Shaped Opacity—Cortical Cataract

Cortical cataract shows as asymmetrical, radial, white spokes with black center. Through ophthalmoscope, black spokes are evident against the red reflex. This forms in outer cortex of lens, progressing faster than nuclear cataract.

TABLE 14–9: Abnormalities in the Optic Disc

Optic Atrophy (Disc Pallor)

Optic atrophy is a white or gray color of the disc due to partial or complete death of the optic nerve. This results in decreased visual acuity, decreased color vision, and decreased contrast sensitivity.

Papilledema (Choked Disc)

Increased intracranial pressure causes venous stasis in the globe, showing redness, congestion, and elevation of the disc; blurred margins; hemorrhages; and absent venous pulsations. This is a serious sign of intracranial pressure, usually caused by a space-occupying mass, e.g., a brain tumor or hematoma. Visual acuity is not affected.

Excessive Cup-Disc Ratio ▶

With primary, open-angle glaucoma, the increased intraocular pressure decreases blood supply to retinal structures. The physiologic cup enlarges to more than half of the disc diameter, vessels appear to plunge over edge of cup, and the vessels are displaced nasally. This is asymptomatic, although the person may experience decreased vision or visual field defects in the late stages of glaucoma.

TABLE 14–10: Abnormalities in Retinal Vessels and Background

Arteriovenous Crossing

Arteriovenous crossing with interruption of blood flow. When vein is occluded, it dilates distal to crossing. This person also has disc edema and hard exudates in a macular star pattern that occur with malignant hypertension.

Narrowed Arteries

This is a generalized decrease in diameter. The light reflex also narrows. It occurs with severe hypertension (shown here) and with occlusion of central retinal artery and retinitis pigmentosa.

Vessel Nicking

Nicking is a localized narrowing in vein caused by arteriole crossing. It is seen with hypertension and arteriosclerosis.

Silverwire Arteries

With hypertension, the arteriole wall thickens and becomes opaque so that no blood is seen inside it.

Copperwire Arteries

The light reflex widens, showing a metallic copper color. This is seen with hypertension.

Diabetic Retinopathy

◀ Microaneurysms

Microaneurysms are round punctate red dots that are localized dilatations of a small vessel. Their edges are smooth and discrete. The vessel itself is too small to view with the ophthalmoscope; only the isolated red dots are seen. This occurs with diabetes.

Dot-Shaped Hemorrhages

Deep intraretinal hemorrhages look splattered on. These occur with diabetes. They may be distinguished from microaneurysms by the blurred irregular edges.

Flame-Shaped Hemorrhages

Flame-shaped hemorrhages are superficial retinal hemorrhages that look linear and spindle shaped. They occur with hypertension.

Soft Exudates

"Cotton wool" areas look like fluffy gray-white cumulus clouds. They are arteriolar microinfarctions that envelop and obscure the vessels. They occur with diabetes, hypertension, subacute bacterial endocarditis, lupus, and papilledema of any cause.

Hard Exudates

These are numerous small yellow-white spots, having distinct edges and a smooth, solid-looking surface (illustrated in figure with microaneurysms on this page). They often form a circular pattern, clustered around a venous microinfarction. They also may form a linear or star pattern. (This is in contrast with the normal drusen, which have a scattered haphazard location [see Fig. 14–34].)

BIBLIOGRAPHY

Bedrossian E: Treatment of hordeolums: styes and chalazia, *Hosp Med* 33(3):59–64, Mar 1997.

Carr L: Case history: cornerstone in the neuro-ophthalmic examination, *Optom Clin* 5(3/4):17–32, 1996.

Deblinger L: Evaluation and management of red eye, *Patient Care* 35(24):36–44, Dec 2001.

Friedman NJ, Pineda R, Kaiser PK: *The Massachusetts Eye and Ear Infirmary illustrated manual of ophthalmology,* Philadelphia, 1998, W.B. Saunders.

Gaasterland DE et al: The advanced glaucoma intervention study (AGIS): 4. Comparison of treatment outcomes within race, *Ophthalmol* 105(7):1146–1164, Jul 1998.

Halle C: Achieve new vision screening objectives, *Nurse Pract* 27(3):15–37, March 2002.

Heffner D: Allergic conjunctivitis, *Lippincotts Prim Care Pract* 1(2):217–219, May–June 1997.

Houde SC: Age-related vision loss in the older adult, *Clin Excell Nurse Pract* 5(4):185–196, Jul 2001.

Hwang MY: Eye health as you grow older, *JAMA* 283(7):956, Feb 2000.

Kamoun L: The red eye, *Top Emerg Med* 22(4):37–51, Dec 2000.

Kane RT, Ouslander JG, Abrass IB: *Essentials of clinical geriatrics,* ed 5, New York, 2003, McGraw-Hill.

Lewis L: Early clues to vision loss, *Patient Care* 33(7):220–237, Apr 1999.

Michel FK, Sulewski ME: Focused assessment of the patient with eye trauma, *Top Emerg Med* 22(4):1–8, Dec 2000.

Modica PA: Afferent pupillary defects and the swinging flashlight test: what you thought you already knew, *Optom Clin* 5(3/4):1–15, 1996.

Molitor L: A woman with unilateral eye pain and malaise, *J Emerg Nurs* 27(5):519–526, Oct 2001.

Rappo PD et al: Eye examination and vision screening in infants, children, and young adults, *Pediatrics* 98(1):153–157, Jul 1996.

Shields SR: How to recognize and treat common eye problems, *Postgrad Med* 108(5):83–96, Oct 2000a.

Shields SR: How to screen for occult disease, *Postgrad Med* 108(5):69–78, Oct 2000b.

Wattx DD, Kokiko J: Air bags and eye injuries: assessment and treatment for ED patients, *J Emerg Nurs* 25(6):572–582, Dec 1999.

Wehenmeyer J, Gallman E: *Neuroscience curriculum,* ed 25, Urbana–Champaign, 2002, University of Illinois.

Wingate S: Treating corneal abrasions, *Nurse Pract* 24(6):53–68, Jun 1999.

Ears

Structure and Function

The ear is the sensory organ for hearing and maintaining equilibrium. The ear has three parts: the external, middle, and inner ear. The external ear is called the **auricle** or **pinna** and consists of movable cartilage and skin (Fig. 15–1). Note the landmarks of the auricle and use these terms to describe your findings. The mastoid process, the bony prominence behind the lobule, is not part of the ear but is an important landmark.

EXTERNAL EAR

The external ear has a characteristic shape and serves to funnel sound waves into its opening, the **external auditory canal** (Fig. 15–2). The canal is a cul-de-sac 2.5 to 3 cm long in the adult and terminates at the eardrum, or tympanic membrane. The canal is lined with glands that secrete cerumen, a yellow waxy material that lubricates and protects the ear. The wax forms a sticky barrier that helps keep foreign bodies from entering and reaching the sensitive tympanic membrane. Cerumen migrates out to the meatus by the movements of chewing and talking.

The outer one third of the canal is cartilage; the inner two thirds consists of bone covered by thin sensitive skin. The canal has a slight S-curve in the adult. The outer one third curves up and toward the back of the head, whereas the inner two thirds angles down and forward toward the nose.

The **tympanic membrane,** or **eardrum,** separates the external and middle ear and is tilted obliquely to the ear canal, facing downward and somewhat forward. It is a translucent membrane with a pearly gray color and a prominent cone of light in the anteroinferior quadrant, which is the reflection of the otoscope light (Fig. 15–3). The drum is oval and slightly concave, pulled in at its center by one of the middle ear ossicles, the **malleus.** The parts of the malleus show through the translucent drum; these are the **umbo,** the **manubrium** (handle), and the **short process.** The small, slack, superior section of the tympanic membrane is called the **pars flaccida.** The remainder of the drum, which is thicker and more taut, is the **pars tensa.** The **annulus** is the outer fibrous rim of the drum.

Lymphatic drainage of the external ear flows to the parotid, mastoid, and superficial cervical nodes.

MIDDLE EAR

The middle ear is a tiny air-filled cavity inside the temporal bone (see Fig. 15–2). It contains tiny ear bones, or auditory ossicles: the **malleus, incus,** and **stapes.** Several openings into the middle ear are present. Its opening to the outer ear is covered by the tympanic membrane. The openings to the inner ear are the oval window at the end of the stapes and the round window. Another opening is the **eustachian tube,** which connects the middle ear with the nasopharynx and allows passage of air. The tube is normally closed, but it opens with swallowing or yawning.

The middle ear has three functions: (1) It conducts sound vibrations from the outer ear to the central hearing appara-

AURICLE, OR PINNA

15–1

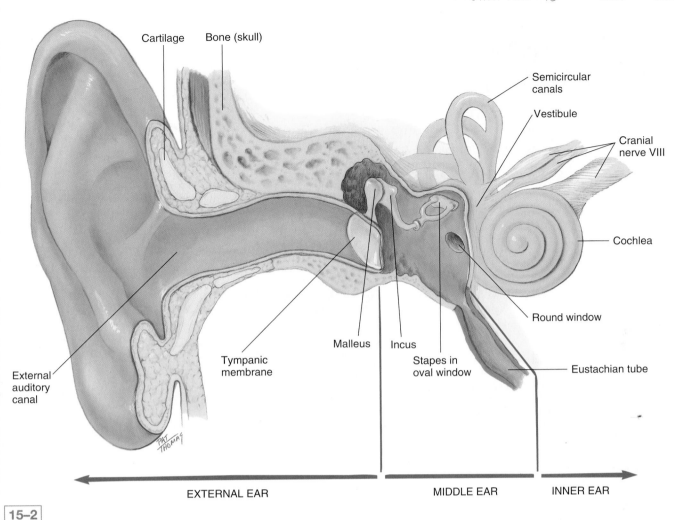

Cartilage

Bone (skull)

Semicircular canals

Vestibule

Cranial nerve VIII

Cochlea

Round window

Malleus

Incus

Stapes in oval window

Eustachian tube

External auditory canal

Tympanic membrane

EXTERNAL EAR

MIDDLE EAR

INNER EAR

15–2

tus in the inner ear; (2) it protects the inner ear by reducing the amplitude of loud sounds; and (3) its eustachian tube allows equalization of air pressure on each side of the tympanic membrane so that the membrane does not rupture (e.g., during altitude changes in an airplane).

Pars flaccida

Posterior fold

Anterior fold

Short process of malleus

Incus

Umbo

Manubrium of malleus

Annulus

Cone of light

Pars tensa

TYMPANIC MEMBRANE

15–3

INNER EAR

The inner ear contains the **bony labyrinth,** which holds the sensory organs for equilibrium and hearing. Within the bony labyrinth, the **vestibule** and the **semicircular canals** compose the vestibular apparatus, and the **cochlea** (Latin for "snail shell") contains the central hearing apparatus. Although the inner ear is not accessible to direct examination, its functions can be assessed.

HEARING

Concerning the function of hearing, the auditory system can be divided into three levels: peripheral, brainstem, and cerebral cortex. At the peripheral level, the ear transmits sound and converts its vibrations into electrical impulses, which can be analyzed by the brain. For example, you hear an alarm bell ringing in the hall. Its sound waves travel instantly to your ears (Fig. 15–4). The *amplitude* is how loud the alarm is; its *frequency* is the pitch (in this case, high) or the number of cycles per second. The sound waves produce vibrations on your tympanic membrane. These vibrations are carried by the middle ear ossicles to your oval window. Then the sound waves travel through your cochlea, which is coiled like a

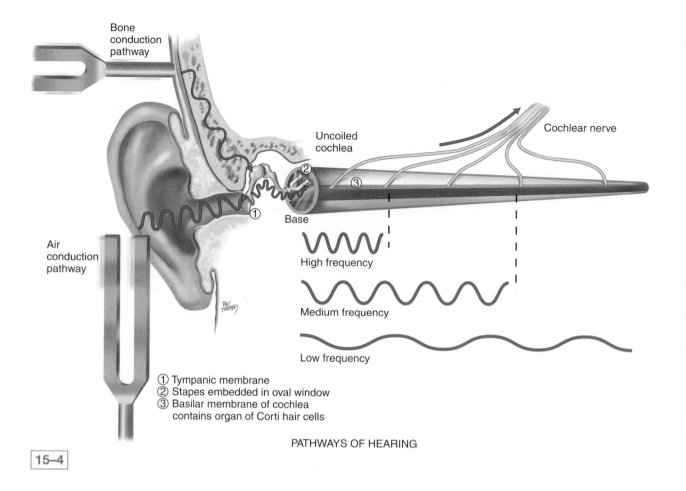

Bone
conduction
pathway

Uncoiled
cochlea

Cochlear nerve

②

③

①

Base

Air
conduction
pathway

High frequency

Medium frequency

Low frequency

① Tympanic membrane
② Stapes embedded in oval window
③ Basilar membrane of cochlea
   contains organ of Corti hair cells

PATHWAYS OF HEARING

15–4

snail's shell, and are dissipated against the round window. Along the way, the **basilar membrane** vibrates at a point specific to the frequency of the sound. In this case, the alarm's high frequency stimulates the basilar membrane at its base near the stapes. The numerous fibers along the basilar membrane are the receptor hair cells of the **organ of Corti,** the sensory organ of hearing. As the hair cells bend, they mediate the vibrations into electric impulses. The electric impulses are conducted by the auditory portion of cranial nerve VIII to the brainstem.

The function at the brainstem level is *binaural interaction,* which permits locating the direction of a sound in space as well as identifying the sound. How does this work? Each ear is actually one half of the total sensory organ. The ears are located on each side of a movable head. The cranial nerve VIII from each ear sends signals to both sides of the brainstem. Areas in the brainstem are sensitive to differences in intensity and timing of the messages from the two ears, depending on the way the head is turned.

Finally, the function of the cortex is to interpret the meaning of the sound and begin the appropriate response. All this happens in the split second it takes you to react to the alarm.

PATHWAYS OF HEARING

The normal pathway of hearing is air conduction (AC) described above; it is the most efficient. An alternate route of hearing is by bone conduction (BC). Here, the bones of the skull vibrate. These vibrations are transmitted directly to the inner ear and to cranial nerve VIII.

HEARING LOSS

Anything that obstructs the transmission of sound impairs hearing. A **conductive** hearing loss involves a mechanical dysfunction of the external or middle ear. It is a partial loss because the person is able to hear if the sound amplitude is increased enough to reach normal nerve elements in the inner ear. Conductive hearing loss may be caused by impacted cerumen, foreign bodies, a perforated tympanic membrane, pus or serum in the middle ear, and otosclerosis (a decrease in mobility of the ossicles).

Sensorineural (or perceptive) loss signifies pathology of the inner ear, cranial nerve VIII, or the auditory areas of the cerebral cortex. A simple increase in amplitude may not enable the person to understand words. Sensorineural hearing loss may be caused by *presbycusis,* a gradual nerve degeneration that occurs with aging, and by ototoxic drugs, which affect the hair cells in the cochlea. A **mixed** loss is a combination of conductive and sensorineural types in the same ear.

EQUILIBRIUM

The labyrinth in the inner ear constantly feeds information to your brain about your body's position in space. It works like a plumb line to determine verticality or depth. The ear's plumb lines register the angle of your head in relation to gravity. If the labyrinth ever becomes inflamed, it feeds the wrong information to the brain, creating a staggering gait and a strong, spinning, whirling sensation called *vertigo.*

DEVELOPMENTAL CONSIDERATIONS

INFANTS AND CHILDREN

The inner ear starts to develop early in the 4th week of gestation. If maternal rubella infection occurs during the first trimester, it can damage the organ of Corti and impair hearing. The infant's eustachian tube is relatively shorter and wider, and its position is more horizontal than the adult's, so it is easier for pathogens from the nasopharynx to migrate through to the middle ear (Fig. 15–5). The lumen is surrounded by lymphoid tissue, which increases during childhood; thus, the lumen is easily occluded. These factors place the infant at greater risk for middle ear infections than the adult.

The infant's and the young child's external auditory canal is shorter and has a slope opposite to that of the adult's (see Fig. 15–17 on p. 355).

THE ADULT

Otosclerosis is a common cause of conductive hearing loss in young adults between the ages of 20 and 40. It is a gradual hardening that causes the foot plate of the stapes to become fixed in the oval window, impeding the transmission of sound and causing progressive deafness.

THE AGING ADULT

In the aging person, cilia lining the ear canal become coarse and stiff. This may cause decreased hearing, since it impedes sound waves traveling toward the tympanic membrane. It also causes cerumen to accumulate and oxidize, which greatly reduces hearing. The cerumen itself is drier because of atrophy of the apocrine glands. Also, a life history of frequent ear infections may result in scarring on the drum.

Impacted cerumen is a common but reversible cause of hearing loss in older people. Data from 226 hospitalized patients 65 years of age or older showed that 35% had impacted cerumen. Following removal of cerumen, 75% of these people had significantly improved hearing ability. This study suggests that nurses could improve the hearing health of older people by routinely performing otoscopic examinations and by performing ear canal irrigations when they find impacted cerumen (Lewis-Cullinan and Janken, 1990).

A person living in a noise-polluted area (e.g., near an airport or a busy highway) has a greater risk of hearing loss. But **presbycusis** is a type of hearing loss that occurs with aging, even in people living in a quiet environment. It is a gradual sensorineural loss caused by nerve degeneration in the inner ear or auditory nerve. Its onset usually occurs in the fifth decade, and then it slowly progresses. The person first notices a high-frequency tone loss; it is harder to hear consonants (high-pitched components of speech) than vowels. This makes words sound garbled. The ability to localize sound is impaired also. This communication dysfunction is accentuated when unfavorable background noise is present (e.g., with music, with dishes clattering, or at a large noisy party).

Lastly, the auditory reaction time increases after age 70 (Kane, Ouslander, and Abrass, 2003). That is, it takes longer for the older adult to process sensory input and to respond to it.

TRANSCULTURAL CONSIDERATIONS

Otitis media, or OM, (middle ear infection) occurs because of obstruction of the eustachian tube and/or passage of nasopharyngeal secretions into the middle ear. Otitis media is one of the most common illnesses in children. The incidence and severity are increased in Native Americans, Alaskan and Canadian Inuits, and Hispanics (Terris, Magit, and Davidson, 1995).

The incidence of otitis media also is increased in premature infants, in those with Down syndrome, and in babies fed by bottle in a supine position. In the supine position the effects of gravity and sucking tend to draw the nasopharyngeal contents directly into the middle ear. Urge the parent to hold

INFANT
Horizontal eustachian tube

ADULT
Sloped eustachian tube

15–5

the baby partly upright against the arm while feeding. Do not prop the bottle or let the baby take a bottle to bed. Encouraging breastfeeding helps prevent this problem.

The most important side effect of acute otitis media is the persistence of fluid in the middle ear after treatment. This middle ear effusion can impair hearing, placing the child at risk for delayed cognitive development.

Cerumen is genetically determined and comes in two major types: (1) dry cerumen, which is gray, flaky, and fre-

quently forms a thin mass in the ear canal; and (2) wet cerumen, which is honey brown to dark brown and moist. Asians and Native Americans have an 84% frequency of dry cerumen, whereas blacks have a 99% and whites have a 97% frequency of wet cerumen (Overfield, 1995). The clinical significance of this occurs when examining or irrigating the ears. The presence and composition of cerumen are not related to poor hygiene. Take caution to avoid mistaking the flaky, dry cerumen for eczematous lesions.

Subjective Data

1. Earaches	**4.** Hearing loss	**7.** Vertigo
2. Infections	**5.** Environmental noise	**8.** Self-care behaviors
3. Discharge	**6.** Tinnitus	

EXAMINER ASKS

RATIONALE

1. Earache. Any **earache** or other pain in ears?
- Location—feel close to the surface or deep in the head?
- Does it hurt when you push on the ear?
- Character—dull, aching or sharp, stabbing? Constant or come and go? Is it affected by changing position of head? Ever had this kind of pain before?
- Any accompanying cold symptoms or sore throat? Any problems with sinuses or teeth?

- Ever been hit on the ear or on the side of the head, or had any sport injury? Ever had any trauma from a foreign body?
- What have you tried to relieve pain?

Otalgia may be directly due to ear disease or may be referred pain from a problem in teeth or oropharynx.

Virus/bacteria from upper respiratory infection may migrate up eustachian tube to involve middle ear.

Trauma may rupture the tympanic membrane.

Assess effect of coping strategies.

2. Infections. Any ear **infections?** As an adult, or in childhood?
- How frequent were they? How were they treated?

A history of chronic ear problems alerts you to possibility of sequelae.

3. Discharge. Any **discharge** from your ears?

- Does it look like pus, or bloody?

- Any odor to the discharge?

- Any relation between the discharge and the ear pain?

Discharge (otorrhea) suggests infection; it may come from canal or may indicate a perforated eardrum. For example:

External otitis—purulent, sanguineous, or watery discharge.

Acute otitis media with perforation—purulent discharge.

Cholesteatoma—dirty yellow/gray discharge, foul odor.

Typically with perforation—ear pain occurs first, stops with a popping sensation, then drainage occurs.

4. Hearing loss. Ever had any trouble hearing?
- Onset—Did the loss come on slowly or all at once?

- Character—Has all your hearing decreased, or just on hearing certain sounds?

Presbycusis has a gradual onset over years, whereas a hearing loss due to trauma is often sudden. Refer any sudden loss in one or both ears *not* associated with upper respiratory infection.

EXAMINER ASKS	RATIONALE
• In what situations do you notice the loss: conversations, using the telephone, listening to TV, at a party?	Loss is apparent when competition from background noise is present, as at a party.
• Do people seem to shout at you?	*Recruitment*—a marked loss occurs when sound is at low intensity, but sound actually may become painful when repeated in a loud voice.
• Do ordinary sounds seem hollow, as if you are hearing in a barrel or under water?	Character of hearing loss when cerumen expands and becomes impacted, as after swimming or showering.
• Recently traveled by airplane?	
• Any family history of hearing loss?	
• Effort to treat—any hearing aid or other device? Anything to help hearing?	
• Coping strategies—how does the loss affect your daily life? Any job problem? Feel embarrassed? Frustrated? How do your family, friends react?	Hearing loss can cause social isolation and can lessen pleasure of leisure activities.

Note to examiner—during history, note these clues from normal conversation, which indicate possible hearing loss

1. Person lip reading or watching your face and lips closely rather than your eyes
2. Frowning or straining forward to hear
3. Posturing of head to catch sounds with better ear
4. Misunderstands your questions, or frequently asks you to repeat
5. Acts irritable or shows startle reflex when you raise your voice (recruitment)
6. Person's speech sounds garbled, possibly vowel sounds distorted
7. Inappropriately loud voice
8. Flat, monotonous tone of voice

5. Environmental noise. Any loud noises at home or on the job? For example, do you live in a noise-polluted area, near an airport or busy traffic area? Now or in the past?	Old trauma to hearing initially goes unnoticed but results in further decibel loss in later years.
• Are you near other noises such as heavy machinery, loud persistent music, gunshots while hunting?	
• Coping strategies—any steps to protect your ears, such as headphones or ear plugs?	
6. Tinnitus. Ever felt ringing, crackling, or buzzing in your ears? When did this occur?	The sound of tinnitus originates within the person. Tinnitus accompanies some hearing loss or ear disorders.
• Seem louder at night?	Tinnitus seems louder when no competition from environment noise exists.
• Are you taking any medications?	Many medications have ototoxic sequelae: aspirin, aminoglycosides (streptomycin, gentamicin, kanamycin, neomycin), ethacrynic acid, furosemide, indomethacin, naproxen, quinine, vancomycin.
7. Vertigo. Ever felt **vertigo,** that is, the room spinning around or yourself spinning? (Vertigo is a true twirling motion.)	True rotational spinning occurs with dysfunction of labyrinth. Objective vertigo—feels like room spins. Subjective vertigo—person feels like she or he spins.
• Ever felt dizzy, like you are not quite steady, like falling or losing your balance? Giddy, lightheaded?	Distinguish true vertigo from dizziness or lightheadedness.

EXAMINER ASKS	RATIONALE
8. Self-care behaviors. How do you clean your ears?	Assess potential trauma from invasive instruments. Cleaning with cotton-tipped applicators can impact cerumen, causing hearing loss.
• Last time you had your hearing checked? • If a hearing loss was noted, did you obtain a hearing aid? How long have you had it? Do you wear it? How does it work? Any trouble with upkeep, cleaning, changing batteries?	Prescribe frequency of hearing assessment according to person's age and/or risk factors.

Additional History for Infants and Children

EXAMINER ASKS	RATIONALE
1. Ear Infections. At what age was the child's first episode? How many ear infections in the last 6 months? How many total? How were these treated? • Has the child had any surgery, such as insertion of ear tubes or removal of tonsils? • Are the infections increasing in frequency, in severity, or staying the same? • Does anyone in the home smoke cigarettes? • Does your child receive child care outside your home? In a day care center or someone else's home? How many children in the group care?	A first episode that occurs within 3 months of life increases risk of recurrent OM. Recurrent OM is 3 episodes in a 6-month period (Fitzgerald, 1999). Passive or secondhand smoke is a risk factor for ear infections. Attendance at group day care and bottle feeding (as opposed to breastfeeding) are also risk factors for otitis media (Tigges, 2000).
2. Does the child seem to be hearing well? • Have you noticed that the infant startles with loud noise? Did the infant babble around 6 months? Does he or she talk? At what age did talking start? Was the speech intelligible? • Ever had the child's hearing tested? If there was a hearing loss, did it follow any diseases in the child, or in the mother during pregnancy? (Note: It is important to catch any problem early, because a child with hearing loss is at risk for delayed speech and social development and learning deficit.)	Children at risk for hearing deficit include those exposed to maternal rubella, syphilis, cytomegalovirus, or toxoplasmosis, or to maternal ototoxic drugs in utero; premature infants; low-birth-weight infants; trauma or hypoxia at birth; and infants with congenital liver or kidney disease. In children the incidence of meningitis, measles, mumps, otitis media, and any illness with persistent high fever may increase risk of hearing deficit.
3. Does the child tend to put objects in the ears? Is the older child or adolescent active in contact sports?	These children are at increased risk for trauma.

Objective Data

PREPARATION

Position the adult sitting up straight with his or her head at your eye level. Occasionally the ear canal is partially filled with cerumen, which obstructs your view of the tympanic membrane. If the eardrum is intact and no current infection is present, a preferred method of cleaning the adult canal is to soften the cerumen with a warmed solution of mineral oil and hydrogen peroxide. Then the canal is irrigated with warm water (body temperature) using a bulb syringe or a low-pulsatile dental irrigator (WaterPik). Direct fluid to the posterior wall. Leave space around the irrigator tip for water to escape. Do not irrigate if the history or the examination suggests perforation or infection.

EQUIPMENT NEEDED

Otoscope with bright light (fresh batteries give off white—not yellow—light)
Pneumatic bulb attachment, sometimes used with infant or young child
Tuning forks in 512, 1024 Hz

NORMAL RANGE OF FINDINGS	ABNORMAL FINDINGS

INSPECT AND PALPATE THE EXTERNAL EAR

Size and Shape

The ears are of equal size bilaterally with no swelling or thickening. Ears of unusual size and shape may be a normal familial trait with no clinical significance.

Microtia—ears smaller than 4 cm vertically.

Macrotia—ears larger than 10 cm vertically.

Edema.

Skin Condition

The skin color is consistent with the person's facial skin color. The skin is intact, with no lumps or lesions. On some people you may note **Darwin's tubercle,** a small painless nodule at the helix. This is a congenital variation and is not significant (see Table 15–2).

Reddened, excessively warm skin indicates inflammation (see Table 15–1, p. 361).

Crusts and scaling occur with otitis externa, eczema, contact dermatitis, and seborrhea.

Enlarged tender lymph nodes in the region indicate inflammation of the pinna or mastoid process.

Red-blue discoloration indicates frostbite.

Tophi, sebaceous cyst, chondrodermatitis, keloid, carcinoma (see Table 15–2).

Tenderness

Move the pinna and push on the tragus. They should feel firm, and movement should produce no pain. Palpating the mastoid process should also produce no pain.

Pain with movement occurs with otitis externa and furuncle.

Pain at the mastoid process may indicate mastoiditis or lymphadenitis of the posterior auricular node.

The External Auditory Meatus

Note the size of the opening to direct your choice of speculum for the otoscope. No swelling, redness, or discharge should be present.

Atresia—absence or closure of the ear canal.

A sticky yellow discharge accompanies otitis externa, or may indicate otitis media if the drum has ruptured.

Some cerumen is usually present. The color varies from gray-yellow to light brown and black, and the texture varies from moist and waxy to dry and desiccated. A large amount of cerumen obscures visualization of the canal and drum.

Impacted cerumen is a common cause of conductive hearing loss.

INSPECT USING THE OTOSCOPE

As you inspect the external ear, note the size of the auditory meatus. Then choose the largest speculum that will fit comfortably in the ear canal, and attach it to the otoscope. Tilt the person's head slightly away from you toward the opposite shoulder. This method brings the obliquely sloping eardrum into better view.

Pull the pinna up and back on an adult or older child; this helps straighten the S-shape of the canal (Fig. 15–6). (Pull the pinna down on an infant and a child under 3 years of age [see Fig. 15–17]). Hold the pinna gently but firmly. Do not release traction on the ear until you have finished the examination and the otoscope is removed.

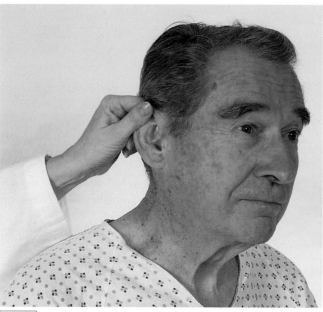

15–6

Hold the otoscope "upside down" along your fingers and have the dorsa (back) of your hand along the person's cheek braced to steady the otoscope (Fig. 15–7). This position feels awkward to you only at first. It soon will feel natural and you will find it useful to prevent forceful insertion. Also your stabilizing hand acts as a protecting lever if the person suddenly moves the head.

15–7

NORMAL RANGE OF FINDINGS	ABNORMAL FINDINGS

Insert the speculum slowly and carefully along the axis of the canal. Watch the insertion; then put your eye up to the otoscope. Avoid touching the inner "bony" section of the canal wall, which is covered by a thin epithelial layer and is sensitive to pain. Sometimes you cannot see anything but canal wall. If so, try to reposition the person's head, apply more traction on the pinna, and re-angle the otoscope to look forward toward the person's nose.

Once it is in place, you may need to rotate the otoscope slightly to visualize all of the drum; do this gently. Lastly, perform the otoscopic examination before you test hearing; ear canals with impacted cerumen give the erroneous impression of pathologic hearing loss.

The External Canal

Note any redness and swelling, lesions, foreign bodies, or discharge. If any discharge is present, note the color and odor. (Also, clean any discharge from the speculum before examining the other ear to avoid contamination with possibly infectious material.) For a person with a hearing aid, note any irritation on the canal wall from poorly fitting earmolds.

> Redness and swelling occur with otitis externa; canal may be completely closed with swelling.
>
> Purulent otorrhea suggests otitis externa, or otitis media if the drum has ruptured.
>
> Frank blood or clear, watery drainage (cerebrospinal fluid [CSF]) following trauma suggests basal skull fracture and warrants immediate referral. CSF feels oily and is positive for glucose on TesTape.
>
> Foreign body, polyp, furuncle, exostosis, (see Table 15–3).

The Tympanic Membrane

COLOR AND CHARACTERISTICS. Systematically explore its landmarks (Fig. 15–8). The normal eardrum is shiny and translucent, with a pearl-gray color. The cone-shaped light reflex is prominent in the anteroinferior quadrant (at 5 o'clock in the right drum and 7 o'clock in the left drum). This is the reflection of your otoscope light. Sections of the malleus are visible through the translucent drum: the umbo, manubrium, and short process. (Infrequently, you also may see the incus behind the drum; it shows as a whitish haze in the upper posterior area.) At the periphery the annulus looks whiter and denser.

> Yellow-amber drum color occurs with serous otitis media.
> Red color occurs with acute otitis media.
> Absent or distorted landmarks.
> Air/fluid level or air bubbles behind drum indicate serous otitis media (see Tables 15–4 and 15–5).

15–8 Normal tympanic membrane, right.

NORMAL RANGE OF FINDINGS	ABNORMAL FINDINGS

POSITION. The eardrum is flat, slightly pulled in at the center, and flutters when the person performs the Valsalva maneuver or holds the nose and swallows (insufflation). You may elicit these maneuvers to assess drum mobility. Avoid them with an aging person because they may disrupt equilibrium. Also avoid middle ear insufflation in a person with upper respiratory infection because it could propel infectious matter into the middle ear.

Retracted drum due to vacuum in middle ear with obstructed eustachian tube.

Bulging drum from increased pressure in otitis media.

Drum hypomobility is an early sign of otitis media (see Table 15–5).

INTEGRITY OF MEMBRANE. Inspect the eardrum and the entire circumference of the annulus for perforations. The normal tympanic membrane is intact. Some adults may show scarring, which is a dense white patch on the drum. This is a sequela of repeated ear infections.

Perforation shows as a dark oval area or as a larger opening on the drum.

Vesicles on drum (see Table 15–5).

TEST HEARING ACUITY

Your screening for a hearing deficit begins during the history; how well does the person hear conversational speech? An audiometer gives a precise quantitative measure of hearing by assessing the person's ability to hear sounds of varying frequency. Since this equipment usually is not available in the clinical setting, you may use alternate screening measures. These are "crude" tests. They are nonquantitative; they are useful to document the *presence* of hearing loss but do not measure the degree of loss. Refer any abnormal findings for more accurate measures with pure tone audiometry.

Voice Test

Test one ear at a time while masking hearing in the other ear to prevent sound transmission around the head. This is done by placing one finger on the tragus and rapidly pushing it in and out of the auditory meatus. Shield your lips so the person cannot compensate for a hearing loss (consciously or unconsciously) by lip reading or using the "good" ear. With your head 30 to 60 cm (1 to 2 ft) from the person's ear, exhale and whisper slowly some two-syllable words, such as Tuesday, armchair, baseball, and fourteen. Normally, the person repeats each word correctly after you say it.

The person is unable to hear whispered words. A whisper is a high-frequency sound and is used to detect high-tone loss.

Tuning Fork Tests

Tuning fork tests measure hearing by air conduction (AC) or by bone conduction (BC), in which the sound vibrates through the cranial bones to the inner ear. The AC route through the ear canal and middle ear is usually the more sensitive route. To activate the tuning fork, hold it by the stem and strike the tines softly on the back of your hand (Fig. 15–9). A hard strike makes the tone too loud, and it takes a long time to fade out.

15–9

NORMAL RANGE OF FINDINGS	ABNORMAL FINDINGS

The **Weber test** is valuable when a person reports hearing better with one ear than the other. Place a vibrating tuning fork in the midline of the person's skull and ask if the tone sounds the same in both ears or better in one (Fig. 15–10). The person should hear the tone by bone conduction through the skull, and it should sound equally loud in both ears.

Sound lateralizes to one ear with a conductive or a sensorineural loss (see Table 15–6).

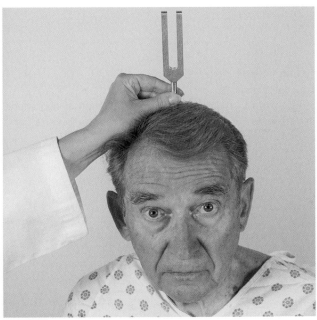

15–10 Weber test.

The **Rinne test** compares air conduction and bone conduction sound (Fig. 15–11). Place the stem of the vibrating tuning fork on the person's mastoid process and ask him or her to signal when the sound goes away. Quickly invert the fork so the vibrating end is near the ear canal; the person should still hear a sound (Fig. 15–12). Normally the sound is heard twice as long by air conduction (next to ear canal) as by bone conduction (through the mastoid process). A normal response is a positive Rinne test, or "AC > BC." Repeat with the other ear.

Ratio of AC to BC is altered with hearing loss (see Table 15–6).

Sound is heard longer by bone conduction with a conductive loss.

15–11 Rinne test.

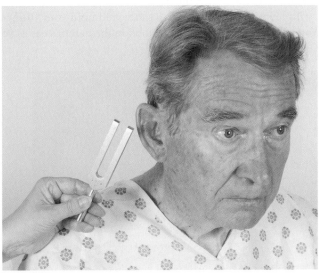

15–12

NORMAL RANGE OF FINDINGS	ABNORMAL FINDINGS

THE VESTIBULAR APPARATUS

The **Romberg test** assesses the ability of the vestibular apparatus in the inner ear to help maintain standing balance. Because the Romberg test also assesses intactness of the cerebellum and proprioception, it is discussed in Chapter 23, Neurologic System (see Fig. 23–17).

 DEVELOPMENTAL CONSIDERATIONS

Infants and Young Children

Examination of the external ear is similar to that described for the adult, with the addition of examination of position and alignment on head. Note the ear position. The top of the pinna should match an imaginary line extending from the corner of the eye to the occiput. Also, the ear should be positioned within 10 degrees of vertical (Fig. 15–13).

Low-set ears or deviation in alignment may indicate mental retardation or a genitourinary malformation.

15–13   Normal alignment

Low-set ears and deviation in alignment

OTOSCOPIC EXAMINATION. In addition to its place in the complete examination, eardrum assessment is mandatory for any infant or child requiring care for illness or fever. For the infant or young child, the timing of the otoscopic examination is best toward the end of the complete examination. Many young children protest vigorously during this procedure no matter how well you prepare, and it is difficult to reestablish cooperation afterward. Save the otoscopic examination until last. Then the parent can hold and comfort the child.

To help prepare the child, let the child hold your funny-looking "flashlight." You may wish to have the child look in the parent's ear as you hold the otoscope (Fig. 15–14).

15–14

NORMAL RANGE OF FINDINGS	ABNORMAL FINDINGS

Positioning of the child is important. You need a clear view of the canal, and you must protect the eardrum from injury in case of sudden head movement. Enlist the aid of a cooperative parent. Prop an infant upright against the parent's chest or shoulder, with the parent's arm around the upper part of the head (Fig. 15–15). A toddler can be held in the parent's lap or may lie on the examining table with his or her arms secured (Fig. 15–16). In each case, the child's head is stabilized to avoid movement against the otoscope.

15–15

15–16

Remember to pull the pinna straight down on an infant or a child under 3 years old. This method will match the slope of the ear canal (Fig. 15–17).

At birth the patency of the ear canal is determined, but the otoscopic examination is not performed because the canal is filled with amniotic fluid and vernix caseosa. After a few days the tympanic membrane is examined. During the first

ADULT

Adult—Pull
Pinna Up and Back

YOUNG CHILD

B

Infant/Child Under 3—Pull
Pinna Straight Down

15–17

few days, the tympanic membrane often looks thickened and opaque. It may look "injected" and have a mild redness due to increased vascularity. The drum also looks injected in infants after crying. The position of the eardrum is more horizontal in the neonate, making it more difficult to see completely and harder to differentiate from the canal wall. By 1 month of age, the drum is in the oblique (more vertical) position as in the older child, and examination is a bit easier.

When examining an infant or young child, a pneumatic bulb attachment enables you to direct a light puff of air toward the drum to assess vibratility (Fig. 15–18). For a secure seal, choose the largest speculum that will fit in the ear canal without causing pain. A rubber tip on the end of the speculum gives a better seal. Give a small pump to the bulb (positive pressure), then release the bulb (negative pressure). Normally the tympanic membrane moves inward with a slight puff and outward with a slight release.

An abnormal response is no movement. Drum hypomobility indicates effusion or a high vacuum in the middle ear. For the newborn's first 6 weeks, drum immobility is the best indicator of middle ear infection.

15–18

Normally the tympanic membrane is intact. In a child being treated for chronic otitis media, you may note the presence of a tympanostomy tube in the central part of the drum. This is inserted surgically to equalize pressure and drain secretions. Finally, although the condition is not normal, it is not uncommon to note a foreign body in a child's canal, such as a small stone or a bead.

Tympanostomy tubes (see Table 15–5).

Foreign body (see Table 15–3).

TEST HEARING ACUITY. Use the developmental milestones mentioned in this section to assess hearing in an infant. Also, attend to the parents' concern over the infant's inability to hear; their assessment is usually well founded.

The room should be silent and the baby contented. Make a loud sudden noise (hand clap or squeeze toy) out of the baby's peripheral range of vision of about 30 cm (12 in). You may need to repeat a few times, but you should note these responses:

Newborn—startle (Moro) reflex, acoustic blink reflex
3 to 4 months—acoustic blink reflex, infant stops movement and appears to "listen," halts sucking, quiets if crying, cries if quiet

6 to 8 months—infant turns head to localize sound, responds to own name

Preschool and school-age child—child must be screened with audiometry

Note that a young child may be unaware of a hearing loss because the child does not know how one "ought" to hear. Note these behavioral manifestations of hearing loss:

Absence of alerting behavior may indicate congenital deafness.

Failure to localize sound.

No intelligible speech by 2 years of age.

NORMAL RANGE OF FINDINGS	ABNORMAL FINDINGS

1. The child is inattentive in casual conversation.
2. The child reacts more to movement and facial expression than to sound.
3. The child's facial expression is strained or puzzled.
4. The child frequently asks to have statements repeated.
5. The child confuses words that sound alike.
6. The child has an accompanying speech problem: Speech is monotonous or garbled; the child mispronounces or omits sounds.
7. The child appears shy and withdrawn and "lives in a world of his or her own."
8. The child frequently complains of earaches.
9. The child hears better at times when the environment is more conducive to hearing.

The Aging Adult

An aging adult may have pendulous earlobes with linear wrinkling because of loss of elasticity of the pinna. Coarse, wiry hairs may be present at the opening of the ear canal. During otoscopy the drum normally may be whiter in color and more opaque, duller than in the younger adult. It also may look thickened.

A high-tone frequency hearing loss is apparent for those affected with presbycusis, the hearing loss that occurs with aging. This condition is revealed in difficulty hearing whispered words in the voice test and in difficulty hearing consonants during conversational speech.

SUMMARY CHECKLIST: Ear Exam

1. Inspect external ear:
Size and shape of auricle
Position and alignment on head
Note skin condition—color, lumps, lesions
Check movement of auricle and tragus for tenderness
Evaluate external auditory meatus—note size, swelling, redness, discharge, cerumen, lesions, foreign bodies

2. Otoscopic examination:
External canal
Cerumen, discharge, foreign bodies, lesions
Redness or swelling of canal wall
3. Inspect tympanic membrane:
Color and characteristics
Note position (flat, bulging, retracted)
Integrity of membrane

4. Test hearing acuity:
Note behavioral response to conversational speech
Voice test
Tuning fork tests—Weber and Rinne

See Health Promotion Guide on CD

Application and Critical Thinking

SAMPLE CHARTING

SUBJECTIVE

States hearing is good, no earaches, infections, discharge, hearing loss, tinnitus, or vertigo.

OBJECTIVE

Pinna—skin intact with no masses, lesions, tenderness, or discharge.
Otoscope—external canals are clear with no redness, swelling, lesions, foreign body, or discharge. Both tympanic membranes are pearly gray in color, with light reflex and landmarks intact, no perforations.
Hearing—whispered words heard bilaterally. Weber test—tone heard midline without lateralization.
Rinne test: AC > BC and = bilaterally.

Continued

FOCUSED ASSESSMENT: CLINICAL CASE STUDY 1

Jamal K. is a 9-month-old black infant who is brought to the clinic by his mother because he "feels hot and was up crying all night."

Past History. Jamal is the third child of Mr. and Mrs. K. Mrs. K. received regular prenatal care. Jamal was born at 37 weeks' gestation; labor and delivery were uncomplicated. Jamal weighed 3200 g at birth, and was discharged 2 days after delivery. Jamal has been bottle fed, with solids introduced at 5 months. Well baby care has been regular, immunizations are up-to-date. Jamal has had two prior episodes of otitis media, no other illnesses.

Social History. Jamal lives with his family in a two-bedroom apartment over their grocery store and shares a bedroom with a 4-year-old brother and a 2-year-old brother. Mr. K. works full time in their grocery store; Mrs. K. provides child care in her own home for her children and for her sister's two young children. Both parents smoke cigarettes, 1 to 2 packs per day.

SUBJECTIVE

1 day PTA—Mrs. K. put Jamal down for nap with a bottle of juice, as is usual for her. Jamal woke up in the middle of the nap crying furiously. Quieted somewhat when held upright but still fussy. Took juice from bottle, refused solid baby food. Temperature 38° C rectally. Crying and fussy all night. Mrs. K. has given no medications to Jamal.

OBJECTIVE

Vital signs—temp 38.4° C (tympanic), pulse 152, resp 36, Wt. 9.2 kg (50th percentile), Ht. 29 in. (75th percentile).

General—alert, active, crying, and fussy. Developmentally appropriate for age.

Skin—warm and dry, no rashes or lesions.

Head—anterior fontanel flat, 1 × 1.5 cm, posterior fontanel closed.

Eyes—no exudate, conjunctivae clear, sclerae white, red reflex present bilaterally.

Ears—both tympanic membranes dull red and bulging, no light reflex, no mobility on pneumatic otoscopy.

Mouth/throat—oral mucosa pink, no lesions or exudate, tonsils 1+.

Neck—supple, no lymphadenopathy.

Heart—regular rate and rhythm, no murmurs.

Lungs—breath sounds clear and equal bilaterally, unlabored.

Abdomen—bowel sounds present, abdomen soft, nontender.

ASSESSMENT

Acute otitis media, both ears

Pain R/T inflammation in TMs

Risk for ear infection injury R/T supine bottle feeding, group child care, secondhand smoke

Deficient knowledge (parents) R/T lack of exposure to risk factors for otitis media

FOCUSED ASSESSMENT: CLINICAL CASE STUDY 2

Todd R. is a 15-year-old high school student who comes to the Health Center to seek care for "cough off and on all winter and earache since last night."

SUBJECTIVE

6 weeks PTA—nonproductive cough throughout day, no fever, no nasal congestion, no chest soreness. Todd's father gave him an over-the-counter decongestant, which helped, but cough continued off/on since. Does not smoke.

1 day PTA—intermittent cough continues, nasal congestion c̄ thick white mucus. Also earache R ear, treated self with heating pad, pain unrelieved. Pain is moderate, not deep and throbbing. Says R ear feels full, "hollow headed," voices sound muffled and far away, switches telephone to L ear to talk. No sore throat, no fever, no chest congestion or soreness.

OBJECTIVE

Vital signs—T 37° C oral, P 76, B/P 106/72.

Ears—L ear, canal, TM normal. R ear and canal normal, R TM retracted, with multiple air bubbles, drum color is yellow/amber. No sinus tenderness.

Nose—turbinates bright red and swollen, mucropurulent discharge.
Throat—not reddened, tonsils 1+.
Neck—1 R anterior cervical node enlarged, firm, movable, tender. All others not palpable.
Lungs—Breath sounds clear to auscultation, resonant to percussion throughout.
Hearing—Weber lateralizes to R.

ASSESSMENT

Serous otitis media, R ear, with mild URI
Transient conductive hearing loss
Disturbed sensory perception (auditory) R/T excessive fluid in middle ear
Pain R/T middle ear pressure

FOCUSED ASSESSMENT: CLINICAL CASE STUDY 3

Emma S., 78 years old, has a medical diagnosis of angina pectoris, which has responded to nitroglycerin prn and periods of rest between activity. She has been independent in her own home, is coping well with activity restrictions through help from neighbors and family. Now hospitalized for evaluation of acute chest pain episode; MI has been ruled out, pain diagnosed as anginal, to be released to own home with a beta-blocking medication and nitroglycerin prn.

Just before this hospitalization, Mrs. S. received a hearing aid following evaluation by audiologist at senior center. Mrs. S. was born in Germany, immigrated to U.S. at age 5, considers English her primary language.

SUBJECTIVE

Since this hospitalization, feels "irritable and nervous." Relates this to worry about heart and also, "I get so mixed up in here, this room is so strange, and I just can't hear the nurses. They talk like cavemen, 'oo-i-ee-uou.'" Tried using her new hearing aid but no relief, "It just kept screeching in my ear, and it made the monitor beep so loud it drove me crazy." States no tinnitus, no vertigo.

OBJECTIVE

Ears—pinna with elongated lobes, but no tenderness to palpation, no discharge, no masses or lesions. Both canals clear of cerumen. Both TM appear gray-white, slightly opaque and dull, although all landmarks visible. No perforation.

Hearing—unable to hear whispered voice bilaterally. Weber test—tone heard midline, although unable to hear 1024 Hz fork, used 512 Hz Rinne test positive, AC > BC, but time reduced overall.

ASSESSMENT

Chest pain/angina pectoris
Deficient knowledge R/T lack of teaching on hearing aid
Disturbed sensory perception (auditory) R/T effects of aging
Anxiety R/T change in cardiovascular health status and inability to communicate effectively

NURSING DIAGNOSES COMMONLY ASSOCIATED WITH THE EARS AND HEARING DISORDERS

RELATED FACTORS (Etiology)	DEFINING CHARACTERISTICS (Symptoms and Signs)
DIAGNOSIS: Disturbed Sensory perception	
Effects of aging	Tinnitus
Neurologic impairment	Abnormal hearing test
Effects of certain antibiotics	Lack of startle reflex
Excessive earwax, fluid, or foreign body in ear	Failure to respond to verbal stimuli
Social isolation	Cupping of ears
Stress	Inattentiveness
Failure to use protective ear devices	Withdrawal
Continuous exposure to excessive noise	Daydreaming
Psychoses	Auditory hallucinations
	Inappropriate responses
	Delayed speech or language development

Continued

RELATED FACTORS (Etiology)	DEFINING CHARACTERISTICS (Symptoms and Signs)
DIAGNOSIS: Impaired Social interaction	
Knowledge/skills deficit about ways to enhance mutuality	Verbalized or observed discomfort
Communication barriers	In social situations
Self-concept disturbances	In receiving or communicating
Limited physical mobility	Observed use of unsuccessful socialization behaviors
Therapeutic isolation	Dysfunctional interaction with peers, family, and/or others
Sociocultural dissonance	
Environmental barriers	

OTHER RELATED NURSING DIAGNOSES

ACTUAL	RISK/WELLNESS
Impaired verbal Communication	**Risk**
Pain	Risk for Infection
	Risk for Trauma related to balance difficulties
	Wellness
	Readiness for enhanced communication
	Health-seeking behavior R/T ways to decrease ear infections in child

 ASSESSMENT VIDEO CRITICAL THINKING QUESTIONS

The Saunders *Physical Examination and Health Assessment* video "Head, Eyes, and Ears" will direct you to consider the following:

1. Describe the following lumps or lesions that may occur on the external ear: sebaceous cyst, keloid, carcinoma, and otitis externa.

2. Contrast the way you would move the pinna to straighten the ear canal of an adult and of a very young child.

Abnormal Findings

TABLE 15–1: Abnormalities of the External Ear

Frostbite

Reddish blue discoloration and swelling of auricle following exposure to extreme cold. Vesicles or bullae may develop, the person feels pain and tenderness, and ear necrosis may ensue.

Reprinted from the Clinical Slide Collection on the Rheumatic Diseases, © 1991, 1995, 1997. Used by permission of the American College of Rheumatology.

Otitis Externa (Swimmer's Ear)

An infection of the outer ear, with severe painful movement of the pinna and tragus, redness and swelling of pinna and canal, scanty purulent discharge, scaling, itching, fever, and enlarged tender regional lymph nodes. Hearing is normal or slightly diminished. More common in hot humid weather. Swimming causes canal to become waterlogged and swell; skinfolds are set up for infection. Prevent by using rubbing alcohol or 2% acetic acid eardrops after every swim.

Branchial Remnant and Ear Deformity

A facial remnant or leftover of the embryological branchial arch usually appears as a skin tag, in this case one containing cartilage. They occur most often in the preauricular area, in front of the tragus. When bilateral, there is increased risk of renal anomalies.

Cerebrospinal Fluid Otorrhea (not illustrated)

Skull fracture of temporal bone causes cerebrospinal fluid to leak from ear canal and pool in concha when the person is supine. Cerebrospinal fluid feels oily and gives a positive glucose reaction on TesTape.

TABLE 15–2: Lumps and Lesions on the External Ear

Darwin's Tubercle

Small painless nodule at the helix. It is a congenital variation and is not significant. Do not mistake it for a tophus.

Sebaceous Cyst

Location is commonly behind lobule, in the postauricular fold. A nodule with central black punctum indicates blocked sebaceous gland. It is filled with waxy sebaceous material and is painful if it becomes infected. Often are multiple.

Tophi

Small, whitish-yellow, hard, nontender nodules in or near helix or antihelix; contain greasy, chalky material of uric acid crystals and are a sign of gout.

Chondrodermatitis Nodularis Helicus

Painful nodules develop on the rim of the helix (where there is no cushioning subcutaneous tissue) as a result of repetitive mechanical pressure or environmental trauma (sunlight). They are small, indurated, dull red, poorly defined, and very painful.

Continued

TABLE 15–2: Lumps and Lesions on the External Ear—cont'd

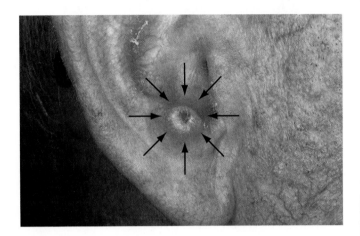

Keloid

Overgrowth of scar tissue, which invades original site of trauma. It is more common in dark-skinned people, although it also occurs in whites. In the ear it is most common at lobule at the site of a pierced ear. Overgrowth shown here is unusually large.

Carcinoma

Ulcerated crusted nodule with indurated base that fails to heal. Bleeds intermittently. Must refer for biopsy. Usually occurs on the superior rim of the pinna, which has the most sun exposure. May occur also in ear canal and show chronic discharge that is either serosanguineous or bloody.

TABLE 15–3: Abnormalities in the Ear Canal

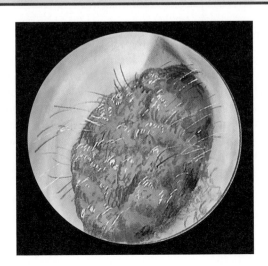

◀ Excessive Cerumen

Excessive cerumen is produced or is impacted due to narrow tortuous canal or to poor cleaning method. May show as round ball partially obscuring drum or totally occluding canal. Even when canal is 90% to 95% blocked, hearing stays normal. But when last 5% to 10% is totally occluded (when cerumen expands after swimming or showering), person experiences ear fullness and sudden hearing loss.

Table continued on following page

TABLE 15–3: Abnormalities in the Ear Canal—cont'd

Otitis Externa

Severe swelling of canal, inflammation, tenderness. Here canal lumen is narrowed to one quarter normal size. (See complete description in Table 15–1.)

Osteoma

Single, stony hard, rounded nodule that obscures the drum; nontender; overlying skin appears normal. Attached to inner third, the bony part, of canal. Benign, but refer for removal.

Foreign Body

Usually it is children who place a foreign body in the ear (here, a stone completely occludes the canal), which is later noted on routine examination. Common objects are beans, corn, jewelry beads, small stones, sponge rubber. Cotton is most common in adults and becomes impacted from cotton-tipped applicators. A trapped live insect is uncommon, but makes the person especially frantic.

Exostosis

More common than osteoma. Small, bony hard, rounded nodules of hypertrophic bone, covered with normal epithelium. They arise near the drum but usually do not obstruct the view of the drum. They are usually multiple and bilateral. They may occur more frequently in cold-water swimmers. The condition needs no treatment, although it may cause accumulation of cerumen, which blocks the canal.

TABLE 15-3: Abnormalities in the Ear Canal—cont'd

Furuncle

Exquisitely painful, reddened, infected hair follicle. Here, it occurs on the tragus but also may be on cartilaginous part of ear canal. Regional lymphadenopathy often accompanies a furuncle.

Polyp

Arises in canal from granulomatous or mucosal tissue; redder than surrounding skin and bleeds easily; bathed in foul purulent discharge; indicates chronic ear disease. Benign, but refer for excision.

TABLE 15-4: Abnormal Findings Seen on Otoscopy

APPEARANCE OF EARDRUM	INDICATES	SUGGESTED CONDITION
Yellow-amber color	Serum or pus	Serous otitis media or chronic otitis media
Prominent landmarks	Retraction of drum	Negative pressure in middle ear from an obstructed eustachian tube
Air/fluid level or air bubbles	Serous fluid	Serous otitis media
Absent or distorted light reflex	Bulging of eardrum	Acute otitis media
Bright red color	Infection in middle ear	Acute purulent otitis media
Blue or dark red color	Blood behind drum	Trauma, skull fracture
Dark oval areas	Perforation	Drum rupture
White dense areas	Scarring	Sequelae of infections
Diminished or absent landmarks	Thickened drum	Chronic otitis media
Black or white dots on drum or canal	Colony of growth	Fungal infection

Reprinted by permission of Elsevier Science Publishing Co., Inc., from Sherman JL, Fields SK: *Guide to patient evaluation,* ed 5, New York, 1988, Medical Examination Publishing.

ABNORMAL FINDINGS

TABLE 15–5: Abnormalities of the Tympanic Membrane

Retracted Drum

Landmarks look more prominent and well defined. Malleus handle looks shorter and more horizontal than normal. Short process is very prominent. Light reflex is absent or distorted. The drum is dull and lusterless and does not move. These signs indicate negative pressure and middle ear vacuum due to obstructed eustachian tube and serous otitis media.

Serous Otitis Media

An amber-yellow drum suggests serum in middle ear that transudates to relieve negative pressure from the blocked eustachian tube. You may note an air/fluid level with fine black dividing line, or air bubbles visible behind drum. Symptoms are feeling of fullness, transient hearing loss, popping sound with swallowing. Also called secretory otitis media, middle ear effusion, glue ear.

Early stage.

Later stage.

Acute Purulent Otitis Media (above)

This results when the middle ear fluid is infected. An absent light reflex due to increasing middle ear pressure is an early sign. Redness and bulging are first noted in superior part of drum (pars flaccida), along with earache and fever. Then fiery red bulging of entire drum occurs; deep throbbing pain; fever; transient hearing loss. Pneumatic otoscopy reveals drum hypomobility.

◀ Perforation

If the acute otitis media is not treated, the drum may rupture from increased pressure. Perforations also occur from trauma (e.g., a slap on the ear). Usually the perforation appears as a round or oval darkened area on the drum, but in this photo the perforation is very large. *Central* perforations occur in the pars tensa. *Marginal* perforations occur at the annulus. Marginal perforations are called *attic perforations* when they occur in superior part of the drum, the pars flaccida.

Continued

TABLE 15-5: Abnormalities of the Tympanic Membrane—cont'd

Insertion of Tympanostomy Tubes

Polyethylene tubes are inserted surgically into the eardrum to relieve middle ear pressure and promote drainage of chronic or recurrent middle ear infections. Number of acute infections tends to decrease because of improved aeration. Tubes extrude spontaneously in 12 to 18 months.

Reprinted from *Atlas of Allergies,* 2nd edition, Fireman, p. 182, 1995, by permission of the publisher, Mosby.

Cholesteatoma

A malignant overgrowth of epidermal tissue may result over the years following a marginal perforation. It has a pearly white, cheesy appearance. Growth of cholesteatoma can erode bone and produce hearing loss.

Scarred Drum

Dense white patches on the eardrum are sequelae of repeated ear infections. They do not necessarily affect hearing.

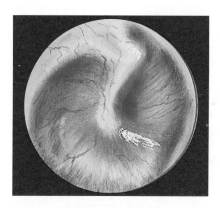

Blue Drum (Hemotympanum)

This indicates blood in the middle ear, as in trauma resulting in skull fracture.

Bullous Myringitis

Small vesicles containing blood on the drum; accompany mycoplasma pneumonia and virus infections. May have blood-tinged discharge and severe otalgia.

Fungal Infection (Otomycosis)

Colony of black or white dots on drum or canal wall suggests a yeast or fungal infection.

TABLE 15–6: Tuning Fork Tests

Weber Test

Normal—Sound is equally loud in both ears; sound does not lateralize.

Conductive loss—Sound lateralizes to "poorer" ear due to background room noise, which masks hearing in normal ear. "Poorer" ear (the one with conductive loss) is not distracted by background noise, thus has a better chance to hear bone-conducted sound. Examples: transient conductive loss with serous or purulent otitis media.

Rinne Test

Normal—Sound is heard twice as long by air conduction (AC) as by bone conduction (BC); a "positive" Rinne, or AC > BC.

Conductive loss—Person hears as long by bone conduction (AC = BC) or even longer (AC < BC), a "negative" finding on the Rinne test.

Continued

TABLE 15–6: Tuning Fork Tests—cont'd

Weber Test

Sensorineural loss

Sensorineural loss—Sound lateralizes to "better" ear or unaffected ear. Poor ear (the one with nerve loss) is unable to perceive the sound.

Rinne Test

Sensorineural loss

Sensorineural loss—Normal ratio of AC > BC is intact but is reduced overall. That is, person hears poorly both ways.

BIBLIOGRAPHY

Abyad A: In-office screening for age-related hearing and vision loss, *Geriatrics* 52(6):51–57, June 1997.

Bluestone CD, Klein JO: *Otitis media in infants and children,* ed 3, Philadelphia, 2001, W.B. Saunders.

Dowell SF et al: Acute otitis media: management and surveillance in an era of pneumococcal resistance, *Nurse Pract* 24(suppl 10):1–9, Oct 1999.

Felis M: Acute otitis externa, Lippincotts *Prim Care Pract* 4(5): 529–533, Sep–Oct 2000.

Fenn AR, Fitzgerald MA: Antimicrobial choices in the treatment of acute otitis media, Lippincotts *Prim Care Pract* 4(5):515–523, Sept–Oct 2000.

Fitzgerald MA: Acute otitis media in an era of drug resistance: implications for NP practice, *Nurse Pract* 24(suppl 10):10–16, Oct 1999.

Green M, Wald ER: Treating childhood respiratory infections in the age of resistance, *Patient Care* 34(13):99–108, Jul 15, 2000.

Jester RW: Dealing with earwax, *Hearing Journal* 54(1):70, Jan 2001.

Kacker A, Gonzales DA, Selesnick SH: The otoscopic examination: what to look for, where to search, *Consultant* 39(9):2397–2406, Sept 1999.

Kane RL, Ouslander JG, Abrass IB: *Essentials of clinical geriatrics,* ed 5, New York, 2003, McGraw-Hill.

La Rosa S: Primary care management of otitis externa, *Nurse Pract* 23(6):125–133, June 1998.

Lewis-Cullinan C, Janken JK: Effect of cerumen removal on the hearing ability of geriatric patients, *J Adv Nurs* 15(5):594–600, 1990.

Lynch JS: Patient education: ear wax, Lippincotts *Prim Care Pract* 4(5):542–543, Sep–Oct 2000.

Naeem Z, Newton V: Prevalence of sensorineural hearing loss in Asian children, *Br J Audiol* 30(5):332–339, Oct 1996.

Overfield T: *Biologic variation in health and illness: race, age, and sex differences,* ed 2, New York, 1995, CRC Press.

Shaw L: Protocol for detection and follow-up of hearing loss, *Clin Nurs Spec* 11(6):240–247, Nov 1997.

Sorrento A, Pichichero ME: Assessing diagnostic accuracy and tympanocentesis skills by nurse practitioners in management of otitis media, *J Am Acad Nurs Pract* 13(11):524–529, Nov 2001.

Takata GS et al: Evidence assessment of management of acute otitis media: the role of antibiotics in treatment of uncomplicated acute otitis media, *Pediatrics* 108 (2 part 1):239–247, Aug 2001.

Terris MH, Magit AE, Davidson TE: Otitis media with effusion in infants and children, *Postgrad Med* 97:137–151, 1995.

Tigges BB: Acute otitis media and pneumococcal resistance: making judicious management decisions, *Nurse Pract* 25(1):69–87, 2000.

Wooldridge WE: Musculoskeletal photo diagnosis: a recurrently tender ear, *J Musculoskel Med* 14(2):78–80, Feb 1997.

Nose, Mouth, and Throat

Structure and Function

NOSE

The **nose** is the first segment of the respiratory system. It warms, moistens, and filters the inhaled air, and it is the sensory organ for smell. The external nose is shaped like a triangle with one side attached to the face (Fig. 16–1). On its leading edge, the superior part is the *bridge* and the free corner is the *tip*. The oval openings at the base of the triangle are the *nares;* just inside, each naris widens into the *vestibule*. The *columella* divides the two nares and is continuous inside with the nasal septum. The *ala* is the lateral outside wing of the nose on either side. The upper third of the external nose is made up of bone; the rest is cartilage.

Inside, the **nasal cavity** is much larger than the external nose would indicate (Fig. 16–2). It extends back over the roof of the mouth. The anterior edge of the cavity is lined with numerous coarse nasal hairs, or vibrissae. The rest of the cavity is lined with a blanket of ciliated mucous membrane. The nasal hairs filter the coarsest matter from inhaled air, whereas the mucous blanket filters out dust and bacteria. Nasal mucosa appears redder than oral mucosa because of the rich blood supply present to warm the inhaled air.

The nasal cavity is divided medially by the **septum** into two slitlike air passages. The anterior part of the septum holds a rich vascular network, *Kiesselbach's plexus,* the most common site of nosebleeds. In many people, the nasal septum is not absolutely straight and may deviate toward one passage.

The lateral walls of each nasal cavity contain three parallel bony projections—the superior, middle, and inferior **turbinates.** They increase the surface area so that more blood vessels and mucous membranes are available to warm, hu-midify, and filter the inhaled air. Underlying each turbinate is a cleft, the **meatus,** which is named for the turbinate above. The sinuses drain into the middle meatus, and tears from the nasolacrimal duct drain into the inferior meatus.

The olfactory receptors (hair cells) lie at the roof of the nasal cavity and in the upper one third of the septum. These receptors for smell merge into the olfactory nerve, cranial nerve I, which transmits to the temporal lobe of the brain. Although it is not necessary for human survival, the sense of smell adds to nutrition by enhancing the pleasure and taste of food.

The **paranasal sinuses** are air-filled pockets within the cranium (Fig. 16–3). They communicate with the nasal cavity and are lined with the same type of ciliated mucous membrane. They lighten the weight of the skull bones, serve as resonators for sound production, and provide mucus, which drains into the nasal cavity. The sinus openings are narrow and easily occluded, which may cause inflammation or sinusitis.

Two pairs of sinuses are accessible to examination: the **frontal** sinuses in the frontal bone above and medial to the orbits, and the **maxillary** sinuses in the maxilla (cheekbone) along the side walls of the nasal cavity. The other two sets are smaller and deeper: the **ethmoid** sinuses between the orbits and the **sphenoid** sinuses deep within the skull in the sphenoid bone.

Only the maxillary and ethmoid sinuses are present at birth. The maxillary sinuses reach full size after all permanent teeth have erupted. The ethmoid sinuses grow rapidly between 6 and 8 years of age and after puberty. The frontal sinuses are absent at birth, are fairly well developed between 7 and 8 years of age, and reach full size after puberty. The sphenoid sinuses are minute at birth and develop after puberty.

16–1

Frontal sinus

Superior turbinate (concha) and meatus

Middle turbinate and meatus

Inferior turbinate and meatus

Vestibule

Hard (bony) palate

Olfactory nerve (c.n.l.)

Sphenoid sinus

Location of the opening of the frontal sinus

Pharyngeal tonsil

Opening of the eustachian tube in nasopharynx

Soft palate

Palatine tonsil in oropharynx

LEFT LATERAL WALL—NASAL CAVITY

16–2

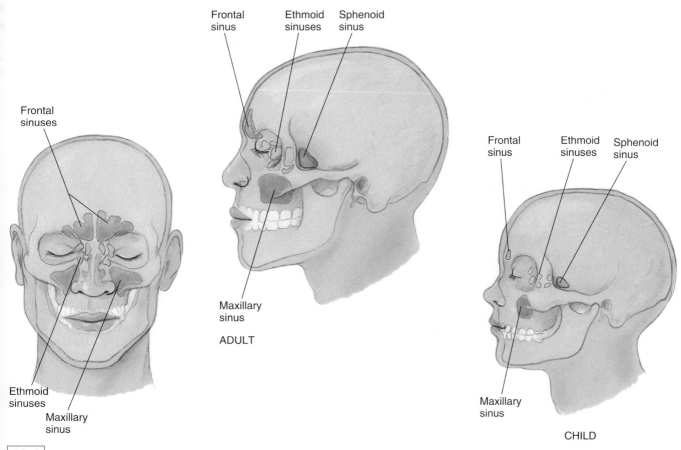

Frontal sinus

Ethmoid sinuses

Sphenoid sinus

Frontal sinuses

Maxillary sinus

ADULT

Ethmoid sinuses

Maxillary sinus

Frontal sinus

Ethmoid sinuses

Sphenoid sinus

Maxillary sinus

CHILD

16–3

MOUTH

The mouth is the first segment of the digestive system and an airway for the respiratory system. The **oral cavity** is a short passage bordered by the lips, palate, cheeks, and tongue. It contains the teeth and gums, tongue, and salivary glands (Fig. 16–4).

The lips are the anterior border of the oral cavity—the transition zone from the outer skin to the inner mucous membrane lining the oral cavity. The arching roof of the mouth is the palate; it is divided into two parts. The anterior **hard palate** is made up of bone and is a whitish color. Posterior to this is the **soft palate,** an arch of muscle that is pinker in color and mobile. The **uvula** is the free projection hanging down from the middle of the soft palate. The cheeks are the side walls of the oral cavity.

The floor of the mouth consists of the horseshoe-shaped mandible bone, the tongue, and underlying muscles. The **tongue** is a mass of striated muscle arranged in a crosswise pattern so that it can change shape and position. The papillae are the rough, bumpy elevations on its dorsal surface. Note the larger vallate papillae in an inverted V shape across the posterior base of the tongue, and do not confuse them with abnormal growths. Underneath, the ventral surface of the tongue is smooth and shiny and has prominent veins. The **frenulum** is a midline fold of tissue that connects the tongue to the floor of the mouth.

The tongue's ability to change shape and position enhances its functions in mastication, swallowing, cleansing the teeth, and the formation of speech. The tongue also functions in taste sensation. Microscopic taste buds are in the papillae at the back and along the sides of the tongue and on the soft palate.

The mouth contains three pairs of salivary glands (Fig. 16–5). The largest, the **parotid** gland, lies within the cheeks in front of the ear extending from the zygomatic arch down to the angle of the jaw. Its duct, Stensen's duct, runs forward to open on the buccal mucosa opposite the second molar. The **submandibular** gland is the size of a walnut. It lies beneath the mandible at the angle of the jaw. Wharton's duct runs up and forward to the floor of the mouth and opens at either side of the frenulum. The smallest, the almond-shaped **sublingual** gland, lies within the floor of the mouth under the tongue. It has many small openings along the sublingual fold under the tongue.

The glands secrete saliva, the clear fluid that moistens and lubricates the food bolus, starts digestion, and cleans and protects the mucosa.

Adults have 32 **permanent** teeth—16 in each arch. Each tooth has three parts: the crown, the neck, and the root. The gums (gingivae) collar the teeth. They are thick fibrous tissues covered with mucous membrane. The gums are different from the rest of the oral mucosa because of their pale pink color and stippled surface.

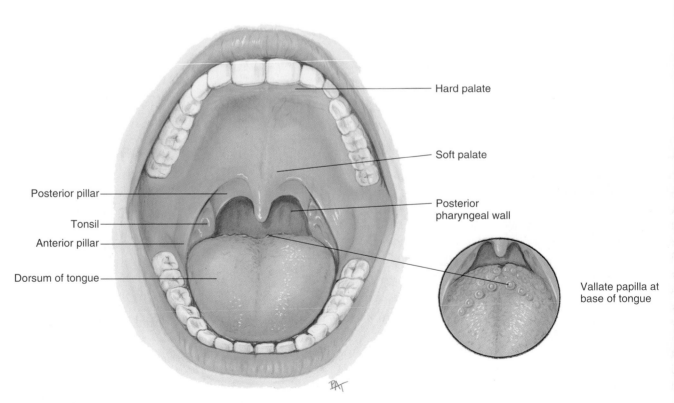

Hard palate

Soft palate

Posterior pillar

Tonsil

Anterior pillar

Dorsum of tongue

Posterior pharyngeal wall

Vallate papilla at base of tongue

ORAL CAVITY

16–4

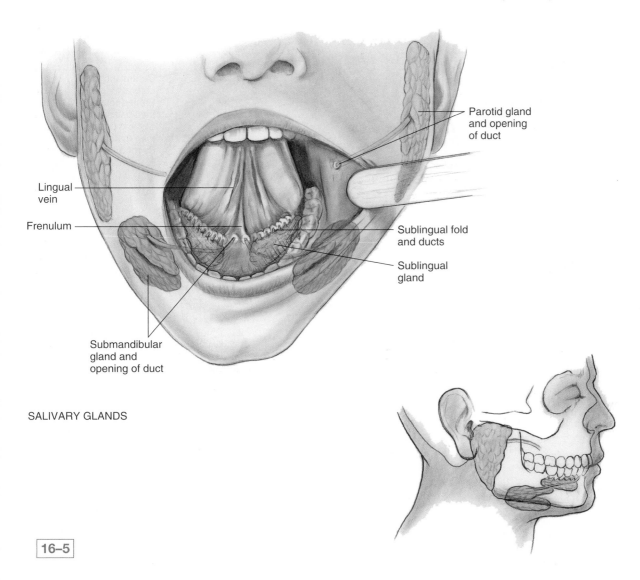

Parotid gland
and opening
of duct

Lingual
vein

Frenulum

Sublingual fold
and ducts

Sublingual
gland

Submandibular
gland and
opening of duct

SALIVARY GLANDS

16–5

THROAT

The throat, or pharynx, is the area behind the mouth and nose. The **oropharynx** is separated from the mouth by a fold of tissue on each side, the anterior tonsillar pillar. Behind the folds are the **tonsils,** each a mass of lymphoid tissue. The tonsils are the same color as the surrounding mucous membrane, although they look more granular, and their surface shows deep crypts. Tonsillar tissue enlarges during childhood until puberty, then involutes. The posterior pharyngeal wall is seen behind these structures. Some small blood vessels may show on it.

The **nasopharynx** is continuous with the oropharynx, although it is above the oropharynx and behind the nasal cavity. The pharyngeal tonsils (adenoids) and the eustachian tube openings are located here (see Fig. 16–2).

The oral cavity and throat have a rich lymphatic network. Review the lymph nodes and their drainage patterns in Chapter 13, and keep this in mind when evaluating the mouth.

 DEVELOPMENTAL CONSIDERATIONS

INFANTS AND CHILDREN

In the infant, salivation starts at 3 months. The baby will drool periodically for a few months before learning to swallow the saliva. This drooling does not herald the eruption of the first tooth, although many parents think it does.

The teeth, both sets, begin development in utero. Children have 20 **deciduous,** or temporary, teeth. These erupt between 6 months and 24 months of age. All 20 teeth should appear by 2½ years of age. The deciduous teeth are lost beginning at age 6 years through age 12. They are replaced by the permanent teeth, starting with the central incisors (Fig. 16–6). The permanent teeth appear earlier in girls than in boys, and they erupt earlier in black children than in white children.

The nose develops during adolescence, along with other secondary sex characteristics. This growth starts at age 12 or 13, reaching full growth at age 16 in females and age 18 in males.

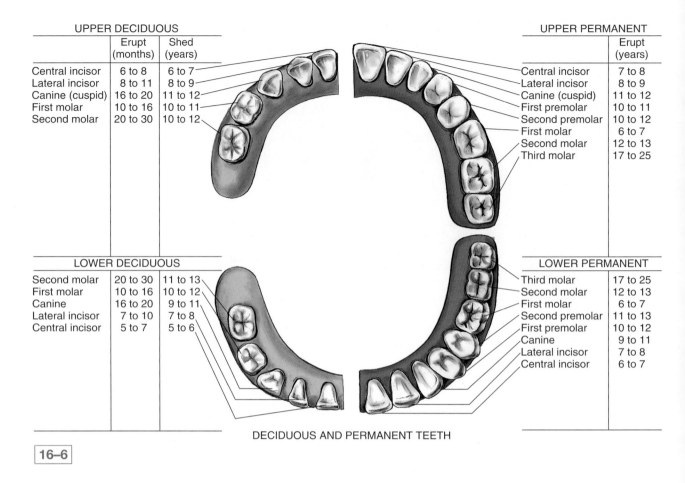

UPPER DECIDUOUS		
	Erupt (months)	Shed (years)
Central incisor	6 to 8	6 to 7
Lateral incisor	8 to 11	8 to 9
Canine (cuspid)	16 to 20	11 to 12
First molar	10 to 16	10 to 11
Second molar	20 to 30	10 to 12

UPPER PERMANENT	
	Erupt (years)
Central incisor	7 to 8
Lateral incisor	8 to 9
Canine (cuspid)	11 to 12
First premolar	10 to 11
Second premolar	10 to 12
First molar	6 to 7
Second molar	12 to 13
Third molar	17 to 25

LOWER DECIDUOUS		
Second molar	20 to 30	11 to 13
First molar	10 to 16	10 to 12
Canine	16 to 20	9 to 11
Lateral incisor	7 to 10	7 to 8
Central incisor	5 to 7	5 to 6

LOWER PERMANENT	
Third molar	17 to 25
Second molar	12 to 13
First molar	6 to 7
Second premolar	11 to 13
First premolar	10 to 12
Canine	9 to 11
Lateral incisor	7 to 8
Central incisor	6 to 7

DECIDUOUS AND PERMANENT TEETH

16–6

THE PREGNANT FEMALE

Nasal stuffiness and epistaxis may occur during pregnancy due to increased vascularity in the upper respiratory tract. Also, the gums may be hyperemic and softened and may bleed with normal toothbrushing. Contrary to superstitious folklore, no evidence exists that pregnancy causes tooth decay or loss.

THE AGING ADULT

A gradual loss of subcutaneous fat starts during later middle adult years, making the nose appear more prominent in some people. The nasal hairs grow coarser and stiffer and may not filter the air as well. The hairs protrude and may cause itching and sneezing. Many older people clip these hairs, thinking them unsightly, but this practice can cause infection. The sense of smell may diminish because of a decrease in the number of olfactory nerve fibers. The decrease in the sensation of smell begins after age 60, and it continues progressively with age (Edelstein, 1996).

In the oral cavity, the soft tissues atrophy and the epithelium thins, especially in the cheek and tongue. This results in loss of taste buds, with about an 80% reduction in taste functioning. Further impairments to taste include a decrease in salivary secretion that is needed to dissolve flavoring agents, and the presence of upper dentures that cover secondary taste sites (Kane, Ouslander, and Abrass, 2003).

Atrophic tissues ulcerate easily, which places the older person at risk for infections such as oral moniliasis. An increased risk of malignant oral lesions is also present.

Many dental changes occur with aging. The tooth surface is abraded. The gums begin to recede and the teeth begin to erode at the gum line. A smooth V-shaped cavity forms around the neck of the tooth, exposing the nerve and making the tooth hypersensitive. Some tooth loss may occur due to bone resorption (osteoporosis), which decreases the inner tooth structure and its outer support. Natural tooth loss is exacerbated by years of inadequate dental care, decay, poor oral hygiene, and tobacco use.

If tooth loss occurs, the remaining teeth drift, causing **malocclusion.** The stress of chewing with maloccluding teeth causes further problems: (1) Excessive bone resorption with further tooth loss occurs; (2) muscle imbalance results from a mandible and maxilla now out of alignment, which produces muscle spasms, tenderness of muscles of mastication, and chronic headaches; and (3) the temporomandibular joint is stressed, leading to osteoarthritis, pain, and inability to fully open the mouth.

A diminished sense of taste and smell decreases the aging person's interest in food and may contribute to malnutrition. Saliva production decreases; saliva acts as a solvent for food flavors and helps move food around the mouth. Decreased saliva also reduces the mouth's self-cleaning property. The major cause of decreased saliva flow is not the aging process itself but the use of medications that have anticholinergic effects. Over 250 medications have a side effect of dry mouth.

The absence of some teeth and trouble with mastication encourage the older person to eat soft foods (usually high in carbohydrates) and to decrease meat and fresh vegetable intake. This produces a risk of nutritional deficit for protein, vitamins, and minerals.

TRANSCULTURAL CONSIDERATIONS

Bifid uvula, a condition in which the uvula is split either completely or partially, occurs in 18% of some Native American groups and in 10% of Asians. The occurrence in whites and blacks is rare. **Cleft lip** and **cleft palate** are most common in Asians and Native Americans and least common in blacks (Overfield, 1995). **Torus palatinus,** a bony ridge running in the middle of the hard palate, is more common in Native Americans, Inuits, and Asians (up to 50%) (Overfield, 1995).

Leukoedema, a grayish white benign lesion occurring on the buccal mucosa, is present in 68% to 90% of blacks but in only 43% of whites (Overfield, 1995). Oral hyperpigmentation also varies according to race. Usually absent at birth, hyperpigmentation increases with age. By 50 years of age, 10% of whites and 50% to 90% of blacks will show oral hyperpigmentation, a condition that is believed to be caused by a lifetime of accumulation of postinflammatory oral changes (Overfield, 1995).

Although it is rare for a white baby to be born with teeth (1 in 3000), the incidence rises to 1 in 11 among Tlingit Indians and to 1 or 2 in 100 among Canadian Inuit infants (Overfield, 1995).

The size of teeth varies widely, with the teeth of whites being the smallest, followed by blacks, then Asians and Native Americans. The largest teeth are found among Inuits and Australian Aborigines (Overfield, 1995). Larger teeth cause some groups to have prognathic, or protruding jaws, a condition that is seen more frequently in blacks and Asians. The condition is normal and does not reflect an orthodontic problem.

Agenesis (absence) of teeth varies by race, with absence of the third molar occurring in 18% to 35% of Asians, 9% to 25% of whites, and 1% to 11% of blacks (Overfield, 1995). Throughout life, whites have more tooth decay than blacks. The differences in tooth decay between blacks and whites occurs because blacks have harder and denser tooth enamel, which makes their teeth less susceptible to the organisms that cause caries.

The incidence of tooth loss and edentulism has decreased substantially in the United States over the past several decades due to fluoridation, improved dental treatment, and better personal care. While the overall prevalence of edentulism has dropped to 10.5% of the population, there remain significant variations among subgroups in the population. Blacks, Hispanics, Native Americans, and Alaska Natives have the poorest oral health of all racial and ethnic groups in the United States. The National Institute of Dental and Craniofacial Research (2001) estimates that fewer than 22% of African-Americans have visited a dentist in the past year, one half the average of the rest of the nation. African-American males have the highest rate of oral cavity and pharyngeal cancers in the United States, a rate that is 40% higher than that of their white counterparts. The 5-year survival rate for oral cancer is also much lower in blacks (34%) than in whites (56%). This may be related to the fact that cancers are usually diagnosed at a much later stage of disease in blacks (Satcher, 2000).

Healthy People 2010 data reveal that 24% of black children 2 to 4 years of age have experienced dental caries in their primary teeth, compared to 15% of white counterparts. Higher levels of gingivitis and periodontal loss of attachment were seen in blacks than in whites. The Surgeon General reports that there are socioeconomic factors influencing dental health. Nearly half of all poor blacks and Hispanics have untreated tooth decay, compared with 27% of poor whites. More than one third of low-income children have at least one untreated decayed tooth by age 9. More than 43% of poor children have tooth decay by the time they reach 17, compared to just 23% of middle-class children. One fourth of low-income children have not visited a dentist before entering kindergarten, and for every child under 18 without medical insurance, there are at least two children without dental insurance (Satcher, 2000).

Subjective Data

Nose
1. Discharge
2. Frequent colds (upper respiratory infections)
3. Sinus pain
4. Trauma
5. Epistaxis (nosebleeds)
6. Allergies
7. Altered smell

Mouth and Throat
1. Sores or lesions
2. Sore throat
3. Bleeding gums
4. Toothache
5. Hoarseness
6. Dysphagia
7. Altered taste
8. Smoking, alcohol consumption
9. Self-care behaviors
   Dental care pattern
   Dentures or appliances

EXAMINER ASKS	RATIONALE

Nose

1. Discharge. Any **nasal discharge** or runny nose? Continuous?
- Is the discharge watery, purulent, mucoid, bloody?

Rhinorrhea occurs with colds, allergies, sinus infection, trauma.

2. Frequent colds. Any unusually **frequent** or **severe colds** (**upper respiratory infections**)? How often do these occur?

Most people have occasional colds; thus, asking this more precise question yields more meaningful data.

3. Sinus pain. Any **sinus pain** or sinusitis? How is this treated?
- Do you have chronic postnasal drip?

4. Trauma. Ever had any **trauma** or a blow to the nose?
- Can you breathe through your nose? Are both sides obstructed or one?

Trauma may cause deviated septum, which may cause nares to be obstructed.

5. Epistaxis (nosebleeds). Any nosebleeds? How often?
- How much bleeding—a teaspoonful or does it pour out?
- Color of the blood—red or brown? Clots?
- From one nostril or both?
- Aggravated by nose-picking or scratching?
- How do you treat the nosebleeds? Are they difficult to stop?

Epistaxis occurs with trauma, vigorous nose blowing, foreign body.

Person should sit up with head tilted forward, pinch nose between thumb and forefinger for 5 to 15 minutes.

6. Allergies. Any **allergies** or hay fever? To what are you allergic (e.g., pollen, dust, pets)?
- How was this determined?
- What type of environment makes it worse? Can you avoid exposure?
- Use inhalers, nasal spray, nose drops? How often? Which type?
- How long have you used this?

"Seasonal" rhinitis if due to pollen; "perennial" if allergen is dust.

Misuse of over-the-counter nasal medications irritates the mucosa, causing rebound swelling, a common problem.

7. Altered smell. Experienced any **change in sense of smell?**

Sense of smell diminished with cigarette smoking or chronic allergies.

Mouth and Throat

1. Sores or lesions. Noticed any **sores** or **lesions** in the mouth, tongue, or gums?
- How long have you had it? Ever had this lesion before?
- Is it single or multiple?
- Does it seem to be associated with stress, season change, food?
- How have you treated the sore? Applied any local medication?

History helps to determine if oral lesions have infectious, traumatic, immunologic, or malignant etiology.

2. Sore throat. How about **sore throats?** How frequently do you get them? Have a sore throat now? When did it start?
- Is it associated with cough, fever, fatigue, decreased appetite, headache, postnasal drip, or hoarseness?
- Is it worse when arising? What is the humidity level in the room where you sleep? Any dust or smoke inhaled at work?
- Usually get a throat culture for the sore throats? Were any documented as streptococcal?
- How have you treated this sore throat: medication, gargling? How effective are these? Have your tonsils or adenoids been taken out?

Untreated strep throat may lead to the complication of rheumatic fever.

3. Bleeding gums. Any **bleeding gums?** How long have you had this?

EXAMINER ASKS	RATIONALE

4. Toothache. Any **toothache**? Do your teeth seem sensitive to hot, cold? Have you lost any teeth?

5. Hoarseness. Any **hoarseness**, voice change? For how long?
- Feel like having to clear your throat? Or, like a "lump in your throat?"
- Use your voice a lot at work, recreation?
- Does the hoarseness seem associated with a cold, sore throat?

A disorder of the larynx due to many causes, such as overuse of the voice, upper respiratory infection, chronic inflammation, lesions, or a neoplasm.

6. Dysphagia. Any difficulty swallowing? How long have you had it?
- Feel like food gets stopped at a certain point?
- Any pain with this?

Dysphagia occurs with many conditions, including gastroesophageal reflux disease, pharyngitis, stroke and other neurologic diseases, esophageal cancer.

7. Altered taste. Any **change in sense of taste**?

8. Smoking, alcohol consumption. Do you smoke? Pipe or cigarettes? Smokeless tobacco? How many packs per day? For how many years?

- When was your last alcohol drink? How much alcohol did you drink that time? How much alcohol do you usually drink?

Chronic tobacco use is associated with tooth loss, coronal and root caries, and periodontal disease in older adults.

Chronic use of tobacco in any form and heavy alcohol consumption highly increase risk of oral and pharyngeal cancers (Shugars and Patton, 1997).

9. Self-care behaviors. Tell me about your daily dental care. How often do you use a toothbrush and floss?
- Last dental examination? Do dental problems affect which foods you eat?
- Do you have a dental appliance: braces, bridge, headgear?
- Wear dentures? All the time? How long have you had this set? How do they fit?
- Any sores or irritation on the palate or gums?
- Any problems with talking—Do the dentures whistle or drop? Can you chew all foods with them? How do you clean them?

Assess self-care behaviors for oral hygiene.

Periodic dental screening is necessary to note caries.

Lesions may arise from ill-fitting dentures, or the presence of dentures may mask the eruption of new lesion.

Additional History for Infants and Children

1. Does the child have any mouth infections or sores, such as thrush or canker sores? How frequently do these occur?

2. Does the child have frequent sore throat, or tonsillitis? How often? How are these treated? Have they ever been documented as streptococcal infections?

3. Did the child's teeth erupt about on time?

- Do the teeth seem straight to you?
- Is the child using a bottle? How often during the day? Does the child go to sleep with a bottle at night?

- Have you noticed any thumb-sucking after the child's secondary teeth came in?
- Have you noticed the child grinding his or her teeth? Does this happen at night?

Eruption is delayed with Down syndrome, cretinism, rickets, and may impair nutrition.

Malocclusion.

Prolonged use of a bottle during day or at bedtime places infant at risk for tooth decay and middle ear infections.

Prolonged thumb-sucking (after age 6 to 7) may affect occlusion.

Bruxism usually occurs in sleep, from dental problems, nervous tension.

4. Self-care behaviors. How are the child's dental habits? Use a toothbrush regularly? How often does the child see a dentist?
- Do you use fluoridated water or fluoride supplement?

Evaluate child's self-care. Early self-care has best compliance.

EXAMINER ASKS	RATIONALE

Additional History for the Aging Adult

1. Any dryness in the mouth? Are you taking any medications? (Note prescribed and over-the-counter medications.)

Xerostomia (dry mouth) is a side effect of many drugs used by older people: antidepressants, anticholinergics, antispasmodics, antihypertensives, antipsychotics, bronchodilators.

2. Have you had any loss of teeth? Can you chew all types of food?

Note a decrease in eating meat, fresh vegetables, and cleansing foods such as apples.

3. Are you able to care for your own teeth or dentures?

Ability to perform self-care may be decreased by physical disability (arthritis), vision loss, confusion, or depression.

4. Noticed a change in your sense of taste or smell?

Some people add condiments to enhance food when taste begins to wane. Note salt and sugar additives especially.

Also, diminished smell may decrease the person's ability to detect food spoilage, natural gas leaks, or smoke from a fire.

Objective Data

PREPARATION

Position the person sitting up straight with his or her head at your eye level. If the person wears dentures, offer a paper towel and ask the person to remove them.

EQUIPMENT NEEDED

Otoscope with short, wide-tipped nasal speculum attachment
Penlight
Two tongue blades
Cotton gauze pad (4 × 4 inches)
Gloves
Occasionally: long-stem light attachment for otoscope

NORMAL RANGE OF FINDINGS	ABNORMAL FINDINGS

INSPECT AND PALPATE THE NOSE

External Nose

Normally, the nose is symmetric, in the midline, and in proportion to other facial features (Fig. 16–7). Inspect for any deformity, asymmetry, inflammation, or skin lesions. If an injury is reported or suspected, palpate gently for any pain or break in contour.

16–7

NORMAL RANGE OF FINDINGS

Test the patency of the nostrils by pushing each nasal wing shut with your finger while asking the person to sniff inward through the other naris. This reveals any obstruction, which later is explored using the nasal speculum. The sense of smell, mediated by cranial nerve I, is usually not tested in a routine examination. The procedure for assessing smell is presented with cranial nerve testing in Chapter 23.

Nasal Cavity

Attach the short wide-tipped speculum to the otoscope head and insert this combined apparatus into the nasal vestibule, avoiding pressure on the nasal septum. Gently lift up the tip of the nose with your finger before inserting.

View each nasal cavity with the person's head erect, then with the head tilted back. Inspect the nasal mucosa, noting its normal red color and smooth moist surface (Fig. 16–8). Note any swelling, discharge, bleeding, or foreign body.

ABNORMAL FINDINGS

Absence of sniff indicates obstruction (e.g., nasal polyps, rhinitis).

Rhinitis—Nasal mucosa is swollen and bright red with an upper respiratory infection.

Discharge is common with rhinitis and sinusitis, varying from watery and copious to thick, purulent, and green-yellow.

With chronic allergy, mucosa looks swollen, boggy, pale, and gray.

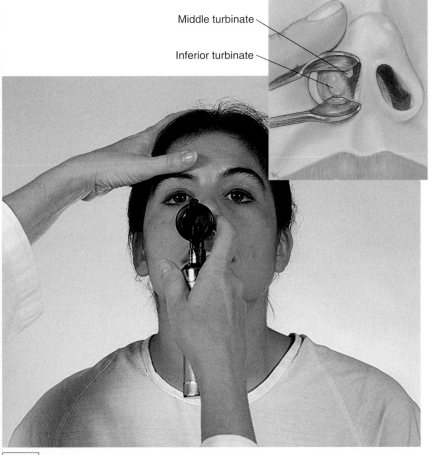

Middle turbinate

Inferior turbinate

16–8

NORMAL RANGE OF FINDINGS

Observe the nasal septum for deviation (Fig. 16–9). A deviated septum is common and is not significant unless airflow is obstructed. (If present in a hospitalized patient, document the deviated septum in the event that the person needs nasal suctioning or a nasogastric tube.) Also note any perforation or bleeding in the septum.

16–9

Inspect the turbinates, the bony ridges curving down from the lateral walls. The superior turbinate will not be in your view, but the middle and inferior turbinates appear the same light red color as the nasal mucosa. Note any swelling but do not try to push the speculum past it. Turbinates are quite vascular and tender if touched.

Note any polyps, which are benign growths that accompany chronic allergy, and distinguish them from the normal turbinates.

PALPATE THE SINUS AREAS

Using your thumbs, press over the frontal sinuses below the eyebrows (Fig. 16–10, A) and over the maxillary sinuses below the cheekbones (Fig. 16–10, B). Take care not to press directly on the eyeballs. The person should feel firm pressure but no pain.

A   B

16–10

ABNORMAL FINDINGS

A deviated septum looks like a hump or shelf in one nasal cavity.

Perforation is seen as a spot of light from penlight shining in other naris.

Epistaxis commonly comes from anterior septum (see Table 16–1 on p. 396).

Polyps are smooth, pale gray, avascular, mobile, and nontender (see Table 16–1).

Sinus areas are tender to palpation in persons with chronic allergies and acute infection (sinusitis).

NORMAL RANGE OF FINDINGS	ABNORMAL FINDINGS

Transillumination

You may use this technique when you suspect sinus inflammation, although it is of limited usefulness. Darken the examining room. Affix a strong narrow light to the end of the otoscope, and hold it under the superior orbital ridge against the location of the frontal sinus area (Fig. 16–11). Cover with your hand. A diffuse red glow is a normal response. It comes from the light shining through the air in the healthy sinus.

An inflamed sinus filled with fluid does not transilluminate.

16–11

You may use the same technique with the maxillary sinuses, providing the person has no upper denture that would impede the light. Ask the person to tilt the head back and open the mouth. Shine the light on each cheek just under the inner corner of the eye. Note a dull glow inside the mouth on the hard palate as the light transmits through the sinuses. Healthy sinuses contain air and may light up symmetrically. But be aware that asymmetry is not a reliable sign of sinus inflammation because many healthy sinuses normally will not transilluminate.

A significant finding is one sinus illuminated and the other clouded. If one has fluid, it looks darker than the healthy one.

INSPECT THE MOUTH

Begin with anterior structures and move posteriorly. Use a tongue blade to retract structures and a bright light for optimal visualization.

Lips

Inspect the lips for color, moisture, cracking, or lesions. Retract the lips and note their inner surface as well (Fig. 16–12). Black persons normally may have bluish lips.

In light-skinned people: circumoral pallor occurs with shock and anemia; cyanosis with hypoxemia and chilling; cherry red lips with carbon monoxide poisoning, acidosis from aspirin poisoning, or ketoacidosis.

Cheilitis (perlèche)—cracking at the corners.

Herpes simplex, other lesions (see Table 16–2).

16–12

NORMAL RANGE OF FINDINGS	ABNORMAL FINDINGS

Teeth and Gums

The condition of the teeth is an index of the person's general health. Your examination should not replace the regular dental examination, but you should note any diseased, absent, loose, or abnormally positioned teeth. The teeth normally look white, straight, and evenly spaced, and clean and free of debris or decay.

Compare the number of teeth with the number expected for the person's age. Ask the person to bite as if chewing something and note alignment of upper and lower jaw. Normal occlusion in the back is the upper teeth resting directly on the lowers; in the front, the upper incisors slightly override the lower incisors.

Normally, the gums look pink or coral with a stippled (dotted) surface. The gum margins at the teeth are tight and well defined. Check for swelling; retraction of gingival margins; and spongy, bleeding, or discolored gums. Black people normally may have a dark melanotic line along the gingival margin.

Abnormal Findings:

Discolored teeth appear brown with excessive fluoride use; yellow with tobacco use.

Grinding down of tooth surface.

Plaque—soft debris.

Caries—decay.

Malocclusion (poor biting relationship), protrusion of upper or lower incisors (see Table 16–3).

Gingival hypertrophy (see Table 16–3), crevices between teeth and gums, pockets of debris.

Gums bleed with slight pressure, indicating gingivitis.

Dark line on gingival margins occurs with lead and bismuth poisoning.

Tongue

Check the tongue for color, surface characteristics, and moisture. The color is pink and even. The dorsal surface is normally roughened from the papillae. A thin white coating may be present. Ask the person to touch the tongue to the roof of the mouth. Its ventral surface looks smooth, glistening, and shows veins. Saliva is present.

Abnormal Findings:

Beefy red swollen tongue. Smooth glossy areas (see Table 16–5).

Enlarged tongue occurs with mental retardation, hypothyroidism, acromegaly; a small tongue accompanies malnutrition.

Dry mouth occurs with dehydration, fever; tongue has deep vertical fissures.

Saliva is decreased while the person is taking anticholinergic and other medication.

Excess saliva and drooling occur with gingivostomatitis and neurologic dysfunction.

With a glove,* hold the tongue using a cotton gauze pad for traction and swing the tongue out and to each side (Fig. 16–13). Inspect for any white patches or lesions—normally none are present. If any occur, palpate these lesions for induration.

16–13

---

*Always wear gloves to examine mucous membranes. This follows Standard Precautions to prevent the spread of possible communicable disease.

NORMAL RANGE OF FINDINGS

Inspect carefully the entire U-shaped area under the tongue. Oral malignancies are most likely to develop here. Note any white patches, nodules, or ulcerations. If lesions are present, or with any person over 50 or with a positive history of smoking or alcohol use, use your gloved hand to palpate the area. Place your other hand under the jaw to stabilize the tissue and to "capture" any abnormality (Fig. 16–14). Note any induration.

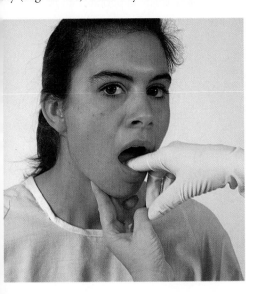

16–14

Buccal Mucosa

Hold the cheek open with a wooden tongue blade, and check the buccal mucosa for color, nodules, or lesions. It looks pink, smooth, and moist, although patchy hyperpigmentation is common and normal in dark-skinned people.

An expected finding is **Stensen's duct,** the opening of the parotid salivary gland. It looks like a small dimple opposite the upper second molar. You also may see a raised occlusion line on the buccal mucosa parallel with the level the teeth meet due to the teeth closing against the cheek.

A larger patch also may be present along the buccal mucosa. This is **leukoedema,** a benign grayish opaque area, more common in blacks and East Indians. When it is mild, the patch disappears as you stretch the cheeks. The severity of the condition increases with age, looking grayish white and thickened. The cause of the condition is unknown. Do not mistake leukoedema for oral infections such as candidiasis (thrush).

Fordyce's granules are small, isolated white or yellow papules on the mucosa of cheek, tongue, and lips (Fig. 16–15). These little sebaceous cysts are painless and not significant.

16–15

Fordyce's granules.

ABNORMAL FINDINGS

Any lesion or ulcer persisting for more than 2 weeks must be investigated.

An indurated area may be a mass or lymphadenopathy, and it must be investigated.

Dappled brown patches are present with Addison's disease (chronic adrenal insufficiency).

Orifice of Stensen's duct looks red with mumps.

Koplik's spots—a prodromal sign of measles.

The chalky white raised patch of **leukoplakia** is abnormal (see Table 16–4).

NORMAL RANGE OF FINDINGS

Palate

Shine your light up to the roof of the mouth. The more anterior hard palate is white with irregular transverse rugae. The posterior soft palate is pinker, smooth, and upwardly movable. A normal variation is a nodular bony ridge down the middle of the hard palate, a **torus palatinus** (Fig. 16–16). This benign growth arises after puberty and is present in 25% of whites and 20% of blacks (Overfield, 1995). It is a more common finding in Native Americans, Inuits, and

The hard palate appears yellow with jaundice. In blacks with jaundice, it may look yellow, muddy yellow, or green-brown.

Oral Kaposi's sarcoma is the most common early lesion in people with AIDS (see Table 16–6).

16–16 Torus palatinus (viewed with a mirror).

Asians. Figure 16–16 uses a mirror to reflect the image of the torus palatinus, which actually lies in the roof of the mouth.

Observe the uvula; it normally looks like a fleshy pendant hanging in the midline (Fig. 16–17). Ask the person to say "ahhh" and note the soft palate and uvula rise in the midline. This tests one function of cranial nerve X, the vagus nerve.

A *bifid* uvula looks like it is split in two; more common in Native Americans (see Table 16–6).

Any deviation to the side or absent movement indicates nerve damage, which also occurs with poliomyelitis and diphtheria.

1+   2+   3+ 4+   Anterior tonsillar pillar

Tonsil

16–17

NORMAL RANGE OF FINDINGS	ABNORMAL FINDINGS

INSPECT THE THROAT

Using your light, observe the oval, rough-surfaced **tonsils** behind the anterior tonsillar pillar (see Fig. 16–17). Their color is the same pink as the oral mucosa, and their surface is peppered with indentations, or crypts. In some people the crypts collect small plugs of whitish cellular debris. This does not indicate infection. However, there should be no exudate on the tonsils. Tonsils are graded in size as follows:

1+   Visible
2+   Halfway between tonsillar pillars and uvula
3+   Touching the uvula
4+   Touching each other

You may normally see 1+ or 2+ tonsils in healthy people, especially in children, because lymphoid tissue is proportionately enlarged until puberty.

Enlarge your view of the posterior pharyngeal wall by depressing the tongue with a tongue blade (Fig. 16–18). Push down halfway back on the tongue; if you push on its tip, the tongue will hump up in back. Press slightly off center to avoid eliciting the gag reflex. You can help the person whose gag reflex is easily triggered by offering a tongue blade to depress his or her own tongue. (Some people can lower their own tongue so the tongue blade is not needed.) Scan the posterior wall for color, exudate, or lesions. When finished, discard the tongue blade.

16–18

Although usually it is not done in the screening examination, touching the posterior wall with the tongue blade elicits the gag reflex. This tests cranial nerves IX and X, the glossopharyngeal and vagus.

Test cranial nerve XII, the hypoglossal nerve, by asking the person to stick out the tongue. It should protrude in the midline. Children enjoy this request! Note any tremor, loss of movement, or deviation to the side.

With an acute infection, tonsils are bright red, swollen, and may have exudate or large white spots.

A white membrane covering the tonsils may accompany infectious mononucleosis, leukemia, and diphtheria.

Tonsils are enlarged to 2+, 3+, or 4+ with an acute infection.

With damage to cranial nerve XII, the tongue deviates *toward* the paralyzed side.

A fine tremor of the tongue occurs with hyperthyroidism; a coarse tremor with cerebral palsy and alcoholism.

NORMAL RANGE OF FINDINGS	ABNORMAL FINDINGS

During the examination, notice any breath odor, *halitosis*. This is common and usually is due to a local cause, such as poor oral hygiene, consumption of odoriferous foods, alcohol consumption, heavy smoking, or dental infection. Occasionally it may indicate a systemic disease.

Diabetic ketoacidosis has a sweet, fruity breath odor; this acetone smell also occurs in children with malnutrition or dehydration. Others are an ammonia breath odor with uremia; a musty odor with liver disease; a foul, fetid odor with dental or respiratory infections; alcohol odor with alcohol ingestion or chemicals; a mouse-like smell of the breath with diphtheria.

 DEVELOPMENTAL CONSIDERATIONS

Infants and Children

Since the oral examination is intrusive for the infant or young child, the timing is best toward the end of the complete examination, along with the ear examination. But if any crying episodes occur earlier, seize the opportunity to examine the open mouth and oropharynx.

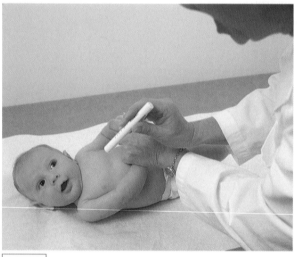

16–19

As with the ear examination, let the parent help position the child. Place the infant supine on the examining table, with the arms restrained (Fig. 16–19). The older infant and toddler may be held on the parent's lap with one of the parent's hands holding the arms down and the other hand restraining the child's head against the parent's chest. Although not often needed, the parent's leg can reach over and capture the child's legs between the parent's own (Fig. 16–20).

16–20

NORMAL RANGE OF FINDINGS	ABNORMAL FINDINGS

Use a game to help prepare the young child. Encourage the preschool child to use a tongue blade to look into a puppet's mouth. Or place a mirror so that the child can look into the mouth while you do. The school-age child is usually co-operative and loves to show off missing or new teeth (Fig. 16–21).

16–21

Be discriminating in your use of the tongue blade. It may be necessary for a full view of oral structures, but it produces a strong gag reflex in the infant. You may avoid the tongue blade completely with a cooperative preschooler and school-age child. Try asking the young child to open the mouth "as big as a lion" and to move the tongue in different directions. To enlarge your view of the oropharynx, ask the child to stick out the tongue and "pant like a dog."

At some point, you will encounter an uncooperative young child who clenches the teeth and refuses to open the mouth. If all your other efforts have failed, slide the tongue blade along the buccal mucosa and turn it between the back teeth. Push down to depress the tongue. This stimulates the gag reflex, and the child opens the mouth wide for a few seconds. You will have a *brief* look at the throat. Make the most of it.

NOSE

The newborn may have milia across the nose. The nasal bridge may be flat in black and Asian children. There should be no nasal flaring or narrowing with breathing.

It is essential to determine the patency of the nares in the immediate newborn period because most newborns are obligate nose-breathers. Nares blocked with amniotic fluid are suctioned gently with a bulb syringe. If obstruction is suspected, a small-lumen (5 to 10 Fr) catheter is passed down each naris to confirm patency.

Nasal flaring in the infant indicates respiratory distress.

A transverse ridge across the nose occurs in a child with chronic allergy from wiping the nose upward with palm (see Table 16–4). Nasal narrowing on inhalation is seen with chronic nasal obstruction and mouth-breathing.

Inability to pass catheter through nasal cavity indicates choanal atresia, which needs immediate intervention (see Table 16–1 on p. 396).

NORMAL RANGE OF FINDINGS

Avoid the nasal speculum when examining the infant and young child. Instead, gently push up the tip of the nose with your thumb while using your other hand to shine the light into the naris. With a toddler, be alert for the possible foreign body lodged in the nasal cavity (see Table 16–1).

Only in children older than 8 years do you need to palpate the child's sinus areas. In younger children, sinus areas are too small for palpation.

MOUTH AND THROAT

A normal finding in infants is the **sucking tubercle,** a small pad in the middle of the upper lip from friction of breast- or bottle-feeding. Note the number of teeth, and whether or not it is appropriate for the child's age. Also note pattern of eruption, position, condition, and hygiene. Use this guide for children under 2 years; the child's age in months minus the number 6 should equal the expected number of deciduous teeth. Normally, all 20 deciduous teeth are in by 2½ years. Saliva is present after 3 months of age and shows in excess with teething children.

Mobility should allow the tongue to extend at least as far as the alveolar ridge.

Note any bruising or laceration on the buccal mucosa or gums of the infant or young child.

On the palate, **Epstein pearls** are a normal finding in newborns and infants (Fig. 16–22). They are small, whitish, glistening, pearly papules along the median raphe of the hard palate and on the gums, where they look like teeth. They are small retention cysts and disappear in the first few weeks.

16–22 Epstein pearls.

Bednar aphthae are traumatic areas or ulcers on the posterior hard palate on either side of the midline. They result from abrasions while sucking.

The tonsils are not visible in the newborn. They gradually enlarge during childhood, remaining proportionately larger until puberty. Tonsils appear still larger if the infant is crying or gagging. Normally the newborn can produce a strong, lusty cry.

Insert your gloved finger into the baby's mouth and palpate the hard and soft palate as the baby sucks. The sucking reflex can be elicited in infants up to 12 months.

ABNORMAL FINDINGS

No teeth by age 1 year.

Discolored teeth appear yellow or yellow-brown with infants taking tetracycline or whose mothers took the drug during the last trimester; appear green or black with excessive iron ingestion, although this reverses when the iron is stopped.

Malocclusion: upper or lower dental arches are out of alignment.

Ankyloglossia, a short lingual frenulum, can limit protrusion and impair speech development (see Table 16–5).

Trauma may indicate child abuse due to forced feeding of bottle or spoon.

A high-arched palate is usually normal in the newborn, but a very narrow or high arch also occurs with Tumer's syndrome, Ehlers-Danlos syndrome, Marfan's syndrome, and Treacher Collins syndrome, or develops in the mouth-breather in chronic allergies.

NORMAL RANGE OF FINDINGS

ABNORMAL FINDINGS

The Pregnant Female

Gum hypertrophy (surface looks smooth and stippling disappears) may occur normally at puberty or during pregnancy (pregnancy gingivitis).

The Aging Adult

The nose may appear more prominent on the face due to a loss of subcutaneous fat. In the edentulous person the mouth and lips fold in, giving a "purse-string" appearance. The teeth may look slightly yellowed, although the color is uniform. Yellowing results from the dentin visible through worn enamel. The surface of the incisors may show vertical cracks from a lifetime of exposure to extreme temperatures. The teeth may look longer as the gum margins recede.

The surfaces look worn down or abraded. Old dental work deteriorates, especially at the gum margins. The teeth loosen with bone resorption and may move with palpation.

The tongue looks smoother due to papillary atrophy. The aging adult's buccal mucosa is thinned and may look shinier, as though it was "varnished."

SUMMARY CHECKLIST: Nose, Mouth, and Throat Exam

Nose

1. Inspect external nose for symmetry, any deformity, or lesions
2. Palpation—Test patency of each nostril
3. Inspect using nasal speculum:
   Color and integrity of nasal mucosa
   Septum—Note any deviation, perforation, or bleeding
   Turbinates—Note color, any exudate, swelling, or polyps

4. Palpate the sinus areas—Note any tenderness

Mouth and Throat

1. Inspect using penlight:
   Lips, teeth and gums, tongue, buccal mucosa—Note color; if structures are intact, any lesions
   Palate and uvula—Note integrity and mobility as person phonates
   Grade tonsils
   Pharyngeal wall—Note color, any exudate, or lesions

2. Palpation:
   When indicated in adults, bimanual palpation of mouth
   With the neonate, palpate for integrity of palate and to assess sucking reflex

See Health Promotion Guide on CD

Application and Critical Thinking

SAMPLE CHARTING

SUBJECTIVE

Nose. No history of discharge, sinus problems, obstruction, epistaxis, or allergy. Colds 1–2/yr, mild. Fractured nose during high school sports, treated by M.D.

Mouth and Throat. No pain, lesions, bleeding gums, toothache, dysphagia, or hoarseness. Occasional sore throat with colds. Tonsillectomy, age 8. Smokes cigarettes 1 PPD × 9 years. Alcohol—1–2 drinks socially, about 2 ×/month. Visits dentist annually, dental hygienist 2 ×/year, flosses daily. No dental appliance.

OBJECTIVE

Nose. Symmetric, no deformity or skin lesions. Nares patent. Mucosa pink, no discharge, lesions, or polyps; no septal deviation or perforation. Sinuses—no tenderness to palpation.

Continued

Mouth. Can clench teeth. Mucosa and gingivae pink, no masses or lesions. Teeth are all present, straight, and in good repair. Tongue smooth, pink, no lesions, protrudes in midline, no tremor.

Throat. Mucosa pink, no lesions or exudate. Uvula rises in midline on phonation. Tonsils out. Gag reflex present.

FOCUSED ASSESSMENT: CLINICAL CASE STUDY 1

Brad D., a 34-year-old electrician, seeks care for "sore throat for 2 days."

SUBJECTIVE

2 days PTA experienced sudden onset of sore throat, swollen glands, fever 101° F, occasional shaking chills, extreme fatigue.

Today—symptoms remain. Cough productive of yellow sputum. Treated self with aspirin for minimal relief. Unable to eat last 2 days because "throat on fire." Taking adequate fluids, on bedrest. Not aware of exposure to other sick persons. Does not smoke.

OBJECTIVE

Ears. Tympanic membranes pearl gray with landmarks intact.

Nose. No discharge. Mucosa pink, no swelling.

Mouth. Mucosa and gingivae pink, no lesions.

Throat. Tonsils 3+. Pharyngeal wall bright red with yellow-white exudate, exudate also on tonsils.

Neck. Enlarged anterior cervical nodes bilaterally, painful to palpation. No other lymph adenopathy.

Chest. Resonant to percussion throughout. Breath sounds clear anterior and posterior. No adventitious sounds.

ASSESSMENT

Pharyngitis
Pain R/T inflammation
Imbalanced nutrition: less than body requirements R/T dysphagia

FOCUSED ASSESSMENT: CLINICAL CASE STUDY 2

Calvin W., a 53-year-old white businessman, is in the hospital awaiting coronary bypass surgery for coronary artery disease. He is allergic to dust and animal hair. As part of a preoperative teaching plan for coughing and deep breathing, a respiratory assessment is performed.

SUBJECTIVE

States understanding of reason for admission to hospital and extent of coronary artery disease. Unaware of details of surgical procedure and postoperative care. Interested: "I do better when I know what I'm dealing with." History of exertional angina after walking one short block or climbing one flight of stairs, treats self with nitroglycerin. Does not smoke. Chronic watery nasal discharge, "comes and goes, but present most of time."

OBJECTIVE

Nose. Only R naris patent. Mucosa gray and boggy bilaterally. L naris has mobile, gray, nontender mass, obstructing view of turbinates and rest of nasal cavity.

Mouth and Throat. Mucosa pink, no lesions. Uvula midline, rises on phonation. Tonsils absent. No lumps or lesions on palpation.

Chest. Thorax symmetric, AP < transverse diameter, respirations 18/min, effortless. Resonant to percussion. Breath sounds are clear. No adventitious sounds.

ASSESSMENT

L nasal mass, possibly polyp
Deficient knowledge for surgery and expected postop course R/T lack of exposure

FOCUSED ASSESSMENT: CLINICAL CASE STUDY 3

Esther V. is a 61-year-old professor who has been admitted to the hospital for chemotherapy for carcinoma of the breast. This is her 5th day in the hospital. An oral assessment is performed when she complains of "soreness and a white coating" in the mouth.

SUBJECTIVE

Felt soreness on tongue and cheeks during night. Now pain persists, and E.V. can see a "white coating" on tongue and cheeks. "I'm worried. Is this more cancer?"

OBJECTIVE

E.V. generally appears restless and overly aware.

Oral mucosa pink. Large white, cheesy patches covering most of dorsal surface of tongue and buccal mucosa. Will scrape off with tongue blade, revealing red eroded area beneath.

Bleeds with slight contact. Posterior pharyngeal wall pink, no lesions. Patches are soft to palpation. No palpable lymph nodes.

ASSESSMENT

Oral lesion, appears as candidiasis
Impaired oral mucous membrane R/T effects of chemotherapy
Pain R/T infectious process
Anxiety R/T threat to health status

NURSING DIAGNOSES COMMONLY ASSOCIATED WITH NOSE, MOUTH, THROAT DISORDERS

RELATED FACTORS (Etiology)	DEFINING CHARACTERISTICS (Symptoms and Signs)

DIAGNOSIS: Impaired **Oral** mucous membrane

Dehydration	Atrophy of gums
Effects of	Coated tongue
Chemotherapy	Dry mouth (xerostomia)
Medication	Edema of mucosa
Radiation to head/neck	Halitosis
Diabetes mellitus	Hemorrhagic gingivitis
Oral cancer	Hyperemia
Immunosuppression	Lack of or decreased salivation
Inadequate oral hygiene	Leukoplakia
Infection	Oral
Lack of knowledge	Lesions
Mouth-breathing	Pain or discomfort
Malnutrition/vitamin deficiency	Plaque
NPO for >24 h	Redness
Chemical trauma	Ulcers
Acidic foods	Vesicles
Alcohol	Purulent drainage
Drugs	Stomatitis
Noxious agents	
Tobacco	
Mechanical trauma	
Braces	
Broken teeth	
Endotracheal tube	
Fractured mandible	
Ill-fitting dentures	
Nasogastric tube	
Vomiting	

Continued

RELATED FACTORS (Etiology)	DEFINING CHARACTERISTICS (Symptoms and Signs)

DIAGNOSIS: Impaired Swallowing

Effects of	Coughing/choking
Cleft lip/palate	Dehydration
Cerebrovascular accident	Evidence of aspiration
Cranial nerve damage (V, VII, IX, X)	Regurgitation of fluids/solids through mouth or nose
Neuromuscular disorder (e.g., cerebral palsy, muscular	Reported pain on swallowing
dystrophy, Guillain-Barré syndrome, myasthenia gravis,	Stasis of food in oral cavity
poliomyelitis), oral/pharyngeal cancer	Weight loss
Excessive/inadequate salivation	
Fatigue	
Limited awareness	
Mechanical obstruction	
Edema	
Tracheostomy tube	
Tumor	
Neuromuscular impairment	
Decreased/absent gag reflex	
Decreased strength of muscles of mastication	
Perceptual impairment	
Facial paralysis	
Reddened, irritated oropharynx	

DIAGNOSIS: Pain

Effects of surgery or trauma	Reports of pain
Experiences during diagnostic tests	Anxiety
Infectious process	Clutching of painful area
Inflammation	Crying or moaning
Muscle spasm	Distraction behavior
Immobility	Focused on self
Obstructive processes	Immobilization
Overactivity	Painful response to palpation
Pressure points	Facial mask of pain
	Changes in posture or gait
	Withdrawal reflex
	Changes in muscle tone—listless to rigid
	Autonomic responses
	Increased blood pressure, pulse, respirations
	Diaphoresis
	Dilated pupils
	Social withdrawal
	Impaired thought process
	Altered time perception
	Feelings of guilt, despair, or helplessness

DIAGNOSIS: Disturbed Sensory perception

Olfactory	
Effects of aging	
Foreign body in nares	Decreased sensitivity to smells
Inflammation of nasal mucosa	Decreased appetite
Neurologic impairment	
Obstruction in nares	

RELATED FACTORS (Etiology)   **DEFINING CHARACTERISTICS** (Symptoms and Signs)

DIAGNOSIS: Disturbed **S**ensory perception—cont'd

Gustatory
    Effects of aging   Decreased sensitivity to tastes
    Effects of trauma to tongue   Decreased appetite
    Inflammation of nasal mucosa   Increased seasoning of foods
    Neurologic impairment
    Side effects of specific medications

OTHER RELATED NURSING DIAGNOSES

ACTUAL   **RISK/WELLNESS**

Ineffective Airway clearance   **Risk**
Impaired verbal Communication   Risk for Aspiration
                                                          Wellness
                                                      Actively seeking knowledge about smoking cessation

 ## ASSESSMENT VIDEO CRITICAL THINKING QUESTIONS

The Saunders *Physical Examination and Health Assessment* video "Nose, Mouth, and Throat" will direct you to consider the following:

1. How may oral self-care affect mouth examination findings?

2. Describe abnormal findings that may be found during inspection of the internal nose.

3. How do mouth examination findings vary among darkly pigmented people?

Abnormal Findings

TABLE 16–1: **Abnormalities of the Nose**

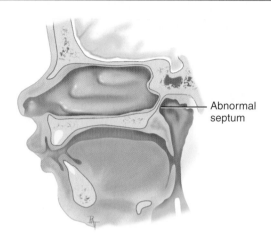

Abnormal septum

Choanal Atresia

A bony or membranous septum between the nasal cavity and the pharynx of the newborn. When the condition is bilateral, it requires the immediate insertion of an oral airway to prevent asphyxia because most newborns are obligate nose-breathers. When the condition is unilateral, the infant may be asymptomatic until the onset of his or her first respiratory infection.

Epistaxis

The most common site of a nosebleed is Kiesselbach's plexus in the anterior septum. It may be spontaneous from a local cause or a sign of underlying illness. Causes include nose-picking, forceful coughing or sneezing, fracture, foreign body, rhinitis, heavy exertion, or a coagulation disorder. Bleeding from the anterior septum is easily controlled and rarely severe. A posterior hemorrhage is less common (<10%) but is more profuse, harder to manage, and more serious.

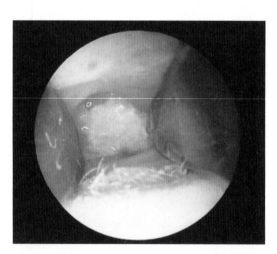

Foreign Body

Children particularly are apt to put an object up the nose (here, yellow plastic foam), producing unilateral mucopurulent drainage and foul odor. Because some risk for aspiration exists, removal should be prompt.

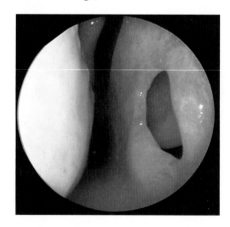

Perforated Septum

A hole in the septum, usually in the cartilaginous part, may be caused by chronic infection, trauma from continual picking of crusts, sniffing cocaine, or nasal surgery. It is seen directly or seen as a spot of light when the penlight is directed into the other naris.

◀ ### Furuncle

A small boil located in the skin or mucous membrane; appears red and swollen and is quite painful. Avoid any manipulation or trauma that may spread the infection.

Continued

TABLE 16-1: **Abnormalities of the Nose—cont'd**

ABNORMAL FINDINGS

Acute Rhinitis

The first sign is a clear, watery discharge, rhinorrhea, which later becomes purulent. This is accompanied by sneezing and swollen mucosa, which causes nasal obstruction. Turbinates are dark red and swollen.

Reprinted from *Atlas of Allergies,* 2nd edition, Fireman, p. 182, 1995, by permission of the publisher Mosby.

Allergic Rhinitis

Rhinorrhea, itching of nose and eyes, lacrimation, nasal congestion, and sneezing are present. Note serous edema and swelling of turbinates to fill the air space. Turbinates are usually pale (although may appear violet), and their surface looks smooth and glistening. May be seasonal or perennial, depending on allergen. Individual has a strong family history of seasonal allergies.

Infected
frontal
sinus

Sinusitis

Facial pain, following upper respiratory infection; signs include red swollen nasal mucosa, swollen turbinates, and purulent discharge. Person also experiences fever, chills, malaise. With maxillary sinusitis, dull throbbing pain occurs in cheeks and teeth on the same side, and pain with palpation is present. With frontal sinusitis, pain is above the supraorbital ridge.

Nasal Polyps

Smooth, pale gray nodules, which are overgrowths of mucosa, most commonly caused by chronic allergic rhinitis. May be stalked. A common site is protrusion from the middle meatus. Often multiple, they are mobile and nontender in contrast to turbinates. They may obstruct air passageways as they get larger. Symptoms include the absence of a sense of smell and a "valve that moves" in the nose as the person breathes.

◀ ## Carcinoma

This appears gray-white and nontender. It may produce slow bloody unilateral discharge, in contrast to the profuse bleeding that accompanies epistaxis. It is not a common lesion.

TABLE 16–2: Abnormalities of the Lips

Cleft Lip

Maxillofacial clefts are the most common congenital deformities of the head and neck. The incidence varies among racial groups, being highest in Native North Americans and in the Japanese (1 in 300 to 400), and lowest in blacks (1 in 1300 to 1800). Although reliable birth registry is not present in all countries, birth records do show a relatively high incidence in Scandinavia and middle European countries, e.g., 1 in 550 in Denmark and Finland, 1 in 575 in Poland and the former Czechoslovakia (Bluestone, Stool, and Kenna, 1996). Early treatment preserves the functions of speech and language formation and deglutition (swallowing).

Herpes Simplex 1

The cold sores are groups of clear vesicles with a surrounding indurated erythematous base. These evolve into pustules, which rupture, weep, and crust, and heal in 4 to 10 days. The most likely site is the lip-skin junction; infection often recurs in same site. Caused by the herpes simplex virus (HSV-1), the lesion is highly contagious and is spread by direct contact. Recurrent herpes infections may be precipitated by sunlight, fever, colds, allergy. It is a very common lesion, affecting 50% of adults.

◄ Angular Cheilitis (Stomatitis, Perlèche)

Erythema, scaling, shallow and painful fissures at the corners of the mouth occur with excess salivation and *Candida* infection. It is often seen in edentulous persons and in those with poorly fitting dentures causing folding in of corners of mouth, creating a warm, moist environment favoring growth of yeast.

Continued

TABLE 16–2: Abnormalities of the Lips—cont'd

Carcinoma

The initial lesion is round and indurated, then it becomes crusted and ulcerated with an elevated border. The vast majority occur between the outer and middle thirds of lip. Any lesion that is still unhealed after 2 weeks should be referred.

Retention "Cyst" (Mucocele)

A round, well-defined translucent nodule that may be very small or up to 1 or 2 cm. It is a pocket of mucus that forms when a duct of a minor salivary gland ruptures. The benign lesion also may occur on the buccal mucosa, on the floor of the mouth, or under the tip of the tongue.

TABLE 16–3: Abnormalities of the Teeth and Gums

Baby Bottle Tooth Decay

Destruction of numerous deciduous teeth may occur in older infants and toddlers who take a bottle of milk, juice, or sweetened drink to bed and prolong bottle feeding past the age of 1 year. Liquid pools around the upper front teeth. Mouth bacteria act on carbohydrates in the liquid, especially sucrose, forming metabolic acids. Acids break down tooth enamel and destroy its protein.

Malocclusion

Upper or lower dental arches are not of alignment and incisors protrude due to developmental problem of mandible or maxilla, or incompatibility between jaw size and tooth size. The condition increases risk of facial deformity, negative body image, chewing problems, or speech dysfluency.

Table continued on following page

TABLE 16–3: Abnormalities of the Teeth and Gums—cont'd

Dental Caries

Progressive destruction of tooth. Decay initially looks chalky white. Later, it turns brown or black and forms a cavity. Early decay is apparent only on x-ray study. Susceptible sites are tooth surfaces where food debris, bacterial plaque, and saliva collect.

Epulis

A nontender, fibrous nodule of the gum, seen emerging between the teeth; an inflammatory response to injury or hemorrhage.

Gingival Hyperplasia

Painless enlargement of the gums, sometimes overreaching the teeth. This occurs with puberty, pregnancy, leukemia, and with long therapeutic use of phenytoin (Dilantin).

Gingivitis

Gum margins are red, swollen, and bleed easily. This case is severe; gingival tissue has desquamated, exposing roots or teeth. Inflammation is usually due to poor dental hygiene or vitamin C deficiency. The condition may occur in pregnancy and puberty because of changing hormonal balance.

TABLE 16–4: Abnormalities of the Buccal Mucosa

Aphthous Ulcers

A "canker sore" is a vesicle at first, then a small, round, "punched-out" ulcer with white base surrounded by a red halo. It is quite painful and lasts for 1 to 2 weeks. The cause is unknown, although it is associated with stress, fatigue, and food allergy. It is common, affecting 20% to 60% of the population.

Koplik's Spots

Small blue-white spots with irregular red halo scattered over mucosa opposite the molars. An early sign, and pathognomonic, of measles.

Leukoplakia

Chalky white, thick, raised patch with well-defined borders. The lesion is firmly attached and does not scrape off. It may occur on the lateral edges of tongue. It is due to chronic irritation, and occurs more frequently with heavy smoking and heavy alcohol use. Lesions are precancerous, and the person should be referred. (Here, the lesion is associated with squamous carcinoma.)

Candidiasis or Monilial Infection

A white, cheesy, curdlike patch on the buccal mucosa and tongue. It scrapes off, leaving raw, red surface that bleeds easily. Termed "thrush" in the newborn. It also occurs after the use of antibiotics, corticosteroids, and in immunosuppressed persons.

TABLE 16–5: Abnormalities of the Tongue

Ankyloglossia

(Tongue-tie.) A short lingual frenulum, here fixing the tongue tip to the floor of the mouth and gums. This limits mobility and will affect speech (pronunciation of a, d, n) if the tongue tip cannot be elevated to the alveolar ridge. A congenital defect.

Fissured or Scrotal Tongue

Deep furrows divide the papillae into small irregular rows. The condition is congenital and is not significant. The incidence increases with age. (Vertical, or longitudinal, fissures also occur with dehydration because of reduced volume of the tongue.)

Geographic Tongue (Migratory Glossitis)

Pattern of normal coating interspersed with bright red, shiny, circular bald areas, having raised pearly borders. Pattern resembles a map, and changes in a few days. Not significant, and its cause is not known.

Smooth, Glossy Tongue (Atrophic Glossitis)

The surface is slick and shiny; the mucosa thins and looks red from decreased papillae. Accompanied by dryness of tongue and burning. Occurs with vitamin B_{12} deficiency (pernicious anemia), folic acid deficiency, and iron deficiency anemia. Here, also note angular cheilitis.

Continued

TABLE 16–5: Abnormalities of the Tongue—cont'd

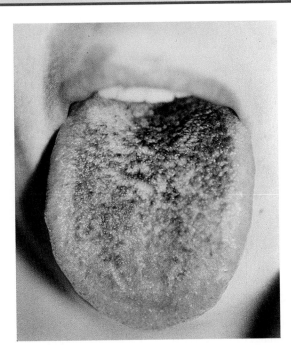

Black Hairy Tongue

This is not really hair but the elongation of filiform papillae and painless overgrowth of mycelial threads of fungus infection on the tongue. It occurs following use of antibiotics, which inhibit normal bacteria and allow proliferation of fungus.

Enlarged Tongue (Macroglossia)

The tongue is enlarged and may protrude from mouth. The condition is not painful but may impair speech development. Here, it occurs with Down syndrome; it also occurs with cretinism, myxedema, acromegaly. Also a transient swelling occurs with local infections.

Carcinoma

An ulcer with rolled edges; indurated. Occurs particularly at sides, base, and under the tongue. When it is in the floor of mouth, it may cause painful movement or limited movement of tongue. Risk of early metastasis is present due to rich lymphatic drainage. Heavy smoking and heavy alcohol use place persons at greater risk.

ABNORMAL FINDINGS

TABLE 16–6: Abnormalities of the Oropharynx

Cleft Palate

A congenital defect, the failure of fusion of the maxillary processes. Wide variation occurs in the extent of cleft formation, from upper lip only, palate only, uvula only, to cleft of the nostril and the hard and soft palates.

Bifid Uvula

The uvula looks partly severed. May indicate a submucous cleft palate, which feels like a notch at the junction of the hard and soft palates. The submucous cleft palate may affect speech development because it prevents necessary air trapping. The incidence of bifid uvula varies among racial groups: It is common in Native Americans, uncommon in whites, and rare in blacks.

Oral Kaposi's Sarcoma

Bruiselike, dark red or violet, confluent macule, usually on the hard palate, may be on soft palate or gingival margin. Oral lesions may be among the earliest lesions to develop with AIDS.

Acute Tonsillitis and Pharyngitis

Bright red throat; swollen tonsils; white or yellow exudate on tonsils and pharynx; swollen uvula; and enlarged, tender anterior cervical and tonsillar nodes. Accompanied by severe sore throat, painful swallowing, fever >101° F of sudden onset.

Caution: One cannot discriminate bacterial from viral infection on clinical data alone; all sore throats need a throat culture. Bacterial pharyngitis caused by group A β-hemolytic streptococcus, if untreated, may lead to the complication of rheumatic fever. This is a serious complex illness characterized by fever, malaise, swollen joints, rash, and scarring on the heart valves.

BIBLIOGRAPHY

Alper C, Myers EN, Eibline DE: *Decision-making in ear, nose, and throat disorders,* Philadelphia, 2001, W.B. Saunders.

Bluestone CD, Stool SE, Kenna MA: *Pediatric otolaryngology,* ed 3, Philadelphia, 1996, W.B. Saunders.

Bromley SM: Smell and taste disorders: a primary care approach, *Am Fam Physician* 61(2):427–438, Jan 15, 2000.

Brothwell DR, Carbonell VM, Goose DH: Congenital absence of teeth in human populations. In Brothwell DR, editor: *Dental anthropology,* New York, 1963, Pergamon Press.

Brown CS, Parker NG, Stegbauer CC: Managing allergic rhinitis, *Nurse Pract* 24(5):107–120, May 1999.

DeRaps PK: The evaluation of the client with acute bacterial rhinosinusitis, Lippincotts *Prim Care Pract* 4(5):490–497, Sep–Oct 2000.

Duchenme TM: Managing sinusitis in children, *Nurse Pract* 25(9):42–55, Sep 2000.

Edell MH et al: Does this patient have strep throat? *JAMA* 284(22):2912–2918, Dec 13, 2000.

Edelstein DR: Aging of the normal nose in adults, *Laryngoscope* 106(9, part 2, suppl 81):1–25, Sep 1996.

Evans WB et al: Managing dysphagia: fundamentals of primary care, *Clin Rev* 8(8):47–71, Aug 1998.

Gaffney KF: Tobacco smoke exposure and pediatric otitis media, Lippincotts *Prim Care Pract* 4(5):508–514, Sep–Oct 2000.

Galvan TJ: Dysphagia: going down and staying down, *Am J Nurs* 101(1):37–43, Jan 2001.

Gawande A: Cold comfort, *New Yorker,* 42–47, Mar 11, 2002.

Gupta A, Hawrych A, Wilson WR: Cocaine-induced sinonasal destruction, *Otolaryngol Heal Neck Surg* 124(4):480, Apr 2001.

Holder R: Preventive dentistry during pregnancy, *Nurse Pract* 24(2):21–24, Feb 1999.

Johnson JT: Examination of the oral cavity: when, how, and what to look for, *Consultant* 39(1):114–120, Jan 1999.

Kane RL, Ouslander JG, Abrass IB: *Essentials of clinical geriatrics,* ed 5, New York, 2003, McGraw-Hill.

Kennedy MM: Influenza viral infections: presentation, prevention, and treatment, *Nurse Pract* 23(9):17–37, Sep 1998.

Klaus BD, Grodesky MJ: Common oral manifestations seen in patients with HIV/AIDS, *Nurse Pract* 23(6):134–139, Jun 1998.

Lash AA: Sjögren's syndrome: pathogenesis, diagnosis, and treatment, *Nurse Pract* 26(8):50–58, Aug 2001.

Leiner S: Acute pharyngitis with lifelong implications, *Nurse Pract* 25(4):119–122, Apr 2000.

Lynch JS, King MS: Chronic nasal obstruction: allergy or infection? Lippincotts *Prim Care Pract* 4(5):455–470, Sep–Oct 2000.

Mackin LA, Antonini CH: Acute sinusitis, Lippincotts *Prim Care Pract* 3(1):65–69, Jan–Feb 1999.

Mulliken RA, Casner MJ: Oral manifestations of systemic disease, *Emerg Med Clin North Am* 18(3):565–575, Aug 2000.

Overfield T: *Biologic variation in health and illness: race, age, and sex differences,* ed 2, New York, 1995, CRC Press.

Satcher D: *Report on oral health,* http://www.surgeongeneral.gov (2000).

Schleicher SM: Diagnosis at a glance—herpes simplex virus infection, *Emerg Med* 31(11):83–84, Nov 1999.

Shugars DC, Patton LL: Detecting, diagnosing, and preventing oral cancer, *Nurse Pract* 22(6):105–132, Jun 1997.

Sparacino LL: Epistaxis management: what's new and what's noteworthy, Lippincotts *Prim Care Pract* 4(5):498–507, Sep–Oct 2000.

Stephenson KN: Acute and chronic pharyngitis across the lifespan, Lippincotts *Prim Care Pract* 4(5):471–489, Sep–Oct 2000.

Swartz M: The oral health of the long-term care patient, *Ann Long Term Care* 8(12):41–46, Dec 2000.

Walpole J: Oral candidiasis, *Am J Nurs Pract* 2(1):37–43, 1998.

CHAPTER 17

Breasts and Regional Lymphatics

Structure and Function

The breasts, or mammary glands, are present in both females and males, although in the male they are rudimentary throughout life. The female breasts are accessory reproductive organs whose function is to produce milk for nourishing the newborn.

SURFACE ANATOMY

The **breasts** lie anterior to the pectoralis major and serratus anterior muscles (Fig. 17–1). The breasts are located between the second and sixth ribs, extending from the side of the sternum to the midaxillary line. The superior lateral corner of breast tissue, called the axillary **tail of Spence,** projects up and laterally into the axilla.

The **nipple** is just below the center of the breast. It is rough, round, and usually protuberant; its surface looks wrinkled and indented with tiny milk duct openings. The **areola** surrounds the nipple for a 1- to 2-cm radius. In the areola are small elevated sebaceous glands, called Montgomery's glands. These secrete a protective lipid material during lactation. The areola also has smooth muscle fibers that cause nipple erection when stimulated. Both the nipple and areola are more darkly pigmented than the rest of the breast surface; the color varies from pink to brown depending on the person's skin color and parity.

INTERNAL ANATOMY

The breast is composed of (1) glandular tissue, (2) fibrous tissue including the suspensory ligaments, and (3) adipose tissue (Fig. 17–2). The **glandular tissue** contains 15 to 20 lobes radiating from the nipple, and these are composed of lobules.

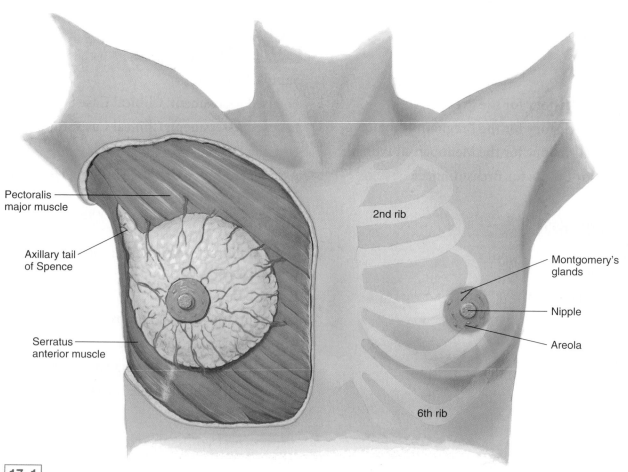

Pectoralis major muscle

Axillary tail of Spence

Serratus anterior muscle

2nd rib

Montgomery's glands

Nipple

Areola

6th rib

17–1

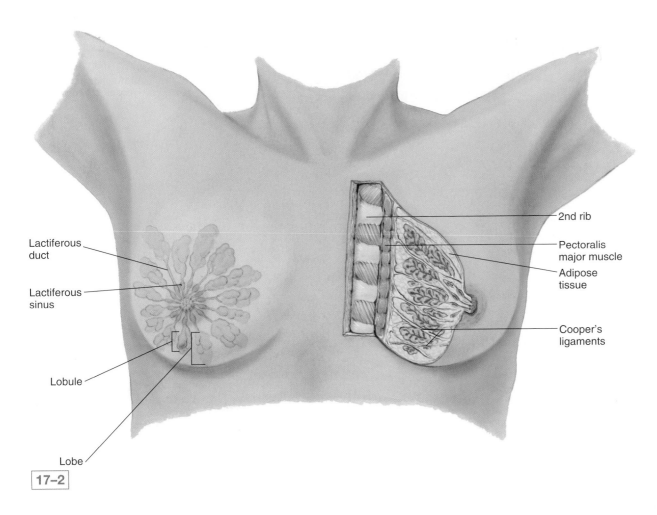

Lactiferous duct

Lactiferous sinus

Lobule

Lobe

2nd rib

Pectoralis major muscle

Adipose tissue

Cooper's ligaments

17–2

Within each lobule are clusters of alveoli that produce milk. Each lobe empties into a lactiferous duct. The 15 to 20 lactiferous ducts form a collecting duct system converging toward the nipple. There, the ducts form ampullae, or lactiferous sinuses, behind the nipple, which are reservoirs for storing milk.

The suspensory ligaments, or **Cooper's ligaments,** are fibrous bands extending vertically from the surface to attach on chest wall muscles. These support the breast tissue. They become contracted in cancer of the breast, producing pits or dimples in the overlying skin.

The lobes are embedded in **adipose tissue.** These layers of subcutaneous and retromammary fat actually provide most of the bulk of the breast. The relative proportion of glandular, fibrous, and fatty tissue varies depending on age, cycle, pregnancy, lactation, and general nutritional state.

The breast may be divided into four quadrants by imaginary horizontal and vertical lines intersecting at the nipple (Fig. 17–3). This makes a convenient map to describe clinical findings. In the upper outer quadrant, note the axillary **tail of Spence,** the cone-shaped breast tissue that projects up into the axilla, close to the pectoral group of axillary lymph nodes. The upper outer quadrant is the site of most breast tumors.

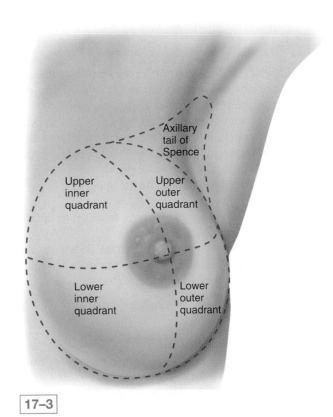

Axillary tail of Spence

Upper inner quadrant

Upper outer quadrant

Lower inner quadrant

Lower outer quadrant

17–3

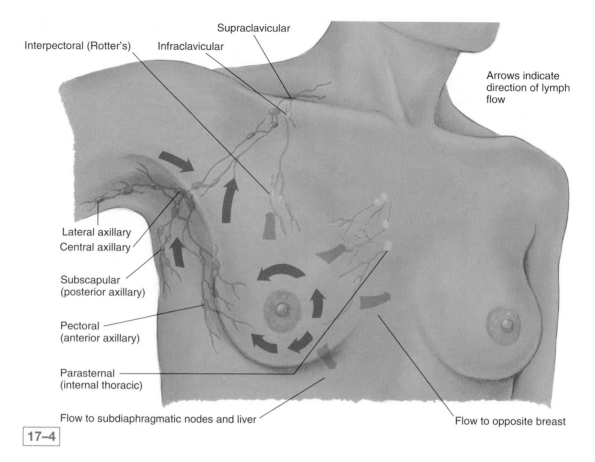

Supraclavicular

Interpectoral (Rotter's)   Infraclavicular

Arrows indicate direction of lymph flow

Lateral axillary
Central axillary

Subscapular (posterior axillary)

Pectoral (anterior axillary)

Parasternal (internal thoracic)

Flow to subdiaphragmatic nodes and liver

Flow to opposite breast

17–4

LYMPHATICS

The breast has extensive lymphatic drainage. Most of the lymph, more than 75%, drains into the ipsilateral axillary nodes. Four groups of axillary nodes are present (Fig. 17–4):

1. **Central axillary nodes**—high up in the middle of the axilla, over the ribs and serratus anterior muscle. These receive lymph from the other three groups of nodes.
2. **Pectoral** (anterior)—along the lateral edge of the pectoralis major muscle, just inside the anterior axillary fold.
3. **Subscapular** (posterior)—along the lateral edge of the scapula, deep in the posterior axillary fold.
4. **Lateral**—along the humerus, inside the upper arm.

From the central axillary nodes, drainage flows up to the infraclavicular and supraclavicular nodes.

A smaller amount of lymphatic drainage does not take these channels but flows directly up to the infraclavicular group, deep into the chest, or into the abdomen, or directly across to the opposite breast.

 DEVELOPMENTAL CONSIDERATIONS

During embryonic life, ventral epidermal ridges, or "milk lines," are present; these curve down from the axilla to the groin bilaterally (Fig. 17–5). The breast develops along the ridge over the thorax, and the rest of the ridge usually atrophies. Occasionally a *supernumerary nipple* (i.e., an extra nip-

ple) persists and is visible somewhere along the track of the mammary ridge (see Fig. 17–8).

At birth, the only breast structures present are the lactiferous ducts within the nipple. No alveoli have developed. Little change occurs until puberty.

Supernumerary nipple

17–5

THE ADOLESCENT

At puberty the estrogen hormones stimulate breast changes. The breasts enlarge, mostly due to extensive fat deposition. The duct system also grows and branches, and masses of small, solid cells develop at the duct endings. These are potential alveoli.

A 1997 study of 17,077 girls in the United States aged 3 through 12 indicates that puberty is occurring earlier than classically used norms (Herman-Giddens et al., 1997). The onset of breast development occurred at an average (mean) age between 8 and 9 years for black girls and by 10 years for white girls. Earlier studies cited breast development begin-

ning at an average age of 10 to 11 years (Harlan, Harlan, and Grillo, 1980; Marshall and Tanner, 1969).

Occasionally, one breast may grow faster than the other, producing a temporary asymmetry. This may cause some distress; reassurance is necessary. Tenderness is common also. Although the age of onset varies widely, the five stages of breast development follow this classic description of Marshall and Tanner's (1969) sexual maturity rating, or **Tanner staging** (Table 17–1).

Full development from stage 2 to stage 5 takes an average of 3 years, although the range is 1.5 to 6 years. During this time, pubic hair develops, and axillary hair appears 2 years after the onset of pubic hair. The beginning of breast develop-

TABLE 17–1: Sexual Maturity Rating in Girls

STAGE

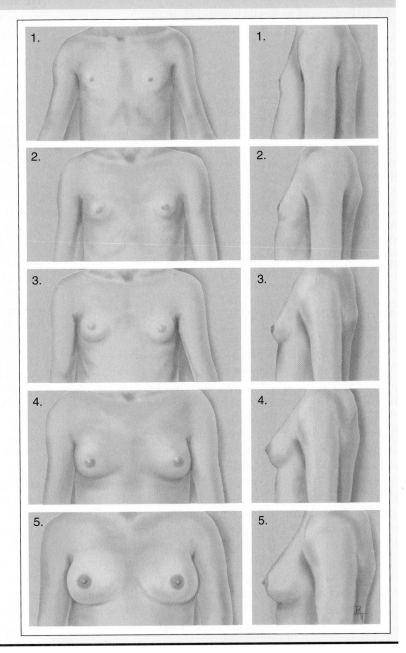

1 **Preadolescent:** Only a small elevated nipple

2 **Breast bud stage:** A small mound of breast and nipple develops; the areola widens

3 The breast and areola enlarge; the nipple is flush with the breast surface

4 The areola and nipple form a secondary mound over the breast

5 **Mature breast:** Only the nipple protrudes; the areola is flush with the breast contour (the areola may continue as a secondary mound in some normal women)

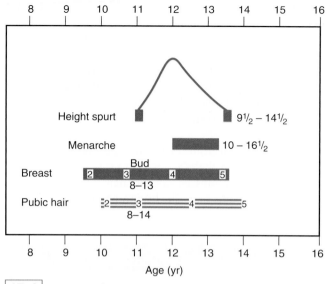

17–6 Patterns of pubertal changes in girls.

ment precedes menarche by about 2 years. Menarche occurs in breast development stage 3 or 4, usually just after the peak of the adolescent growth spurt, which occurs around age 12. Note the relationship of these events (Fig. 17–6). This knowledge aids in assessing the development of adolescent girls and increasing their knowledge about their own development.

Breasts of the nonpregnant woman change with the ebb and flow of hormones during the monthly menstrual cycle. Nodularity increases from midcycle up to menstruation. During the 3 to 4 days before menstruation, the breasts feel full, tight, heavy, and occasionally sore. The breast volume is smallest on days 4 to 7 of the menstrual cycle.

THE PREGNANT FEMALE

During pregnancy, breast changes start during the 2nd month and are an early sign of pregnancy for most women. Pregnancy stimulates the expansion of the ductal system and supporting fatty tissue as well as development of the true secretory alveoli. Thus the breasts enlarge and feel more nodular. The nipples are larger, darker, and more erectile. The areolae become larger and grow a darker brown as pregnancy progresses, and the tubercles become more prominent. (The brown color fades after lactation, but the areolae never return to the original color.) A venous pattern is prominent over the skin surface (see Fig. 27–4 on p. 815).

After the 4th month, **colostrum** may be expressed. This thick yellow fluid is the precursor for milk, containing the same amount of protein and lactose but practically no fat. The breasts produce colostrum for the first few days after delivery. It is rich with antibodies that protect the newborn against infection, so breastfeeding is important. Milk production (lactation) begins 1 to 3 days postpartum. The whitish color is from emulsified fat and calcium caseinate.

THE AGING FEMALE

After menopause, ovarian secretion of estrogen and progesterone decreases, which causes the breast glandular tissue to atrophy. This is replaced with fibrous connective tissue. The fat envelope atrophies also, beginning in the middle years and becoming marked in the eighth and ninth decades. These changes decrease breast size and elasticity so the breasts droop and sag, looking flattened and flabby. Drooping is accentuated by the kyphosis in some older women.

The decreased breast size makes inner structures more prominent. A breast lump may have been present for years but is suddenly palpable. Around the nipple the lactiferous ducts are more palpable and feel firm and stringy because of fibrosis and calcification. The axillary hair decreases.

THE MALE BREAST

The male breast is a rudimentary structure consisting of a thin disk of undeveloped tissue underlying the nipple. The areola is well developed, although the nipple is relatively very small. During adolescence, it is common for the breast tissue to temporarily enlarge, producing **gynecomastia**. This condition is usually unilateral and temporary. Reassurance is necessary for the adolescent male, whose attention is riveted on his body image. Gynecomastia may reappear in the aging male and may be due to testosterone deficiency.

TRANSCULTURAL CONSIDERATIONS

Marshall and Tanner's data on sexual maturity are derived from studies of white British females and do not generalize to other racial groups. The 1997 study of secondary sexual characteristics in 17,077 young American girls shows that black girls begin puberty about 1 to 1.5 years earlier than white girls and start menstruating about 8.5 months earlier (Herman-Giddens et al., 1997). The onset of breast development occurred at an average (mean) age of 8.87 years for black girls and 9.96 years for white girls (Hispanic ethnicity occurs in both groups). At age 7, 27.2% of black girls and 6.7% of white girls had begun breast and/or pubic hair development, and at age 8 this increased to 48.3% of black girls and 14.7% of white girls. Menses began at an average age of 12.16 years for black girls and at 12.88 years for white girls.

Breast Cancer. The incidence of breast cancer varies with different cultural groups. The development of breast cancer is slightly more likely in white women than in black women. However, black women are more likely to die of breast cancer, possibly because diagnosis occurs at an advanced stage when the disease is harder to treat and cure (American Cancer Society [ACS], 2002). Asian, Hispanic, and Native American women have a lower risk of developing breast cancer (ACS, 2002). This racial difference in mortality may relate to insufficient use of early-detection procedures, including mammograms and breast self-examinations. However, the use of these preventive measures may be related more to socioeconomic factors than directly related to ethnicity (Qureshi et al., 2000). Factors that influence breast cancer screening mammography include lack of access to healthcare, insurance problems, and a lack of engaging in other healthy behaviors.

Some studies have found that a diet rich in certain fats has a strong promoting effect on breast cancer (Weisburger, 1997), and that breast cancer is less common in countries where the diet is low in total fat, low in polyunsaturated fat, and low in saturated fat (ACS, 2002). Other studies of U.S. women have not found a risk due to dietary fat. It is possible that the breast cancer risk in differing countries may be confounded by other factors, such as genetics, intake of other nutrients, and activity. Although the relationship of breast cancer to dietary fat is not clear at this time, it is known that intake of dietary fat increases risk of heart disease and should be limited (ACS, 2002).

Subjective Data

Breast
1. Pain
2. Lump
3. Discharge
4. Rash
5. Swelling
6. Trauma

7. History of breast disease
8. Surgery
9. Self-care behaviors
   Perform breast self-
      examination
   Last mammogram

Axilla
1. Tenderness, lump, or swelling
2. Rash

In Western culture the female breasts signify more than their primary purpose of lactation. Women are surrounded by messages that feminine norms of beauty and desirability are enhanced by and dependent on the size of the breasts and their appearance. More recently, women leaders have tried to refocus this attitude, stressing women's self-worth as individual human beings, not as stereotyped sexual objects. The intense cultural emphasis is gradually changing, yet the breasts still are crucial to a woman's self-concept and her perception of her femininity. Matters pertaining to the breast affect a woman's body image and generate deep emotional responses.

This emotionality may take strong forms that you observe as you discuss the woman's history. One woman may be acutely embarrassed talking about the breasts, as evidenced by lack of eye contact, minimal response, nervous gestures, or inappropriate humor. Another woman may talk wryly and disparagingly about the size or development of her breasts. A young adolescent is acutely aware of her own development in relation to her peers. Or, a woman who has found a breast lump may come to you with fear, high anxiety, and even panic. Although a high percentage of breast lumps are benign, many women initially assume the worst possible outcome—cancer, disfigurement, and death. While you are collecting the subjective data, tune in to cues for these behaviors that call for a straightforward and reasoned attitude.

EXAMINER ASKS	RATIONALE
Breast	
1. Pain. Any **pain** or tenderness in the breasts? When did you first notice it?	Mastalgia occurs with trauma, inflammation, infection, and benign breast disease.
• Where is the pain? Localized or all over?	
• Is the painful spot sore to touch? Do you feel a burning or pulling sensation?	
• Is the pain cyclic? Any relation to your menstrual period?	Cyclic pain is common with normal breasts, use of oral contraceptives, and benign breast (fibrocystic) disease.
• Is the pain brought on by strenuous activity, especially involving one arm; a change in activity; manipulation during sex; part of underwire bra; exercise?	Is pain related to specific cause?

EXAMINER ASKS	RATIONALE

2. Lump. Ever noticed a **lump** or **thickening** in the breast? Where?
- When did you first notice it? Changed at all since then?
- Does the lump have any relation to your menstrual period?
- Noticed any change in the overlying skin: redness, warmth, dimpling, swelling?

The presence of any lump must be carefully explored. A lump that is present for many years and is exhibiting no change may not be serious but still should be explored. Approach any recent change or new lump with suspicion.

3. Discharge. Any **discharge** from the nipple?
- When did you first notice this?
- What color is the discharge?
- Consistency—thick or runny?
- Odor?

Galactorrhea. Note use of medications that may cause clear nipple discharge: oral contraceptives, phenothiazines, diuretics, digitalis, steroids, reserpine, methyldopa, calcium channel blockers.

Bloody or blood-tinged discharge always is significant. Any discharge in the presence of a lump is significant.

4. Rash. Any **rash** on the breast?
- When did you first notice this?
- Where did it start? On the nipple, areola, or surrounding skin?

Paget's disease starts with a small crust on the nipple apex, then spreads to areola.

Eczema or other dermatitis rarely starts at nipple unless it is due to breast-feeding. It usually starts on the areola or surrounding skin and then spreads to the nipple.

5. Swelling. Any **swelling** in the breasts? In one spot or all over?
- Related to your menstrual period, pregnancy, or breastfeeding?
- Any change in bra size?

6. Trauma. Any **trauma** or injury to the breasts?
- Did it result in any swelling, lump, or break in skin?

A lump from an injury is due to local hematoma or edema and should resolve shortly. Or, trauma may cause a woman to feel the breast and find a lump that really was there before.

7. History of breast disease. Any **history of breast disease** yourself?
- What type? How was this diagnosed?
- When did this occur?
- How is it being treated?

A history of breast cancer increases the risk of recurrent cancer (see Table 17–2 on p. 416).

The presence of fibrocystic disease makes it more difficult to examine the breasts; the general lumpiness of the breast conceals a new lump.

- Any breast cancer in your family? Who? Sister, mother, maternal grandmother, maternal aunts, daughter?
- At what age did this relative have breast cancer?

The finding of breast cancer occurring before menopause in certain family members increases risk for this woman (see Table 17–2).

8. Surgery. Ever had **surgery** on the breasts? Was this a biopsy? What were the biopsy results?
- Mastectomy? Mammoplasty—augmentation or reduction?

9. Self-care behaviors.
- Have you ever been taught **breast self-examination?**
- (**If so.**) How often do you perform it? What helps you remember? That is an excellent way to be in charge of your own health. I would like you to show me your technique after we do your examination.

The monthly practice of breast self-examination (BSE), and routine clinical breast examination and mammograms are complementary screening measures. With good BSE practice, a woman knows how

EXAMINER ASKS	RATIONALE
• (**If not.**) This will be an excellent way that you can take charge of your own health. You can make breast self-examination a very routine health habit, just like brushing your teeth. I will teach you the technique after we do your examination. • Ever had **mammography**, a screening x-ray examination of the breasts? When was the last x-ray?	her breasts normally feel and can detect any change more easily. Mammography can reveal cancers too small to be detected by the woman or by the most experienced examiner. However, mammography does not detect *all* palpable lumps, and interval lumps may become palpable between mammograms (Cole, 1998). Women ages 20 to 39 should perform monthly BSE and have a clinical breast exam (CBE) every 3 years; women 40 and older should perform monthly BSE, with an annual mammogram and an annual CBE conducted close to the same time (ACS, 2002).

Axilla

1. Tenderness, lump, or swelling. Any **tenderness** or **lump** in the underarm area?
• Where? When did you first notice this?

2. Rash. Any axillary **rash**? Please describe it.
• Seem to be a reaction to deodorant?

Breast tissue extends up into the axilla. Also, the axilla contains numerous lymph nodes.

Additional History for the Preadolescent

1. Have you noticed your breasts changing?
• How long has this been happening?

2. Many girls notice other changes in their bodies too that come with growing up. What have you noticed?
• What do you think about all this?

Developing breasts are the most obvious sign of puberty. This is the focus of attention for most girls, especially in comparison to their peers. Assess each adolescent's perception of her own development and provide teaching and reassurance as indicated.

Additional History for the Pregnant Female

1. Have you noticed any enlargement or fullness in the breasts?
• Is there any tenderness or tingling?

• Do you have a history of inverted nipples?

2. Are you planning to breast-feed your baby?

Breast changes are expected and normal during pregnancy. Assess the woman's knowledge and provide reassurance.
Inverted nipples may need special care in preparation for breastfeeding.

In addition to providing the perfect food and antibodies for the baby, promoting bonding, and providing relaxation, lactation is also associated with a slight reduction in the risk of breast cancer (ACS, 2002).

Additional History for the Menopausal Woman

1. Have you noticed any change in the breast contour, size, or firmness? (Note: Change may not be as apparent to obese woman or to the woman whose earlier pregnancies already have produced breast changes.)

Decreased estrogen level causes decreased firmness. Rapid decrease in estrogen level causes actual shrinkage.

EXAMINER ASKS	RATIONALE

Risk Factor Profile for Breast Cancer

Breast cancer is the second major cause of death from cancer in women. However, early detection and improved treatment have increased survival rates. The 5-year survival rate for localized breast cancer has increased from 78% in the 1940s to 98% today. If the cancer has spread regionally, the survival rate is 76% to 88% (ACS, 2002).

TABLE 17–2: Breast Cancer Risk Factors

RISK FACTORS THAT CANNOT BE CHANGED	LIFESTYLE-RELATED RISK FACTORS
Female gender, age >50	Nulliparity or first child after age 30*
Personal history of breast cancer	Current oral contraceptive use*
Mutation of BRCA1 and BRCA2 genes	Long-term use combined hormone replacement therapy (HRT)
First-degree relative with breast cancer (mother, sister, daughter)	Not breast-feeding*
Previous breast biopsy with *atypical hyperplasia,* or *breast disease without atypia* or *usual hyperplasia*	Alcohol intake of 2 to 5 drinks daily
Previous breast irradiation	Obesity (especially after menopause) and high-fat diet
Menstruation before age 12* or menopause after age 50*	Physical inactivity (new research area)
White race*	

*Slightly higher risk.
Data adapted from American Cancer Society:
http://www.cancer.org/docroot/CRI/content/CRI_2_4_2X_What_are_the_risk_factors_for_breast_cancer_5.asp [accessed August 2002].

The best way to detect a person's risk for breast cancer is by asking the right history questions. Table 17–2 highlights risk factors for breast cancer, and from these you can fashion your questions. Be aware, however, that about 70% of breast cancers occur in women with no identifiable risk factors except gender and age (Love and Lindsey, 2000). Just because a woman does not report the cited risk factors does not mean that you or she should fail to consider breast cancer seriously.

Objective Data

PREPARATION

The woman is sitting up, disrobed to the waist, facing the examiner. An alternative draping method is to use a short gown, open at the back, and lift it up to the woman's shoulders during inspection. During palpation when the woman is supine, cover one breast with the gown while examining the other. Be aware that many women are embarrassed to have their breasts examined; use a sensitive but matter-of-fact approach.

Following your examination, be prepared to teach the woman breast self-examination.

EQUIPMENT NEEDED

Small pillow
Ruler marked in centimeters
Pamphlet or teaching aid for BSE

NORMAL RANGE OF FINDINGS	ABNORMAL FINDINGS

INSPECT THE BREASTS

General Appearance
Note symmetry of size and shape (Fig. 17–7). It is common to have a slight asymmetry in size; often the left breast is slightly larger than the right.

A sudden increase in the size of one breast signifies inflammation or new growth.

NORMAL RANGE OF FINDINGS	ABNORMAL FINDINGS

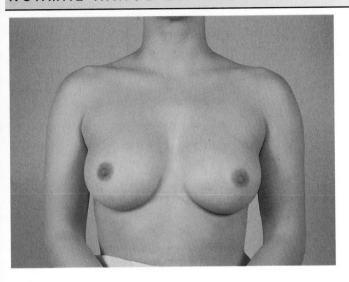

17-7

Skin

The skin normally is smooth and of even color. Note any localized areas of redness, bulging, or dimpling. Also, note any skin lesions or focal vascular pattern. A fine blue vascular network is visible normally during pregnancy. Pale linear striae, or stretch marks, often follow pregnancy.

Normally no edema is present. Edema exaggerates the hair follicles, giving a "pig-skin" or "orange-peel" look (also called *peau d'orange*).

Hyperpigmentation.
Redness and heat with inflammation.
Unilateral dilated superficial veins in a nonpregnant woman.

Edema (see Table 17–3 p. 430).

Lymphatic Drainage Areas

Observe the axillary and supraclavicular regions. Note any bulging, discoloration, or edema.

Nipple

The nipples should be symmetrically placed on the same plane on the two breasts. Nipples usually protrude, although some are flat and some are inverted. They tend to stay in their original condition. Distinguish a recently retracted nipple from one that has been inverted for many years or since puberty. Normal nipple inversion may be unilateral or bilateral and usually can be pulled out (i.e., it is not fixed).

Note any dry scaling, any fissure or ulceration, and bleeding or other discharge.

A normal variation in about 1% of men and women is a **supernumerary nipple** (Fig. 17–8). An extra nipple along the embryonic "milk line" on the thorax or abdomen is a congenital finding. Usually, it is 5 to 6 cm below the breast near the midline and has no associated glandular tissue. It looks like a mole, although a close look reveals a tiny nipple and areola. It is not significant; merely distinguish it from a mole.

Deviation in pointing (see Table 17–3).

Recent nipple retraction signifies acquired disease (see Table 17–3).

Explore any discharge, especially in the presence of a breast mass.

Rarely, glandular tissue, a supernumerary breast, or polymastia is present.

17-8 Supernumerary nipple and areolar complex.

NORMAL RANGE OF FINDINGS

ABNORMAL FINDINGS

Maneuvers to Screen for Retraction

Direct the woman to change position while you check the breasts for skin retraction signs. First ask her to lift the arms slowly over the head. Both breasts should move up symmetrically (Fig. 17–9).

Retraction signs are due to fibrosis in the breast tissue, usually caused by growing neoplasms. The fibrosis shortens with time, causing contrasting signs with the normally loose breast tissue.

Note a lag in movement of one breast.

17–9

Next ask her to push her hands onto her hips (Fig. 17–10) and to push her two palms together (Fig. 17–11). These maneuvers contract the pectoralis major muscle. A slight lifting of both breasts will occur.

Note a dimpling or a pucker, which indicates skin retraction (see Table 17–3).

17–10

17–11

Ask the woman with large pendulous breasts to lean forward while you support her forearms. Note the symmetric free-forward movement of both breasts (Fig. 17–12).

NORMAL RANGE OF FINDINGS

Note fixation to chest wall or skin retraction (see Table 17–3).

17–12

INSPECT AND PALPATE THE AXILLAE

Examine the axillae while the woman is sitting. Inspect the skin, noting any rash or infection. Lift the woman's arm and support it yourself, so that her muscles are loose and relaxed. Use your right hand to palpate the left axilla (Fig. 17–13). Reach your fingers high into the axilla. Move them firmly down in four directions: down the chest wall in a line from the middle of the axilla, along the anterior border of the axilla, along the posterior border, and along the inner aspect of the upper arm. Move the woman's arm through range-of-motion to increase the surface area you can reach.

Usually nodes are not palpable, although you may feel a small, soft, nontender node in the central group. Expect some tenderness when palpating high in the axilla. Note any enlarged and tender lymph nodes.

Nodes enlarge with any local infection of the breast, arm, or hand, and with breast cancer metastases.

17–13

PALPATE THE BREASTS

Help the woman to a supine position. Tuck a small pad under the side to be palpated and raise her arm over her head. These maneuvers will flatten the breast tissue and displace it medially. Any significant lumps will then feel more distinct (Fig. 17–14).

17-14

Use the pads of your first three fingers and make a gentle rotary motion on the breast. Choose one of two patterns for palpation: (1) You may start at the nipple and palpate out to the periphery as if following spokes on a wheel (Fig. 17–15); or (2) start at the nipple and palpate in concentric circles, increasing out to the periphery. With either pattern, move in a clockwise direction, taking care to examine every square inch of the breast. Also, take care to palpate the tail of Spence extending from the upper outer quadrant into the axilla. It does not matter which method of palpation you use, but be consistent and thorough.

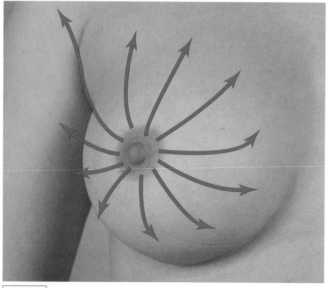

17-15 A, Spokes-on-a-wheel pattern of palpation.

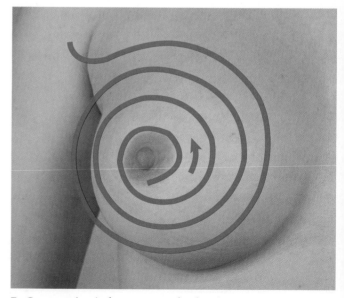

B, Concentric-circles pattern of palpation.

NORMAL RANGE OF FINDINGS

In nulliparous women, normal breast tissue feels firm, smooth, and elastic. After pregnancy, the tissue feels softer and looser. Premenstrual engorgement is normal due to increasing progesterone. This consists of a slight enlargement, a tenderness to palpation, and a generalized nodularity; the lobes feel prominent and their margins more distinct.

Also, normally you may feel a firm transverse ridge of compressed tissue in the lower quadrants. This is the **inframammary ridge,** and it is especially noticeable in large breasts. Do not confuse it with an abnormal lump.

After palpating over the four breast quadrants, palpate the nipple (Fig. 17–16). Note any induration or subareolar mass. Use your thumb and forefinger to apply gentle pressure or a stripping action to the nipple. Starting at the outside of the areola, "milk" your fingers toward the nipple—repeat, from a few different directions. If any discharge appears, note its color and consistency.

17–16

For the woman with large pendulous breasts, you may palpate using a bimanual technique (Fig. 17–17). The woman is in a sitting position, leaning forward. Support the inferior part of the breast with one hand. Use your other hand to palpate the breast tissue against your supporting hand.

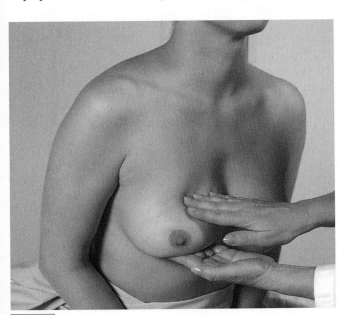

17–17

ABNORMAL FINDINGS

Heat, redness, and swelling in nonlactating and nonpostpartum breasts indicate inflammation.

Except in pregnancy and lactation, discharge is abnormal (see Table 17–6). Note the number of discharge droplets and the quadrant(s) producing them. Blot the discharge on a white tissue to ascertain its color. Test any abnormal discharge for the presence of blood.

NORMAL RANGE OF FINDINGS

If the woman mentions a breast lump that she has discovered herself, examine the unaffected breast first to learn a baseline of normal consistency for this individual. If you do feel a lump or mass, note these characteristics (Fig. 17–18):

1. **Location**—Using the breast as a clock face, describe the distance in centimeters from the nipple (e.g., "7:00, 2 cm from the nipple"). Or diagram the breast in the woman's record and mark in the location of the lump.
2. **Size**—Judge in centimeters in three dimensions: width × length × thickness.
3. **Shape**—State if the lump is oval, round, lobulated, or indistinct.
4. **Consistency**—State if the lump is soft, firm, or hard.
5. **Movable**—Is the lump freely movable, or is it fixed when you try to slide it over the chest wall?
6. **Distinctness**—Is the lump solitary or multiple?
7. **Nipple**—Is it displaced or retracted?
8. **Note the skin over the lump**—Is it erythematous, dimpled, or retracted?
9. **Tenderness**—Is the lump tender to palpation?
10. **Lymphadenopathy**—Are any regional lymph nodes palpable?

See Tables 17–4 and 17–5 for description of common breast lumps using these characteristics.

17–18

A procedure called the *friction-free examination* incorporates hot, soapy lather applied to the breasts before palpation. The soap acts as a lubricant and greatly enhances the breast features. Talcum powder also can be used. Some high-risk breast clinics advocate this technique as a valuable tool for detection of lumps because the details are so clearly defined. The heat also enhances detection of any nipple secretions. Following the examination, the breasts are cleaned with a hot wet towel.

TEACH THE BREAST SELF-EXAMINATION

Finish your own assessment first, then teach the self-examination. You need to focus your skill and concentration on the examination, and you may be diverted by teaching at the same time. The same is true for the woman. She waits to hear that your examination of her affirms that she is healthy. Once reassured, she can relax about the findings and concentrate on your teaching.

Help each woman establish a regular schedule of self-care. The best time to conduct BSE is right after the menstrual period, or the 4th through 7th day of the menstrual cycle, when the breasts are the smallest and least congested. Advise the pregnant or menopausal woman who is not having menstrual periods to select a familiar date to examine her breasts each month, for example, her birthdate or the day the rent is due.

NORMAL RANGE OF FINDINGS	ABNORMAL FINDINGS

Stress that a regular monthly self-examination will familiarize the woman with her own breasts and their normal variation. This is a positive step that will reassure her of her healthy state. Emphasize the absence of lumps (not the presence of them). However, do encourage her to report any unusual finding promptly.

While teaching, focus on the positive aspects of BSE. Avoid citing frightening mortality statistics about breast cancer. This may generate excessive fear and denial that actually obstructs a woman's self-care action. Rather, be selective in your choice of factual material:

The majority of women will never get breast cancer.
The great majority of breast lumps are benign.
Early detection of breast cancer is important; if the cancer is not invasive, the survival rate is close to 100%.

Emphasize self-care through knowledge of risk factors, regular performance of BSE to increase confidence in detecting abnormalities, and early referral for any suspicious findings.

Keep your teaching simple! The simpler the plan, the more likely the person is to comply. Describe the correct technique and rationale and the expected findings to note as the woman inspects her own breasts (Fig. 17–19). Teach the

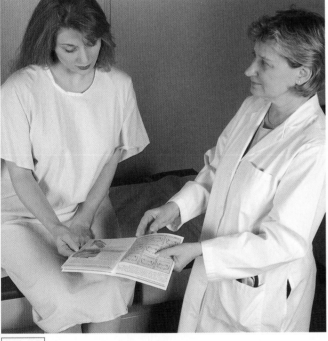

17–19

woman to do this in front of a mirror while she is disrobed to the waist. At home, she can start palpation in the shower, where soap and water assist palpation. Then palpation should be performed while lying supine. Encourage the woman to palpate her own breasts while you are there to monitor her technique. Use the return demonstration to assess her technique and understanding of the procedure.

Many examiners use a simulated breast model so that the woman can palpate a "lump." Pamphlets are helpful reinforcers; just be sure they conform to the method you teach (e.g., circular approach versus radiating line approach to palpation). Give the woman two pamphlets to take home and encourage her to give one to a relative or friend. This may promote discussion, which is reinforcing.

THE MALE BREAST

Your examination of the male breast can be much more abbreviated, but do not omit it. Inspect the chest wall, noting the skin surface and any lumps or swelling. Palpate the nipple area for any lump or tissue enlargement (Fig. 17–20). It should feel even, with no nodules.

17–20

The normal male breast has a flat disk of undeveloped breast tissue beneath the nipple. **Gynecomastia** is an enlargement of this breast tissue, making it clinically distinguishable from the other tissues in the chest wall (Fig. 17–21). It feels like a smooth, firm, movable disk. This occurs normally during puberty. It usually affects only one breast and is temporary. The adolescent male is acutely aware of his body image. Reassure him that this change is normal, common, and temporary.

An obese male has an increase of fatty, not glandular, tissue.

Gynecomastia also occurs with use of anabolic steroids, some medications, and some disease states. See Table 17-8.

17–21 Adolescent gynecomastia.

 DEVELOPMENTAL CONSIDERATIONS

Infants and Children

In the neonate of either sex, the breasts may be enlarged and visible due to maternal estrogen crossing the placenta. They may secrete a clear or white fluid, called "witch's milk." These signs are not significant and are resolved within a few days to a few weeks.

Note the position of the nipples on the prepubertal child. They should be symmetric, just lateral to the midclavicular line, between the fourth and fifth ribs. The nipple is flat, and the areola is darker pigmented.

Premature thelarche is early breast development with no other hormone-dependent signs (pubic hair, menses).

The Adolescent

Adolescent breast development usually begins on an average between 8 and 10 years of age. Expect some asymmetry during growth. (Distinguish breast development from extra adipose tissue present in obese children.) Record the stage of development using Tanner's staging described on p. 411. Use the chart to teach the adolescent normal developmental stages and to assure her of her own normal progress.

Note precocious development, occurring before age 8. It is usually normal but also occurs with thyroid dysfunction, stilbestrol ingestion, or ovarian or adrenal tumor.

Note delayed development, occurring with hormonal failure or anorexia nervosa beginning before puberty, or with severe malnutrition.

With maturing adolescents, palpate the breasts as you would with the adult. The breasts normally feel firm and uniform. Note any mass.

At this age a mass is almost always a benign fibroadenoma or a cyst (see Table 17–4).

Teach BSE now, so that the technique will become a natural, comfortable habit by the time the girl becomes an adult and will be at higher risk.

NORMAL RANGE OF FINDINGS	ABNORMAL FINDINGS

The Pregnant Female

A delicate blue vascular pattern is visible over the breasts. The breasts increase in size, as do the nipples. Jagged linear stretch marks, or striae, may develop if the breasts have a large increase. The nipples also become darker and more erectile. The areolae widen; grow darker; and contain the small, scattered, elevated Montgomery's glands. On palpation, the breasts feel more nodular, and thick yellow colostrum can be expressed after the first trimester.

The Lactating Female

Colostrum changes to milk production around the 3rd postpartum day. At this time, the breasts may become engorged, appearing enlarged, reddened, and shiny and feeling warm and hard. Frequent nursing helps drain the ducts and sinuses and stimulate milk production. Nipple soreness is normal, appearing around the twentieth nursing, lasting 24 to 48 hours, then disappearing rapidly. The nipples may look red and irritated. They may even crack but will heal rapidly if kept dry and exposed to air. Again, frequent nursings are the best treatment for nipple soreness.

> One section of the breast surface appearing red and tender indicates a plugged duct (see Table 17–7).

The Aging Female

On inspection, the breasts look pendulous, flattened, and sagging. Nipples may be retracted but can be pulled outward. On palpation, the breasts feel more granular, and the terminal ducts around the nipple feel more prominent and stringy. Thickening of the inframammary ridge at the lower breast is normal, and it feels more prominent with age.

Reinforce the value of the breast self-examination. Women over 50 years have an increased risk of breast cancer. Older women may have problems with arthritis, limited range of motion, or decreased vision that may inhibit self-care. Suggest aids to the self-examination; for example, talcum powder helps fingers glide over skin.

> Since atrophy causes shrinkage of normal glandular tissue, cancer detection is somewhat easier. Any palpable lump that cannot be positively identified as a normal structure should be referred.

SUMMARY CHECKLIST: Breasts and Regional Lymphatics

1. Inspect breasts as the woman sits, raises arms overhead, pushes hands on hips, leans forward
2. Inspect the supraclavicular and infraclavicular areas
3. Palpate the axillae and regional lymph nodes
4. With woman supine, palpate the breast tissue, including tail of Spence, the nipples, and areolae
5. Teach BSE

 See Health Promotion Guide on CD

Application and Critical Thinking

SAMPLE CHARTING

FEMALE

SUBJECTIVE

States no breast pain, lump, discharge, rash, swelling, or trauma. No history of breast disease herself, does have mother with fibrocystic disease. No history of breast surgery. Never been pregnant. Performs BSE monthly.

OBJECTIVE

Inspection. Breasts symmetrical. Skin smooth with even color and no rash or lesions. Arm movement shows no dimpling or retractions. No nipple discharge, no lesions.
Palpation. Breast contour and consistency firm and homogeneous. No masses or tenderness. No lymphadenopathy.

MALE

SUBJECTIVE

No pain, lump, rash, or swelling.

OBJECTIVE

No masses or tenderness. No lymphadenopathy.

FOCUSED ASSESSMENT: CLINICAL CASE STUDY 1

J.G. is a 32-year-old white female high school teacher, married, with no children. She reports good health until finding "lump in right breast 2 weeks ago."

SUBJECTIVE

2 weeks PTA—noticed lump in R breast on self-examination. Lump firm, nonmovable area "the size of a quarter," in upper outer quadrant of breast, tender on touch only. No skin changes, no nipple discharge, on no medications. Last breast exam by MD 3 months before was reported normal. Did not notice lump on previous self-exam 1 month before. No history of breast disease in self or family.

2 days PTA—saw MD, who confirmed presence of lump and recommended biopsy as outpatient. Last menstrual period 1/25/(2 ½ weeks PTA). States the last 2 days has been so nervous has been unable to sleep well or to concentrate at work. "I just know it's cancer."

OBJECTIVE

Voice trembling and breathless during history. Sitting posture stiff and rigid. B/P 148/78. 37°-92-16.
Inspection. Breasts symmetric, nipples everted. No skin lesions, no dimpling, no retraction, no fixation.
Palpation. Left breast firm, no mass, no tenderness, no discharge. Right breast firm, with 2 cm × 2 cm × 1 cm mass at 10:00 position, 5 cm from the nipple. Lump is firm, oval, with smooth discrete borders, non-movable, tender to palpation. No other mass. No discharge. No lymphadenopathy.

ASSESSMENT

Lump in R breast
Anxiety R/T threat to health status

FOCUSED ASSESSMENT: CLINICAL CASE STUDY 2

D.B. is a 62-year-old black female bank comptroller, married, with no children. History of hypertension, managed by diuretic medication and diet. No other health problems until yearly company physical exam 3 days PTA, when MD "found a lump in my right breast."

SUBJECTIVE

3 days PTA—MD noted lump in R breast during yearly physical exam. MD did not describe lump but told D.B. it was "serious" and needed immediate biopsy. D.B. has not felt it herself. States has noted no skin changes, no nipple discharge. No previous history of breast disease. Mother died age 54 of breast cancer, no other relative with breast disease. D.B. has had no full-term pregnancies; two spontaneous abortions, ages 28, 31. Menopause completed at age 52.

Aware of BSE but has never performed it. "I feel so bad. If only I had been doing it. I should have found this myself." Married 43 years. States husband supportive, but "I just can't talk to him about this. I can't even go near him now."

OBJECTIVE

Inspection. Breasts symmetric when sitting, arms down. Nipples flat. No lesions, no discharge. As lifts arms, left breast elevates, right breast stays fixed. Dimple in right breast, 9:00 position, apparent at rest and with muscle contraction. Leaning forward reveals left breast falls free, right breast flattens.
Palpation. Left breast feels soft and granular throughout, no mass. Right breast soft and granular, with large, stony hard mass in outer quadrant. Lump is 5 cm × 4 cm × 2 cm, at 9:00 position, 3 cm from nipple. Borders irregular, mass fixed to tissues, no pain with palpation.

One firm, palpable lymph node in center of right axilla. No palpable nodes on the left.

ASSESSMENT

Lump in R breast
Ineffective coping R/T effects of breast lump

NURSING DIAGNOSES COMMONLY ASSOCIATED WITH BREAST DISORDERS

RELATED FACTORS (Etiology)	DEFINING CHARACTERISTICS (Symptoms and Signs)
DIAGNOSIS: Ineffective Breastfeeding	
Prematurity	Unsatisfactory breastfeeding process
Infant receiving supplemental feedings with artificial nipple	Actual or perceived inadequate milk supply
Poor infant sucking reflex	Infant inability to attach onto maternal breast correctly
Nonsupportive partner/family	Nonsustained suckling at the breast
Deficient knowledge	Persistence of sore nipples beyond first week of breastfeeding
Interruption of breastfeeding	Observable signs of inadequate infant intake
Maternal anxiety or ambivalence	Insufficient emptying of each breast per feeding
	Insufficient opportunity for suckling at the breast
	Infant arching and crying at the breast, resisting latching on
DIAGNOSIS: Ineffective Coping	
Effects of acute or chronic illness	Change in communication pattern
Loss of control over body part or body system	Inability to meet or be responsible for basic needs
Lack of support systems	Fear of pain, death
Low self-esteem	Frequent headaches
Major change in lifestyle	Emotional tension
Unrealistic perceptions	Insomnia
Situational or maturational crisis	Verbalizes inability to cope or inability to ask for help
Knowledge deficit about	Inability to perform expected roles
Disease process	Physical inactivity
Therapeutic regimen	Stress-related disorders
Prognosis	Ulcers
Separation from or loss of significant other	Hypertension
Sensory overload	Irritable bowel
	Substance abuse
	Inappropriate use of defense mechanisms
	Withdrawal
	Depression
	Overeating
	Blaming
	Scapegoating
	Manipulative behavior
	Self-pity
	Chronic anxiety
	Indecisiveness

RELATED FACTORS (Etiology)

DEFINING CHARACTERISTICS (Symptoms and Signs)

DIAGNOSIS: Deficient knowledge: Breast self-examination

Lack of exposure or recall	Expresses inaccurate perception of potential problem
Information misinterpretation	Repeatedly requests information
Unfamiliarity with information resources	Inadequate performance of examination
Lack of interest in learning	Verbalizes the problem
Denial	Inaccurate use of health-related vocabulary
Effects of aging	Inability to explain therapeutic regimen or describe personal health status
Sensory deficits	
Language barrier	
Cognitive limitations	
Inadequate economic resources	

OTHER RELATED NURSING DIAGNOSES

ACTUAL

Anxiety
Disturbed Body image (see example in Chapter 13)
Interrupted Breastfeeding

RISK/WELLNESS

Risk
Risk for Loneliness
Wellness
Effective Breastfeeding
Increasing Compliance with prescribed regimen
Actively seeking Knowledge about BSE

ASSESSMENT VIDEO CRITICAL THINKING QUESTIONS

The Saunders *Physical Examination and Health Assessment* video "Breasts and Regional Lymphatics" will direct you to consider the following:

1. How do breast assessment findings differ between older women and younger adult women?
2. How should you modify breast palpation in a woman with large, pendulous breasts?

3. Which conditions may be associated with a breast lump? Nipple rash? Enlarged axillary lymph nodes?
4. How does breast examination in men differ from that in women?

ABNORMAL FINDINGS

Abnormal Findings

TABLE 17–3: Signs of Retraction and Inflammation in the Breast

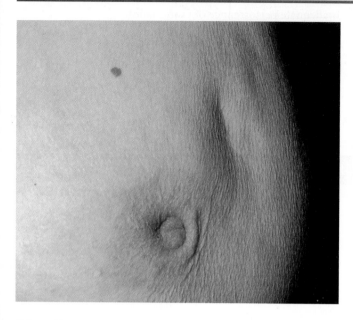

Dimpling

The shallow dimple (also called a skin tether) shown here is a sign of skin retraction. Cancer causes fibrosis, which contracts the suspensory ligaments. The dimple may be apparent at rest, with compression, or with lifting of the arms. Also note the distortion of the areola here as the fibrosis pulls the nipple toward it.

Edema (Peau d'Orange)

Lymphatic obstruction produces edema. This thickens the skin and exaggerates the hair follicles, giving a pig-skin or orange-peel look. This condition suggests cancer. Edema usually begins in the skin around and beneath the areola, the most dependent area of the breast. Also note nipple infiltration here.

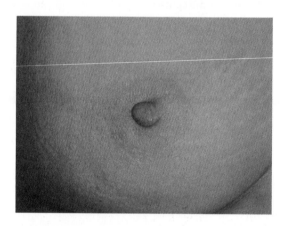

Deviation in Nipple Pointing

An underlying cancer causes fibrosis in the mammary ducts, which pulls the nipple angle toward it. Here, note that the swelling behind the right nipple and the nipple tilts laterally.

Fixation

Asymmetry, distortion, or decreased mobility with the elevated arm maneuver. As cancer becomes invasive, the fibrosis fixes the breast to the underlying pectoral muscles. Here, note the right breast is held against the chest wall.

Nipple Retraction

The retracted nipple looks flatter and broader, like an underlying crater. A recent retraction suggests cancer, which causes fibrosis of the whole duct system and pulls in the nipple. It also may occur with benign lesions such as ectasia of the ducts. Do not confuse retraction with the normal long-standing type of nipple inversion, which has no broadening and is not fixed.

TABLE 17–4: Breast Lump

◀ ## Benign Breast Disease (Formerly Fibrocystic Breast Disease)

Multiple tender masses. "Fibrocystic disease" is a meaningless term because it covers too many entities. Actually, six diagnostic categories exist, based on symptoms and physical findings (Love and Lindsey, 2000):

- Swelling and tenderness (cyclic discomfort)
- Mastalgia (severe pain, both cyclic and noncyclic)
- Nodularity (significant lumpiness, both cyclic and noncyclic)
- Dominant lumps (including cysts and fibroadenomas)
- Nipple discharge (including intraductal papilloma and duct ectasia)
- Infections and inflammations (including subareolar abscess, lactational mastitis, breast abscess, and Mondor's disease)

About 50% of all women have some form of benign breast disease. Nodularity occurs bilaterally; regular, firm nodules that are mobile, well demarcated, and feel rubbery, like small water balloons. Pain may be dull, heavy, and cyclic or just before menses as nodules enlarge. Some women have nodularity but no pain, and vice versa. Cysts are discrete, fluid-filled sacs. Dominant lumps and nipple discharge must be investigated carefully and may need biopsy to rule out cancer. Nodularity itself is not premalignant, but may produce difficulty in detecting other cancerous lumps.

Cancer

Solitary unilateral nontender mass. Single focus in one area, although it may be interspersed with other nodules. Solid, hard, dense, and fixed to underlying tissues or skin as cancer becomes invasive. Borders are irregular and poorly delineated. Grows constantly. Often painless, although the person may have pain. Most common in upper outer quadrant. Usually found in women 30 to 80 years of age; increased risk in ages 40 to 44 and in women older than 50 years. As cancer advances, signs include firm or hard irregular axillary nodes; skin dimpling; nipple retraction, elevation, and discharge.

Fibroadenoma

Solitary nontender mass. A category of benign breast disease that deserves mention due to its frequency and characteristic appearance. Solid, firm, rubbery, and elastic. Round, oval, or lobulated; 1 to 5 cm. Freely movable, slippery; fingers slide it easily through tissue. Most common between 15 and 30 years of age, but can occur up to age 55 years. Grows quickly and constantly. Benign, although it must be diagnosed by biopsy.

TABLE 17–5: Differentiating Breast Lumps

	FIBROADENOMA	BENIGN BREAST DISEASE	CANCER
Likely age	15–30, can occur up to 55	30–55, decreases after menopause	30–80, risk increases after 50
Shape	Round, lobular	Round, lobular	Irregular, star-shaped
Consistency	Usually firm, rubbery	Firm to soft, rubbery	Firm to stony hard
Demarcation	Well demarcated, clear margins	Well demarcated	Poorly defined
Number	Usually single	Usually multiple, may be single	Single
Mobility	Very mobile, slippery	Mobile	Fixed
Tenderness	Usually none	Tender, usually increases before menses, may be noncyclic	Usually none, can be tender
Skin retraction	None	None	Usually
Pattern of growth	Grows quickly and constantly	Size may increase or decrease rapidly	Grows constantly
Risk to health	None; they are benign—must diagnose by biopsy	Benign, although general lumpiness may mask other cancerous lump	Serious, needs early treatment

TABLE 17–6: Abnormal Nipple Discharge

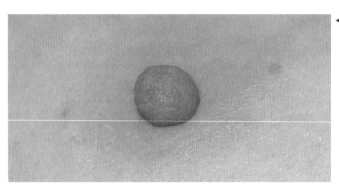

◀ Mammary Duct Ectasia

Pastelike matter in subareolar ducts produces sticky, purulent discharge that may be white, gray, brown, green, or bloody. A light green, single duct discharge is shown here. Caused by stagnation of cellular debris and secretions in the ducts, leading to obstruction, inflammation, and infection. Occurs in women who have lactated; usually occurs in perimenopause.

Itching, burning, or drawing pain occurs around nipple. May have subareolar redness and swelling. Ducts are palpable as rubbery, twisted tubules under areola. May have palpable mass, soft or firm, poorly delineated. Not malignant, but needs biopsy.

Carcinoma

Bloody nipple discharge that is unilateral and from a single duct requires further investigation. Although there was no palpable lump associated with the discharge shown here, mammography revealed a 1-cm, centrally located, ill-defined mass.

Intraductal Papilloma

Serous or serosanguineous discharge, which is spontaneous, unilateral, or from a single duct. Lesion consists of tiny tumors, 2 to 3 mm. Often there is a palpable nodule in the underlying duct (highlighted here). Papillomas affect women 40 to 60 years of age; most are benign. Refer any bloody discharge for careful evaluation, including biopsy, to rule out cancer.

TABLE 17-6: Abnormal Nipple Discharge—cont'd

Paget's Disease (Intraductal Carcinoma) ▶

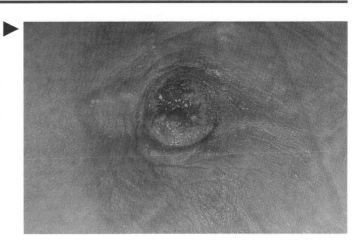

Early lesion has unilateral, clear, yellow discharge and dry, scaling crusts, friable at nipple apex. Spreads outward to areola with erythematous halo on areola and crusted, eczematous, retracted nipple. Later lesion shows nipple reddened, excoriated, ulcerated, with bloody discharge when surface is eroded, and an erythematous plaque surrounding the nipple. Symptoms include tingling, burning, itching.

Except for the redness and occasional cracking due to initial breastfeeding, any dermatitis of the nipple area must be carefully explored and referred immediately.

TABLE 17-7: Disorders Occurring During Lactation

Mastitis

This is uncommon; an inflammatory mass before abscess formation. Usually occurs in single quadrant. Area is red, swollen, tender, very hot, and hard, here forming outward from areola upper edge, in right breast. Also the woman has a headache, malaise, fever, chills and sweating, increased pulse, flulike symptoms. May occur during first 4 months of lactation from infection or from stasis due to plugged duct. Treat with rest, local heat to area, antibiotics, and frequent nursing to keep breast as empty as possible. Must not wean now or the breast will become engorged and the pain will increase. Mother's antibiotic not harmful to infant. Usually resolves in 2 to 3 days.

Plugged Duct

A fairly common and not serious condition. One milk duct is clogged. One section of the breast is tender; may be reddened. No infection. It is important to keep breast as empty as possible and milk flowing. The woman should nurse her baby frequently, on affected side first to ensure complete emptying, and manually express any remaining milk. A plugged duct usually resolves in less than 1 day.

Breast Abscess ▶

A rare complication of generalized infection, e.g., mastitis if untreated. A pocket of pus accumulates in one local area. Here extensive nipple edema, and abscess is "pointing" at 3:00 on areolar margin. Must temporarily discontinue nursing on affected breast; manually express milk and discard. Continue to nurse on unaffected side. Treat with antibiotics, surgical incision, and drainage.

ABNORMAL FINDINGS

TABLE 17–8: Abnormalities in the Male Breast

Gynecomastia

Noninflammatory enlargement of male breast tissue. This is physiologic at puberty, unilateral, usually mild and transient. Gynecomastia occurs commonly in aging males due to changing hormone levels. It is bilateral and may be tender.

It also occurs bilaterally from hormone stimulation, e.g., on estrogen for cancer of prostate; Cushing's syndrome; cirrhosis of liver as unable to metabolize estrogen completely; leukemia occasionally; and sometimes with medication—digitalis, isoniazid, spironolactone, phenothiazines, and marijuana; testicular tumor, lung cancer; adrenal disease; and thyrotoxicosis.

Carcinoma

Less than 1% of all breast cancer occurs in men. The lesion is a hard, irregular, nontender mass, most often directly under the areola, fixed to the area, and may have nipple retraction. Mass is noticeable early due to minimal breast tissue. There is also early spread to axillary lymph nodes due to minimal breast tissue. The ulcerating mass shown here had been present for $3^{1}/_{2}$ years and is advanced carcinoma.

BIBLIOGRAPHY

American Cancer Society: www.cancer.org/docroot/CRI/content/CRI_2_4_2X_What_are_the_risk_factors_for_breast_cancer_5.asp [accessed Aug 2002].

Apantaku LM: Breast cancer diagnosis and screening, *Am Fam Physician* 62(3):596–606, Aug 1, 2000.

Appling SE: Mastitis, Lippincotts *Prim Care Pract* 2(2):184–188, Mar–Apr 1998.

Appling SE: Prevention, early detection, and treatment of breast cancer: a collaborative approach, Lippincotts *Prim Care Pract* 2(2):111–120, Mar-Apr 1998.

Arnold GJ, Neiheisel MB: A comprehensive approach to evaluating nipple discharge, *Nurse Pract* 22(7):96–111, Jul 1997.

Bell KK, Rawlings NL: Promoting breast-feeding by managing common lactation problems, *Nurse Pract* 23(6):102–123, Jun 1998.

Chiechi LM, Secreto G: Factors of risk for breast cancer influencing post-menopausal long-term hormone replacement therapy, *Tumori* 86(1):12–16, Jan–Feb 2000.

Colditz GA, Rosner B: Cumulative risk of breast cancer to age 70 years according to risk factor status: data from the Nurses' Health Study, *Am J Epidemiol* 152(10):950–964, Nov 15, 2000.

Cole CF: Issues in breast imaging, Lippincotts *Prim Care Pract* 2(2):141–148, Mar–Apr 1998.

Coleman EA, Heard JK: Clinical breast examination: an illustrated educational review and update, *Clin Excellence Nurse Pract* 5(4):197–204, Jul 2001.

Facione NC, Katapodi M: Culture as an influence on breast cancer screening and early detection, *Semin Oncol Nurs* 16(3):238–247, Aug 2000.

Facione NC et al: The self-reported likelihood of patient delay in breast cancer, *Prev Med* 34(4):397–407, Apr 2002.

Friedenreich CM, Courneya KS, Bryant HE: Relation between intensity of physical activity and breast cancer risk reduction, *Med Sci Sports Exerc* 33(9):1538–1545, Sep 2001.

Hall IJ et al: Body size and breast cancer risk in black women and white women, *Am J Epidemiol* 151(8):754–764, Apr 15, 2000.

Harlan WR, Harlan EA, Grillo GP: Secondary sex characteristics of girls 12 to 17 years of age: the U.S. Health Examination Survey, *J Pediatr* 96(6):1074–1078, 1980.

Herman-Giddens ME et al: Secondary sexual characteristics and menses in young girls seen in office practice: a study from the pediatric research in office settings network, *Pediatrics* 99(4):505–512, Apr 1997.

Johnson P: Breast lumps in the adolescent female, *J Pediatr Health Care* 16(1):43–48, Jan–Feb 2002.

Judkins AF, Akins J: Breast cancer: initial diagnosis and current treatment options, *Nurs Clin North Am* 36(3):527–542, Sep 2001.

Love S, Lindsey K: *Dr. Susan Love's breast book,* ed 3, Cambridge, MA, 2000, Perseus Publishing.

Machia J: Breast cancer: risk, prevention, and tamoxifen, *Am J Nurs* 101(4):26–36, Apr 2001.

Marchant DJ: *Breast disease.* Philadelphia, 1997, W.B. Saunders.

Marsden J: Hormone-replacement therapy and breast cancer, *Lancet Oncol* 3(5):303–311, May 2002.

Marshall WA, Tanner JM: Variations in pattern of pubertal changes in girls, *Arch Dis Child* 44:291–303, Jun 1969.

McCance KL, Jorde LB: Evaluating the genetic risk of breast cancer, *Nurs Pract* 23(8):14–29, Aug 1998.

Morrison C: The significance of nipple discharge: diagnosis and treatment regimes, *Lippincotts Prim Care Pract* 2(2):129–140, Mar–Apr 1998.

Nelson MT: Breast cancer diagnosis: screening and diagnosis, *Postgrad Med* 108(5):195–198, Oct 2000.

Poole K, Lyne PA: The cues to diagnosis: describing the monitoring activities of women undergoing diagnostic investigations for breast disease, *J Adv Nurs* 31(4):752–758, Apr 2000.

Qureshi M et al: Differences in breast cancer screening rates: an issue of ethnicity or socioeconomics? *J Womens Health Gender Based Med* 9(9):1025–1031, Nov 2000.

Resnick B, Belcher AE: Breast reconstruction, *Am J Nurs* 102(4):26–43, Apr 2002.

Sloand E: Pediatric and adolescent breast health, *Lippincott's Prim Care Pract* 2(2):170–175, Mar–Apr 1998.

Smith ED, Phillips JM, Price MM: Screening and early detection among racial and ethnic minority women, *Semin Oncol Nurs* 17(3):159–170, Aug 2001.

Tanner JM: *Growth at adolescence,* ed 2, Oxford, England, 1962, Blackwell Scientific.

Weisburger JH: Dietary fat and risk of chronic disease: mechanistic insights from experimental studies, *J Am Diet Assoc* 97(suppl 7):S16–S23, Jul 1997.

Ziegfeld CR: Differential diagnosis of a breast mass, Lippincotts *Prim Care Pract* 2(2):121–128, Mar–Apr 1998.

Thorax and Lungs

Structure and Function

POSITION AND SURFACE LANDMARKS

The **thoracic cage** is a bony structure with a conical shape, which is narrower at the top (Fig. 18–1). It is defined by the **sternum,** 12 pairs of **ribs** and 12 thoracic **vertebrae.** Its "floor" is the **diaphragm,** a musculotendinous septum that separates the thoracic cavity from the abdomen. The first seven ribs attach directly to the sternum via their costal cartilages; ribs 8, 9, and 10 attach to the costal cartilage above, and ribs 11 and 12 are "floating," with free palpable tips. The **costochondral junctions** are the points at which the ribs join their cartilages. They are not palpable.

ANTERIOR THORACIC LANDMARKS

Surface landmarks on the thorax are signposts for underlying respiratory structures. Knowledge of landmarks will help you localize a finding and will facilitate communication of your findings to others.

SUPRASTERNAL NOTCH. Feel this hollow U-shaped depression just above the sternum, in between the clavicles.

STERNUM. The "breastbone" has three parts—the manubrium, the body, and the xiphoid process. Walk your fingers down the manubrium a few centimeters until you feel a distinct bony ridge, the manubriosternal angle.

MANUBRIOSTERNAL ANGLE. Often called the sternal angle or the "angle of Louis," this is the articulation of the manubrium and body of the sternum, and it is continuous with the second rib. The angle of Louis is a useful place to start counting ribs, which helps localize a respiratory finding horizontally. Identify the angle of Louis, palpate lightly to the second rib, and slide down to the second intercostal space. Each intercostal space is numbered by the rib above it. Continue counting down the ribs in the middle of the hemithorax, not close to the sternum where the costal cartilages lie too close together to count. You can palpate easily down to the 10th rib.

The angle of Louis also marks the site of tracheal bifurcation into the right and left main bronchi; it corresponds with the upper border of the atria of the heart, and it lies above the fourth thoracic vertebra on the back.

COSTAL ANGLE. The right and left costal margins form an angle where they meet at the xiphoid process. Usually 90 degrees or less, this angle increases when the rib cage is chronically overinflated, as in emphysema.

POSTERIOR THORACIC LANDMARKS

Counting ribs and intercostal spaces on the back is a bit harder due to the muscles and soft tissue surrounding the ribs and spinal column (Fig. 18–2).

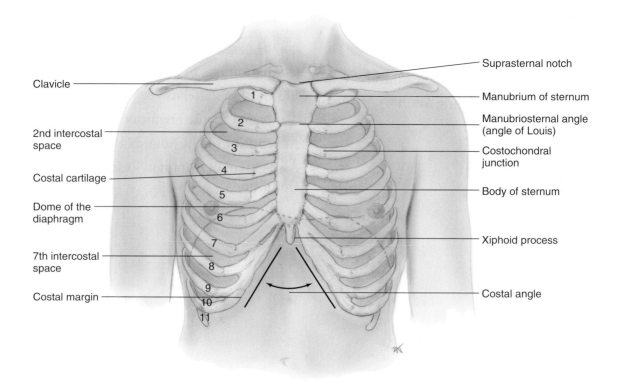

Clavicle

2nd intercostal space

Costal cartilage

Dome of the diaphragm

7th intercostal space

Costal margin

Suprasternal notch

Manubrium of sternum

Manubriosternal angle (angle of Louis)

Costochondral junction

Body of sternum

Xiphoid process

Costal angle

18–1   ANTERIOR THORACIC CAGE

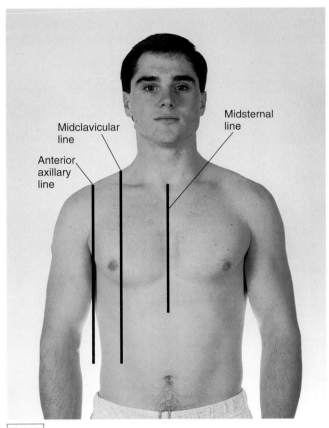

18–2 POSTERIOR THORACIC CAGE

VERTEBRA PROMINENS. Start here. Flex your head and feel for the most prominent bony spur protruding at the base of the neck. This is the spinous process of C7. If two bumps seem equally prominent, the upper one is C7 and the lower one is T1.

SPINOUS PROCESSES. Count down these knobs on the vertebrae, which stack together to form the spinal column. Note that the spinous processes align with their same numbered ribs only down to T4. After T4, the spinous processes angle downward from their vertebral body and overlie the vertebral body and rib below.

INFERIOR BORDER OF THE SCAPULA. The scapulae are located symmetrically in each hemithorax. The lower tip is usually at the seventh or eighth rib.

TWELFTH RIB. Palpate midway between the spine and the person's side to identify its free tip.

REFERENCE LINES

Use the reference lines to pinpoint a finding vertically on the chest. On the anterior chest, note the **midsternal** line and the **midclavicular** line. The midclavicular line bisects the center of each clavicle at a point halfway between the palpated sternoclavicular and acromioclavicular joints (Fig. 18–3).

18–3

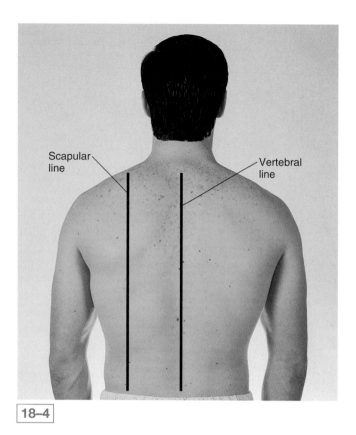

Scapular line

Vertebral line

18–4

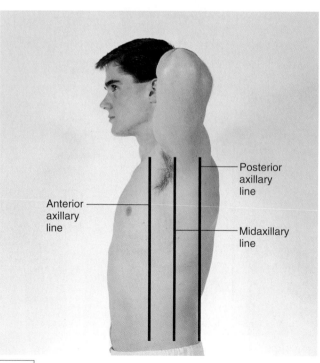

Anterior axillary line

Posterior axillary line

Midaxillary line

18–5

The posterior chest wall has the **vertebral** (or midspinal) line and the **scapular** line, which extends through the inferior angle of the scapula when the arms are at the sides of the body (Fig. 18–4).

Lift up the person's arm 90 degrees, and divide the lateral chest by three lines: The **anterior axillary** line extends down from the anterior axillary fold where the pectoralis major muscle inserts; the **posterior axillary** line continues down from the posterior axillary fold where the latissimus dorsi muscle inserts; and the **midaxillary** line runs down from the apex of the axilla and lies between and parallel to the other two (Fig. 18–5).

THE THORACIC CAVITY

The **mediastinum** is the middle section of the thoracic cavity containing the esophagus, trachea, heart, and great vessels. The right and left **pleural cavities,** on either side of the mediastinum, contain the lungs.

LUNG BORDERS. In the anterior chest, the **apex,** or highest point, of lung tissue is 3 or 4 cm above the inner third of the clavicles. The **base,** or lower border, rests on the diaphragm at about the sixth rib in the midclavicular line. Laterally, lung tissue extends from the apex of the axilla down to the seventh or eighth rib. Posteriorly, the location of C7 marks the apex of lung tissue, and T10 usually corresponds to the base. Deep inspiration expands the lungs, and their lower border drops to the level of T12.

LOBES OF THE LUNGS

The lungs are paired but not precisely symmetric structures (Fig. 18–6). The right lung is shorter than the left lung because of the underlying liver. The left lung is narrower than the right lung because the heart bulges to the left. The right lung has three lobes, and the left lung has two lobes. These lobes are not arranged in horizontal bands like dessert layers in a parfait glass. Rather, they stack in diagonal sloping segments and are separated by **fissures** that run obliquely through the chest.

ANTERIOR. On the anterior chest, the **oblique** (the major, or diagonal) fissure crosses the fifth rib in the midaxillary line and terminates at the sixth rib in the midclavicular line. The right lung also contains the **horizontal** (minor) fissure, which divides the right upper and middle lobes. This fissure extends from the fifth rib in the right midaxillary line to the third intercostal space or fourth rib at the right sternal border.

POSTERIOR. The most remarkable point about the posterior chest is that it is almost all lower lobe (Fig. 18–7). The upper lobes occupy a smaller band of tissue from their apices at T1 down to T3 or T4. At this level, the lower lobes begin, and their inferior border reaches down to the level of T10 on expiration and to T12 on inspiration. Note that the right middle lobe does not project onto the posterior chest at all. If the person abducts the arms and places the hands on the back of the head, the division between upper and lower lobes corresponds to the medial border of the scapulae.

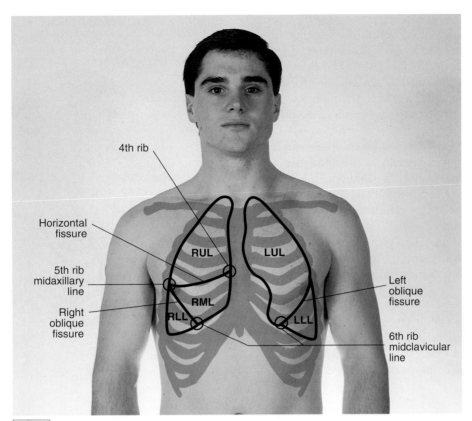

4th rib

Horizontal
fissure

5th rib
midaxillary
line

Right
oblique
fissure

RUL

LUL

RML

RLL   LLL

Left
oblique
fissure

6th rib
midclavicular
line

18–6

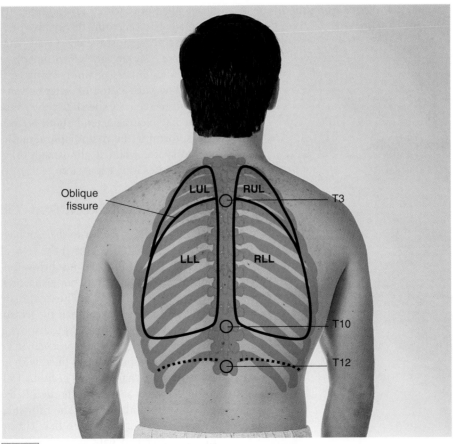

Oblique
fissure

LUL   RUL   T3

LLL   RLL

T10

T12

18–7

LATERAL. Laterally, lung tissue extends from the apex of the axilla down to the seventh or eighth rib. The right upper lobe extends from the apex of the axilla down to the horizontal fissure at the fifth rib (Fig. 18–8). The right middle lobe extends from the horizontal fissure down and forward to the sixth rib at the midclavicular line. The right lower lobe continues from the fifth rib to the eighth rib in the midaxillary line.

The left lung contains only two lobes, upper and lower (Fig. 18–9). These are seen laterally as two triangular areas separated by the oblique fissure. The left upper lobe extends from the apex of the axilla down to the fifth rib at the midaxillary line. The left lower lobe continues down to the eighth rib in the midaxillary line.

Using these landmarks, take a grease pencil and try tracing the outline of each lobe on a willing partner. Take special note of the three points that commonly confuse beginning examiners:

1. The left lung has no middle lobe.
2. The anterior chest contains mostly upper and middle lobe with very little lower lobe.
3. The posterior chest contains almost all lower lobe.

PLEURAE

The thin, slippery **pleurae** form an envelope between the lungs and the chest wall (Fig. 18–10). The **visceral** pleura lines the outside of the lungs, dipping down into the fissures. It is continuous with the **parietal** pleura lining the inside of the chest wall and diaphragm.

18–9

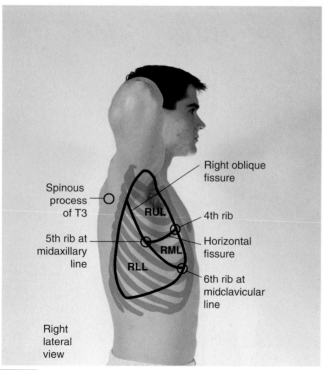

18–8

The inside of the envelope, the pleural cavity, is a potential space filled only with a few milliliters of lubricating fluid. It normally has a vacuum, or negative pressure, which holds the lungs tightly against the chest wall. The lungs slide smoothly and noiselessly up and down during respiration, lubricated by a few milliliters of fluid. Think of this as similar to two glass slides with a drop of water between them; although it is difficult to separate the slides, they slide smoothly back and forth. The pleurae extend about 3 cm below the level of the lungs, forming the **costodiaphragmatic recess.** This is a potential space; when it abnormally fills with air or fluid, it compromises lung expansion.

TRACHEA AND BRONCHIAL TREE

The **trachea** lies anterior to the esophagus and is 10 to 11 cm long in the adult. It begins at the level of the cricoid cartilage in the neck and bifurcates just below the sternal angle into the right and left main bronchi. Posteriorly, tracheal bifurcation is at the level of T4 or T5. The right main bronchus is shorter, wider, and more vertical than the left main bronchus.

The **trachea** and **bronchi** transport gases between the environment and the lung parenchyma. They constitute the *dead space,* or space that is filled with air but is not available for gaseous exchange. This is about 150 ml in the adult. The bronchial tree also protects alveoli from small particulate matter in the inhaled air. The bronchi are lined with goblet cells, which secrete mucus that entraps the particles. The bronchi are lined with cilia, which sweep particles upward where they can be swallowed or expelled.

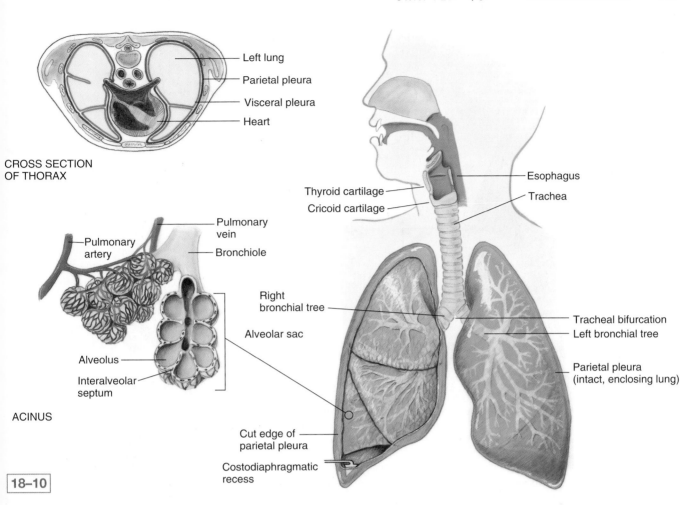

CROSS SECTION OF THORAX

- Left lung
- Parietal pleura
- Visceral pleura
- Heart

- Pulmonary vein
- Pulmonary artery
- Bronchiole
- Right bronchial tree
- Alveolar sac
- Alveolus
- Interalveolar septum

ACINUS

- Thyroid cartilage
- Cricoid cartilage
- Esophagus
- Trachea
- Tracheal bifurcation
- Left bronchial tree
- Parietal pleura (intact, enclosing lung)
- Cut edge of parietal pleura
- Costodiaphragmatic recess

18–10

An **acinus** is a functional respiratory unit that consists of the bronchioles, alveolar ducts, alveolar sacs, and the alveoli. Gaseous exchange occurs across the respiratory membrane in the alveolar duct and in the millions of alveoli. Note how the alveoli are clustered like grapes around each alveolar duct. This creates millions of interalveolar septa (walls) that increase tremendously the working space available for gas exchange. This bunched arrangement creates a surface area for gas exchange that is as large as a tennis court.

MECHANICS OF RESPIRATION

There are four major functions of the respiratory system: (1) supplying oxygen to the body for energy production; (2) removing carbon dioxide as a waste product of energy reactions; (3) maintaining homeostasis (acid-base balance) of arterial blood; and (4) maintaining heat exchange (less important in humans).

By supplying oxygen to the blood and eliminating excess carbon dioxide, respiration maintains the pH or the acid-base balance of the blood. The body tissues are bathed by blood that normally has a narrow acceptable range of pH. Although a number of compensatory mechanisms regulate the pH, the lungs help maintain the balance by adjusting the level of carbon dioxide through respiration. That is, hypoventilation (slow, shallow breathing) causes carbon dioxide to build up in the blood, and hyperventilation (rapid, deep breathing) causes carbon dioxide to be blown off.

CONTROL OF RESPIRATIONS

Normally our breathing pattern changes without our awareness in response to cellular demands. This involuntary control of respirations is mediated by the respiratory center in the brain stem (pons and medulla). The major feedback loop is humoral regulation, or the change in carbon dioxide and oxygen levels in the blood, and, less importantly, the hydrogen ion level. The *normal stimulus to breathe* for most of us is an increase of carbon dioxide in the blood, or **hypercapnia**. A decrease of oxygen in the blood (**hypoxemia**) also increases respirations but is less effective than hypercapnia.

CHANGING CHEST SIZE

Respiration is the physical act of breathing; air rushes into the lungs as the chest size increases (inspiration) and is expelled from the lungs as the chest recoils (expiration). The mechanical expansion and contraction of the chest cavity alters the size of the thoracic container in two dimensions: (1) The vertical diameter lengthens or shortens, which is accomplished

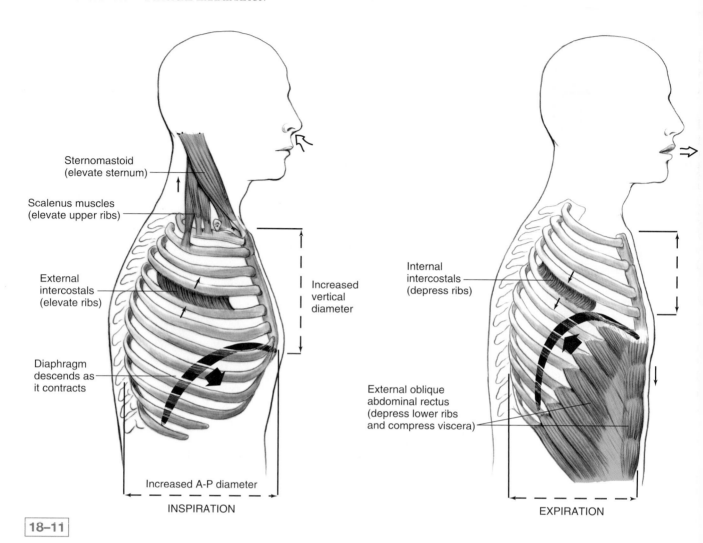

Sternomastoid
(elevate sternum)

Scalenus muscles
(elevate upper ribs)

External
intercostals
(elevate ribs)

Diaphragm
descends as
it contracts

Increased
vertical
diameter

Increased A-P diameter

INSPIRATION

Internal
intercostals
(depress ribs)

External oblique
abdominal rectus
(depress lower ribs
and compress viscera)

EXPIRATION

 18–11

by downward or upward movement of the diaphragm; and (2) the anteroposterior diameter increases or decreases, which is accomplished by elevation or depression of the ribs (Fig. 18–11).

In inspiration, increasing the size of the thoracic container creates a slightly negative pressure in relation to the atmosphere, so air rushes in to fill the partial vacuum. The major muscle responsible for this increase is the diaphragm. During inspiration, contraction of the bell-shaped diaphragm causes it to descend and flatten. This lengthens the vertical diameter. Intercostal muscles lift the sternum and elevate the ribs, making them more horizontal. This increases the anteroposterior diameter.

Expiration is primarily passive. As the diaphragm relaxes, elastic forces within the lung, chest cage, and abdomen cause it to dome up. All this squeezing creates a relatively positive pressure within the alveoli, and the air flows out.

Forced inspiration, such as that following heavy exercise or occurring pathologically with respiratory distress, commands the use of the accessory neck muscles to heave up the sternum and rib cage. These neck muscles are the sternomastoids, the scaleni, and the trapezii. In forced expiration, the abdominal muscles contract powerfully to push the abdominal viscera forcefully in and up against the diaphragm, making it dome upward, and making it squeeze against the lungs.

DEVELOPMENTAL CONSIDERATIONS

INFANTS AND CHILDREN

During the first 5 weeks of fetal life, the primitive lung bud emerges; by 16 weeks, the conducting airways reach the same number as in the adult; at 32 weeks, **surfactant,** the complex lipid substance needed for sustained inflation of the air sacs, is present in adequate amounts; and by birth the lungs have 70 million primitive alveoli ready to start the job of respiration.

Breath is life. When the newborn inhales the first breath, the lusty cry that follows reassures straining parents that their baby is all right (Fig. 18–12). The baby's body systems all develop in utero, but the respiratory system alone does not function until birth. Birth demands its instant performance.

When the cord is cut, blood is cut off from the placenta, and it gushes into the pulmonary circulation. Relatively less resistance exists in the pulmonary arteries than in the aorta, so the foramen ovale in the heart closes just after birth. (See the discussion of fetal circulation in Chapter 19.) The ductus arteriosus (linking the pulmonary artery and the aorta) contracts and closes some hours later, and pulmonary and systemic circulation are functional.

Respiratory development continues throughout childhood, with increases in diameter and length of airways, and increases in size and number of alveoli, reaching the adult range of 300 million by adolescence.

The relatively smaller size and immaturity of children's pulmonary systems, as well as the presence of older caregivers who smoke, result in enormously increased risks to child health. "Each year, among American children, tobacco is associated with an estimated 284 to 360 deaths from lower respiratory tract illnesses and fires initiated by smoking materials . . . 529,000 physician visits for asthma, 1.3 to 2 million visits for coughs, and in children younger than 5 years of age, 260,000 to 436,000 episodes of bronchitis and 115,000 to 190,000 episodes of pneumonia" (DiFranza and Lew, 1996).

THE PREGNANT FEMALE

The enlarging uterus elevates the diaphragm 4 cm during pregnancy. This decreases the vertical diameter of the thoracic cage, but this decrease is compensated for by an increase in the horizontal diameter. The increase in estrogen level relaxes the chest cage ligaments. This allows an increase in the transverse diameter of the chest cage by 2 cm, and the costal angle widens. The total circumference of the chest cage increases by 6 cm. Although the diaphragm is elevated, it is not fixed. It moves with breathing even more during pregnancy, which results in an increase in tidal volume (Cunningham et al., 2001).

The growing fetus increases the oxygen demand on the mother's body. This is met easily by the increasing tidal volume (deeper breathing). Little change occurs in the respiratory rate. An increased awareness of the need to breathe develops, even early in pregnancy, and some pregnant women may interpret this as dyspnea even though structurally nothing is wrong.

THE AGING ADULT

The costal cartilages become calcified, which produces a less mobile thorax. Respiratory muscle strength declines after age 50 and continues to decrease into the 70s. A more significant change is the decrease in elastic properties within the lungs, making them less distensible and lessening their tendency to collapse and recoil. In all, the aging lung is a more rigid structure that is harder to inflate.

These changes result in an increase in small airway closure, and that yields a *decreased vital capacity* (the maximum amount of air that a person can expel from the lungs after first filling the lungs to maximum) and an *increased residual volume* (the amount of air remaining in the lungs even after the most forceful expiration).

With aging, histologic changes (i.e., a gradual loss of intraalveolar septa and a decreased number of alveoli) also occur, so less surface area is available for gas exchange. Also the lung bases become less ventilated due to closing off of a number of airways. This increases the older person's risk of dyspnea with exertion beyond his or her usual workload.

The histologic changes also increase the older person's risk of postoperative pulmonary complications. That is, the older person has a greater risk of postoperative atelectasis and infection due to a decreased ability to cough, a loss of protective airway reflexes, and increased secretions (Bezanson, 1997).

TRANSCULTURAL CONSIDERATIONS

The incidence of **tuberculosis** (TB) is higher in Asian-Americans, and this occurs primarily in those who have recently immigrated to the United States from countries with a high endemic rate of TB (Makinodan and Harada, 1996). Their TB incidence peaks in the first 2 months of entry to the United States. Relative to the risk for the U.S. general population, the risk is increased by 112 times for newly arrived Vietnamese, 60 times for newly arrived Filipinos, 37 times for those from mainland China, and 28 times for those from Korea.

Biocultural differences in the **size of the thoracic cavity** significantly influence pulmonary functioning as determined by vital capacity and forced expiratory volume. In descending order, the largest chest volumes are found in whites, blacks, Asians, and Native Americans. Even when the shorter height of Asians is considered, their chest volume remains significantly lower than that of whites and blacks.

Some biocultural differences are present even before birth. The **lecithin/sphingomyelin ratio** is a laboratory measurement of the amniotic fluid that indicates fetal pulmonary maturation. The ratio is used to calculate the risk of respiratory distress syndrome in premature infants. This ratio differs between blacks and whites, as does the pulmonary maturity it predicts (Richardson and Torday, 1994). Blacks have higher ratios than whites from 23 to 42 weeks of gestation. Lung maturity, mea-

18–12

sured by a lecithin/sphingomyelin ratio of 2.0, is reached 1 week earlier in blacks than in whites (i.e., at 34 versus 35 weeks). The risk of respiratory distress syndrome is 40% to 50% for a ratio score between 1.5 and 1.9 for premature white infants but not for premature blacks. Premature black infants have a much lower risk of respiratory distress syndrome at the same low ratio scores. When the lecithin/sphingomyelin ratio is determined before induction of labor or elective cesarean section, the racial difference should be considered in making the decision (Overfield, 1995).

Subjective Data

1. Cough	4. Past history of respiratory infections	6. Environmental exposure
2. Shortness of breath		7. Self-care behaviors
3. Chest pain with breathing	5. Smoking history	

EXAMINER ASKS	RATIONALE
1. Cough. Do you have a **cough?** When did it start? Gradual or sudden? • How long have you had it? • How often do you cough? At any special time of day or just on arising? Cough wake you up at night?	Some conditions have a characteristic timing of a cough: Continuous throughout day—associated with acute illness, e.g., respiratory infection Afternoon/evening—may reflect exposure to irritants at work Night—postnasal drip, sinusitis Early morning—chronic bronchial inflammation of smokers Chronic bronchitis is characterized by a history of productive cough for 3 months of the year for 2 years in a row.
• Do you cough up any phlegm or sputum? How much? What color is it?	Hemoptysis.
• Cough up any blood? Does this look like streaks or frank blood? Does the sputum have a foul odor?	Although sputum is not diagnostic alone, some conditions have characteristic sputum production: white or clear mucoid—colds, bronchitis, viral infections; yellow or green—bacterial infections; rust colored—tuberculosis, pneumococcal pneumonia; pink, frothy—pulmonary edema, some sympathomimetic medications have a side effect of pink-tinged mucus.
• How would you describe your cough: hacking, dry, barking, hoarse, congested, bubbling?	Although not mutually exclusive, some conditions have a characteristic cough: mycoplasma pneumonia—hacking; early heart failure—dry; croup—barking; colds, bronchitis, pneumonia—congested.
• Cough seem to come with anything: activity, position (lying), fever, congestion, talking, anxiety? • Activity make it better or worse? • What treatment have you tried? Prescription or over-the-counter medications, vaporizer, rest, position change?	Assess effectiveness of coping strategies.
• Does the cough bring on anything: chest pain, ear pain? Is it tiring? Are you concerned about it?	Note severity.

EXAMINER ASKS	RATIONALE
2. Shortness of breath. Ever had any **shortness of breath** or hard-breathing spells? What brings it on? How severe is it? How long does it last?	Determine exactly how much activity precipitates the shortness of breath—state specific number of blocks walked, number of stairs.
• Is it affected by position, like lying down?	Orthopnea is difficulty breathing when supine. State number of pillows the person sleeps with to achieve comfort, e.g., "two-pillow orthopnea."
• Occur at any specific time of day or night?	Paroxysmal nocturnal dyspnea is awakening from sleep with shortness of breath and needing to be upright to achieve comfort. Diaphoresis. Cyanosis.
• Shortness of breath episodes associated with night sweats? • Or cough, chest pain, or bluish color around lips or nails? Wheezing sound? • Episodes seem to be related to food, pollen, dust, animals, season, or emotion? • What do you do in a hard-breathing attack? Take a special position, or use pursed-lip breathing? Use any oxygen, inhalers, or medications? • How does the shortness of breath affect your work or home activities? Getting better or worse or staying about the same?	Asthma attacks are associated with a specific allergen. Assess effect of coping strategies and the need for more teaching. Assess effect on activities of daily living.
3. Chest pain with breathing. Any **chest pain with breathing?** Please point to the exact location. • When did it start? Constant or does it come and go? • Describe the pain: burning, stabbing? • Brought on by respiratory infection, coughing, or trauma? Is it associated with fever, deep breathing, unequal chest inflation? • What have you done to treat it? Medication or heat application?	
4. Past history of respiratory infections. Any **past history** of breathing trouble or lung diseases like bronchitis, emphysema, asthma, pneumonia? • Any unusually frequent or unusually severe colds? • Any family history of allergies, tuberculosis, or asthma?	Consider sequelae following these conditions. Since most people have had some colds, it is more meaningful to ask about excess number or severity. Assess possible risk factors.
5. Smoking history. Do you **smoke** cigarettes or cigars? At what age did you start? How many packs per day do you smoke now? For how long? • Have you ever tried to quit? What helped? Why do you think it did not work? What activities do you associate with smoking? • Live with someone who smokes?	State number of packs per day and the number of years smoked. Most people already know they should quit smoking. Instead of admonishing, assess smoking behavior and ways to modify daily smoking activities.
6. Environmental exposure. Are there any **environmental conditions** that may affect your breathing? Where do you work? At a factory, chemical plant, coal mine, farming, outdoors in a heavy traffic area?	Pollution exposure. Farmers may be at risk for grain inhalation, pesticide inhalation. People in the rural Midwest have a risk of histoplasmosis exposure; those in the Southwest and Mexico have a risk of coccidioidomycosis. Coal miners have a risk of pneumoconiosis. Stone cutters, miners, potters—silicosis. Other irritants: asbestos, beryllium.

EXAMINER ASKS	RATIONALE
• Do anything to protect your lungs, such as wear a mask or have the ventilatory system checked at work? Do anything to monitor your exposure? Have periodic examinations, pulmonary function tests, x-ray examination?	Assess **self-care** measures.
• Do you know what specific symptoms to note that may signal breathing problems?	General symptoms: cough, shortness of breath. Exposure to some gases produces specific symptoms: carbon monoxide—dizziness, headache, fatigue; sulfur dioxide—cough, congestion.
7. Self-care behaviors. Last tuberculosis skin test, chest x-ray study, pneumonia or influenza immunization?	Self-care measures.

Additional History for Infants and Children

1. Has the child had any frequent or very severe colds?	Limit of four to six uncomplicated upper respiratory infections per year is expected in early childhood.
2. Is there any history of allergy in the family? • (For child under 2 years of age): At what age were new foods introduced? Was the child breast-fed or bottle-fed?	Consider new foods as possible allergens. Consider formula as allergen.
3. Does the child have a cough? Seem congested? Have noisy breathing or wheezing? (Further questions similar to those listed in the section on adults.)	Screen for onset and follow course of childhood chronic respiratory problems: asthma, bronchitis.
4. What measures have you taken to child-proof your home? Yard? Is there any possibility of the child inhaling or swallowing toxic substances?	Self-care behaviors. Young child is at risk for accidental aspiration, poisoning, and injury.
• Has anyone taught you emergency care measures in case of accidental choking or a hard-breathing spell?	Assess knowledge level of parent and caregivers.
5. Any smokers in the home or in the car with child?	Second-hand smoke enormously increases the risk of upper and lower respiratory infections in children (DiFranza and Lew, 1996).

Additional History for the Aging Adult

1. Have you noticed any shortness of breath or fatigue with your daily activities?	Some older adults have a less efficient respiratory system (decreased vital capacity, less surface area for gas exchange), so they experience less tolerance for activity.
2. Tell me about your usual amount of physical activity.	Assess self-care behaviors. May have reduced capacity to perform exercise because of pulmonary function deficits of aging. Sedentary or bedridden people are at risk for respiratory dysfunction.
3. (For those with a history of chronic obstructive pulmonary disease, lung cancer, or tuberculosis): How are you getting along each day? Any weight change in the last 3 months? How much?	Assess coping strategies.
• How about energy level? Do you tire more easily? How does your illness affect you at home? At work?	Activities may decrease because of increasing shortness of breath or pain.

EXAMINER ASKS	RATIONALE
4. Do you have any chest pain with breathing?	Some older adults feel pleuritic pain less intensely than younger adults.
• Any chest pain after a bout of coughing? After a fall?	Precisely localized sharp pain (when person points to it with one finger)—consider fractured rib or muscle injury.

Objective Data

PREPARATION

Ask the person to sit upright and the male to disrobe to the waist. For the female, leave the gown on and open at the back. When examining the anterior chest, lift up the gown and drape it on her shoulders rather than removing it completely. This promotes comfort by giving her the feeling of being somewhat clothed. These provisions will ensure further comfort: a warm room, a warm diaphragm endpiece, and a private examination time with no interruptions.

For smooth choreography in a complete examination, begin the respiratory examination just after palpating the thyroid gland when you are standing behind the person. Perform the inspection, palpation, percussion, and auscultation on the posterior and lateral thorax. Then move to face the person and repeat the four maneuvers on the anterior chest. This avoids repetitiously moving front-to-back around the person.

Finally, clean your stethoscope endpiece with an alcohol swab. Since your stethoscope touches many people, it could be a possible vector for both aerobic and anaerobic bacteria (Assadian et al., 1998). Cleaning with an alcohol swab is very effective.

EQUIPMENT NEEDED

Stethoscope
Small ruler, marked in centimeters
Marking pen
Alcohol swab

NORMAL RANGE OF FINDINGS	ABNORMAL FINDINGS

INSPECT THE POSTERIOR CHEST

Thoracic Cage

Note the **shape and configuration** of the chest wall. The spinous processes should appear in a straight line. The thorax is symmetric, in an elliptical shape, with downward sloping ribs, about 45 degrees relative to the spine. The scapulae are placed symmetrically in each hemithorax.

Skeletal deformities may limit thoracic cage excursion: scoliosis, kyphosis (see Table 18–4 on p. 470).

The anteroposterior diameter should be less than the transverse diameter. The ratio of anteroposterior to transverse diameter is from 1 : 2 to 5 : 7.

Anteroposterior = transverse diameter, or "barrel chest." Ribs are horizontal, chest appears as if held in continuous inspiration. This occurs in chronic emphysema due to hyperinflation of the lungs (see Table 18–4).

The neck muscles and trapezius muscles should be developed normally for age and occupation.

Neck muscles are hypertrophied in chronic obstructive pulmonary disease (COPD) from aiding in forced respirations.

Note the **position** the person takes to breathe. This includes a relaxed posture and the ability to support one's own weight with arms comfortably at the sides or in the lap.

People with COPD often sit in a tripod position, leaning forward with arms braced against their knees, chair, or bed. This gives them leverage so that their rectus abdominis, intercostal, and accessory neck muscles all can aid in expiration.

Assess the **skin color and condition.** Color should be consistent with person's genetic background, with allowance for sun-exposed areas on the chest and the back. No cyanosis or pallor should be present. Note any lesions. Inquire as to any change in a nevus on the back, for example, where the person may have difficulty monitoring (see Chapter 12, "Skin, Hair, and Nails").

PALPATE THE POSTERIOR CHEST

Symmetric Expansion

Confirm **symmetric chest expansion** by placing your warmed hands on the posterolateral chest wall with thumbs at the level of T9 or T10. Slide your hands medially to pinch up a small fold of skin between your thumbs (Fig. 18–13).

18–13

Ask the person to take a deep breath. Your hands serve as mechanical amplifiers; as the person inhales deeply, your thumbs should move apart symmetrically. Note any lag in expansion.

Unequal chest expansion occurs with marked atelectasis or pneumonia; with thoracic trauma, such as fractured ribs; or with pneumothorax.

Pain accompanies deep breathing when the pleurae are inflamed.

Tactile Fremitus

Assess **tactile (or vocal) fremitus.** Fremitus is a palpable vibration. Sounds generated from the larynx are transmitted through patent bronchi and through the lung parenchyma to the chest wall, where you feel them as vibrations.

Use either the palmar base (the ball) of the fingers or the ulnar edge of one hand, and touch the person's chest while he or she repeats the words "ninety-nine" or "blue moon." These are resonant phrases that generate strong vibrations. Start over the lung apices and palpate from one side to another (Fig. 18–14).

| NORMAL RANGE OF FINDINGS | ABNORMAL FINDINGS |

18–14

Fremitus varies among persons but symmetry is most important; the vibrations should feel the same in the corresponding area on each side. However, just between the scapulae, fremitus may feel stronger on the right side than on the left side because the right side is closer to the bronchial bifurcation. Avoid palpating over the scapulae because bone damps out sound transmission.

The following factors affect the normal intensity of tactile fremitus:

- *Relative location of bronchi to the chest wall.*
  Normally, fremitus is most prominent between the scapulae and around the sternum, sites where the major bronchi are closest to the chest wall. Fremitus normally decreases as you progress down because more and more tissue impedes sound transmission.
- *Thickness of the chest wall.*
  Fremitus feels greater over a thin chest wall than over an obese or heavily muscular one where thick tissue damps the vibration.
- *Pitch and intensity.*
  A loud, low-pitched voice generates more fremitus than a soft, high-pitched one.

Note any areas of abnormal fremitus. Sound is conducted better through a uniformly dense structure than through a porous one, which changes in shape and solidity (as does the lung tissue during normal respiration). Thus conditions that increase the density of lung tissue make a better conducting medium for sound vibrations and increase tactile fremitus.

Decreased fremitus occurs when anything obstructs transmission of vibrations, e.g., obstructed bronchus, pleural effusion or thickening, pneumothorax, or emphysema. Any barrier that comes between the sound and your palpating hand will decrease fremitus.

Increased fremitus occurs with compression or consolidation of lung tissue, e.g., lobar pneumonia. This is present only when the bronchus is patent and when the consolidation extends to the lung surface. Note that only gross changes increase fremitus. Small areas of early pneumonia do not significantly affect fremitus.

Rhonchal fremitus is palpable with thick bronchial secretions.

Pleural friction fremitus is palpable with inflammation of the pleura (see Table 18–6).

Using the fingers, gently **palpate the entire chest wall.** This enables you to note any areas of tenderness, to note skin temperature and moisture, to detect any superficial lumps or masses, and to explore any skin lesions noted on inspection.

Crepitus is a coarse crackling sensation palpable over the skin surface. It occurs in subcutaneous emphysema when air escapes from the lung and enters the subcutaneous tissue, as following open thoracic injury or surgery.

PERCUSS THE POSTERIOR CHEST

Lung Fields

Determine the **predominent note over the lung fields.** Start at the apices and percuss the band of normally resonant tissue across the tops of both shoulders (Fig. 18–15). Then, percussing in the interspaces, make a side-to-side comparison all the way down the lung region. Percuss at 5-cm intervals. Avoid the damping effect of the scapulae and ribs.

| 18–15 | Sequence for percussion.

Resonance predominates in healthy lung tissue in the adult (Fig. 18–16). However, resonance is a relative term and has no constant standard. The resonant note may be modified somewhat in the athlete with a heavily muscular chest wall and in the heavily obese adult in whom subcutaneous fat produces scattered dullness.

Hyperresonance is found when too much air is present, as in emphysema or pneumothorax.

A **dull** note signals abnormal density in the lungs, as with pneumonia, pleural effusion, atelectasis, or tumor.

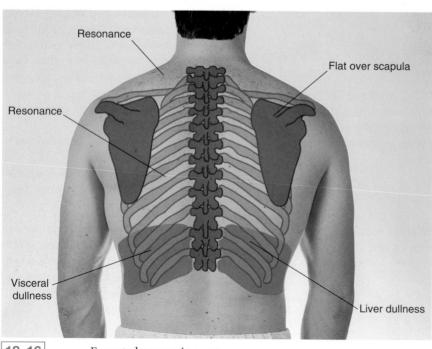

| 18–16 | Expected percussion notes.

NORMAL RANGE OF FINDINGS	ABNORMAL FINDINGS

The depth of penetration of percussion has limits. Percussion sets into motion only the outer 5 to 7 cm tissue. It will not penetrate to reveal any change in density deeper than that. Also, an abnormal finding must be 2 to 3 cm wide to yield an abnormal percussion note. Lesions smaller than that are not detectable by percussion.

Diaphragmatic Excursion

Determine **diaphragmatic excursion** (Fig. 18–17, *A*). Percuss to map out the lower lung border, both in expiration and in inspiration. First, ask the person to "exhale and hold it" briefly while you percuss down the scapular line until the sound changes from resonant to dull on each side. This estimates the level of the diaphragm separating the lungs from the abdominal viscera. It may be somewhat higher on the right side (about 1 to 2 cm) due to the presence of the liver. Mark the spot.

A

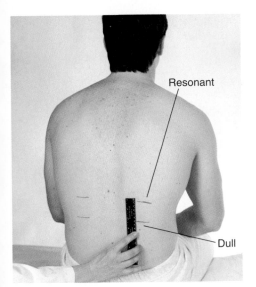

Resonant

Dull

B

18–17

Now ask the person to "take a deep breath and hold it." Continue percussing down from your first mark and mark the level where the sound changes to dull on this deep inspiration. Measure the difference. This diaphragmatic excursion should be equal bilaterally and measure about 3 to 5 cm in adults, although it may be up to 7 to 8 cm in well-conditioned people (Fig. 18–17, B).

Often, the beginning examiner becomes so involved in the subtle differences of percussion notes that she or he extends the patient's limits of breathholding. Always hold your own breath when you ask your patient to. When you run out of air, the other person surely has too, especially if that person has a respiratory problem.

AUSCULTATE THE POSTERIOR CHEST

The passage of air through the tracheobronchial tree creates a characteristic set of noises that are audible through the chest wall. These noises also may be modified by obstruction within the respiratory passageways or by changes in the lung parenchyma, the pleura, or the chest wall.

Breath Sounds

Evaluate the presence and quality of **normal breath sounds.** The person is sitting, leaning forward slightly, with arms resting comfortably across the lap. Instruct the person to breathe through the mouth, a little bit deeper than usual, but to stop if he or she begins to feel dizzy. Be careful to monitor the breathing throughout the examination, and offer times for the person to rest and breathe normally. The person is usually willing to comply with your instructions in an effort to please you and to be a "good patient." Watch that he or she does not hyperventilate to the point of fainting.

Use the flat diaphragm endpiece of the stethoscope and hold it firmly on the person's chest wall. Listen to at least one full respiration in each location. Side-to-side comparison is most important.

Do not confuse background noise with lung sounds. Become familiar with these extraneous noises that may be confused with lung pathology if not recognized:

1. Examiner's breathing on stethoscope tubing
2. Stethoscope tubing bumping together
3. Patient shivering
4. Patient's hairy chest; movement of hairs under stethoscope sounds like crackles (rales) (see p. 474)—minimize this by pressing harder or by wetting the hair with a damp cloth
5. Rustling of paper gown or paper drapes

While standing behind the person, listen to the following lung areas—posterior from the apices at C7 to the bases (around T10), and laterally from the axilla down to the seventh or eighth rib. Use the sequence illustrated in Fig. 18–18.

An abnormally high level of dullness, as well as absence of excursion, occurs with pleural effusion or atelectasis of the lower lobes.

NORMAL RANGE OF FINDINGS | ABNORMAL FINDINGS

18-18

Continue to visualize approximate locations of the lobes of each lung so that you correlate your findings to anatomical areas. As you listen, think (1) What AM I hearing over this spot? and (2) What should I EXPECT to be hearing? You should expect to hear three types of normal breath sounds in the adult and older child: **bronchial** (sometimes called tracheal or tubular), **bronchovesicular,** and **vesicular.** Study the description of the characteristics of these normal breath sounds in Table 18–1.

TABLE 18–1: Characteristics of Normal Breath Sounds

	PITCH	AMPLITUDE	DURATION	QUALITY	NORMAL LOCATION
BRONCHIAL (TRACHEAL)	High	Loud	Inspiration < expiration	Harsh, hollow tubular	Trachea and larynx
BRONCHOVESICULAR	Moderate	Moderate	Inspiration = expiration	Mixed	Over major bronchi where fewer alveoli are located: posterior, between scapulae especially on right; anterior, around upper sternum in first and second intercostal spaces
VESICULAR	Low	Soft	Inspiration > expiration	Rustling, like the sound of the wind in the trees	Over peripheral lung fields where air flows through smaller bronchioles and alveoli

NORMAL RANGE OF FINDINGS

Note the normal location of the three types of breath sounds on the chest wall of the adult and older child (Figs. 18–19 and 18–20).

Bronchovesicular   Vesicular

18–19

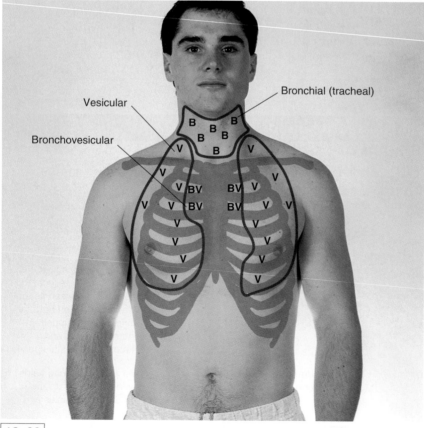

Vesicular   Bronchial (tracheal)

Bronchovesicular

18–20

ABNORMAL FINDINGS

Decreased or **absent breath sounds** occur

1. When the bronchial tree is obstructed at some point by secretions, mucous plug, or a foreign body
2. In emphysema due to loss of elasticity in the lung fibers and decreased force of inspired air; also the lungs are already hyperinflated so the inhaled air does not make as much noise
3. When anything obstructs transmission of sound between the lung and your stethoscope, such as pleurisy or pleural thickening, or air (pneumothorax) or fluid (pleural effusion) in the pleural space

A silent chest means no air is moving in or out, which is an ominous sign.

Increased breath sounds mean that sounds are louder than they should be, e.g., bronchial sounds are abnormal when they are heard over an abnormal location, the peripheral lung fields. They have a high-pitched tubular quality, with a prolonged expiratory phase and a distinct pause between inspiration and expiration. They sound very close to your stethoscope, as if they were right *in* the tubing close to your ear. They occur when consolidation (e.g., pneumonia) or compression (e.g., fluid in the intrapleural space) yields a dense lung area that enhances the transmission of sound from the bronchi. When the inspired air reaches the alveoli, it hits solid lung tissue that conducts sound more efficiently to the surface.

NORMAL RANGE OF FINDINGS	ABNORMAL FINDINGS

Adventitious Sounds

Note the presence of any **adventitious sounds.** These are added sounds that are *not* normally heard in the lungs. If present, they are heard as being superimposed on the breath sounds. They are caused by moving air colliding with secretions in the tracheobronchial passageways, or by the popping open of previously deflated airways. Sources differ as to the classification and nomenclature of these sounds (see Table 18–7), but **crackles** (or rales) and **wheeze** (or rhonchi) are terms commonly used by most examiners.

Study Table 18–7 on p. 474 for a complete description of these abnormal adventitious breath sounds.

One type of adventitious sound, **atelectatic crackles,** is not pathologic. They are short, popping, crackling sounds that sound like fine crackles but do not last beyond a few breaths. When sections of alveoli are not fully aerated (as in people who are asleep, or in the elderly), they deflate slightly and accumulate secretions. Crackles are heard when these sections are expanded by a few deep breaths. Atelectatic crackles are heard only in the periphery, usually in dependent portions of the lungs, and disappear after the first few breaths or after a cough.

In the past, persons were asked to "take a deep breath and blow it out hard" to screen for the presence of wheezing. However, this maneuver is futile because it is known that wheezing may occur on maximal forced exhalation in normal people (King et al., 1989).

During normal tidal flow, wheezing indicates asthma.

Voice Sounds

Determine the quality of **voice sounds** or **vocal resonance.** The spoken voice can be auscultated over the chest wall just as it can be felt in tactile fremitus described earlier. Ask the person to repeat a phrase while you listen over the chest wall. Normal voice transmission is soft, muffled, and indistinct; you can hear sound through the stethoscope but cannot distinguish exactly what is being said. Pathology that increases lung density enhances transmission of voice sounds.

Consolidation or compression of lung tissue will enhance the voice sounds.

Eliciting the voice sounds is usually not done in the routine examination. Rather, these are supplemental maneuvers that are performed if you suspect lung pathology based on earlier data. When they are performed, you are testing for possible presence of **bronchophony, egophony,** and **whispered pectoriloquy** (Table 18–2).

NORMAL RANGE OF FINDINGS

ABNORMAL FINDINGS

TABLE 18–2: **Voice Sounds**		
TECHNIQUE	NORMAL FINDING	ABNORMAL FINDING
BRONCHOPHONY Ask the person to repeat "ninety-nine" while you listen with the stethoscope over the chest wall; listen especially if you suspect pathology	Normal voice transmission is soft, muffled, and indistinct; you can hear sound through the stethoscope but cannot distinguish exactly what is being said	Pathology that increases lung density will enhance transmission of voice sounds; you auscultate a clear "ninety-nine" The words are more distinct than normal and sound close to your ear

EGOPHONY (Greek: the voice of a goat) Auscultate the chest while the person phonates a long "ee-ee-ee-ee" sound	Normally, you should hear "eeeeee" through your stethoscope	Over areas of consolidation or compression, the spoken "eeee" sound changes to a bleating long "aaaaa" sound If this is present, record, "E → A changes"
WHISPERED PECTORILOQUY Ask the person to whisper a phrase like "one-two-three" as you auscultate	The normal response is faint, muffled, and almost inaudible	With only small amounts of consolidation, the whispered voice is transmitted very clearly and distinctly, although still somewhat faint; it sounds as if the person is whispering right into your stethoscope, "one-two-three"

INSPECT THE ANTERIOR CHEST

Note the **shape and configuration** of the chest wall. The ribs are sloping downward with symmetric interspaces. The costal angle is within 90 degrees. Development of abdominal muscles is as expected for the person's age, weight, and athletic condition.

Barrel chest has horizontal ribs and costal angle >90 degrees.

Hypertrophy of abdominal muscles occurs in chronic emphysema.

NORMAL RANGE OF FINDINGS	ABNORMAL FINDINGS
Note the person's **facial expression.** The facial expression should be relaxed and benign, indicating an unconscious effort of breathing.	Tense, strained, tired facies accompany COPD.
	The person with COPD may purse the lips in a whistling position. By exhaling slowly and against a narrow opening, the pressure in the bronchial tree remains positive, and fewer airways collapse.
Assess the **level of consciousness.** The level of consciousness should be alert and cooperative.	Cerebral hypoxia may be reflected by excessive drowsiness or by anxiety, restlessness, and irritability.
Note skin **color and condition.** The lips and nail beds are free of cyanosis or unusual pallor. The nails are of normal configuration. Explore any skin lesions.	Clubbing of distal phalanx occurs with chronic respiratory disease. Cutaneous angiomas (spider nevi) associated with liver disease or portal hypertension may be evident on the chest.
Assess the quality of **respirations.** Normal relaxed breathing is automatic and effortless, regular and even, and produces no noise. The chest expands symmetrically with each inspiration. Note any localized lag on inspiration.	Noisy breathing occurs with severe asthma or chronic bronchitis. Unequal chest expansion occurs when part of the lung is obstructed or collapsed, as with pneumonia, or when guarding to avoid postoperative incisional pain or pleurisy pain.
No retraction or bulging of the interspaces should occur on inspiration.	Retraction suggests obstruction of respiratory tract or increased inspiratory effort is needed, as with atelectasis. Bulging indicates trapped air as in the forced expiration associated with emphysema or asthma.
Normally, accessory muscles are not used to augment respiratory effort. However, with very heavy exercise, the accessory neck muscles (scalene, sternomastoid, trapezius) are used momentarily to enhance inspiration.	Accessory muscles must be used in acute airway obstruction and massive atelectasis. Rectus abdominis and internal intercostal muscles are used to force expiration in COPD.
The respiratory rate is within normal limits for the person's age (see Table 10–3) and the pattern of breathing is regular. Occasional sighs normally punctuate breathing.	Tachypnea and hyperventilation, bradypnea and hypoventilation, periodic breathing (see Table 18–5).

NORMAL RANGE OF FINDINGS	ABNORMAL FINDINGS

PALPATE THE ANTERIOR CHEST

Palpate **symmetric chest expansion.** Place your hands on the anterolateral wall with the thumbs along the costal margins and pointing toward the xiphoid process (Fig. 18–21).

Ask the person to take a deep breath. Watch your thumbs move apart symmetrically, and note smooth chest expansion with your fingers. Any limitation in thoracic expansion is easier to detect on the anterior chest because greater range of motion exists with breathing here.

An abnormally wide costal angle with little inspiratory variation occurs with emphysema.

A lag in expansion occurs with atelectasis, pneumonia, and postoperative guarding.

A palpable grating sensation with breathing indicates pleural friction fremitus (see Table 18–6).

18–21 Palpate anterior chest.

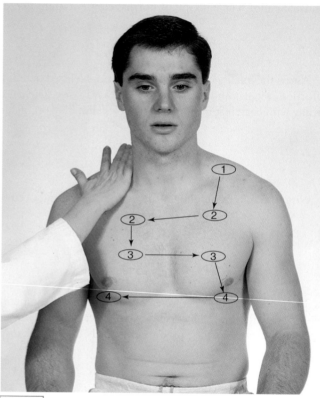

18–22 Assess tactile fremitus.

Assess **tactile (vocal) fremitus.** Begin palpating over the lung apices in the supraclavicular areas (Fig. 18–22). Compare vibrations from one side to the other as the person repeats "ninety-nine." Avoid palpating over female breast tissue because breast tissue normally damps the sound.

Palpate the anterior chest wall to note any tenderness (normally none is present) and to detect any superficial lumps or masses (again, normally none are present). Note skin mobility and turgor, and note skin temperature and moisture.

PERCUSS THE ANTERIOR CHEST

Begin percussing the apices in the supraclavicular areas. Then, percussing the interspaces and comparing one side to the other, move down the anterior chest.

Interspaces are easier to palpate on the anterior chest than on the back. Do not percuss directly over female breast tissue because this would produce a dull note. Shift the breast tissue over slightly using the edge of your stationary hand. In females with large breasts, percussion may yield little useful data. With all people, use the sequence illustrated in Figure 18–23.

NORMAL RANGE OF FINDINGS

ABNORMAL FINDINGS

18–23 Sequence for percussion and auscultation.

Note the borders of cardiac dullness normally found on the anterior chest and do not confuse these with suspected lung pathology (Fig. 18–24). In the right hemithorax the upper border of liver dullness is located in the fifth intercostal space in the right midclavicular line. On the left, tympany is evident over the gastric space.

Lungs are hyperinflated with chronic emphysema, resulting in hyperresonance where you would expect cardiac dullness.

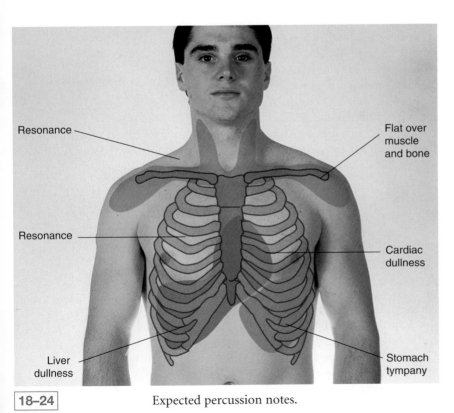

Resonance

Flat over muscle and bone

Resonance

Cardiac dullness

Liver dullness

Stomach tympany

18–24 Expected percussion notes.

AUSCULTATE THE ANTERIOR CHEST

Breath Sounds

Auscultate the lung fields over the anterior chest from the apices in the supra-clavicular areas down to the sixth rib. Progress from side to side as you move downward, and listen to one full respiration in each location. Use the sequence indicated for percussion. Do not place your stethoscope directly over the female breast. Displace the breast and listen directly over the chest wall.

Evaluate normal breath sounds, noting any abnormal breath sounds and any adventitious sounds. If the situation warrants, assess the voice sounds on the anterior chest.

Study Table 18–8 for a complete description of abnormal respiratory conditions.

Measurement of Pulmonary Function Status

The **forced expiratory time** is the number of seconds it takes for the person to exhale from total lung capacity to residual volume. It is a screening measure of airflow obstruction. Although the test usually is not performed in the respiratory assessment, it is useful when you wish to screen for pulmonary function.

Ask the person to inhale the deepest breath possible and then to blow it all out hard, as quickly as possible, with the mouth open. Listen with your stethoscope over the sternum. The normal time for full expiration is 4 seconds or less.

A forced expiration of 6 seconds or more occurs with obstructive lung disease. Refer this person for more precise pulmonary function studies.

The **pulse oximeter** is a noninvasive method to assess arterial oxygen saturation (SpO_2). A sensor attached to the person's finger or ear has a diode that emits light and a detector that measures the relative amount of light absorbed by oxyhemoglobin (HbO_2) and unoxygenated (reduced) hemoglobin (Hb). The pulse oximeter compares the ratio of light emitted to light absorbed and converts this ratio into the percentage of oxygen saturation. Since it only measures light absorption of pulsatile flow, the result is arterial oxygen saturation. A healthy person with no lung disease and no anemia normally has an SpO_2 of 97% to 98%. However, every SpO_2 result must be evaluated in the context of the person's hemoglobin level, acid-base balance, and ventilatory status.

The **12-minute distance (12MD) walk** is a simple, inexpensive, clinical measure of functional status in people with COPD (Larson et al., 1996). The 12MD is used as an outcome measure for people in pulmonary rehabilitation because it mirrors conditions that are used in everyday life. Locate a flat-surfaced corridor that has little foot traffic, is wide enough to permit comfortable turns, and has a controlled environment. Ensure that the person is wearing comfortable shoes, and equip him or her with a pulse oximeter to monitor oxygen saturation. Ask the person to set his or her own pace to cover as much ground as possible in 12 minutes, and assure the person it is all right to slow down or to stop to rest at any time. Use a stopwatch to time the walk.

Ask the person to stop the walk if you notice an SpO_2 below 85% to 88% or if extreme breathlessness occurs.

DEVELOPMENTAL CONSIDERATIONS

Infants and Children

To prepare, let the parent hold an infant supported against the chest or shoulder. Do not let the usual sequence of the physical examination restrain you; seize the opportunity with a sleeping infant to inspect and then to listen to lung sounds next. This way you can concentrate on the breath sounds before the baby wakes up and possibly cries. Infant crying does not have to be a problem for you though, because it actually enhances palpation of tactile fremitus and auscultation of breath sounds.

A child may sit upright on the parent's lap. Offer the stethoscope and let the child handle it. This reduces any fear of the equipment. Promote the child's participation; school-age children usually are delighted to hear their own breath sounds when you place the stethoscope properly. While listening to breath

NORMAL RANGE OF FINDINGS	ABNORMAL FINDINGS

sounds, ask the young child to take a deep breath and "blow out" your penlight while you hold the stethoscope with your other hand. Time your letting go of the penlight button so the light goes off after the child blows. Or, ask the child to "pant like a dog" while you auscultate.

INSPECTION. The infant has a rounded thorax with an equal anteroposterior-to-transverse chest diameter (Fig. 18–25). By age 6, the thorax reaches the adult ratio of 1:2 (anteroposterior-to-transverse diameter). The newborn's chest circumference is 30 to 36 cm and is 2 cm smaller than the head circumference until 2 years of age. The chest wall is thin with little musculature. The ribs and the xiphoid are prominent; you can see as well as feel the sharp tip of the xiphoid process. The thoracic cage is soft and flexible.

Note a barrel shape persisting after age 6, which may develop with chronic asthma or cystic fibrosis.

18–25 Round thorax in an infant.

In newborn males and females, the breasts may look enlarged by the 2nd or 3rd day due to maternal estrogen. Occasionally a white fluid, sometimes referred to by the slang expression "witch's milk," can be expressed. This resolves within a week.

In some children, "Harrison groove" occurs normally. This is a horizontal groove in the rib cage at the level of the insertion of the diaphragm, extending from the sternum to the midaxillary line.

Harrison groove also occurs with rickets from the pull of the diaphragm on weakened ribs.

The newborn's first respiratory assessment is part of the **Apgar scoring system** to measure the successful transition to extrauterine life (Table 18–3). The five standard parameters are scored at 1 minute and at 5 minutes after birth. A 1-minute Apgar with a total score of 7 to 10 indicates a newborn in good condition, needing only suctioning of the nose and mouth and otherwise routine care.

In the immediate newborn period, depressed respirations are due to maternal drugs, interruption of the uterine blood supply, or obstruction of the tracheobronchial tree with mucus or fluid.

A 1-minute Apgar with a total score of 3 to 6 indicates a moderately depressed newborn needing more resuscitation and subsequent close observation. A score of 0 to 2 indicates a severely depressed newborn needing full resuscitation, ventilatory assistance, and subsequent intensive care.

NORMAL RANGE OF FINDINGS   **ABNORMAL FINDINGS**

TABLE 18–3: Apgar Scoring System

	2	1	0	
HEART RATE	Over 100	Slow (below 100)	Absent	_____
RESPIRATORY EFFORT	Good, sustained cry; regular respirations	Slow, irregular, shallow	Absent	_____
MUSCLE TONE	Active motion, spontaneous flexion	Some flexion of extremities; some resistance to extension	Limp, flaccid	_____
REFLEX IRRITABILITY (response to catheter nares)	Sneeze, cough, cry	Grimace, frown	No response	_____
COLOR	Completely pink	Body pink, extremities pale	Cyanotic, pale	_____
			Total score	_____

The infant breathes through the nose rather than the mouth and is an obligate nose-breather until 3 months. Slight flaring of the lower costal margins may occur with respirations, but normally no flaring of the nostrils and no sternal retractions or intercostal retractions occur. The diaphragm is the newborn's major respiratory muscle. Intercostal muscles are not well developed. Thus you observe the abdomen bulge with each inspiration but see little thoracic expansion.

Count the respiratory rate for 1 full minute. Normal rates for the newborn are 30 to 40 breaths per minute but may spike up to 60 per minute. Obtain the most accurate respiratory rate by counting when the infant is asleep, because infants reach rapid rates with very little excitation when awake. The respiratory pattern may be irregular when extremes in room temperature occur or with feeding or sleeping. Brief periods of apnea less than 10 or 15 seconds are common. This periodic breathing is more common in premature infants.

PALPATION. Palpate symmetric chest expansion by encircling the infant's thorax with both hands. Further palpation should yield no lumps, masses, or crepitus, although you may feel the costochondral junctions in some normal infants.

PERCUSSION. Percussion is of limited usefulness in the newborn and especially in the premature newborn because the adult's fingers are too large in relation to the tiny chest. The percussion note of hyperresonance occurs normally in the infant and young child due to the relatively thin chest wall. Anything less than hyperresonance would have the same clinical significance as dullness in the adult. If measured, diaphragmatic excursion measures about one to two rib interspaces in children.

AUSCULTATION. Auscultation normally yields bronchovesicular breath sounds in the peripheral lung fields of the infant and young child up to age 5 to 6. Their relatively thin chest walls with underdeveloped musculature do not damp off the sound as do the thicker walls of adults, so breath sounds are louder and harsher.

Marked retractions of sternum and intercostal muscles indicate increased inspiratory effort, as in atelectasis, pneumonia, asthma, and acute airway obstruction.

Rapid respiratory rates accompany pneumonia, fever, pain, heart disease, and anemia.

In an infant, tachypnea of 50 to 100 per minute during sleep may be an early sign of heart failure.

Asymmetric expansion occurs with diaphragmatic hernia or pneumothorax.

Crepitus is palpable around a fractured clavicle, which may occur with difficult forceps delivery.

Rachitic rosary—prominent round knobs at costochondral junctions—is seen in infants with rickets or scurvy.

Diminished breath sounds occur with pneumonia, atelectasis, pleural effusion, or pneumothorax.

NORMAL RANGE OF FINDINGS

Fine crackles are the adventitious sounds commonly heard in the immediate newborn period due to opening of the airways and clearing of fluid. Since the newborn's chest wall is so thin, transmission of sounds is enhanced and is heard easily all over the chest, making localization of breath sounds a problem. Even bowel sounds are easily heard in the chest. Try using the smaller pediatric diaphragm endpiece, or place the bell over the infant's interspaces and not over the ribs. Use the pediatric diaphragm on an older infant or toddler (Fig. 18–26).

18–26

The Pregnant Female

The thoracic cage may appear wider, and the costal angle may feel wider than in the nonpregnant state. Respirations may be deeper, although this can be quantified only with pulmonary function tests.

The Aging Adult

The chest cage commonly shows an increased anteroposterior diameter, giving a round barrel shape, and **kyphosis** or an outward curvature of the thoracic spine (see Table 18–4). The person compensates by holding the head extended and tilted back. You may palpate marked bony prominences because of decreased subcutaneous fat. Chest expansion may be somewhat decreased with the older person, although it still should be symmetric. The costal cartilages become calcified with aging, resulting in a less mobile thorax.

The older person may fatigue easily, especially during auscultation when deep mouth breathing is required. Take care that this person does not hyperventilate and become dizzy. Allow brief rest periods or quiet breathing. If the person does feel faint, holding the breath for a few seconds will restore equilibrium.

The Acutely Ill Person

Ask a second examiner to hold the person's arms and to support him or her in the upright position. If no one else is available, you need to roll the person from side to side, examining the uppermost half of the thorax. This obviously prevents you from comparing findings from one side to another. Also, side flexion of the trunk alters percussion findings because the ribs of the upward side may flex closer together.

ABNORMAL FINDINGS

Persistent fine crackles that are scattered over the chest occur with pneumonia, bronchiolitis, or atelectasis.

Crackles only in upper lung fields occur with cystic fibrosis; crackles only in lower lung fields occur with heart failure.

Expiratory wheezing occurs with lower airway obstruction, e.g., asthma or bronchiolitis. When unilateral, it may be foreign body aspiration.

Persistent peristaltic sounds with diminished breath sounds on the same side may indicate diaphragmatic hernia.

Stridor is a high-pitched inspiratory crowing sound heard without the stethoscope, occurring with upper airway obstruction, e.g., croup, foreign body aspiration, or acute epiglottitis.

SUMMARY CHECKLIST: Thorax and Lung Exam

1. Inspection
Thoracic cage
Respirations
Skin color and condition
Person's position
Facial expression
Level of consciousness

2. Palpation
Confirm symmetric expansion
Tactile fremitus
Detect any lumps, masses, tenderness

3. Percussion
Percuss over lung fields
Estimate diaphragmatic excursion

4. Auscultation
Assess normal breath sounds
Note any abnormal breath sounds
If so, perform bronchophony,
  whispered pectoriloquy,
  egophony
Note any adventitious sounds

 See Health Promotion Guide on CD

Application and Critical Thinking

SAMPLE CHARTING

SUBJECTIVE

No cough, shortness of breath, or chest pain with breathing. No past history of respiratory diseases. Has "one or no" colds per year. Has never smoked. Works in well-ventilated office—smoking co-workers are restricted to smoke in lounge. Last TB skin test 4 years PTA, negative. Never had chest x-ray.

OBJECTIVE

Inspection. AP < transverse diameter. Respirations 16/min, relaxed and even.
Palpation. Chest expansion symmetric. Tactile fremitus equal bilaterally. No tenderness to palpation. No lumps or lesions.
Percussion. Resonant to percussion over lung fields. Diaphragmatic excursion 5 cm and = bilaterally.
Auscultation. Vesicular breath sounds clear over lung fields. No adventitious sounds.

FOCUSED ASSESSMENT: CLINICAL CASE STUDY

Thomas G. is a 58-year-old, thin, white, male traffic patrolman who appears older than stated age. Face is anxious and tense, although in no acute distress at this time. Seeks care for "increasing SOB and fatigue in last couple months."

SUBJECTIVE

1 year PTA—noticed more "winded" than usual when walking >3–4 blocks. Early morning cough present daily × 10 years, but now increased sputum production to 2 T per morning, frothy white.

6 mo. PTA—had a "cold" with severe harsh coughing, productive of ½ cup thick white sputum/day. Noted midsternal chest pain (mild) with cough. Lasted 2 weeks. Treated self with humidifier and OTC cough syrup—minimal relief.

3 mo. PTA—noticed increasing SOB with less activity. Fatigue and SOB when working outside during traffic rush hours. Unable to take evening walks (usually 2–3 blocks) due to SOB and fatigue. Has two-pillow orthopnea. Wakes 3–4 times during night.

Now—feels he is "worse and needs some help." Continues with 2-pillow orthopnea. Unable to walk > two blocks or climb > one flight stairs without resting. Unable to blow out birthday candles on cake last week. Morning cough productive of ¼ cup thin white sputum, cough continues sporadically during day.

No chest pain, hemoptysis, night sweats, or paroxysmal nocturnal dyspnea. No history of allergies, hospitalizations, or injuries to chest. No family history of TB, allergies, asthma, or cancer. Smokes cigarettes 2 packs per day × 30 years. Alcohol < one 6-pack beer/week summer months only.

OBJECTIVE

Inspection. Sitting on side of bed with arms propped on bedside table. Resp. resting 24/min, regular, shallow with prolonged expiration; resp. 34/min ambulating. Increased use of accessory muscles, AP = transverse diameter with widening of costal angle, slightly flushed face, tense expression.

Palpation. Minimal but symmetric chest expansion. Tactile fremitus = bilaterally. No lumps, masses, or tenderness to palpation.
Percussion. Diaphragmatic excursion is 1 cm and = bilaterally. Hyperresonance over lung fields.
Auscultation. Breath sounds diminished. Expiratory wheeze throughout posterior chest, R > L. No crackles.

ASSESSMENT

Chronic and increasing SOB
Ineffective airway clearance R/T bronchial secretions and obstruction
Activity intolerance R/T imbalance between oxygen supply and demand
Disturbed sleep pattern R/T dyspnea and decreased mobility
Anxiety R/T change in health status

NURSING DIAGNOSES COMMONLY ASSOCIATED WITH THE THORAX AND LUNGS/ RESPIRATORY DISORDERS

RELATED FACTORS (Etiology)	DEFINING CHARACTERISTICS (Symptoms and Signs)
DIAGNOSIS: Activity intolerance	
Imbalance between oxygen supply and demand	Increased or decreased heart rate, blood pressure, respirations
Deconditioned status	Exertional discomfort or dyspnea
Pain	Redness, cyanosis, or pallor of skin during activity
Fatigue	Dizziness during activity
Bedrest	Requiring frequent rest periods
Sedentary lifestyle	Worried or uneasy facial expression
Electrolyte imbalance	Verbal report of fatigue or weakness
Hypovolemia	Impaired ability to change position or stand or walk without support
Malnourishment	Weakness
Interrupted sleep	Confusion
Impaired sensory or motor function	
Effects of aging	
Generalized weakness	
Side effects of sedatives, tranquilizers, or narcotics	
Immobility	
Depression	
Lack of motivation	
DIAGNOSIS: Ineffective Breathing pattern	
Decreased energy, lung expansion	Abnormal blood gases
Effect of	Altered chest excursion
Anesthesia	Assumption of three-point position
Medication (narcotics, sedatives, tranquilizers)	Cough
Obesity	Cyanosis
Fatigue	Dyspnea
Immobility, inactivity	Fremitus
Impairment	Nasal flaring
Cognitive	Pursed-lip breathing and prolonged expiratory phase
Musculoskeletal	Respiratory rate, depth changes
Neuromuscular	Shortness of breath
Perceptual	Tachypnea
Inflammatory processes	Use of accessory muscles
Pain	
Tracheobronchial obstruction	
Anxiety	

Table continued on following page

RELATED FACTORS (Etiology)

DEFINING CHARACTERISTICS (Symptoms and Signs)

DIAGNOSIS: Ineffective Airway clearance

Decreased energy, fatigue
Effects of
   Anesthesia
   Infection
   Medication (narcotics, sedatives, tranquilizers)
Inability to cough effectively
Perceptual or cognitive impairment
Presence of artificial airway
Tracheobronchial secretions or obstruction
Aspiration of foreign matter
Environmental pollutants
Inhalation of toxic fumes or substances
Trauma

Absent or adventitious sounds
Air hunger
Change in respiratory rate or depth
Cough, effective or ineffective, with or without spasm
Cyanosis
Diaphoresis
Dyspnea
Fever
Nasal flaring
Restlessness
Stridor
Substernal, intercostal retraction
Tachycardia
   Tachypnea
Anxiety

DIAGNOSIS: Impaired Gas exchange

Altered
   Blood flow
   Oxygen-carrying capacity of blood
   Oxygen supply
Alveolar-capillary membrane changes
Aspiration of foreign matter
Decreased surfactant production
Effects of
   Anesthesia
   Medications (narcotics, sedatives, tranquilizers)
Hypoventilation or hyperventilation
Inhalation of toxic fumes or substances

Clubbing of fingers
Confusion
Cyanosis
Fatigue and lethargy
Hypercapnia
Hypoxia
Inability to move secretions
Irritability
Restlessness
Somnolence
Tachycardia
Use of accessory muscles

DIAGNOSIS: Excess Fluid volume

Compromised regulatory mechanisms
   Aldosterone
   Antidiuretic hormone
   Renin-angiotensin
Effects of
   Age extremes
   Medications
   Pregnancy
Excessive fluid or sodium intake

Abnormal breath sounds, rales
Changes in
   Respiratory pattern
   Blood pressure
   Central venous pressure
   Mental status
   Pulmonary artery pressure
   Specific gravity
   Edema
Pulmonary congestion on x-ray study
Shortness of breath, orthopnea
Restlessness and anxiety
Altered electrolytes
Anasarca
Azotemia
Intake greater than output
Jugular vein distention
Nausea and/or vomiting
Oliguria
Positive finding of hepatojugular reflex
S_3 heart sound
Weight gain

RELATED FACTORS (Etiology)

DEFINING CHARACTERISTICS (Symptoms and Signs)

DIAGNOSIS: Anxiety

RELATED FACTORS (Etiology)	DEFINING CHARACTERISTICS (Symptoms and Signs)
Threat to or change in health status, relationships, role functioning, self-concept, socioeconomic status Threat of death Lack of knowledge Loss of control Actual or perceived loss of significant others Situational or maturational crises Unmet needs Unconscious conflict about essential values and goals of life Feelings of failure Disruptive family life Interpersonal transmission and contagion	Trembling Increased blood pressure Rapid respiration and pulse Feelings of helplessness, apprehensiveness, inadequacy, dread, worry Focus on self Irritability Restlessness Inability to concentrate Crying Change in appetite Diaphoresis Lack of eye contact Extraneous movements, foot shuffling, hand or arm movements Nausea Headache Increased wariness Lack of awareness of surroundings Regret Uncertainty Change in sleeping patterns Agitated Worried Feeling of dread Difficulty expressing self Change in voice quality Fear of unspecific consequences Expressed concern regarding changes in life events

OTHER RELATED NURSING DIAGNOSES

ACTUAL

Fatigue (see Chapter 19)
Impaired Home maintenance (see Chapter 14)
Pain (see Chapter 16)
Ineffective Role performance
Self-care deficit
Disturbed Sleep pattern
Altered Tissue perfusion
Impaired spontaneous Ventilation
Dysfunctional Ventilatory weaning response

RISK/WELLNESS

Risk
Risk for Infection
Wellness
Health-seeking behavior about smoking cessation strategies

ASSESSMENT VIDEO CRITICAL THINKING QUESTIONS

The Saunders *Physical Examination and Health Assessment* video "Thorax and Lungs" will direct you to consider the following:

1. Which conditions are associated with a productive cough?
2. Describe the characteristics of the following adventitious sounds: fine crackles, coarse crackles, wheezes, and rhonchi.
3. What assessment findings are normal variations in a pregnant woman?
4. Which nursing diagnoses are most appropriate for a person with wheezes, dyspnea, and tachypnea?

Abnormal Findings

TABLE 18–4: Configurations of the Thorax

Normal Adult (for Comparison)

The thorax has an elliptical shape with an anteroposterior-to-transverse diameter of 1:2 or 5:7.

Barrel Chest

Note equal anteroposterior-to-transverse diameter and that ribs are horizontal instead of the normal downward slope. This is associated with normal aging and also with chronic emphysema and asthma due to hyperinflation of lungs.

Pectus Excavatum

A markedly sunken sternum and adjacent cartilages (also called funnel breast). Depression begins at second intercostal space, becoming depressed most at junction of xiphoid with body of sternum. More noticeable on inspiration. Congenital, usually not symptomatic. When severe, sternal depression may cause embarrassment and a negative self-concept. Surgery may be indicated.

Pectus Carinatum

A forward protusion of the sternum, with ribs sloping back at either side and vertical depressions along costochondral junctions (pigeon breast). Less common than pectus excavatum, this minor deformity requires no treatment. If severe, surgery may be indicated.

TABLE 18-4: Configurations of the Thorax—cont'd

Scoliosis

A lateral S-shaped curvature of the thoracic and lumbar spine, usually with involved vertebrae rotation. Note unequal shoulder and scapular height and unequal hip levels, rib interspaces flared on convex side. More prevalent in adolescent age groups, especially girls. Mild deformities are asymptomatic. If severe (>45 degrees) deviation is present, scoliosis may reduce lung volume, then person is at risk for impaired cardiopulmonary function. Primary impairment is cosmetic deformity, negatively affecting self-image. Refer early for treatment, often surgery.

Kyphosis

An exaggerated posterior curvature of the thoracic spine (humpback) that causes significant back pain and limited mobility. Severe deformities impair cardiopulmonary function. Compensation may occur by hyperextension of head to maintain level of vision.

Kyphosis has been associated with aging, especially the familiar "dowager's hump" of postmenopausal osteoporotic women. However, it is common well before menopause. It is related to physical fitness; women with adequate exercise habits are less likely to have kyphosis (Cutler et al., 1993).

TABLE 18-5: Respiration Patterns*

Inspiration　Expiration

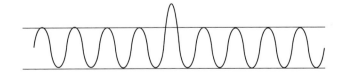

Normal Adult (for Comparison)

Rate—10 to 20 breaths per minute.
Depth—500 ml to 800 ml.
Pattern—even.
The ratio of pulse to respirations is fairly constant, about 4:1. Both values increase as a normal response to exercise, fear, or fever.
Depth—air moving in and out with each respiration.

Sigh

Occasional sighs punctuate the normal breathing pattern and are purposeful to expand alveoli. Frequent sighs may indicate emotional dysfunction. Frequent sighs also may lead to hyperventilation and dizziness.

*Assess the (1) rate, (2) depth (tidal volume), and (3) pattern.

Table continued on following page

ABNORMAL FINDINGS

TABLE 18–5: Respiration Patterns—cont'd

Tachypnea

Rapid shallow breathing. Increased rate >24 per minute. This is a normal response to fever, fear, or exercise. Rate also increases with respiratory insufficiency, pneumonia, alkalosis, pleurisy, and lesions in the pons.

Hyperventilation

Increase in both rate and depth. Normally occurs with extreme exertion, fear, or anxiety. Also occurs with diabetic ketoacidosis (Kussmaul's respirations), hepatic coma, salicylate overdose (producing a respiratory alkalosis to compensate for the metabolic acidosis), lesions of the midbrain, and alteration in blood gas concentration (either an increase in carbon dioxide or decrease in oxygen). Hyperventilation blows off carbon dioxide, causing a decreased level in the blood (alkalosis).

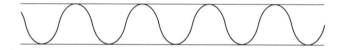

Bradypnea

Slow breathing. A decreased but regular rate (less than 10 per minute), as in drug-induced depression of the respiratory center in the medulla, increased intracranial pressure, and diabetic coma.

Hypoventilation

An irregular shallow pattern caused by an overdose of narcotics or anesthetics. May also occur with prolonged bed rest or conscious splinting of the chest to avoid respiratory pain.

Cheyne-Stokes Respiration

A cycle in which respirations gradually wax and wane in a regular pattern, increasing in rate and depth and then decreasing. The breathing periods last 30 to 45 seconds, with periods of apnea (20 seconds) alternating the cycle. The most common cause is severe heart failure; other causes are renal failure, meningitis, drug overdose, and increased intracranial pressure. Occurs normally in infants and aging persons during sleep.

Biot's Respiration

Similar to Cheyne-Stokes respiration, except that the pattern is irregular. A series of normal respirations (3 to 4) is followed by a period of apnea. The cycle length is variable, lasting anywhere from 10 seconds to 1 minute. Seen with head trauma, brain abscess, heat stroke, spinal meningitis, and encephalitis.

Normal inspiration | Prolonged expiration | Air trapping

◀ Chronic Obstructive Breathing

Normal inspiration and prolonged expiration to overcome increased airway resistance. In a person with chronic obstructive lung disease, any situation calling for increased heart rate (exercise) may lead to dyspneic episode (air trapping), because then the person does not have enough time for full expiration.

TABLE 18–6: Abnormal Tactile Fremitus

Increased Tactile Fremitus

Occurs with conditions that increase the density of lung tissue, thereby making a better conducting medium for vibrations, e.g., compression or consolidation (pneumonia). There must be a patent bronchus, and consolidation must extend to lung surface for increased fremitus to be apparent.

Decreased Tactile Fremitus

Occurs when anything obstructs transmission of vibrations, e.g., an obstructed bronchus, pleural effusion or thickening, pneumothorax, and emphysema. Any barrier that gets in the way of the sound and your palpating hand decreases fremitus.

Rhonchal Fremitus

Vibration felt when inhaled air passes through thick secretions in the larger bronchi. This may decrease somewhat by coughing.

Pleural Friction Fremitus

Produced when inflammation of the parietal or visceral pleura causes a decrease in the normal lubricating fluid. Then the opposing surfaces make a coarse grating sound when rubbed together during breathing. Although this sound is best detected by auscultation, it may sometimes be palpable and feels like two pieces of leather grating together. It is synchronous with respiratory excursion. Also called a palpable friction rub.

ABNORMAL FINDINGS

TABLE 18–7: Adventitious Lung Sounds

SOUND	DESCRIPTION	MECHANISM	CLINICAL EXAMPLE

(1) Discontinuous Sounds

These are discrete, crackling sounds.

SOUND	DESCRIPTION	MECHANISM	CLINICAL EXAMPLE
Crackles—fine (formerly called rales) 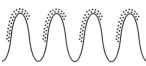 *Inspiration Expiration*	Discontinuous, high-pitched, short crackling, popping sounds heard during inspiration that are not cleared by coughing; you can simulate this sound by rolling a strand of hair between your fingers near your ear, or by moistening your thumb and index finger and separating them near your ear	Inhaled air collides with previously deflated airways; airways suddenly pop open, creating crackling sound as gas pressures between the two compartments equalize (Forgacs, 1978a)	*Late inspiratory crackles* occur with restrictive disease: pneumonia, heart failure, and interstitial fibrosis *Early inspiratory crackles* occur with obstructive disease: chronic bronchitis, asthma, and emphysema *Posturally induced crackles* (PICs) are fine crackles that appear with a change from sitting to the supine position, or with a change from supine to supine with legs elevated. PICs that appear after acute myocardial infarction have been associated with increased mortality (Deguchi et al., 1993)
Crackles—coarse (coarse rales)	Loud, low-pitched, bubbling and gurgling sounds that start in early inspiration and may be present in expiration; may decrease somewhat by suctioning or coughing but will reappear shortly—sounds like opening a Velcro fastener	Inhaled air collides with secretions in the trachea and large bronchi	Pulmonary edema, pneumonia, pulmonary fibrosis, and the terminally ill who have a depressed cough reflex
Atelectatic crackles (atelectatic rales)	Sounds like fine crackles, but do not last and are not pathologic; disappear after the first few breaths; heard in axillae and bases (usually dependent) of lungs	When sections of alveoli are not fully aerated, they deflate and accumulate secretions. Crackles are heard when these sections reexpand with a few deep breaths	In aging adults, bedridden persons, or in persons just aroused from sleep
Pleural friction rub	A very superficial sound that is coarse and low pitched; it has a grating quality as if two pieces of leather are being rubbed together; sounds just like crackles, but *close* to the ear; sounds louder if you push the stethoscope harder onto the chest wall; sound is inspiratory and expiratory	Caused when pleurae become inflamed and lose their normal lubricating fluid; their opposing roughened pleural surfaces rub together during respiration; heard best in anterolateral wall where greatest lung mobility exists	Pleuritis, accompanied by pain with breathing (rub disappears after a few days if pleural fluid accumulates and separates pleurae)

Continued

TABLE 18–7: Adventitious Lung Sounds—cont'd

SOUND	DESCRIPTION	MECHANISM	CLINICAL EXAMPLE
(2) Continuous Sounds These are connected, musical sounds.			
Wheeze—high-pitched (sibilant)	High-pitched, musical squeaking sounds that sound polyphonic (multiple notes as in a musical chord); predominate in expiration but may occur in both expiration and inspiration	Air squeezed or compressed through passageways narrowed almost to closure by collapsing, swelling, secretions, or tumors; the passageway walls oscillate in apposition between the closed and barely open positions; the resulting sound is similar to a vibrating reed (Forgacs, 1978a)	Diffuse airway obstruction from acute asthma or chronic emphysema
Wheeze—low-pitched (sonorous rhonchi)	Low-pitched; monophonic single note, musical snoring, moaning sounds; they are heard throughout the cycle, although they are more prominent on expiration; may clear somewhat by coughing	Airflow obstruction as described by the vibrating reed mechanism above; the pitch of the wheeze cannot be correlated to the size of the passageway that generates it	Bronchitis, single bronchus obstruction from airway tumor
Stridor	High-pitched, monophonic, inspiratory, crowing sound, louder in neck than over chest wall	Originating in larynx or trachea, upper airway obstruction from swollen, inflamed tissues or lodged foreign body	Croup and acute epiglottitis in children, and foreign inhalation, obstructed airway may be life threatening

TABLE 18–8: Assessment of Common Respiratory Conditions

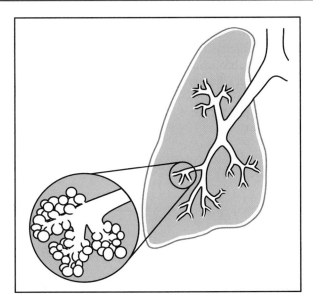

◀ Normal Lung (for comparison)

Inspection Anteroposterior < transverse diameter, relaxed posture, normal musculature; rate 10 to 18 breaths per minute, regular, no cyanosis or pallor.

Palpation Symmetric chest expansion. Tactile fremitus present and equal bilaterally, diminishing toward periphery. No lumps, masses, or tenderness.

Percussion Resonant. Diaphragmatic excursion 3 to 5 cm and equal bilaterally.

Auscultation Vesicular over peripheral fields. Bronchovesicular parasternally (anterior) and between scapulae (posterior). Infant and young child—bronchovesicular throughout.

Adventitious Sounds None.

Table continued on following page

ABNORMAL FINDINGS

TABLE 18–8: Assessment of Common Respiratory Conditions—cont'd

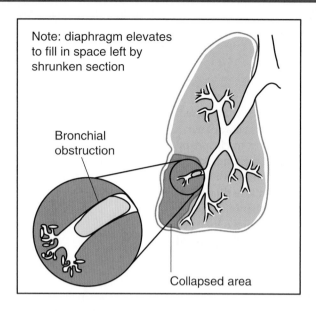

Note: diaphragm elevates to fill in space left by shrunken section

Bronchial obstruction

Collapsed area

◀ Atelectasis (Collapse)

Condition Collapsed shrunken section of alveoli, or an entire lung, due to (1) airway obstruction (e.g., the bronchus is completely blocked by thick exudate, aspirated foreign body, or tumor), the alveolar air beyond it is gradually absorbed by the pulmonary capillaries, and the alveolar walls cave in; (2) compression on the lung; and (3) lack of surfactant (hyaline membrane disease).

Inspection Cough. Lag on expansion on affected side. Increased respiratory rate and pulse. Possible cyanosis.

Palpation Chest expansion decreased on affected side. Tactile fremitus decreased or absent over area. With large collapse, tracheal shift toward affected side.

Percussion Dull over area (remainder of thorax sometimes may have hyperresonant note).

Auscultation Breath sounds decreased vesicular or absent over area. Voice sounds variable, usually decreased or absent over affected area.

Adventitious Sounds None if bronchus is obstructed. Occasional fine crackles if bronchus is patent.

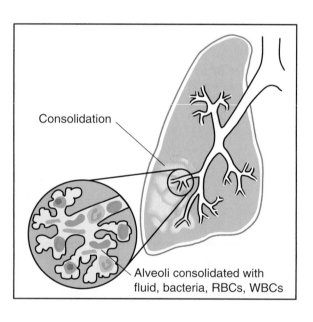

Consolidation

Alveoli consolidated with fluid, bacteria, RBCs, WBCs

◀ Lobar Pneumonia

Condition Infection in lung parenchyma leaves alveolar membrane edematous and porous, so red blood cells and white blood cells pass from blood to alveoli. Alveoli progressively fill up (become consolidated) with bacteria, solid cellular debris, fluid, and blood cells, all of which replace alveolar air. This results in decreased surface area of the respiratory membrane, which causes hypoxemia.

Inspection Increased respiratory rate. Guarding and lag on expansion on affected side. Children—sternal retraction, nasal flaring.

Palpation Chest expansion decreased on affected side. Tactile fremitus increased if bronchus patent, decreased if bronchus obstructed.

Percussion Dull over lobar pneumonia.

Auscultation Breath sounds louder with patent bronchus, as if coming directly from larynx. Voice sounds have increased clarity, bronchophony, egophony, whispered pectoriloquy present. Children—diminished breath sounds may occur early in pneumonia.

Adventitious Sounds Crackles, fine to medium.

Continued

TABLE 18–8: Assessment of Common Respiratory Conditions—cont'd

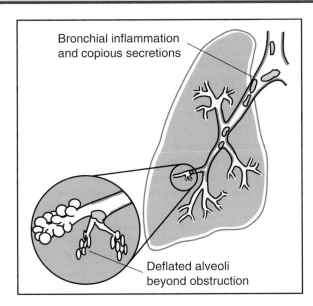

Bronchial inflammation and copious secretions

Deflated alveoli beyond obstruction

◄ Bronchitis

Condition Proliferation of mucous glands in the passageways, resulting in excessive mucus secretion. Inflammation of bronchi with partial obstruction of bronchi by secretions or constrictions. Sections of lung distal to obstruction may be deflated. Bronchitis may be acute or chronic with recurrent productive cough. Chronic bronchitis is usually caused by cigarette smoking.

Inspection Hacking, rasping cough productive of thick mucoid sputum. Chronic—dyspnea, fatigue, cyanosis, possible clubbing of fingers.

Palpation Tactile fremitus normal.

Percussion Resonant.

Auscultation Normal vesicular. Voice sounds normal. Chronic—prolonged expiration.

Adventitious Sounds Crackles over deflated areas. May have wheeze.

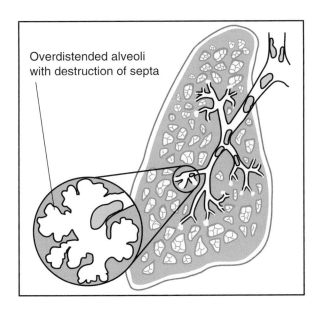

Overdistended alveoli with destruction of septa

◄ Emphysema

Condition Caused by destruction of pulmonary connective tissue (elastin, collagen); characterized by permanent enlargement of air sacs distal to terminal bronchioles and rupture of interalveolar walls. This increases airway resistance, especially on expiration—producing a hyperinflated lung and an increase in lung volume. Cigarette smoking accounts for 80% to 90% of cases of emphysema.

Inspection Increased anteroposterior diameter. Barrel chest. Use of accessory muscles to aid respiration. Tripod position. Shortness of breath, especially on exertion. Respiratory distress. Tachypnea.

Palpation Decreased tactile fremitus and chest expansion.

Percussion Hyperresonant. Decreased diaphragmatic excursion.

Auscultation Decreased breath sounds. May have prolonged expiration. Muffled heart sounds secondary to overdistention of lungs.

Adventitious Sounds Usually none; occasionally, wheeze.

Table continued on following page

TABLE 18–8: Assessment of Common Respiratory Conditions—cont'd

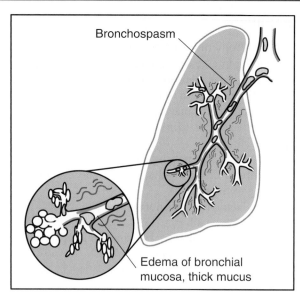

Bronchospasm

Edema of bronchial mucosa, thick mucus

◀ Asthma (Reactive Airway Disease)

Condition An allergic hypersensitivity to certain inhaled allergens (pollen), irritants (tobacco, ozone), microorganisms, stress, or exercise that produces a complex response characterized by bronchospasm, and inflammation, edema in walls of bronchioles, and secretion of highly viscous mucus into airways. These factors greatly increase airway resistance, especially during expiration, and produce the symptoms of wheezing, dyspnea, and chest tightness.

Inspection During severe attack: increased respiratory rate, shortness of breath with audible wheeze, use of accessory neck muscles, cyanosis, apprehension, retraction of intercostal spaces. Expiration labored, prolonged. When chronic may have barrel chest.

Palpation Tactile fremitus decreased, tachycardia.

Percussion Resonant. May be hyperresonant if chronic.

Auscultation Diminished air movement. Breath sounds decreased, with prolonged expiration. Voice sounds decreased.

Adventitious Sounds Bilateral wheezing on expiration, sometimes inspiratory and expiratory wheezing.

Pleural fluid
☐ transudative
▨ exudative
▨ empyemic
■ hemothorax
☐ chylothorax

◀ Pleural Effusion (Fluid) or Thickening

Condition Collection of excess fluid in the intrapleural space, with compression of overlying lung tissue. Effusion may contain watery capillary fluid (transudative), protein (exudative), purulent matter (empyemic), blood (hemothorax), or milky lymphatic fluid (chylothorax). Gravity settles fluid in dependent areas of thorax. Presence of fluid subdues all lung sounds.

Inspection Increased respirations, dyspnea; may have dry cough, tachycardia, cyanosis, abdominal distention.

Palpation Tactile fremitus decreased or absent. Tracheal shift away from affected side. Chest expansion decreased on affected side.

Percussion Dull to flat. No diaphragmatic excursion on affected side.

Auscultation Breath sounds decreased or absent. Voice sounds decreased or absent. When remainder of lung is compressed near the effusion, may have bronchial breath sounds over the compression along with bronchophony, egophony, whispered pectoriloquy.

Adventitious Sounds None.

Continued

TABLE 18–8: Assessment of Common Respiratory Conditions—cont'd

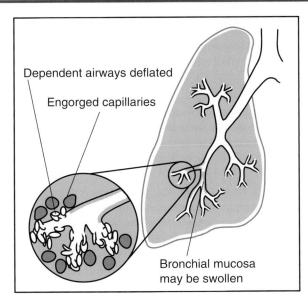

◄ Heart Failure

Condition Pump failure with increasing pressure of cardiac overload causes pulmonary congestion or an increased amount of blood present in pulmonary capillaries. Dependent air sacs are deflated. Pulmonary capillaries engorged. Bronchial mucosa may be swollen.

Inspection Increased respiratory rate, shortness of breath on exertion, orthopnea, paroxysmal nocturnal dyspnea, nocturia, ankle edema, pallor in light-skinned people.

Palpation Skin moist, clammy. Tactile fremitus normal.

Percussion Resonant.

Auscultation Normal vesicular. Heart sounds include S_3 gallop.

Adventitious Sounds Crackles at lung bases.

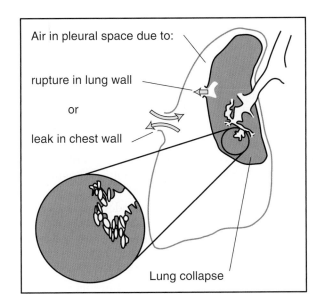

◄ Pneumothorax

Condition Free air in pleural space causes partial or complete lung collapse. Air in pleural space neutralizes the usual negative pressure present, thus lung collapses. Usually unilateral. Pneumothorax can be (1) **spontaneous** (air enters pleural space through rupture in lung wall; (2) **traumatic** (air enters through opening or injury in chest wall); or (3) **tension** (trapped air in pleural space increases, compressing lung and shifting mediastinum to the unaffected side).

Inspection Unequal chest expansion. If large, tachypnea, cyanosis, apprehension, bulging in interspaces.

Palpation Tactile fremitus decreased or absent. Tracheal shift to opposite side (unaffected side). Chest expansion decreased on affected side. Tachycardia, decreased BP.

Percussion Hyperresonant. Decreased diaphragmatic excursion.

Auscultation Breath sounds decreased or absent. Voice sounds decreased or absent.

Adventitious Sounds None.

Table continued on following page

TABLE 18–8: Assessment of Common Respiratory Conditions—cont'd

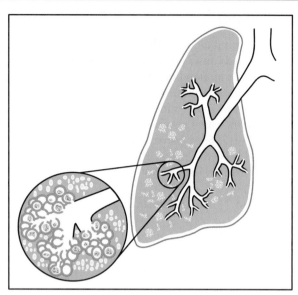

◀ *Pneumocystis carinii* Pneumonia

Condition This virulent form of pneumonia is a protozoal infection associated with AIDS. The parasite *P. carinii* is common in the United States and harmless to most people, except to the immunocompromised, in whom a diffuse interstitial pneumonitis ensues. Cysts containing the organism and macrophages form in alveolar spaces, alveolar walls thicken, and the disease spreads to bilateral interstitial infiltrates of foamy, protein-rich fluid.

Inspection Anxiety, shortness of breath, dyspnea on exertion, malaise are common; also tachypnea; fever; a dry, nonproductive cough; intercostal retractions in children; cyanosis.

Palpation Decreased chest expansion.

Percussion Dull over areas of diffuse infiltrate.

Auscultation Breath sounds may be diminished.

Adventitious Sounds Crackles may be present, but often are absent.

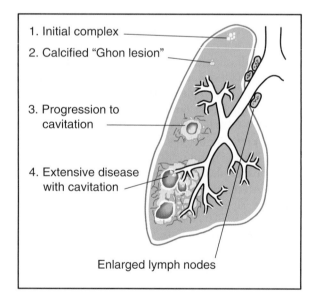

1. Initial complex
2. Calcified "Ghon lesion"
3. Progression to cavitation
4. Extensive disease with cavitation

Enlarged lymph nodes

◀ Tuberculosis

Condition Inhalation of tubercle bacilli into the alveolar wall starts: (1) Initial complex is acute inflammatory response—macrophages engulf bacilli but do not kill them. Tubercle forms around bacilli; (2) Scar tissue forms, lesion calcifies and shows on x-ray; (3) Reactivation of previously healed lesion. Dormant bacilli now multiply, producing necrosis, cavitation, and caseous lung tissue (cheeselike); (4) Extensive destruction as lesion erodes into bronchus, forming air-filled cavity. Apex usually has the most damage.

Subjective Initially asymptomatic, showing as positive skin test or on x-ray. Progressive tuberculosis involves weight loss, anorexia, easy fatigability, low-grade afternoon fevers, night sweats. May have pleural effusion, recurrent lower respiratory infections.

Inspection Cough initially nonproductive, later productive of purulent, yellow-green sputum, may be blood tinged. Dyspnea, orthopnea, fatigue, weakness.

Palpation Skin moist at night from night sweats.

Percussion Resonant initially. Dull over any effusion.

Auscultation Normal or decreased vesicular breath sounds.

Adventitious Sounds Crackles over upper lobes common, persist following full expiration and cough.

Continued

TABLE 18–8: Assessment of Common Respiratory Conditions—cont'd

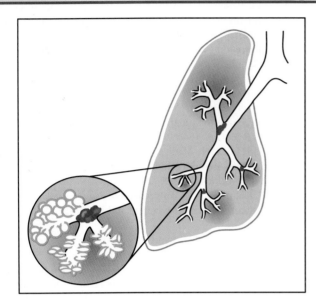

◀ Pulmonary Embolism

Condition Undissolved materials (e.g., thrombus, or air bubbles, fat globules) originating in legs or pelvis, detach and travel through venous system returning blood to right heart, and lodge to occlude pulmonary vessels. Over 95% arise from deep vein thrombi in lower legs due to stasis of blood, vessel injury, or hypercoaguability. Pulmonary occlusion results in ischemia of down-stream lung tissue, increased pulmonary artery pressure, decreased cardiac output, and hypoxia. Rarely, a saddle embolus in bifurcation of pulmonary arteries leads to sudden death from hypoxia. More often, small to medium pulmonary branches occlude, leading to dyspnea. These may resolve by fibrolytic activity.

Subjective Chest pain, worse on deep inspiration, dyspnea.

Inspection Apprehensive, restless, anxiety, mental status changes, cyanosis, tachypnea, cough, hemoptysis, $PaO_2 <80$ on pulse oximetry. Arterial blood gases show respiratory alkalosis.

Palpation Diaphosesis, hypotension.

Auscultation Tachycardia, accentuated pulmonic component of S_2 heart sound.

Adventitious Sounds Crackles, wheezes.

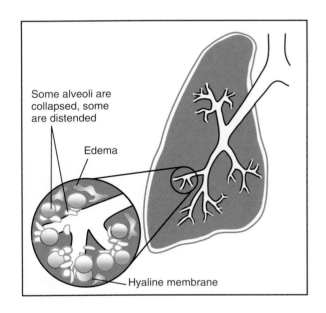

Some alveoli are collapsed, some are distended

Edema

Hyaline membrane

◀ Acute Respiratory Distress Syndrome (ARDS)

Condition An acute pulmonary insult (trauma, gastric acid aspiration, shock, sepsis) damages alveolar capillary membrane, leading to increased permeability of pulmonary capillaries and alveolar epithelium, and to pulmonary edema. Gross examination (autopsy) would show dark red, firm, airless tissue, with some alveoli collapsed, and hyaline membranes lining the distended alveoli.

Subjective Acute onset of dyspnea, apprehension.

Inspection Restlessness, disorientation, rapid shallow breathing, productive cough, thin frothy sputum, retractions of intercostal spaces and sternum. Decreased PaO_2, blood gases show respiratory alkalosis, x-rays show diffuse pulmonary infiltrates, a late sign is cyanosis.

Palpation Hypotension.

Auscultation Tachycardia.

Adventitious Sounds Crackles, rhonchi.

BIBLIOGRAPHY

Assadian O, Assadian A, Aspock C, Killer W: The stethoscope as a potential source of transmission of bacteria, *Infect Control Hosp Epidemiol* 19(5):298–299, May 1998.

Autio L, Rosenow D: Effectively managing asthma in young and middle adulthood, *Nurse Pract* 24(1):100–113, Jan 1999.

Avila PC: Differential diagnosis of wheezing in children, *Lippincotts Prim Care Pract* 2(6):559–577, Nov–Dec 1998.

Bezanson J: Respiratory care of older adults after cardiac surgery, *J Cardiovasc Nurs* 12(1):71–83, Oct 1997.

Boldt MD, Kiresuk T: Community-acquired pneumonia in adults, *Nurse Pract* 26(11):14–25, Nov 2001.

Brocato C: Breathing room: tips for the assessment and management of respiratory emergencies, *JEMS* 26(2):44–53, Feb 2001.

Carlson-Catalano J: Clinical validation of ineffective breathing pattern, ineffective airway clearance, and impaired gas exchange, *Image* 30(3):243–248, 1998.

Chernecky C, Shelton B: Pulmonary complications in patients with cancer, *Am J Nurs* 101(5):24A–24H, May 2001.

Chiramannil A: Lung cancer, *Am J Nurs* 98(4):46–47, Apr 1998.

Christie F: Pulmonary embolism, *Am J Nurs* 98(11):36–37, Nov 1998.

Cunningham FG, Gant NF, Leveno KJ: *Williams obstetrics,* ed 21, Norwalk, CT, 2001, Appleton-Lange.

Cutler WB, Friedmann E, Genovese-Stone E: Prevalence of kyphosis in a healthy sample of pre- and postmenopausal women, *Am J Phys Med Rehabil* 72(4):219–225, 1993.

Deguchi F et al: Prognostic significance of posturally induced crackles: long term follow-up of patients after recovery from acute myocardial infarction, *Chest* 103:1457–1462, 1993.

DiFranza JR, Lew RA: Morbidity and mortality in children associated with the use of tobacco products by other people, *Pediatrics* 97(4):560–568, Apr 1996.

Emde K, Rush C: Suspecting pulmonary embolism, *Am J Nurs* 101(9):19–30, Sep 2001.

Ferguson GT et al: Office spirometry for lung health assessment in adults, *Respir Care* 45(5):513–530, May 2000.

Forgacs P: The functional basis of pulmonary sounds, *Chest* 73:399–405, 1978a.

Forgacs P: *Lung sounds,* London, 1978b, Ballière Tindall.

Fowler C: Preventing and managing exercise-induced asthma, *Nurse Pract* 26(3):25–35, Mar 2001.

Garvey C: Pulmonary rehabilitation for the elderly client, *Top Adv Pract Nurs* 1(2):6p, Summer 2001.

Goolsby MJ: Viral upper respiratory infections, *J Am Acad Nurse Pract* 13(2):50–54, Feb 2001.

Karnath B, Boyars MC: Pulmonary auscultation, *Hosp Physician* 38(1):22–26, Jan 2002.

Kearney K: Epiglottitis, *Am J Nurs* 101(8):37–38, Aug 2001.

King RP, Thompson BT, Johnson DC: Wheezing on maximal forced exhalation in the diagnosis of atypical asthma, *Ann Intern Med* 110(6):451–455, 1989.

Kwiatkowski M, Jain M: Current trends and treatments in chronic obstructive pulmonary disease, *Lippincotts Prim Care Pract* 2(6):545–558, Nov–Dec 1998.

Larson JL et al: Reliability and validity of the 12-minute distance walk in patients with chronic obstructive pulmonary disease, *Nurs Res* 45(4):203–210, Jul–Aug 1996.

Lehrer S: *Understanding lung sounds,* ed 3, Philadelphia, 2002, W.B. Saunders Company.

Leiner S: Acute bronchitis in adults: commonly diagnosed but poorly defined, *Nurse Pract* 22(1):104–117, Jan 1997.

Loudon RG: The lung exam, *Clin Chest Med* 8:265–272, 1987.

Mackin LA: Screening for tuberculosis in the primary care setting, Lippincotts *Prim Care Pract* 2(6):599–610, Nov–Dec 1998.

Makinodan T, Harada N: Medical health outcome studies in the Asian and Pacific Islander American population, *Asian Am Pacific Islander J Health* 4(1–3):97–104, 1996.

Marchese TW, Diamond FB: Comprehensive assessment of the respiratory system, *J Nurse Midwifery* 40(2):150–162, Mar–Apr 1995.

Marion BS: A turn for the better: prone positioning of patients with ARDS, *Am J Nurs* 101(5):26–35, May 2001.

McDermott TD, Chestnut T, Schumann L: A comparison of conventional percussion and auscultation percussion in the detection of pleural effusions of hospitalized patients, *J Am Acad Nurs Pract* 9(10):483–486, Oct 1997.

Nelson RS et al: Rapid clinical diagnosis of pulmonary abnormalities in HIV-seropositive patients by auscultatory percussion, *Chest* 105(2):402–407, Feb 1994.

O'Hanlon-Nichols T: The adult pulmonary system, *Am J Nurs* 98(2):39–45, Feb 1998.

Overfield T: *Biologic variation in health and illness: race, age, and sex differences,* ed 2, New York, 1995, CRC Press.

Owen C: New directions in asthma management, *Am J Nurs* 99(3):26–34, Mar 1999.

Page A: Improving pediatric asthma outcomes using self-management skills, *Nurse Pract* 25(11):16–38, Nov 2000.

Prisco MK: Update your understanding of influenza, *Nurse Pract* 27(6):32–41, Jun 2002.

Richardson DK, Torday JS: Racial differences in predictive value of the lecithin/sphingomyelin ratio, *Am J Obstet Gynecol* 170:1273, 1994.

Seppa Y et al: Severity assessment of lower respiratory tract infection in elderly patients in primary care, *Arch Int Med* 161(22):2709–2713, 2001.

Stein P et al: Asymmetry of the calves in the assessment of patients with suspected acute pulmonary embolism, *Chest* 107(4):936–939, Apr 1995.

Straus SE et al: The accuracy of patient history, wheezing, and laryngeal measurements in diagnosing obstructive airway disease, *JAMA* 283(14):1853–1857, Apr 12, 2000.

Walsek C, Boler AM, Zwerski S: Lower respiratory tract infections in the pediatric patient, *Lippincotts Prim Care Pract* 3(1):93–107, Jan–Feb 1999.

Wintermeyer SF: Occupational asthma, *Lippincotts Prim Care Pract* 2(6):614–624, Nov–Dec 1998.

Heart and Neck Vessels

Structure and Function

The cardiovascular system consists of the **heart,** a muscular pump, and the **blood vessels.** The blood vessels are arranged in two continuous loops, the *pulmonary circulation* and the *systemic circulation* (Fig. 19–1). When the heart contracts, it pumps blood simultaneously into both loops.

POSITION AND SURFACE LANDMARKS

The **precordium** is the area on the anterior chest overlying the heart and great vessels (Fig. 19–2). The great vessels are the major arteries and veins connected to the heart. The heart and the great vessels are located between the lungs in the middle third of the thoracic cage, called the **mediastinum.** The heart extends from the second to the fifth intercostal space and from the right border of the sternum to the left midclavicular line.

Think of the heart as an upside-down triangle in the chest. The "top" of the heart is the broader *base,* and the "bottom" is the *apex,* which points down and to the left. During con-traction, the apex beats against the chest wall, producing an apical impulse. This is palpable in most people, normally at the fifth intercostal space, 7 to 9 cm from the midsternal line.

Inside the body, the heart is rotated so that its right side is anterior and its left side is mostly posterior. Of the heart's four chambers, the right ventricle forms the greatest area of anterior cardiac surface (Fig. 19–3). The left ventricle lies behind the right ventricle and forms the apex and slender area of the left border. The right atrium lies to the right and above the right ventricle and forms the right border. The left atrium is located posteriorly, with only a small portion, the left atrial appendage, showing anteriorly.

The **great vessels** lie bunched above the base of the heart. The **superior** and **inferior vena cava** return unoxygenated venous blood to the right side of the heart. The **pulmonary artery** leaves the right ventricle, bifurcates, and carries the venous blood to the lungs. The **pulmonary veins** return the freshly oxygenated blood to the left side of the heart, and the **aorta** carries it out to the body. The aorta ascends from the left ventricle, arches back at the level of the sternal angle, and descends behind the heart.

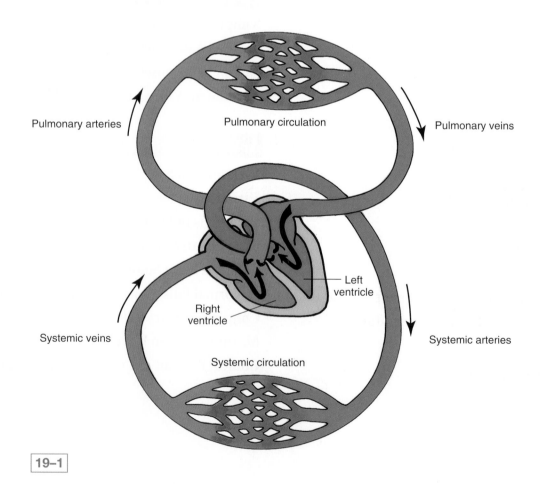

Pulmonary arteries

Pulmonary circulation

Pulmonary veins

Left ventricle

Right ventricle

Systemic veins

Systemic arteries

Systemic circulation

19–1

19–2

Precordium

Apex

Base

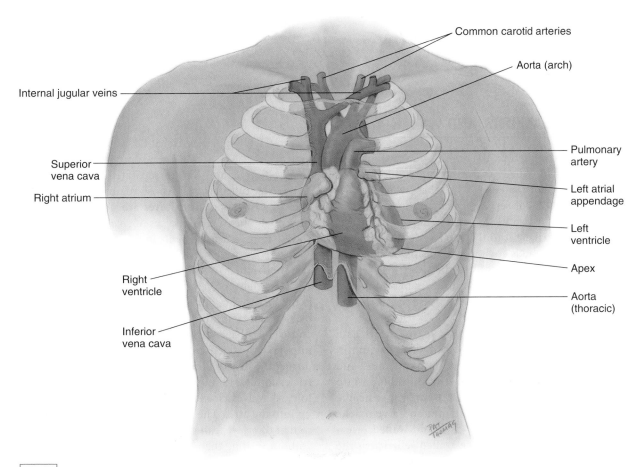

19–3

Common carotid arteries

Aorta (arch)

Internal jugular veins

Pulmonary artery

Superior vena cava

Left atrial appendage

Right atrium

Left ventricle

Apex

Right ventricle

Aorta (thoracic)

Inferior vena cava

Superior vena cava

Pulmonary arteries

Pulmonic valve

Right atrium

Tricuspid (AV) valve

Right ventricle

Inferior vena cava

Aorta (thoracic)

Aorta (arch)

Pulmonary artery

Cut edge of pericardium

Pulmonary veins

Left atrium

Aortic valve

Mitral (AV) valve

Chordae tendineae

Papillary muscle

Left ventricle

Endocardium

Myocardium

19–4

HEART WALL, CHAMBERS, AND VALVES

The **heart wall** has numerous layers. The **pericardium** is a tough, fibrous, double-walled sac that surrounds and protects the heart (see its cut edge in Fig. 19–4). It has two layers that contain a few milliliters of serous *pericardial fluid.* This ensures smooth, friction-free movement of the heart muscle. The pericardium is adherent to the great vessels, esophagus, sternum, and pleurae and is anchored to the diaphragm. The **myocardium** is the muscular wall of the heart; it does the pumping. The **endocardium** is the thin layer of endothelial tissue that lines the inner surface of the heart chambers and valves.

The common metaphor is to think of the heart as a pump. But consider that the heart is actually *two* pumps; the right side of the heart pumps blood into the lungs, and the left side of the heart simultaneously pumps blood into the body. The two pumps are separated by an impermeable wall, the septum. Each side has an **atrium** and a **ventricle.** The atrium (Latin for "anteroom") is a thin-walled reservoir for holding blood, and the thick-walled ventricle is the muscular pumping chamber. (It is common to use the following abbreviations to refer to the chambers: *RA,* right

atrium; *RV,* right ventricle; *LA,* left atrium; and *LV,* left ventricle.)

The four **chambers** are separated by swinging doorlike structures, called *valves,* whose main purpose is to prevent backflow of blood. The valves are unidirectional; they can only open one way. The valves open and close *passively* in response to pressure gradients in the moving blood.

There are four **valves** in the heart (Fig. 19–4). The two **atrioventricular** (AV) valves separate the atria and the ventricles. The right AV valve is the **tricuspid,** and the left AV valve is the bicuspid or **mitral** valve (so named, because it resembles a bishop's mitred cap). The valves' thin leaflets are anchored by collagenous fibers (**chordae tendineae**) to papillary muscles embedded in the ventricle floor. The AV valves open during the heart's filling phase, or **diastole,** to allow the ventricles to fill with blood. During the pumping phase, or **systole,** AV valves close to prevent regurgitation of blood back up into the atria. The papillary muscles contract at this time, so that the valve leaflets meet and unite to form a perfect seal without turning themselves inside out.

The **semilunar** (SL) valves are set between the ventricles and the arteries. Each valve has three cusps that look like half-moons. The SL valves are the **pulmonic** valve in the right side of the heart and the **aortic** valve in the left side of the heart. They open during pumping, or **systole,** to allow blood to be ejected from the heart.

Note that no valves are present between the vena cava and the right atrium, nor between the pulmonary veins and the left atrium. For this reason, abnormally high pressure in the left side of the heart gives a person symptoms of pulmonary congestion, and abnormally high pressure in the right side of the heart shows in the neck veins and abdomen.

DIRECTION OF BLOOD FLOW

Think of an unoxygenated red blood cell being drained downstream into the vena cava. It is swept along with the flow of venous blood and follows the route illustrated in Fig. 19–5.

1. From liver to right atrium (RA) via inferior vena cava; Superior vena cava drains venous blood from the head and upper extremities
   From RA, venous blood travels through tricuspid valve to right ventricle (RV)
2. From RV, venous blood flows through pulmonic valve to pulmonary artery
   Pulmonary artery delivers unoxygenated blood to lungs
3. Lungs oxygenate blood
   Pulmonary veins return fresh blood to LA
4. From LA, arterial blood travels through mitral valve to LV
   LV ejects blood through aortic valve into aorta
5. Aorta delivers oxygenated blood to body

Remember that the circulation is a continuous loop. The blood is kept moving along by continually shifting pressure gradients. The blood flows from an area of higher pressure to one of lower pressure.

19–5

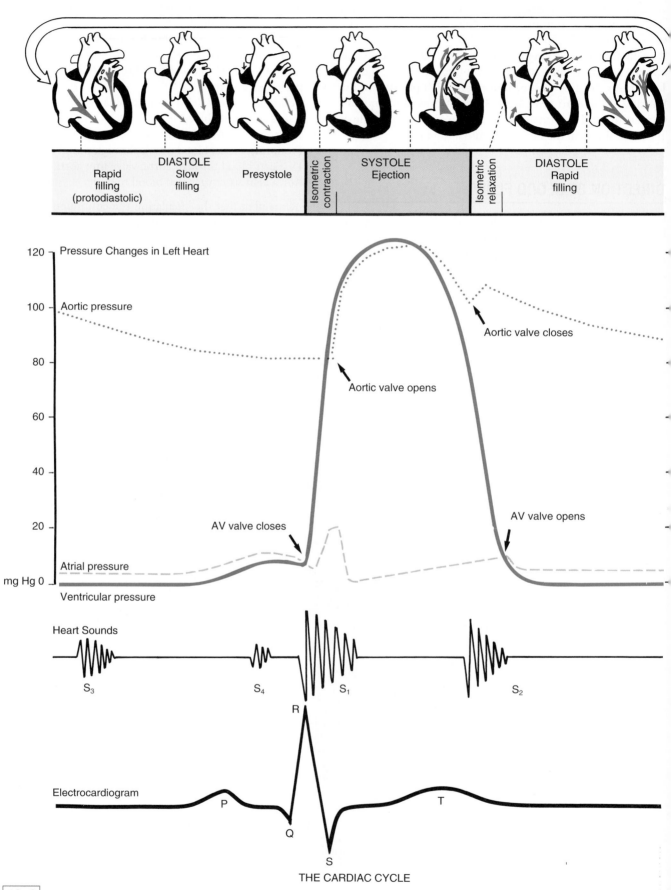

DIASTOLE

Rapid filling (protodiastolic)

Slow filling

Presystole

Isometric contraction

SYSTOLE
Ejection

Isometric relaxation

DIASTOLE
Rapid filling

Pressure Changes in Left Heart

120

100 — Aortic pressure

80

60

40

20

mg Hg 0

Ventricular pressure

Atrial pressure

AV valve closes

Aortic valve opens

Aortic valve closes

AV valve opens

Heart Sounds

S_3 S_4 S_1 S_2

Electrocardiogram

R

P

Q

S

T

THE CARDIAC CYCLE

19–6

CARDIAC CYCLE

The rhythmic movement of blood through the heart is the **cardiac cycle.** It has two phases, **diastole** and **systole.** In **diastole,** the ventricles relax and fill with blood. This takes up two thirds of the cardiac cycle. The heart's contraction is **systole.** During systole, blood is pumped from the ventricles and fills the pulmonary and systemic arteries. This is one third of the cardiac cycle.

DIASTOLE. In diastole, the ventricles are relaxed, and the AV valves, (i.e., the tricuspid and mitral) are open (Fig. 19–6). (Opening of the normal valve is acoustically silent.) The pressure in the atria is higher than that in the ventricles, so blood pours rapidly into the ventricles. This first passive filling phase is called *early* or *protodiastolic filling.*

Toward the end of diastole, the atria contract and push the last amount of blood (about 25% of stroke volume) into the ventricles. This active filling phase is called *presystole,* or *atrial systole,* or sometimes the "atrial kick." It causes a small rise in left ventricular pressure. (Note that atrial systole occurs during ventricular diastole, a confusing but important point.)

SYSTOLE. Now so much blood has been pumped into the ventricles that ventricular pressure is finally higher than that in the atria, so the mitral and tricuspid valves swing shut. The closure of the AV valves contributes to the first heart sound (S_1) and signals the beginning of systole. The AV valves close to prevent any regurgitation of blood back up into the atria during contraction.

For a very brief moment, all four valves are closed. The ventricular walls contract. This contraction against a closed system works to build pressure inside the ventricles to a high level (*isometric contraction*). Consider first the left side of the heart. When the pressure in the ventricle finally exceeds pressure in the aorta, the aortic valve opens and blood is ejected rapidly.

After the ventricle's contents are ejected, its pressure falls. When pressure falls below pressure in the aorta, some blood flows backward toward the ventricle, causing the aortic valve to swing shut. This closure of the semilunar valves causes the second heart sound (S_2) and signals the end of systole.

DIASTOLE AGAIN. Now all four valves are closed and the ventricles relax (called *isometric* or *isovolumic relaxation*). Meanwhile, the atria have been filling with blood delivered from the lungs. Atrial pressure is now higher than the relaxed ventricular pressure. The mitral valve drifts open and diastolic filling begins again.

EVENTS IN THE RIGHT AND LEFT SIDES. The same events are happening in the right side of the heart, but pressures in the right side of the heart are much lower than those of the left side because less energy is needed to pump blood to its destination, the pulmonary circulation. Also, events occur just slightly later in the right side of the heart due to the route of myocardial depolarization. As a result, two distinct components to each of the heart sounds exist, and sometimes you can hear them separately. In the first heart sound, the mitral component (M_1) closes just before the tricuspid component (T_1). And with S_2, aortic closure (A_2) occurs slightly before pulmonic closure (P_2).

HEART SOUNDS

Events in the cardiac cycle generate sounds that can be heard through a stethoscope over the chest wall. These include normal heart sounds and, occasionally, extra heart sounds and murmurs (Fig. 19–7).

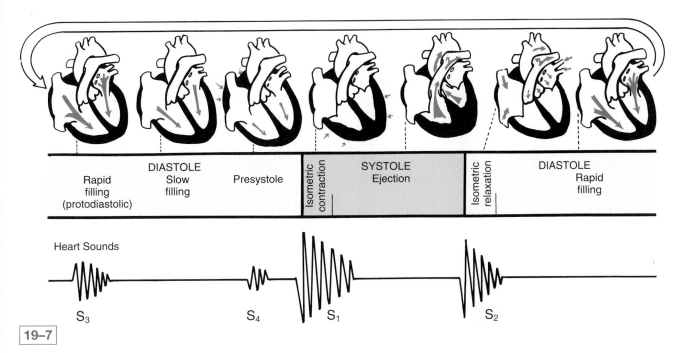

19–7

NORMAL HEART SOUNDS

The **first heart sound** (S_1) occurs with closure of the AV valves and thus signals the beginning of systole. The mitral component of the first sound (M_1) slightly precedes the tricuspid component (T_1), but you usually hear these two components fused as one sound. You can hear S_1 over all the precordium, but usually it is loudest at the apex.

The **second heart sound** (S_2) occurs with closure of the semilunar valves and signals the end of systole. The aortic component of the second sound (A_2) slightly precedes the pulmonic component (P_2). Although it is heard over all the precordium, S_2 is loudest at the base.

EFFECT OF RESPIRATION. The volume of right and left ventricular systole is just about equal, but this can be affected by respiration. To learn this, consider the phrase:

MoRe to the Right heart,
Less to the Left

That means that during inspiration, intrathoracic pressure is decreased. This pushes more blood into the vena cava, increasing venous return to the right side of the heart, which increases right ventricular stroke volume. The increased volume prolongs right ventricular systole and delays pulmonic valve closure.

Meanwhile on the left side, a greater amount of blood is sequestered in the lungs during inspiration. This momentarily decreases the amount returned to the left side of the heart, decreasing left ventricular stroke volume. The decreased volume shortens left ventricular systole and allows the aortic valve to close a bit earlier. When the aortic valve closes significantly earlier than the pulmonic valve, you can hear the two components separately. This is a *split* S_2.

EXTRA HEART SOUNDS

THIRD HEART SOUND (S_3). Normally diastole is a silent event. However, in some conditions, ventricular filling creates vibrations that can be heard over the chest. These vibrations are S_3. The S_3 occurs when the ventricles are resistant to filling during the early rapid filling phase (protodiastole). This occurs immediately after S_2, when the AV valves open and atrial blood first pours into the ventricles. (See a complete discussion of S_3 in Table 19–6 on p. 522.)

FOURTH HEART SOUND (S_4). The S_4 occurs at the end of diastole, at presystole, when the ventricle is resistant to filling. The atria contract and push blood into a noncompliant ventricle. This creates vibrations that are heard as S_4. The S_4 occurs just before S_1.

MURMURS

Blood circulating through normal cardiac chambers and valves usually makes no noise. However, some conditions create turbulent blood flow and collision currents. These result in a murmur, much like a pile of stones or a sharp turn in a stream creates a noisy water flow. A murmur is a gentle, blowing, swooshing sound that can be heard on the chest wall. Conditions resulting in a murmur are as follows:

1. Velocity of blood increases (flow murmur) (e.g., in exercise, thyrotoxicosis)
2. Viscosity of blood decreases (e.g., in anemia)
3. Structural defects in the valves (narrowed valve, incompetent valve) or unusual openings occur in the chambers (dilated chamber, wall defect)

CHARACTERISTICS OF SOUND

All heart sounds are described by:

1. Frequency (pitch)—heart sounds are described as high pitched or low pitched, although these terms are relative because all are low-frequency sounds, and you need a good stethoscope to hear them
2. Intensity (loudness)—loud or soft
3. Duration—very short for heart sounds; silent periods are longer
4. Timing—systole or diastole

CONDUCTION

Of all organs, the heart has a unique ability—automaticity. The heart can contract by itself, independent of any signals or stimulation from the body. The heart contracts in response to an electrical current conveyed by a conduction system (Fig. 19–8). Specialized cells in the sinoatrial (SA) node near the superior vena cava initiate an electrical impulse. (Because the SA node has an intrinsic rhythm, it is the "pacemaker.") The current flows in an orderly sequence, first across the atria to the AV node low in the atrial septum. There, it is delayed slightly so that the atria have time to contract before the ventricles are stimulated. Then, the impulse travels to the bundle of His, the right and left bundle branches, and then through the ventricles.

The electrical impulse stimulates the heart to do its work, which is to contract. A small amount of electricity spreads to the body surface, where it can be measured and recorded on the electrocardiograph (ECG). The ECG waves are arbitrarily labeled PQRST, which stand for the following elements:

P wave—depolarization of the atria
PR interval—from the beginning of the P wave to the beginning of the QRS complex (the time necessary for atrial depolarization plus time for the impulse to travel through the AV node to the ventricles)
QRS complex—depolarization of the ventricles
T wave—repolarization of the ventricles

Electrical events slightly *precede* the mechanical events in the heart. The ECG juxtaposed on the cardiac cycle is illustrated in Figure 19–6.

Conduction system

Electrocardiograph (ECG) wave

19–8

PUMPING ABILITY

In the resting adult, the heart normally pumps between 4 and 6 L of blood per minute throughout the body. This **cardiac output** equals the volume of blood in each systole (called the stroke volume) times the number of beats per minute (rate). This is described as:

$$CO = SV \times R$$

The heart can alter its cardiac output to adapt to the metabolic needs of the body. Preload and afterload affect the heart's ability to increase cardiac output.

Preload is the venous return that builds during diastole. It is the length to which the ventricular muscle is stretched at the end of diastole just before contraction (Fig. 19–9).

When the volume of blood returned to the ventricles is increased (as when exercise stimulates skeletal muscles to contract and force more blood back to the heart), the muscle bundles are stretched beyond their normal resting state to accommodate. The force of this switch is the preload. According to the Frank-Starling law, the greater the stretch, the stronger is the heart's contraction. This increased contractility results in an increased volume of blood ejected (increased stroke volume).

Preload

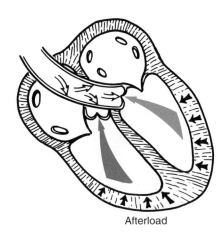

Afterload

19–9

Afterload is the opposing pressure the ventricle must generate to open the aortic valve against the higher aortic pressure. It is the resistance against which the ventricle must pump its blood. Once the ventricle is filled with blood, the ventricular end diastolic pressure is 5 to 10 mm Hg, whereas that in the aorta is 70 to 80 mm Hg. To overcome this difference, the ventricular muscle *tenses* (isovolumic contraction). After the aortic valve opens, rapid ejection occurs.

THE NECK VESSELS

Cardiovascular assessment includes the survey of vascular structures in the neck—the carotid artery and the jugular veins (Fig. 19–10). These vessels reflect the efficiency of cardiac function.

THE CAROTID ARTERY PULSE

Chapter 10 describes the pulse as a pressure wave generated by each systole pumping blood into the aorta. The carotid artery is a central artery—that is, it is close to the heart. Its timing closely coincides with ventricular systole. (Assessment of the peripheral pulses is found in Chapter 20, and blood pressure assessment is found in Chapter 10.)

The **carotid artery** is located in the groove between the trachea and the sternomastoid muscle, medial to and along-side that muscle. Note the characteristics of its waveform (Fig. 19–11): a smooth rapid upstroke, a summit that is rounded and smooth, and a downstroke that is more gradual and that has a dicrotic notch caused by closure of the aortic valve (marked D in the figure).

JUGULAR VENOUS PULSE AND PRESSURE

The **jugular veins** empty unoxygenated blood directly into the superior vena cava. Since no cardiac valve exists to separate the superior vena cava from the right atrium, the jugular veins give information about activity on the right side of the heart. Specifically, they reflect filling pressure and volume changes. Since, volume and pressure increase when the right side of the heart fails to pump efficiently, the jugular veins expose this.

Two jugular veins are present in each side of the neck (see Fig. 19–10). The larger **internal jugular** lies deep and medial to the sternomastoid muscle. It is usually not visible, although its diffuse pulsations may be seen in the sternal notch when the person is supine. The **external jugular** vein is more superficial; it lies lateral to the sternomastoid muscle, above the clavicle.

Although an arterial pulse is caused by a forward propulsion of blood, the jugular pulse is different. The jugular pulse results from a backwash, a waveform moving backward caused by events upstream. The jugular pulse has five components (Fig. 19–12):

Right external jugular vein

Right common carotid artery

Sternomastoid muscle

Left external jugular vein

Left common carotid artery

Left internal jugular vein

Sternomastoid muscle and clavicle cut

Superior vena cava

Aorta

NECK VESSELS

19–10

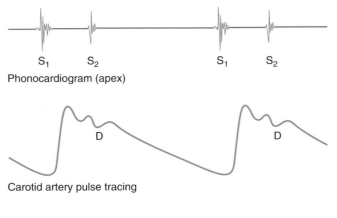

Phonocardiogram (apex)

Carotid artery pulse tracing

ECG

ARTERIAL PULSE

19–11

Jugular Pulse	Reflects	Results from	Jugular Pulse	Reflects	Results from
A wave	Atrial contraction	Some blood flows backward to the vena cava during right atrial contraction	X descent	Atrial relaxation	Right ventricle contracts (systole) and pulls bottom of atria downward
C wave	Ventricular contraction	Backflow from bulging upward of tricuspid valve when it closes at beginning of ventricular systole (not from neighboring carotid artery pulsation)	V wave	Passive atrial filling	Increasing volume of atrial filling and increased pressure
			Y descent	Passive ventricular filling	Tricuspid valve opens and blood flows from RA to RV

Phonocardiogram

Jugular venous pulse

ECG

VENOUS PULSE

19–12

DEVELOPMENTAL CONSIDERATIONS

INFANTS AND CHILDREN

The fetal heart functions early; it begins to beat at the end of 3 weeks' gestation. The lungs are nonfunctional, but the fetal circulation compensates for this (Fig. 19–13). Oxygenation takes place at the placenta, and the arterial blood is returned to the right side of the heart. There is no point in pumping all this freshly oxygenated blood through the lungs, so it is rerouted in two ways. First, about two thirds of it is shunted through an opening in the atrial septum, the **foramen ovale,** into the left side of the heart, where it is pumped out through the aorta. Second, the rest of the oxygenated blood is pumped by the right side of the heart out via the pulmonary artery, but it is detoured through the **ductus arteriosus** to the aorta. Because they are both pumping into the systemic circulation,

the right and left ventricles are equal in weight and muscle wall thickness.

Inflation and aeration of the lungs at birth produces circulatory changes. Now the blood is oxygenated through the lungs rather than through the placenta. The foramen ovale closes within the 1st hour because of the new lower pressure in the right side of the heart than in the left side. The ductus arteriosus closes later, usually within 10 to 15 hours of birth. Now, the left ventricle has the greater workload of pumping into the systemic circulation, so that when the baby has reached 1 year of age, the left ventricle's mass increases to reach the adult ratio of 2:1, left ventricle to right ventricle.

The heart's position in the chest is more horizontal in the infant than in the adult; thus the apex is higher, located at the fourth left intercostal space (Fig. 19–14). It reaches the adult position when the child reaches age 7.

FETAL CIRCULATION

19–13

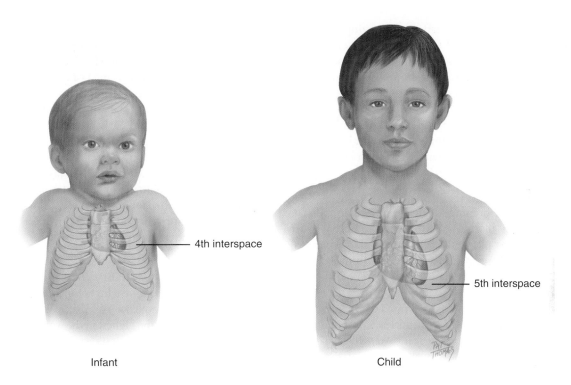

4th interspace

5th interspace

Infant

Child

19–14 HEART'S POSITION IN THE CHEST

THE PREGNANT FEMALE

Blood volume increases by 30% to 40% during pregnancy, with the most rapid expansion occurring during the second trimester. This creates an increase in stroke volume and cardiac output and an increased pulse rate of 10 to 15 beats per minute. Despite the increased cardiac output, arterial blood pressure decreases in pregnancy due to peripheral vasodilation. The blood pressure drops to its lowest point during the second trimester, then rises after that. The blood pressure varies with the person's position, as described on p. 514.

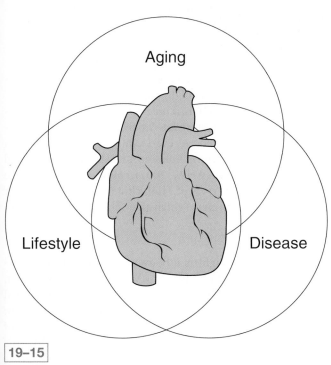

19–15

THE AGING ADULT

It is difficult to isolate the "aging process" of the cardiovascular system *per se* because it is so closely interrelated with lifestyle, habits, and diseases. We now know that lifestyle is a modifying factor in the development of cardiovascular disease; smoking, diet, alcohol use, exercise patterns, and stress have an influence on coronary artery disease. Lifestyle also affects the aging process; cardiac changes once thought to be due to aging are partially due to the secondary lifestyle accompanying aging (Fig. 19–15).

What is left to be attributed to the aging process alone? When studies exclude people with clinical or occult heart disease (Lakatta, Gerstenblith, Weisfeldt, 1997), the following hemodynamic "aging process" emerges.

Hemodynamic Changes with Aging

- From age 20 to 60, systolic blood pressure tends to increase by about 20 mm Hg, and by another 20 mm Hg between ages 60 and 80, (Wei, 1992). This is due to stiffening of the large arteries, which, in turn is due to calcification of vessel walls (arteriosclerosis). This stiffening creates an increase in pulse wave velocity because the less compliant arteries cannot store the volume ejected.
- The overall size of the heart does not increase with age, but left ventricular wall thickness increases somewhat. This is an adaptive mechanism to accommodate the vascular stiffening mentioned earlier that creates an increased workload on the heart.
- No significant change in diastolic pressure occurs with age. A rising systolic pressure with a relatively constant diastolic pressure results in an increase in pulse pressure (the difference between the two).
- No change in resting heart rate occurs with aging.

- Cardiac output at rest is not changed with aging.
- There is a decreased ability of the heart to augment cardiac output with exercise. This is shown by a decreased maximum heart rate with exercise and diminished sympathetic response. Noncardiac factors also cause a decrease in maximum work performance with aging: decrease in skeletal muscle performance, increase in muscle fatigue, increased sense of dyspnea. Chronic exercise conditioning will modify many of the aging changes in cardiovascular function (Lakatta et al., 1997).

ARRHYTHMIAS. The presence of supraventricular and ventricular arrhythmias increases with age. Ectopic beats are common in aging people; while these are usually asymptomatic in healthy older people, they may compromise cardiac output and blood pressure when disease is present (Lakatta et al., 1997).

Tachyarrhythmias may not be tolerated as well in older people. The myocardium is thicker and less compliant, and early diastolic filling is impaired at rest (Wei, 1992). Thus, it may not tolerate a tachycardia as well because of shortened diastole. Also, tachyarrhythmias may further compromise a vital organ whose function has already been affected by aging or disease. For example, a ventricular tachycardia produces a 40% to 70% decrease in cerebral blood flow. Although a younger person may tolerate this, an older person with cerebrovascular disease may experience syncope (Lakatta et al., 1997).

ECG. Age-related changes in the ECG occur due to histologic changes in the conduction system. These include:

- Prolonged P-R interval (first-degree AV block) and prolonged Q-T interval, but the QRS interval is unchanged
- Left axis deviation due to age-related mild LV hypertrophy and fibrosis in left bundle branch
- Increased incidence of bundle branch block (Lakatta et al., 1997).

Although the hemodynamic changes associated with aging alone do not seem severe or portentous, the fact remains that the incidence of cardiovascular disease increases with age. The incidence of coronary artery disease increases sharply with advancing age and accounts for about half of the deaths of older people. Hypertension (systolic >160 mm Hg and diastolic >95 mm Hg) and heart failure also increase with age (Wei, 1992). Certainly, lifestyle habits (smoking, lack of exercise, diet) play a significant role in the acquisition of heart disease. Also, increasing the physical activity of older adults—even at a moderate level—is associated with a reduced risk of death from cardiovascular diseases and respiratory illnesses (Kushi et al., 1997). Both points underscore the need for health teaching as an important treatment parameter.

TRANSCULTURAL CONSIDERATIONS

The prevalence of heart disease and stroke is higher among black adults than in other racial groups: 40.5% for men and 39.6% for women, as opposed to 30.0% for white men and 23.8% for white women, and 28.8% for Mexican-American men and 26.6% for Mexican-American women. Also, black and Mexican-American women have higher cardiovascular risk factors than do white women of the same socioeconomic status. These differences in prevalence by ethnicity and socioeconomic group show the crucial need to improve screening, early detection, and early treatment among black and Mexican-American groups (American Heart Association [AHA], 2002).

The major risk factors for heart disease and stroke are high blood pressure, smoking, high cholesterol levels, obesity, and diabetes. In addition, for some women, the use of oral contraceptives and postmenopausal endogenous hormones are risk factors (Anderson and Kessenich, 2001).

HIGH BLOOD PRESSURE (HBP). Blacks, Mexican-Americans, and Native Americans have a higher incidence of hypertension than whites. The prevalence of HBP in blacks in the United States is listed among the highest in the world (AHA, 2002). The prevalence of HBP in U.S. adults age 20 and older is, for whites, 25.2% for men and 20.5% for women; for blacks, 36.7% for men and 36.6% for women; and for Mexican-Americans, 24.2% for men and 22.4% for women. The prevalence of HBP in Native Americans age 45 and older is 26.8% for men and 27.5% for women. Data available on Asian/Pacific Islanders show a lower prevalence of HBP among these groups—9.7% for men and 8.4% for women (AHA, 2002).

SMOKING. In adults, more black men (28.7%) and Native American men (40.9%) smoke than white men (25.5%). The usage rates for Hispanics and Asian/Pacific Islanders are just slightly less than for white men. When looking at youth as a subclass (age 18 to 24), whites from lower educational levels show higher smoking rates than blacks and Mexican-American youth from similar backgrounds; 77% of young white men and 61% of young white women are smokers, as opposed to 35% of minority youth (AHA, 2002).

SERUM CHOLESTEROL. During childhood ages 4-19, black children and adolescents have higher total cholesterol, higher low-density lipoprotein (LDL) cholesterol, and higher high-density lipoprotein (HDL) cholesterol (the "good" cholesterol) than white and Mexican-American children and adolescents. These differences reverse during adulthood when blacks have lower serum cholesterol levels than whites and Mexican-Americans (AHA, 2002). However, black men tend to have higher rates of HDL cholesterol than white or Mexican-American men, which may help reduce coronary artery disease risk.

OBESITY. Overweight is a body mass index (BMI) of 25 kg/m^2 or higher, and obesity is a BMI of 30 kg/m^2 or higher. These levels have reached epidemic proportions in the United States. The following adults age 18 and older are overweight: 62.4% of white men and 43% of white women; 64.1% of black men and 64.5% of black women; 64.7% of Hispanic men and 56.8% of Hispanic women; and 35.2% of Asian/Pacific Islander men and 25.2% of Asian/Pacific Islander women (AHA, 2002).

DIABETES. The prevalence of diabetes increased in the United States from 4.9% in 1990 to 6.5% in 1998—this represents a 33.3% increase. The increases occurred in men and women, all age and ethnic groups, and all educational levels (AHA, 2002). In Native Americans, the rates are particularly high. For those over age 45, 43.5% of men and 52.4% of women have diabetes. This increases the risk of complications of diabetes as well, including kidney disease, blindness, and amputation. The risk of diabetes is almost twice as high for blacks and Mexican-Americans than for whites. Adults age 20 and older having diabetes include 8.1% of Mexican-American men and 11.4% of Mexican-American women; 7.6% of black men and 9.5% of black women; and 5.4% of white men and 4.7% of white women (AHA, 2002).

Among Japanese men in the United States 40 years of age or older, researchers find the diabetes rate to be as high as 10% to 14%, and Japanese living in the United States have, as a group, more than twice the incidence of diabetes as Japanese living in Japan. Japanese-, Chinese-, and Filipino-Americans who are born in the United States have higher death rates from diabetes than their native-born counterparts. The blame for what these statistics reveal is being placed on the high-fat content of a typical American diet. Japanese diets in the United States, for example, are much higher in both animal and total fat content than those in Japan.

Subjective Data

1. Chest pain	**5.** Fatigue	**9.** Past cardiac history
2. Dyspnea	**6.** Cyanosis or pallor	**10.** Family cardiac history
3. Orthopnea	**7.** Edema	**11.** Personal habits (cardiac risk
4. Cough	**8.** Nocturia	factors)

EXAMINER ASKS	RATIONALE
1. Chest pain. Any **chest pain** or tightness? • Onset: When did it start? How long have you had it *this* time? Had this type of pain before? How often? • Location: where did the pain start? Does the pain radiate to any other spot? • Character: How would you describe it? Crushing, stabbing, burning, vise-like? (Allow the person to offer adjectives before you suggest them.) (Note if uses clenched fist to describe pain.) • Pain brought on by: activity—what type; rest; emotional upset; after eating; during sexual intercourse; with cold weather? • Any associated symptoms: sweating, ashen gray or pale skin, heart skips beat, shortness of breath, nausea or vomiting, racing of heart? • Pain made worse by moving the arms or neck, breathing, lying flat? • Pain relieved by rest or nitroglycerin? How many tablets? **2. Dyspnea.** Any shortness of breath? • What type of activity and how much brings on shortness of breath? How much activity brought it on 6 months ago? • Onset: Does the shortness of breath come on unexpectedly? • Duration: constant or does it come and go? • Seem to be affected by position: lying down? • Awaken you from sleep at night? • Does the shortness of breath interfere with activities of daily living?	Angina, an important cardiac symptom, occurs when heart's vascular supply cannot keep up with metabolic demand. Chest pain also may have pulmonary, musculoskeletal, or gastrointestinal origin; it is important to differentiate. "Clenched fist" sign is characteristic of angina. Diaphoresis, pallor. Palpitations, dyspnea, nausea, tachycardia. Try to differentiate pain of cardiac versus noncardiac origin. **Dyspnea.** Dyspnea on exertion (DOE)—Quantify exactly, for example, DOE after walking two level blocks. Paroxysmal. Constant or intermittent. Recumbent. Paroxysmal nocturnal dyspnea (PND) occurs with heart failure. Lying down increases volume of intrathoracic blood, and the weakened heart cannot accommodate the increased load. Classically, the person awakens after 2 hours of sleep, arises, and flings open a window with the perception of needing fresh air.

EXAMINER ASKS | **RATIONALE**

3. Orthopnea. How many pillows do you use when sleeping or lying down?

Orthopnea is the need to assume a more upright position to breathe. Note the exact number of pillows used.

4. Cough. Do you have a **cough?**
- Duration: How long have you had it?
- Frequency: Is it related to time of day?
- Type: dry, hacking, barky, hoarse, or congested?
- Do you cough up mucus? Color? Any odor? Blood tinged?

Sputum production, mucoid or purulent. Hemoptysis is often a pulmonary disorder but also occurs with mitral stenosis.

- Associated with: activity, position (lying down), anxiety, talking?
- Does activity make it better or worse (sit, walk, exercise)?
- Relieved by rest or medication?

5. Fatigue. Do you seem to tire easily? Able to keep up with your family and co-workers?
- Onset: When did fatigue start? Sudden or gradual? Has any *recent* change occurred in energy level?
- Fatigue related to time of day: all day, morning, evening?

Fatigue due to decreased cardiac output is worse in the evening, whereas fatigue from anxiety or depression occurs all day or is worse in the morning.

6. Cyanosis or pallor. Ever noted your facial skin turn blue or ashen?

Cyanosis or **pallor** occurs with myocardial infarction or low cardiac output states due to decreased tissue perfusion.

7. Edema. Any swelling of your feet and legs?
- Onset: When did you first notice this?
- Any recent change?
- What time of day does the swelling occur? Do your shoes feel tight at the end of day?

Edema is dependent when due to heart failure.

Cardiac edema is worse at evening and better in morning after elevating legs all night.

- How much swelling would you say there is? Are both legs equally swollen?
- Does the swelling go away with: rest, elevation, after a night's sleep?
- Any associated symptoms, such as shortness of breath? If so, does the shortness of breath occur before leg swelling or after?

8. Nocturia. Do you awaken at night with an urgent need to urinate? How long has this been occurring? Any recent change?

Nocturia—Recumbency at night promotes fluid reabsorption and excretion; this occurs with heart failure in the person who is ambulatory during the day.

9. Past cardiac history. Any **past history** of: hypertension, elevated blood cholesterol or triglycerides, heart murmur, congenital heart disease, rheumatic fever or unexplained joint pains as child or youth, recurrent tonsillitis, anemia?
- Ever had heart disease? When was this? Treated by medication or heart surgery?
- Last ECG, stress ECG, serum cholesterol measurement, other heart tests?

10. Family cardiac history. Any **family history** of: hypertension, obesity, diabetes, coronary artery disease (CAD), sudden death at younger age?

EXAMINER ASKS	RATIONALE
11. Personal habits (cardiac risk factors).	**Risk factors for coronary artery disease**—Collect data regarding elevated serum cholesterol, elevated blood pressure, blood sugar levels above 130 or known diabetes mellitus, obesity, cigarette smoking, low activity level and length of any hormone replacement therapy for postmenopausal women.

11. Personal habits (cardiac risk factors).

- Nutrition: Please describe your usual daily diet. (Note if this diet is representative of the basic food groups, the amount of calories, cholesterol, and any additives such as salt.) What is your usual weight? Has there been any recent change?
- Smoking: Do you smoke cigarettes or other tobacco? At what age did you start? How many packs per day? For how many years have you smoked this amount? Have you ever tried to quit? If so, how did this go?
- Alcohol: How much alcohol do you usually drink each week, or each day? When was your last drink? What was the number of drinks that episode? Have you ever been told you had a drinking problem?
- Exercise: What is your usual amount of exercise each day or week? What type of exercise (state type or sport)? If a sport, what is your usual amount (light, moderate, heavy)?
- Drugs: Do you take any antihypertensives, beta-blockers, calcium channel blockers, digoxin, diuretics, aspirin/anticoagulants, over-the-counter, or street drugs?

Additional History for Infants

1. How was the mother's health during pregnancy: any unexplained fever, rubella first trimester, other infection, hypertension, drugs taken?

2. Have you noted any cyanosis while nursing, crying? Is the baby able to eat, nurse, or finish bottle without tiring?

> To screen for heart disease in infant, note fatigue during feeding. Infant with heart failure takes fewer ounces each feeding; becomes dyspneic with sucking; may be diaphoretic, then falls into exhausted sleep; awakens after a short time hungry again.

3. Growth: Has this baby grown as expected by growth charts and about the same as siblings or peers?

> Poor weight gain.

4. Activity: Were this baby's motor milestones achieved as expected? Is the baby able to play without tiring? How many naps does the baby take each day? How long does a nap last?

Additional History for Children

1. Growth: Has this child grown as expected by growth charts?

> Poor weight gain.

2. Activity: Is this child able to keep up with siblings or age-mates? Is the child willing or reluctant to go out to play? Is the child able to climb stairs, ride a bike, walk a few blocks? Does the child squat to rest during play or to watch television, or assume a knee-chest position while sleeping?
Have you noted "blue spells" during exercise?

> Fatigue. Record specific limitations.
>
> Cyanosis.

3. Has the child had any unexplained joint pains or unexplained fever?

4. Does the child have frequent headaches, nosebleeds?

5. Does the child have frequent respiratory infections? How many per year? How are they treated? Have any of these proved to be streptococcal infections?

EXAMINER ASKS	RATIONALE

6. Family history: Does the child have a sibling with heart defect?

7. Past history: Is anyone in the child's family known to have chromosomal abnormalities, such as Down syndrome?

Additional History for the Pregnant Female

1. Have you had any high blood pressure during this or earlier pregnancies?
- What was your usual blood pressure level before pregnancy? How has your blood pressure been monitored during the pregnancy?
- If high blood pressure, what treatment has been started?
- Any associated symptoms: weight gain, protein in urine, swelling in feet, legs, or face?

2. Have you experienced any faintness or dizziness with this pregnancy?

Additional History for the Aging Adult

1. Do you have any known heart or lung disease: hypertension, CAD, chronic emphysema, or bronchitis?
- What efforts to treat this have been started?
- Usual symptoms changed recently? Does your illness interfere with activities of daily living?

2. Do you take any medications for your illness such as digitalis? Aware of side effects? Have you recently stopped taking your medication? Why?

Noncompliance may be related to side effects or lack of finances.

3. Environment: Does your home have any stairs? How often do you need to climb them? Does this have any effect on activities of daily living?

Objective Data

PREPARATION

To evaluate the carotid arteries, the person can be sitting up. To assess the jugular veins and the precordium, the person should be supine with the head and chest slightly elevated.

Stand on the person's right side; this will facilitate your hand placement and auscultation of the precordium.

The room must be warm—chilling makes the person uncomfortable, and shivering interferes with heart sounds. Take scrupulous care to ensure *quiet;* heart sounds are very soft, and any ambient room noise masks them.

Ensure the female's privacy by keeping her breasts draped. The female's left breast overrides part of the area you will need to examine. Gently displace the breast upward, or ask the woman to hold it out of the way.

When performing a regional cardiovascular assessment, use this order:

1. Pulse and blood pressure (see Chapter 10)
2. Extremities (see "Peripheral Vascular Assessment," Chapter 20)
3. Neck vessels
4. Precordium

The logic of this order is that you will begin observations peripherally and move in toward the heart. For choreography of these steps in the complete physical examination, see Chapter 28.

EQUIPMENT NEEDED

Marking pen
Small centimeter ruler
Stethoscope with diaphragm and bell endpieces
Alcohol swab (to clean endpiece)

NORMAL RANGE OF FINDINGS	ABNORMAL FINDINGS

THE NECK VESSELS

Palpate the Carotid Artery

Located central to the heart, the carotid artery yields important information on cardiac function.

Palpate each carotid artery medial to the sternomastoid muscle in the neck (Fig. 19–16). Avoid excessive pressure on the carotid sinus area higher in the neck; excessive vagal stimulation here could slow down the heart rate, especially in older adults. Take care to palpate gently. Palpate only one carotid artery at a time to avoid compromising arterial blood to the brain.

Carotid sinus hypersensitivity is the condition in which pressure over the carotid sinus leads to a decreased heart rate, decreased BP, and cerebral ischemia with syncope. This may occur in older adults with hypertension or occlusion of the carotid artery.

19–16

Feel the contour and amplitude of the pulse. Normally the contour is smooth with a rapid upstroke and slower downstroke, and the normal strength is 2+ or moderate (see Chapter 20). Your findings should be the same bilaterally.

Diminished pulse feels small and weak (decreased stroke volume).
Increased pulse feels full and strong (hyperkinetic states) (see Table 20–1).

Auscultate the Carotid Artery

For persons middle-aged or older, or who show symptoms or signs of cardiovascular disease, auscultate each carotid artery for the presence of a **bruit** (pronounced BRU′-ee) (Fig. 19–17). This is a blowing, swishing sound indicating blood flow turbulence; normally none is present.

A bruit indicates turbulence due to a local vascular cause, such as atherosclerotic narrowing.

19–17

NORMAL RANGE OF FINDINGS

Keep the neck in a neutral position. Lightly apply the bell of the stethoscope over the carotid artery at three levels: (1) the angle of the jaw, (2) the midcervical area, and (3) the base of the neck (see Fig. 19–17). Avoid compressing the artery because this could create an artificial bruit, and it could compromise circulation if the carotid artery is already narrowed by atherosclerosis. Ask the person to take a breath, exhale, and hold it briefly while you listen so that tracheal breath sounds do not mask or mimic a carotid artery bruit. (Holding the breath on inhalation will also tense the levator scapulae muscles, which makes it hard to hear the carotids.) Sometimes you can hear normal heart sounds transmitted to the neck; do not confuse these with a bruit.

Inspect the Jugular Venous Pulse

From the jugular veins you can assess the **central venous pressure** (CVP) and thus judge the heart's efficiency as a pump. Although the external jugular vein is easier to see, the internal (especially the right) jugular vein is attached more directly to the superior vena cava and thus is more reliable for assessment. You cannot see the internal jugular vein itself, but you can see its pulsation.

Position the person supine anywhere from a 30- to a 45-degree angle, wherever you can best see the pulsations. In general, the higher the venous pressure is, the higher the position you need. Remove the pillow to avoid flexing the neck; the head should be in the same plane as the trunk. Turn the person's head slightly away from the examined side, and direct a strong light tangentially onto the neck to highlight pulsations and shadows.

Note the external jugular veins overlying the sternomastoid muscle. In some persons, the veins are not visible at all; whereas in others, they are full in the supine position. As the person is raised to a sitting position, these external jugulars flatten and disappear, usually at 45 degrees.

Now look for pulsations of the internal jugular veins in the area of the suprasternal notch or around the origin of the sternomastoid muscle around the clavicle. You must be able to distinguish internal jugular vein pulsation from that of the carotid artery. It is easy to confuse them because they lie close together. Use the guidelines shown in Table 19-1.

ABNORMAL FINDINGS

A carotid bruit is audible when the lumen is occluded by one half to two thirds. Bruit loudness increases as the atherosclerosis worsens until the lumen is occluded by two thirds. After that, bruit loudness decreases. When the lumen is completely occluded, the bruit disappears. Thus absence of a bruit does not ensure absence of a carotid lesion.

A murmur sounds much the same but is caused by a cardiac disorder. Some aortic valve murmurs (aortic stenosis) radiate to the neck and must be distinguished from a local bruit.

Unilateral distention of external jugular veins is due to local cause (kinking or aneurysm).

Full distended external jugular veins above 45 degrees signify increased CVP as with heart failure.

TABLE 19–1 Characteristics of Jugular Versus Carotid Pulsations		
	INTERNAL JUGULAR PULSE	CAROTID PULSE
1. **Location**	Lower, more lateral, under or behind the sternomastoid muscle	Higher and medial to this muscle
2. **Quality**	Undulant and diffuse, two visible waves per cycle	Brisk and localized, one wave per cycle
3. **Respiration**	Varies with respiration; its level descends during inspiration when intrathoracic pressure is decreased	Does not vary
4. **Palpable**	No	Yes
5. **Pressure**	Light pressure at the base of the neck easily obliterates	No change
6. **Position of person**	Level of pulse drops and disappears as the person is brought to a sitting position	Unaffected

NORMAL RANGE OF FINDINGS	ABNORMAL FINDINGS

Estimate the Jugular Venous Pressure

Think of the jugular veins as a CVP manometer attached directly to the right atrium. You can "read" the CVP at the highest level of pulsations (Fig. 19–18). Use the angle of Louis (sternal angle) as an arbitrary reference point, and compare it with the highest level of venous pulsation. Hold a vertical ruler on the sternal angle. Align a straight edge on the ruler like a T-square, and adjust the level of the horizontal straight edge to the level of pulsation. Read the level of intersection on the vertical ruler; normal jugular venous pulsation is 2 cm or less above the sternal angle. Also state the person's position, for example, "internal jugular vein pulsations 3 cm above sternal angle when elevated 30 degrees."

Elevated pressure is a level of pulsation that is more than 3 cm above the sternal angle while at 45 degrees. This occurs with heart failure.

19–18

If you cannot find the internal jugular veins, use the external jugular veins and note the point where they look collapsed. Be aware that the technique of estimating venous pressure is difficult and is not always a reliable predictor of CVP. Consistency in grading among examiners is difficult to achieve.

If venous pressure is elevated, or if you suspect heart failure, perform **hepatojugular reflux** (Fig. 19–19). Position the person comfortably supine and instruct him or her to breathe quietly through an open mouth. Hold your right hand on the right upper quadrant of the person's abdomen just below the rib cage. Watch the level of jugular pulsation as you push in with your hand. Exert firm sustained pressure for 30 seconds. This empties venous blood out of the liver sinusoids and adds its volume to the venous system. If the heart is able to pump this additional volume (i.e., if no elevated CVP is present), the jugular veins will rise for a few seconds, then recede back to previous level.

If heart failure is present, the jugular veins will elevate and stay elevated as long as you push.

19–19   Hepatojugular reflux

NORMAL RANGE OF FINDINGS	ABNORMAL FINDINGS

THE PRECORDIUM

Inspect the Anterior Chest

Arrange tangential lighting to accentuate any flicker of movement.

PULSATIONS. You may or may not see the **apical impulse,** the pulsation created as the left ventricle rotates against the chest wall during systole. When visible, it occupies the fourth or fifth intercostal space, at or inside the midclavicular line. It is easier to see in children and in those with thinner chest walls.

A **heave** or **lift** is a sustained forceful thrusting of the ventricle during systole. It occurs with ventricular hypertrophy due to increased workload. A right ventricular heave is seen at the sternal border; a left ventricular heave is seen at the apex (see Table 19–7).

Palpate the Apical Impulse

(This used to be called the *point of maximal impulse,* or PMI. Since some abnormal conditions may cause a maximal impulse to be felt elsewhere on the chest, use the term **apical impulse** specifically for the apex beat.)

Localize the apical impulse precisely using one finger pad (Fig. 19–20, *A*). Asking the person to "exhale and then hold it" aids the examiner in locating the pulsation. You may need to roll the person midway to the left to find it; note that this also displaces the apical impulse farther to the left (Fig. 19–20, *B*).

A

B

19–20 The apical impulse.

Note:

- *Location*—The apical impulse should occupy only one interspace, the fourth or fifth, and be at or medial to the midclavicular line
- *Size*—Normally 1 cm × 2 cm
- *Amplitude*—Normally a short, gentle tap
- *Duration*—Short, normally occupies only first half of systole

Cardiac enlargement:

- Left ventricular dilatation (volume overload) displaces impulse down and to left, and increases size more than one space.
- Increased force and duration but no change in location occurs with left ventricular hypertrophy and no dilatation (pressure overload) (see Table 19–7).

Not palpable with pulmonary emphysema due to overriding lungs.

The apical impulse is palpable in about half of adults. It is not palpable in obese persons or in persons with thick chest walls. With high cardiac output states (anxiety, fever, hyperthyroidism, anemia), the apical impulse increases in amplitude and duration.

NORMAL RANGE OF FINDINGS

ABNORMAL FINDINGS

Palpate Across the Precordium

Using the palmar aspects of your four fingers, gently palpate the apex, the left sternal border, and the base, searching for any other pulsations (Fig. 19–21). Normally none occur. If any are present, note the timing. Use the carotid artery pulsation as a guide, or auscultate as you palpate.

19–21

A **thrill** is a palpable vibration. It feels like the throat of a purring cat. The thrill signifies turbulent blood flow and accompanies loud murmurs. Absence of a thrill, however, does not necessarily rule out the presence of a murmur.

Accentuated first and second heart sounds and extra heart sounds also may cause abnormal pulsations.

Percussion

Percussion is used to outline the heart's borders, but it often has been displaced by the chest x-ray or echocardiogram. These are much more accurate in detecting heart enlargement. When the right ventricle enlarges, it does so in the anteroposterior diameter, which is better seen on x-ray film. Also, percussion is of limited usefulness with the female breast tissue or in an obese person or a person with a muscular chest wall.

However, there are times when your percussing hands are the only tools you have with you, such as in an outpatient setting, extended care facility, or the person's home. When you need to search for cardiac enlargement, place your stationary finger in the person's fifth intercostal space over on the left side of the chest near the anterior axillary line. Slide your stationary hand toward yourself, percussing as you go, and note the change of sound from resonance over the lung to dull (over the heart). Normally, the left border of cardiac dullness is at the midclavicular line in the fifth interspace and slopes in toward the sternum as you progress upward, so that by the second interspace the border of dullness coincides with the left sternal border. The right border of dullness normally matches the sternal border.

Cardiac enlargement is due to increased ventricular volume or wall thickness; it occurs with hypertension, CAD, heart failure, and cardiomyopathy.

Auscultation

Identify the auscultatory areas where you will listen. These include the four traditional valve "areas" (Fig. 19–22). The valve areas are not over the actual anatomic locations of the valves but are the sites on the chest wall where sounds produced by the valves are best heard. The sound radiates with the direction of blood flow. The valve areas are:

- Second right interspace—aortic valve area
- Second left interspace—pulmonic valve area
- Left lower sternal border—tricuspid valve area
- Fifth interspace at around left midclavicular line—mitral valve area

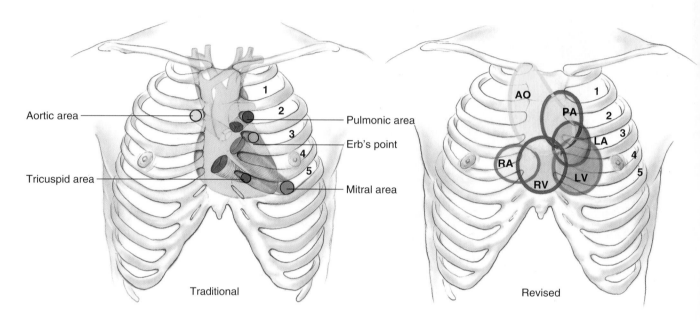

AUSCULTATORY AREAS

19–22

Do not limit your auscultation to only four locations. Sounds produced by the valves may be heard all over the precordium. (For this reason, many experts even discourage the naming of the valve areas.) Thus, learn to inch your stethoscope in a Z pattern, from the base of the heart across and down, then over to the apex. Or start at the apex and work your way up. Include the sites shown in Figure 19–22.

Recall the characteristics of a good stethoscope (see Chapter 9). Clean the endpieces with an alcohol swab; you will use both endpieces. Although all heart sounds are low frequency, the diaphragm is for relatively higher pitched sounds, and the bell is for relatively lower pitched ones.

Before you begin, alert the person: "I always listen to the heart in a number of places on the chest. Just because I am listening a long time, it does not necessarily mean that something is wrong."

After you place the stethoscope, try closing your eyes briefly to tune out any distractions. Concentrate, and listen selectively to *one sound at a time.* Consider that at least two, and perhaps three or four, sounds may be happening in less than 1 second. You cannot process everything at once. Begin with the diaphragm endpiece and use the following routine: (1) Note the rate and rhythm, (2) identify S_1 and S_2, (3) assess S_1 and S_2 separately, (4) listen for extra heart sounds, and (5) listen for murmurs.

NORMAL RANGE OF FINDINGS	ABNORMAL FINDINGS

NORMAL RANGE OF FINDINGS

NOTE THE RATE AND RHYTHM

The rate ranges normally from 60 to 100 beats per minute. (Review the full discussion of the pulse in Chapter 10 and the normal rates across age groups.) The rhythm should be regular, although **sinus arrhythmia** occurs normally in young adults and children. With sinus arrhythmia, the rhythm varies with the person's breathing, increasing at the peak of inspiration and slowing with expiration. Note any other irregular rhythm. If one occurs, check if it has any pattern, or if it is totally irregular.

When you notice any irregularity, check for a **pulse deficit** by auscultating the apical beat while simultaneously palpating the radial pulse. Count a serial measurement (one after the other) of apical beat and radial pulse. Normally, every beat you hear at the apex should perfuse to the periphery and be palpable. The two counts should be identical. When different, subtract the radial rate from the apical and record the remainder as the pulse deficit.

IDENTIFY S_1 AND S_2.

This is important because S_1 is the start of systole and thus serves as the reference point for the timing of all other cardiac sounds. Usually, you can identify S_1 instantly because you hear a pair of sounds close together (lub-dup), and S_1 is the first of the pair. This guideline works, except in the cases of the tachyarrhythmias (rates >100 per minute). Then the diastolic filling time is shortened, and the beats are too close together to distinguish. Other guidelines to distinguish S_1 from S_2 are:

- S_1 is louder than S_2 at the apex; S_2 is louder than S_1 at the base.
- S_1 coincides with the carotid artery pulse. Feel the carotid gently as you auscultate at the apex; the sound you hear as you feel each pulse is S_1 (Fig. 19–23).
- S_1 coincides with the R wave (the upstroke of the QRS complex) if the person is on an ECG monitor.

19–23

LISTEN TO S_1 AND S_2 SEPARATELY

Note whether each heart sound is normal, accentuated, diminished, or split. Inch your diaphragm across the chest as you do this.

ABNORMAL FINDINGS

Premature beat—an isolated beat is early, or a pattern occurs in which every third or fourth beat sounds early.

Irregularly irregular—no pattern to the sounds; beats come rapidly and at random intervals.

A **pulse deficit** signals a weak contraction of the ventricles; it occurs with atrial fibrillation, premature beats, and heart failure.

NORMAL RANGE OF FINDINGS

FIRST HEART SOUND (S₁). Caused by closure of the AV valves, S₁ signals the beginning of systole. You can hear it over the entire precordium, although it is loudest at the apex (Fig. 1.metimes the two sounds are equally loud at the apex, because S₁ is lower pitched than S₂.)

You can hear S₁ with the diaphragm with the person in any position and equally well in inspiration and expiration. A split S₁ is normal, but it occurs rarely. A split S₁ means you are hearing the mitral and tricuspid components separately. It is audible in the tricuspid valve area, the left lower sternal border. The split is very rapid, with the two components only 0.03 second apart.

SECOND HEART SOUND (S₂). The S₂ is associated with closure of the semilunar valves. You can hear it with the diaphragm, over the entire precordium, although S₂ is loudest at the base (Fig. 19–25).

SPLITTING OF S₂. A split S₂ is a normal phenomenon that occurs toward the end of inspiration in some people. Recall that closure of the aortic and pulmonic valves is nearly synchronous. Because of the effects of respiration on the heart described earlier, inspiration separates the timing of the two valves' closure, and the aortic valve closes 0.06 second before the pulmonic valve. Instead of one DUP, you hear a split sound—T-DUP (Fig. 19–26). During expiration, synchrony returns, and the aortic and pulmonic components fuse together. A split S₂ is heard only in the pulmonic valve area, the second left interspace.

SPLITTING OF THE SECOND HEART SOUND

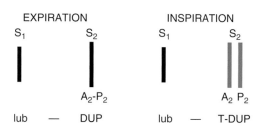

ABNORMAL FINDINGS

Causes of accentuated or diminished S₁ (see Table 19–2).

Both heart sounds are diminished with conditions that place an increased amount of tissue between the heart and your stethoscope: emphysema (hyperinflated lungs), obesity, pericardial fluid.

Accentuated or diminished S₂ (see Table 19–3).

NORMAL RANGE OF FINDINGS

When you first hear the split S_2, do *not* be tempted to ask the person to hold his or her breath so that you can concentrate on the sounds. Breath-holding will only equalize ejection times in the right and left sides of the heart and cause the split to go away. Instead, concentrate on the split as you watch the person's chest rise up and down with breathing. The split S_2 occurs about every fourth heartbeat, fading in with inhalation and fading out with exhalation.

FOCUS ON SYSTOLE, THEN ON DIASTOLE, AND LISTEN FOR ANY EXTRA HEART SOUNDS
Listen with the diaphragm, then switch to the bell, covering all auscultatory areas (Fig. 19–27). Usually, these are silent periods. When you do detect an extra heart sound, listen carefully to note its timing and characteristics. During systole, the **midsystolic click** (which is associated with mitral valve prolapse) is the most common extra sound (see Table 19–5). The third and fourth heart sounds occur in diastole; either may be normal or abnormal (see Table 19–6).

19–27

LISTEN FOR MURMURS
A murmur is a blowing, swooshing sound that occurs with turbulent blood flow in the heart or great vessels. Except for the innocent murmurs described, murmurs are abnormal. If you hear a murmur, describe it by indicating these following characteristics:

TIMING. It is crucial to define the murmur by its occurrence in systole or diastole. You must be able to identify S_1 and S_2 accurately to do this. Try to further describe the murmur as being in early, mid-, or late systole or diastole; throughout the cardiac event (termed pansystolic or holosystolic/pandiastolic or holodiastolic); and whether it obscures or muffles the heart sounds.

ABNORMAL FINDINGS

A **fixed split** is unaffected by respiration; the split is always there.

A **paradoxical split** is the opposite of what you would expect; the sounds fuse on inspiration and split on expiration (see Table 19–4).

A pathologic S_3 (ventricular gallop) occurs with heart failure and volume overload; a pathologic S_4 (atrial gallop) occurs with CAD (see Table 19–6 for a full description).

Study Tables 19–8 and 19–9 for a complete description of murmurs due to congenital defects and acquired valvular defects.

A systolic murmur may occur with a normal heart or with heart disease; a diastolic murmur always indicates heart disease.

NORMAL RANGE OF FINDINGS	ABNORMAL FINDINGS

LOUDNESS. Describe the intensity in terms of six "grades." For example, record a grade ii murmur as "ii/vi."

Grade i—Barely audible, heard only in a quiet room and then with difficulty
Grade ii—Clearly audible, but faint
Grade iii—Moderately loud, easy to hear
Grade iv—Loud, associated with a thrill palpable on the chest wall
Grade v—Very loud, heard with one corner of the stethoscope lifted off the chest wall
Grade vi—Loudest, still heard with entire stethoscope lifted just off the chest wall

PITCH. Describe the pitch as high, medium, or low. The pitch depends on the pressure and the rate of blood flow producing the murmur.

PATTERN. The intensity may follow a pattern during the cardiac phase, growing louder (crescendo), tapering off (decrescendo), or increasing to a peak and then decreasing (crescendo-decrescendo, or diamond shaped). Since the whole murmur is just milliseconds long, it takes practice to diagnose any pattern.

QUALITY. Describe the quality as musical, blowing, harsh, or rumbling.

> The murmur of mitral stenosis is rumbling, whereas that of aortic stenosis is harsh (see Table 19–9).

LOCATION. Describe the area of maximum intensity of the murmur (where it is best heard) by noting the valve area or intercostal spaces.

RADIATION. The murmur may be transmitted downstream in the direction of blood flow and may be heard in another place on the precordium, the neck, the back, or the axilla.

POSTURE. Some murmurs disappear or are enhanced by a change in position.
  Some murmurs are common in healthy children or adolescents and are termed *innocent* or *functional*. **Innocent** indicates having no valvular or other pathologic cause; **functional** is due to increased blood flow in the heart (e.g., in anemia, fever, pregnancy, hyperthyroidism). The contractile force of the heart is greater in children. This increases blood flow velocity. The increased velocity plus a smaller chest measurement makes an audible murmur.
  The innocent murmur is generally soft (grade ii), midsystolic, short, crescendo-decrescendo, and with a vibratory or musical quality ("vooot" sound like fiddle strings). Also, the innocent murmur is heard at the second or third left intercostal space and disappears with sitting, and the young person has no associated signs of cardiac dysfunction.
  Although it is important to distinguish innocent murmurs from pathologic ones, it is best to suspect all murmurs as pathologic until they are proved otherwise. Diagnostic tests such as ECG, phonocardiogram, and echocardiogram are needed to establish an accurate diagnosis.

NORMAL RANGE OF FINDINGS	ABNORMAL FINDINGS
CHANGE POSITION. After auscultating in the supine position, roll the person toward his or her left side. Listen with the bell at the apex for the presence of any diastolic filling sounds (i.e., the S₃ or S₄) (Fig. 19–28).	S_3 and S_4, and the murmur of mitral stenosis sometimes may be heard only when on the left side.

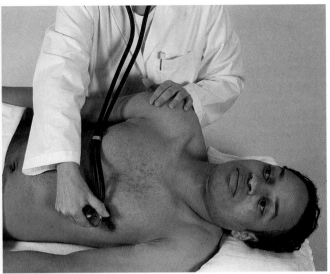

19–28

Ask the person to sit up, lean forward slightly, and exhale. Listen with the diaphragm firmly pressed at the base, right, and left sides. Check for the soft, high-pitched, early diastolic murmur of aortic or pulmonic regurgitation (Fig. 19–29).

Murmur of aortic regurgitation sometimes may be heard only when the person is leaning forward in the sitting position.

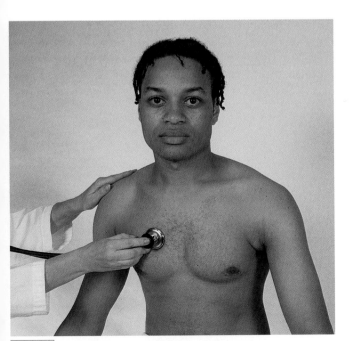

19–29

NORMAL RANGE OF FINDINGS	ABNORMAL FINDINGS

 DEVELOPMENTAL CONSIDERATIONS

Infants

The transition from fetal to pulmonic circulation occurs in the immediate new-born period. Fetal shunts normally close within 10 to 15 hours but may take up to 48 hours. Thus, you should assess the cardiovascular system during the first 24 hours and again in 2 to 3 days.

Note any extracardiac signs that may reflect heart status (particularly in the skin), liver size, and respiratory status. The skin color should be pink to pinkish brown, depending on the infant's genetic heritage. If cyanosis occurs, determine its first appearance—at or shortly after birth versus after the neonatal period. Normally, the liver is not enlarged, and the respirations are not labored. Also, note the expected parameters of weight gain throughout infancy.

Palpate the apical impulse to determine the size and position of the heart. Since the infant's heart has a more horizontal placement, expect to palpate the apical impulse at the fourth intercostal space just lateral to the midclavicular line. It may or may not be visible.

The heart rate is best auscultated because radial pulses are hard to count accurately. Use the small (pediatric size) diaphragm and bell (Fig. 19–30). The heart rate may range from 100 to 180 per minute immediately after birth, then

Failure of shunts to close, e.g., patent ductus arteriosus (PDA), atrial septal defect (ASD; see Table 19–8).

Cyanosis signals oxygen desaturation of congenital heart disease. Cyanosis at or just after birth suggests tetralogy of Fallot, transposition of great vessels, severe septal defect, severe pulmonic stenosis, or tricuspid atresia.

The most important signs of heart failure in an infant are persistent tachycardia, tachypnea, and liver enlargement. Engorged veins, gallop rhythm, and pulsus alternans also are signs. Respiratory crackles (rales) is an important sign in adults but not in infants.

Failure to thrive occurs with cardiac disease.

The apex is displaced with:

- Cardiac enlargement, shifts to the left
- Pneumothorax, shifts away from affected side
- Diaphragmatic hernia, shifts usually to right because this hernia occurs more often on the left
- Dextrocardia, a rare anomaly in which the heart is located on right side of chest

Persistent tachycardia is >200 per minute in newborns, or >150 per minute in infants.

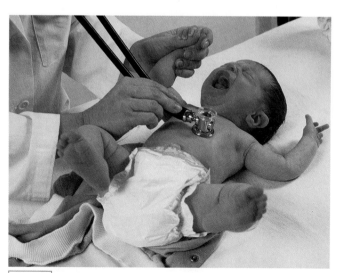

19–30

NORMAL RANGE OF FINDINGS	ABNORMAL FINDINGS

stabilize to an average of 120 to 140 per minute. Infants normally have wide fluctuations with activity, from 170 per minute or more with crying or being active to 70 to 90 per minute with sleeping. Variations are greatest at birth and are even more so with premature babies (see Table 10–3).

Expect the heart rhythm to have sinus arrhythmia, the phasic speeding up or slowing down with the respiratory cycle.

Rapid rates make it more challenging to evaluate heart sounds. Expect heart sounds to be louder in infants than in adults because of the infant's thinner chest wall. Also, S_2 has a higher pitch and is sharper than S_1. Splitting of S_2 just after the height of inspiration is common, not at birth, but beginning a few hours after birth.

Murmurs in the immediate newborn period do not necessarily indicate congenital heart disease. Murmurs are relatively common in the first 2 to 3 days because of fetal shunt closure. These murmurs are usually grade i or ii, are systolic, accompany no other signs of cardiac disease, and disappear in 2 to 3 days. The murmur of PDA is a continuous machinery murmur, which disappears by 2 to 3 days. On the other hand, absence of a murmur in the immediate newborn period does not ensure a perfect heart; congenital defects can be present that are not signaled by an early murmur. It is best to listen frequently and to note and describe any murmur according to the characteristics listed on p. 510.

Children

Note any extracardiac or cardiac signs that may indicate heart disease: poor weight gain, developmental delay, persistent tachycardia, tachypnea, dyspnea on exertion, cyanosis, and clubbing. Note that clubbing of fingers and toes usually does not appear until late in the 1st year, even with severe cyanotic defects.

The apical impulse is sometimes visible in children with thin chest walls. Note any obvious bulge or any heave—these are not normal.

Palpate the apical impulse: in the fourth intercostal space to the left of the midclavicular line until age 4; at the fourth interspace at the midclavicular line from age 4 to 6; and in the fifth interspace to the right of the midclavicular line at age 7 (Fig. 19–31).

ABNORMAL FINDINGS (column):

Bradycardia is <90 per minute in newborns or <60 in older infants or children. This causes a serious drop in cardiac output because the small muscle mass of their hearts cannot increase stroke volume significantly.

Investigate any irregularity except sinus arrhythmia.

Fixed split S_2 indicates ASD (see Table 19–8).

Persistent murmur after 2 to 3 days, holosystolic murmurs or those that last into diastole, and those that are loud—all warrant further evaluation.

A precordial bulge to the left of the sternum with a hyperdynamic precordium signals cardiac enlargement. The bulge occurs because the cartilaginous rib cage is more compliant.

A substernal heave occurs with right ventricular enlargement, and an apical heave occurs with left ventricular hypertrophy.

The apical impulse moves laterally with cardiac enlargement.

Thrill (palpable vibration).

19–31

The average heart rate slows as the child grows older, although it is still variable with rest or activity (see Table 10–2).

The heart rhythm remains characterized by sinus arrhythmia. Physiologic S_3 is common in children (see Table 19–6). It occurs in early diastole, just after S_2, and is a dull soft sound that is best heard at the apex.

A **venous hum**—due to turbulence of blood flow in the jugular venous system—is common in normal children and has no pathologic significance. It is a continuous, low-pitched, soft hum that is heard throughout the cycle, although it is loudest in diastole. Listen with the bell over the supraclavicular fossa at the medial third of the clavicle, especially on the right, or over the upper anterior chest. The venous hum is usually not affected by respiration, may sound louder when the child stands, and is easily obliterated by occluding the jugular veins in the neck with your fingers. The latter maneuver helps differentiate the insignificant venous hum from other organic cardiac murmurs (e.g., PDA).

Heart murmurs that are innocent (or functional) in origin are very common through childhood. Some authors say they have a 30% occurrence, and some authors say nearly all children may demonstrate a murmur at some time. Most innocent murmurs have these characteristics: soft, relatively short systolic ejection murmur; medium pitch; vibratory; best heard at the left lower sternal or mid-sternal border, with no radiation to the apex, base, or back.

It is important to distinguish innocent murmurs from pathologic ones. This may involve referral to another examiner or the performance of diagnostic tests such as the ECG or echocardiogram.

For the child whose murmur has been shown to be innocent, it is very important that the parents understand this completely. They need to believe that this murmur is just a "noise" and has no pathologic significance. Otherwise, the parents may become overprotective and limit activity for the child, which may result in the child developing a negative self-concept.

The Pregnant Female

The vital signs usually yield an increase in resting pulse rate of 10 to 15 beats per minute and a drop in blood pressure from the normal prepregnancy level. The blood pressure decreases to its lowest point during the second trimester and then slowly rises during the third trimester. The blood pressure varies with position. It is usually lowest in left lateral recumbent position, a bit higher when supine (except for some who experience hypotension when supine), and highest when sitting (Cunningham et al., 2001).

Inspection of the skin often shows a mild hyperemia in light-skinned women because the increased cutaneous blood flow tries to eliminate the excess heat generated by the increased metabolism. Palpation of the apical impulse is higher and lateral compared with the normal position, as the enlarging uterus elevates the diaphragm and displaces the heart up and to the left and rotates it on its long axis.

Auscultation of the heart sounds shows changes due to the increased blood volume and workload:

- Heart sounds
  Exaggerated splitting of S_1 and increased loudness of S_1
  A loud, easily heard S_3
- Heart murmurs
  A systolic murmur in 90% which disappears soon after delivery
  A soft, diastolic murmur heard transiently in 19%
  A continuous murmur arising from breast vasculature in 10% (Cunningham et al., 2001).

The last-mentioned murmur is termed a **mammary souffle** (pronounced SOOF′ f′l), which occurs near term or when the mother is lactating; it is due to in-

Suspect pregnancy-induced hypertension with a sustained rise of 30 mm Hg systolic or 15 mm Hg diastolic under basal conditions.

NORMAL RANGE OF FINDINGS	ABNORMAL FINDINGS

creased blood flow through the internal mammary artery. The murmur is heard in the second, third, or fourth intercostal space; it is continuous, although it is accented in systole. You can obliterate it by pressure with the stethoscope or one finger lateral to the murmur. This distinguishes it from the murmur of aortic stenosis, aortic insufficiency, or PDA.

The ECG has no changes except for a slight left axis deviation due to the change in the heart's position.

The Aging Adult

A gradual rise in systolic blood pressure is common with aging; the diastolic blood pressure stays fairly constant with a resulting widening of pulse pressure. Some older adults experience **orthostatic hypotension,** a sudden drop in blood pressure when rising to sit or stand.

Use caution in palpating and auscultating the carotid artery. Avoid pressure in the carotid sinus area, which could cause a reflex slowing of the heart rate. Also, pressure on the carotid artery could compromise circulation if the artery is already narrowed by atherosclerosis.

When measuring jugular venous pressure, view the right internal jugular vein. The aorta stiffens, dilates, and elongates with aging, which may compress the left neck veins and obscure pulsations on the left side (Fleg, 1990).

The chest often increases in anteroposterior diameter with aging. This makes it more difficult to palpate the apical impulse and to hear the splitting of S_2. The S_4 often occurs in older people with no known cardiac disease. Systolic murmurs are common, occurring in over 50% of aging people (Fleg, 1990).

Occasional premature ectopic beats are common and do not necessarily indicate underlying heart disease. When in doubt, obtain an ECG. However, consider that the ECG only records for one isolated minute in time and may need to be supplemented by a test of 24-hour ambulatory heart monitoring.

The S_3 is associated with heart failure and is always abnormal over age 35 (see Table 19–10).

SUMMARY CHECKLIST: Heart and Neck Vessels Exam

1. Neck
Carotid pulse—Observe and palpate
Observe jugular venous pulse
Estimate jugular venous pressure

2. Precordium
Inspection and palpation
1. Describe location of apical impulse
2. Note any heave (lift) or thrill

Auscultation
1. Identify anatomic areas where you listen
2. Note rate and rhythm of heartbeat
3. Identify S_1 and S_2 and note any variation
4. Listen in systole and diastole for any extra heart sounds

5. Listen in systole and diastole for any murmurs
6. Repeat sequence with bell
7. Listen at the apex with person in left lateral position
8. Listen at the base with person in sitting position

See Health Promotion Guide on CD

Application and Critical Thinking

SAMPLE CHARTING

SUBJECTIVE

No chest pain, dyspnea, orthopnea, cough, fatigue, or edema. No past history of hypertension, abnormal blood tests, heart murmur, or rheumatic fever in self. Last ECG 2 yrs. PTA, result normal. No stress ECG or other heart tests.

Continued

Family history: father with obesity, smoking, and hypertension, treated $\bar{c}$ diuretic medication. No other family history significant for cardiovascular disease.

Personal habits: diet balanced in 4 food groups, 2 to 3 c. regular coffee/day; no smoking; alcohol, 1 to 2 beers occasionally on weekend; exercise, runs 2 miles, 3 to 4 ×/week; no prescription or OTC medications or street drugs.

OBJECTIVE

Neck. Carotids 2+ and = bilaterally. Internal jugular vein pulsations present when supine, and disappear when elevated to a 45° position.

Precordium. Inspection. No visible pulsations, no heave or lift.

Palpation. Apical impulse in 5th ics at left midclavicular line, no thrill.

Auscultation. Rate 68 beats per minute, rhythm regular, S_1–S_2 are normal, not diminished or accentuated, no S_3, no S_4 or other extra sounds, no murmurs.

FOCUSED ASSESSMENT: CLINICAL CASE STUDY

Mr. N.V. is a 53-year-old white male woodcutter admitted to the CCU at University Medical Center (UMC) with chest pain.

SUBJECTIVE

1 year PTA—N.V. admitted to UMC with crushing substernal chest pain, radiating to L shoulder, accompanied by nausea, vomiting, diaphoresis.

Diagnosed as MI, hospitalized 7 days, discharged with nitroglycerin prn for anginal pain.

Did not return to work. Activity included walking 1 mile/day, hunting. Had occasional episodes of chest pain with exercise, relieved by rest.

1 day PTA—had increasing frequency of chest pain, about every 2 hours, lasting few minutes, saw pain as warning to go to MD.

Day of admission—severe substernal chest pain ("like someone sitting on my chest") unrelieved by rest. Saw personal MD, while in office had episode of chest pain as last year's, accompanied by diaphoresis, no N & V or SOB, relieved by 1 nitroglycerin. Transferred to UMC by paramedics. No further pain since admission 2 hours ago.

Family hx.—mother died of MI at age 57.

Personal habits—smokes $1\frac{1}{2}$ pack cigarettes daily × 34 years, no alcohol, diet—trying to limit fat and fried food, still high in added salt.

OBJECTIVE

Extremities. Skin pink, no cyanosis. Upper extrem.—capillary refill sluggish, no clubbing. Lower extrem.—no edema, no hair growth 10 cm below knee bilaterally.

Pulses—

carotid	brachial	radial	femoral	popliteal	P.T.	D.P.	
2+	2+	2+	2+	0	0	1+	all = bilaterally

B/P R arm 104/66

Neck. External jugulars flat. Internal jugular pulsations present when supine and absent when elevated to 45°.

Precordium. Inspection. Apical impulse visible 5th ics, 7 cm left of midsternal line, no heave.

Palpation. Apical impulse palpable in 5th and 6th ics. No thrill.

Auscultation. Apical rate 92 regular, S_1–S_2 are normal, not diminished or accentuated, no S_3 or S_4, grade iii/vi systolic murmur present at left lower sternal border.

ASSESSMENT

Substernal chest pain
Systolic murmur
Ineffective tissue perfusion R/T interruption in flow
Decreased cardiac output R/T reduction in stroke volume

NURSING DIAGNOSES COMMONLY ASSOCIATED WITH CARDIOVASCULAR DISORDERS

RELATED FACTORS (Etiology)	DEFINING CHARACTERISTICS (Symptoms and Signs)

DIAGNOSIS: Decreased Cardiac output

Reduction in stroke volume as a result of
  Electrical malfunction (alteration in conduction, rate, or
    rhythm)
  Mechanical malfunction (alteration in afterload, inotropic
    changes in heart, or preload)
  Structural problems secondary to congenital abnomalities,
    trauma
	Abnormal heart sounds
	Altered blood gases
	Changes in mental status
	Cool, clammy skin
	Cough
	Crackles (rales)
	Cyanosis or pallor
	Decreased peripheral pulses
	Dyspnea
	Dysrhythmias, electrocardiographic changes
	Edema, dependent
	Fatigue
	Frothy sputum
	Jugular vein distention
	Orthopnea
	Restlessness
	Syncope
	Tachycardia
	Urine output decreased
	Variations in hemodynamic readings
	Weight gain, sudden

DIAGNOSIS: Ineffective Tissue perfusion

Exchange problems
Hypervolemia
Hypovolemia
Interruption of flow
	Cardiopulmonary
	  Chest pain (relieved by rest)
	  Increased heart rate
	  Increased respiratory rate
	  Shortness of breath
	Cerebral
	  Alteration in thought processes
	  Blurred vision
	  Changes in level of consciousness
	  Confusion
	  Restlessness
	  Syncope/vertigo

DIAGNOSIS: Dysfunctional Grieving

Effects of loss of function or body part Absence of anticipatory grieving Actual or perceived loss of health or social status, signifi- cant other, or valued object Multiple losses or crises Changes in lifestyle Decreased support system Thwarted grieving in response to a loss Lack of resolution of previous grieving response Ambivalent feelings toward loss	Changes in sleep patterns Feelings of anger, guilt, worthlessness, denial, sorrow Decreased interest in personal appearance Interference with life functioning Difficulty in expressing loss Fear of future Absence of emotion Suicidal thoughts Social withdrawal Weight loss Amenorrhea Decreased level of activity Reliving of past experiences Alteration in concentration Developmental regression Hyperactivity

Continued

RELATED FACTORS (Etiology)	DEFINING CHARACTERISTICS (Symptoms and Signs)

DIAGNOSIS: Fatigue

Decreased/increased metabolic energy production	Verbalization of an unremitting and overwhelming lack of energy
Increased energy requirements to perform activities of daily living	Inability to maintain usual routines
Overwhelming psychological or emotional demands	Increase in physical complaints
Excessive social and/or role demands	Inability to concentrate
States of discomfort	Decreased performance
Altered body chemistry	Accident prone
Medications	Lethargy or listlessness
Drug withdrawal	Disinterest in surroundings/introspection
Chemotherapy	Decreased libido

OTHER RELATED NURSING DIAGNOSES

ACTUAL	RISK/WELLNESS
Activity intolerance (see Chapter 18)	**Risk**
Anxiety (see Chapter 18)	Risk for Injury
Ineffective Breathing pattern	**Wellness**
Ineffective Coping	Health-seeking behavior R/T learning a low-fat diet
Fear	
Fluid volume deficit	
Fluid volume excess	
Impaired Home maintenance (see Chapter 14)	
Impaired physical Mobility	
Noncompliance	
Pain (see Chapter 14)	
Powerlessness	
Ineffective Role performance	
Self-care deficit	
Ineffective Sexuality patterns	

 ## ASSESSMENT VIDEO CRITICAL THINKING QUESTIONS

The Saunders *Physical Examination and Health Assessment* video "Cardiovascular System: Heart and Neck Vessels" will direct you to consider the following:

1. What cardiac risk factors are important to explore during the health history? How do they affect cardiovascular function?

2. How would you modify your technique when assessing an older adult's neck vessels?

3. How do you describe sinus arrhythmia and what does it signify?

4. What heart sounds should you expect to hear in a person with aortic stenosis?

Abnormal Findings

TABLE 19–2: Variations in S_1

The intensity of S_1 depends on three factors: (1) position of AV valve at the start of systole, (2) structure of the valve leaflets, and (3) how quickly pressure rises in the ventricle.

	FACTOR	EXAMPLES
Loud (Accentuated) S_1 S_1 S_2	1. Position of AV valve at start of systole—wide open and no time to drift together 2. Change in valve structure—calcification of valve, needs increasing ventricular pressure to close the valve against increased atrial pressure	Hyperkinetic states where blood velocity is increased: exercise, fever, anemia, hyperthyroidism Mitral stenosis with leaflets still mobile
Faint (Diminished) S_1 S_1 S_2	1. Position of AV valve—delayed conduction from atria to ventricles. Mitral valve drifts shut before ventricular contraction closes it 2. Change in valve structure—extreme calcification, which limits mobility 3. More forceful atrial contraction into noncompliant ventricle; delays or diminishes ventricular contraction	First-degree heart block (prolonged PR interval) Mitral insufficiency Severe hypertension—systemic or pulmonary
Varying Intensity of S_1 S_1 S_2 S_1 S_2	1. Position of AV valve varies before closing from beat to beat 2. Atria and ventricles beat independently	Atrial fibrillation—irregularly-irregular rhythm Complete heart block with changing PR interval
Split S_1 S_1 S_2 T M	Mitral and tricuspid components are heard separately	Normal but uncommon

TABLE 19–3: Variations in S₂

	CONDITION	EXAMPLE

Accentuated S₂

	1. Higher closing pressure	Systemic hypertension, ringing or booming S_2
	2. Exercise and excitement increase pressure in aorta	
	3. Pulmonary hypertension	Mitral stenosis, heart failure
	4. Semilunar valves calcified but still mobile	Aortic or pulmonic stenosis

Diminished S₂

	1. A fall in systemic blood pressure causes a decrease in valve strength	Shock
	2. Semilunar valves thickened and calcified, with decreased mobility	Aortic or pulmonic stenosis

TABLE 19–4: Variations in Split S₂

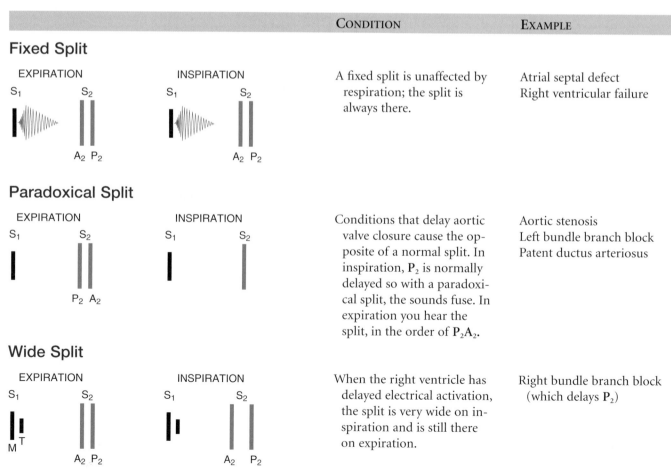

Normal Splitting

EXPIRATION
S_1 S_2
A_2-P_2

INSPIRATION
S_1 S_2
A_2 P_2

	CONDITION	EXAMPLE

Fixed Split

EXPIRATION
S_1 S_2
A_2 P_2

INSPIRATION
S_1 S_2
A_2 P_2

| A fixed split is unaffected by respiration; the split is always there. | Atrial septal defect Right ventricular failure |

Paradoxical Split

EXPIRATION
S_1 S_2
P_2 A_2

INSPIRATION
S_1 S_2

| Conditions that delay aortic valve closure cause the opposite of a normal split. In inspiration, P_2 is normally delayed so with a paradoxical split, the sounds fuse. In expiration you hear the split, in the order of P_2A_2. | Aortic stenosis Left bundle branch block Patent ductus arteriosus |

Wide Split

EXPIRATION
S_1 S_2
M ^{T}
A_2 P_2

INSPIRATION
S_1 S_2
A_2 P_2

| When the right ventricle has delayed electrical activation, the split is very wide on inspiration and is still there on expiration. | Right bundle branch block (which delays P_2) |

TABLE 19–5: Systolic Extra Sounds

Early systolic	Mid-/late systolic
Ejection click	Midsystolic (mitral) click
Aortic prosthetic valve sounds	

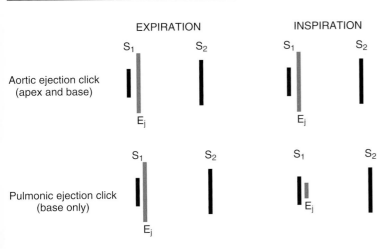

Ejection Click

The ejection click occurs early in systole at the start of ejection, because it results from opening of the semilunar valves. Normally, the SL valves open silently, but in the presence of stenosis (e.g., aortic stenosis, pulmonic stenosis) their opening makes a sound. It is short and high pitched, with a click quality, and is heard better with the diaphragm.

The aortic ejection click is heard at the second right interspace and apex, and may be loudest at the apex. Its intensity does not change with respiration. The pulmonic ejection click is best heard in the second left interspace and often grows softer with inspiration.

Aortic Prosthetic Valve Sounds

As a sequela of modern technologic intervention for heart problems, some people now have *iatrogenically* induced heart sounds. The opening of an aortic ball-in-cage prosthesis (e.g., Starr-Edwards prosthesis) produces an early systolic sound. This sound is less intense with a tilting disk prosthesis (e.g., Bjork-Shiley prosthesis) and is absent with a tissue prosthesis (e.g., porcine).

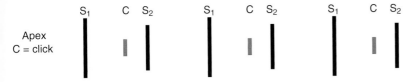

Midsystolic Click

Although it is systolic, this is not an ejection click. It is associated with **mitral valve prolapse,** in which the mitral valve leaflets not only close with contraction but balloon back up into the left atrium. During ballooning, the sudden tensing of the valve leaflets and the chordae tendineae creates the click.

The sound occurs in mid- to late systole and is short and high pitched, with a click quality. It is best heard with the diaphragm, at the apex, but also may be heard at the left lower sternal border. The click usually is followed by a systolic murmur. The click and murmur move with postural change; when the person assumes a squatting position, the click may move closer to S_2, and the murmur may sound louder and delayed. The Valsalva maneuver also moves the click closer to S_2.

TABLE 19–6: Diastolic Extra Sounds

Early diastole	Mid-diastole	Late diastole
Opening snap	Third heart sound	Fourth heart sound
Mitral prosthetic valve sound	Summation sound ($S_3 + S_4$)	Pacemaker-induced sound

Opening Snap

Normally the opening of the AV valves is silent. In the presence of stenosis, increasingly higher atrial pressure is required to open the valve. The deformed valve opens with a noise: the opening snap. It is sharp and high pitched, with a snapping quality. It sounds after S_2 and is best heard with the diaphragm at the third or fourth left interspace at the sternal border, less well at the apex.

The opening snap usually is not an isolated sound. As a sign of mitral stenosis, the opening snap usually ushers in the low-pitched diastolic rumbling murmur of that condition.

Mitral Prosthetic Valve Sound

An iatrogenic sound, the opening of a ball-in-cage mitral prosthesis gives an early diastolic sound: an opening click just after S_2. It is loud, is heard over the whole precordium, and is loudest at the apex and left lower sternal border.

Third Heart Sound

The S_3 is a ventricular filling sound. It occurs in early diastole during the rapid filling phase. Your hearing quickly accommodates to the S_3, so it is best heard when you listen initially. It sounds after S_2 but later than an opening snap would be. It is a dull, soft sound, and it is low pitched, like "distant thunder." It is heard best in a quiet room, at the apex, with the bell held lightly (just enough to form a seal), and with the person in the left lateral position.

The S_3 can be confused with a split S_2. Use these guidelines to distinguish the S_3:

- *Location*—The S_3 is heard at the apex or left lower sternal border; the split S_2 at the base.
- *Respiratory variation*—The S_3 does not vary in timing with respirations; the split S_2 does.
- *Pitch*—The S_3 is lower pitched; the pitch of the split S_2 stays the same.

The S_3 may be normal (physiologic) or abnormal (pathologic). The **physiologic** S_3 is heard frequently in children and young adults; it occasionally may persist after age 40, especially in women. The normal S_3 usually disappears when the person sits up.

In adults, the S_3 is usually abnormal. The **pathologic** S_3 is also called a **ventricular gallop** or an S_3 **gallop,** and it persists when sitting up. The S_3 indicates decreased compliance of the ventricles, as in heart failure. The S_3 may be the earliest sign of heart failure. The S_3 may originate from either the left or the right ventricle; a left-sided S_3 is heard at the apex in the left lateral position, and a right-sided S_3 is heard at the left lower sternal border with the person supine and is louder in inspiration.

The S_3 occurs also with conditions of volume overload, such as mitral regurgitation and aortic or tricuspid regurgitation. The S_3 is also found in high cardiac output states in the absence of heart disease, such as hyperthyroidism, anemia, and pregnancy. When the primary condition is corrected, the gallop disappears.   *Continued*

TABLE 19-6: Diastolic Extra Sounds—cont'd

$S_4 \; S_1$ S_2 $S_4 \; S_1$ S_2

daLUB   –   dup   daLUB   –   dup

Fourth Heart Sound

The S_4 is a ventricular filling sound. It occurs when the atria contract late in diastole. It is heard immediately before S_1. This is a very soft sound, of very low pitch. You need a good bell, and you must listen for it. It is heard best at the apex, with the person in left lateral position.

A **physiologic** S_4 may occur in adults older than 40 or 50 with no evidence of cardiovascular disease, especially after exercise.

A **pathologic** S_4 is termed an **atrial gallop** or an S_4 **gallop.** It occurs with decreased compliance of the ventricle (e.g., coronary artery disease, cardiomyopathy) and with systolic overload (afterload), including outflow obstruction to the ventricle (aortic stenosis) and systemic hypertension. A left-sided S_4 occurs with these conditions. It is heard best at the apex, in the left lateral position.

A right-sided S_4 is less common. It is heard at the left lower sternal border and may increase with inspiration. It occurs with pulmonary stenosis or pulmonary hypertension.

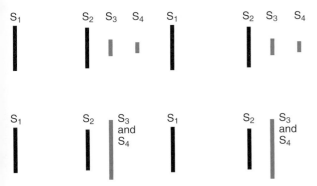

Summation Sound

When both the pathologic S_3 and S_4 are present, a quadruple rhythm is heard. Often, in cases of cardiac stress, one response is tachycardia. During rapid rates, the diastolic filling time shortens and the S_3 and S_4 move closer together. They sound superimposed in mid-diastole, and you hear one loud, prolonged, summated sound, often louder than either S_1 or S_2.

EXTRACARDIAC SOUNDS

S_1 S_2 S_1

Pericardial Friction Rub

Inflammation of the precordium gives rise to a friction rub. The sound is high pitched and scratchy, like sandpaper being rubbed. It is best heard with the diaphragm, with the person sitting up and leaning forward, and with the breath held in expiration.

A friction rub can be heard any place on the precordium but usually is best heard at the apex and left lower sternal border, places where the pericardium comes in close contact with the chest wall. Timing may be systolic and diastolic. The friction rub of pericarditis is common during the 1st week following a myocardial infarction and may last only a few hours.

TABLE 19–7: Abnormal Pulsations on the Precordium

Base

A **thrill** in the second and third right interspaces occurs with severe aortic stenosis and systemic hypertension.

A **thrill** in the second and third left interspaces occurs with pulmonic stenosis and pulmonic hypertension.

Left Sternal Border

A **lift** (**heave**) occurs with right ventricular hypertrophy, as found in pulmonic valve disease, pulmonic hypertension, and chronic lung disease. You feel a diffuse lifting impulse during systole at the left lower sternal border. It may be associated with retraction at the apex, because the left ventricle is rotated posteriorly by the enlarged right ventricle.

Apex

Cardiac enlargement displaces the apical impulse laterally and over a wider area when left ventricular hypertrophy and dilatation are present. This is **volume overload,** as in mitral regurgitation, aortic regurgitation, and left-to-right shunts.

Apex

The apical impulse is increased in force and duration but is not necessarily displaced to the left when left ventricular hypertrophy occurs alone without dilatation. This is **pressure overload,** as found in aortic stenosis or systemic hypertension.

TABLE 19–8: Congenital Heart Defects

DESCRIPTION	CLINICAL DATA

Patent Ductus Arteriosus (PDA)

Persistence of the channel joining left pulmonary artery to aorta. This is normal in the fetus and usually closes spontaneously within hours of birth.

S: Usually no symptoms in early childhood; growth and development are normal.

O: Blood pressure has wide pulse pressure and bounding peripheral pulses due to rapid runoff of blood into low-resistance pulmonary bed during diastole. Thrill often palpable at left upper sternal border. The continuous murmur heard in systole and diastole is called a machinery murmur.

Atrial Septal Defect (ASD)

Abnormal opening in the atrial septum, resulting usually in left-to-right shunt and causing large increase in pulmonary blood flow.

S: Defect is remarkably well tolerated. Symptoms in infant are rare; growth and development normal. Children and young adults have mild fatigue and DOE.

O: Sternal lift often present. S_2 has fixed split, with P_2 often louder than A_2. Murmur is systolic, ejection, medium pitch, best heard at base in second left interspace. Murmur caused not by shunt itself but by increased blood flow through pulmonic valve.

Ventricular Septal Defect (VSD)

Abnormal opening in septum between the ventricles, usually subaortic area. The size and exact position vary considerably.

S: Small defects are asymptomatic. Infants with large defects have poor growth, slow weight gain; later look pale, thin, delicate. May have feeding problems; DOE; frequent respiratory infections; and when the condition is severe, heart failure.

O: Loud, harsh holosystolic murmur, best heard at left lower sternal border, may be accompanied by thrill. Large defects also have soft diastolic murmur at apex (mitral flow murmur) due to increased blood flow through mitral valve.

S = subjective data; O = objective data.

Table continued on following page

TABLE 19–8: Congenital Heart Defects—cont'd

DESCRIPTION	CLINICAL DATA

Tetralogy of Fallot

Four components: (1) right ventricular outflow stenosis, (2) VSD, (3) right ventricular hypertrophy, and (4) overriding aorta. *Result:* shunts a lot of venous blood directly into aorta away from pulmonary system, so blood never gets oxygenated.

S: Severe cyanosis, not in first months of life but develops as infant grows and RV outflow (i.e., pulmonic) stenosis gets worse. Cyanosis with crying and exertion at first, then at rest. Uses squatting posture after starts walking. DOE common. Development is slowed.

O: Thrill palpable at left lower sternal border. S_1 normal; S_2 has A_2 loud and P_2 diminished or absent. Murmur is systolic, loud, crescendo-decrescendo.

Coarctation of the Aorta

Severe narrowing of descending aorta, usually at the junction of the ductus arteriosus and the aortic arch, just distal to the origin of the left subclavian artery. Results in increased work load on left ventricle. Associated with defects of aortic valve in most cases, as well as associated patent ductus arteriosus; and associated ventricular septal defect (Braunwald, 1997).

S: In infants with associated lesions or symptoms, diagnosis occurs in first few months as symptoms of heart failure develop. For asymptomatic children and adolescents, growth and development are normal. Diagnosis usually accidental due to blood pressure findings. Adolescents may complain of vague lower extremity cramping that is worse with exercise.

O: Upper extremity hypertension over 20 mm Hg higher than lower extremity measures is a hallmark of coarctation. Another important sign is absent or greatly diminished femoral pulses. A systolic murmur is heard best at the left sternal border, radiating to the back.

S = subjective data; O = objective data.

TABLE 19–9: Murmurs Due to Valvular Defects

Midsystolic Ejection Murmurs

Due to forward flow through semilunar valves

SYSTOLE   DIASTOLE

S1   S2   S1   S2   S1   S2

DESCRIPTION	CLINICAL DATA

Aortic Stenosis

Calcification of aortic valve cusps restricts forward flow of blood during systole; LV hypertrophy develops.

S: Fatigue, DOE, palpitation, dizziness, fainting, anginal pain.
O: Pallor, slow diminished radial pulse, low blood pressure, and auscultatory gap are common. Apical impulse sustained and displaced to left. Thrill in systole over second and third right interspaces and right side of neck. S_1 normal, often ejection click present, often paradoxical split S_2, S_4 present with LV hypertrophy.
Murmur: Loud, harsh, midsystolic, crescendo-decrescendo, loudest at second right interspace, radiates widely to side of neck, down left sternal border, or apex.

Pulmonic Stenosis

Calcification of pulmonic valve restricts forward flow of blood.

O: Thrill in systole at second and third left interspace, ejection click often present after S_1, diminished S_2 and usually with wide split, S_4 common with RV hypertrophy.
Murmur: Systolic, medium pitch, coarse, crescendo-decrescendo (diamond shape), best heard at second left interspace, radiates to left and neck.

S = subjective data; O = objective data.

Table continued on following page

ABNORMAL FINDINGS

TABLE 19–9: Murmurs Due to Valvular Defects—cont'd

Pansystolic Regurgitant Murmurs

Due to backward flow of blood from area of higher
pressure to one of lower pressure

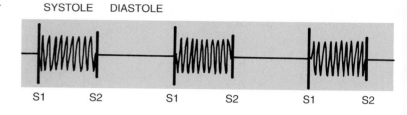

SYSTOLE   DIASTOLE

S1   S2   S1   S2   S1   S2

DESCRIPTION	CLINICAL DATA

Mitral Regurgitation

Stream of blood regurgitates back into LA
during systole through incompetent mitral
valve. In diastole, blood passes back into
LV again along with new flow; results in LV
dilatation and hypertrophy.

S: Fatigue, palpitation, orthopnea, PND
O: Thrill in systole at apex. Lift at apex.
   Apical impulse displaced down and to left.
   S_1 diminished, S_2 accentuated, S_3 at apex
   often present.
Murmur: Pansystolic, often loud, blowing,
   best heard at apex, radiates well to left
   axilla.

Tricuspid Regurgitation

Backflow of blood through incompetent tricuspid valve into RA.

O: Engorged pulsating neck veins, liver enlarged. Lift at sternum if RV hypertrophy
   present, often thrill at left lower sternal
   border.
Murmur: Soft, blowing, pansystolic, best
   heard at left lower sternal border, increases
   with inspiration.

S = subjective data; O = objective data.

Continued

TABLE 19–9: Murmurs Due to Valvular Defects—cont'd

Diastolic Rumbles of AV Valves

Filling murmurs at low pressures, best heard with bell lightly touching skin

SYSTOLE DIASTOLE

OS OS OS

S1 S2 S1 S2 S1 S2

DESCRIPTION	CLINICAL DATA

Mitral Stenosis

Calcified mitral valve will not open properly, impedes forward flow of blood into LV during diastole. Results in LA enlarged and LA pressure increased.

S: Fatigue, palpitations, DOE, orthopnea, occasional PND or pulmonary edema.
O: Diminished, often irregular arterial pulse. Lift at apex, diastolic thrill common at apex. S_1 accentuated; opening snap after S_2 heard over wide area of precordium, followed by murmur.
Murmur: Low-pitched diastolic rumble, best heard at apex, with person in left lateral position; does not radiate.

Tricuspid Stenosis

Calcification of tricuspid valve impedes forward flow into RV during diastole.

O: Diminished arterial pulse, jugular venous pulse prominent.
Murmur: Diastolic rumble; best heard at left lower sternal border; louder in inspiration.

S = subjective data; O = objective data.

Table continued on following page

TABLE 19–9: Murmurs Due to Valvular Defects—cont'd

Early Diastolic Murmurs

Due to SL valve incompetence

Aortic Regurgitation

DESCRIPTION	CLINICAL DATA

Stream of blood regurgitates back through incompetent aortic valve into LV during diastole. LV dilatation and hypertrophy due to increased LV stroke volume. Rapid ejection of large stroke volume into poorly filled aorta, then rapid runoff in diastole as part of blood pushed back into LV.

S: Only minor symptoms for many years, then rapid deterioration: DOE, PND, angina, dizziness.
O: Bounding "water-hammer" pulse in carotid, brachial, and femoral arteries. Blood pressure has wide pulse pressure. Pulsations in cervical and suprasternal area, apical impulse displaced to left and down, apical impulse feels brief.
Murmur starts almost simultaneously with S_2: soft high pitched, blowing diastolic, decrescendo, best heard at third left interspace at base, as person sits up and leans forward, radiates down.

Pulmonic Regurgitation

Backflow of blood through incompetent pulmonic valve, from pulmonary artery to RV.

Murmur has same timing and characteristics as that of aortic regurgitation, and is hard to distinguish on physical examination.

S = subjective data; O = objective data.

TABLE 19–10: Clinical Portrait of Heart Failure

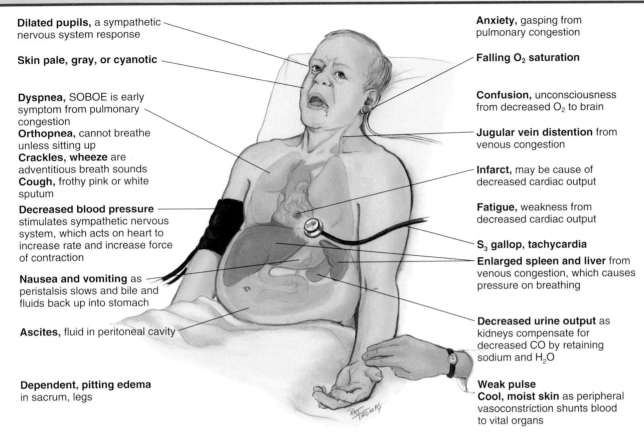

Dilated pupils, a sympathetic nervous system response

Skin pale, gray, or cyanotic

Dyspnea, SOBOE is early symptom from pulmonary congestion
Orthopnea, cannot breathe unless sitting up
Crackles, wheeze are adventitious breath sounds
Cough, frothy pink or white sputum

Decreased blood pressure stimulates sympathetic nervous system, which acts on heart to increase rate and increase force of contraction

Nausea and vomiting as peristalsis slows and bile and fluids back up into stomach

Ascites, fluid in peritoneal cavity

Dependent, pitting edema in sacrum, legs

Anxiety, gasping from pulmonary congestion

Falling O_2 saturation

Confusion, unconsciousness from decreased O_2 to brain

Jugular vein distention from venous congestion

Infarct, may be cause of decreased cardiac output

Fatigue, weakness from decreased cardiac output

S_3 gallop, tachycardia

Enlarged spleen and liver from venous congestion, which causes pressure on breathing

Decreased urine output as kidneys compensate for decreased CO by retaining sodium and H_2O

Weak pulse
Cool, moist skin as peripheral vasoconstriction shunts blood to vital organs

Decreased cardiac output occurs when the heart fails as a pump, and the circulation becomes backed up and congested.

Signs and symptoms of heart failure come from two basic mechanisms: (1) the heart's inability to pump enough blood to meet the metabolic demands of the body, and (2) the kidney's compensatory mechanisms of abnormal retention of sodium and water to compensate for the decreased cardiac output. This increases blood volume and venous return, which causes further congestion.

Onset of heart failure may be: (1) *acute,* as following a myocardial infarction when direct damage to the heart's contracting ability has occurred; or (2) *chronic,* as with hypertension, when the ventricles must pump against chronically increased pressure.

BIBLIOGRAPHY

American Heart Association: *2002 heart and stroke statistical update.* Available at www.americanheart.org/downloadable/heart/.

Anderson J, Kessenich CR: Women and coronary heart disease, *Nurse Pract* 26(8):12–33, Aug 2001.

Asprey DP: Evaluation of children with heart murmurs, Lippincotts *Prim Care Pract* 2(5):505–513, Sep–Oct 1998.

Beattie S: Management of chronic stable angina, *Nurse Pract* 24(5): 44–61, May 1999.

Behrman RE, editor: *Nelson textbook of pediatrics,* ed 16, Philadelphia, 2000, W.B. Saunders.

Braunwald E: *Heart disease: a textbook of cardiovascular medicine,* ed 5, Philadelphia, 1997, W.B. Saunders.

Caboral M, Mitchell J: New guidelines for heart failure: focus on prevention, *Nurse Pract* 28(1):13–25, Jan 2003.

Campbell C: Comprehensive cardiovascular assessment, *J Nurse Midwifery* 40(2):137–149, Mar–Apr 1995.

Chorzempa A, Tabloski P: Post myocardial infarction treatment in the older adult, *Nurse Pract* 26(3):36–51, Mar 2001.

Colgan J: Syncope: a fall from grace, *Prog Cardiovasc Nurs* 17(2):66–70, Spring 2002.

Collins AS: More than a pump: the endocrine functions of the heart, *Am J Crit Care* 10(2):94–96, Mar 2001.

Connolly K: New directions in heart failure management, *Nurse Pract* 25(7):23–43, July 2000.

Cunningham FG et al: *Williams obstetrics,* ed 21, Norwalk, CT, 2001, Appleton-Century-Crofts.

Daly TM, Dempster JS: Mitral valve prolapse, *J Am Acad Nurse Pract* 8(9):437–443, Sep 1996.

Evangelista JK, Parsons M, Renneburg AK: Chest pain in children: diagnosis through history and physical examination, *J Pediatr Health Care* 14(1):3–8, 2000.

Fleg JL: Diagnostic evaluations. In Abrams WB, Berkow R, editors: *The Merck manual of geriatrics,* Rahway, NJ, 1990, Merck, Sharp, and Dohme.

Fleury J, Keller C: Cardiovascular risk assessment in elderly individuals, *J Gerontol Nurs* 26(5):30–37, May 2000.

Garrett AP: Assessing cardiovascular status in the older adult with cognitive impairments, *J Cardiovasc Nurs* 11(4):1–11, Jul 1997.

Greenland P, Smith SC, Grundy SM: Improving coronary heart disease risk assessment in asymptomatic people: role of traditional risk factors and noninvasive cardiovascular tests, *Circulation* 104(15):1863–1867, Oct 9, 2001.

Grenier M et al: Clinical comparison of acoustic and electronic stethoscopes and design of a new electronic stethoscope, *Am J Cardiol* 81(5):653–656, Mar 1, 1998.

Halm MA, Penque S: Heart disease in women, *Am J Nurs* 99(4):26–32, Apr 1999.

Hanson MJ: Modifiable risk factors for coronary heart disease in women, *Am J Critical Care* 3(3):177–186, 1994.

Hill B, Geraci SA: A diagnostic approach to chest pain based on history and ancillary evaluation, *Nurse Pract* 23(4):20–47, Apr 1998.

Houde SC, Melillo KD: Physical activity and exercise counseling in primary care, *Nurse Pract* 25(8):8–39, Aug 2000.

Howes DG: Cardiovascular disease and women, Lippincotts *Prim Care Pract* 2(5):514–524, Sep–Oct 1998.

Karz JR, Kraft P, Fox K: Assessing a murmur, saving a life: current trends in the management of hypertrophic cardiomyopathy, *Nurse Pract* 21(11):62–74, Nov 1996.

Kushi LH et al: Physical activity and mortality in postmenopausal women, *JAMA* 277(16):1287–1292, Apr 23/30, 1997.

Lakatta EG, Gerstenblith G, Weisfeldt ML: The aging heart: structure, function, and disease. In Braunwald E, editor: *Heart disease: a textbook of cardiovascular medicine,* ed 5, Philadelphia, 1997, W.B. Saunders.

Mangione S, Nieman LZ: Cardiac auscultatory skills of internal medicine and family practice trainees, *JAMA* 278(9):717–722, Sep 3, 1997.

Marolf GA, Kuhn A, White RD: Exercise testing in special populations: athletes, women, and the elderly, *Prim Care* 28(1):55–72, Mar 2001.

Meyer N: Using physiologic and pharmacologic stress testing in the evaluation of coronary artery disease, *Nurse Pract* 24(4):70–82, Apr 1999.

Moody LY: Pediatric cardiovascular assessment and referral in the primary care setting, *Nurse Pract* 22(1):120–134, Jan 1997.

Office of Minority Health: *Heart disease, stroke, and minorities: closing the gap.* Public Health Service, Department of Health and Human Services, Washington, DC, 1990, Government Printing Office.

O'Hanlon-Nichols T: The adult cardiovascular system, *Am J Nurs* 97(12):34–40, Dec 1997.

Perloff JK: *Physical examination of the heart and circulation,* ed 3, Philadelphia, 2000, W.B. Saunders.

Reisz WG, Robinson, DJ: Evaluating nontraumatic chest pain, *Lippincotts Prim Care Pract* 2(5):455–471, Sep–Oct 1998.

Stampfer MJ et al: Primary prevention of coronary heart disease in women through diet and lifestyle, *N Eng J Med* 343:16–22, Jul 6, 2000.

Tilkian AG, Conover MB: *Understanding heart sounds and murmurs,* ed 3, Philadelphia, 1993, W.B. Saunders.

Wei JY: Age and the cardiovascular system, *N Engl J Med* 327(14): 1735–1739, Dec 10, 1992.

Weidner G: Why do men get more heart disease than women: an international perspective, *J Am College Health* 48(6):291–294, May 2000.

Wimbush FB, Peters RM: Identification of cardiovascular risk: use of a cardiovascular-specific genogram, *Public Health Nurs* 17(3): 148–154, May–Jun 2000.

CHAPTER 20

Peripheral Vascular System and Lymphatic System

![icon] Structure and Function

The vascular system consists of the vessels of the body. Vessels are tubes for transporting fluid, such as the blood or lymph. Any disease in the vascular system creates problems with delivery of oxygen and nutrients to the tissues and/or elimination of waste products from cellular metabolism.

ARTERIES

The heart pumps freshly oxygenated blood through the arteries to all body tissues. The pumping heart makes this a high-pressure system. The artery walls are strong, tough, and tense to withstand pressure demands. Arteries contain elastic fibers, which allow their walls to stretch with systole and recoil with diastole. Arteries also contain muscle fibers (vascular smooth muscle, or VSM), which control the amount of blood delivered to the tissues. The VSM contracts or dilates, which changes the diameter of the arteries to control the rate of blood flow.

Each heartbeat creates a pressure wave, which makes the arteries expand and then recoil. It is the recoil that propels blood through like a wave. All arteries have this pressure wave, or **pulse**, throughout their length, but you can feel it only at body sites where the artery lies close to the skin and over a bone. The arteries described in the following sections are accessible to examination.

TEMPORAL ARTERY. The temporal artery is palpated in front of the ear, as discussed in Chapter 13 with the head and neck.

CAROTID ARTERY. The carotid artery is palpated in the groove between the sternomastoid muscle, and the trachea and is covered in Chapter 19 with the great vessels.

ARTERIES IN THE ARM. The major artery supplying the arm is the **brachial** artery, which runs in the biceps-triceps furrow of the upper arm and surfaces at the antecubital fossa in the elbow medial to the biceps tendon (Fig. 20–1). Immediately below the elbow, the brachial artery bifurcates into the **ulnar** and **radial** arteries. These run distally and form two arches supplying the hand; these are called the *superficial* and *deep palmar arches.* The radial pulse lies just medial to the radius at the wrist; the ulnar artery is in the same relation to the ulna, but it is deeper and often difficult to feel.

ARTERIES IN THE LEG. The major artery to the leg is the **femoral** artery, passing under the inguinal ligament (Fig. 20–2). The femoral artery travels down the thigh. At the lower thigh, it courses posteriorly; then it is termed the **popliteal** artery. Below the knee, the popliteal artery divides. The anterior tibial artery travels down the front of the leg on to the dorsum of the foot, where it becomes the **dorsalis pedis.** In back of the leg, the **posterior tibial** artery travels down behind the medial malleolus and in the foot forms the plantar arteries.

The function of the arteries is to supply oxygen and essential nutrients to the tissues. *Ischemia* is a deficient supply of oxygenated arterial blood to a tissue caused by obstruction of a blood vessel. A complete blockage leads to death of the distal tissue. A partial blockage creates an insufficient supply, and the ischemia may be apparent only at exercise when oxygen needs increase.

VEINS

The course of veins parallels that of arteries, but the body has more veins, and they lie closer to the skin surface. The following veins are accessible to examination.

20–1

20–2   Arteries in the leg.

JUGULAR VEINS. Assessment of the jugular veins is presented in Chapter 19.

VEINS IN THE ARM. Each arm has two sets of veins: superficial and deep. The superficial veins are in the subcutaneous tissue and are responsible for most of the venous return.

VEINS IN THE LEG. The legs have three types of veins (Fig. 20–3).

1. The **deep veins** run alongside the deep arteries and conduct most of the venous return from the legs. These are the **femoral** and **popliteal** veins. As long as these veins remain intact, the superficial veins can be excised without harming the circulation.
2. The **superficial veins** are the **great** and **small saphenous** veins. The great saphenous vein, inside the leg, starts at the medial side of the dorsum of the foot. You can see it ascend

in front of the medial malleolus; then it crosses the tibia obliquely and ascends along the medial side of the thigh. The small saphenous vein, outside the leg, starts on the lateral side of the dorsum of the foot, ascends behind the lateral malleolus, up the back of the leg, where it joins the popliteal vein.
3. **Perforators** (not illustrated) are connecting veins that join the two sets. They also have one-way valves that route blood from the superficial into the deep veins.

VENOUS FLOW

Veins drain the deoxygenated blood and its waste products from the tissues and return it to the heart. Unlike the arteries, veins are a low-pressure system. Because veins do not have a pump to generate their blood flow, the veins need a mechanism to keep blood moving (Fig. 20–4). This is accomplished by (1) the contracting skeletal muscles that milk the blood

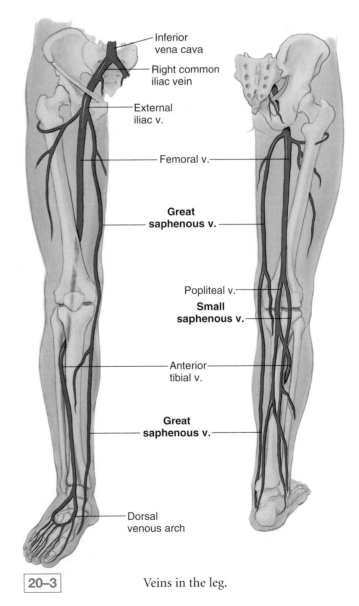

20–3   Veins in the leg.

② Inspiration: ⬇Thoracic pressure   ⬆ Abdominal pressure

①   Skeletal muscle pressure

③   Intraluminal valves

Open   Closed

20–4   MECHANISMS OF VENOUS FLOW

proximally, back toward the heart; (2) the pressure gradient caused by breathing, in which inspiration makes the thoracic pressure decrease and the abdominal pressure increase; and (3) the intraluminal valves, which ensure unidirectional flow. Each valve is a paired semilunar pocket that opens toward the heart and closes tightly when filled to prevent backflow of blood.

In the legs, this mechanism is called the "calf pump," or "peripheral heart." While walking, the calf muscles alternately contract (systole) and relax (diastole). In the contraction phase, the gastrocnemius and soleus muscles squeeze the veins and direct the blood flow proximally. Because of the valves, venous blood flows just one way—toward the heart.

Besides the presence of intraluminal valves, venous structure differs from arterial structure. Because venous pressure is lower, walls of the veins are thinner than those of the arteries. Veins have a larger diameter and are more distensible;

they can expand and hold more blood when blood volume increases. This is a compensatory mechanism to reduce stress on the heart. Because of this ability to stretch, veins are called **capacitance vessels.**

Efficient venous return is dependent on contracting skeletal muscles, competent valves in the veins, and patent lumen. Problems with any of these three elements lead to venous stasis. At risk for venous disease are people who undergo prolonged standing, sitting, or bedrest, because they do not benefit from the milking action that walking accomplishes. Hypercoagulable states and vein wall trauma are other factors that increase risk for venous disease. Also, dilated and tortuous (varicose) veins create *incompetent valves,* wherein the lumen is so wide the valve cusps cannot approximate. This condition increases venous pressure, which further dilates the vein. Some people have a genetic predisposition to varicose veins, but obesity and pregnancy are increased risk factors.

LYMPHATICS

The lymphatics form a completely separate vessel system, which retrieves excess fluid from the tissue spaces and returns it to the bloodstream (Fig. 20–5). During circulation of the blood, somewhat more fluid leaves the capillaries than the veins can absorb. Without lymphatic drainage, fluid would build up in the interstitial spaces and produce edema.

The vessels drain into two main trunks, which empty into the venous system at the subclavian veins (see Fig. 20–5):

1. The **right lymphatic duct** empties into the right subclavian vein. It drains the right side of the head and neck, right arm, right side of thorax, right lung and pleura, right side of the heart, and right upper section of the liver.
2. The **thoracic duct** drains the rest of the body. It empties into the left subclavian vein.

The functions of the lymphatic system are (1) to conserve fluid and plasma proteins that leak out of the capillaries, (2) to form a major part of the immune system that defends the body against disease, and (3) to absorb lipids from the intestinal tract.

The processes of the immune system are complicated and not fully understood. The immune system detects and eliminates foreign pathogens, both those that come in from the environment and those arising from inside (abnormal or mutant cells). It accomplishes this by phagocytosis (digestion) of the substances by neutrophils and monocytes/macrophages, and by production of specific antibodies or specific immune responses by the lymphocytes.

The lymphatic vessels have a unique structure. Lymphatic capillaries start as microscopic open-ended tubes, which siphon interstitial fluid. The capillaries converge to form vessels. The vessels, like veins, drain into larger ones. The vessels have valves, so flow is one way from the tissue spaces into the bloodstream. The many valves make the vessels look beaded. The flow of lymph is slow compared with that of the blood. Lymph flow is propelled by contracting skeletal muscles, by

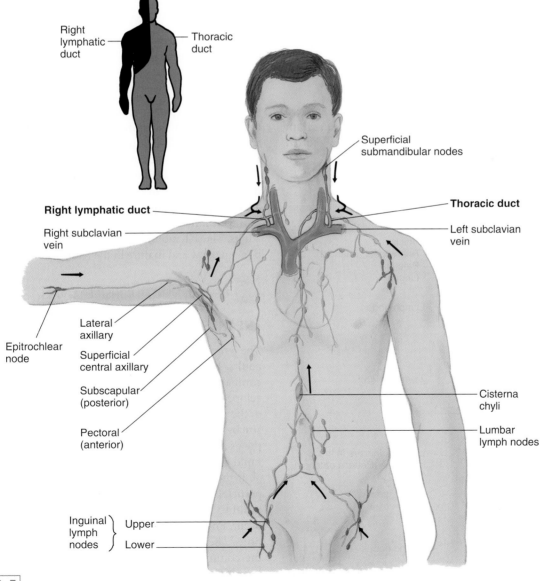

20–5   LYMPHATIC DUCTS AND DRAINAGE PATTERNS

pressure changes secondary to breathing, and by contraction of the vessel walls themselves.

Lymph nodes are small oval clumps of lymphatic tissue located at intervals along the vessels. Most nodes are arranged in groups, both deep and superficial in the body. Nodes filter the fluid before it is returned to the bloodstream and filter out microorganisms that could be harmful to the body. The pathogens are exposed to lymphocytes in the lymph nodes. The lymphocytes mount an antigen-specific response to eliminate the pathogens. With local inflammation, the nodes in that area become swollen and tender.

The superficial groups of nodes are accessible to inspection and palpation and give clues to the status of the lymphatic system:

- **Cervical nodes** drain the head and neck and are described in Chapter 13.
- **Axillary nodes** drain the breast and upper arm. They are described in Chapter 17.
- The **epitrochlear node** is in the antecubital fossa and drains the hand and lower arm.
- The **inguinal nodes** in the groin drain most of the lymph of the lower extremity, the external genitalia, and the anterior abdominal wall.

RELATED ORGANS

The spleen, tonsils, and thymus aid the lymphatic system (Fig. 20–6). The **spleen** is located in the left upper quadrant of the abdomen. It has four functions: (1) to destroy old red blood cells, (2) to produce antibodies, (3) to store red blood cells, and (4) to filter microorganisms from the blood.

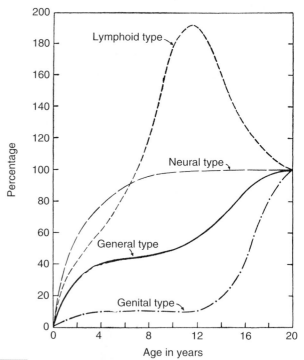

20–7 Comparison of growth rates of three types of tissues and the body as a whole.

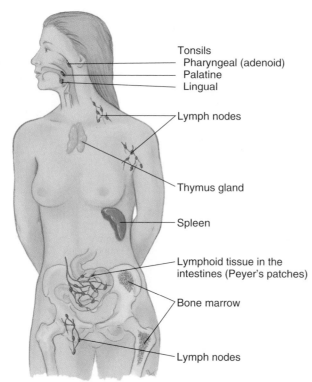

RELATED ORGANS IN IMMUNE SYSTEM

20–6

The **tonsils** (palatine, adenoid, and lingual) are located at the entrance to the respiratory and gastrointestinal tracts and respond to local inflammation.

The **thymus** is the flat, pink-gray gland located in the superior mediastinum behind the sternum and in front of the aorta. It is relatively large in the fetus and young child and atrophies after puberty. It is important in developing the T-lymphocytes of the immune system in children, but it serves no function in adults. The T-lymphocytes and B-lymphocytes originate in the bone marrow and mature in the lymphoid tissue.

 DEVELOPMENTAL CONSIDERATIONS

INFANTS AND CHILDREN

The lymphatic system has the same function in children as in adults. Lymphoid tissue has a unique growth pattern when compared with other body systems (Fig. 20–7). It is well developed at birth and grows rapidly until age 10 and 11. By age 6, the lymphoid tissue reaches adult size; it surpasses adult size by puberty, and then it slowly atrophies. It is possible that the excessive antigen stimulation in children causes the early rapid growth.

Lymph nodes are relatively large in children, and the superficial ones often are palpable even when the child is healthy. With infection, excessive swelling and hyperplasia occur. Enlarged tonsils are familiar signs in respiratory infections. The excessive lymphoid response also may account for the common childhood symptom of abdominal pain with seemingly unrelated problems such as upper respiratory infections (Johnson et al., 1978). Possibly the inflammation of mesenteric lymph nodes produces the abdominal pain.

THE PREGNANT FEMALE

Hormonal changes cause vasodilatation and the resulting drop in blood pressure described in Chapter 19. The growing uterus obstructs drainage of the iliac veins and the inferior vena cava. This condition causes low blood flow and increases venous pressure. This, in turn, causes dependent edema, varicosities in the legs and vulva, and hemorrhoids.

THE AGING ADULT

Peripheral blood vessels grow more rigid with age, resulting in a condition called *arteriosclerosis*. This condition produces the rise in systolic blood pressure discussed in Chapter 10. Do not confuse this process with another one, *atherosclerosis*, or the deposition of fatty plaques on the intima of the arteries.

Aging produces a progressive enlargement of the intramuscular calf veins. Prolonged bed rest, prolonged sitting, and heart failure increase the risk of deep venous thrombosis and subsequent pulmonary embolism. These conditions are common in aging and also occur following myocardial infarction (MI). However, care for MI now includes early mobilization and low-dose anticoagulant medication, which reduce the risk of pulmonary embolism (Braunwald, 1997).

Loss of lymphatic tissue leads to fewer numbers of lymph nodes in older people and to a decrease in the size of remaining nodes.

Subjective Data

1. Leg pain or cramps
2. Skin changes on arms or legs
3. Swelling
4. Lymph node enlargement
5. Medications

EXAMINER ASKS	RATIONALE
1. Leg pain or cramps. Any leg pain (cramps)? Where? • Describe the type of pain; is it burning, aching, cramping, stabbing? Did this come on gradually or suddenly? • Is it aggravated by activity, walking? • How many blocks (stairs) does it take to produce this pain? • Has this amount changed recently? • Is the pain worse with elevation? Worse with cool temperatures? • Does the pain wake you up at night? • Any recent change in exercise, a new exercise, increasing exercise? • What relieves this pain: dangling, walking, rubbing? Is the leg pain associated with any skin changes? • Is it associated with any change in sexual function (males)? • Any past history of vascular problems, heart problems, diabetes, obesity, pregnancy, smoking, trauma, prolonged standing, or bed rest? **2. Skin changes on arms or legs.** Any **skin changes** in arms or legs? What color: redness, pallor, blueness, brown discolorations? • Any change in temperature—excess warmth or coolness? • Do your leg veins look bulging and crooked? How have you treated these? Do you use support hose? • Any leg sores or ulcers? Where on the leg? Any pain with the leg ulcer?	Peripheral vascular disease (PVD)—see Table 20–3, History Profiles, p. 556. *Claudication distance* is the number of blocks walked or stairs climbed to produce pain. Note sudden decrease in claudication distance, or pain suddenly not relieved by rest. Night leg pain is common in aging adults. It may indicate the ischemic rest pain of PVD, severe night muscle cramping (usually the calf), or the restless leg syndrome. Pain of musculoskeletal origin rather than vascular. Aortoiliac occlusion is associated with impotence (Leriche's syndrome). Coolness is associated with arterial disease. Varicose veins. Leg ulcers occur with chronic arterial and chronic venous disease.

EXAMINER ASKS	RATIONALE
3. Swelling in the arms or legs. Swelling in one or both legs? When did this swelling start? • What time of day is the swelling at its worst: morning, or after up most of day? • Does the swelling come and go, or is it constant? • What seems to bring it on: trauma, standing all day, sitting? • What relieves swelling: elevation, support hose? • Is swelling associated with pain, heat, redness, ulceration, hardened skin?	**Edema** is bilateral when caused by a systemic problem such as heart failure, or unilateral when due to a local obstruction or inflammation.
4. Lymph node enlargement. Any "swollen glands" (lumps, kernels)? Where in body? How long have you had them? • Any recent change? • How do they feel to you: hard, soft? • Are the swollen glands associated with pain, or local infection?	**Enlarged lymph nodes** occur with infectious diseases, immunologic diseases, and malignant diseases.
5. Medications. What medications are you taking (e.g., oral contraceptives, hormone replacement)?	

Objective Data

PREPARATION

During a complete physical examination, examine the arms at the very beginning when you are checking the vital signs—the person is sitting. Examine the legs directly after the abdominal examination while the person is still supine. Then stand the person up to evaluate the leg veins.

Examination of the arms and legs includes peripheral vascular characteristics (following here), the skin (see Chapter 12), musculoskeletal findings (see Chapter 22), and neurologic findings (see Chapter 23). A method of integrating these steps is discussed in Chapter 28.

Room temperature should be about 22° C (72° F) and draftless to prevent vasodilatation or vasoconstriction.

Use inspection and palpation. Compare your findings with the opposite extremity.

EQUIPMENT NEEDED

Occasionally need: paper tape measure
Tourniquet or blood pressure cuff
Stethoscope
Doppler ultrasonic stethoscope

NORMAL RANGE OF FINDINGS	ABNORMAL FINDINGS

INSPECT AND PALPATE THE ARMS

Lift both the person's hands in your hands. Inspect, then turn the person's hands over, noting color of skin and nailbeds; temperature, texture, and turgor of skin; and the presence of any lesions, edema, or clubbing. Use the *profile sign* (viewing the finger from the side) to detect early clubbing. The normal nail bed angle is 160 degrees. (See Chapter 12, "Skin, Hair, and Nails," for a full discussion of skin color, lesions, and clubbing.)

With the person's hands near the level of his or her heart, check **capillary refill.** This is an index of peripheral perfusion and cardiac output. Depress and blanch the nail beds; release and note the time for color return. Usually, the vessels refill within a fraction of a second. Consider it normal if the color returns in less than 1 or 2 seconds. Note conditions that can skew your findings: a cool room, decreased body temperature, cigarette smoking, peripheral edema, and anemia.

Flattening of angle and clubbing (diffuse enlargement of terminal phalanges) occur with congenital cyanotic heart disease, cor pulmonale, and subacute bacterial endocarditis.

Refill lasting more than 1 or 2 seconds signifies vasoconstriction or decreased cardiac output (hypovolemia, heart failure, shock). The hands are cold, clammy, and pale.

NORMAL RANGE OF FINDINGS

The two arms should be symmetric in size.

Note the presence of any scars on hands and arms. Many occur normally with usual childhood abrasions or with occupations involving hand tools.

Palpate both radial pulses, noting rate, rhythm, elasticity of vessel wall, and equal force (Fig. 20–8). Grade the force (amplitude) on a four-point scale:

4+, bounding
3+, increased
2+, **normal**
1+, weak
0, absent

20–8

It usually is not necessary to palpate the ulnar pulses. If indicated, palpate along the medial side of the inner forearm (Fig. 20–9), although the ulnar pulses often are not palpable in the normal person.

20–9

ABNORMAL FINDINGS

Edema of upper extremities occurs when lymphatic drainage is obstructed, which may occur following breast surgery (see Table 20–2).

Needle tracks in antecubital fossae occur with intravenous drug use; linear scars in wrists may signify past self-inflicted injury.

Full, bounding pulse (3+ or 4+) occurs with hyperkinetic states (exercise, anxiety, fever), anemia, and hyperthyroidism. Weak, "thready" pulse occurs with shock and peripheral arterial disease. See Table 20–1 on p. 554 for illustrations of these and irregular pulse rhythms.

NORMAL RANGE OF FINDINGS

ABNORMAL FINDINGS

Palpate the brachial pulses—their force should be equal bilaterally (Fig. 20–10).

20–10

Check the epitrochlear lymph node in the depression above and behind the medial condyle of the humerus. Do this by "shaking hands" with the person and reaching your other hand under the person's elbow to the groove between the biceps and triceps muscles, above the medial epicondyle (Fig. 20–11). This node is not palpable normally.

An enlarged epitrochlear node occurs with infection of the hand or forearm.

20–11

The **modified Allen test** is used to evaluate the adequacy of collateral circulation prior to cannulating the radial artery (Fig. 20–12). (A) Firmly occlude both the ulnar and radial arteries of one hand while the person makes a fist several times. This causes the hand to blanch. (B) Ask the person to open the hand without hyperextending it; then release pressure on the ulnar artery while maintaining pressure on the radial artery. Adequate circulation is suggested by a return to the hand's normal color in approximately 2 to 5 seconds. Although this test is simple and useful, it is relatively crude and subject to error—that is, you must occlude both arteries uniformly with 11 pounds of pressure for the test to be accurate (Fuhrman et al., 1992; Gelberman and Blasingame, 1981).

(C) Pallor persists or a sluggish return to color suggests occlusion of the collateral circulation. Avoid radial artery cannulation until plethysmography has shown adequate circulation.

| NORMAL RANGE OF FINDINGS | ABNORMAL FINDINGS |

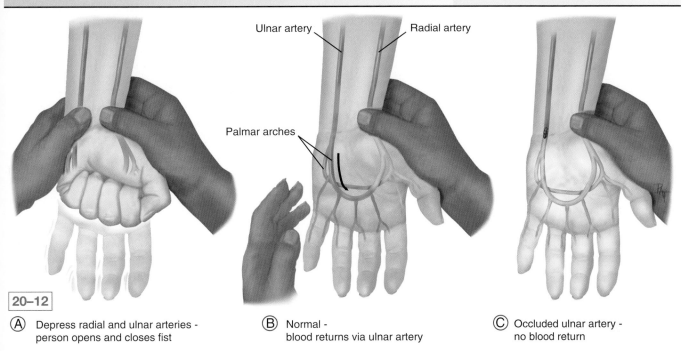

20–12

(A) Depress radial and ulnar arteries - person opens and closes fist

(B) Normal - blood returns via ulnar artery

(C) Occluded ulnar artery - no blood return

INSPECT AND PALPATE THE LEGS

Uncover the legs while keeping the genitalia draped. Inspect both legs together, noting skin color, hair distribution, venous pattern, size (swelling or atrophy), and any skin lesions or ulcers.

Normally hair covers the legs. Even if leg hair is shaved, you will still note hair on the dorsa of the toes.

The venous pattern normally is flat and barely visible. Note obvious varicosities, although these are best assessed while standing.

Both legs should be symmetric in size without any swelling or atrophy. If the lower legs look asymmetric or if deep venous thrombosis is suspected, measure the calf circumference with a nonstretchable tape measure (Fig. 20–13). Measure at the widest point, taking care to measure the other leg in exactly the same place—the same number of centimeters down from the patella or other landmark. If lymphedema is suspected, measure also at the ankle, distal calf, knee, and thigh. Record your findings in centimeters.

20–13

Pallor with vasoconstriction; erythema with vasodilatation; cyanosis.

Malnutrition: thin, shiny atrophic skin, thick-ridged nails, loss of hair, ulcers, gangrene. Malnutrition, pallor, and coolness occur with arterial insufficiency.

Diffuse bilateral edema occurs with systemic illnesses.

Unilateral swelling indicates a local acute problem. Asymmetry of calves of 1 cm or more is abnormal; refer the person to determine if deep venous thrombosis is present.

Asymmetry of 1 to 3 cm occurs with mild lymphedema; 3 to 5 cm with moderate lymphedema; and more than 5 cm with severe lymphedema (see Table 20–2).

NORMAL RANGE OF FINDINGS

In the presence of skin discoloration, skin ulcers, or gangrene, note the size and the exact location.

Palpate for temperature along the legs down to the feet, comparing symmetric spots (Fig. 20–14). The skin should be warm and equal bilaterally. Bilateral cool feet may be due to environmental factors such as cool room temperature, apprehension, and cigarette smoking. If any increase in temperature is present higher up the leg, note if it is gradual or abrupt.

20–14

Flex the person's knee, then gently compress the gastrocnemius (calf) muscle anteriorly against the tibia; no tenderness should be present. Or you may sharply dorsiflex the foot toward the tibia. Flexing the knee first exerts pressure on the posterior tibial vein. Normally this does not cause pain.

Palpate the inguinal lymph nodes. It is not unusual to find palpable nodes that are small (1 cm or less), movable, and nontender.

Palpate these peripheral arteries in both legs: femoral, popliteal, dorsalis pedis, and posterior tibial. Grade the force on the four-point scale. Locate the **femoral arteries** just below the inguinal ligament halfway between the pubis and anterior superior iliac spines (Fig. 20–15). To help expose the femoral area, particularly in obese people, ask the person to bend his or her knees to the side in a froglike position. Press firmly and then slowly release, noting the pulse tap under your fingertips. Should this pulse be weak or diminished, auscultate the site for a bruit.

ABNORMAL FINDINGS

Brown discoloration occurs with chronic venous stasis due to hemosiderin deposits (a by-product of red blood cell degradation).

Venous ulcers occur usually at medial malleolus because of bacterial invasion of poorly drained tissues (see Table 20–4 on p. 557).

With arterial deficit, ulcers occur on tips of toes, metatarsal heads, and lateral malleoli.

A unilateral cool foot or leg or a sudden temperature drop as you move down the leg occurs with arterial deficit.

Calf pain with these maneuvers is a positive **Homans' sign,** which occurs in about 35% of cases of deep vein thrombosis. It is not specific for this condition because it occurs also with superficial phlebitis, Achilles tendinitis, gastrocnemius and plantar muscle injury, and lumbosacral disorders.

Enlarged nodes, tender, or fixed in area.

A bruit occurs with turbulent blood flow, indicating partial occlusion (see Table 20–5).

NORMAL RANGE OF FINDINGS	ABNORMAL FINDINGS

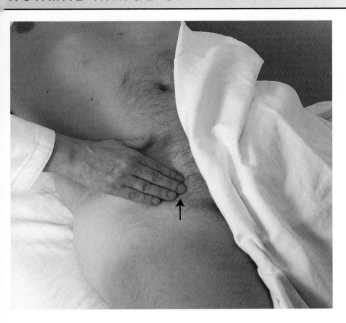

20–15

The **popliteal pulse** is a more diffuse pulse and can be difficult to localize. With the leg extended but relaxed, anchor your thumbs on the knee, and curl your fingers around into the popliteal fossa (Fig. 20–16). Press your fingers forward hard to compress the artery against the bone (the lower edge of the femur or the upper edge of the tibia). Often it is just lateral to the medial tendon.

20–16

If you have difficulty, turn the person prone and lift up the lower leg (Fig. 20–17). Let the leg relax against your arm and press in deeply with your two thumbs. Often a normal popliteal pulse is impossible to palpate.

20–17

NORMAL RANGE OF FINDINGS

ABNORMAL FINDINGS

For the **posterior tibial** pulse, curve your fingers around the medial malleolus (Fig. 20–18). You will feel the tapping right behind it in the groove between the malleolus and the Achilles tendon. If you cannot, try passive dorsiflexion of the foot to make the pulse more accessible.

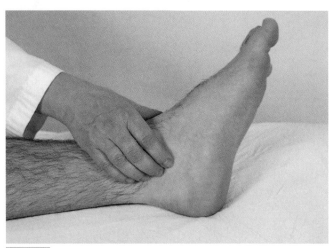

20–18 Posterior tibial pulse.

The **dorsalis pedis** pulse requires a very light touch. Normally it is just lateral to and parallel with the extensor tendon of the big toe (Fig. 20–19). Do not mistake the pulse in your own fingertips for that of the person.

20–19 Dorsalis pedis pulse.

In adults over 45 years, occasionally either the dorsalis pedis or the posterior tibial pulse may be hard to find, but not both on the same foot.

Check for pretibial edema. Firmly depress the skin over the tibia or the medial malleolus for 5 seconds and release (Fig. 20–20, *A*). Normally, your finger should leave no indentation, although a pit commonly is seen if the person has been standing all day or during pregnancy.

If pitting edema is present, grade it on the following scale:

1+ Mild pitting, slight indentation, no perceptible swelling of the leg
2+ Moderate pitting, indentation subsides rapidly
3+ Deep pitting, indentation remains for a short time, leg looks swollen
4+ Very deep pitting, indentation lasts a long time, leg is very swollen

Bilateral, dependent, pitting edema occurs with heart failure, diabetic neuropathy, and hepatic cirrhosis (Fig. 20–20, *B*).

Unilateral edema occurs with occlusion of a deep vein. Unilateral or bilateral edema occurs with lymphatic obstruction. With these factors, it is "brawny" or nonpitting and feels hard to the touch.

NORMAL RANGE OF FINDINGS

20–20 **A,** Check pretibial edema.

This scale is subjective and qualitative. The amount of pressure used is arbitrary, as is the judgment of the depth and rate of pitting. Clinicians need a standard quantified scale in order to ensure consistent clinical measurements and management. Many classify the edema by measuring the depth of the pitting in centimeters ($1+ = 1$ cm, $2+ = 2$ cm, etc.) (Welsh, Arzouman, and Holm, 1996).

Some measure with a millimeter scale, others by an increase in weight; still others try to quantify the rate of time the pitting remains after release of pressure. Check with your institution to determine a consistently used scale.

Ask the person to stand so that you can assess the venous system. Note any visible, dilated, and tortuous veins.

Manual Compression Test

While the person is still standing, test the length of the varicose vein to determine if its valves are competent (Fig. 20–21). Place one hand on the lower part of the varicose vein, and compress the vein with your other hand about 15 to 20 cm higher. Competent valves will prevent a wave transmission and your distal fingers will feel no change.

1 Compress vein

2 No wave—COMPETENT
VALVES
Wave felt—INCOMPETENT
VALVES

MANUAL COMPRESSION TEST   20–21

ABNORMAL FINDINGS

20–20 **B,** Pitting edema.

Varicosities occur in the saphenous veins (see Table 20–4).

A palpable wave transmission occurs when the valves are incompetent.

NORMAL RANGE OF FINDINGS	ABNORMAL FINDINGS

ADDITIONAL TECHNIQUES

THE TRENDELENBURG TEST. When varicosities are present in the legs, use the Trendelenburg test to determine valve competence (Fig. 20–22). Return the person to supine position, elevate the involved leg 90 degrees until the veins empty, and place a tourniquet high on the thigh. Help the person to stand up, and watch for venous filling. The saphenous veins should fill slowly from below in about 30 seconds.

Rapid filling of veins from above indicates incompetent valves.

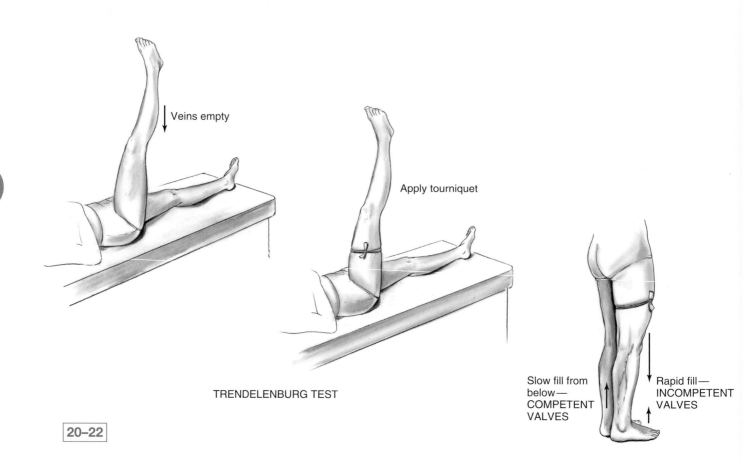

Veins empty

Apply tourniquet

TRENDELENBURG TEST

Slow fill from below— COMPETENT VALVES

Rapid fill— INCOMPETENT VALVES

20–22

After 30 seconds, take the tourniquet off. Now observe whether or not the varicose veins fill suddenly from above. Normally no sudden filling occurs.

Sudden filling after removing the tourniquet indicates retrograde flow past incompetent saphenous valves.

Color Changes

If you suspect an arterial deficit, raise the legs about 30 cm (12 inches) off the table and ask the person to wag the feet to drain off venous blood (Fig. 20–23). The skin color now reflects only the contribution of arterial blood. A light-skinned person's feet normally will look a little pale but still should be pink. A dark-skinned person's feet are more difficult to evaluate, but the soles should reveal extreme color change.

Elevational pallor (marked) indicates arterial insufficiency.

NORMAL RANGE OF FINDINGS	ABNORMAL FINDINGS

20–23

Now have the person sit up with the legs over the side of the table (Fig. 20–24). Compare the color of both feet. Note the time it takes for color to return to the feet. Normally, this is 10 seconds or less. Note also the time it takes for the superficial veins around the feet to fill—the normal time is about 15 seconds. This test is unreliable if the person has concomitant venous disease with incompetent valves.

Dependent rubor (deep blue-red color) occurs with severe arterial insufficiency. Chronic hypoxia produces a loss of vasomotor tone and a pooling of blood in the veins.

Delayed venous filling occurs with arterial insufficiency.

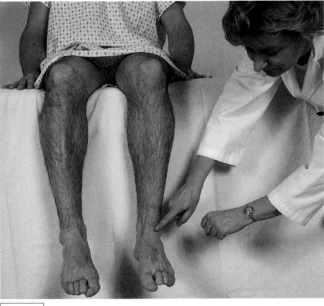

20–24

Test the lower legs for strength (see Chapter 22). Test the lower legs for sensation (see Chapter 23).

Motor loss occurs with severe arterial deficit.

Sensory loss occurs with arterial deficit, especially diabetes.

NORMAL RANGE OF FINDINGS	ABNORMAL FINDINGS

The Doppler Ultrasonic Stethoscope

Use this device to detect a weak peripheral pulse, to monitor blood pressure in infants or children, or to measure a low blood pressure or blood pressure in a lower extremity (Fig. 20–25). The Doppler stethoscope magnifies pulsatile sounds from the heart and blood vessels. Position the person supine, with the legs externally rotated so you can reach the medial ankles easily. Place a drop of coupling gel on the end of the handheld transducer. Place the transducer over a pulse site, swiveled at a 45-degree angle. Apply very light pressure; locate the pulse site by the swishing, whooshing sound.

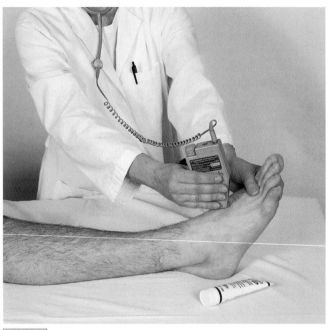

20–25

The Ankle-Brachial Index (ABI)

Use of the Doppler stethoscope is a noninvasive way to determine the extent of peripheral vascular disease. Apply a regular arm blood pressure cuff above the ankle and determine the systolic pressure in either the posterior tibial or dorsalis pedis artery. Then divide that figure by the systolic pressure of the brachial artery. (Take brachial systolic pressures in both arms and use the higher measurement.) The normal ankle pressure is slightly greater than or equal to the brachial pressure; thus, a normal ABI is usually 1.0 to 1.2. For example,

$$\frac{132 \text{ ankle systolic pressure}}{124 \text{ arm systolic pressure}} = 1.06 \text{ or } 106\%, \text{ indicating no flow reduction}$$

In people with diabetes mellitus, the ABI may be less reliable because of calcification (which makes their arteries noncompressible) and may give a falsely high measurement (Cantwell-Gab, 1996).

An ABI of 90% or less indicates the presence of peripheral vascular disease:

- 0.90 to 0.70—mild claudication
- 0.70 to 0.40—moderate to severe claudication
- 0.40 to 0.30—severe claudication, usually with rest pain except in the presence of diabetic neuropathy
- <0.30—ischemia, with impending loss of tissue

NORMAL RANGE OF FINDINGS	ABNORMAL FINDINGS

 DEVELOPMENTAL CONSIDERATIONS

Infants and Children

Transient acrocyanosis and skin mottling at birth are discussed in Chapter 12. Pulse force should be normal and symmetric. Pulse force also should be the same in the upper and lower extremities.

Weak pulses occur with vasoconstriction of diminished cardiac output.

Full, bounding pulses occur with patent ductus arteriosus due to the large left-to-right shunt.

Diminished or absent femoral pulses while upper extremity pulses are normal suggest coarctation of aorta.

Palpable lymph nodes occur often in normal infants and children. They are small, firm (shotty), mobile, and nontender. They may be the sequelae of past infection, such as inguinal nodes from a diaper rash or cervical nodes from a respiratory infection. Vaccinations also can produce local lymphadenopathy. Note characteristics of any palpable nodes and whether they are local or generalized.

Enlarged, warm, tender nodes indicate current infection. Look for source of infection.

The Pregnant Female

Expect diffuse bilateral pitting edema in the lower extremities, especially at the end of the day and into the third trimester. Varicose veins in the legs also are common in the third trimester.

The Aging Adult

The dorsalis pedis and posterior tibial pulse may become more difficult to find. Trophic changes associated with arterial insufficiency (thin, shiny skin, thick-ridged nails, loss of hair on lower legs) also occur normally with aging.

SUMMARY CHECKLIST: Peripheral Vascular Exam

1. Inspect arms for color, size, any lesions
2. Palpate pulses: radial, brachial
3. Check epitrochlear node
4. Inspect legs for color, size, any lesions, trophic skin changes
5. Palpate temperature of feet and legs
6. Palpate inguinal nodes
7. Palpate pulses: femoral, popliteal, posterior tibial, dorsalis pedis

See Health Promotion Guide on CD

Application and Critical Thinking

SAMPLE CHARTING

SUBJECTIVE

No leg pain, no skin changes, no swelling or lymph node enlargement. No past history of heart or vascular problems, diabetes, or obesity. Does not smoke. On no medications.

OBJECTIVE

Inspection. Extremities have pink-tan color without redness, cyanosis, or any skin lesions. Extremity size is symmetric without swelling or atrophy.

Palpation. Temperature is warm and = bilaterally. All pulses present, 2+ and = bilaterally. No lymphadenopathy.

Continued

FOCUSED ASSESSMENT: CLINICAL CASE STUDY

James K. is a 43-year-old married white male city sanitation worker, admitted to University Medical Center today for "bypass surgery tomorrow to fix my aorta and these black toes."

SUBJECTIVE

6 yrs PTA: motorcycle accident with handle bars jammed into groin. Treated and released at local hospital. No apparent injury, although M.D. now thinks accident may have precipitated present stenosis of aorta.

1 yr PTA: radiating pain in right calf on walking 1 mile. Pain relieved by stopping walking.

3 months PTA: problems with sex, unable to maintain erection during intercourse.

1 month PTA: leg pain present after walking two blocks. Numbness and tingling in right foot and calf. Tips of three toes on right foot look black. Saw M.D. Diagnostic studies showed stenosis of aorta "below vessels that go to my kidneys."

Present: leg pain at rest, constant and severe, worse at night, partially relieved by dangling leg over side of bed.

Past history: no history of heart or vessel disease, hypertension, diabetes, obesity.

Personal habits: smokes cigarettes three packs/day X 23 years. Now cut down to 1 ppd.

Walking is part of occupation, although has been driving city truck last 3 months due to leg pain. On no medications.

OBJECTIVE

Inspection. Lower extremity size = bilaterally with no swelling or atrophy. No varicosities. Color L leg pink, R leg pink when supine, but marked pallor to R foot on elevation. Black gangrene at tips of R 2nd, 3rd, 4th toes. Leg hair present but absent on involved toes.

Palpation. R foot cool and temperature gradually warms as proceed palpating up R leg.

Pulses. Femorals, both 1+; popliteals, both O; posterior tibial, both O but present with Doppler; dorsalis pedis O, but left dorsalis pedis is present with Doppler, and right is not present with Doppler.

ASSESSMENT

Ischemic rest pain R leg
Ineffective tissue perfusion R/T interruption of flow
Impaired tissue integrity R/T altered circulation
Activity intolerance R/T leg pain
Sexual dysfunction R/T effects of disease

NURSING DIAGNOSES COMMONLY ASSOCIATED WITH PERIPHERAL VASCULAR SYSTEM AND LYMPHATIC DISORDERS

RELATED FACTORS (Etiology)	DEFINING CHARACTERISTICS (Symptoms and Signs)
DIAGNOSIS: Ineffective Tissue perfusion (peripheral)	
Exchange problems	Altered sensory or motor function
Hypervolemia	Burning
Hypovolemia	Changes in hair pattern
Interruption of flow	Claudication
	Coolness of skin
	Diminished pulse quality
	Edema
	Erythema
	Extremity pain
	Inflammation
	Pallor
	Positive Homans' sign
	Tissue necrosis
	Trophic skin changes
	Ulcerated skin/poorly healing areas

RELATED FACTORS (Etiology)

DEFINING CHARACTERISTICS (Symptoms and Signs)

DIAGNOSIS: Disturbed Sensory perception (tactile)

Circulatory impairment	Paresthesias
Inflammation	Hyperesthesias
Effects of anesthesia	Anesthesias
Nutritional deficiencies	
Effects of aging	
Effects of burns	
Neurologic impairment	
Pain	
Persistent tactile stimulation	

OTHER RELATED NURSING DIAGNOSES

ACTUAL

RISK/WELLNESS

Activity intolerance (see Chapter 18)

Disturbed Body image

Fatigue (see Chapter 19)

Impaired bed Mobility

Pain (see Chapters 16 and 22)

Risk for Peripheral neurovascular dysfunction

Sexual dysfunction (see Chapter 26)

Disturbed Sleep pattern

Impaired Tissue integrity

Impaired Walking

Risk

Risk for Infection

Risk for Peripheral neurovascular dysfunction

Wellness

Health-seeking behavior about beginning an exercise
  program

 ASSESSMENT VIDEO CRITICAL THINKING QUESTIONS

The Saunders *Physical Examination and Health Assessment* video "Cardiovascular System: Peripheral Vascular System and Lymphatics" will direct you to consider the following:

1. Which assessment findings are you likely to see in a patient who seeks care because of leg pain or cramps?
2. How do ulcers caused by chronic arterial insufficiency compare to those of chronic venous insufficiency?

3. How may aging affect your findings when examining an older adult's peripheral vascular and lymphatic systems?
4. What nursing diagnoses commonly are related to abnormal findings in the peripheral vascular system?

Abnormal Findings

TABLE 20–1: Variations in Arterial Pulse

DESCRIPTION	ASSOCIATED WITH

Weak, "Thready" Pulse—1+

Hard to palpate, need to search for it, may fade in and out, easily obliterated by pressure.

Decreased cardiac output; peripheral arterial disease; aortic valve stenosis

Full, Bounding Pulse—3+ or 4+

Easily palpable, pounds under your fingertips.

Hyperkinetic states (exercise, anxiety, fever), anemia, hyperthyroidism

Water-Hammer (Corrigan's) Pulse—4+

Greater than normal force, then collapses suddenly.

Aortic valve regurgitation; patent ductus arteriosus

Pulsus Bigeminus

Rhythm is coupled, every other beat comes early, or normal beat followed by premature beat. Force of premature beat is decreased due to shortened cardiac filling time.

Conduction disturbance, e.g., premature ventricular contraction, premature atrial contraction

Pulsus Alternans

Rhythm is regular, but force varies with alternating beats of large and small amplitude.

Heart failure

Pulsus Paradoxus

Beats have weaker amplitude with inspiration, stronger with expiration. Best determined during blood pressure measurement; reading decreases (>10 mm Hg) during inspiration and increases with expiration.

Any condition that blocks venous return to the right side of the heart, or blocks left ventricular filling, e.g., cardiac tamponade; constrictive pericarditis, pulmonary embolism

Pulsus Bisferiens

Each pulse has two strong systolic peaks, with a dip in between. Best assessed at the carotid artery.

Aortic valve stenosis plus regurgitation

TABLE 20–2: Peripheral Vascular Disease in the Arms

◀ Raynaud's Syndrome

Episodes of abrupt progressive tricolor change of the fingers in response to cold, vibration, or stress: first white (pallor) from arteriospasm and resulting deficit in supply; then blue (cyanosis) due to slight relaxation of the spasm that allows a slow trickle of blood through the capillaries and increased oxygen extraction of hemoglobin; finally red (rubor) due to return of blood into the dilated capillary bed or reactive hyperemia.

May have cold, numbness, or pain along with pallor or cyanosis stage; then burning, throbbing pain, swelling along with rubor. Lasts minutes to hours; occurs bilaterally.

◀ Lymphedema

Removal of lymph nodes with breast surgery, or damage to lymph nodes and channels with radiation therapy for breast cancer; can impede drainage of lymph. Protein-rich lymph builds up in the interstitial spaces, which further raises local colloid oncotic pressure and promotes more fluid leakage. Stagnant lymphatic fluid can lead to infection, delayed wound healing, chronic inflammation, and fibrosis of surrounding tissue. Chronic lymphedema is unilateral swelling, nonpitting brawny edema, with overlying skin indurated, and is psychologically demoralizing as a threat to body image and constant reminder of the cancer.

TABLE 20–3: History Profiles of Pain of Peripheral Vascular Disease

SYMPTOM ANALYSIS	CHRONIC ARTERIAL SYMPTOMS	ACUTE ARTERIAL SYMPTOMS
Location	Deep muscle pain, usually in calf, but may be lower leg or dorsum of foot	Varies, distal to occlusion, may involve entire leg
Character	Intermittent claudication, feels like "cramp," "numbness and tingling," "feeling of cold"	Throbbing
Onset and duration	Chronic pain, onset gradual following exertion	Sudden onset (within 1 hr)
Aggravating factors	Activity (walking, stairs) "Claudication distance" is specific number of blocks, stairs it takes to produce pain Elevation (Rest pain indicates severe involvement)	
Relieving factors	Rest (usually within 2 min; e.g., standing) Dangling (severe involvement)	
Associated symptoms	Cool pale skin	Six Ps: pain, pallor, pulselessness, paresthesia, poikilothermia (coldness), paralysis (indicates severe)
Those at risk	Older adults, more males than females, inherited predisposition, history of hypertension, smoking, diabetes, hypercholesterolemia, obesity, vascular disease	History of vascular surgery; arterial invasive procedure; abdominal aneurysm (emboli); trauma, including injured arteries, chronic atrial fibrillation
	CHRONIC VENOUS SYMPTOMS	ACUTE VENOUS SYMPTOMS
Location	Calf, lower leg	Calf
Character	Aching, tiredness, feeling of fullness	Intense, sharp; deep muscle tender to touch
Onset and duration	Chronic pain, increases at end of day	Sudden onset (within 1 hr)
Aggravating factors	Prolonged standing, sitting	Pain may increase with sharp dorsiflexion of foot
Relieving factors	Elevation, lying, walking	
Associated symptoms	Edema, varicosities, weeping ulcers at ankles	Red, warm, swollen leg
Those at risk	Job with prolonged standing or sitting; obesity; pregnancy; prolonged bed rest; history of heart failure, varicosities, or thrombophlebitis; veins crushed by trauma or surgery	

TABLE 20–4: Peripheral Vascular Disease in the Legs

CHRONIC ARTERIAL INSUFFICIENCY	CHRONIC VENOUS INSUFFICIENCY

Arteriosclerosis—Ischemic Ulcer

Buildup of fatty plaques on intima (atherosclerosis) plus hardening and calcification of arterial wall (arteriosclerosis).

S: Deep muscle pain in calf or foot, claudication (pain with walking), pain at rest indicates worsening of condition.

O: Coolness, pallor, elevational pallor, and dependent rubor; diminished pulses; systolic bruits; trophic skin; signs of malnutrition (thin, shiny skin, thick-ridged nails, absence of hair, atrophy of muscles); xanthoma formation; distal gangrene.

Ulcers occur at toes, metatarsal heads, heels, lateral ankle, and are characterized by pale ischemic base, well-defined edges, and no bleeding.

Diabetes hastens changes described above, with generalized dysfunction in all arterial areas: peripheral, coronary, cerebral, retina, kidney. Peripheral involvement is associated with diabetic neuropathy and local infection.

Venous (Stasis) Ulcer

Following acute deep vein thrombosis or following chronic incompetent valves in deep veins.

S: Aching pain in calf or lower leg, worse at end of the day, worse with prolonged standing or sitting.

O: Firm brawny edema; coarse, thickened skin; pulses normal; brown pigment discoloration; petechiae; dermatitis. Venous stasis causes increased venous pressure, which then causes red blood cells (RBCs) to leak out of veins and into the skin. As these RBCs break down, they leave hemosiderin (iron deposits) behind, which are the brown pigment deposits.

Ulcers occur at medial malleolus and are characterized by bleeding, uneven edges.

S, Subjective data; *O*, objective data.

Table continued on following page

ABNORMAL FINDINGS

TABLE 20–4: Peripheral Vascular Disease in the Legs—cont'd

CHRONIC VENOUS DISEASE	ACUTE VENOUS DISEASE

Superficial Varicose Veins

Incompetent valves permit reflux of blood, producing dilated, tortuous veins. Unremitting hydrostatic pressure causes distal valves to be incompetent and causes worsening of the varicosity.

Over age 45, occurrence is three times more common in women than in men.

S: Aching, heaviness in calf, easy fatigability, night leg or foot cramps.
O: Dilated, tortuous veins.

Deep Vein Thrombophlebitis

A deep vein is occluded by a thrombus, causing inflammation, blocked venous return, cyanosis, and edema. Cause may be prolonged bed rest; history of varicose veins; trauma; infection; cancer; and, in younger women, the use of oral estrogenic contraceptives (Dockery, 1997).

S: Sudden onset of intense, sharp, deep muscle pain, may increase with sharp dorsiflexion of foot.
O: Increased warmth; swelling (to compare swelling, observe the usual shoe size as in above photo); redness; dependent cyanosis is mild or may be absent; tender to palpation; Homans' sign is present only in few cases.

Requires emergency referral due to risk of pulmonary embolism.

TABLE 20–5: Peripheral Artery Disease

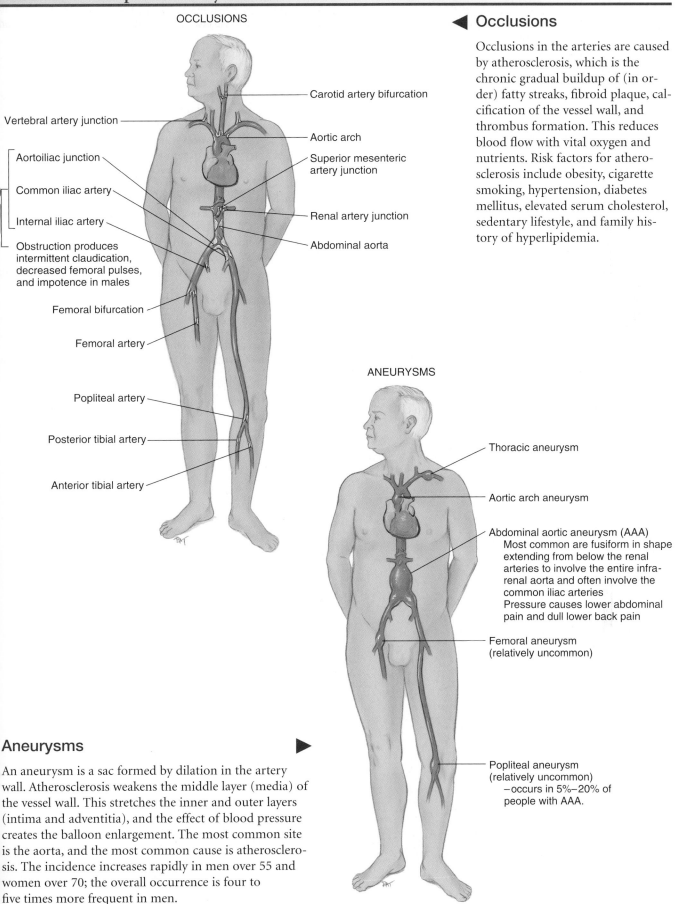

OCCLUSIONS

- Carotid artery bifurcation
- Vertebral artery junction
- Aortic arch
- Aortoiliac junction
- Superior mesenteric artery junction
- Common iliac artery
- Internal iliac artery
- Renal artery junction
- Obstruction produces intermittent claudication, decreased femoral pulses, and impotence in males
- Abdominal aorta
- Femoral bifurcation
- Femoral artery
- Popliteal artery
- Posterior tibial artery
- Anterior tibial artery

ANEURYSMS

- Thoracic aneurysm
- Aortic arch aneurysm
- Abdominal aortic aneurysm (AAA)
  Most common are fusiform in shape extending from below the renal arteries to involve the entire infra-renal aorta and often involve the common iliac arteries
  Pressure causes lower abdominal pain and dull lower back pain
- Femoral aneurysm (relatively uncommon)
- Popliteal aneurysm (relatively uncommon) –occurs in 5%–20% of people with AAA.

◀ Occlusions

Occlusions in the arteries are caused by atherosclerosis, which is the chronic gradual buildup of (in order) fatty streaks, fibroid plaque, calcification of the vessel wall, and thrombus formation. This reduces blood flow with vital oxygen and nutrients. Risk factors for atherosclerosis include obesity, cigarette smoking, hypertension, diabetes mellitus, elevated serum cholesterol, sedentary lifestyle, and family history of hyperlipidemia.

Aneurysms ▶

An aneurysm is a sac formed by dilation in the artery wall. Atherosclerosis weakens the middle layer (media) of the vessel wall. This stretches the inner and outer layers (intima and adventitia), and the effect of blood pressure creates the balloon enlargement. The most common site is the aorta, and the most common cause is atherosclerosis. The incidence increases rapidly in men over 55 and women over 70; the overall occurrence is four to five times more frequent in men.

BIBLIOGRAPHY

Barach P: Pulsus paradoxus, *Hosp Physician* 36(1):49–50, Jan 2000.

Braun CM, Colucci AM, Patterson RB: Components of an optimal exercise program for the treatment of patients with claudication, *J Vasc Nurs* 17(2):32–36, June 1999.

Braunwald E: *Heart disease: a textbook of cardiovascular medicine,* ed 6, Philadelphia, 2001, W.B. Saunders.

Cameron BL: Making diabetes management routine, *Am J Nurs* 102(2):26–40, Feb 2002.

Cantwell-Gab K: Identifying chronic peripheral arterial disease, *Am J Nurs* 96(7):40–47, Jul 1996.

Dockery GL: *Cutaneous disorders of the lower extremity,* Philadelphia, 1997, W.B. Saunders.

Fahey VA: *Vascular nursing,* ed 3, Philadelphia, 1999, W.B. Saunders.

Fuhrman TM et al: Evaluation of collateral circulation of the hand, *J Clin Monit* 8(1):28–32, Jan 1992.

Gelberman RH, Blasingame JP: The timed Allen test, *J Trauma* 21(6):477–479, June 1981.

Goodall S, Al-Khaffaf H: Assessing vascular disease: a review of primary care practice, *J Community Nurs* 16(2):16–21, Feb 2002.

Habermann TM, Steensma DP: Lymphadenopathy, *Mayo Clin Proc* 75(7):723–732, Jul 2000.

Heitman B, Irizarry A: Infectious disease causes of lymphadenopathy: localized versus diffuse, Lippincotts *Prim Care Pract* 3(1):19–38, Jan–Feb 1999.

Johnson TR, Moore WM, Jeffries JE: *Children are different: developmental physiology,* ed 2, Columbus, OH, 1978, Ross Labs.

Kennedy D, Setnik G, Li J: Physical examination findings in deep venous thrombosis, *Emerg Med Clin North Am* 19(4):869–876, Nov 2001.

McDermott MM: Ankle brachial index as a predictor of outcomes in peripheral arterial disease, *J Lab Clin Med* 133(1):33–40, Jan 1999.

Morrison C, Gordon S, Yeo TP: Hodgkin's disease in primary care, *Nurse Pract* 25(7):44–62, July 2000.

Perrodin JP: Noninvasive assessment of the peripheral vascular system: hand-held Doppler, oscillometry, and air plethysmography, *Acute Care Perspect* 10(3):13–15, Fall 2001.

Price J, Purtell JR: Prevention and treatment of lymphedema after breast cancer, *Am J Nurs* 97(9):34–37, Sep 1997.

Rosen CL, Tracy JA: The diagnosis of lower extremity deep venous thrombosis, *Emerg Med Clin North Am* 19(4):895–912, Nov 2001.

Samdani S, Lachmann E, Nagler W: Unilateral extremity swelling in female patients with cancer, *J Womens Health Gender Based Med* 10(4):319–326, May 2001.

Urbano FL: Homans' sign in the diagnosis of deep venous thrombosis, *Hosp Physician* 37(3):22–24, Mar 2001.

Urbano FL: Raynaud's phenomenon, *Hosp Physician* 37(9):27–30, Sep 2001.

Weiner SD, Reis ED, Kerstein MD: Peripheral arterial disease: medical management in primary care practice, *Geriatrics* 56(4):20–30, Apr 2001.

Welsh JR, Arzouman JM, Holm K: Nurses' assessment and documentation of peripheral edema, *Clin Nurs Spec* 10(1):7–10, Jan 1996.

Abdomen

Structure and Function

SURFACE LANDMARKS

The **abdomen** is a large oval cavity extending from the diaphragm down to the brim of the pelvis. It is bordered in back by the vertebral column and paravertebral muscles, and at the sides and front by the lower rib cage and abdominal muscles (Fig. 21–1). Four layers of large, flat muscles form the ventral abdominal wall. These are joined at the midline by a tendinous seam, the **linea alba.** One set, the **rectus abdominis,** forms a strip extending the length of the midline, and its edge is often palpable.

INTERNAL ANATOMY

Inside the abdominal cavity, all the internal organs are the **viscera.** It is important that you know the location of these organs so well that you could draw a map of them on the skin (Fig. 21–2). You must be able to visualize each organ that you listen to or palpate through the abdominal wall.

The **solid viscera** are those that maintain a characteristic shape (liver, pancreas, spleen, adrenal glands, kidneys, ovaries, and uterus). The liver fills most of the right upper quadrant (RUQ) and extends over to the left midclavicular line. The lower edge of the liver and the right kidney may be palpable normally. The ovaries normally are palpable only on bimanual examination during the pelvic examination.

The shape of the **hollow viscera** (stomach, gallbladder, small intestine, colon, and bladder) depends on the contents. They usually are not palpable, although you may feel a colon distended with feces or a bladder distended with urine. The stomach is just below the diaphragm, between the liver and spleen. The gallbladder rests under the posterior surface of the liver, just lateral to the right midclavicular line. Note that the small intestine is located in all four quadrants. It extends from the stomach's pyloric valve to the ileocecal valve in the right lower quadrant (RLQ), where it joins the colon.

The **spleen** is a soft mass of lymphatic tissue on the posterolateral wall of the abdominal cavity, immediately under the diaphragm (Fig. 21–3). It lies obliquely with its long axis behind and parallel to the 10th rib, lateral to the midaxillary line. Its width extends from the 9th to the 11th rib, about 7 cm. It is not palpable normally. If it becomes enlarged, its lower pole moves downward and toward the midline.

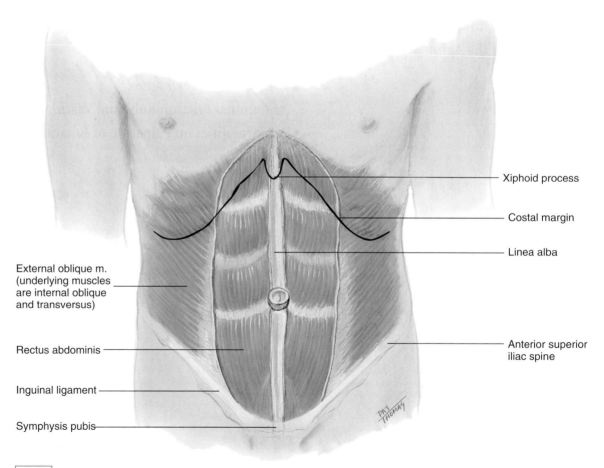

External oblique m. (underlying muscles are internal oblique and transversus)

Rectus abdominis

Inguinal ligament

Symphysis pubis

Xiphoid process

Costal margin

Linea alba

Anterior superior iliac spine

21–1

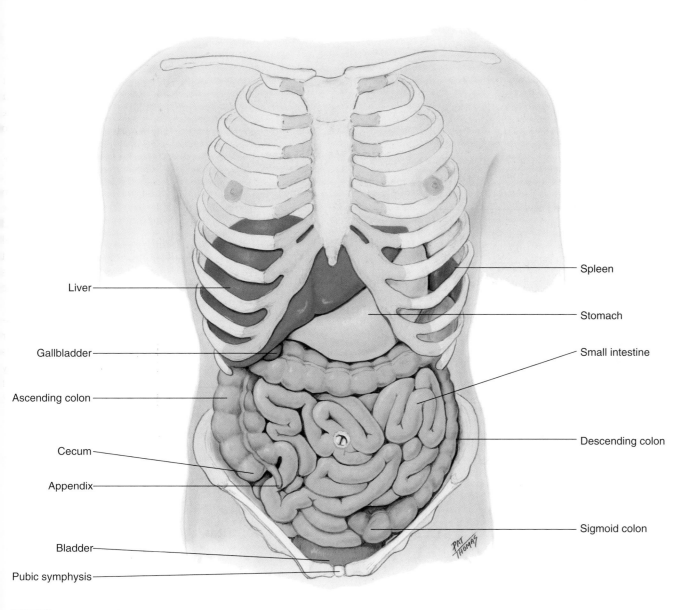

Liver

Gallbladder

Ascending colon

Cecum

Appendix

Bladder

Pubic symphysis

Spleen

Stomach

Small intestine

Descending colon

Sigmoid colon

PAT THOMAS

21–2

10th rib

Spleen

Midaxillary line

21–3

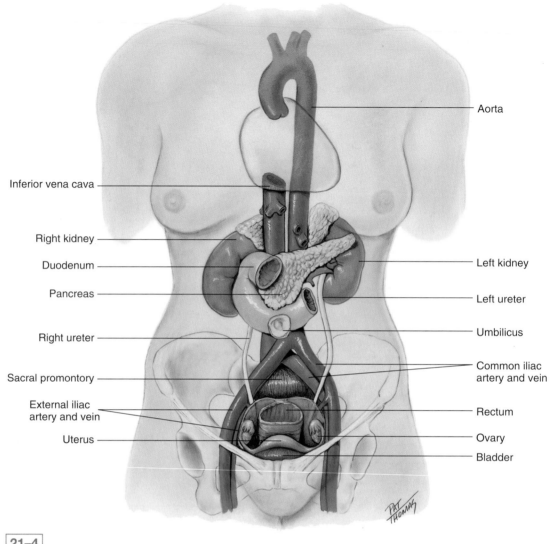

Aorta

Inferior vena cava

Right kidney

Duodenum

Pancreas

Left kidney

Left ureter

Right ureter

Umbilicus

Sacral promontory

Common iliac
artery and vein

External iliac
artery and vein

Rectum

Uterus

Ovary

Bladder

21–4

The **aorta** is just to the left of midline in the upper part of the abdomen (Fig. 21–4). It descends behind the peritoneum and at 2 cm below the umbilicus, it bifurcates into the right and left common iliac arteries opposite the 4th lumbar vertebra. You can palpate the aortic pulsations easily in the upper anterior abdominal wall. The right and left iliac arteries become the femoral arteries in the groin area. Their pulsations are easily palpated as well, at a point halfway between the anterior superior iliac spine and the symphysis pubis.

The **pancreas** is a soft, lobulated gland located behind the stomach. It stretches obliquely across the posterior abdominal wall to the left upper quadrant.

The bean-shaped **kidneys** are retroperitoneal, or posterior to the abdominal contents (Fig. 21–5). They are well protected by the posterior ribs and musculature. The 12th rib forms an angle with the vertebral column, the **costovertebral angle.** The left kidney lies here at the 11th and 12th ribs. Because of the placement of the liver, the right kidney rests 1 to 2 cm lower than the left kidney and sometimes may be palpable.

For convenience in description, the abdominal wall is divided into **four quadrants** by a vertical and a horizontal line

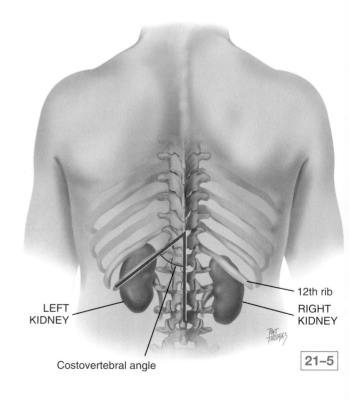

12th rib

LEFT
KIDNEY

RIGHT
KIDNEY

Costovertebral angle

21–5

bisecting the umbilicus (Fig. 21–6). (An older, more complicated scheme divided the abdomen into nine regions. Although the old system generally is not used, some regional names persist, such as *epigastric* for the area between the costal margins, *umbilical* for the area around the umbilicus, and *hypogastric* or *suprapubic* for the area above the pubic bone.)

The anatomic location of the organ by quadrants is

Right Upper Quadrant (RUQ)
Liver
Gallbladder
Duodenum
Head of pancreas
Right kidney and adrenal
Hepatic flexure of colon
Part of ascending and
  transverse colon

Left Upper Quadrant (LUQ)
Stomach
Spleen
Left lobe of liver
Body of pancreas
Left kidney and adrenal
Splenic flexure of colon
Part of transverse and
  descending colon

Right Lower Quadrant (RLQ)
Cecum
Appendix
Right ovary and tube
Right ureter
Right spermatic cord

Left Lower Quadrant (LLQ)
Part of descending colon
Sigmoid colon
Left ovary and tube
Left ureter
Left spermatic cord

Midline
Aorta
Uterus (if enlarged)
Bladder (if distended)

DEVELOPMENTAL CONSIDERATIONS

INFANTS AND CHILDREN

In the newborn, the umbilical cord shows prominently on the abdomen. It contains two arteries and one vein. The liver takes up proportionately more space in the abdomen at birth than in later life. In normal full-term neonates, the lower edge may be palpated 0.5 to 2.5 cm below the right costal margin. Age-related values of expected liver span are listed in the Objective Data section. The urinary bladder is located higher in the abdomen than in the adult. It lies between the symphysis and the umbilicus. Also during early childhood, the abdominal wall is less muscular, so the organs may be easier to palpate.

THE PREGNANT FEMALE

Nausea and vomiting, or "morning sickness," is an early sign of pregnancy for 50% to 75% of pregnant women, starting between the first and second missed periods. The cause is unknown but may be due to hormone changes such as the production of human chorionic gonadotropin (hCG). Another symptom is "acid indigestion" or heartburn (pyrosis) caused by esophageal reflux. Gastrointestinal motility decreases, which prolongs gastric emptying time. The decreased motility also causes more water to be reabsorbed from the colon, which leads to constipation. The constipation, as well as increased venous pressure in the lower pelvis, may lead to hemorrhoids.

The enlarging uterus displaces the intestines upward and posteriorly. Bowel sounds are diminished. The appendix is

21–6 Four quadrants

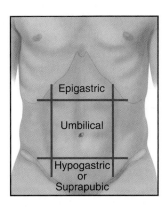

displaced upward and to the right, which may complicate diagnosis of a possible appendicitis. Skin changes on the abdomen, such as striae and linea nigra, are discussed later in this chapter and in Chapter 12.

THE AGING ADULT

Aging alters the appearance of the abdominal wall. During and after middle age, some fat accumulates in the suprapubic area in females due to decreased estrogen levels. Males also show some fat deposits in the abdominal area, resulting in the "spare tire," or "bay window." This accentuates in adults with a more sedentary lifestyle.

With further aging, adipose tissue is redistributed away from the face and extremities and to the abdomen and hips. The abdominal musculature relaxes.

Changes of aging occur in the gastrointestinal system but do not significantly affect function as long as no disease is present.

- Salivation decreases, causing the aging person to have a dry mouth and a decreased sense of taste. Further changes involving the mouth and dentition are discussed in Chapter 16.
- Esophageal emptying is delayed. If an aging person is fed in the supine position, this increases risk of aspiration.
- Gastric acid secretion decreases with aging. This may cause pernicious anemia (because it interferes with vitamin B_{12} absorption), iron deficiency anemia, and malabsorption of calcium.
- The incidence of gallstones increases with age, occurring in 10% to 20% of middle-aged and older adults, being more common in females.
- Liver size decreases with age, particularly after 80 years, although most liver function remains normal. Drug metabolism by the liver is impaired, in part because by age 60 to 80 years, blood flow through the liver is decreased by 55% to 60% (Katzung, 1998). Therefore, the liver metabolism that is responsible for the enzymatic oxidation, reduction, and hydrolysis of drugs is substantially decreased with age. This is clinically significant because prolonged liver metabolism causes increased side effects. For example, older people taking benzodiazepines scored lower on functional status measures and had increased risk of hip fracture (Reid et al., 1998).

- Aging persons frequently report constipation. However, a greater number use laxatives regularly (up to 30% of healthy older people) than actually are constipated (<10% of healthy, ambulatory, aged people). Reasons for the disparity in perceived and actual constipation include a mistaken opinion about how often a healthy person should defecate (true constipation is having a bowel movement less often than every 3rd day) and confusing the passage of hard or small stools, the feeling of incomplete evacuation, or the need to strain at stool for constipation (Stone, Wyman, and Salisbury, 1999).

Of those aging people who actually are constipated, two thirds have been found to have slowed passage in the distal colon and delayed rectal emptying. Common causes of constipation include decreased physical activity, inadequate intake of water, a low-fiber diet, side effects of medications, irritable bowel syndrome, bowel obstruction, hypothyroidism, inadequate toilet facilities (i.e., difficulty ambulating to the toilet may cause the person to deliberately retain the stool until it becomes hard and difficult to pass), and colorectal dysmotility.

TRANSCULTURAL CONSIDERATIONS

Lactase is the digestive enzyme necessary for the absorption of the carbohydrate lactose (milk sugar). In some racial groups, lactase activity is high at birth but declines to low levels by adulthood. These people are *lactose intolerant* (or lactase deficient) and experience abdominal pain, bloating, and flatulence when milk products are consumed. The incidence of lactose intolerance is 70% to 90% in blacks, Native Americans, Asians, and Mediterranean groups. However, in Europeans and Americans of northern and western European descent, the level of lactase activity remains high through adulthood, and the incidence of milk intolerance is only about 15% (Ganong, 1995).

Subjective Data

1. Appetite	4. Abdominal pain	7. Past abdominal history
2. Dysphagia	5. Nausea/vomiting	8. Medications
3. Food intolerance	6. Bowel habits	9. Nutritional assessment

EXAMINER ASKS	RATIONALE
1. Appetite. • Any change in **appetite?** Is this a loss of appetite? • Any change in weight? How much weight gained or lost? Over what time period? Is the weight loss due to diet?	Anorexia is a loss of appetite for food that occurs with gastrointestinal disease or as a side effect to some medications, with pregnancy, or with psychological disorders.

EXAMINER ASKS	RATIONALE

2. Dysphagia.

- Any difficulty swallowing? When did you first notice this?

Dysphagia occurs with disorders of the throat or esophagus.

3. Food intolerance.

- Are there any foods you cannot eat? What happens if you do eat them: allergic reaction, heartburn, belching, bloating, indigestion?
- Do you use antacids? How often?

Food intolerance, e.g., lactase deficiency resulting in bloating or excessive gas after taking milk products.
Pyrosis (heartburn), a burning sensation in esophagus and stomach, due to reflux of gastric acid.
Eructation (belching).

4. Abdominal pain.

- Any **abdominal pain?** Please point to it.
- Is the pain in one spot or does it move around?
- How did it start? How long have you had it?
- Constant or does it come and go? Occur before or after meals? Does it peak? When?
- How would you describe the character: cramping (colic type), burning in pit of stomach, dull, stabbing, aching?
- Is the pain relieved by food, or worse after eating?
- Is the pain associated with: menstrual period or irregularities, stress, dietary indiscretion, fatigue, nausea and vomiting, gas, fever, rectal bleeding, frequent urination, vaginal or penile discharge?
- What makes the pain worse: food, position, stress, medication, activity?
- What have you tried to relieve pain: rest, heating pad, change in position, medication?

Abdominal pain may be *visceral* from an internal organ (dull, general, poorly localized), *parietal* from inflammation of overlying peritoneum (sharp, precisely localized, aggravated by movement), or *referred* from a disorder in another site (see Table 21–2 on p. 593).

Aggravating factors.
Alleviating factors.

5. Nausea/vomiting.

- Any **nausea** or **vomiting?** How often? How much comes up? What is the color? Is there an odor?

- Is it bloody?

- Is the nausea and vomiting associated with colicky pain, diarrhea, fever, chills?
- What foods did you eat in the last 24 hours? Where? At home, school, restaurant? Is there anyone else in the family with same symptoms in last 24 hours?

Nausea/vomiting is a common side effect of many medications and occurs with gastrointestinal disease as well as early pregnancy.
Hematemesis occurs with stomach or duodenal ulcers and esophageal varices.

Consider food poisoning.

6. Bowel habits.

- How often do you have a **bowel movement?**
- What is the color? Consistency?
- Any diarrhea or constipation? How long?
- Any recent change in bowel habits?
- Use laxatives? Which ones? How often do you use them?

Assess usual **bowel habits.**
Black stools may be tarry due to passage of occult blood (melena) from gastrointestinal bleeding or nontarry from injection of iron medications.
Red blood in stools occurs with gastrointestinal bleeding or localized bleeding around the anus.

7. Past abdominal history.

- Any **past history** of gastrointestinal problems: ulcer, gallbladder disease, hepatitis/jaundice, appendicitis, colitis, hernia?
- Ever had any operations in the abdomen? Please describe.
- Any problems after surgery?
- Any abdominal x-ray studies? How were the results?

EXAMINER ASKS	RATIONALE

8. Medications.
- What **medications** are you currently taking?
- How about alcohol—how much would you say you drink each day? Each week? When was your last alcoholic drink?
- How about cigarettes—do you smoke? How many packs per day? For how long?

Peptic ulcer disease has risk factors that include frequent use of nonsteroidal antiinflammatory drugs (NSAIDs), alcohol, smoking, and *Helicobacter pylori* infection.

9. Nutritional assessment.
- Now I would like to ask you about your diet. Please tell me all the food you ate yesterday, starting with breakfast.

Nutritional assessment, via 24-hour recall (see Chapter 8 for a complete discussion).

Additional History for Infants and Children

1. Are you breast- or bottle-feeding the baby? If bottle-feeding, how does baby tolerate the formula?

2. What table foods have you introduced? How does the infant tolerate the food?

With allergies, consider a new food as a possible allergen. Adding only one new food at a time to the infant's diet helps identify any possible allergies.

3. How often does your toddler/child eat? Does he or she eat regular meals? How do you feel about your child's eating problems?
- Please describe all that your child had to eat yesterday, starting with breakfast. What foods does the child eat for snacks?

- Does toddler/child ever eat nonfoods: grass, dirt, paint chips?

Irregular eating patterns, although common at this age, can be a source of parental anxiety. As long as child shows normal growth and development and only nutritious foods are offered, parents may be reassured.

Pica: Although a toddler may attempt nonfoods at some time, he or she should recognize edibles by age 2.

4. Does your child have constipation: How long?
- What are the number of stools/day? Stools/week?
- How much water, juice is in the diet?
- Does the constipation seem to be associated with toilet training?
- What have you tried to treat the constipation?

5. Does the child have abdominal pain? Please describe what you have noticed and when it started.

This symptom is hard to assess with young children. Many conditions of unrelated organ systems are associated with vague abdominal pain (e.g., otitis media). Young children do not have the capacity to articulate specific symptoms and often focus on "the tummy." Abdominal pain accompanies inflammation of the bowel, as well as constipation, urinary tract infection, and anxiety.

6. For the overweight child: How long has weight been a problem?
- At what age did the child first seem overweight? Did any change in diet pattern occur then?
- Describe the diet pattern now.
- Do any others in family have similar problem?
- How does child feel about his or her own weight?

Alteration in nutrition: more than body overweight requirements.

Family history of obesity.
Assess body image.

EXAMINER ASKS	RATIONALE

Additional History for Adolescents

1. What do you eat at regular meals? Do you eat breakfast? What do you eat for snacks?

Adolescent takes control of eating and may reject family values, e.g., skipping breakfast, consuming junk foods, soda pop. The only control parents have is to control what food is in the house.

• How many calories do you figure you consume?

You probably cannot change adolescent eating pattern, but you can supply nutritional facts.

2. What is your exercise pattern?

Boys need an average 4000 cal/day to maintain weight; more calories are needed if exercise is pursued. Girls need 20% fewer calories and the same nutrients as boys. Fast food is a problem because it is high in fat, calories, and salt and has no fiber.

3. If weight is less than body requirements: How much have you lost? By diet, exercise, or how?

Screen any extremely thin teenage girl for *anorexia nervosa,* a serious psychosocial disorder that includes loss of appetite, voluntary starvation, and grave weight loss. This person may augment weight loss by purging (self-induced vomiting) and use of laxatives.

• How do you feel? Tired, hungry? How do you think your body looks?

Denial of these feelings is common. Though thin, this person insists she looks fat, "disgusting." Distorted body image.

• What is your activity pattern?

The anorectic may participate in normal activity and exercise but often is hyperactive.

• Is the weight loss associated with any other body change, such as menstrual irregularity?

Amenorrhea is common with anorexia nervosa.

• What do your parents say about your eating? Your friends?

This is a family problem involving control issues. Anyone at risk warrants immediate referral to a physician or psychologist.

Additional History for the Aging Adult

1. How do you acquire your groceries and prepare your meals?

Assess if at risk for nutritional deficit due to limited access to grocery store, limited income, limited cooking facilities, physical disability (impaired vision, decreased mobility, decreased strength, neurologic deficit).

2. Do you eat alone or share meals with others?

Assess if at risk for nutritional deficit if living alone; may not bother to prepare all meals; social isolation; depression.

EXAMINER ASKS	RATIONALE
3. Please tell me all that you had to eat yesterday, starting with breakfast.	Note: 24-hour recall may not be sufficient because pattern may vary from day to day. Attempt week-long diary of intake. Food pattern may be different at the end of the month if monthly income (e.g., social security check) runs out.
• Do you have any trouble swallowing these foods? • What do you do right after eating: walk, take a nap?	
4. How often do your bowels move? • If the person reports constipation: What do you mean by constipation? How much liquid is in your diet? How much bulk or fiber? • Do you take anything for constipation, such as laxatives? Which ones? How often? • What medications do you take?	Consider gastrointestinal side effects, e.g., nausea, upset stomach, anorexia, dry mouth.

Objective Data

PREPARATION

The lighting should include a strong overhead light and a secondary stand light. Expose the abdomen so that it is fully visible. Drape the genitalia and female breasts.

   The following measures will enhance abdominal wall relaxation:

- The person should have emptied the bladder, saving a urine specimen if needed.
- Keep the room warm to avoid chilling and tensing of muscles.
- Position the person supine, with the head on a pillow, the knees bent or on pillow, and the arms at the sides or across the chest. (Note: Discourage the person from placing his or her arms over the head because this tenses abdominal musculature.)
- To avoid abdominal tensing, the stethoscope endpiece must be warm, your hands must be warm, and your fingernails must be very short.
- Inquire about any painful areas. Examine such an area last to avoid any muscle guarding.
- Finally, learn to use distraction: Enhance muscle relaxation through breathing exercises; emotive imagery; your low, soothing voice; and the person relating his or her abdominal history while you palpate.

EQUIPMENT NEEDED

Stethoscope
Small centimeter ruler
Skin-marking pen
Alcohol swab (to clean endpiece)

NORMAL RANGE OF FINDINGS	ABNORMAL FINDINGS
INSPECT THE ABDOMEN **Contour** Stand on the person's right side and look down on the abdomen. Then stoop or sit to gaze across the abdomen. Your head should be slightly higher than the abdomen. Determine the profile from the rib margin to the pubic bone. The contour describes the nutritional state and normally ranges from flat to rounded (Fig. 21–7).	Scaphoid abdomen, protuberant abdomen, abdominal distention (see also Table 21–3, p. 594).

NORMAL RANGE OF FINDINGS	ABNORMAL FINDINGS

Flat

Scaphoid

Rounded

Protuberant

21-7

Symmetry

Shine a light across the abdomen toward you, or shine it lengthwise across the person. The abdomen should be symmetric bilaterally (Fig. 21–8). Note any localized bulging, visible mass, or asymmetric shape. Even small bulges are highlighted by shadow. Step to the foot of the examination table to recheck symmetry.

Bulges, masses.

Hernia—protrusion of abdominal viscera through abnormal opening in muscle wall (see Table 21–4, p. 596).

21-8

Ask the person to take a deep breath to further highlight any change. The abdomen should stay smooth and symmetric. Or ask the person to perform a sit-up without pushing up with his or her hands.

Note any localized bulging.

Hernia, enlarged liver or spleen may show.

Umbilicus

Normally it is midline and inverted, with no sign of discoloration, inflammation, or hernia. It becomes everted and pushed upward with pregnancy.

Everted with acites, or underlying mass (see Table 21–3).
Deeply sunken with obesity.
Enlarged and everted with umbilical hernia.
Bluish periumbilical color occurs with intraabdominal bleeding (Cullen's sign).

Skin

The surface is smooth and even, with homogeneous color. This is a good area to judge pigment because it is often protected from sun.

Redness with localized inflammation.

NORMAL RANGE OF FINDINGS

One common pigment change is **striae** (lineae albicantes), silvery white, linear, jagged marks about 1 to 6 cm long (Fig. 21–9). They occur when elastic fibers in the reticular layer of the skin are broken following rapid or prolonged stretching, as in pregnancy or excessive weight gain. Recent striae are pink or blue; then they turn silvery white.

21–9   Striae.

Moles, circumscribed brown macular or papular areas, are common on the abdomen.

Normally, no lesions are present, although you may note well-healed surgical scars. If a scar is present, draw its location in the person's record, indicating the length in centimeters (Fig. 21–10). (Note infrequently, a person forgets a past operation while providing the history. If you note a scar now, ask about it.) A surgical scar alerts you to the possible presence of underlying adhesions and excess fibrous tissue.

21–10

Jaundice (shows best in natural daylight).
Skin glistening and taut occurs with ascites.

Striae also occur with ascites.

Striae look purple-blue with Cushing's syndrome (excess adrenocortical hormone causes the skin to be fragile and easily broken from normal stretching).

Unusual color or change in shape of mole (see Chapter 12).
Petechiae.

Cutaneous angiomas (spider nevi) occur with portal hypertension or liver disease.
Lesions, rashes (see Chapter 12).

NORMAL RANGE OF FINDINGS	ABNORMAL FINDINGS

Veins usually are not seen, but a fine venous network may be visible in thin persons.

Good skin turgor reflects healthy nutrition. Gently pinch up a fold of skin; then release to note the skin's immediate return to original position.

Pulsation or Movement
Normally, you may see the pulsations from the aorta beneath the skin in the epigastric area, particularly in thin persons with good muscle wall relaxation. Respiratory movement also shows in the abdomen, particularly in males. Finally, waves of peristalsis sometimes are visible in very thin persons. They ripple slowly and obliquely across the abdomen.

Hair Distribution
The pattern of pubic hair growth normally has a diamond shape in adult males and an inverted triangle shape in adult females (see Chapters 24 and 26).

Demeanor
A comfortable person is relaxed quietly on the examining table and has a benign facial expression and slow, even respirations.

AUSCULTATE BOWEL SOUNDS AND VASCULAR SOUNDS

Depart from the usual examination sequence and auscultate the abdomen next. This is done because percussion and palpation can increase peristalsis, which would give a false interpretation of bowel sounds. Use the diaphragm endpiece because bowel sounds are relatively high pitched. Hold the stethoscope lightly against the skin; pushing too hard may stimulate more bowel sounds (Fig. 21–11). Begin in the RLQ at the ileocecal valve area, because bowel sounds are always present here normally.

21–11

ABNORMAL FINDINGS column:

Prominent, dilated veins occur with portal hypertension, cirrhosis, ascites, or vena caval obstruction. Veins are more visible with malnutrition due to thinned adipose tissue.

Poor turgor occurs with dehydration, which often accompanies gastrointestinal disease.

Marked pulsation of the aorta occurs with widened pulse pressure (e.g., hypertension, aortic insufficiency, thyrotoxicosis) and with aortic aneurysm.
Marked visible peristalsis, together with a distended abdomen, indicates intestinal obstruction.

Patterns alter with endocrine or hormone abnormalities and with chronic liver disease.

Restlessness and constant turning to find a comfortable position occur with the colicky pain of gastroenteritis or bowel obstruction.
Absolute stillness, resisting any movement, occurs with the pain of peritonitis.
Knees flexed up; facial grimacing; and rapid, uneven respirations also indicate pain.

NORMAL RANGE OF FINDINGS	ABNORMAL FINDINGS

Bowel Sounds

Note the character and frequency of bowel sounds. Bowel sounds originate from the movement of air and fluid through the small intestine. Depending on the time elapsed since eating, a wide range of normal sounds can occur. Bowel sounds are high pitched, gurgling, cascading sounds, occurring irregularly anywhere from 5 to 30 times per minute. Do not bother to count them. Judge if they are normal, hypoactive, or hyperactive.

One type of hyperactive bowel sounds is fairly common. This is the hyperperistalsis when you feel your "stomach growling," termed *borborygmus*. A perfectly "silent abdomen" is uncommon; you must listen for 5 minutes by your watch before deciding bowel sounds are completely absent.

Two distinct patterns of abnormal bowel sounds may occur:

1. **Hyperactive sounds** are loud, high-pitched, rushing, tinkling sounds that signal increased motility.
2. **Hypoactive or absent sounds** follow abdominal surgery or with inflammation of the peritoneum (see Table 21–5).

Vascular Sounds

As you listen to the abdomen, note the presence of any vascular sounds or **bruits.** Using firmer pressure, check over the aorta, renal arteries, iliac, and femoral arteries, especially in people with hypertension (Fig. 21–12). Usually, no such sound is present.

Note location, pitch, and timing of a vascular sound.

A systolic bruit is a pulsatile blowing sound and occurs with stenosis or occlusion of an artery.

Venous hum and peritoneal friction rub are rare (see Table 21–6).

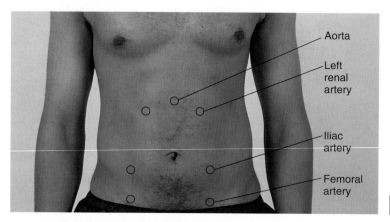

Aorta

Left renal artery

Iliac artery

Femoral artery

21-12

PERCUSS GENERAL TYMPANY, LIVER SPAN, AND SPLENIC DULLNESS

Percuss to assess the relative density of abdominal contents, to locate organs, and to screen for abnormal fluid or masses.

General Tympany

First, percuss lightly in all four quadrants to determine the prevailing amount of tympany and dullness (Fig. 21–13). Tympany should predominate because air in the intestines rises to the surface when the person is supine.

Dullness occurs over a distended bladder, adipose tissue, fluid, or a mass.

Hyperresonance is present with gaseous distention.

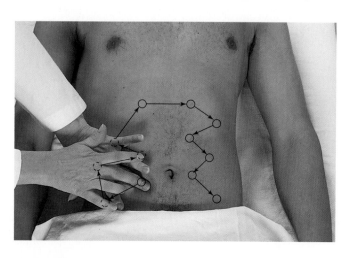

21-13

NORMAL RANGE OF FINDINGS	ABNORMAL FINDINGS

Liver Span

Next, percuss to map out the boundaries of certain organs. Measure the height of the liver in the right midclavicular line. (For a consistent placement of the midclavicular line landmark, remember to palpate the acromioclavicular and the sternoclavicular joints and judge the line at a point midway between the two.)

Begin in the area of lung resonance, and percuss down the interspaces until the sound changes to a dull quality (Fig. 21–14). Mark the spot, usually in the fifth intercostal space. Then find abdominal tympany and percuss up in the midclavicular line. Mark where the sound changes from tympany to a dull sound, normally at the right costal margin.

21–14

Measure the distance between the two marks; the normal liver span in the adult ranges from 6 to 12 cm (Fig. 21–15). The height of the liver span correlates with the height of the person; taller people have longer livers. Also males have a larger liver span than females of the same height. Overall, the mean liver span is 10.5 cm for males and 7 cm for females.

An enlarged liver span indicates liver enlargement or **hepatomegaly.**

Accurate detection of liver borders is confused by dullness above the fifth intercostal space, which occurs with lung disease, e.g., pleural effusion or consolidation. Accurate detection at the lower border is confused when dullness is pushed up with ascites or pregnancy or with gas distention in colon, which obscures lower border.

21–15

NORMAL RANGE OF FINDINGS

One variation occurs in people with chronic emphysema, in which the liver is displaced downward by the hyperinflated lungs. Although you hear a dull percussion note well below the right costal margin, the overall span is still within normal limits.

Clinical estimation of liver span is important to screen for hepatomegaly and to monitor changes in liver size. However, this measurement is a gross estimate; the liver span may be underestimated because of inaccurate detection of the upper border.

SCRATCH TEST. One final technique is the *scratch test,* which may help define the liver border when the abdomen is distended or the abdominal muscles are tense. Place your stethoscope over the liver. With one fingernail, scratch short strokes over the abdomen, starting in the RLQ and moving progressively up toward the liver (Fig. 21–16). When the scratching sound in your stethoscope becomes magnified, you will have crossed the border from over a hollow organ to a solid one.

21–16

Splenic Dullness

Often the spleen is obscured by stomach contents, but you may locate it by percussing for a dull note from the 9th to 11th intercostal space just behind the left midaxillary line (Fig. 21–17). The area of splenic dullness normally is not wider than 7 cm in the adult and should not encroach on the normal tympany over the gastric air bubble.

A dull note forward of the midaxillary line indicates enlargement of the spleen, as occurs with mononucleosis, trauma, and infection.

21–17

NORMAL RANGE OF FINDINGS

Now percuss in the lowest interspace in the left *anterior* axillary line. Tympany should result. Ask the person to take a deep breath. Normally, tympany remains through full inspiration.

Costovertebral Angle Tenderness

Indirect fist percussion causes the tissues to vibrate instead of producing a sound. To assess the kidney, place one hand over the 12th rib at the costovertebral angle on the back (Fig. 21–18). Thump that hand with the ulnar edge of your other fist. The person normally feels a thud but no pain. (Although this step is explained here with percussion techniques, its usual sequence in a complete examination is with thoracic assessment, when the person is sitting up and you are standing behind.)

21–18

Special Procedures

At times, you may suspect that a person has ascites (free fluid in the peritoneal cavity) because of a distended abdomen, bulging flanks, and an umbilicus that is protruding and displaced downward. You can differentiate ascites from gaseous distention by performing two percussion tests.

FLUID WAVE. First, test for a **fluid wave** by standing on the person's right side. Place the ulnar edge of another examiner's hand or the patient's own hand firmly on the abdomen in the midline (Fig. 21–19). (This will stop transmission across the skin of the upcoming tap.) Place your left hand on the person's right flank. With your right hand, reach across the abdomen and give the left flank a firm strike. If ascites is present, the blow will generate a fluid wave through the abdomen and you will feel a distinct tap on your left hand. If the abdomen is distended from gas or adipose tissue, you will feel no change.

21–19

Fluid wave.

ABNORMAL FINDINGS

In this site, the *anterior* axillary line, a change in percussion from tympany to a dull sound with full inspiration is a **positive spleen percussion sign,** indicating splenomegaly. This method will detect mild to moderate splenomegaly before the spleen becomes palpable, as in mononucleosis, malaria, or hepatic cirrhosis.

Sharp pain occurs with inflammation of the kidney or paranephric area.

Ascites occurs with heart failure, portal hypertension, cirrhosis, hepatitis, pancreatitis, and cancer.

A positive fluid wave test occurs with large amounts of ascitic fluid.

NORMAL RANGE OF FINDINGS

SHIFTING DULLNESS.   The second test for ascites is percussing for **shifting dull-ness.** In a supine person, ascitic fluid settles by gravity into the flanks, displacing the air-filled bowel upward. You will hear a tympanitic note as you percuss over the top of the abdomen because gas-filled intestines float over the fluid (Fig. 21–20). Then percuss down the side of the abdomen. If fluid is present, the note will change from tympany to dull as you reach its level. Mark this spot.

Tympany
Dullness

21–20

Now turn the person onto the right side (roll the person toward you) (Fig. 21–21). The fluid will gravitate to the dependent (in this case, right) side, displacing the lighter bowel upward. Begin percussing the upper side of the abdomen and move downward. The sound changes from tympany to a dull sound as you reach the fluid level, but this time the level of dullness is higher, upward toward the umbilicus. This *shifting level of dullness* indicates the presence of fluid.

Shifting dullness is positive with a large volume of ascitic fluid: It will not detect less than 500 ml of fluid.

Tympany

Shifting level
of dullness

21–21

Both tests, fluid wave and shifting dullness, are not reliable. Ultrasound study is the definitive tool.

| NORMAL RANGE OF FINDINGS | ABNORMAL FINDINGS |

PALPATE SURFACE AND DEEP AREAS

Perform palpation to judge the size, location, and consistency of certain organs and to screen for an abnormal mass or tenderness. Review comfort measures on p. 570. Since most people are naturally inclined to protect the abdomen, you need to use additional measures to enhance complete muscle relaxation.

1. Bend the person's knees.
2. Keep your palpating hand low and parallel to the abdomen. Holding the hand high and pointing down would make anyone tense up.
3. Teach the person to breathe slowly (in through the nose, and out through the mouth).
4. Keep your own voice low and soothing. Conversation may relax the person.
5. Try "emotive imagery." For example, you might say, "Now I want you to imagine you are dozing on the beach, with the sun warming your muscles and the sound of the waves lulling you to sleep. Let yourself relax."
6. With a very ticklish person, keep the person's hand under your own with your fingers curled over his or her fingers. Move both hands around as you palpate; people are not ticklish to themselves.
7. Alternatively, perform palpation just after auscultation. Keep the stethoscope in place and curl your fingers around it, palpating as you pretend to auscultate. People do not perceive a stethoscope as a ticklish object. You can slide the stethoscope out when the person is used to being touched.

Light and Deep Palpation

Begin with **light palpation.** With the first four fingers close together, depress the skin about 1 cm (Fig. 21–22). Make a gentle rotary motion, sliding the fingers and skin together. Then lift the fingers (do not drag them) and move clockwise to the next location around the abdomen. The objective here is not to search for organs but to form an overall impression of the skin surface and superficial musculature. Save the examination of any identified tender areas until last. This method avoids pain and the resulting muscle rigidity that would obscure deep palpation later in the examination.

Muscle guarding.
Rigidity.
Large masses.
Tenderness.

21–22

NORMAL RANGE OF FINDINGS

As you circle the abdomen, discriminate between voluntary muscle guarding and involuntary rigidity. **Voluntary guarding** occurs when the person is cold, tense, or ticklish. It is bilateral, and you will feel the muscles relax slightly during exhalation. Use the relaxation measures to try to eliminate this type of guarding, or it will interfere with deep palpation. If the rigidity persists, it is probably involuntary.

Now perform **deep palpation** using the same technique described earlier, but push down about 5 to 8 cm (2 to 3 inches) (Fig. 21–23). Moving clockwise, explore the entire abdomen.

21–23

To overcome the resistance of a very large or obese abdomen, use a bimanual technique. Place your two hands on top of each other (Fig. 21–24). The top hand does the pushing; the bottom hand is relaxed and can concentrate on the sense of palpation. With either technique, note the location, size, consistency, and mobility of any palpable organs and the presence of any abnormal enlargement, tenderness, or masses.

21–24

ABNORMAL FINDINGS

Involuntary rigidity is a constant board-like hardness of the muscles. It is a protective mechanism accompanying acute inflammation of the peritoneum. It may be unilateral, and the same area usually becomes painful when the person increases intraabdominal pressure by attempting a sit-up.

NORMAL RANGE OF FINDINGS

Making sense of what you are feeling is more difficult than it looks. Inexperienced examiners complain that the abdomen "all feels the same," as if they are pushing their hand into a soft sofa cushion. It helps to memorize the anatomy and visualize what is under each quadrant as you palpate. Also remember that some structures are normally palpable, as illustrated in Figure 21–25.

Mild tenderness normally is present when palpating the sigmoid colon. Any other tenderness should be investigated.

ABNORMAL FINDINGS

Tenderness occurs with local inflammation, with inflammation of the peritoneum or underlying organ, and with an enlarged organ whose capsule is stretched.

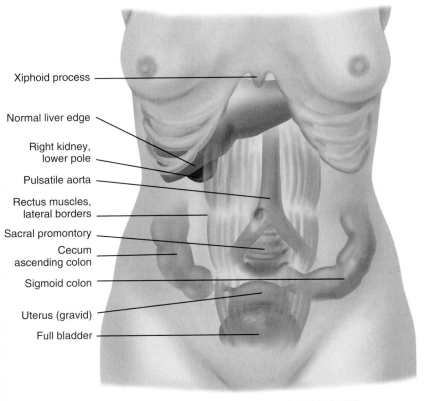

Xiphoid process

Normal liver edge

Right kidney, lower pole

Pulsatile aorta

Rectus muscles, lateral borders

Sacral promontory

Cecum ascending colon

Sigmoid colon

Uterus (gravid)

Full bladder

NORMALLY PALPABLE STRUCTURES

21–25

If you identify a mass, first distinguish it from a normally palpable structure or an enlarged organ. Then note the following:

1. Location
2. Size
3. Shape
4. Consistency (soft, firm, hard)
5. Surface (smooth, nodular)
6. Mobility (including movement with respirations)
7. Pulsatility
8. Tenderness

NORMAL RANGE OF FINDINGS

Liver

Next, palpate for specific organs, beginning with the liver in the RUQ (Fig. 21–26). Place your left hand under the person's back parallel to the 11th and 12th ribs and lift up to support the abdominal contents. Place your right hand on the RUQ, with fingers parallel to the midline. Push deeply down and under the right costal margin. Ask the person to take a deep breath. It is normal to feel the edge of the liver bump your fingertips as the diaphragm pushes it down during inhalation. It feels like a firm regular ridge. Often, the liver is not palpable and you feel nothing firm.

21–26

HOOKING TECHNIQUE. An alternative method of palpating the liver is to stand up at the person's shoulder and swivel your body to the right so that you face the person's feet (Fig. 21–27). Hook your fingers over the costal margin from above. Ask the person to take a deep breath. Try to feel the liver edge bump your fingertips.

21–27

Spleen

Normally, the spleen is not palpable and must be enlarged three times its normal size to be felt. To search for it, reach your left hand over the abdomen and behind the left side at the 11th and 12th ribs (Fig. 21–28, A). Lift up for support.

ABNORMAL FINDINGS

Except with a depressed diaphragm, a liver palpated more than 1 to 2 cm below the right costal margin is enlarged. Record the number of centimeters it descends and note its consistency (hard, nodular) and tenderness (see Table 21–7.)

NORMAL RANGE OF FINDINGS

Place your right hand obliquely on the LUQ with the fingers pointing toward the left axilla and just inferior to the rib margin. Push your hand deeply down and under the left costal margin and ask the person to take a deep breath. You should feel nothing firm.

A

B

21-28

When enlarged, the spleen slides out and bumps your fingertips. It can grow so large that it extends into the lower quadrants. When this condition is suspected, start low so you will not miss it. An alternative position is to roll the person onto his or her right side to displace the spleen more forward and downward (Fig. 21-28, B). Then palpate as described earlier.

ABNORMAL FINDINGS

The spleen enlarges with mononucleosis and trauma (see Table 21-7). If you feel an enlarged spleen, refer the person but do not continue to palpate it. An enlarged spleen is friable and can rupture easily with overpalpation.

Describe the number of centimeters it extends below the left costal margin.

NORMAL RANGE OF FINDINGS

Kidneys

Search for the right kidney by placing your hands together in a "duck-bill" position at the person's right flank (Fig. 21–29, A). Press your two hands together firmly (you need deeper palpation than that used with the liver or spleen) and ask the person to take a deep breath. In most people, you will feel no change. Occasionally, you may feel the lower pole of the right kidney as a round, smooth mass slide between your fingers. Either condition is normal.

Enlarged kidney.
Kidney mass.

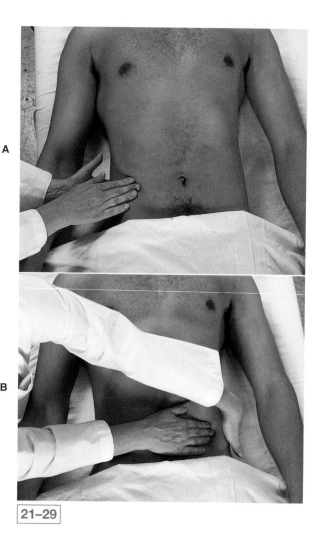

A

B

21–29

The left kidney sits 1 cm higher than the right kidney and is not palpable normally. Search for it by reaching your left hand across the abdomen and behind the left flank for support (Fig. 21–29, B). Push your right hand deep into the abdomen and ask the person to breathe deeply. You should feel no change with the inhalation.

Aorta

Using your opposing thumb and fingers, palpate the aortic pulsation in the upper abdomen slightly to the left of midline (Fig. 21–30). Normally, it is 2.5 to 4 cm wide in the adult and pulsates in an anterior direction.

Widened with aneurysm (see Tables 21–6 and 21–7).

Prominent lateral pulsation with aortic aneurysm.

NORMAL RANGE OF FINDINGS	ABNORMAL FINDINGS

21-30

Special Procedures

REBOUND TENDERNESS (BLUMBERG'S SIGN). Assess rebound tenderness when the person reports abdominal pain or when you elicit tenderness during palpation. Choose a site away from the painful area. Hold your hand 90 degrees, or perpendicular, to the abdomen. Push down slowly and deeply; then lift up *quickly* (Fig. 21–31, *A*, *B*). This makes structures that are indented by palpation rebound suddenly. A normal, or negative, response is no pain on release of pressure. Perform this test at the end of the examination, because it can cause severe pain and muscle rigidity.

Pain on release of pressure confirms rebound tenderness, which is a reliable sign of peritoneal inflammation. Peritoneal inflammation accompanies appendicitis.

21-31   Rebound tenderness.

INSPIRATORY ARREST (MURPHY'S SIGN). Normally, palpating the liver causes no pain. In a person with inflammation of the gallbladder, or cholecystitis, pain occurs. Hold your fingers under the liver border. Ask the person to take a deep breath. A normal response is to complete the deep breath without pain.

When the test is positive, as the descending liver pushes the inflamed gallbladder onto the examining hand, the person feels sharp pain and abruptly stops inspiration midway.

NORMAL RANGE OF FINDINGS

ILIOPSOAS MUSCLE TEST. Perform the iliopsoas muscle test when the acute abdominal pain of appendicitis is suspected. With the person supine, lift the right leg straight up, flexing at the hip (Fig. 21–32); then push down over the lower part of the right thigh as the person tries to hold the leg up. When the test is negative, the person feels no change.

When the iliopsoas muscle is inflamed (which occurs with an inflamed or perforated appendix), pain is felt in the right lower quadrant.

21–32 Iliopsoas muscle test.

OBTURATOR TEST. The obturator test also is performed when appendicitis is suspected. With the person supine, lift the right leg, flexing at the hip and 90 degrees at the knee (Fig. 21–33). Hold the ankle and rotate the leg internally and externally. A negative or normal response is no pain.

A perforated appendix irritates the obturator muscle, producing pain.

21–33 Obturator test.

 DEVELOPMENTAL CONSIDERATIONS

The Infant

INSPECTION. The contour of the abdomen is protuberant because of the immature abdominal musculature. The skin contains a fine, superficial venous pattern. This may be visible in lightly pigmented children up to the age of puberty.

Scaphoid shape occurs with dehydration. Dilated veins.

Inspect the umbilical cord throughout the neonatal period. At birth, it is white and contains two umbilical arteries and one vein surrounded by mucoid connective tissue, called Wharton's jelly. The umbilical stump dries within a week, hardens, and falls off by 10 to 14 days. Skin covers the area by 3 to 4 weeks.

The presence of only one artery signals the risk of congenital defects.
Inflammation.
Drainage after cord falls off.

NORMAL RANGE OF FINDINGS	ABNORMAL FINDINGS

The abdomen should be symmetric, although two bulges are common. You may note an **umbilical hernia.** It appears at 2 to 3 weeks and is especially prominent when the infant cries. The hernia reaches maximum size at 1 month (up to 2.5 cm or 1 inch) and usually disappears by 1 year. Another common variation is **diastasis recti,** a separation of the rectus muscles with a visible bulge along the midline. The condition is more common with black infants, and it usually disappears by early childhood.

Refer any umbilical hernia larger than 2.5 cm (see Table 21–4); continuing to grow after 1 month; or lasting for more than 2 years in a white child or for more than 7 years in a black child.

Refer diastasis recti lasting more than 6 years.

The abdomen shows respiratory movement. The only other abdominal movement you should note is occasional peristalsis, which may be visible because of the thin musculature.

Marked peristalsis with pyloric stenosis (see Table 21–4).

AUSCULTATION.   Auscultation yields only bowel sounds, the metallic tinkling of peristalsis. No vascular sounds should be heard.

Bruit.
Venous hum.

PERCUSSION.   Percussion finds tympany over the stomach (the infant swallows some air with feeding) and dullness over the liver. Percussing the spleen is not done. The abdomen sounds tympanitic, although it is normal to percuss dullness over the bladder. This dullness may extend up to the umbilicus.

PALPATION.   Aid palpation by flexing the baby's knees with one hand while palpating with the other (Fig. 21–34). Alternatively, you may hold the upper back and flex the neck slightly with one hand. Offer a pacifier to a crying baby.

The liver fills the RUQ. It is normal to feel the liver edge at the right costal margin or 1 to 2 cm below. Normally, you may palpate the spleen tip and both kidneys as well as the bladder. Also easily palpated are the cecum in the RLQ, and the sigmoid colon, which feels like a sausage in the left inguinal area.

Make note of the newborn's first stool, a sticky, greenish-black meconium stool within 24 hours of birth. By the fourth day, stools of breast-fed babies are golden-yellow, pasty, and smell like sour milk, whereas those of formula-fed babies are brown-yellow, firmer, and more fecal smelling.

21–34

The Child
Under age 4 years, the abdomen looks protuberant when the child is both supine and standing. After age 4 years, the potbelly remains when standing because of lumbar lordosis, but the abdomen looks flat when supine. Normal movement on the abdomen includes respirations, which remain abdominal until 7 years of age.

A scaphoid abdomen is associated with dehydration or malnutrition.

Under 7 years of age, the absence of abdominal respirations occurs with inflammation of the peritoneum.

| NORMAL RANGE OF FINDINGS | ABNORMAL FINDINGS |

To palpate the abdomen, position the young child on the parent's lap as you sit knee-to-knee with the parent (Fig. 21–35). Flex the knees up, and elevate the head slightly. The child can "pant like a dog" to further relax abdominal muscles. Hold your entire palm flat on the abdominal surface for a moment before starting palpation. This accustoms the child to being touched. If the child is very ticklish, hold his or her hand under your own as you palpate; or apply the stethoscope and palpate around it.

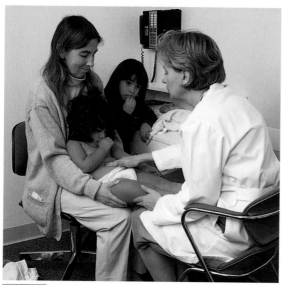

21–35

The liver remains easily palpable 1 to 2 cm below the right costal margin. The edge is soft and sharp and moves easily. On the left, the spleen also is easily palpable with a soft, sharp, movable edge. Usually you can feel 1 to 2 cm of the right kidney and the tip of the left kidney.

TABLE 21–1: Expected Liver Span by Percussion Through Childhood and Adolescence

| AGE | MEAN ESTIMATED LIVER SPAN (CM) | |
	MALES	FEMALES
6 mo	2.4	2.8
1 yr	2.8	3.1
2 yr	3.5	3.6
3 yr	4.0	4.0
4 yr	4.4	4.3
5 yr	4.8	4.5
6 yr	5.1	4.8
8 yr	5.6	5.1
10 yr	6.1	5.4
12 yr	6.5	5.6
14 yr	6.8	5.8
16 yr	7.1	6.0
18 yr	7.4	6.1
20 yr	7.7	6.3

Modified from Lawson EE, Grand RJ, Neff RK, Cohen LF: Clinical estimation of liver span in infants and children, *Am J Dis Child* 132:474–476, 1978. Copyright 1978, American Medical Association.

NORMAL RANGE OF FINDINGS	ABNORMAL FINDINGS

In assessing abdominal tenderness, remember that the young child often answers this question affirmatively no matter how the abdomen actually feels. Use objective signs to aid assessment, such as a cry changing in pitch as you palpate, facial grimacing, moving away from you, and guarding.

The school-age child has a slim abdominal shape as she or he loses the pot-belly. This slimming trend continues into adolescence. See Table 21–1 for age-related values of liver span by percussion.

The adolescent easily is embarrassed with exposure of the abdomen, and adequate draping is necessary. The physical findings are the same as those listed for the adult.

The Aging Adult

On inspection, you may note increased deposits of subcutaneous fat on the abdomen and hips, as it is redistributed away from the extremities. The abdominal musculature is thinner and has less tone than that of the younger adult, so in the absence of obesity you may note peristalsis.

Because of the thinner, softer abdominal wall, the organs may be easier to palpate (in the absence of obesity). The liver is easier to palpate. Normally, you will feel the liver edge at or just below the costal margin. With distended lungs and a depressed diaphragm, the liver is palpated lower, descending 1 to 2 cm below the costal margin with inhalation. The kidneys are easier to palpate.

Abdominal rigidity with acute abdominal conditions is less common in aging persons.

With an acute abdomen, the aging person often complains of less pain than a younger person would.

SUMMARY CHECKLIST: Abdomen Exam

1. Inspection
Contour
Symmetry
Umbilicus
Skin
Pulsation or movement
Hair distribution
Demeanor

2. Auscultation
Bowel sounds
Note any vascular sounds

3. Percussion
Percuss all four quadrants
Percuss borders of liver, spleen

4. Palpation
Light palpation in all four quadrants
Deeper palpation in all four quadrants
Palpate for liver, spleen, kidneys

See Health Promotion Guide on CD

Application and Critical Thinking

SAMPLE CHARTING

SUBJECTIVE

States appetite is good with no recent change, no dysphagia, no food intolerance, no pain, no nausea/vomiting. Has one formed BM/day. Takes vitamins, no other prescribed or over-the-counter medication. No history of abdominal disease, injury, or surgery. Diet recall of last 24 hours listed at end of history.

OBJECTIVE

Inspection. Abdomen flat, symmetric with no apparent masses. Skin smooth with no striae, scars, or lesions.
Auscultation. Bowel sounds present, no bruits.
Percussion. Tympany predominates in all four quadrants, liver span is 8 cm in right midclavicular line. Splenic dullness located at 10th intercostal space in left midaxillary line.
Palpation. Abdomen soft, no organomegaly, no masses, no tenderness.

Continued

FOCUSED ASSESSMENT: CLINICAL CASE STUDY 1

George E. is a 58-year-old unemployed divorced white male with chronic alcoholism who enters the chemical dependency treatment center.

SUBJECTIVE

States last 6 months has been drinking 1 pint whiskey/day. Last alcohol use 1 week PTA, with "5 or 6" drinks that episode. Estranged from family, lives alone. Makes a few meals on hot plate. States never has appetite. Has fatigue and weakness.

OBJECTIVE

Inspection. Appears older than stated age. Oriented, although verbal response time slowed. Weight loss of 12 lb in last 3 mo.
Abdomen protuberant, symmetric, no visible masses. Poor skin turgor. Dilated venous pattern over abdominal wall. Hair sparse in axillary, pubic area.
Auscultation. Bowel sounds present. No vascular sounds.
Percussion. Tympany predominates over abdomen. Liver span is 16 cm in right midclavicular line. No fluid wave. No shifting dullness.
Palpation. Soft. Liver palpable 10 cm below right costal margin, smooth and nontender. No other organomegaly or masses.

ASSESSMENT

Alcohol dependence, severe, with physiologic dependence
Imbalanced nutrition: less than body requirements R/T impaired absorption
Ineffective coping R/T effects of chronic alcoholism
Social isolation

FOCUSED ASSESSMENT: CLINICAL CASE STUDY 2

Edith J. is a 63-year-old retired homemaker with a history of lung cancer with metastases to the liver.

SUBJECTIVE

Feeling "puffy and bloated" for the past week. States unable to get comfortable. Also short of breath "all the time now." Difficulty sleeping. "I feel like crying all the time now."

OBJECTIVE

Inspection. Weight increase of 8 lb in 1 week. Abdomen is distended with everted umbilicus and bulging flanks. Girth at umbilicus is 85 cm. Prominent dilated venous pattern present over abdomen.
Auscultation. Bowel sounds present, no vascular sounds.
Percussion. When supine, tympany present at dome of abdomen, dullness over flanks. Shifting dullness present. Positive fluid wave present. Liver span is 12 cm in right midclavicular line.
Palpation. Abdominal wall firm, able to feel liver with deep palpation at 6 cm below right costal margin. Liver feels firm, nodular, nontender. 4+ pitting edema in both ankles.

ASSESSMENT

Anticipatory grieving
Ascites
Ineffective breathing pattern R/T increased intraabdominal pressure
Pain R/T distended abdomen
Risk for impaired skin integrity: R/T ascites, edema, and faulty metabolism
Disturbed sleep pattern

FOCUSED ASSESSMENT: CLINICAL CASE STUDY 3

Dan G. is a 17-year-old black male high school student who enters the emergency department with abdominal pain for 2 days.

SUBJECTIVE

Two days PTA Dan noted general abdominal pain in umbilical region. Now pain is sharp and severe, and Dan points to location in right lower quadrant. No BM for 2 days. Nausea and vomiting off and on 1 day.

OBJECTIVE

Inspection. BP 112/70 Temp 38° C, pulse 116, resp 18.
Lying on side with knees drawn up under chin. Resists any movement. Face tight and occasionally grimacing. Cries out with any sudden movement.
Auscultation. No bowel sounds present. No vascular sounds.
Percussion. Tympany. Percussion over RLQ leads to tenderness.
Palpation. Abdominal wall is rigid and boardlike. Extreme tenderness to palpation in RLQ. Rebound tenderness is present in RLQ. Positive iliopsoas muscle test.

ASSESSMENT

Acute abdominal pain in RLQ
Nausea

NURSING DIAGNOSES COMMONLY ASSOCIATED WITH ABDOMINAL DISORDERS

RELATED FACTORS (Etiology)	DEFINING CHARACTERISTICS (Symptoms and Signs)
DIAGNOSIS: Constipation	
Less than adequate dietary intake and bulk	Frequency less than usual pattern
Neuromuscular or musculoskeletal impairment	Hard, formed stools
Pain/discomfort on defecation	Palpable mass
Effects of	Straining at stool
Diagnostic procedures	Less than usual amount of stool
Pregnancy	Decreased bowel sounds
Aging	Gas pain and flatulence
Medication	Abdominal or back pain
Stress or anxiety	Reported feeling of abdominal or rectal fullness or pressure
Weak abdominal musculature	Impaired appetite
Immobility or less-than-adequate physical activity	Headache
Chronic use of laxatives and enemas	Nausea
Gastrointestinal lesions	Irritability
Ignoring urge to defecate	Palpable hard stool on rectal examination
Fear of rectal or cardiac pain	
DIAGNOSIS: Diarrhea	
Effects of	Abdominal pain
Medications	Anorexia
Radiation	Change in color or odor of stool
Surgical intervention	Chills
Infectious process	Cramping
Inflammatory process	Fatigue
Malabsorption syndrome	Increased frequency of bowel sounds
Stress and anxiety	Loose, liquid stools
Dietary alterations	Increased frequency of stool
Food intolerances	Irritated anal area
Increased caffeine consumption	Fever
Excessive use of laxatives	Malaise
Allergies	Muscle weakness
Nutritional disorders	Thirst
Ingestion of contaminated water or food	Urgency
Hyperosmolar tube feeding	Weight loss

Continued

RELATED FACTORS (Etiology)	DEFINING CHARACTERISTICS (Symptoms and Signs)

DIAGNOSIS: Urinary retention

Diminished or absent sensory and/or motor impulses	Bladder distention
Effects of some medications	Diminished force of urinary stream
Anesthetics	Dribbling
Opiates	Dysuria
Psychotropics	Hesitancy
Strong sphincter	High residual urine
Urethral blockage associated with fecal impaction, postpartum edema, prostate hypertrophy, or surgical swelling	Nocturia
	Sensation of bladder fullness
Anxiety (fear of postoperative pain)	Small, frequent voiding or absence of urine output

DIAGNOSIS: Ineffective Tissue perfusion (renal, gastrointestinal)

Exchange problems	Renal
Hypervolemia	Diminished urine output
Hypovolemia	Edema
Interruption of flow	Gastrointestinal
	Constipation
	Nausea and vomiting
	Pain

OTHER RELATED NURSING DIAGNOSES

ACTUAL	RISK/WELLNESS
Constipation	**Risk**
Perceived Constipation	Risk for Constipation
Bowel Incontinence	Risk for Infection
Functional urinary Incontinence	Risk for imbalanced Nutrition: more than body requirements
Reflex urinary Incontinence	
Stress urinary Incontinence	**Wellness**
Total urinary Incontinence	Health-seeking behavior regarding weight-loss diet
Urge urinary Incontinence	
Nausea	
Imbalanced Nutrition: less than body requirements	
Imbalanced Nutrition: more than body requirements	
Pain	
Impaired Urinary elimination	

ASSESSMENT VIDEO CRITICAL THINKING QUESTIONS

The Saunders *Physical Examination and Health Assessment* video "Abdomen" will direct you to consider the following:
1. Describe common sites of referred abdominal pain.
2. What bowel sounds would you expect to hear in a patient with diarrhea?

3. What abnormal findings can be detected by light palpation of the abdomen?
4. What should you suspect if your palpation detects an enlarged spleen? What should you do next?

Abnormal Findings

TABLE 21–2: Common Sites of Referred Abdominal Pain

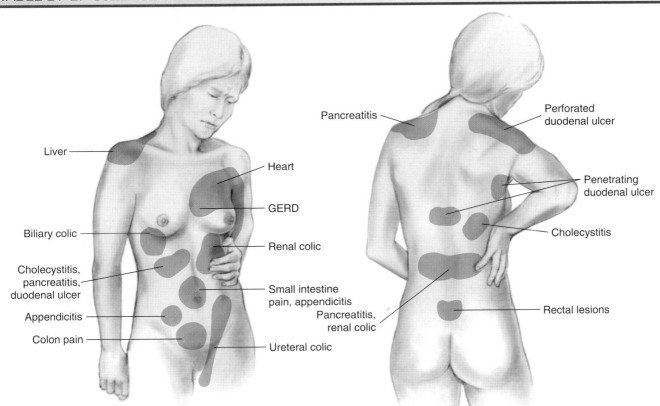

When a person gives a history of abdominal pain, the pain's location may not necessarily be directly over the involved organ. That is because the human brain has no felt image for internal organs. Rather, pain is referred to a site where the organ was located in fetal development. Although the organ migrates during fetal development, its nerves persist in referring sensations from the former location. The following are examples, not a complete list.

Liver. Hepatitis may have mild-to-moderate, dull pain in right upper quadrant or epigastrium, along with anorexia, nausea, malaise, low-grade fever.

Esophagus. Gastroesophageal reflux disease (GERD) is a complex of symptoms of esophagitis, including burning pain in mid-epigastrium or behind lower sternum that radiates upward, or "heartburn." Occurs 30 to 60 minutes after eating; aggravated by lying down or bending over.

Gallbladder. Cholecystitis is biliary colic, sudden pain in right upper quadrant that may radiate to right or left scapula, and which builds over time, lasting 2 to 4 hours, following ingestion of fatty foods, alcohol, or caffeine. Associated with nausea and vomiting, and positive Murphy's sign or sudden stop in inspiration with RUQ palpation.

Pancreas. Pancreatitis has acute, boring midepigastric pain radiating to the back and sometimes to the left scapula or flank, severe nausea, and vomiting.

Duodenum. Duodenal ulcer typically has dull, aching, gnawing pain, does not radiate, may be relieved by food, and may awaken the person from sleep.

Stomach. Gastric ulcer pain is dull, aching, gnawing epigastric pain, usually brought on by food, radiates to back or substernal area. Pain of perforated ulcer is burning epigastric pain of sudden onset that refers to one or both shoulders.

Appendix. Appendicitis typically starts as dull, diffuse pain in periumbilical region that later shifts to severe, sharp, persistent pain and tenderness localized in RLQ (McBurney's point). Pain is aggravated by movement, coughing, deep breathing; associated with anorexia, then nausea and vomiting, fever.

Kidney. Kidney stones prompt a sudden onset of severe, colicky flank or lower abdominal pain.

Small intestine. Gastroenteritis has diffuse, generalized abdominal pain, with nausea, diarrhea.

Colon. Large bowel obstruction has moderate, colicky pain of gradual onset in lower abdomen, bloating. Irritable bowel syndrome (IBS) has sharp or burning, cramping pain over a wide area; does not radiate. Brought on by meals, relieved by bowel movement.

TABLE 21–3: Abdominal Distention*

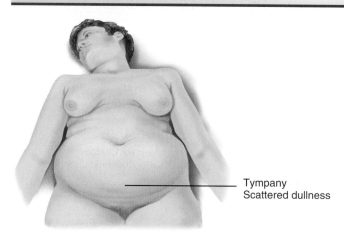

Obesity

Inspection. Uniformly rounded. Umbilicus sunken (it adheres to peritoneum, and layers of fat are superficial to it).
Auscultation. Normal bowel sounds.
Percussion. Tympany. Scattered dullness over adipose tissue.
Palpation. Normal. May be hard to feel through thick abdominal wall.

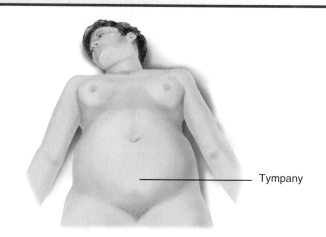

Air or Gas

Inspection. Single round curve.
Auscultation. Depends on cause of gas, e.g., decreased or absent bowel sounds with ileus; hyperactive with early intestinal obstruction.
Percussion. Tympany over large area.
Palpation. May have muscle spasm of abdominal wall.

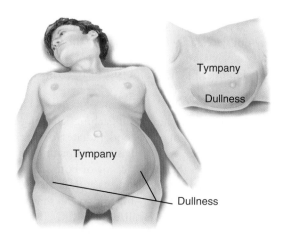

Ascites

Inspection. Single curve. Everted umbilicus. Bulging flanks when supine. Taut, glistening skin, recent weight gain, increase in abdominal girth.
Auscultation. Normal bowel sounds over intestines. Diminished over ascitic fluid.
Percussion. Tympany at top where intestines float. Dull over fluid. Produces fluid wave and shifting dullness.
Palpation. Taut skin and increased intraabdominal pressure limit palpation.

Ovarian Cyst (Large)

Inspection. Curve in lower half of abdomen, midline. Everted umbilicus.
Auscultation. Normal bowel sounds over upper abdomen where intestines pushed superiorly.
Percussion. Top dull over fluid. Intestines pushed superiorly. Large cyst produces fluid wave and shifting dullness.
Palpation. Transmits aortic pulsation while ascites does not.

*A mnemonic device to recall the common causes of abdominal distention is the seven Fs: fat, flatus, fluid, fetus, feces, fetal growth, and fibroid.

Continued

TABLE 21–3: Abdominal Distention—cont'd

Fetal
heart tones

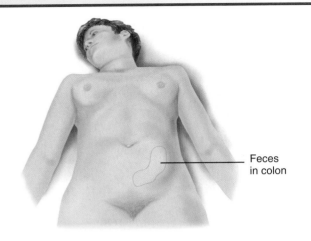

Feces
in colon

Pregnancy*

Inspection. Single curve. Umbilicus protruding. Breasts engorged.
Auscultation. Fetal heart tones. Bowel sounds diminished.
Percussion. Tympany over intestines. Dull over enlarging uterus.
Palpation. Fetal parts. Fetal movements.

Feces

Inspection. Localized distention.
Auscultation. Normal bowel sounds.
Percussion. Tympany predominates. Scattered dullness over fecal mass.
Palpation. Plastic- or ropelike mass with feces in intestines.

Tumor

Inspection. Localized distention.
Auscultation. Normal bowel sounds.
Percussion. Dull over mass if reaches up to skin surface.
Palpation. Define borders. Distinguish from enlarged organ or normally palpable structure.

*Obviously a normal finding, pregnancy is included for comparison of conditions causing abdominal distention.

TABLE 21-4: Abnormalities on Inspection

◀ Umbilical Hernia

Umbilical hernia is a soft, skin-covered mass, which is the protrusion of the omentum or intestine through a weakness or incomplete closure in the umbilical ring. It is accentuated by increased intraabdominal pressure as with crying, coughing, vomiting, or straining, but the bowel rarely incarcerates or strangulates. It is more common in black, Chinese, and premature infants. Most umbilical hernias resolve spontaneously by 1 year; parents should avoid affixing a belt or coin at the hernia because this will not help closure and may cause contact dermatitis.

In an adult, it occurs with pregnancy, chronic ascites, or from chronic intrathoracic pressure (e.g., asthma, chronic bronchitis).

Epigastric Hernia (not illustrated)

A small, fatty nodule at epigastrium in midline, through the linea alba. Usually one can feel it rather than observe it. May be palpable only when standing.

Incisional Hernia (not illustrated)

A bulge near an old operative scar that may not show when person is supine but is apparent when the person increases intra-abdominal pressure by a sit-up, stand, or Valsalva maneuver.

Diastasis Recti (not illustrated)

Diastasis recti, or a midline longitudinal ridge, is a separation of the abdominal rectus muscles. Ridge is revealed when intraabdominal pressure is increased by raising head while supine. Occurs congenitally and as a result of pregnancy or marked obesity in which prolonged distention or a decrease in muscle tone has occurred. It is not clinically significant.

TABLE 21–5: Abnormal Bowel Sounds

◀ Succussion Splash

Unrelated to peristalsis, this is a very loud splash auscultated over the upper abdomen when the infant is rocked side to side. It indicates increased air and fluid in the stomach, as seen with pyloric obstruction or large hiatus hernia.

Marked peristalsis, together with projectile vomiting in the newborn, suggests pyloric stenosis, an obstruction of the stomach's pyloric sphincter. Pyloric stenosis is a congenital defect and appears in the 2nd or 3rd week. After feeding, pronounced peristaltic waves cross from left to right, leading to projectile vomiting. Then one can palpate an olive-sized mass in the RUQ midway between the right costal margin and umbilicus. Refer promptly because of the risk of weight loss.

Hypoactive Bowel Sounds

Diminished or absent bowel sounds signal decreased motility due to inflammation as seen with peritonitis, from paralytic ileus as following abdominal surgery, or from late bowel obstruction. Occurs also with pneumonia.

Hyperactive Bowel Sounds

Loud, gurgling sounds, "borborygmi," signal increased motility. They occur with early mechanical bowel obstruction (high pitched), gastroenteritis, brisk diarrhea, laxative use, and subsiding paralytic ileus.

TABLE 21–6: Abdominal Friction Rubs and Vascular Sounds

Peritoneal Friction Rub

Vascular Sounds

◀ Peritoneal Friction Rub

A rough, grating sound, like two pieces of leather rubbed together, indicates peritoneal inflammation. Occurs rarely. Usually occurs over organs with a large surface area in contact with the peritoneum.

Liver—friction rub over lower right rib cage, due to abscess or metastatic tumor.

Spleen—friction rub over lower left rib cage in left anterior axillary line, from abscess, infection, or tumor.

Vascular Sounds

Arterial—a **bruit** indicates turbulent blood flow, as found in constricted, abnormally dilated, or tortuous vessels. Listen with the bell. Occurs with the following three conditions:

Aortic aneurysm—murmur is harsh, systolic, or continuous and accentuated with systole. Note in person with hypertension.

Renal artery stenosis—murmur is midline or toward flank, soft, low-to-medium pitch.

Partial occlusion of femoral arteries

Venous hum—occurs rarely. Heard in periumbilical region. Originates from inferior vena cava. Medium pitch, continuous sound, pressure on bell may obliterate it. May have palpable thrill. Occurs with portal hypertension and cirrhotic liver.

TABLE 21–7: Abnormalities on Palpation of Enlarged Organs

Enlarged Liver

An enlarged, smooth, and nontender liver occurs with fatty infiltration, portal obstruction or cirrhosis, high obstruction of inferior vena cava, and lymphocytic leukemia.

The liver feels enlarged and smooth but is tender to palpation with early heart failure, acute hepatitis, or hepatic abscess.

Enlarged Nodular Liver

An enlarged and nodular liver occurs with late portal cirrhosis, metastatic cancer, or tertiary syphilis.

Continued

TABLE 21–7: Abnormalities on Palpation of Enlarged Organs—cont'd

Enlarged Gallbladder

An enlarged, tender gallbladder suggests acute cholecystitis. Feel it behind the liver border as a smooth and firm mass like a sausage, although it may be difficult to palpate due to involuntary rigidity of abdominal muscles. The area is exquisitely painful to fist percussion, and inspiratory arrest (Murphy's sign) is present.

An enlarged, nontender gallbladder also feels like a smooth, sausagelike mass. It occurs when the gallbladder is filled with stones, as with common bile duct obstruction.

Enlarged Spleen

Since any enlargement superiorly is stopped by the diaphragm, the spleen enlarges down and to the midline. When extreme, it can extend down to the left pelvis. It retains the splenic notch on the medial edge. When splenomegaly occurs with acute infections (mononucleosis), it is moderately enlarged and soft, with rounded edges. When due to a chronic cause, the enlargement is firm or hard, with sharp edges. An enlarged spleen is usually not tender to palpation; it is tender only if the peritoneum is also inflamed.

Enlarged Kidney

Enlarged with hydronephrosis, cyst, or neoplasm. May be difficult to distinguish an enlarged kidney from an enlarged spleen because they have a similar shape. Both extend forward and down. However, the spleen may have a sharp edge, whereas the kidney never does. The spleen retains the splenic notch, whereas the kidney has no palpable notch. Percussion over the spleen is dull, whereas over the kidney it is tympanitic due to the overriding bowel.

Aortic Aneurysm

Most aortic aneurysms (more than 95%) are located below the renal arteries and extend to the umbilicus. About 80% of these are palpable during routine physical examination and feel like a pulsating mass in the upper abdomen just to the left of midline. You will hear a bruit. Femoral pulses are present but decreased.

Additional information on abdominal aneurysm is illustrated in Table 20–5.

BIBLIOGRAPHY

Alexander IM: Viral hepatitis: primary care diagnosis and management, *Nurse Pract* 23(10):13–45, Oct 1998.

Bode C, Bode JC: Alcohol's role in gastrointestinal tract disorders, *Alcohol Health Res World* 21(1):76–96, 1997.

Brenner H et al: Relation of smoking and alcohol and coffee consumption to active *Helicobacter pylori* infection: cross sectional study, *BMJ* 315(7121):1489–1492, Dec 1997.

Carlson E: Irritable bowel syndrome, *Nurse Pract* 23(1):82–93, Jan 1998.

Cozad J: Infectious mononucleosis, *Nurse Pract* 21(3):14–28, Mar 1996.

Ganong WF: *Review of medical physiology,* ed 17, Norwalk, CT, 1995, Appleton & Lange.

Iosue K: Chronic hepatitis: latest treatment options, *Nurse Pract* 27(4):32–49, Apr 2002.

Katzung BG: *Basic and clinical pharmacology,* ed 17, Norwalk, CT, 1998, Appleton & Lange.

Knowdley KV: Update on therapy for hepatobiliary diseases, *Nurse Pract* 21(7):78–88, July 1996.

Lawson EE et al: Clinical estimation of liver span in infants and children, *Am J Dis Child* 132:474–476, 1978.

Lo Buono C: Evaluation of the acute abdomen, *Patient Care* 34(14):26–36, Jul 30, 2000.

McManus TJ: *Helicobacter pylori:* an emerging infectious disease, *Nurse Pract* 25(8):40–53, Aug 2000.

O'Hanlon-Nichols T: Basic assessment series: gastrointestinal system, *Am J Nurs* 98(4):48–53, Apr 1998.

Pisarra VH: Recognizing the various presentations of appendicitis, *Nurse Pract* 24(8):42–53, Aug 1999.

Ray SW et al: Managing gastroesophageal reflux disease, *Nurse Pract* 27(5):36–55, May 2002.

Reid LD, Johnson RE, Gettman DA: Benzodiazepine exposure and functional status in older people, *J Am Geriatr Soc* 46(1):71–76, Jan 1998.

Shaw B: Comprehensive assessment of gastrointestinal disorders, *J Nurse Midwifery* 40(2):216–230, Mar–Apr 1995.

Spiller RC: ABC of the upper gastrointestinal tract: anorexia, nausea, vomiting, and pain, *BMJ* 323(7325):1354–1357, Dec 8, 2001.

Stone JK, Wyman JF, Salisbury SA: *Clinical gerontological nursing—a guide to advanced practice,* ed 2, Philadelphia, 1999, W.B. Saunders.

Stone R: Primary care diagnosis of acute abdominal pain, *Nurse Pract* 21(12):19–39, Dec 1996.

CHAPTER 22

Musculoskeletal System

Structure and Function

The musculoskeletal system consists of the body's **bones, joints,** and **muscles.** Humans need this system (1) for *support* to stand erect, and (2) for *movement.* The musculoskeletal system also functions (3) to encase and *protect* the inner vital organs (e.g., brain, spinal cord, heart), (4) to *produce* the red blood cells in the bone marrow (hematopoiesis), and (5) as a *reservoir* for *storage* of essential minerals, such as calcium and phosphorus in the bones.

COMPONENTS OF THE MUSCULOSKELETAL SYSTEM

The skeleton is the bony framework of the body. It has 206 bones, which support the body like the posts and beams of a building. **Bone** and cartilage are specialized forms of connective tissue. Bone is hard, rigid, and very dense. Its cells are continually turning over and remodeling. The **joint** (or articulation) is the place of union of two or more bones. Joints are the functional units of the musculoskeletal system because they permit the mobility needed for activities of daily living.

NONSYNOVIAL OR SYNOVIAL JOINTS

In **nonsynovial** joints, the bones are united by fibrous tissue or cartilage and are immovable (e.g., the sutures in the skull) or only slightly movable (e.g., the vertebrae). **Synovial** joints are freely movable because they have bones that are separated from each other and are enclosed in a joint cavity (Fig. 22–1). This cavity is filled with a lubricant, or synovial fluid. Just like grease on gears, synovial fluid allows sliding of opposing surfaces, and this sliding permits movement.

In synovial joints, a layer of resilient **cartilage** covers the surface of opposing bones. Cartilage is avascular; it receives nourishment from synovial fluid that circulates during joint movement. It is a very stable connective tissue with a slow cell turnover. It has a tough, firm consistency, yet is flexible. This cartilage cushions the bones and gives a smooth surface to facilitate movement.

The joint is surrounded by a fibrous capsule and is supported by ligaments. **Ligaments** are fibrous bands running directly from one bone to another that strengthen the joint and help prevent movement in undesirable directions. A **bursa** is an enclosed sac filled with viscous synovial fluid, much like a joint. Bursae are located in areas of potential friction (e.g., subacromial bursa of the shoulder, prepatellar bursa of the knee) and help muscles and tendons glide smoothly over bone.

MUSCLES

Muscles account for 40% to 50% of the body's weight. When they contract, they produce movement. Muscles are of three types: skeletal, smooth, and cardiac. This chapter is concerned with **skeletal,** or voluntary, muscles, those under conscious control.

Tibia

Cartilage

Synovial membrane

Synovial cavity

Capsular ligament

} **Synovial joint**

Tendo calcaneus
(Achilles tendon)

Talus

Bursae

Extensor tendon

Flexor muscles

Flexor tendon

22–1

Flexion

Extension

Abduction

Adduction

Pronation

Supination

Circumduction

Rotation

Elevation ↑
Depression ↓

Eversion   Inversion

← Protraction
→ Retraction

22–2

SKELETAL MUSCLE MOVEMENTS

Each **skeletal muscle** is composed of bundles of muscle fibers, or **fasciculi.** The skeletal muscle is attached to bone by a **tendon**—a strong fibrous cord. Skeletal muscles produce the following movements (Fig. 22–2):

1. Flexion—bending a limb at a joint
2. Extension—straightening a limb at a joint
3. Abduction—moving a limb away from the midline of the body
4. Adduction—moving a limb toward the midline of the body
5. Pronation—turning the forearm so that the palm is down
6. Supination—turning the forearm so that the palm is up
7. Circumduction—moving the arm in a circle around the shoulder
8. Inversion—moving the sole of the foot inward at the ankle
9. Eversion—moving the sole of the foot outward at the ankle
10. Rotation—moving the head around a central axis
11. Protraction—moving a body part forward and parallel to the ground
12. Retraction—moving a body part backward and parallel to the ground
13. Elevation—raising a body part
14. Depression—lowering a body part

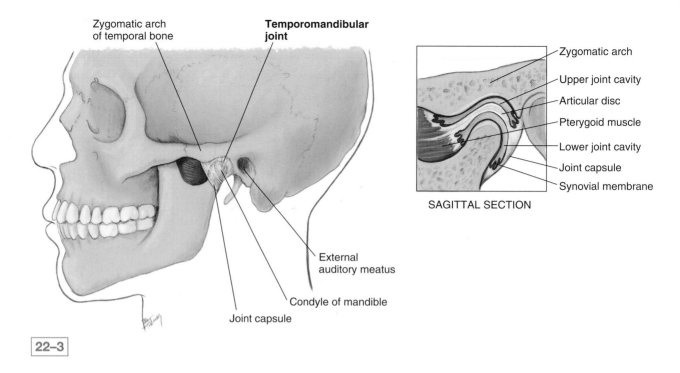

Zygomatic arch
of temporal bone

**Temporomandibular
joint**

Zygomatic arch

Upper joint cavity

Articular disc

Pterygoid muscle

Lower joint cavity

Joint capsule

Synovial membrane

SAGITTAL SECTION

External
auditory meatus

Condyle of mandible

Joint capsule

22–3

TEMPOROMANDIBULAR JOINT

The temporomandibular joint (TMJ) is the articulation of
the mandible and the temporal bone (Fig. 22–3). You can feel
it in the depression anterior to the tragus of the ear. The TMJ
permits jaw function for speaking and chewing. The joint allows three motions: (1) hinge action to open and close the
jaws, (2) gliding action for protrusion and retraction, and (3)
gliding for side-to-side movement of the lower jaw.

SPINE

The **vertebrae** are 33 connecting bones stacked in a vertical
column (Fig. 22–4). You can feel their spinous processes in a
furrow down the midline of the back. The furrow has paravertebral muscles mounded on either side down to the
sacrum, where it flattens. Humans have 7 cervical, 12 thoracic, 5 lumbar, 5 sacral, and 3 to 4 coccygeal vertebrae. The
following surface landmarks will orient you to their levels:

- The spinous processes of C7 and T1 are prominent at the
  base of the neck.
- The inferior angle of the scapula normally is at the level of
  the interspace between T7 and T8.
- An imaginary line connecting the highest point on each iliac crest crosses L4.
- An imaginary line joining the two symmetric dimples that
  overlie the posterior superior iliac spines crosses the
  sacrum.

T1

C7

T7
T8

Scapula

L1

T12

Iliac crest

Posterior
superior
iliac spine

L4

S2

Coccyx

LANDMARKS OF THE SPINE

22–4

A lateral view shows that the vertebral column has four curves (a double **S** shape) (Fig. 22–5). The cervical and lumbar curves are concave (inward), and the thoracic and sacrococcygeal curves are convex. The balanced or compensatory nature of these curves, together with the resilient intervertebral disks, allows the spine to absorb a great deal of shock.

The **intervertebral disks** are elastic fibrocartilaginous plates that constitute one-quarter of the length of the column (Fig. 22–6). Each disk center has a **nucleus pulposus,** made of soft, semifluid, mucoid material that has the consistency of toothpaste in the young adult. The disks cushion the spine like a shock absorber and help it move. As the spine moves, the elasticity of the disks allows compression on one side, with compensatory expansion on the other. Sometimes compression can be too great. The disk then can rupture and the nucleus pulposus can herniate out of the vertebral column, compressing on the spinal nerves and causing pain.

The unique structure of the spine enables both up-right posture and flexibility for motion. The motions of the vertebral column are flexion (bending forward), extension (bending back), abduction (to either side), and rotation.

22–5

22–6

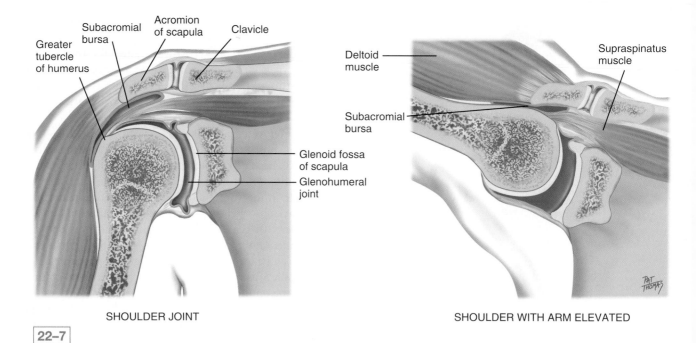

Greater tubercle of humerus
Subacromial bursa
Acromion of scapula
Clavicle
Glenoid fossa of scapula
Glenohumeral joint

SHOULDER JOINT

22–7

Deltoid muscle
Supraspinatus muscle
Subacromial bursa

SHOULDER WITH ARM ELEVATED

SHOULDER

The **glenohumeral joint** is the articulation of the humerus with the glenoid fossa of the scapula (Fig. 22–7). Its ball-and-socket action allows great mobility of the arm on many axes. The joint is enclosed by a group of four powerful muscles and tendons that support and stabilize it. Together these are called the **rotator cuff** of the shoulder. The large **subacromial bursa** helps during abduction of the arm, so that the greater tubercle of the humerus moves easily under the acromion process of the scapula.

The bones of the shoulder have palpable landmarks to guide your examination (Fig. 22–8). The scapula and the clavicle connect to form the shoulder girdle. You can feel

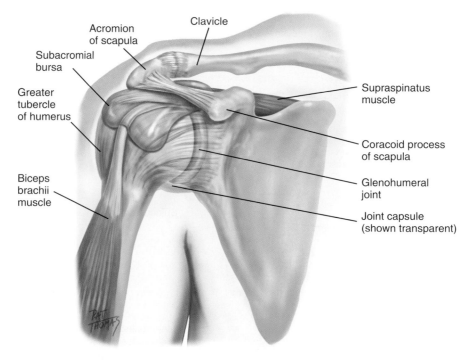

Subacromial bursa
Acromion of scapula
Clavicle
Greater tubercle of humerus
Supraspinatus muscle
Biceps brachii muscle
Coracoid process of scapula
Glenohumeral joint
Joint capsule (shown transparent)

BONY LANDMARKS OF THE SHOULDER

22–8

RIGHT ELBOW - POSTERIOR VIEW

22-9

ELBOW

The elbow joint contains the three bony articulations of the humerus, radius, and ulna of the forearm (Fig. 22–9). Its hinge action moves the forearm (radius and ulna) on one plane, allowing flexion and extension. The olecranon bursa lies between the olecranon process and the skin.

Palpable landmarks are the **medial** and **lateral epicondyles** of the humerus and the large **olecranon process** of the ulna in between them. The sensitive ulnar nerve runs between the olecranon process and the medial epicondyle.

The radius and ulna articulate with each other at two radioulnar joints, one at the elbow and one at the wrist. These move together to permit pronation and supination of the hand and forearm.

WRIST AND CARPALS

Of the body's 206 bones, over half are in the hands and feet. The wrist or **radiocarpal joint** is the articulation of the radius (on the thumb side) and a row of carpal bones (Fig. 22–10). Its condyloid action permits movement in two planes at right angles: flexion and extension, and side-to-side deviation. You can feel the groove of this joint on the dorsum of the wrist.

The **midcarpal** joint is the articulation between the two parallel rows of carpal bones. It allows flexion, extension, and some rotation. The **metacarpophalangeal** and the **interphalangeal** joints permit finger flexion and extension. The flexor tendons of the wrist and hand are enclosed in synovial sheaths.

the bump of the scapula's **acromion process** at the very top of the shoulder. Move your fingers in a small circle outward, down, and around. The next bump is the **greater tubercle** of the humerus a few centimeters down and laterally, and from that the **coracoid process** of the scapula is a few centimeters medially. These surround the deeply situated joint.

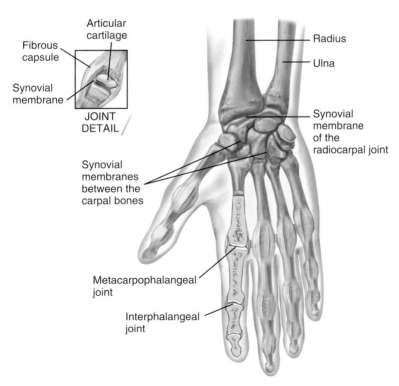

BONES OF THE HAND - PALMAR VIEW

22-10

Anterior superior iliac spine

Greater trochanter of femur

Articular capsule

Iliopectineal bursa

Pubis

Obturator foramen

Ischial tuberosity

Head of femur

Acetabulum

HIP JOINT

22–11

HIP

The hip joint is the articulation between the acetabulum and the head of the femur (Fig. 22–11). As in the shoulder, ball-and-socket action permits a wide range of motion on many axes. The hip has somewhat less range of motion (ROM) than the shoulder, but it has more stability as befits its weight-bearing function. Hip stability is due to powerful muscles that spread over the joint, a strong fibrous articular capsule, and the very deep insertion of the head of the femur. Three bursae facilitate movement.

Palpation of these bony landmarks will guide your examination. You can feel the entire iliac crest, from the **anterior superior iliac spine** to the posterior. The **ischial tuberosity** lies under the gluteus maximus muscle and is palpable when the hip is flexed. The **greater trochanter** of the femur is nor-

Femur

Medial collateral ligament

Medial meniscus

Gastrocnemius muscle

Suprapatellar bursa

Prepatellar bursa

Patella

Infrapatellar fat pad

Patellar ligament

Tibia

Femur

Suprapatellar bursa

Prepatellar bursa

Patella

Infrapatellar fat pad

Subcutaneous infrapatellar bursa

Deep infrapatellar bursa

Tibia

Meniscus

Joint capsule

LEFT KNEE - MEDIAL VIEW

SAGITTAL SECTION

22–12

mally the width of the person's palm below the iliac crest and halfway between the anterior superior iliac spine and the ischial tuberosity. Feel it when the person is standing, in a flat depression on the upper lateral side of the thigh.

KNEE

The knee joint is the articulation of three bones—the femur, the tibia, and the patella (kneecap), in one common articular cavity (Fig. 22–12). It is the largest joint in the body and is complex. It is a hinge joint, permitting flexion and extension of the lower leg on a single plane.

The knee's synovial membrane is the largest in the body. It forms a sac at the superior border of the patella, called the **suprapatellar pouch,** which extends up as much as 6 cm behind the quadriceps muscle. Two wedge-shaped cartilages, called the **medial** and **lateral menisci,** cushion the tibia and femur. The joint is stabilized by two sets of ligaments. The **cruciate ligaments** (not shown) crisscross within the knee; they give anterior and posterior stability and help control rotation. The **collateral ligaments** connect the joint at both sides; they give medial and lateral stability and prevent dislocation. Numerous bursae prevent friction. One, the **prepatellar bursa,** lies between the patella and the skin. The **infrapatellar fat pad** is a small, triangular fat pad below the patella behind the patellar ligament.

Landmarks of the knee joint start with the large **quadriceps** muscle, which you can feel on your anterior and lateral thigh (Fig. 22–13). The muscle's four heads merge into a common tendon that continues down to enclose the round bony patella. Then the tendon inserts down on the **tibial tuberosity,** which you can feel as a bony prominence in the midline. Move to the sides and a bit superiorly and note the lateral and medial condyles of the tibia. Superior to these on either side of the patella are the medial and lateral epicondyles of the femur.

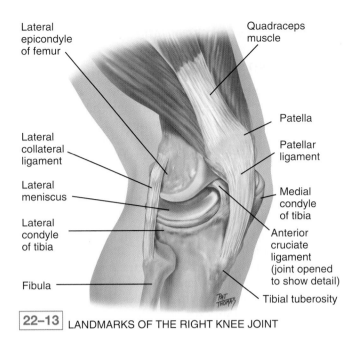

22–13   LANDMARKS OF THE RIGHT KNEE JOINT

ANKLE AND FOOT

The ankle or **tibiotalar joint** is the articulation of the tibia, fibula, and talus (Fig. 22–14). It is a hinge joint, limited to flexion (dorsiflexion) and extension (plantar flexion) on one plane. Landmarks are two bony prominences on either side—the **medial malleolus** and the **lateral malleolus.** Strong, tight medial and lateral ligaments extend from each malleolus onto the foot. These help the lateral stability of the ankle joint, although they may be torn in eversion or inversion sprains of the ankle.

Joints distal to the ankle give additional mobility to the foot. The subtalar joint permits inversion and eversion of the foot. The foot has a longitudinal arch, with weight-bearing distributed between the parts that touch the ground—the heads of the metatarsals and the calcaneus (heel).

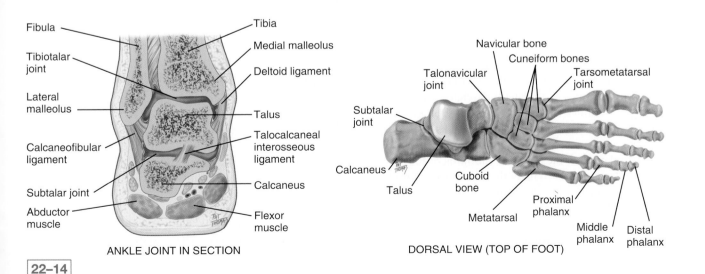

ANKLE JOINT IN SECTION

DORSAL VIEW (TOP OF FOOT)

22–14

DEVELOPMENTAL CONSIDERATIONS

INFANTS AND CHILDREN

By 3 months' gestation, the fetus has formed a "scale model" of the skeleton that is made up of cartilage. During succeeding months in utero, the cartilage ossifies into true bone and starts to grow. Bone growth continues after birth—rapidly during infancy and then steadily during childhood—until adolescence, when both boys and girls experience a rapid growth spurt.

Long bones grow in two dimensions. They increase in width or diameter by deposition of new bony tissue around the shafts. Lengthening occurs at the **epiphyses,** or growth plates. These specialized growth centers are transverse disks located at the ends of long bone. Any trauma or infection at this location puts the growing child at risk for bone deformity. This longitudinal growth continues until closure of the epiphyses; the last closure occurs at about age 20.

Skeletal contour changes are apparent at the vertebral column. At birth the spine has a single **C**-shaped curve. At 3 to 4 months, raising the baby's head from prone position develops the anterior curve in the cervical neck region. From 1 year to 18 months, standing erect develops the anterior curve in the lumbar region.

Whereas the skeleton contributes to linear growth, muscles and fat are significant for weight increase. Individual muscle fibers grow through childhood, but growth is marked during the adolescent growth spurt. Then muscles respond to increased secretion of growth hormone, to adrenal androgens, and in boys, to further stimulation by testosterone. Muscles vary in size and strength in different people. This is due to genetic programming, nutrition, and exercise. All through life, muscles increase with use and atrophy with disuse.

THE PREGNANT FEMALE

Increased levels of circulating hormones (estrogen, relaxin from the corpus luteum, and corticosteroids) presumably cause increased mobility in the joints. Increased mobility in the sacroiliac, sacrococcygeal, and symphysis pubis joints in the pelvis may contribute to the noticeable changes in maternal posture. The most characteristic change in posture is progressive **lordosis.** Lordosis compensates for the enlarging fetus; otherwise, the center of balance would shift forward. Lordosis compensates by shifting the weight farther back on the lower extremities. This shift in balance in turn creates strain on the low back muscles, which is felt as low back pain during late pregnancy in some women.

Anterior flexion of the neck and slumping of the shoulder girdle are other postural changes that compensate for the lordosis. These upper back changes may put pressure on the ulnar and median nerves during the third trimester. Nerve pressure creates aching, numbness, and weakness in the upper extremities in some women.

THE AGING ADULT

With aging, loss of bone matrix (resorption) occurs more rapidly than new bone growth (deposition). The net effect is a loss of bone density, or **osteoporosis.** Although some degree of osteoporosis is nearly universal, females experience it more than males, and whites more than blacks.

Postural changes are evident with aging, and decreased height is the most noticeable. Long bones do not shorten with age. Decreased height is due to shortening of the vertebral column. This is caused by loss of water content and thinning of the intervertebral disks, which occurs more in the middle years, and a decrease in height of individual vertebrae, which occurs in later years from osteoporosis. Both men and women can expect a progressive decrease in height beginning at age 40 in males and age 43 in females, although this is not significant until age 60 (Cline et al., 1989). A greater decrease occurs in the 70s and 80s due to osteoporotic collapse of the vertebrae. The result is a shortening of the trunk and comparatively long extremities. Other postural changes are kyphosis, a backward head tilt to compensate for kyphosis, and a slight flexion of hips and knees.

The distribution of subcutaneous fat changes through life. Usually, men and women gain weight in their 40s and 50s. The contour is different, even if the weight is the same as when younger. They begin to lose fat in the face and deposit it in abdomen and hips. In the 80s and 90s, fat further decreases in the periphery, which is especially noticeable in the forearms, although it is still apparent over the abdomen and hips.

Loss of subcutaneous fat leaves bony prominences more marked (e.g., tips of vertebrae, ribs, iliac crests), and body hollows deeper (e.g., cheeks, axillae). An absolute loss in muscle mass occurs; some muscles decrease in size, and some atrophy, producing weakness. The contour of muscles becomes more prominent, and muscle bundles and tendons feel more distinct.

It has become more apparent that lifestyle affects musculoskeletal changes. A sedentary lifestyle hastens musculoskeletal changes of aging. However, physical exercise increases skeletal mass. This helps prevent or delay osteoporosis. Physical activity delays or prevents bone loss in postmenopausal and older women (Ebrahim et al., 1997; Gregg et al., 1998).

TRANSCULTURAL CONSIDERATIONS

The long bones of blacks are significantly longer, narrower, and denser than those of whites (Overfield, 1995). Measurement of bone density by race and sex reveals that black males have the densest bones, thus accounting for the relatively low incidence of osteoporosis in this population. Bone density in the Chinese, Japanese, and Inuits is below that of white Americans (Overfield, 1995).

Curvature of the long bones varies widely among culturally diverse groups. Native Americans have anteriorly convex femurs, blacks have markedly straight femurs, and in whites

TABLE 22–1: Biocultural Variations in the Musculoskeletal System

BONE	VARIATIONS
Frontal	Thicker in black males than in white males.
Parietal occiput	Thicker in white males than in black males.
Palate	Tori (protuberances) along the suture line of the hard palate; problematic for denture wearers. Incidence: blacks—20%; whites—24%; Asians—up to 50%; Native Americans—up to 50%.
Mandible	Tori (protuberances) on the lingual surface of the mandible near the canine and premolar teeth; problematic for denture wearers; most common in Asians and Native Americans; incidence exceeds 50% in some Inuit groups.
Humerus	Torsion or rotation of proximal end with muscle pull; whites have a greater incidence than blacks; torsion in blacks is symmetric; torsion in whites greater on the right side than on the left side.
Radius	Length at the wrist variable.
Ulna	Ulna or radius may be longer. Equal length in Swedes—61%; in Chinese—16%. Ulna longer than radius in Swedes—16%; in Chinese—48%. Radius longer than ulna in Swedes—23%; in Chinese—10%.
Vertebrae	Twenty-four vertebrae (cervical, thoracic, lumbar) are found in 85% to 93% of all people. Racial and sex differences reveal 23 or 25 vertebrae in select groups; 11% of black females have 23, and 12% of Inuit and Native American males have 25. Increased number is related to lower back pain and lordosis.
Pelvis	Hip width is 1.6 cm (0.6 in) smaller in black women than in white women; Asian women have significantly smaller pelvises.
Femur	The femur has a convex anterior curve in Native Americans, is straight in blacks, and has an intermediate curve in whites.
Second tarsal	Second toe longer than the great toe—incidence: whites—8%–34%; blacks—8%–12%; Vietnamese—31%; Melanesians—21%–57%. Clinical significance for joggers and athletes, who reported increased foot problems.
Height	White males are 1.27 cm (0.5 in) taller than black males and 7.6 cm (2.9 in) taller than Asian males. White females have the same height as black females. Asian females are 4.14 cm (1.6 in) shorter than white or black females.
Composition of long bones	Longer, narrower, and denser in blacks than whites; bone density in whites is greater than in Chinese, Japanese, and Inuits. Osteoporosis incidence is lowest in black males; highest in white females.

MUSCLE	VARIATIONS
Peroneus tertius	Responsible for dorsiflexion of foot—muscle absent in 3%–10% of Asians, Native Americans, and whites; in 10%–15% of blacks; and in 24% of Berbers (Sahara desert). No clinical significance because the tibialis anterior also dorsiflexes the foot.
Palmaris longus	Responsible for wrist flexion—muscle absent in 12%–20% of whites; in 2%–12% of Native Americans; in 5% of blacks; and in 3% of Asians. No clinical significance because three other muscles are also responsible for flexion.

Data from Overfield T: *Biologic variation in health and illness: race, age, and sex differences,* ed 2, New York, 1995, CRC Press; Andrews MM, Boyle JS, editors: *Transcultural concepts in nursing care,* ed. 4, Philadelphia, 2003, Lippincott Williams & Wilkins.

the femoral curvature is intermediate. This characteristic is related to both genetics and body weight. Thin blacks and whites have less curvature than average, whereas obese blacks and whites display increased curvatures. It is possible that the heavier density of the bones of blacks helps to protect them from increased curvature due to obesity.

Table 22–1 summarizes reported biocultural variations occurring in the musculoskeletal system.

Subjective Data

1. Joints
   Pain
   Stiffness
   Swelling, heat, redness
   Limitation of movement
2. Muscles
   Pain (cramps)
   Weakness
3. Bones
   Pain
   Deformity
   Trauma (fractures, sprains, dislocations)
4. Functional assessment (ADL)
5. Self-care behaviors

EXAMINER ASKS	RATIONALE

1. Joints.

- Any problems with your joints? Any **pain?**

- Location: Which joints? On one side or both sides?

- Quality: What does the pain feel like: aching, stiff, sharp or dull, shooting? Severity: How strong is the pain?
- Onset: When did this pain start?
- Timing: What time of day does the pain occur? How long does it last? How often does it occur?

- Is the pain aggravated by movement, rest, position, weather? Is the pain relieved by rest, medications, application of heat or ice?

- Is the pain associated with chills, fever, recent sore throat, trauma, repetitive activity?

- Any **stiffness** in your joints?

- Any **swelling, heat, redness** in the joints?
- Any **limitation of movement** in any joint? Which joint?
- Which activities give you problems? (See Functional Assessment, p. 644.)

2. Muscles.

- Any problems in the muscles, such as any **pain** or **cramping?** Which muscles?
- If in calf muscles: Is the pain with walking? Does it go away with rest?

- Are your muscle aches associated with fever, chills, the "flu"?
- Any **weakness** in muscles?
- Location: Where is the weakness? How long have you noticed weakness?

- Do the muscles look smaller there?

3. Bones.

- Any **bone pain?** Is the pain affected by movement?
- Any **deformity** of any bone or joint? Is the deformity due to injury or trauma? Does the deformity affect ROM?
- Any **accidents** or **trauma** ever affected the bones or joints: fractures, joint strain, sprain, dislocation? Which ones?
- When did this occur? What treatment was given? Any problems or limitations now as a result?
- Any back pain? In which part of your back? Is pain felt anywhere else, like shooting down leg?
- Any numbness and tingling? Any limping?

RATIONALE

Joint pain and loss of function are the most common musculoskeletal concerns that prompt a person to seek care.

Rheumatoid arthritis (RA) involves symmetric joints; other musculoskeletal illnesses involve isolated or unilateral joints.

Exquisitely tender with acute inflammation.

RA pain is worse in morning when the person gets up; osteoarthritis is worse later on in the day; tendinitis is worse in morning, improves during the day.

Movement increases most joint pain except in RA, in which movement decreases pain.

Joint pain 10 to 14 days after an untreated strep throat suggests rheumatic fever.

Joint injury occurs from trauma, repetitive motion.

RA stiffness occurs in morning and after rest periods.

Suggests acute inflammation.

Decreased ROM may be due to joint problems (injury to cartilage or capsule) or to muscle contracture.

Muscle pain is usually felt as cramping or aching.

Suggests intermittent claudication (see Chapter 20).

Viral illness often includes myalgia.

Weakness may involve musculoskeletal or neurologic systems (see also Chapter 23).

Atrophy.

Fracture causes sharp pain that increases with movement. Other bone pain usually feels "dull" and "deep" and is unrelated to movement.

EXAMINER ASKS	RATIONALE

4. Functional assessment (ADL).

Do your joint (muscle, bone) problems create any limits on your usual activities of daily living (ADLs)? Which ones? (Note: Ask about each category; if the person answers "yes," ask specifically about each activity in category.)

- Bathing—getting in and out of the tub, turning faucets?
- Toileting—urinating, moving bowels, able to get self on/off toilet, wipe self?
- Dressing—doing buttons, zipper, fasten opening behind neck, pulling dress or sweater over head, pulling up pants, tying shoes, getting shoes that fit?
- Grooming—shaving, brushing teeth, brushing or fixing hair, applying makeup?
- Eating—preparing meals, pouring liquids, cutting up foods, bringing food to mouth, drinking?
- Mobility—walking, walking up or down stairs, getting in/out of bed, getting out of house?
- Communicating—talking, using phone, writing?

Functional assessment is important to screen the safety of independent living, the need for home health care services, and quality of life.

Assess any self-care deficit.

Impaired physical mobility.

Impaired verbal communication.

5. Self-care behaviors.

Any occupational hazards that could affect the muscles and joints? Does your work involve heavy lifting? Or any repetitive motion or chronic stress to joints? Any efforts to alleviate these?

- Tell me about your exercise program. Describe the type of exercise, frequency, the warm-up program.
- Any pain during exercise? How do you treat it?
- Have you had any recent weight gain? Please describe your usual daily diet. (Note the person's usual caloric intake, all four food groups, daily amount of protein, calcium.)
- Are you taking any medications for musculoskeletal system: aspirin, anti-inflammatory, muscle relaxant, pain reliever?
- If person has chronic disability or crippling illness: How has your illness affected
  - Your interaction with family
  - Your interaction with friends
  - The way you view yourself

Assess risk for back pain or carpal tunnel syndrome.

Self-care behaviors.

Assess for
- Self-esteem disturbance
- Loss of independence
- Body image disturbance
- Role performance disturbance
- Social isolation

Additional History for Infants and Children

1. Were you told about any trauma to infant during labor and delivery? Did the baby come head first? Was there a need for forceps?

Traumatic delivery increases risk for fractures, (e.g., humerus, clavicle).

2. Did the baby need resuscitation?

Period of anoxia may result in hypotonia of muscles.

3. Were the baby's motor milestones achieved at about the same time as siblings or age-mates?

4. Has your child ever broken any bones? Any dislocations? How were these treated?

5. Have you ever noticed any bone deformity? Spinal curvature? Unusual shape of toes or feet? At what age? Have you ever sought treatment for any of these?

EXAMINER ASKS	RATIONALE

Additional History for Adolescents

1. Involved in any sports at school or after school? How frequently (times per week)?

Assess safety of sport for child. Note if child's height and weight are adequate for the particular sport (e.g., football).

2. Do you use any special equipment? Does any training program exist for your sport?

Use of safety equipment and presence of adult supervision decreases risk of sports injuries.

3. What is the nature of your daily warm-up?

Lack of adequate warm-up increases risk of sports injury.

4. What do you do if you get hurt?

Students may not report injury or pain for fear of limiting participation in sport.

5. How does your sport fit in with other school demands and other activities?

Additional History for the Aging Adult

Use the functional assessment history (pp. 90–91) questions to elicit any loss of function, self-care deficit, or safety risk that may occur as a process of aging or musculoskeletal illness. (If needed, review the section on functional assessment in Chapter 6 for further details.)

1. Any change in weakness over the past months or years?

2. Any increase in falls or stumbing over the past months or years?

3. Do you use any mobility aids to help you get around: cane, walker?

Objective Data

PREPARATION

The purpose of the musculoskeletal examination is to assess function for ADL, as well as to screen for any abnormalities. You already will have considerable data regarding ADL through the history. Note additional ADL data as the person goes through the motions necessary for an examination: gait, posture, how the person sits in a chair, raises from chair, takes off jacket, manipulates small object such as a pen, raises from supine.

A **screening** musculoskeletal examination suffices for most people:

- Inspection and palpation of joints integrated with each body region
- Observation of ROM as person proceeds through motions described earlier
- Age-specific screening measures, such as Ortolani's sign for infants, or scoliosis screening for adolescents

A **complete** musculoskeletal examination, as described in this chapter, is appropriate for persons with articular disease, a history of musculoskeletal symptoms, or any problems with ADL.

EQUIPMENT NEEDED

Tape measure
Goniometer, to measure joint angles
Skin marking pen

Make the person comfortable before and throughout the examination. Drape for full visualization of the body part you are examining without needlessly exposing the person.

Take an orderly approach—head to toe, proximal to distal.

The joint to be examined should be supported at rest. Muscles must be soft and relaxed to assess the joints under them accurately. Take care when examining any inflamed area where rough manipulation could cause pain and muscle spasm. To avoid this, use firm support, gentle movement, and gentle return to a relaxed state.

Compare corresponding paired joints. Expect symmetry of structure and function, as well as normal parameters for that joint.

NORMAL RANGE OF FINDINGS	ABNORMAL FINDINGS

ORDER OF THE EXAMINATION

Inspection

Note the **size** and **contour** of the joint. Inspect the skin and tissues over the joints for **color, swelling,** and any **masses** or **deformity.** Presence of swelling is significant and signals joint irritation.

Swelling may be due to excess joint fluid (effusion), thickening of the synovial lining, inflammation of surrounding soft tissue (bursae, tendons) or bony enlargement.

Deformities include **dislocation** (one or more bones in a joint being out of position), **subluxation** (partial dislocation of a joint), **contracture** (shortening of a muscle leading to limited ROM of joint), or **ankylosis** (stiffness or fixation of a joint).

Palpation

Palpate each joint, including its skin for temperature, its muscles, bony articulations, and area of joint capsule. Notice any heat, tenderness, swelling, or masses. Joints normally are not tender to palpation. If any tenderness does occur, try to localize it to specific anatomic structures (e.g., skin, muscles, bursae, ligaments, tendons, fat pads, or joint capsule).

The synovial membrane normally is not palpable. When thickened, it feels "doughy" or "boggy." A small amount of fluid is present in the normal joint, but it is not palpable.

Palpable fluid is abnormal. Because fluid is contained in an enclosed sac, if you push on one side of the sac, the fluid will shift and cause a visible bulging on another side.

Range of Motion (ROM)

Ask for **active ROM** while stabilizing the body area proximal to that being moved. Familiarize yourself with the type of each joint and its normal ROM so that you can recognize limitations. If you see a limitation, gently attempt **passive motion.** Anchor the joint with one hand while your other hand slowly moves it to its limit. The normal ranges of active and passive motion should be the same.

If any limitation or any increase in ROM occurs, use a goniometer to measure the angles precisely (Fig. 22–15). First extend the joint to neutral or 0 degrees. Center the 0 point of the goniometer on the joint. Keep the fixed arm of the goniometer on the 0 line and use the movable arm to measure; then flex the joint and measure through the goniometer to determine the angle of greatest flexion.

22–15

Joint motion normally causes no tenderness, pain, or crepitation. Do not confuse crepitation with the normal discrete "crack" heard as a tendon or ligament slips over bone during motion, such as when you do a knee bend.

Crepitation is an audible and palpable crunching or grating that accompanies movement. It occurs when the articular surfaces in the joints are roughened, as with rheumatoid arthritis (see Table 22–3, p. 648).

Muscle Testing

Test the strength of the prime mover muscle groups for each joint. Repeat the motions you elicited for active ROM. Now ask the person to flex and hold as you apply opposing force. Muscle strength should be equal bilaterally and should fully resist your opposing force. (Note: Muscle status and joint status are interdependent and should be interpreted together. Chapter 23 discusses the examination of muscles for size and development, tone, and presence of tenderness.)

A wide variability of strength exists among people. You may wish to use a grading system from no voluntary movement to full strength, as shown in Table 22–2.

TABLE 22–2: Grading Muscle Strength			
GRADE	DESCRIPTION	PERCENT NORMAL	ASSESSMENT
5	Full ROM against gravity, full resistance	100	Normal
4	Full ROM against gravity, some resistance	75	Good
3	Full ROM with gravity	50	Fair
2	Full ROM with gravity eliminated (passive motion)	25	Poor
1	Slight contraction	10	Trace
0	No contraction	0	Zero

ROM = range of motion.

TEMPOROMANDIBULAR JOINT

With the person seated, **inspect** the area just anterior to the ear. Place the tips of your first two fingers in front of each ear and ask the person to open and close the mouth. Drop your fingers into the depressed area over the joint, and note smooth motion of the mandible. An audible and palpable snap or click occurs in many normal people as the mouth opens (Fig. 22–16).

Ask the person to perform these motions (Fig. 22–17):

Swelling looks like a round bulge over the joint, although it must be moderate or marked to be visible.

Crepitus and pain occur with temporomandibular joint dysfunction.

NORMAL RANGE OF FINDINGS   **ABNORMAL FINDINGS**

22–16

22–17

Instructions to Person
- Open mouth maximally.

- Partially open mouth, protrude lower jaw, and move it side to side.
- Stick out lower jaw.

Motion and Expected Range
Vertical motion. You can measure the space between the upper and lower incisors. Normal is 3 to 6 cm, or three fingers inserted sideways.
Lateral motion. Normal extent is 1 to 2 cm.
Protrude without deviation.

Lateral motion may be lost earlier and more significantly than vertical.

Palpate the contracted temporalis and masseter muscles as the person clenches the teeth. Compare right and left sides for size, firmness, and strength. Ask the person to move the jaw forward and laterally against your resistance, and to open mouth against your resistance. This also tests the integrity of cranial nerve V (trigeminal).

NORMAL RANGE OF FINDINGS	ABNORMAL FINDINGS

CERVICAL SPINE

Inspect the alignment of head and neck. The spine should be straight and the head erect. **Palpate** the spinous processes and the sternomastoid, trapezius, and paravertebral muscles. They should feel firm, with no muscle spasm or tenderness.

Ask the person to follow these motions (Fig. 22–18):*

Head tilted to one side.
Asymmetry of muscles.
Tenderness and hard muscles with muscle spasm.

A

B

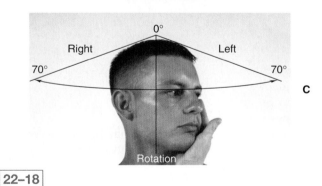

C

22–18

*Do not attempt if you suspect neck trauma.

NORMAL RANGE OF FINDINGS	ABNORMAL FINDINGS

Instructions to Person

- Touch chin to chest.
- Lift the chin toward the ceiling.
- Touch each ear toward the corresponding shoulder. Do not lift up the shoulder.
- Turn the chin toward each shoulder.

Motion and Expected Range

Flexion of 45 degrees (Fig. 22–18, *A*).

Hyperextension of 55 degrees.

Lateral bending of 40 degrees (Fig. 22–18, *B*).

Rotation of 70 degrees (Fig. 22–18, *C*).

Limited ROM.

Pain with movement.

Repeat the motions while applying opposing force. The person normally can maintain flexion against your full resistance. This also tests integrity of cranial nerve XI (spinal).

The person cannot hold flexion.

UPPER EXTREMITY

Shoulders

Inspect and compare both shoulders posteriorly and anteriorly. Check the size and contour of the joint and compare shoulders for equality of bony landmarks. Normally, no redness, muscular atrophy, deformity, or swelling is present. Check the anterior aspect of the joint capsule and the subacromial bursa for abnormal swelling.

Redness.
Inequality of bony landmarks.
Atrophy, shows as lack of fullness.
Dislocated shoulder loses the normal rounded shape and looks flattened laterally.
Swelling from excess fluid is best seen anteriorly. Considerable fluid must be present to cause a visible distention because the capsule normally is so loose (see Table 22–4).

If the person reports any shoulder pain, ask that he or she point to the spot with the hand of the unaffected side. Be aware that shoulder pain may be from local causes or it may be referred pain due to a hiatal hernia or a cardiac or pleural condition, which could be potentially serious. Pain from a local cause is reproducible during the examination by palpation or motion.

Swelling of subacromial bursa is localized under deltoid muscle and may be accentuated when the person tries to abduct the arm.

While standing in front of the person, **palpate** both shoulders, noting any muscular spasm or atrophy, swelling, heat, or tenderness. Start at the clavicle and methodically explore the acromioclavicular joint, scapula, greater tubercle of the humerus, area of the subacromial bursa, the biceps groove, and the anterior aspect of the glenohumeral joint. Palpate the pyramid-shaped axilla; no adenopathy or masses should be present.

Swelling.
Hard muscles with muscle spasm.
Tenderness or pain.

NORMAL RANGE OF FINDINGS

Test ROM by asking the person to perform four motions (Fig. 22–19). Cup one hand over the shoulder during ROM to note any crepitation; normally none is present.

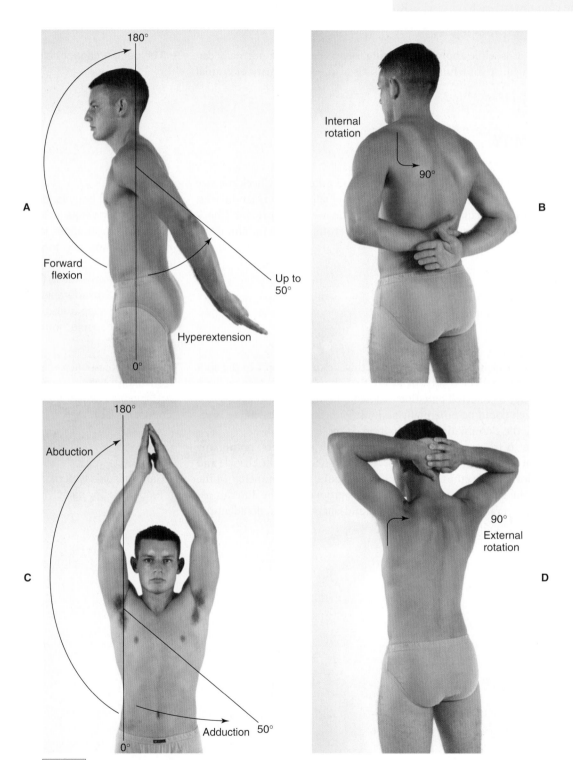

22–19

NORMAL RANGE OF FINDINGS

ABNORMAL FINDINGS

Instructions to Person | **Motion and Expected Range**

- With arms at sides and elbows extended, move both arms forward and up in wide vertical arcs, then move them back.

Forward flexion of 180 degrees. Hyperextension up to 50 degrees (Fig. 22–19, *A*).

- Rotate arms internally behind back, place back of hands as high as possible toward the scapulae.

Internal rotation of 90 degrees (Fig. 22–19, *B*).

- With arms at sides and elbows extended, raise both arms in wide arcs in the coronal plane. Touch palms together above head.
- Touch both hands behind the head with elbows flexed and rotated posteriorly.

Abduction of 180 degrees. Adduction of 50 degrees (Fig. 22–19, *C*).

External rotation of 90 degrees (Fig. 22–19, *D*).

Test the strength of the shoulder muscles by asking the person to shrug the shoulders, flex forward and up, and abduct against your resistance. The shoulder shrug also tests the integrity of cranial nerve XI, the spinal accessory.

Elbow

Inspect the size and contour of the elbow in both flexed and extended positions. Look for any deformity, redness, or swelling. Check the olecranon bursa and the normally present hollows on either side of the olecranon process for abnormal swelling.

22-20

Palpate with the elbow flexed about 70 degrees and as relaxed as possible (Fig. 22–20). Use your left hand to support the person's left forearm and palpate the extensor surface of the elbow—the olecranon process and the medial and lateral epicondyles of humerus—with your right thumb and fingers.

With your thumb in the lateral groove and your index and middle fingers in the medial groove, palpate either side of the olecranon process using varying pressure. Normally, present tissues and fat pads feel fairly solid. Check for any synovial thickening, swelling, nodules, or tenderness.

ABNORMAL FINDINGS (column)

Limited ROM.

Asymmetry.

Pain with motion.

Crepitus with motion.

Rotator cuff lesions may cause limited ROM, pain, and muscle spasm during abduction, whereas forward flexion stays fairly normal.

Subluxation of the elbow shows the forearm dislocated posteriorly.

Swelling and redness of olecranon bursa are localized and easy to observe because of the close proximity of the bursa to skin.

Effusion or synovial thickening shows first as a bulge or fullness in groove on either side of the olecranon process, and it occurs with gouty arthritis.

Epicondyles, head of radius, and tendons are common sites of inflammation and local tenderness, or "tennis elbow."

Soft, boggy, or fluctuant swelling in both grooves occurs with synovial thickening or effusion.

Local heat or redness (signs of inflammation) can extend beyond synovial membrane.

Palpate the area of the olecranon bursa for heat, swelling, tenderness, consistency, or nodules.

Subcutaneous nodules are raised, firm, and nontender, and overlying skin moves freely. Common sites are in the olecranon bursa and along extensor surface of the ulna. These nodules occur with RA (see Table 22–5).

Test ROM by asking the person to do the following:

Instructions to Person	**Motion and Expected Range**
• Bend and straighten the elbow (Fig. 22–21).	Flexion of 150 to 160 degrees; extension at 0. Some normal people lack 5 to 10 degrees of full extension, and others have 5 to 10 degrees of hyperextension.
• Movement of 90 degrees in pronation and supination (Fig. 22–22).	Hold the hand midway; then touch front and back sides of hand to table.

160°

Flexion

0°
Extension

22–21

0°

Pronation 90°   90° Supination

22–22

While testing **muscle strength**, stabilize the person's arm with one hand (Fig. 22–23). Have the person flex the elbow against your resistance applied just proximal to the wrist. Then ask the person to extend the elbow against your resistance.

22–23

NORMAL RANGE OF FINDINGS

Wrist and Hand

Inspect the hands and wrists on the dorsal and palmar sides, noting position, contour, and shape. The normal functional position of the hand shows the wrist in slight extension. This way the fingers can flex efficiently, and the thumb can oppose them for grip and manipulation. The fingers lie straight in the same axis as the forearm. Normally, no swelling or redness, deformity, or nodules are present.

The skin looks smooth with knuckle wrinkles present and no swelling or lesions. Muscles are full, with the palm showing a rounded mound proximal to the thumb (the **thenar eminence**) and a smaller rounded mound proximal to the little finger.

Palpate each joint in the wrist and hands. Facing the person, support the hand with your fingers under it and palpate the wrist firmly with both your thumbs on its dorsum (Fig. 22–24). Make sure the person's wrist is relaxed and in straight alignment. Move your palpating thumbs side to side to identify the normal depressed areas that overlie the joint space. Use gentle but firm pressure. Normally the joint surfaces feel smooth, with no swelling, bogginess, nodules, or tenderness.

22–24

Palpate the metacarpophalangeal joints with your thumbs, just distal to and on either side of the knuckle (Fig. 22–25).

Use your thumb and index finger in a pinching motion to palpate the sides of the interphalangeal joints (Fig. 22–26). Normally, no synovial thickening, tenderness, warmth, or nodules are present.

22–25

22–26

ABNORMAL FINDINGS

Subluxation of wrist.
Ulnar deviation; fingers list to ulnar side.
Ankylosis; wrist in extreme flexion.
Dupuytren's contracture; flexion contracture of finger(s).

Swan-neck or boutonnière deformity in fingers.
Atrophy of the thenar eminence (see Table 22–6).

Ganglion in wrist.
Synovial swelling on dorsum.
Generalized swelling.
Tenderness.

Heberden's and Bouchard's nodules are hard and nontender and occur with osteoarthritis (see Table 22–6).

NORMAL RANGE OF FINDINGS

ABNORMAL FINDINGS

Test ROM (Fig. 22–27) by asking the person to do the following:

Instructions to Person
- Bend the hand up at the wrist.

- Bend hand down at the wrist.
- Bend the fingers up and down at metacarpophalangeal joints.
- With palms flat on table, turn them outward and in.

Motion and Expected Range
Hyperextension of 70 degrees (Fig. 22–27, *A*).

Palmar flexion of 90 degrees.
Flexion of 90 degrees. Hyperextension of 30 degrees (Fig. 22–27, *B*).
Ulnar deviation of 50–60 degrees, and radial deviation of 20 degrees (Fig. 22–27, *C*).

Loss of ROM here is the most common and the most significant type of functional loss of the wrist.
Limited motion.
Pain on movement.

A

B

C

D

E

F

22–27

NORMAL RANGE OF FINDINGS	ABNORMAL FINDINGS

* Spread fingers apart; make a fist.   Abduction of 20 degrees; fist tight. The responses should be equal bilaterally (Fig. 22–27, *D, E*).

* Touch the thumb to each finger and to the base of little finger.   The person is able to perform, and the responses are equal bilaterally (Fig. 22–27, *F*).

For **muscle testing,** position the person's forearm supinated (palm up) and resting on a table (Fig. 22–28). Stabilize by holding your hand at the person's midforearm. Ask the person to flex the wrist against your resistance at the palm.

22–28

PHALEN'S TEST. Ask the person to hold both hands back to back while flexing the wrists 90 degrees. Acute flexion of the wrist for 60 seconds produces no symptoms in the normal hand (Fig. 22–29).

Phalen's test reproduces numbness and burning in a person with carpal tunnel syndrome (see Table 22–6).

22–29   Phalen's test.

NORMAL RANGE OF FINDINGS	ABNORMAL FINDINGS

TINEL'S SIGN. Direct percussion of the location of the median nerve at the wrist produces no symptoms in the normal hand (Fig. 22–30).

In carpal tunnel syndrome, percussion of the median nerve produces burning and tingling along its distribution, which is a positive Tinel's sign.

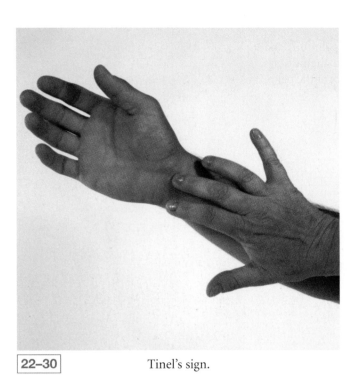

22–30   Tinel's sign.

LOWER EXTREMITY

Hip

Wait to **inspect** the hip joint together with the spine a bit later in the examination as the person stands. At that time, note symmetric levels of iliac crests, gluteal folds, and equally sized buttocks. A smooth, even gait reflects equal leg lengths and functional hip motion.

Help the person into a supine position and **palpate** the hip joints. The joints should feel stable and symmetric, with no tenderness or crepitance.

Pain with palpation.
Crepitation.

Assess **ROM** (Fig. 22–31) by asking the person to do the following:

Instructions to Person	Motion and Expected Range
• Raise each leg with knee extended.	Hip flexion of 90 degrees (Fig. 22–31, *A*).
• Bend each knee up to the chest while keeping the other leg straight.	Hip flexion of 120 degrees. The opposite thigh should remain on the table (Fig. 22–31, *B*).
• Flex knee and hip to 90 degrees. Stabilize by holding the thigh with one hand and the ankle with the other hand. Swing the foot outward. Swing the foot inward. (Foot and thigh move in opposite directions.)	Internal rotation of 40 degrees. External rotation of 45 degrees (Fig. 22–31, *C*).

Limited motion.
Pain with motion.
Flexion flattens the lumbar spine; if this reveals a flexion deformity in the opposite hip, it represents a positive *Thomas test.*

Limited internal rotation of hip is an early and reliable sign of hip disease.

NORMAL RANGE OF FINDINGS	ABNORMAL FINDINGS

A

B

C

D

22–31

* Swing leg laterally, then medially, with knee straight. Stabilize pelvis by pushing down on the opposite anterior superior iliac spine.
* When standing (later in examination), swing straight leg back behind body. Stabilize pelvis to eliminate exaggerated lumbar lordosis. The most efficient way is to ask person to bend over the table and to support the trunk on the table. Or the person can lie prone on the table.

Abduction of 40 to 45 degrees. Adduction of 20 to 30 degrees (Fig. 22–31, *D*).

Hyperextension of 15 degrees when stabilized.

Limitation of abduction of the hip while supine is the most common motion dysfunction found in hip disease.

Knee

The person should remain supine with legs extended, although some examiners prefer the knees to be flexed and dangling for **inspection.** The skin normally looks smooth, with even coloring and no lesions.

Shiny and atrophic skin.
Swelling or inflammation (see Table 22–7).
Lesions (e.g., psoriasis).

NORMAL RANGE OF FINDINGS

ABNORMAL FINDINGS

Inspect lower leg alignment. The lower leg should extend in the same axis as the thigh.

Angulation deformity:

- Genu varum (bowlegs) (see p. 640)
- Genu valgum (knock knees)
- Flexion contracture

Inspect the knee's shape and contour. Normally, distinct concavities, or hollows, are present on either side of the patella. Check them for any sign of fullness or swelling. Note other locations, such as the prepatellar bursa and the suprapatellar pouch, for any abnormal swelling.

Hollows disappear, then they may bulge with synovial thickening or effusion.

Check the quadriceps muscle in the anterior thigh for any atrophy. Since it is the prime mover of knee extension, this muscle is important for joint stability during weight-bearing.

Atrophy occurs with disuse or chronic disorders. First, it appears in the medial part of the muscle, although it is difficult to note because the vastus medialis is relatively small.

Enhance **palpation** with the knee in the supine position with complete relaxation of the quadriceps muscle. Start high on the anterior thigh, about 10 cm above the patella. Palpate with your left thumb and fingers in a grasping fashion (Fig. 22–32). Proceed down toward the knee, exploring the region of the suprapatellar pouch. Note the consistency of the tissues. The muscles and soft tissues should feel solid, and the joint should feel smooth, with no warmth, tenderness, thickening, or nodularity.

Feels fluctuant or boggy with synovitis of suprapatellar pouch.

22–32

When swelling occurs, you need to distinguish whether it is due to soft tissue swelling or increased fluid in the joint. The tests for the bulge sign and ballottement of the patella aid this assessment.

BULGE SIGN. For swelling in the suprapatellar pouch, the bulge sign confirms the presence of small amounts of fluid as you try to move the fluid from one side of the joint to the other. Firmly stroke up on the medial aspect of the knee two

NORMAL RANGE OF FINDINGS	ABNORMAL FINDINGS

or three times to displace any fluid (Fig. 22–33, *A*). Tap the lateral aspect (Fig. 22–33, *B*). Watch the medial side in the hollow for a distinct bulge from a fluid wave. Normally, none is present.

The bulge sign occurs with very small amounts of effusion, 4 to 8 ml, from fluid flowing across the joint (Fig. 22-33, *C*).

A

B

C

22–33   Bulge sign.

BALLOTTEMENT OF THE PATELLA. This test is reliable when larger amounts of fluid are present. Use your left hand to compress the suprapatellar pouch to move any fluid into the knee joint. With your right hand, push the patella sharply against the femur. If no fluid is present, the patella is already snug against the femur (Fig. 22–34, *A*).

If fluid has collected, your tap on the patella moves it through the fluid, and you will hear a tap as the patella bumps up on the femoral condyles (Fig. 22-34, *B*).

A

22–34   A, Ballottement.

B

Continue palpation and explore the tibiofemoral joint (Fig. 22–35). Note smooth joint margins and absence of pain. Palpate the infrapatellar fat pad and the patella. Check for crepitus by holding your hand on the patella as the knee is flexed and extended. Some crepitus in an otherwise asymptomatic knee is not uncommon.

Irregular bony margins occur with osteoarthritis.

Pain at joint line.

Pronounced crepitus is significant and it occurs with degenerative diseases of the knee.

22–35

NORMAL RANGE OF FINDINGS	ABNORMAL FINDINGS

Check ROM (Fig. 22–36) by asking the person to do the following:

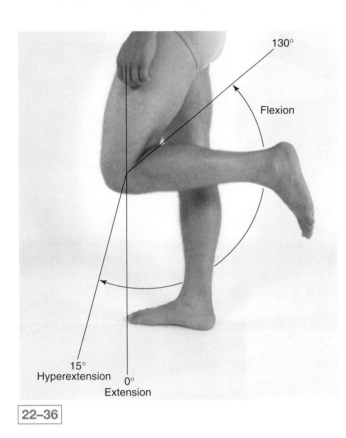

130°

Flexion

15°
Hyperextension   0°
Extension

22–36

Instructions to Person
- Bend each knee.
- Extend each knee.

- Check knee ROM during ambulation.

Motion and Expected Range
Flexion of 130 to 150 degrees.
A straight line of 0 degrees in some persons; a hyperextension of 15 degrees in others.

Limited ROM.
Contracture.
Pain with motion.
Limp.
Sudden locking—the person is unable to extend the knee fully. This usually occurs with a painful and audible "pop" or "click." Sudden buckling, or "giving way," occurs with ligament injury, which causes weakness and instability.

Check **muscle strength** by asking the person to maintain knee flexion while you oppose by trying to pull the leg forward. Muscle extension is demonstrated by the person's success in rising from a seated position in a low chair or by rising from a squat without using the hands for support.

SPECIAL TEST FOR MENISCAL TEARS. *MCMURRAY'S TEST.* Perform this test when the person has reported a history of trauma followed by locking, giving way, or local pain in the knee. Position the person supine, as you stand on the affected side. Hold the heel and flex the knee and hip. Place your other hand on the knee with fingers on the medial side. Rotate the leg in and out to loosen the joint. Externally rotate the leg and push a valgus (inward) stress on the knee. Then slowly extend the knee. Normally the leg extends smoothly with no pain (Fig. 22–37).

NORMAL RANGE OF FINDINGS	ABNORMAL FINDINGS

If you hear or feel a "click," McMurray's test is positive for a torn meniscus.

22–37   McMurray's test.

Ankle and Foot

Inspect while the person is in a sitting, non–weight-bearing position, as well as when standing and walking. Compare both feet, noting position of feet and toes, contour of joints, and skin characteristics. The foot should align with the long axis of the lower leg; an imaginary line would fall from midpatella to between the first and second toes.

Weight-bearing should fall on the middle of the foot, from the heel, along the midfoot, to between the second and third toes. Most feet have a longitudinal arch, although that can vary normally from "flat feet" to a high instep.

The toes point straight forward and lie flat. The ankles (malleoli) are smooth bony prominences. Normally the skin is smooth, with even coloring and no lesions. Note the locations of any calluses or bursal reactions because they reveal areas of abnormal friction. Examining well-worn shoes helps assess areas of wear and accommodation.

Support the ankle by grasping the heel with your fingers while palpating with your thumbs (Fig. 22–38). Explore the joint spaces. They should feel smooth and depressed, with no fullness, swelling, or tenderness.

Hallux valgus (see Table 22–8).
Hammer toes. Claw toes.
Swelling or inflammation.
Calluses. Ulcers.

Swelling or inflammation.
Tenderness.

22–38

NORMAL RANGE OF FINDINGS	ABNORMAL FINDINGS

Palpate the metatarsophalangeal joints between your thumb on the dorsum and your fingers on the plantar surface (Fig. 22–39).

Swelling or inflammation; tenderness.

22–39

Using a pinching motion of your thumb and forefinger, palpate the interphalangeal joints on the medial and lateral sides of the toes.

Test ROM (Fig. 22–40) by asking the person to do the following:

22–40

Instructions to Person	**Motion and Expected Range**	
• Point toes toward the floor.	Plantar flexion of 45 degrees.	Limited ROM.
• Point toes toward your nose.	Dorsiflexion of 20 degrees (Fig. 22–40, *A*).	
		Pain with motion.
• Turn soles of feet out, then in. (Stabilize the ankle with one hand, hold heel with the other to test the subtalar joint.)	Eversion of 20 degrees. Inversion of 30 degrees (Fig. 22–40, *B*).	
• Flex and straighten toes.		

Assess **muscle strength** by asking the person to maintain dorsiflexion and plantar flexion against your resistance.

Unable to hold flexion.

NORMAL RANGE OF FINDINGS	ABNORMAL FINDINGS

SPINE

The person should be standing, draped in a gown open at the back. Place yourself far enough back so that you can see the entire back. **Inspect** and note if the spine is straight by following an imaginary vertical line from the head through the spinous processes and down through the gluteal cleft, and by noting equal horizontal positions for the shoulders, scapulae, iliac crests, and gluteal folds, and equal spaces between arm and lateral thorax on the two sides (Fig. 22–41, A). The person's knees and feet should be aligned with the trunk and should be pointing forward.

A difference in shoulder elevation and in level of scapulae and iliac crests occur with scoliosis (see Table 22–9).

B

22–41

From the side, note the normal convex thoracic curve and concave lumbar curve (Fig. 22–41, B). An enhanced thoracic curve, or kyphosis, is common in aging people. A pronounced lumbar curve, or lordosis, is common in obese people.

Lateral tilting and forward bending occur with a herniated nucleus pulposus (see Table 22–9).

NORMAL RANGE OF FINDINGS	ABNORMAL FINDINGS

Palpate the spinous processes. Normally they are straight and not tender. Palpate the paravertebral muscles; they should feel firm with no tenderness or spasm.

Check **ROM** of the spine by asking the person to bend forward and touch the toes (Fig. 22–42). Look for flexion of 75 to 90 degrees and smoothness and symmetry of movement. Note that the concave lumbar curve should disappear with this motion, and the back should have a single convex **C**-shaped curve.

Spinal curvature.
Tenderness. Spasm of paravertebral muscles.

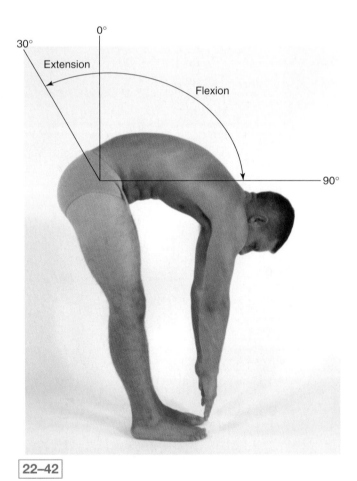

22–42

If you suspect a spinal curvature during inspection, this may be more clearly seen when the person touches the toes. While the person is bending over, mark a dot on each spinous process. When the person resumes standing, the dots should form a straight vertical line.

If the dots form a slight S-shape when the person stands, a spinal curve is present.

NORMAL RANGE OF FINDINGS	ABNORMAL FINDINGS

Stabilize the pelvis with your hands. Check ROM (Fig. 22–43) by asking the person to do the following:

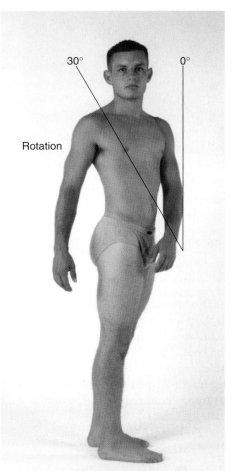

22–43

Instructions to Person	**Motion and Expected Range**	
• Bend sideways.	Lateral bending of 35 degrees (Fig. 22–43, A).	Limited ROM.
• Bend backward.	Hyperextension of 30 degrees.	
• Twist shoulders to one side, then the other.	Rotation of 30 degrees, bilaterally (Fig. 22–43, B).	Pain with motion.

These maneuvers reveal only gross restriction. Movement is still possible even if some spinal fusion has occurred.

NORMAL RANGE OF FINDINGS	ABNORMAL FINDINGS

STRAIGHT LEG RAISING OR LASEGUE'S TEST. These maneuvers reproduce back and leg pain and help confirm the presence of a herniated nucleus pulposus. Straight leg raising while keeping the knee extended normally produces no pain. Raise the affected leg just short of the point where it produces pain. Then dorsiflex the foot (Fig. 22–44).

Positive if the test reproduces sciatic pain. If lifting the affected leg reproduces sciatic pain, it confirms the presence of a herniated nucleus pulposus.

22–44

Raise the unaffected leg while leaving the other leg flat. Inquire about the involved side.

If lifting the unaffected leg reproduces sciatic pain, it strongly suggests a herniated nucleus pulposus.

MEASURE LEG LENGTH DISCREPANCY. Perform this measurement if you need to determine if one leg is shorter than the other. For *true leg length,* measure between *fixed* points, from the anterior iliac spine to the medial malleolus, crossing the medial side of the knee (Fig. 22–45). Normally these measurements are equal or within 1 cm, indicating no true bone discrepancy.

Sometimes the true leg length is equal, but the legs still look unequal. For *apparent leg length,* measure from a nonfixed point (the umbilicus) to a fixed point (medial malleolus) on each leg.

Unequal leg lengths.

True leg lengths are equal, but apparent leg lengths unequal—this condition occurs with pelvic obliquity or adduction or flexion deformity in the hip.

22–45

 DEVELOPMENTAL CONSIDERATIONS

Review the developmental milestones discussed in Chapter 2. Keep handy a concise chart of the usual sequence of motor development so that you can refer to expected findings for the age of each child you are examining. Use the Denver II test to screen the fine and gross motor skills for the child's age.

NORMAL RANGE OF FINDINGS	ABNORMAL FINDINGS

Since some overlap exists between the musculoskeletal and neurologic examinations, assessment of muscle tone, resting posture, and motor activity are discussed in the next chapter.

Infants

Examine the infant fully undressed and lying on the back. Take care to place the newborn on a warming table to maintain body temperature.

FEET AND LEGS. Start with the feet and work your way up the extremities. Note any *positional deformities,* a residual of fetal positioning. Often the newborn's feet are not held straight but in a varus (apart) or valgus (together) position. It is important to distinguish whether this position is flexible (and thus usually self-correctable) or fixed. Scratch the outside of the bottom of the foot. If the deformity is self-correctable, the foot assumes a normal right angle to the lower leg. Or immobilize the heel with one hand and gently push the forefoot to the neutral position with the other hand. If you can move it to neutral position, it is flexible.

> A true deformity is fixed and assumes a right angle only with forced manipulation or not at all.

Note the relationship of the forefoot to the hindfoot. Commonly, the hindfoot is in alignment with the lower leg and just the forefoot angles inward. This forefoot adduction is *metatarsus adductus.* It is usually present at birth and usually resolves spontaneously by age 3 years.

> Metatarsus varus—adduction and inversion of forefoot.
> Talipes equinovarus (see Table 22–10).

Check for *tibial torsion,* a twisting of the tibia. Place both feet flat on the table, and push to flex up the knees. With the patella and the tibial tubercle in a straight line, place your fingers on the malleoli. In an infant, note that a line connecting the four malleoli is parallel to the table.

> More than 20 degrees of deviation; or if lateral malleolus is anterior to medial malleolus, it indicates tibial torsion.

Tibial torsion may originate from intrauterine positioning and then may be exacerbated at a later age by continuous sitting in a reverse tailor position, the "TV squat." This is sitting with the buttocks on the floor and the lower legs splayed back and out on either side.

HIPS. Check the hips for *congenital dislocation.* The most reliable method is **Ortolani's maneuver,** which should be done at every professional visit until the infant is 1 year old. With the infant supine, flex the knees holding your thumbs on the inner mid-thighs, and your fingers outside on the hips touching the greater trochanters. Adduct the legs until your thumbs touch (Fig. 22–46, *A*). Then gently lift and *abduct,* moving the knees apart and down so their lateral aspects touch the table (Fig. 22–46, *B*). This normally feels smooth and has no sound.

> With a dislocated hip, the head of the femur is not cupped in the acetabulum but rests posterior to it.
> Hip instability feels like a clunk as the head of the femur pops back into place. This is a *positive Ortolani's sign* and warrants referral.

A

B

22–46   Ortolani's maneuver.

NORMAL RANGE OF FINDINGS	ABNORMAL FINDINGS

The **Allis test** also is used to check for hip dislocation by comparing leg lengths (Fig. 22–47). Place the baby's feet flat on the table and flex the knees up. Scan the tops of the knees; normally they are at the same elevation.

Finding one knee significantly lower than the other is a positive indication of Allis' sign and suggests hip dislocation.

22–47   Allis test.

Note the gluteal folds. Normally they are equal on both sides. However, some asymmetry may occur in normal children.

Unequal gluteal folds may accompany hip dislocation after 2 to 3 months of age.

HANDS AND ARMS. Inspect the hands, noting shape, number, and position of fingers and palmar creases.

Polydactyly is the presence of extra fingers or toes. Syndactyl is webbing between adjacent fingers or toes (see Table 22–6).

A simian crease is a single palmar crease that occurs with Down syndrome, accompanied by short broad fingers, incurving of little fingers, and low-set thumbs.

Palpate the length of the clavicles because the clavicle is the bone most frequently fractured during birth. The clavicles should feel smooth, regular, and without crepitus. Also note equal ROM of arms during Moro's reflex.

Fractured clavicle: Note irregularity at the fracture site, crepitus, and angulation. The site has rapid callus formation with a palpable lump within a few weeks. Observe limited arm ROM and unilateral response to Moro's reflex.

BACK. Lift up the infant and examine the back. Note the normal single C curve of the newborn's spine (Fig. 22–48). By 2 months of age, the infant can lift the head while prone. This builds the concave cervical spinal curve and indicates normal forearm strength. Inspect the length of the spine for any tuft of hair, dimple in midline, cyst, or mass. Normally, none are present.

A tuft of hair over a dimple in the midline may indicate spina bifida.

NORMAL RANGE OF FINDINGS

22–48

Observe ROM through spontaneous movement of extremities.

Test muscle strength by lifting up the infant with your hands under the axillae (Fig. 22–49). A baby with normal muscle strength wedges securely between your hands.

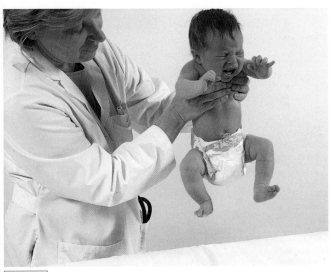

22–49

Preschool- and School-Age Children

Once the infant learns to crawl and then to walk, the waking hours show perpetual motion. This is convenient for your musculoskeletal assessment; you can observe the muscles and joints during spontaneous play before a table-top examination. Most young children enjoy showing off their physical accomplishments. For specific motions, coax the toddler: "Show me how you can walk to Mom," "climb the step stool." Ask the preschooler to hop on one foot or to jump.

BACK. While the child is standing, note the posture. From behind, you should note a "plumb line" from the back of the head, along the spine, to the middle of the sacrum. Shoulders are level within 1 cm, and scapulae are symmetric. From the side, lordosis is common throughout childhood, appearing more pronounced in children with a protuberant abdomen.

ABNORMAL FINDINGS

A small dimple in the midline—anywhere from the head to the coccyx—suggests dermoid sinus.

Mass, such as meningocele.

A baby who starts to "slip" between your hands shows weakness of the shoulder muscles.

Lordosis is marked with muscular dystrophy and rickets.

NORMAL RANGE OF FINDINGS

LEGS AND FEET.   Anteriorly, note the leg position. A "bowlegged" stance *(genu varum)* is a lateral bowing of the legs (Fig. 22–50, *A*). It is present when you measure a persistent space of more than 2.5 cm between the knees when the medial malleoli are together. Genu varum is normal for 1 year after the child begins walking. The child may walk with a waddling gait. This resolves with growth; no treatment is indicated.

Genu varum also occurs with rickets.

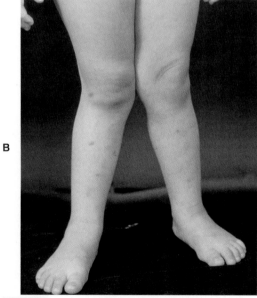

22–50   A, Genu varum. B, Genu valgum.

"Knock knees" *(genu valgum)* are present when there is more than 2.5 cm between the medial malleoli when the knees are together (Fig. 22–50, *B*). It occurs normally between 2 and 3¹/₂ years of age. Also, treatment is not indicated. (Note: To remember the two conditions, remember to link the r's and g's: genu varum—knees apart; genu valgum—knees together.)

Genu valgum also occurs with rickets, poliomyelitis, and syphilis.

NORMAL RANGE OF FINDINGS

Often, parents tell you they are concerned about the child's foot development. The most common questions are about "flatfeet" and "pigeon toes." Flatfoot (*pes planus*) is pronation, or turning in, of the medial side of the foot. The young child may look flatfooted because the normal longitudinal arch is concealed by a fat pad until age 3 years. When standing begins, the child takes a broad-based stance, which causes pronation. Thus pronation is common between 12 and 30 months. You can see it best from behind the child, where the medial side of the foot drops down and in.

Pigeon toes, or toeing in, are demonstrated when the child tends to walk on the lateral side of the foot, and the longitudinal arch looks higher than normal. It often starts as a forefoot adduction, which usually corrects spontaneously by age 3 years, as long as the foot is flexible.

Check the child's gait while walking away from and returning to you. Let the child wear socks, because a cold tile floor will distort the usual gait. From 1 to 2 years of age, expect a broad-based gait, with arms out for balance. Weight-bearing falls on the inside of the foot. From 3 years of age, the base narrows and the arms are closer to the sides. Inspect the shoes for spots of greatest wear to aid your judgment of the gait. Normally the shoes wear more on the outside of the heel and the inside of the toe.

Check the **Trendelenburg's sign** to screen progressive subluxation of the hip (Fig. 22–51). Watching from behind, ask the child to stand on one leg, then the other. Watch the iliac crests; they should stay level when weight is shifted.

22–51

The child may sit for the remainder of the examination. Start with the feet and hands of the child from 2 to 6 years of age because the child is happy to show these off, and proceed through the examination described earlier.

Particularly, check the arm for full ROM and presence of pain. Look for subluxation of the elbow (head of the radius). This occurs most often between 2 and 4 years of age as a result of forceful removal of clothing or dangling while adults suspend the child by the hands.

ABNORMAL FINDINGS

Pronation beyond 30 months.

Toeing in from forefoot adduction that is fixed, or lasts beyond age 3 years.
Toeing in from tibial torsion.

Limp, usually caused by trauma, fatigue, or hip disease.
Abnomal gait patterns (see Chapter 23).

The sign occurs with subluxation of one hip. When the child stands on the good leg, the pelvis looks level. When the child stands on the affected leg, the pelvis drops toward the "good" side.

Inability to supinate the hand while the arm is flexed, together with pain in elbow, indicates subluxation of the head of the radius.

NORMAL RANGE OF FINDINGS

Palpate the bones, joints, and muscles of the extremities as described in the adult examination.

Adolescents

Proceed with the musculoskeletal examination you provide for the adult, except pay special note to spinal posture. Kyphosis is common during adolescence because of chronic poor posture. **Screen for scoliosis** with the *forward bend test* starting at age 10 to 12 (Fig. 22–52). Seat yourself behind the standing child, and ask the child to stand with the feet shoulder-width apart and bend forward slowly to touch the toes. Expect a straight vertical spine while standing and also while bending forward. Posterior ribs should be symmetric, with equal elevation of shoulders, scapulae, and iliac crests. You may wish to mark each spinous process with a felt marker. The lineup of ink dots highlights even a subtle curve.

Be aware of the risk of sports-related injuries with the adolescent, because sports participation and competition often peak with this age group.

ABNORMAL FINDINGS

Pain or tenderness in extremities is usually caused by trauma or infection.

Fractures are usually due to trauma and are exhibited as an inability to use the area, a deformity, or an excess motion in the involved bone with pain and crepitation.

Enlargement of the tibial tubercles with tenderness suggests Osgood-Schlatter disease (see Table 22–7).

Scoliosis is most apparent during the preadolescent growth spurt. Asymmetry suggests scoliosis—ribs hump up on one side as child bends forward, and with unequal landmark elevation (see Table 22–9).

A   B

22–52

NORMAL RANGE OF FINDINGS	ABNORMAL FINDINGS

The Pregnant Female

Proceed through the examination described in the adult section. Expected postural changes in pregnancy include progressive lordosis and, toward the third trimester, anterior cervical flexion, kyphosis, and slumped shoulders (Fig. 22–53, A). When the pregnancy is at term, the protuberant abdomen and the relaxed mobility in the joints create the characteristic "waddling" gait (Fig. 22–53, B).

A   B

22–53

22–54

The Aging Adult

Postural changes include a decrease in height, more apparent in the eighth and ninth decades (Fig. 22–54). "Lengthening of the arm-trunk axis" describes this shortening of the trunk with comparatively long extremities. Kyphosis is common, with a backward head tilt to compensate. This creates the outline of a figure 3 when you view this older adult from the left side. Slight flexion of hips and knees is also common.

NORMAL RANGE OF FINDINGS	ABNORMAL FINDINGS

Contour changes include a decrease of fat in the body periphery and fat deposition over the abdomen and hips. The bony prominences become more marked.

For most older adults, ROM testing proceeds as described earlier. ROM and muscle strength are much the same as with the younger adult, provided no musculoskeletal illnesses or arthritic changes are present.

FUNCTIONAL ASSESSMENT. For those with advanced aging changes, arthritic changes, or musculoskeletal disability, perform a **functional assessment for ADL.** This applies the ROM and muscle strength assessments to the accomplishment of specific activities. You need to determine adequate and safe performance of functions essential for independent home life.

Instructions to Person	Common Adaptation for Aging Changes*
1. Walk (with shoes on).	Shuffling pattern; swaying; arms out to help balance; broader base of support; person may watch feet.
2. Climb up stairs.	Person holds hand rail; may haul body up with it; may lead with favored (stronger) leg.
3. Walk down stairs.	Holds hand rail, sometimes with both hands. If the person is weak, he or she may descend sideways, lowering the weaker leg first. If the person is unsteady, he or she may watch feet.
4. Pick up object from floor.	Person often bends at waist instead of bending knees; holds furniture to support while bending and straightening.
5. Rise up from sitting in chair.	Person uses arms to push off chair arms, upper trunk leans forward before body straightens, feet planted wide in broad base of support.
6. Rise up from lying in bed.	May roll to one side, push with arms to lift up torso, grab bedside table to increase leverage.

*Data from Bowers AC, Thompson JM, 1992.

SUMMARY CHECKLIST: Musculoskeletal Exam

For each joint to be examined:
1. **Inspection**
   Size and contour of joint
   Skin color and characteristics
2. **Palpation of joint area**
   Skin
   Muscles
   Bony articulations
   Joint capsule

3. **ROM**
   Active
   Passive (if limitation in active ROM is present)
   Measure with goniometer (if abnormality in ROM is present)

4. **Muscle testing**

Application and Critical Thinking

SAMPLE CHARTING

SUBJECTIVE

States no joint pain, stiffness, swelling, or limitation. No muscle pain or weakness. No history of bone trauma or deformity. Able to manage all usual daily activities with no physical limitations. Occupation involves no musculoskeletal risk factors. Exercise pattern is brisk walk 1 mile 5×/week.

OBJECTIVE

Joints and muscles symmetric; no swelling, masses, deformity; normal spinal curvature. No tenderness to palpation of joints; no heat, swelling, or masses. Full ROM; movement smooth, no crepitance, no tenderness. Muscle strength—able to maintain flexion against resistance and without tenderness.

FOCUSED ASSESSMENT: CLINICAL CASE STUDY

M.T. is a 45-year-old white female salesperson with a diagnosis of rheumatoid arthritis 3 years PTA, who seeks care now for "swelling and burning pain in my hands" for 1 day.

SUBJECTIVE

M.T. was diagnosed as having rheumatoid arthritis at age 41, by staff at this agency. Since that time, her "flare-ups" seem to come every 6 to 8 months. Acute episodes involve hand joints and are treated with aspirin, which gives relief. Typically experiences morning stiffness, lasting $\frac{1}{2}$ to 1 hour. Joints feel warm, swollen, tender. Has had weight loss of 15 pounds over last 4 years and feels fatigued much of the time. States should rest more, but "I can't take the time." Daily exercises have been prescribed but doesn't do them regularly. Takes aspirin for acute flare-ups, feels better in a few days, decreases dose by herself.

OBJECTIVE

Body joints within normal limits with exception of joints of wrist and hands. Radiocarpal, metacarpophalangeal, and proximal interphalangeal joints are red, swollen, tender to palpation. Spindle-shaped swelling of proximal interphalangeal joints of third digit right hand and second digit left hand; ulnar deviation of metacarpophalangeal joints.

ASSESSMENT

Acute pain R/T inflammation
Impaired physical mobility R/T inflammation
Deficient knowledge about aspirin treatment R/T lack of exposure
Noncompliance with exercise program R/T lack of perceived benefits of treatment
Noncompliance with advised rest periods R/T lack of perceived benefits of treatment

NURSING DIAGNOSES COMMONLY ASSOCIATED WITH THE MUSCULOSKELETAL DISORDERS

RELATED FACTORS (Etiology)	DEFINING CHARACTERISTICS (Symptoms and Signs)
DIAGNOSIS: Impaired Physical mobility	
Neuromuscular impairment	Reluctance to attempt movement
Sensory-perceptual impairment	Imposed restrictions on movement
Fatigue, decreased strength and endurance	Limited range of motion
Intolerance to activity	Decreased muscle strength, control, or mass
Effects of trauma or surgery	Inability to move purposefully within the environment
Inflammation	Impaired coordination
Pain	Falling or stumbling
Obesity	
Side effects of sedatives, narcotics, or tranquilizers	

Continued

RELATED FACTORS (Etiology)　　　　　　　　　　**DEFINING CHARACTERISTICS** (Symptoms and Signs)

DIAGNOSIS: Impaired Physical mobility—cont'd

Depression
Severe anxiety
Fear of movement
Architectural barriers
Lack of assistive devices

DIAGNOSIS: Risk for Disuse syndrome

Presence of risk factors such as:
　Paralysis
　Mechanical immobilization
　Prescribed immobilization
　Severe pain
　Altered level of consciousness

DIAGNOSIS: Risk for Trauma

Balancing difficulties
Pain
Reduced large, small muscle coordination
Reduced mobility of arms, legs
Weakness
Insufficient finances to purchase safety equipment or to
　make repairs
Lack of safety precautions, safety education
Fatigue
Visual, hearing impairment
History of
　Previous trauma
　Substance abuse

DIAGNOSIS: Pain

Inflammation
Muscle spasm
Effects of surgery or trauma
Immobility
Pressure points
Infectious process
Overactivity
Obstructive processes

Clutching of painful area
Trembling
Facial mask of pain
Changes in posture or gait
Change in muscle tone: listless to rigid
Reports of pain
Anxiety
Immobilization
Positive response to palpation
Withdrawal reflex
Autonomic responses
　Increased blood pressure, pulse, respirations
　Diaphoresis
　Dilated pupils
Crying or moaning
Fatigue
Distraction behavior—pacing, restlessness
Focused on self
Depression

OTHER RELATED NURSING DIAGNOSES

ACTUAL

Activity intolerance (see Chapter 18)

Disturbed Body image

Deficient Diversional activity

Delayed Growth and development

Impaired Home maintenance (see Chapter 14)

Chronic Pain

Self-care deficit

Impaired Skin integrity (see Chapter 12)

Disturbed Sleep pattern

RISK/WELLNESS

Risk

Risk for Disuse syndrome

Risk for disproportionate Growth

Risk for Injury

Risk for impaired Skin integrity

Wellness

Health-seeking behavior R/T knowledge about community resources

Health-seeking behavior R/T knowledge about disease process

Maintaining current Mobility

Progressing toward previous Mobility status

Increasing own responsibility for Self-care

ASSESSMENT VIDEO CRITICAL THINKING QUESTIONS

The Saunders *Physical Examination and Health Assessment* video "Musculoskeletal System" will direct you to consider the following:

1. What other assessment findings can you expect to see in a patient who reports joint pain?

2. What abnormal findings may commonly be detected during assessment of the wrists and hands?

3. When are genu varum and genu valgum considered normal? What abnormal conditions may also cause them?

4. How does musculoskeletal assessment of an adolescent differ from that of an adult?

Abnormal Findings

TABLE 22–3: Abnormalities Affecting Multiple Joints

INFLAMMATORY CONDITIONS

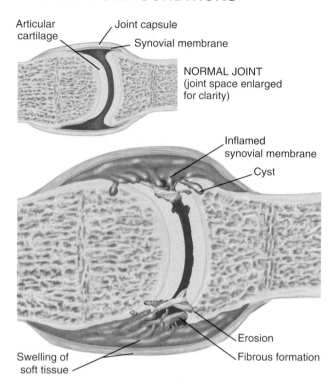

Rheumatoid Arthritis (RA)

This is a chronic, systemic inflammatory disease of joints and surrounding connective tissue. Inflammation of synovial membrane leads to thickening; then to fibrosis, which limits motion; and finally to bony ankylosis. The disorder is symmetrical and bilateral and is characterized by heat, redness, swelling, and painful motion of the affected joints. RA is associated with fatigue, weakness, anorexia, weight loss, low-grade fever, and lymphadenopathy. Associated signs are described in the following tables, especially Table 22–6.

Ankylosing Spondylitis (not illustrated)

Chronic progressive inflammation of spine, sacroiliac, and larger joints of the extremities, leading to bony ankylosis and deformity. A form of RA, this affects primarily men by a 10:1 ratio, in late adolescence or early adulthood. Spasm of paraspinal muscles pulls spine into forward flexion, obliterating cervical and lumbar curves. Thoracic curve exaggerated into single kyphotic rounding. Also includes flexion deformities of hips and knees.

DEGENERATIVE CONDITIONS

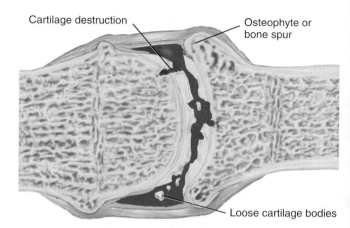

Osteoarthritis (Degenerative Joint Disease)

Noninflammatory, localized, progressive disorder involving deterioration of articular cartilages and subchondral bone, and formation of new bone (osteophytes) at joint surfaces. Aging increases incidence; nearly all adults over 60 have some radiographic signs of osteoarthritis. Asymmetric joint involvement commonly affects hands, knees, hips, and lumbar and cervical segments of the spine. Affected joints have stiffness, swelling with hard, bony protuberances, pain with motion, and limitation of motion (see Table 22–6).

Osteoporosis

Decrease in skeletal bone mass occurring when rate of bone resorption is greater than that of bone formation. The weakened bone state increases risk for stress fractures, especially at wrist, hip, and vertebrae. Occurs primarily in postmenopausal white women. Osteoporosis risk also is associated with smaller height and weight, younger age at menopause, lack of physical activity, and lack of estrogen replacement therapy.

TABLE 22–4: Abnormalities of the Shoulder

ABNORMAL FINDINGS

Atrophy

Loss of muscle mass is exhibited as a lack of fullness surrounding the deltoid muscle. In this case, atrophy is due to axillary nerve palsy. Atrophy also occurs from disuse, muscle tissue damage, or motor nerve damage.

Dislocated Shoulder

Anterior dislocation (95%) is exhibited when hunching the shoulder forward and the tip of the clavicle dislocates. It occurs with trauma involving abduction, extension, and rotation (e.g., falling on an outstretched arm or diving into a pool).

Joint Effusion

Swelling from excess fluid in the joint capsule, here from rheumatoid arthritis. Best observed anteriorly. Fluctuant to palpation. Considerable fluid must be present to cause a visible distention because the capsule normally is so loose.

Tear of Rotator Cuff

Characteristic "hunched" position and limited abduction of arm. Occurs from traumatic adduction while arm is held in abduction, or from fall on shoulder, throwing, or heavy lifting. Positive drop arm test: If the arm is passively abducted at the shoulder, the person is unable to sustain the position and the arm falls to the side.

◀ Frozen Shoulder—Adhesive Capsulitis

Fibrous tissues form in the joint capsule, causing stiffness, progressive limitation of motion, and pain. Motion limited in abduction and external rotation; unable to reach overhead. It may lead to atrophy of shoulder girdle muscles. Gradual onset; unknown cause. It is associated with prolonged bed rest or shoulder immobility. May resolve spontaneously.

Subacromial Bursitis (not illustrated)

Inflammation and swelling of subacromial bursa over the shoulder cause limited ROM and pain with motion. Localized swelling under deltoid muscle may increase by partial passive abduction of the arm. Caused by direct trauma, strain during sports, local or systemic inflammatory process, or repetitive motion with injury.

TABLE 22–5: Abnormalities of the Elbow

Olecranon Bursitis

Large soft knob, or "goose egg," and redness due to inflammation of olecranon bursa. Localized and easy to see because bursa lies just under skin.

Gouty Arthritis

Joint effusion or synovial thickening, seen first as bulge or fullness in grooves on either side of olecranon process. Redness and heat can extend beyond area of synovial membrane. Soft, boggy, or fluctuant fullness to palpation. Limited extension of elbow.

Subcutaneous Nodules

Raised, firm, nontender nodules that occur with rheumatoid arthritis. Common sites are in the olecranon bursa and along extensor surface of arm. The skin slides freely over the nodules.

Epicondylitis—Tennis Elbow

Chronic disabling pain at lateral epicondyle of humerus, radiates down extensor surface of forearm. Pain can be located with one finger. Resisting extension of the hand will increase the pain. Occurs with activities combining excessive pronation and supination of forearm with an extended wrist (e.g., racquet sports or using a screwdriver).

Medial epicondylitis is more rare and is due to activity of forced palmar flexion of wrist against resistance.

TABLE 22–6: Abnormalities of the Wrist and Hand

Ganglion Cyst

Round, cystic, nontender nodule overlying a tendon sheath or joint capsule, usually on dorsum of wrist. Flexion makes it more prominent. A common benign tumor; it does not become malignant.

Ankylosis

Wrist in extreme flexion, due to severe rheumatoid arthritis. This is a functionally useless hand, because when the wrist is palmar flexed, a good deal of power is lost from the fingers, and the thumb cannot oppose the fingers.

Colles' Fracture (not illustrated)

Nonarticular fracture of distal radius, with or without fracture of ulna at styloid process. Usually from a fall on an outstretched hand; occurs more often in older women. Wrist looks puffy, with "silver fork" deformity, a characteristic hump when viewed from the side.

Carpal Tunnel Syndrome With Atrophy of Thenar Eminence

Atrophy occurs from interference with motor function, due to compression of the median nerve inside the carpal tunnel. Caused by chronic repetitive motion; occurs between 30 and 60 years of age and is five times more common in women than in men. Symptoms of carpal tunnel syndrome include pain, burning and numbness, positive findings on Phalen's test, positive indication of Tinel's sign, and often atrophy of thenar muscles.

Dupuytren's Contracture

Chronic hyperplasia of the palmar fascia causes flexion contractures of the digits, first in the fourth digit, then the fifth digit, and then the third digit. Note the bands that extend from the midpalm to the digits, and the puckering of palmar skin. The condition occurs commonly in men past 40 years of age and is usually bilateral. It occurs with diabetes, epilepsy, and alcoholic liver disease, and as an inherited trait. The contracture is painless but impairs hand function.

Table continued on following page

TABLE 22–6: Abnormalities of the Wrist and Hand—cont'd

CONDITIONS CAUSED BY CHRONIC RHEUMATOID ARTHRITIS

Swan-Neck and Boutonnière Deformity

Flexion contracture resembles curve of a **swan's neck.** Note flexion contracture of metacarpophalangeal joint, then hyperextension of the proximal interphalangeal joint, and flexion of the distal interphalangeal joint. It occurs with chronic rheumatoid arthritis and is often accompanied by ulnar drift of the fingers.

In **boutonnière deformity** the knuckle looks as if it is being pushed through a buttonhole. It is a relatively common deformity and includes flexion of proximal interphalangeal joint with compensatory hyperextension of distal interphalangeal joint.

Reprinted from the Clinical Slide Collection on the Rheumatic Diseases, © 1991, 1995, 1997. Used by permission of the American College of Rheumatology.

Ulnar Deviation or Drift

Fingers drift to the ulnar side because of stretching of the articular capsule and muscle imbalance. Also note subluxation and swelling in the joints, and muscle atrophy on the dorsa of the hands. This is caused by chronic rheumatoid arthritis.

Continued

TABLE 22–6: Abnormalities of the Wrist and Hand—cont'd

Degenerative Joint Disease or Osteoarthritis

Osteoarthritis is characterized by hard, nontender nodules, 2 to 3 mm or more. These osteophytes (bony over-growths) of the distal interphalangeal joints are called Heberden's nodes, and those of the proximal interphalangeal joints are called Bouchard's nodes.

Acute Rheumatoid Arthritis

Painful swelling and stiffness of joints, with fusiform or spindle-shaped swelling of the soft tissue of proximal interphalangeal joints. Fusiform swelling is usually symmetric, the hands are warm, and the veins are engorged. The inflamed joints have a limited range of motion.

Syndactyly

Webbed fingers are a congenital deformity, usually requiring surgical separation. The metacarpals and phalanges of the webbed fingers are different lengths, and the joints do not line up. To leave the fingers fused would thus limit their flexion and extension.

Polydactyly

Extra digits are a congenital deformity, usually occurring at the fifth finger or the thumb. Surgical removal is considered for cosmetic appearance. The sixth finger shown here was not removed, because it had full ROM and sensation and a normal appearance.

TABLE 22–7: Abnormalities of the Knee

Mild Synovitis

Loss of normal hollows on either side of the patella, which are replaced by mild distention. Occurs with synovial thickening or effusion (excess fluid). Also note mild distention of the suprapatellar pouch.

Prepatellar Bursitis

Localized swelling on anterior knee between patella and skin. A tender fluctuant mass indicates swelling; in some cases, infection spreads to surrounding soft tissue. The condition is limited to the bursa, and the knee joint itself is not involved. Overlying skin may be red, shiny, atrophic, or coarse and thickened.

◀ Swelling of Menisci

Localized soft swelling due to cyst in lateral meniscus shows at the midpoint of the anterolateral joint line. Semiflexion of the knee makes swelling more prominent.

Osgood-Schlatter Disease (not illustrated)

Painful swelling of the tibial tubercle just below the knee, probably due to repeated stress on the patellar tendon. Occurs most in puberty during rapid growth and most often in males. Pain increases with kicking, running, bike riding, stair climbing, or kneeling. The condition is usually self-limited, and symptoms resolve with rest.

Chondromalacia Patellae (not illustrated)

Degeneration of articular surface of patellae. The condition occurs most often in females, and its cause is unknown. May produce mild effusion. Joint motion is painless, but crepitus may be present. Pain starts with kneeling.

TABLE 22–8: Abnormalities of the Ankle and Foot

Achilles Tenosynovitis

Inflammation of a tendon sheath near the ankle (here, the Achilles tendon) produces a superficial linear swelling and a localized tenderness along the route of the sheath. Movement of the involved tendon usually causes pain.

Tophi With Chronic Gout

Hard, painless nodule (tophi) over metatarsophalangeal joint of first toe. Tophi are collections of sodium urate crystals due to chronic gout in and around the joint that cause extreme swelling and joint deformity. They sometimes burst with a chalky discharge.

Acute Gout

Acute episode of gout usually involves first the metatarsophalangeal joint. Clinical findings consist of redness, swelling, heat, and extreme tenderness. Gout is a metabolic disorder of disturbed purine metabolism, associated with elevated serum uric acid. It occurs primarily in men over 40 years of age.

Table continued on following page

TABLE 22–8:   Abnormalities of the Ankle and Foot—cont'd

◄ Hallux Valgus With Bunion and Hammer Toes

Hallux valgus is a common deformity from rheumatoid arthritis. It is a lateral or outward deviation of the great toe with medial prominence of the head of the first metatarsal. The **bunion** is the inflamed bursa that forms at the pressure point. The great toe loses power to push off while walking; this stresses the second and third metatarsal heads, and they develop calluses and pain. Chronic sequelae include corns, calluses, hammer toes, and joint subluxation.

Note the **hammer toe** deformities in the second, third, fourth, and fifth toes. Often associated with hallux valgus, hammer toe includes hyperextension of the metatarsophalangeal joint and flexion of the proximal interphalangeal joint.

Corns (thickening of soft tissue) develop on the dorsum over the bony prominence due to prolonged pressure from shoes.

Callus (not illustrated)

Hypertrophy of the epithelium develops because of prolonged pressure, commonly on the plantar surface of the first metatarsal head in the hallux valgus deformity. The condition is not painful.

Plantar Wart (not illustrated)

Vascular papillomatous growth is probably due to a virus and occurs on the sole of the foot, commonly at the ball. The condition is extremely painful.

Ingrown Toenail (not illustrated)

A misnomer; the nail does not grow in, but the soft tissue grows over the nail and obliterates the groove. It occurs almost always on the great toe on the medial or lateral side. It is due to trimming the nail too short or toe-crowding in tight shoes. The area becomes infected when the nail grows and its corner penetrates the soft tissue.

TABLE 22–9: Abnormalities of the Spine

◀ Scoliosis

Lateral curvature of thoracic and lumbar segments of the spine, usually with some rotation of involved vertebral bodies.

Functional scoliosis is flexible; it is apparent with standing and disappears with forward bending. It may be compensatory for other abnormalities such as leg length discrepancy.

Structural scoliosis is fixed; the curvature shows both on standing and on bending forward. Note rib hump with forward flexion. When the person is standing, note unequal shoulder elevation, unequal scapulae, obvious curvature, and unequal hip level. At greatest risk are females 10 years of age through adolescence, during the peak of the growth spurt.

Herniated Nucleus Pulposus ▶

The nucleus pulposus (at the center of the intervertebral disk) ruptures into the spinal canal and puts pressure on the local spinal nerve root. Usually occurs from stress, such as lifting, twisting, continuous flexion with lifting, or fall on buttocks. Occurs mostly in men 20 to 45 years of age. Lumbar herniations occur mainly in interspaces L4 to L5 and L5 to S1. Note: sciatic pain, numbness, and paresthesia of involved dermatome; listing away from affected side; decreased mobility; low back tenderness; and decreased motor and sensory function in leg. Straight leg raising tests reproduce sciatic pain.

TABLE 22–10: Common Congenital or Pediatric Abnormalities

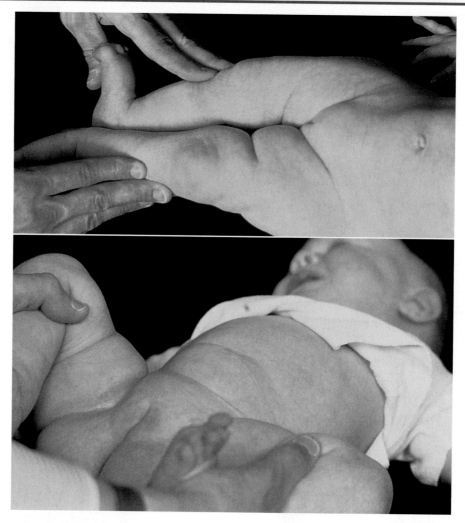

Congenital Dislocated Hip

Head of the femur is displaced out of the cup-shaped acetabulum.

The degree of the condition varies; subluxation may occur as stretched ligaments allow partial displacement of femoral head, and acetabular dysplasia may develop because of excessive laxity of hip joint capsule.

Occurrence is 1:500 to 1:1000 births; common in girls by 7:1 ratio. Signs include limited abduction of flexed thigh, positive indications of Ortolani's and Barlow's signs, asymmetric skin creases or gluteal folds, limb length discrepancy, and positive indication of Trendelenburg's sign in older children.

Continued

TABLE 22-10: Common Congenital or Pediatric Abnormalities—cont'd

Talipes Equinovarus (Clubfoot) ▶

Congenital, rigid, and fixed malposition of foot, including (1) inversion, (2) forefoot adduction, and (3) foot pointing downward (equinus). A common birth defect, with an incidence of 1:1000 to 3:1000 live births. Males are affected twice as frequently as females.

◀ Spina Bifida

Incomplete closure of posterior part of vertebrae results in a neural tube defect. Seriousness varies from skin defect along the spine to protrusion of the sac containing meninges, spinal fluid, or malformed spinal cord. The most serious type is myelomeningocele (shown here), in which the meninges and neural tissue protrude. In these cases the child is usually paralyzed below the level of the lesion.

Coxa Plana (Legg-Calvé-Perthes Syndrome) (not illustrated)

Avascular necrosis of the femoral head, occurring primarily in males between 3 and 12 years of age, with peak at age 6 years. In initial inflammatory stage, interruption of blood supply to femoral epiphysis occurs, halting growth. Revascularization and healing occur later, but significant residual deformity and dysfunction may be present.

BIBLIOGRAPHY

Abbruzzese LD: The Tinetti performance oriented mobility assessment tool, *Am J Nurs* 98(12):16J–16L, Dec 1998.

Allison M, Keller C: Physical activity in the elderly: benefits and intervention strategies, *Nurse Pract* 22(8):53–69, Aug 1997.

Arcuni SE: Rotator cuff pathology and subacromial impingement, *Nurse Pract* 25(5):58–77, May 2000.

Arendt EA: Gender differences in musculoskeletal health, *J Gender Specific Med* 3(7):58–64, Oct 2000.

Barry ME: Ankle sprains, *Am J Nurs* 101(10):40–42, Oct 2001.

Childs S: Acute ankle injury, *Lippincotts Prim Care Pract* 3(4):428–437, Jul–Aug 1999.

Clarke J: Organizing the approach to musculoskeletal misuse syndrome, *Nurse Pract* 26(7):11–27, 2001.

Cline MG et al: Decline of height with age in adults in a general population sample: estimating maximum height and distinguishing birth cohort effects from actual loss of stature with aging, *Hum Biol* 61(3):415–425, June 1989.

Cote P et al: A study of the diagnostic accuracy and reliability of the scoliometer and Adam's forward bend test, *Spine* 23(7):796–803, Apr 1, 1998.

Crowther CL: Approach to knee problems in primary care, *Lippincotts Prim Care Pract* 3(4):355–375, July–Aug 1999.

Dodds TA et al: A validation of the Functional Independence Measurement and its performance among rehabilitation inpatients, *Arch Phys Rehabil* 74:531–536, 1993.

Douglas S: Sciatic pain and piriformis syndrome, *Nurse Pract* 22(5):166–180, May 1997.

Ebrahim S et al: Randomized placebo-controlled trial of brisk walking in the prevention of postmenopausal osteoporosis, *Age Aging* 26(4):253–260, May 1997.

Ensrud KE et al: Correlates of kyphosis in older women, *J Am Geriatr Soc* 45(6):682–687, June 1997.

Granger CV et al: Reliability of a brief outpatient functional outcome assessment measure, *Am J Phys Med Rehabil* 74(6):469–475, Nov–Dec 1995.

Gregg EW et al: Physical activity and osteoporotic fracture risk in older women, *Ann Intern Med* 129(2):81–88, Jul 15, 1998.

Kaufmann JA: Low back pain: diagnosis and management in primary care, *Lippincotts Prim Care Pract* 3(4):376–393, Jul-Aug 1999.

Lawson MT: Evaluating and managing osteoporosis in men, *Nurse Pract* 26(5):26–51, 2001.

Lewis T, Tesh AS, Lyles KW: Caring for the patient with Paget's disease of the bone, *Nurse Pract* 24(7):50–65, 1999.

Maldonado A: Comprehensive assessment of common musculoskeletal disorders, *J Nurse Midwifery* 40(2):202–215, Mar-Apr 1995.

Maurizio SJ, Robers JL: Recognizing and treating fibromyalgia, *Nurse Pract* 22(12):18–33, Dec 1997.

McClung BL: Using osteoporosis management to reduce fractures in elderly women, *Nurse Pract* 24(3):26–49, 1999.

Muscari ME: Preventing sports injuries, *Am J Nurs* 98(7):58–60, July 1998.

O'Hanlon-Nichols T: A review of the adult musculoskeletal system, *Am J Nurs* 98(6):48–52, June 1998.

Onieal M: Common wrist and elbow injuries in primary care, *Lippincotts Prim Care Pract* 3(4):441–450, Jul-Aug 1999.

Overfield T: *Biologic variation in health and illness: race, age, and sex differences,* ed 2, New York, 1995, CRC Press.

Ramsburg KL: Rheumatoid arthritis, *Am J Nurs* 100(11):40–48, Nov 2000.

Ross C: A comparison of osteoarthritis and rheumatoid arthritis: diagnosis and treatment, *Nurse Pract* 22(9):20–41, Sep 1997.

Schmitt M: Evaluation of the elbow, *Patient Care for the Nurse Pract* 2(5):32–41, May 1999.

Szer IS: Musculoskeletal pain in adolescents: growing pains or something else? *Consultant* 40(6):1061–1065, May 2000.

Urquhart BS: Anterior shoulder dislocation, *Am J Nurs* 101(2):33–35, Feb 2001.

Woodhead GA, Moss MM: Osteoporosis: diagnosis and prevention, *Nurse Pract* 23(11):18–37, Nov 1998.

Yim-Chiplis PK, Talbot LA: Defining and measuring balance in adults, *Biological Research for Nursing* 1(4):321–331, April 2000.

Neurologic System

http://evolve.elsevier.com/Jarvis/

Structure and Function

The nervous system can be divided into two parts—central and peripheral. The **central nervous system** (CNS) includes the brain and spinal cord. The **peripheral nervous system** includes the 12 pairs of cranial nerves, the 31 pairs of spinal nerves, and all their branches. The peripheral nervous system carries sensory messages *to* the CNS from sensory receptors, motor messages *from* the CNS out to muscles and glands, as well as autonomic messages that govern the internal organs and blood vessels.

THE CENTRAL NERVOUS SYSTEM (CNS)

CEREBRAL CORTEX. The cerebral cortex is the cerebrum's outer layer of nerve cell bodies, which looks like "gray matter" because it lacks myelin. The cerebral cortex is the center for humans' highest functions, governing thought, memory, reasoning, sensation, and voluntary movement (Fig. 23–1). Each half of the cerebrum is a **hemisphere;** the left hemisphere is dominant in most (95 percent) people, including those who are left-handed.

Each hemisphere is divided into four **lobes:** frontal, parietal, temporal, and occipital. The lobes have certain areas that mediate specific functions.

- The **frontal** lobe has areas concerned with personality, behavior, emotions, and intellectual function.
- The precentral gyrus of the frontal lobe initiates voluntary movement.
- The **parietal** lobe's postcentral gyrus is the primary center for sensation.
- The **occipital** lobe is the primary visual receptor center.
- The **temporal** lobe behind the ear has the primary auditory reception center.
- **Wernicke's area** in the temporal lobe is associated with language comprehension. When damaged in the person's dominant hemisphere, *receptive aphasia* results. The person hears sound, but it has no meaning, like hearing a foreign language.
- **Broca's area** in the frontal lobe mediates motor speech. When injured in the dominant hemisphere, *expressive aphasia* results; the person cannot talk. The person can understand language and knows what he or she wants to say, but can produce only a garbled sound.

Damage to any of these specific cortical areas produces a corresponding loss of function: motor weakness, paralysis, loss of sensation, or impaired ability to understand and process language. Damage occurs when the highly specialized

Precentral gyrus— primary motor area

Central sulcus

Postcentral gyrus— primary sensory area

Frontal lobe personality behavior emotion intellectual functions

Parietal lobe sensation

Broca's area motor speech

Wernicke's area speech comprehension

Occipital lobe visual reception

Lateral sulcus

Temporal lobe hearing taste smell

Cerebellum motor coordination equilibrium balance

CEREBRAL CORTEX

23–1

Plane of
coronal section B

Thalamus

Midbrain

Pons

Cerebellum

Medulla

Spinal cord

Hypothalamus

Pituitary

Brain stem

Basal ganglia

Hypothalamus

A Medial view of right hemisphere

B Coronal section

COMPONENTS OF THE CENTRAL NERVOUS SYSTEM

23–2

neurologic cells are deprived of their blood supply, such as when a cerebral artery becomes occluded, or when vascular bleeding or vasospasm occurs.

BASAL GANGLIA. The basal ganglia are bands of gray matter buried deep within the two cerebral hemispheres that form the subcortical associated motor system (the extrapyramidal system) (Fig. 23–2). They control automatic associated movements of the body, e.g., the arm swing alternating with the legs during walking.

THALAMUS. The thalamus is the main relay station for the nervous system. Sensory pathways of the spinal cord and brain stem form **synapses** (sites of contact between two neurons) on their way to the cerebral cortex.

HYPOTHALAMUS. The hypothalamus is a major control center with many vital functions: temperature, heart rate, and blood pressure control, sleep center, anterior and posterior pituitary gland regulator, and coordinator of autonomic nervous system activity and emotional status.

CEREBELLUM. The cerebellum is a coiled structure located under the occipital lobe that is concerned with motor coordination of voluntary movements, equilibrium, and muscle tone. It does not initiate movement but coordinates and smooths it, e.g., the complex and quick coordination of many different muscles needed in playing the piano, swimming, or

juggling. It is like a "black box" in that it adjusts and corrects the voluntary movements, but operates entirely below the conscious level.

BRAIN STEM. The brain stem is the central core of the brain consisting of mostly nerve fibers. It has three areas:

1. **Midbrain**—the most anterior part of the brain stem that still has the basic tubular structure of the spinal cord. It merges into the thalamus and hypothalamus. It contains many motor neurons and tracts.
2. **Pons**—the enlarged area containing ascending and descending fiber tracts.
3. **Medulla**—the continuation of the spinal cord in the brain that contains all ascending and descending fiber tracts connecting the brain and spinal cord. It has vital autonomic centers (respiration, heart, gastrointestinal function), as well as nuclei for cranial nerves VIII through XII. Pyramidal decussation (crossing of the motor fibers) occurs here (see p. 665).

SPINAL CORD. The spinal cord is the long cylindrical structure about as big around as the little finger that occupies the upper two thirds of the vertebral canal. It is the main highway for ascending and descending fiber tracts that connect the brain to the spinal nerves, and it mediates reflexes. Its nerve cell bodies, or gray matter, are arranged in a butterfly shape with anterior and posterior "horns."

PATHWAYS OF THE CNS

Crossed representation is a notable feature of the nerve tracts; the *left* cerebral cortex receives sensory information from and controls motor function to the *right* side of the body, while the *right* cerebral cortex likewise interacts with the *left* side of the body. Knowledge of where the fibers cross the midline will help you interpret clinical findings.

Sensory Pathways

Millions of sensory receptors are embroidered into the skin, mucous membranes, muscles, tendons, and viscera. They monitor conscious sensation, internal organ functions, body position, and reflexes. Sensation travels in the afferent fibers in the peripheral nerve, then through the posterior (dorsal) root, and then into the spinal cord. There, it may take one of two routes—the spinothalamic tract or the posterior (dorsal) columns (Fig. 23–3).

SPINOTHALAMIC TRACT. The spinothalamic tract contains sensory fibers that transmit the sensations of pain, temperature, and crude or light touch. The fibers enter the dorsal root of the spinal cord and synapse with a second sensory neuron. The second-order neuron fibers cross to the opposite side and ascend up the spinothalamic tract to the thalamus. Fibers carrying pain and temperature sensations ascend the *lateral* spinothalamic tract, whereas those of crude touch form the *anterior* spinothalamic tract. At the thalamus, the fibers synapse with a third sensory neuron, which carries the message to the sensory cortex for full interpretation.

POSTERIOR (DORSAL) COLUMNS. These fibers conduct the sensations of position, vibration, and finely localized touch.

- **Position** (proprioception)—Without looking, you know where your body parts are in space and in relation to each other
- **Vibration**—Feeling vibrating objects
- **Finely localized touch** (stereognosis)—Without looking, you can identify familiar objects by touch

These fibers enter the dorsal root and proceed immediately up the same side of the spinal cord to the brain stem. At the medulla, they synapse with a second sensory neuron and then cross. They travel to the thalamus, synapse again, and

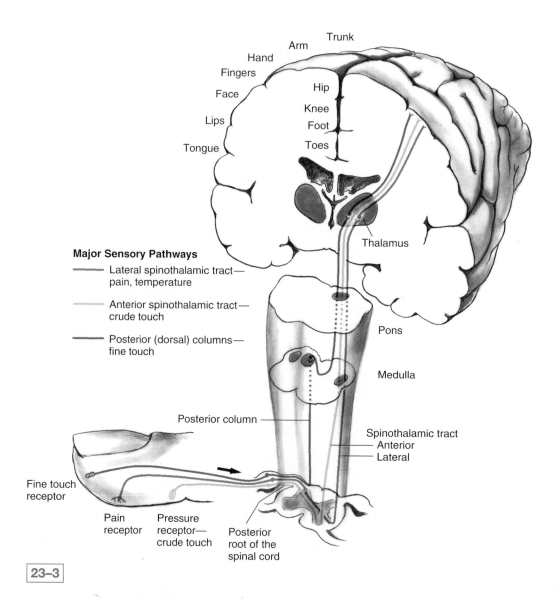

Major Sensory Pathways

——— Lateral spinothalamic tract— pain, temperature

——— Anterior spinothalamic tract— crude touch

——— Posterior (dorsal) columns— fine touch

23–3

proceed to the sensory cortex, which localizes the sensation and makes full discrimination.

The sensory cortex is arranged in a specific pattern forming a corresponding "map" of the body. Pain in the right hand is perceived at its specific spot on the left cortex map. Some organs are absent from the brain map, such as the heart, liver, or spleen. You know you have one but you have no "felt image" of it. Pain originating in these organs is referred, because no felt image exists in which to have pain. Pain is felt "by proxy" by another body part that does have a felt image. For example, pain in the heart is referred to the chest, shoulder, and left arm, which were its neighbors in fetal development. Pain originating in the spleen is felt on the top of the left shoulder.

Motor Pathways

CORTICOSPINAL OR PYRAMIDAL TRACT. (Fig. 23–4). The area has been named "pyramidal" because it crosses through the pyramids of the medulla. Motor nerve fibers originate in the motor cortex and travel to the brain stem, where they cross to the opposite side *(pyramidal decussation)* and then pass down in the lateral column of the spinal cord. At each cord level, they synapse with a lower motor neuron contained in the anterior horn of the spinal cord. Ten percent of corticospinal fibers do *not* cross, and these descend in the anterior column of the spinal cord. Corticospinal fibers mediate voluntary movement, particularly very skilled, discrete, purposeful movements, such as writing.

The corticospinal tract is a newer, "higher," motor system that humans have that permits very skilled and purposeful movements. The tract's origin in the motor cortex is arranged in a specific pattern called *somatotopic organization.* It is another body map, this one of a person, or *homunculus,* hanging "upside down" (see Fig. 23–1). Body parts are not equally represented on the map, and the homunculus looks distorted. It is more like an electoral map than a geographic map. That is, body parts whose movements are relatively more important to humans (e.g., the hand) occupy proportionally more space on the brain map.

EXTRAPYRAMIDAL TRACTS. The extrapyramidal tracts include all the motor nerve fibers originating in the motor cortex, basal ganglia, brain stem, and spinal cord that are *outside*

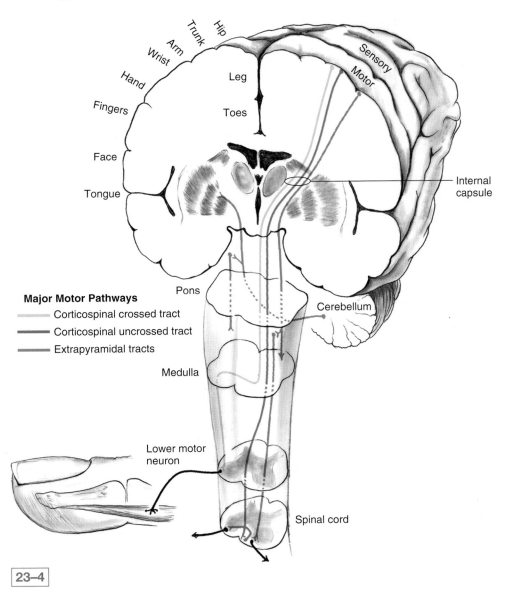

Major Motor Pathways
— Corticospinal crossed tract
— Corticospinal uncrossed tract
— Extrapyramidal tracts

23–4

the pyramidal tract. This is a phylogenetically older, "lower," more primitive motor system. These subcortical motor fibers maintain muscle tone and control body movements, especially gross automatic movements, such as walking.

CEREBELLAR SYSTEM. This complex motor system coordinates movement, maintains equilibrium, and helps maintain posture. The cerebellum receives information about the position of muscles and joints, the body's equilibrium, and what kind of motor messages are being sent from the cortex to the muscles. The information is integrated, and the cerebellum uses feedback pathways to exert its control back on the cortex or down to lower motor neurons in the spinal cord. This entire process occurs on a subconscious level.

UPPER AND LOWER MOTOR NEURONS

Upper motor neurons are a complex of all the descending motor fibers that can influence or modify the lower motor neurons. Upper motor neurons are located completely within the CNS. The neurons convey impulses from motor areas of the cerebral cortex to the lower motor neurons in the anterior horn cells of the spinal cord. Examples of upper motor neurons are corticospinal, corticobulbar, and extrapyramidal tracts. Examples of upper motor neuron diseases are cerebrovascular accident, cerebral palsy, and multiple sclerosis.

Lower motor neurons are located mostly in the peripheral nervous system. The cell body of the lower motor neuron is located in the anterior gray column of the spinal cord, but the nerve fiber extends from here to the muscle. The lower motor neuron is the "final common pathway," because it funnels many neural signals here, and it provides the final direct contact with the muscles. Any movement must be translated into action by lower motor neuron fibers. Examples of lower motor neurons are cranial nerves and spinal nerves of the peripheral nervous system. Examples of lower motor neuron diseases are spinal cord lesions, poliomyelitis, and amyotrophic lateral sclerosis.

THE PERIPHERAL NERVOUS SYSTEM

A **nerve** is a bundle of fibers *outside* the CNS. The peripheral nerves carry input to the CNS via their sensory afferent fibers and deliver output from the CNS via the efferent fibers.

REFLEX ARC

Reflexes are basic defense mechanisms of the nervous system. They are involuntary, operating below the level of conscious control and permitting a quick reaction to potentially painful or damaging situations. Reflexes also help the body maintain balance and appropriate muscle tone. There are four types of reflexes: (1) **deep tendon reflexes** (myotatic), e.g., patellar or knee jerk; (2) **superficial,** e.g., corneal reflex, abdominal reflex; (3) **visceral** (organic), e.g., pupillary response to light and accommodation; and (4) **pathologic** (abnormal), e.g., Babinski's or extensor plantar reflex.

REFLEX ARC

23–5

The fibers that mediate the reflex are carried by a specific spinal nerve. In the most simple reflex, tapping the tendon stretches the muscle spindles in the muscle, which activates the sensory afferent nerve. The sensory afferent fibers carry the message from the receptor and travel through the dorsal root into the spinal cord (Fig. 23–5). They synapse in the cord with the motor neuron in the anterior horn. Motor efferent fibers leave via the ventral root and travel to the muscle.

The deep tendon (myotatic or stretch) reflex has five components: (1) an intact sensory nerve (afferent); (2) a functional synapse in the cord; (3) an intact motor nerve fiber (efferent); (4) the neuromuscular junction; and (5) a competent muscle.

CRANIAL NERVES

Cranial nerves enter and exit the brain rather than the spinal cord (Fig. 23–6 and Table 23–1). The 12 pairs of cranial nerves supply primarily the head and neck, except the vagus nerve (Lat. *vagus,* or wanderer, as in "vagabond"), which travels to the heart, respiratory muscles, stomach, and gallbladder.

SPINAL NERVES

The 31 pairs of **spinal nerves** arise from the length of the spinal cord and supply the rest of the body. They are named for the region of the spine from which they exit: 8 cervical, 12 thoracic, 5 lumbar, 5 sacral, and 1 coccygeal. They are "mixed" nerves because they contain both sensory and motor fibers. The nerves enter and exit the cord through roots—sensory afferent fibers through the posterior or dorsal roots, and motor efferent fibers through the anterior or ventral roots.

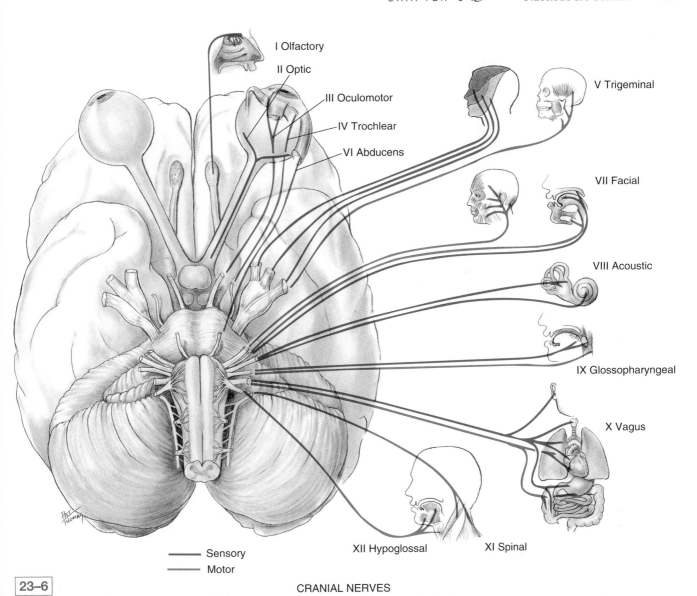

I Olfactory

II Optic

III Oculomotor

IV Trochlear

VI Abducens

V Trigeminal

VII Facial

VIII Acoustic

IX Glossopharyngeal

X Vagus

XII Hypoglossal

XI Spinal

—— Sensory

—— Motor

23-6

CRANIAL NERVES

TABLE 23–1: Cranial Nerves

CRANIAL NERVE	TYPE	FUNCTION
I: Olfactory	Sensory	Smell
II: Optic	Sensory	Vision
III: Oculomotor	Mixed*	Motor—most EOM movement, raise eyelids Parasympathetic—pupil constriction, lens shape
IV: Trochlear	Motor	Down and inward movement of eye
V: Trigeminal	Mixed	Motor—muscles of mastication Sensory—sensation of face and scalp, cornea, mucous membranes of mouth and nose
VI: Abducens	Motor	Lateral movement of eye
VII: Facial	Mixed	Motor—facial muscles, close eye, labial speech Sensory—taste (sweet, salty, sour, bitter) on anterior two-thirds of tongue Parasympathetic—saliva and tear secretion
VIII: Acoustic	Sensory	Hearing and equilibrium
IX: Glossopharyngeal	Mixed	Motor—pharynx (phonation and swallowing) Sensory—taste on posterior one-third of tongue, pharynx (gag reflex) Parasympathetic—parotid gland, carotid reflex
X: Vagus	Mixed	Motor—pharynx and larynx (talking and swallowing) Sensory—general sensation from carotid body, carotid sinus, pharynx, viscera Parasympathetic—carotid reflex
XI: Spinal	Motor	Movement of trapezius and sternomastoid muscles
XII: Hypoglossal	Motor	Movement of tongue

*Mixed refers to a nerve carrying a combination of fibers: motor + sensory; motor + parasympathetic; or motor + sensory + parasympathetic.

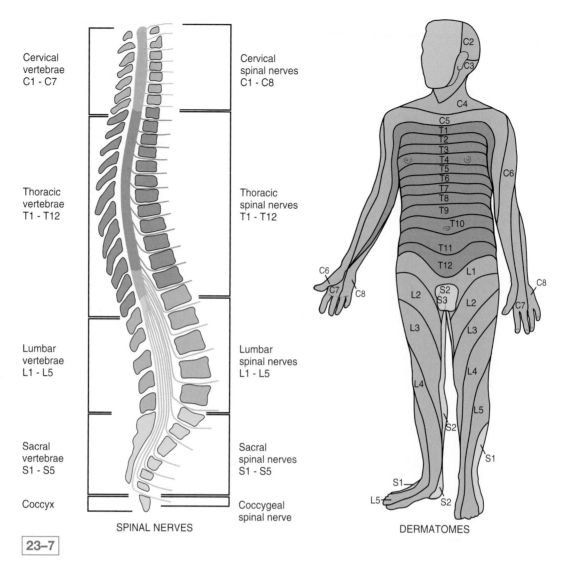

Cervical
vertebrae
C1 - C7

Thoracic
vertebrae
T1 - T12

Lumbar
vertebrae
L1 - L5

Sacral
vertebrae
S1 - S5

Coccyx

SPINAL NERVES

Cervical
spinal nerves
C1 - C8

Thoracic
spinal nerves
T1 - T12

Lumbar
spinal nerves
L1 - L5

Sacral
spinal nerves
S1 - S5

Coccygeal
spinal nerve

DERMATOMES

23–7

The nerves exit the spinal cord in an orderly ladder. Each nerve innervates a particular segment of the body. **Dermal segmentation** is the cutaneous distribution of the various spinal nerves.

A **dermatome** is a circumscribed skin area that is supplied mainly from one spinal cord segment through a particular spinal nerve (Fig. 23–7). The dermatomes overlap, which is a form of biologic insurance. That is, if one nerve is severed, most of the sensations can be transmitted by the one above and the one below. While you may not need to memorize all dermatome segments, the following are useful landmarks:

- The **thumb, middle finger,** and **fifth finger** are each in the dermatomes of C6, C7, and C8.
- The **nipple** is at the level of T4.
- The **umbilicus** is at the level of T10.
- The **groin** is in the region of L1.

AUTONOMIC NERVOUS SYSTEM

The peripheral nervous system is composed of cranial nerves and spinal nerves. These nerves carry fibers that can be divided functionally into two parts—somatic and autonomic.

The somatic fibers innervate the skeletal (voluntary) muscles; the autonomic fibers innervate smooth (involuntary) muscles, cardiac muscle, and glands. The autonomic system mediates unconscious activity. Although a description of the autonomic system is beyond the scope of this book, its overall function is to maintain homeostasis of the body.

 DEVELOPMENTAL CONSIDERATIONS

INFANTS

The neurologic system is not completely developed at birth. Motor activity in the newborn is under the control of the spinal cord and medulla. Very little cortical control exists, and the neurons are not yet myelinated. Movements are directed primarily by primitive reflexes. As the cerebral cortex develops during the 1st year, it inhibits these reflexes, and they disappear at predictable times. Persistence of the primitive reflexes is an indication of CNS dysfunction.

The infant's sensory and motor development proceeds along with the gradual acquisition of myelin, because myelin is needed to conduct most impulses. The process of myelinization follows a cephalocaudal and proximodistal order (head, neck, trunk, and extremities). This is just the order we observe the infant gaining motor control (lifts head, lifts head and shoulders, rolls over, moves whole arm, uses hands, walks). As the milestones are achieved, each is more complex and coordinated. Milestones occur in an orderly sequence, although the exact age of occurrence may vary.

Sensation also is rudimentary at birth. The newborn needs a strong stimulus and then responds by crying and with whole body movements. As myelinization develops, the infant is able to localize the stimulus more precisely and to make a more accurate motor response.

THE AGING ADULT

The aging process causes a general atrophy with a steady loss of neurons in the brain and spinal cord. The loss of neurons causes a decrease in weight and volume so that by 80 years, the brain has decreased in weight by 15 percent (Waxman, 1999). Neuron loss leads many people over 65 to show signs that, in the younger adult, would be considered abnormal, such as general loss of muscle bulk, loss of muscle tone in the face, in the neck, and around the spine, decreased muscle strength, impaired fine coordination and agility, loss of vibratory sense at the ankle, decreased or absent Achilles reflex,

loss of position sense at the big toe, pupillary miosis, irregular pupil shape, and decreased pupillary reflexes.

The velocity of nerve conduction decreases between 5 and 10 percent with aging, making the reaction time slower in some older persons. An increased delay at the synapse also occurs, so the impulse takes longer to travel. As a result, touch and pain sensation, taste, and smell may be diminished.

The motor system may show a general slowing down of movement. Muscle strength and agility decrease. A generalized decrease occurs in muscle bulk, which is most apparent in the dorsal hand muscles. Muscle tremors may occur in the hands, head, and jaw, along with possible repetitive facial grimacing (dyskinesias).

Aging has a progressive decrease in cerebral blood flow and oxygen consumption. In some people this causes dizziness and a loss of balance with position change. These people need to be taught to get up slowly. Otherwise they have an increased risk for falls and resulting injuries. Additionally, older people may forget they fell, which makes it hard to diagnose the cause of the injury.

When they are in good health, aging people walk about as well as they did during their middle and younger years, except more slowly and more deliberately. Some survey the ground for obstacles or uneven terrain. Some show a hesitation and a slightly wayward path.

Subjective Data

1. Headache	**6.** Weakness	**11.** Significant past history
2. Head injury	**7.** Incoordination	**12.** Environmental/occupational hazards
3. Dizziness/vertigo	**8.** Numbness or tingling	
4. Seizures	**9.** Difficulty swallowing	
5. Tremors	**10.** Difficulty speaking	

EXAMINER ASKS	RATIONALE
1. Headache. Any unusually frequent or severe headaches? • When did this start? How often does it occur? • Where in your head do you feel the headaches? Do the headaches seem to be associated with anything? (Headache history fully discussed in Chapter 13.)	
2. Head injury. Ever had any **head injury**? Please describe. • What part of your head was hit? • Did you have a loss of consciousness? For how long?	
3. Dizziness/vertigo. Ever feel lightheaded, a swimming sensation, like feeling faint? • When have you noticed this? How often does it occur? Does it occur with activity, change in position? • Do you ever feel a sensation called **vertigo**, a rotational spinning sensation? (Note—Distinguish vertigo from dizziness.) Do you feel as if the room spins (objective vertigo)? Or do you feel that you are spinning (subjective vertigo)? Did this come on suddenly or gradually?	Syncope is a sudden loss of strength, a temporary loss of consciousness due to lack of cerebral blood flow, a faint. True vertigo is rotational spinning caused by neurologic dysfunction or a problem in the vestibular apparatus or the vestibular nuclei in the brain stem.

EXAMINER ASKS	RATIONALE
4. Seizures. Ever had any convulsions? When did they start? How often do they occur?	**Seizures** occur with epilepsy, a paroxysmal disease characterized by altered or loss of consciousness, involuntary muscle movements, and sensory disturbances. *Aura* is a subjective sensation that precedes a seizure; it could be auditory, visual, or motor.
• Course and duration—When a seizure starts, do you have any warning sign? What type of sign? • Motor activity—Where in your body do the seizures begin? Do the seizures travel through your body? On one side or both? Does your muscle tone seem tense or limp? • Any associated signs: color change in face or lips, loss of consciousness, for how long, automatisms (eyelid fluttering, eye rolling, lip smacking), incontinence? • Postictal phase—After the seizure, are you told you spend time sleeping or have any confusion, weakness, headache, or muscle ache? • Precipitating factors—Does anything seem to bring on the seizures: activity, discontinuing medication, fatigue, stress? • Are you on any medication? • Coping strategies—How have the seizures affected daily life, occupation?	
5. Tremors. Any shakes or **tremors** in the hands or face? When did these start? • Do they seem to grow worse with anxiety, intention, or rest? • Are they relieved with rest, activity, alcohol? Do they affect daily activities?	Tremor is an involuntary shaking, vibrating, or trembling.
6. Weakness. Any **weakness** or problem moving any body part? Is this generalized or local? Does it occur with anything?	Paresis is a partial or incomplete paralysis. Paralysis is a loss of motor function due to a lesion in the neurologic or muscular system or loss of sensory innervation.
7. Incoordination. Any problem with **coordination?** Any problem with balance when walking? Do you list to one side? Any falling? Which way? Do your legs seem to give way? Any clumsy movement?	Dysmetria is the inability to control range of motion of muscles.
8. Numbness or tingling. Any **numbness or tingling** in any body part? Does it feel like pins and needles? When did this start? Where do you feel it? Does it occur with activity?	Paresthesia is an abnormal sensation, e.g., burning, tingling.
9. Difficulty swallowing. Any problem **swallowing?** Occur with solids or liquids? Have you experienced excessive saliva, drooling?	
10. Difficulty speaking. Any problem **speaking:** with forming words or with saying what you intended to say? When did you first notice this? How long did it last?	
11. Significant past history. Past history of: stroke (cerebrovascular accident), spinal cord injury, meningitis or encephalitis, congenital defect, or alcoholism?	
12. Environmental/occupational hazards. Are you exposed to any environmental/occupational hazards: insecticides, organic solvents, lead? • Are you taking any medications now? • How much alcohol do you drink? Each week? Each day? • How about other mood-altering drugs: marijuana, cocaine, barbiturates, tranquilizers?	Review anticonvulsants, antitremor, antivertigo, pain medication.

EXAMINER ASKS	RATIONALE

Additional History for Infants and Children

1. Did you (the mother) have any health problems during the pregnancy: any infections or illnesses, medications taken, toxemia, hypertension, alcohol or drug use, diabetes?

Prenatal history may affect infant's neurologic development.

2. Please tell me about this baby's birth. Was the baby at term or premature? Birth weight?
- Any birth trauma? Did the baby breathe immediately?
- Were you told the baby's Apgar scores?
- Any congenital defects?

3. Reflexes—What have you noticed about the baby's behavior? Do the baby's sucking and swallowing seem coordinated? When you touch the cheek, does the baby turn his or her head toward touch? Does the baby startle with a loud noise or shake of crib? Does the baby grasp your finger?

4. Does the child seem to have any problem with balance? Have you noted any unexplained falling, clumsy or unsteady gait, progressive muscular weakness, problem with going up or down stairs, problem with getting up from lying position?

If occurs, may not be noticed until starts to walk in late infancy.
Screens for muscular dystrophy.

5. Has this child had any seizures? Please describe. Did the seizure occur with a high fever? Did any loss of consciousness occur—how long? How many seizures occurred with this same illness (if occurred with high fever)?

Seizures may occur with high fever in infants and toddlers. Or, seizures may be sign of neurologic disease.

6. Did this child's motor or developmental milestones seem to come at about the right age? Does this child seem to be growing and maturing normally to you? How does this child's development compare to siblings or to age-mates?

7. Do you know if your child has had any environmental exposure to lead?

Chronically elevated lead levels may cause a developmental delay, a loss of a newly acquired skill, or no clinical signs may be present.

8. Have you been told about any learning problems in school: problems with attention span, cannot concentrate, hyperactive?

9. Any family history of: seizure disorder, cerebral palsy, muscular dystrophy?

Additional History for the Aging Adult

1. Any problem with dizziness? Does this occur when you first sit or stand up, when you move your head, when you get up and walk just after eating?

Diminished cerebral blood flow and diminished vestibular response may produce staggering with position change, which increases risk of falls.
Micturition syncope.

- (For men) Do you ever get up at night and then feel faint while standing to urinate?
- How does dizziness affect your daily activities? Are you able to drive safely and to maneuver within your house safely?
- What safety modifications have you applied at home?

2. Have you noticed any decrease in memory, change in mental function? Have you felt any confusion? Did this seem to come on suddenly or gradually?

EXAMINER ASKS	RATIONALE
3. Have you ever noticed any tremor? Is this in your hands or face? Is this worse with: anxiety, activity, rest? Does the tremor seem to be relieved with: alcohol, activity, rest? Does the tremor interfere with daily or social activities?	Senile tremor is relieved by alcohol, although this is not a recommended treatment. Assess if the person is abusing alcohol in effort to relieve tremor.
4. Have you ever had any sudden vision change, fleeting blindness? Did this occur along with weakness? Did you have any loss of consciousness?	Screen symptoms of stroke.

Objective Data

PREPARATION

Perform a **screening neurologic examination** (items identified in following sections) on seemingly well persons who have no significant subjective findings from the history.

Perform a **complete neurologic examination** on persons who have neurologic concerns (e.g., headache, weakness, loss of coordination) or who have shown signs of neurologic dysfunction.

Perform a **neurologic recheck** examination on persons with demonstrated neurologic deficits who require periodic assessments (e.g., hospitalized persons or those in extended care), using the examination sequence beginning on page 700.

Integrate the steps of the neurologic examination with the examination of each particular part of the body, as much as you are able. For example, test cranial nerves while assessing the head and neck (recall Chapters 13 through 16) and superficial abdominal reflexes while assessing the abdomen. When recording your findings, however, consider all neurologic data as a functional unit, and record them all together.

Use the following sequence for the complete neurologic examination.

1. Mental status (see Chapter 7)
2. Cranial nerves
3. Motor system
4. Sensory system
5. Reflexes

Position the person sitting up with the head at your eye level.

EQUIPMENT NEEDED

Penlight
Tongue blade
Cotton swab
Cotton ball
Tuning fork (128 Hz or 256 Hz)
Percussion hammer
(Possibly) familiar aromatic substances, e.g., peppermint, coffee, vanilla

NORMAL RANGE OF FINDINGS	ABNORMAL FINDINGS

TEST CRANIAL NERVES

Cranial Nerve I—Olfactory Nerve

Do not test routinely. Test the sense of smell in those who report loss of smell, those with head trauma, and those with abnormal mental status, and when the presence of an intracranial lesion is suspected. First, assess patency by occluding one nostril at a time and asking the person to sniff. Then, with the person's eyes closed, occlude one nostril and present an aromatic substance. Use familiar, conveniently obtainable, and non-noxious smells, such as coffee, toothpaste, orange, vanilla, soap, or peppermint. Alcohol swabs smell familiar and are easy to find but are irritating.

One cannot test smell when air passages are occluded with upper respiratory infection or with sinusitis.

Anosmia—decrease or loss of smell occurs bilaterally with tobacco smoking, allergic rhinitis, and cocaine use.

NORMAL RANGE OF FINDINGS	ABNORMAL FINDINGS

Normally, a person can identify an odor on each side of the nose. Smell normally is decreased bilaterally with aging. Any asymmetry in the sense of smell is important.

Unilateral loss of smell in the absence of nasal disease is *neurogenic anosmia* (see Table 23–3 on p. 708).

Cranial Nerve II—Optic Nerve
Test visual acuity and test visual fields by confrontation (see Chapter 14).

Using the ophthalmoscope, examine the ocular fundus to determine the color, size, and shape of the optic disc (see Chapter 14).

Visual field loss (see Table 14–2). Papilledema with increased intracranial pressure; optic atrophy (see Table 14–11).

Cranial Nerves III, IV, and VI—Oculomotor, Trochlear, and Abducens Nerves
Palpebral fissures are usually equal in width or nearly so.

Ptosis (drooping) occurs with myasthenia gravis, dysfunction of cranial nerve III, or Horner's syndrome (see Table 14–4). (See Table 14–9.)

Check pupils for size, regularity, equality, direct and consensual light reaction, and accommodation (see Chapter 14).

Assess extraocular movements by the cardinal positions of gaze (see Chapter 14).

Strabismus (deviated gaze) or limited movement (see Table 14–3).

Nystagmus is a back-and-forth oscillation of the eyes. End-point nystagmus, a few beats of horizontal nystagmus at extreme lateral gaze, occurs normally. Assess any other nystagmus carefully, noting:

- Presence of nystagmus in one or both eyes.
- *Pendular* movement (oscillations move equally left to right) or *jerk* (a quick phase in one direction, then a slow phase in the other). Classify the jerk nystagmus in the direction of the quick phase.
- Amplitude. Judge whether the degree of movement is fine, medium, or coarse.
- Frequency. Is it constant, or does it fade after a few beats?
- Plane of movement: horizontal, vertical, rotary, or a combination.

Nystagmus occurs with disease of the vestibular system, cerebellum, or brain stem.

Cranial Nerve V—Trigeminal Nerve
MOTOR FUNCTION. Assess the muscles of mastication by palpating the temporal and masseter muscles as the person clenches the teeth (Fig. 23–8). Muscles should feel equally strong on both sides. Next, try to separate the jaws by pushing down on the chin; normally you cannot.

Decreased strength on one or both sides.

Asymmetry in jaw movement.

Pain with clenching of teeth.

23–8

NORMAL RANGE OF FINDINGS	ABNORMAL FINDINGS

SENSORY FUNCTION. With the person's eyes closed, test light touch sensation by touching a cotton wisp to these designated areas on person's face: forehead, cheeks, and chin (Fig. 23–9). Ask the person to say "Now," whenever the touch is felt. This tests all three divisions of the nerve: (1) ophthalmic, (2) maxillary, and (3) mandibular.

Decreased or unequal sensation.

23–9

CORNEAL REFLEX. (Omit this test, unless the person has abnormal facial sensation or abnormalities of facial movement.) Remove any contact lenses. With the person looking forward, bring a wisp of cotton in from the side (to minimize defensive blinking) and lightly touch the cornea, not the conjunctiva (Fig. 23–10). Normally, the person will blink bilaterally. The corneal reflex may be decreased or absent in those who have worn contact lenses. This procedure tests the sensory afferent in cranial nerve V and the motor efferent in cranial nerve VII.

No blink occurs with a lesion of cranial nerve V or cranial nerve VII paralysis.

23–10

NORMAL RANGE OF FINDINGS

ABNORMAL FINDINGS

Cranial Nerve VII—Facial Nerve

MOTOR FUNCTION. Note mobility and facial symmetry as the person responds to these requests: smile (Fig. 23–11), frown, close eyes tightly (against your attempt to open them), lift eyebrows, show teeth, and puff cheeks (Fig. 23–12). Then, press the person's puffed cheeks in, and note that the air should escape equally from both sides.

Muscle weakness is shown by loss of the nasolabial fold, drooping of one side of the face, lower eyelid sagging, and escape of air from only one cheek that is pressed in.

Loss of movement and asymmetry of movement occur with both central nervous system lesions (e.g., brain attack or stroke) and peripheral nervous system lesions (e.g., Bell's palsy).

23–11

23–12

SENSORY FUNCTION. Do not test routinely. Test only when you suspect facial nerve injury. When indicated, test sense of taste by applying to the tongue a cotton applicator covered with a solution of sugar, salt, or lemon juice (sour). Ask the person to identify the taste.

Cranial Nerve VIII—Acoustic (Vestibulocochlear) Nerve

Test hearing acuity by the ability to hear normal conversation, by the whispered voice test, and by Weber and Rinne tuning fork tests (see Chapter 15).

Cranial Nerves IX and X—Glossopharyngeal and Vagus Nerves

MOTOR FUNCTION. Depress the tongue with a tongue blade, and note pharyngeal movement as the person says "ahhh" or yawns; the uvula and soft palate should rise in the midline, and the tonsillar pillars should move medially.

Absence or asymmetry of soft palate movement.
Uvula deviates to side.
Asymmetry of tonsillar pillar movement.

Touch the posterior pharyngeal wall with a tongue blade, and note the gag reflex. Also note that the voice sounds smooth and not strained.

Hoarse or brassy voice occurs with vocal cord dysfunction; nasal twang occurs with weakness of soft palate.

SENSORY FUNCTION. Cranial nerve IX does mediate taste on the posterior one third of the tongue, but technically this sensation is too difficult to test.

NORMAL RANGE OF FINDINGS	ABNORMAL FINDINGS

Cranial Nerve XI—Spinal Accessory Nerve

Examine the sternomastoid and trapezius muscles for equal size. Check equal strength by asking the person to rotate the head forcibly against resistance applied to the side of the chin (Fig. 23–13). Then ask the person to shrug the shoulders against resistance (Fig. 23–14). These movements should feel equally strong on both sides.

Atrophy.
Muscle weakness or paralysis.

23–13

23–14

Cranial Nerve XII—Hypoglossal Nerve

Inspect the tongue. No wasting or tremors should be present. Note the forward thrust in the midline as the person protrudes the tongue. Also ask the person to say "light, tight, dynamite," and note that lingual speech (sounds of letters l, t, d, n) is clear and distinct.

Atrophy. Fasciculations.
Tongue deviates to side with lesions of the hypoglossal nerve (when this occurs, deviation is toward the paralyzed side).

INSPECT AND PALPATE THE MOTOR SYSTEM

Muscles

SIZE. As you proceed through the examination, inspect all muscle groups for size. Compare the right side with the left. Muscle groups should be within the normal size limits for age and should be symmetric bilaterally. When muscles in the extremities look asymmetric, measure each in centimeters and record the difference. A difference of 1 cm or less is not significant. Note that it is difficult to assess muscle mass in very obese people.

Atrophy—abnormally small muscle with a wasted appearance; occurs with disuse, injury, lower motor neuron disease such as polio, diabetic neuropathy.
Hypertrophy—increased size and strength; occurs with isometric exercise.

NORMAL RANGE OF FINDINGS

STRENGTH. (See Chapter 22, Musculoskeletal System.) Test the power of homologous muscles simultaneously. Test muscle groups of the extremities, neck, and trunk.

TONE. Tone is the normal degree of tension (contraction) in voluntarily relaxed muscles. It shows as a mild resistance to passive stretch. To test muscle tone, move the extremities through a passive range of motion. First, persuade the person to relax completely, to "go loose like a rag doll." Move each extremity smoothly through a full range of motion. Support the arm at the elbow and the leg at the knee (Fig. 23–15). Normally, you will note a mild, even resistance to movement.

23–15

INVOLUNTARY MOVEMENTS. Normally, no involuntary movements occur. If they are present, note their location, frequency, rate, and amplitude. Note if the movements can be controlled at will.

Cerebellar Function

BALANCE TESTS

GAIT. Observe as the person walks 10 to 20 feet, turns, and returns to the starting point. Normally, the person moves with a sense of freedom. The gait is smooth, rhythmic, and effortless; the opposing arm swing is coordinated; the turns are smooth. The step length is about 15 inches from heel to heel.

ABNORMAL FINDINGS

Paresis or weakness is diminished strength; paralysis or plegia is absence of strength.

Limited range of motion.
Pain with motion.
Flaccidity—decreased resistance, hypotonic.
Spasticity and rigidity—types of increased resistance (see Table 23–4).

Tic, tremor, fasciculation, myoclonus, chorea, and athetosis (see Table 23–5).

Stiff, immobile posture. Staggering or reeling. Wide base of support.
Lack of arm swing or rigid arms.
Unequal rhythm of steps. Slapping of foot. Scraping of toe of shoe.
Ataxia—uncoordinated or unsteady gait (see Table 23–6).

NORMAL RANGE OF FINDINGS	ABNORMAL FINDINGS
Ask the person to walk a straight line in a heel-to-toe fashion (tandem walking) (Fig. 23–16). This decreases the base of support and will accentuate any problem with coordination. Normally, the person can walk straight and stay balanced.	Crooked line of walk. Widens base to maintain balance. Staggering, reeling, loss of balance. An ataxia that did not appear with regular gait may appear now. Inability to tandem walk is sensitive for an upper motor neuron lesion, such as multiple sclerosis.

23–16 Tandem walking.

THE ROMBERG TEST. Ask the person to stand up with feet together and arms at the sides. Once in a stable position, ask the person to close the eyes and to hold the position (Fig. 23–17). Wait about 20 seconds. Normally, a person can maintain posture and balance even with the visual orienting information blocked, although slight swaying may occur. (Stand close to catch the person in case he or she falls.)	Sways, falls, widens base of feet to avoid falling. *Positive* Romberg sign is loss of balance that occurs when closing the eyes. You eliminate the advantage of orientation with the eyes, which had compensated for sensory loss. A positive Romberg sign occurs with cerebellar ataxia (multiple sclerosis, alcohol intoxication), loss of proprioception, and loss of vestibular function.

NORMAL RANGE OF FINDINGS	ABNORMAL FINDINGS

23-17 Romberg test.

Ask the person to perform a shallow knee bend or to hop in place, first on one leg, then the other (Fig. 23–18). This demonstrates normal position sense, muscle strength, and cerebellar function. Note that some individuals cannot hop because of aging or obesity.

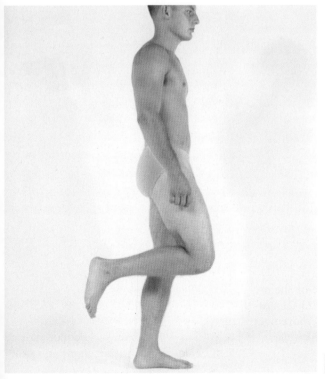

23-18

NORMAL RANGE OF FINDINGS	ABNORMAL FINDINGS

COORDINATION AND SKILLED MOVEMENTS

RAPID ALTERNATING MOVEMENTS (RAM). Ask the person to pat the knees with both hands, lift up, turn hands over, and pat the knees with the backs of the hands (Fig. 23–19). Then ask the person to do this faster. Normally, this is done with equal turning and a quick rhythmic pace.

Lack of coordination.

Slow, clumsy, and sloppy response is termed *dysdiadochokinesia* and occurs with cerebellar disease.

23–19

Alternatively, ask the person to touch the thumb to each finger on the same hand, starting with the index finger, then reverse direction (Fig. 23–20). Normally, this can be done quickly and accurately.

Lack of coordination.

23–20

FINGER-TO-FINGER TEST. With the person's eyes open, ask that he or she use the index finger to touch your finger, then his or her own nose (Fig. 23–21). After a few times move your finger to a different spot. The person's movement should be smooth and accurate.

NORMAL RANGE OF FINDINGS	ABNORMAL FINDINGS

ABNORMAL FINDINGS

Dysmetria is clumsy movement with overshooting the mark and occurs with cerebellar disorders.

Past-pointing is a constant deviation to one side.

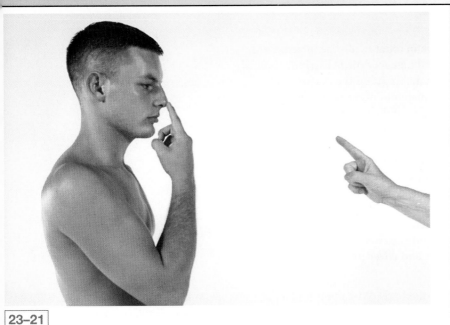

23–21

FINGER-TO-NOSE TEST. Ask the person to close the eyes and to stretch out the arms. Ask the person to touch the tip of his or her nose with each index finger, alternating hands and increasing speed. Normally this is done with accurate and smooth movement.

Misses nose. Worsening of coordination when the eyes are closed occurs with cerebellar disease.

HEEL-TO-SHIN TEST. Test lower extremity coordination by asking the person, who is in a supine position, to place the heel on the opposite knee, and run it down the shin from the knee to the ankle (Fig. 23–22). Normally, the person moves the heel in a straight line down the shin.

Lack of coordination.
Heel falls off shin.

23–22

NORMAL RANGE OF FINDINGS	ABNORMAL FINDINGS

ASSESS THE SENSORY SYSTEM

Ask the person to identify various sensory stimuli in order to test the intactness of the peripheral nerve fibers, the sensory tracts, and higher cortical discrimination.

Ensure validity of sensory system testing by making sure the person is alert, cooperative, and comfortable and has an adequate attention span. Otherwise, you may get misleading and invalid results. Testing of the sensory system can be fatiguing. You may need to repeat the examination later or to break it into parts when the person is tired.

You do not need to test the entire skin surface for every sensation. Routine screening procedures include testing superficial pain, light touch, and vibration in a few distal locations, and testing stereognosis. This will suffice for all who have not demonstrated any neurologic symptoms or signs. Complete testing of the sensory system is warranted in those with neurologic symptoms (e.g., localized pain, numbness, and tingling) or when you discover abnormalities (e.g., motor deficit). Then, test all sensory modalities and cover most dermatomes of the body.

Compare sensations on symmetric parts of the body. When you find a definite decrease in sensation, map it out by systematic testing in that area. Proceed from the point of decreased sensation toward the sensitive area. By asking the person to tell you where the sensation changes, you can map the exact borders of the deficient area. Draw your results on a diagram.

Avoid asking leading questions, "Can you feel this pinprick?" This creates an expectation of how the person should feel the sensation, which is called *suggestion*. Instead, use unbiased directions.

The person's eyes should be closed during each of the tests. Take time to explain what will be happening and exactly how you expect the person to respond.

Spinothalamic Tract

PAIN. Pain is tested by the person's ability to perceive a pinprick. Break a tongue blade lengthwise, forming a sharp point at the fractured end and a dull spot at the rounded end. Lightly apply the sharp point or the dull end to the person's body in a random, unpredictable order (Fig. 23–23). Ask the person to say "sharp" or "dull," depending on the sensation felt. (Note that the sharp edge is used to test for pain; the dull edge is used as a general test of the person's responses.)

Let at least 2 seconds elapse between each stimulus to avoid *summation*. With summation, frequent consecutive stimuli are perceived as one strong stimulus.

Note if the topographic pattern of sensory loss is distal, i.e., over the hands and feet in a "glove and stocking" distribution, or if it is over a specific dermatome.

Hypalgesia—decreased pain sensation.

Analgesia—absent pain sensation.

Hyperalgesia—increased pain sensation.

A   B

23–23

NORMAL RANGE OF FINDINGS	ABNORMAL FINDINGS

TEMPERATURE. Test temperature sensation only when pain sensation is abnormal; otherwise, you may omit it because the fiber tracts are much the same. Fill two test tubes, one with hot water and one with cold water, and apply the bottom ends to the person's skin in a random order. Ask the person to say which temperature is felt. Alternatively, you could place the flat side of the tuning fork on the skin; its metal always feels cool.

LIGHT TOUCH. Apply a wisp of cotton to the skin. Stretch a cotton ball to make a long end and brush it over the skin in a random order of sites and at irregular intervals (Fig. 23–24). This prevents the person from responding just from repetition. Include the arms, forearms, hands, chest, thighs, and legs. Ask the person to say "now" or "yes" when touch is felt. Compare symmetric points.

Hypoesthesia—decreased touch sensation.

Anesthesia—absent touch sensation.

Hyperesthesia—increased touch sensation.

23–24

Posterior Column Tract

VIBRATION. Test the person's ability to feel vibrations of a tuning fork over bony prominences. Use a low-pitch tuning fork (128 Hz or 256 Hz) because its vibration has a slower decay. Strike the tuning fork on the heel of your hand, and hold the base on a bony surface of the fingers and great toe (Fig. 23–25). Ask the person to indicate when the vibration starts and stops. If the person feels the normal vibration or buzzing sensation on these distal areas, you may assume proximal spots are normal and proceed no further. If no vibrations are felt, move proximally and test ulnar processes, and ankles, patellae, and iliac crests. Compare the right side with the left side. If you find a deficit, note whether it is gradual or abrupt.

Unable to feel vibration. Loss of vibration sense occurs with peripheral neuropathy, e.g., diabetes and alcoholism. Often, this is the first sensation lost.

Peripheral neuropathy is worse at the feet and gradually improves as you move up the leg, as opposed to a specific nerve lesion, which has a clear zone of deficit for its dermatome.

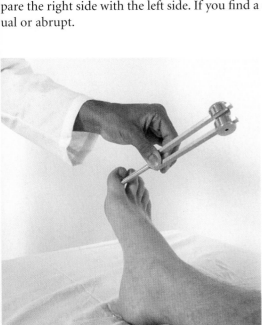

23–25

NORMAL RANGE OF FINDINGS	ABNORMAL FINDINGS

POSITION (KINESTHESIA). Test the person's ability to perceive passive movements of the extremities. Move a finger or the big toe up and down, and ask the person to tell you which way it is moved (Fig. 23–26). The test is done with the eyes closed, but to be sure it is understood, have the person watch a few trials first. Vary the order of movement up or down. Hold the digit by the sides, since upward or downward pressure on the skin may provide a clue as to how it has been moved. Normally, a person can detect movement of a few millimeters.

Loss of position sense.

23–26

TACTILE DISCRIMINATION (FINE TOUCH). The following tests also measure the discrimination ability of the sensory cortex. As a prerequisite, the person needs a normal or near-normal sense of touch and position sense.

Problems with tactile discrimination occur with lesions of the sensory cortex or posterior column.

STEREOGNOSIS. Test the person's ability to recognize objects by feeling their forms, sizes, and weights. With the eyes closed, place a familiar object (paper clip, key, coin, cotton ball, or pencil) in the person's hand and ask the person to identify it (Fig. 23–27). Normally, a person will explore it with the fingers and correctly name it. Test a different object in each hand; testing the left hand assesses right parietal lobe functioning.

Astereognosis—inability to identify object correctly. Occurs in sensory cortex lesions, e.g., brain attack (stroke).

23–27 Stereognosis.

NORMAL RANGE OF FINDINGS	ABNORMAL FINDINGS

GRAPHESTHESIA. Graphesthesia is the ability to "read" a number by having it traced on the skin. With the person's eyes closed, use a blunt instrument to trace a single digit number or a letter on the palm (Fig. 23–28). Ask the person to tell you what it is. Graphesthesia is a good measure of sensory loss if the person cannot make the hand movements needed for stereognosis, as occurs in arthritis.

Inability to distinguish number occurs with lesions of the sensory cortex.

23–28 Graphesthesia.

TWO-POINT DISCRIMINATION. Test the person's ability to distinguish the separation of two simultaneous pin points on the skin. Apply the two points of an opened paper clip lightly to the skin in ever-closing distances. Note the distance at which the person no longer perceives two separate points. The level of perception varies considerably with the region tested; it is most sensitive in the fingertips (2 to 8 mm) and least sensitive on the upper arms, thighs, and back (40 to 75 mm).

An increase in the distance it normally takes to identify two separate points occurs with sensory cortex lesions.

EXTINCTION. Simultaneously touch both sides of the body at the same point. Ask the person to state how many sensations are felt and where they are. Normally, both sensations are felt.

The ability to recognize only one of the stimuli occurs with sensory cortex lesion; the stimulus is extinguished on the side *opposite* the cortex lesion.

POINT LOCATION. Touch the skin, and withdraw the stimulus promptly. Tell the person, "Put your finger where I touched you." You can perform this test simultaneously with light touch sensation.

With a sensory cortex lesion, the person cannot localize the sensation accurately, even though light touch sensation may be retained.

TEST THE REFLEXES

Stretch, or Deep Tendon Reflexes (DTRs)

Measurement of the stretch reflexes reveals the intactness of the reflex arc at specific spinal levels as well as the normal override on the reflex of the higher cortical levels.

For an adequate response, the limb should be relaxed and the muscle partially stretched. Stimulate the reflex by directing a short, snappy blow of the reflex hammer onto the muscle's insertion tendon. Use a relaxed hold on the hammer. As with the percussion technique, the action takes place at the wrist. Strike a brief, well-aimed blow, and bounce up promptly; do not let the hammer rest on the tendon. Use the pointed end of the reflex hammer when aiming at a smaller

NORMAL RANGE OF FINDINGS

target such as your thumb on the tendon site; use the flat end when the target is wider or to diffuse the impact and prevent pain.

Use just enough force to get a response. Compare right and left sides—The responses should be equal. The reflex response is graded on a 4-point scale:

4+	Very brisk, hyperactive with clonus, indicative of disease
3+	Brisker than average, may indicate disease
2+	Average, normal
1+	Diminished, low normal
0	No response

This is a subjective scale and requires some clinical practice. Even then the scale is not completely reliable because no standard exists to say *how* brisk a reflex should be to warrant a grade of 3+. Also, a wide range of normal exists in reflex responses. Healthy people may have diminished reflexes or they may have brisk ones. Your best plan is to interpret the DTRs *only* within the context of the rest of the neurologic exam.

Sometimes the reflex response fails to appear. Try further encouragement of relaxation, varying the person's position, or increasing the strength of the blow. **Reinforcement** is another technique to relax the muscles and enhance the response (Fig. 23–29). Ask the person to perform an isometric exercise in a muscle group somewhat away from the one being tested. For example, to enhance a patellar reflex, ask the person to lock the fingers together and "pull." To enhance a biceps response, ask the person to clench the teeth or to grasp the thigh with the opposite hand.

Clonus is a set of short jerking contractions of the same muscle.

Hyperreflexia is the exaggerated reflex seen when the monosynaptic reflex arc is released from the influence of higher cortical levels. This occurs with upper motor neuron lesions, e.g., a brain attack.

Hyporeflexia, which is the absence of a reflex, is a lower motor neuron problem. It occurs with interruption of sensory afferents or destruction of motor efferents and anterior horn cells, e.g., spinal cord injury.

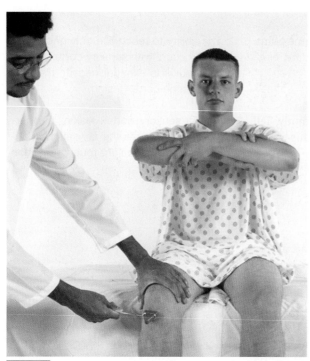

23–29   Reinforcement.

NORMAL RANGE OF FINDINGS	ABNORMAL FINDINGS

BICEPS REFLEX (C5 TO C6). Support the person's forearm on yours; this position relaxes, as well as partially flexes, the person's arm. Place your thumb on the biceps tendon and strike a blow on your thumb. You can feel as well as see the normal response, which is contraction of the biceps muscle and flexion of the forearm (Fig. 23–30).

23–30

TRICEPS REFLEX (C7 TO C8). Tell the person to let the arm "just go dead" as you suspend it by holding the upper arm. Strike the triceps tendon directly just above the elbow (Fig. 23–31). The normal response is extension of the forearm. Alternately, hold the person's wrist across the chest to flex the arm at the elbow, and tap the tendon.

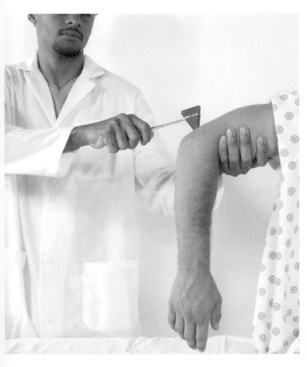

23–31 Triceps reflex.

NORMAL RANGE OF FINDINGS	ABNORMAL FINDINGS

BRACHIORADIALIS REFLEX (C5 TO C6). Hold the person's thumbs to suspend the forearms in relaxation. Strike the forearm directly, about 2 to 3 cm above the radial styloid process (Fig. 23–32). The normal response is flexion and supination of the forearm.

23–32   Brachioradialis reflex.

QUADRICEPS REFLEX ("KNEE JERK") (L2 TO L4). Let the lower legs dangle freely to flex the knee and stretch the tendons. Strike the tendon directly just below the patella (Fig. 23–33). Extension of the lower leg is the expected response. You also will palpate contraction of the quadriceps.

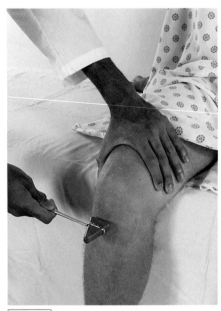

23–33

For the person in the supine position, use your own arm as a lever to support the weight of one leg against the other leg (Fig. 23–34). This maneuver also flexes the knee.

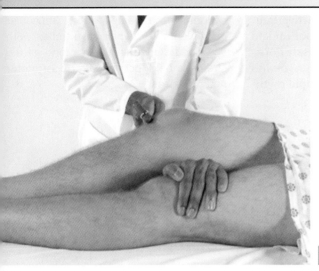

23–34

ACHILLES REFLEX ("ANKLE JERK") (L5 TO S2). Position the person with the knee flexed and the hip externally rotated. Hold the foot in dorsiflexion, and strike the Achilles tendon directly (Fig. 23–35). Feel the normal response as the foot plantar flexes against your hand.

23–35

For the person in the supine position, flex one knee and support that lower leg against the other leg so that it falls "open." Dorsiflex the foot and tap the tendon (Fig. 23–36).

23–36

NORMAL RANGE OF FINDINGS

CLONUS. Test for clonus, particularly when the reflexes are hyperactive. Support the lower leg in one hand. With your other hand, move the foot up and down a few times to relax the muscle. Then stretch the muscle by briskly dorsiflexing the foot. Hold the stretch (Fig. 23–37). With a normal response, you feel no further movement. When clonus is present, you will feel and see rapid rhythmic contractions of the calf muscle and movement of the foot.

23–37

Superficial Reflexes
Here, the receptors are in the skin rather than the muscles.

ABDOMINAL REFLEXES—UPPER (T8 TO T10), LOWER (T10 TO T12). Have the person assume a supine position, with the knees slightly bent. Use the handle end of the reflex hammer, a wood applicator tip, or the end of a split tongue blade to stroke the skin. Move from the side of the abdomen toward the midline at both the upper and lower abdominal levels (Fig. 23–38). The normal response is ipsilateral contraction of the abdominal muscle with an observed deviation of the umbilicus toward the stroke. When the abdominal wall is very obese, pull the skin to the opposite side, and feel it contract toward the stimulus.

23–38

CREMASTERIC REFLEX (L1 TO L2). On the male, lightly stroke the inner aspect of the thigh with the reflex hammer or tongue blade (see Fig. 23–38). Note elevation of the ipsilateral testicle.

ABNORMAL FINDINGS

Clonus is repeated reflex muscular movements. A hyperactive reflex with sustained clonus (lasting as long as the stretch is held) occurs with upper motor neuron disease.

Superficial reflexes are absent with diseases of the pyramidal tract, e.g., they are absent on the contralateral side with brain attack.

NORMAL RANGE OF FINDINGS

PLANTAR REFLEX (L4 TO S2). Position the thigh in slight external rotation. With the reflex hammer, draw a light stroke up the lateral side of the sole of the foot and inward across the ball of the foot, like an upside-down J (Fig. 23–39, *A*). The normal response is plantar flexion of all the toes and inversion and flexion of the forefoot.

ABNORMAL FINDINGS

Except in infancy, the abnormal response is dorsiflexion of the big toe and fanning of all toes, which is a **positive Babinski sign,** also called "upgoing toes" (Fig. 23–39, *B*). This occurs with upper motor neuron disease of the corticospinal (or pyramidal) tract.

A
B

23–39 | A, Plantar reflex

 DEVELOPMENTAL CONSIDERATIONS

Infants (Birth to 12 Months)

The neurologic system shows dramatic growth and development during the 1st year of life. Assessment includes noting that milestones you normally would expect for each month have indeed been achieved, and that the early, more primitive reflexes are eliminated from the baby's repertory when they are supposed to be.

At birth, the newborn is very alert, with the eyes open, and demonstrates strong, urgent sucking. The normal cry is loud, lusty, and even angry. The next 2 or 3 days may be spent mostly sleeping as the baby recovers from the birth process. After that, the pattern of sleep and waking activity is highly variable; it depends on the baby's individual body rhythm as well as external stimuli.

The behavioral assessment should include your observations of the infant's spontaneous waking activity, responses to environmental stimuli, and social interaction with the parents and others.

By 2 months of age, the baby smiles responsively and recognizes the parent's face. Babbling occurs at 4 months, and one or two words (mama, dada) are used nonspecifically after 9 months.

The cranial nerves cannot be tested directly, but you can infer their proper functioning by the maneuvers shown in Table 23–2.

Failure to attain a skill by expected time.
Persistence of reflex behavior beyond the normal time.

A high-pitched, shrill cry or cat-sounding screech occurs with CNS damage.
A weak, groaning cry or expiratory grunt occurs with respiratory distress.

Lethargy, hyporeactivity, hyperirritability, and parent's report of significant change in behavior all warrant referral.

TABLE 23–2: Testing Cranial Nerve Function of Infants

CRANIAL NERVE	RESPONSE
II, III, IV, VI	Optical blink reflex—shine light in open eyes, note rapid closure
	Size, shape, equality of pupils
	Regards face or close object
	Eyes follow movement
V	Rooting reflex, sucking reflex
VII	Facial movements (e.g., wrinkling forehead and nasolabial folds) symmetric when crying or smiling
VIII	Loud noise yields Moro reflex (until 4 mo)
	Acoustic blink reflex—infant blinks in response to a loud hand clap 30 cm (12 in) from head (avoid making air current)
	Eyes follow direction of sound
IX, X	Swallowing, gag reflex
	Coordinated sucking and swallowing
XII	Pinch nose, infant's mouth will open and tongue rise in midline

NORMAL RANGE OF FINDINGS	ABNORMAL FINDINGS

THE MOTOR SYSTEM

Observe spontaneous motor activity for smoothness and symmetry. Smoothness of movement suggests proper cerebellar function, as does the coordination involved in sucking and swallowing. To screen gross and fine motor coordination, use the Denver II test with its age-specific developmental milestones. You also can assess movement by testing the reflexes listed in the following section. Note their smoothness of response and symmetry. Also, note whether their presence or absence is appropriate for the infant's age.

Assess muscle tone by first observing resting posture. The newborn favors a flexed position; extremities are symmetrically folded inward, the hips are slightly abducted, and the fists are tightly flexed (Fig. 23–40). Infants born by breech delivery, however, do not have flexion in the lower extremities.

23–40

After 2 months of age, flexion gives way to gradual extension, beginning with the head and continuing in a cephalocaudal direction. Now is the time to check for spasticity; none should be present. Test for spasticity by flexing the infant's knees onto the abdomen and then quickly releasing them. They will unfold but not too quickly. Also, gently push the head forward—The baby should comply.

The fists normally are held in tight flexion for the first 3 months. Then the fists open for part of the time. A purposeful reach for an object with both hands occurs around 4 months of age, a transfer of an object from hand to hand at 7 months of age, a grasp using fingers and opposing thumb at 9 months of age, and a purposeful release at 10 months of age. Babies are normally ambidextrous for the first 18 months.

Head control is an important milestone in motor development. You can incorporate the following two movements into every infant assessment to check the muscle tone necessary for head control.

First, with the baby supine, pull to a sit holding the wrists and note head control (Fig. 23–41). The newborn will hold the head almost in the same plane as the body, and it will balance briefly when the baby reaches a sitting position, then flop forward. (Even a premature infant shows some head flexion.) At 4 months of age, the head stays in line with the body and does not flop.

Abnormal Findings

Delay in motor activity occurs with brain damage, mental retardation, peripheral neuromuscular damage, prolonged illness, and parental neglect.

Abnormal postures:

Frog position—hips abducted and almost flat against the table, externally rotated (only normal after breech delivery).

Opisthotonos—head arched back, stiffness of neck, and extension of arms and legs; occurs with meningeal or brain stem irritation and kernicterus (see Table 23–10).

Extension of limbs may occur with intracranial hemorrhage.

Any type of continual asymmetry, e.g., asymmetry of upper limbs occurs with brachial plexus palsy.

Spasticity is an early sign of cerebral palsy. After releasing flexed knees, legs will quickly extend and adduct, even to a "scissoring" motion when spasticity is present. Also, the baby often resists head flexion and extends back against your hand when spasticity is present.

Note persistent one-hand preference in baby younger than 18 months of age, which may indicate a motor deficit on the opposite side.

Because development progresses in a cephalocaudal direction, head lag is an early sign of brain damage.

After 6 months of age, refer any baby with failure to hold head in midline when sitting.

NORMAL RANGE OF FINDINGS	ABNORMAL FINDINGS

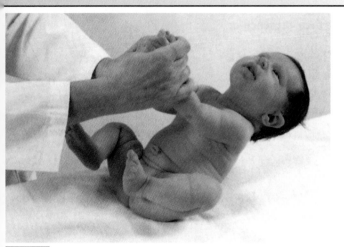

23–41

Second, lift up the baby in a prone position, with one hand supporting the chest (Fig. 23–42). The term newborn holds the head at an angle of 45 degrees or less from horizontal, the back is straight or slightly arched, and the elbows and knees are partly flexed. At 3 months of age, the baby raises the head and arches the back, as in a swan dive. This is the *Landau reflex,* which persists until 1¹/₂ years of age.

Assess muscle strength by noting the strength of sucking and of spontaneous motor activity. Normally, no tremors are present, and no continual over-shooting of the mark occurs when reaching.

Head lag, a limp, floppy trunk, and dangling arms and legs.

Absence of the reflex indicates motor weakness, upper motor neuron disease, or mental retardation.

23–42

THE SENSORY SYSTEM

You will perform very little sensory testing with infants and toddlers. The newborn normally has hypoesthesia and requires a strong stimulus to elicit a response. The baby responds to pain by crying and a general reflex withdrawal of all limbs. By 7 to 9 months of age, the infant can localize the stimulus and shows more specific signs of withdrawal. Other sensory modalities are not tested.

Unusually rapid withdrawal is *hyperesthesia,* which occurs with spinal cord lesions, CNS infections, increased intracranial pressure, peritonitis.

No withdrawal is decreased sensation, which occurs with decreased consciousness, mental deficiency, spinal cord or peripheral nerve lesions.

NORMAL RANGE OF FINDINGS

REFLEXES

Infantile automatisms are reflexes that have a predictable timetable of appearance and departure. The reflexes most commonly tested are listed in the following section. For the screening examination, you can just check the rooting, grasp, tonic neck, and Moro reflexes.

ROOTING REFLEX. Brush the infant's cheek near the mouth. Note whether the infant turns the head toward that side and opens the mouth (Fig. 23–43). Appears at birth and disappears at 3 to 4 months.

23–43

SUCKING REFLEX. Touch the lips and offer your gloved little finger to suck. Note strong sucking reflex. The reflex is present at birth and disappears at 10 to 12 months.

PALMAR GRASP. Place the baby's head midline to ensure symmetric response. Offer your finger from the baby's ulnar side, away from the thumb. Note tight grasp of all the baby's fingers (Fig. 23–44). Sucking enhances grasp. Often, you can pull baby to a sit from grasp. The reflex is present at birth, is strongest at 1 to 2 months, and disappears at 3 to 4 months.

The palmar grasp reflex is absent with brain damage and with local muscle or nerve injury.

Persistence of palmar grasp reflex after 4 months of age occurs with frontal lobe lesion.

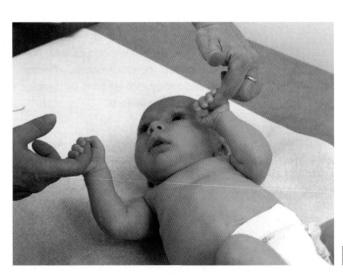

23–44

NORMAL RANGE OF FINDINGS

PLANTAR GRASP. Touch your thumb at the ball of the baby's foot. Note that the toes curl down tightly (Fig. 23–45). The reflex is present at birth and disappears at 8 to 10 months.

23–45

BABINSKI'S REFLEX. Stroke your finger up the lateral edge and across the ball of the infant's foot. Note fanning of toes (positive Babinski's reflex) (Fig. 23–46). The reflex is present at birth and disappears (changes to the adult response) by 24 months of age (variable).

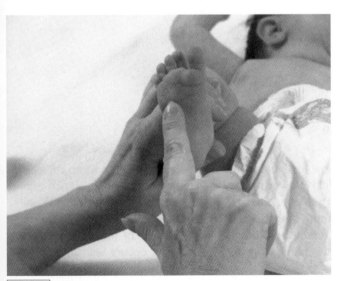

23–46

ABNORMAL FINDINGS

Positive Babinski's reflex after 2 or $2\frac{1}{2}$ years of age occurs with pyramidal tract disease.

NORMAL RANGE OF FINDINGS	ABNORMAL FINDINGS

TONIC NECK REFLEX. With the baby supine, relaxed, or sleeping, turn the head to one side with the chin over shoulder. Note ipsilateral extension of the arm and leg, and flexion of the opposite arm and leg; this is the "fencing" position. If you turn the infant's head to the opposite side, positions will reverse (Fig. 23–47). The reflex appears by 2 to 3 months, decreases at 3 to 4 months, and disappears by 4 to 6 months.

Persistence later in infancy occurs with brain damage.

23–47

MORO REFLEX. Startle the infant by jarring the crib, making a loud noise, or supporting the head and back in a semi-sitting position and quickly lowering the infant to 30 degrees. The baby looks as if he or she is hugging a tree. That is, symmetric abduction and extension of the arms and legs, fanning fingers, and curling of the index finger and thumb to C position occur. The infant then brings in both arms and legs (Fig. 23–48). The reflex is present at birth, and disappears at 1 to 4 months.

Absence of the Moro reflex in the newborn or persistence after 5 months of age indicates severe CNS injury.

Absence of movement in just one arm occurs with fracture of the humerus or clavicle and with brachial nerve palsy.

Absence in one leg occurs with a lower spinal cord problem or a dislocated hip.

A hyperactive Moro reflex occurs with tetany or CNS infection.

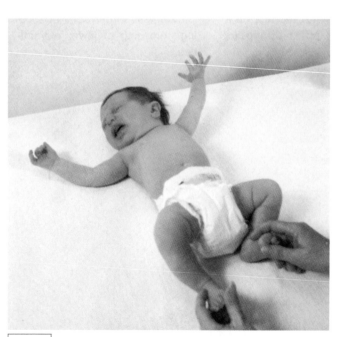

23–48 Moro reflex.

NORMAL RANGE OF FINDINGS

ABNORMAL FINDINGS

PLACING REFLEX. Hold the infant upright under the arms, close to a table. Let the dorsal "top" of foot touch the underside of table. Note flexing of hip and knee, followed by extension at the hip, to place foot on table (Fig. 23–49). Reflex appears at 4 days after birth.

23–49

STEPPING REFLEX. Hold the infant upright under the arms, with the feet on a flat surface. Note regular alternating steps (Fig. 23–50). The reflex disappears before voluntary walking.

Extensor thrust, or "scissoring"; crossing of lower extremities.

23–50

NORMAL RANGE OF FINDINGS	ABNORMAL FINDINGS

Preschool- and School-Age Children

Use the same sequence of neurologic assessment as with the adult, with the omissions or modifications mentioned in the following section.

Assess the child's general behavior during play activities, reaction to parent, and cooperation with parent and with you. Complete details are described in Chapter 7, Mental Status Assessment.

Smell and taste are almost never tested, but if you need to test the child's sense of smell (cranial nerve I), use a scent familiar to the child such as peanut butter or orange peel. When testing visual fields (cranial nerve II) and cardinal positions of gaze (cranial nerves III, IV, VI), you often need to gently immobilize the head, or the child will track with the whole head. Make a game out of asking the child to imitate your funny "faces" (cranial nerve VII); thus, the child has fun and you win a friend.

Much of the motor assessment can be derived from watching the child undress and dress and manipulate buttons. This indicates muscle strength, symmetry, joint range of motion, and fine motor skills. Use the Denver II to screen gross and fine motor skills that are appropriate for the child's specific age. Be familiar with developmental milestones described in Chapter 2 for each age.

Note the child's gait during both walking and running. Allow for the normal wide-based gate of the toddler and the normal knock-kneed walk of the preschooler. Normally, the child can balance on one foot for about 5 seconds by 4 years of age, can balance for 8 to 10 seconds at 5 years of age, and can hop at 4 years. Children enjoy performing these tests (Fig. 23–51).

Muscle hypertrophy or atrophy occurs with muscular dystrophy.
Muscle weakness.
Incoordination.

Causes of motor delay are listed earlier in the infant section.

Staggering, falling.

Weakness climbing up or down stairs occurs with muscular dystrophy.

Broad-based gait beyond toddlerhood, scissor gait (see Table 23–6).

Failure to hop after 5 years of age indicates incoordination of gross motor skill.

23–51

NORMAL RANGE OF FINDINGS

Observe the child as he or she rises from a supine position on the floor to a sitting position, and then to a stand. Note the muscles of the neck, abdomen, arms, and legs. Normally, the child curls up in the midline to sit up, then pushes off with both hands against the floor to stand (Fig. 23–52, *A*).

ABNORMAL FINDINGS

Weak pelvic muscles are a sign of muscular dystrophy; from the supine position, the child will roll to one side, bend forward to all four extremities, plant hands on legs, and literally "climb" up him- or herself. This is *Gower's sign* (Fig. 23–52, *B*).

A

B

23–52

Assess fine coordination by using the finger-to-nose test if you can be sure the young child understands your directions. Demonstrate the procedure first, then ask the child to do the test with the eyes open, then with the eyes closed. Fine coordination is not fully developed until the child has reached 4 or 6 years of age. Consider it normal if a younger child can bring the finger to within 2 to 5 cm (1 to 2 in) of the nose.

Testing sensation is very unreliable in toddlers and preschoolers. You may test light touch by asking the child to close the eyes and then to point to the spot where you touch or tickle. Testing of vibration, position, stereognosis, graphesthesia, or two-point discrimination usually is not done on a child younger than 6 years of age. Also, do not test for perception of superficial pain. In children older than 6 years of age, you may perform sensory testing as with adults. Use a fractured tongue blade if you need to test superficial pain.

The DTRs usually are not tested in children younger than 5 years of age due to lack of cooperation in relaxation. When you need to test DTRs in a young child, use your finger to percuss the tendon. Use a reflex hammer only with an older child. Coax the child to relax, or distract and percuss discreetly when the child is not paying attention. The knee jerk is present at birth, then the ankle jerk and brachial reflex appear, and the triceps reflex is present at 6 months.

Failure of the finger-to-nose test with the eyes open indicates gross incoordination; failure of the test with the eyes closed indicates minor incoordination or lack of position sense.

Sensory loss occurs with decreased consciousness, mental deficiency, or spinal cord or peripheral nerve dysfunction.

Hyperactivity of DTRs occurs with upper motor neuron lesion, hypocalcemia, and hyperthyroidism, and with muscle spasm associated with early poliomyelitis.

Decreased or absent reflexes occur with a lower motor neuron lesion, muscular dystrophy, and flaccidity or flaccid paralysis.

Clonus may occur with fatigue, but it usually indicates hyperreflexia.

NORMAL RANGE OF FINDINGS	ABNORMAL FINDINGS

The Aging Adult

Use the same examination as used with the younger adult. Be aware that some aging adults show a slower response to your requests, especially to those calling for coordination of movements. The conditions discussed in the following sections are normal variants due to aging.

Although the cranial nerves mediating taste and smell are not usually tested, they may show some decline in function.

Any decrease in muscle bulk is most apparent in the hand, as seen by guttering between the metacarpals. These dorsal hand muscles often look wasted, even with no apparent arthropathy. The grip strength remains relatively good.

Senile tremors occasionally occur. These benign tremors include an intention tremor of the hands, head nodding (as if saying yes or no), and tongue protrusion. *Dyskinesias* are the repetitive stereotyped movements in the jaw, lips, or tongue that may accompany senile tremors. No associated rigidity is present.

The gait may be slower and more deliberate than that in the younger person, and it may deviate slightly from a midline path.

The rapid alternating movements, e.g., pronating and supinating the hands on the thigh, may be more difficult to perform by the aging adult.

After 65 years of age, loss of the sensation of vibration at the ankle malleolus is common and is usually accompanied by loss of the ankle jerk. Position sense in the big toe may be lost, although this is less common than vibration loss. Tactile sensation may be impaired. The aging person may need stronger stimuli for light touch and especially for pain.

The DTRs are less brisk. Those in the upper extremities are usually present, but the ankle jerks are commonly lost. Knee jerks may be lost, but this occurs less often. Because aging people find it difficult to relax their limbs, always use reinforcement when eliciting the DTRs.

The plantar reflex may be absent or difficult to interpret. Often, you will not see a definite normal flexor response. However, you still should consider a definite extensor response to be abnormal.

The superficial abdominal reflexes may be absent, probably because of stretching of the musculature through pregnancy or obesity.

NEUROLOGIC RECHECK

Some hospitalized persons have head trauma or a neurologic deficit due to a systemic disease process. These people must be monitored closely for any improvement or deterioration in neurologic status and for any indication of increasing intracranial pressure. Signs of increasing intracranial pressure signal impending cerebral disaster and death and require early and prompt intervention.

Use an abbreviation of the neurologic examination in the following sequence:

1. Level of consciousness
2. Motor function
3. Pupillary response
4. Vital signs

LEVEL OF CONSCIOUSNESS. A *change* in the level of consciousness is the single most important factor in this examination. It is the earliest and most sensitive index of change in neurologic status. Note the ease of *arousal* and the state of awareness, or *orientation*. Assess orientation by asking questions about:

Hand muscle atrophy is worsened with disuse and degenerative arthropathy.

Distinguish senile tremors from tremors of parkinsonism. The latter includes rigidity and slowness and weakness of voluntary movement.

Absence of a rhythmic reciprocal gait pattern is seen in parkinsonism and hemiparesis (see Table 23–6).

Note any difference in sensation between right and left sides, which may indicate a neurologic deficit.

A change in consciousness may be subtle. Note any decreasing level of consciousness, disorientation, memory loss, uncooperative behavior, or even complacency in a previously combative person.

NORMAL RANGE OF FINDINGS

ABNORMAL FINDINGS

- Person—own name, occupation, names of workers around person, their occupations
- Place—where person is, nature of building, city, state
- Time—day of week, month, year

Vary the questions during repeat assessments so that the person is not merely memorizing answers. Note the quality and the content of the verbal response; articulation, fluency, manner of thinking; and any deficit in language comprehension or production (see Chapter 7).

When the person is intubated and cannot speak, you will have to ask questions that require a nod or shake of the head, "Is this a hospital?" "Are you at home?" "Are we in Texas?"

A person is fully alert when his or her eyes open at your approach or spontaneously; when he or she is oriented to person, place, and time; and when he or she is able to follow verbal commands appropriately.

Review Table 7–3, Levels of Consciousness, Chapter 7.

If the person is not fully alert, increase the amount of stimulus used in this order:

1. Name called
2. Light touch on person's arm
3. Vigorous shake of shoulder
4. Pain applied (pinch nail bed, pinch trapezius muscle, rub your knuckles on the person's sternum)

Record the stimulus used as well as the person's response to it.

MOTOR FUNCTION. Check the voluntary movement of each extremity by giving the person specific commands. (This procedure also tests level of consciousness by noting the person's ability to follow commands.)

Ask the person to lift the eyebrows, frown, bare teeth. Note symmetric facial movements and bilateral nasolabial folds (cranial nerve VII).

You can check upper arm strength by checking hand grasps. Ask the person to squeeze your fingers. Offer your two fingers, one on top of the other, so that a strong hand grasp does not hurt your knuckles (Fig. 23–53). Be judicious about asking the person to squeeze your hands; some persons with diffuse brain damage, especially frontal lobe injury, have a grasp that is a reflex only.

23–53

NORMAL RANGE OF FINDINGS	ABNORMAL FINDINGS

Alternatively, ask the person to lift each hand or to hold up one finger. You also can check upper extremity strength by palmar drift. Ask the person to extend both arms forward or halfway up, palms up, eyes closed, and hold for 10 to 20 seconds (Fig. 23–54). Normally, the arms stay steady with no downward drift.

23–54

Check lower extremities by asking the person to do straight leg raises. Ask the person to lift one leg at a time straight up off the bed (Fig. 23–55). Full strength allows the leg to be lifted 90 degrees. If multiple trauma, pain, or equipment preclude this motion, ask the person to push one foot at a time against your hand's resistance, "like putting your foot on the gas pedal of your car" (Fig. 23–56).

For the person with decreased level of consciousness, note if movement occurs spontaneously and as a result of noxious stimuli such as pain or suctioning. An attempt to push away your hand after such stimuli is called *localizing* and is characterized as purposeful movement.

Any abnormal posturing, decorticate rigidity, or decerebrate rigidity indicates diffuse brain injury (see Table 23–10).

23–55

23–56

PUPILLARY RESPONSE. Note the size, shape, and symmetry of both pupils. Shine a light into each pupil and note the direct and consensual light reflex. Both pupils should constrict briskly. (Allow for the effects of any medication that could affect pupil size and reactivity.) When recording, pupil size is best expressed in millimeters. Tape a millimeter scale onto a tongue blade and hold it next to the person's eyes for the most accurate measurement (Fig. 23–57).

In a brain-injured person, a sudden, unilateral, dilated and nonreactive pupil is ominous. Cranial nerve III runs parallel to the brain stem. When increasing intracranial pressure pushes the brain stem down (uncal herniation), it puts pressure on cranial nerve III, causing pupil dilatation.

| NORMAL RANGE OF FINDINGS | ABNORMAL FINDINGS |

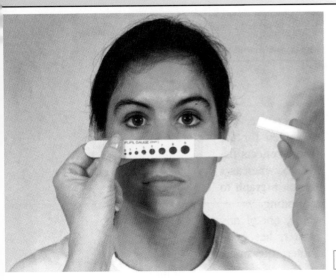

23–57

VITAL SIGNS. Measure the temperature, pulse, respiration, and blood pressure as often as the person's condition warrants. Although they are vital to the overall assessment of the critically ill person, pulse and blood pressure are notoriously unreliable parameters of CNS deficit. Any changes are late consequences of rising intracranial pressure.

THE GLASGOW COMA SCALE (GCS). Since the terms describing levels of consciousness are ambiguous, the Glasgow Coma Scale was developed as an accurate and reliable *quantitative* tool (Fig. 23–58). The GCS is a standardized, objective assessment that defines the level of consciousness by giving it a numeric value.

The **Cushing reflex** shows signs of increasing intracranial pressure: blood pressure—sudden elevation with widening pulse pressure; pulse—decreased rate, slow and bounding.

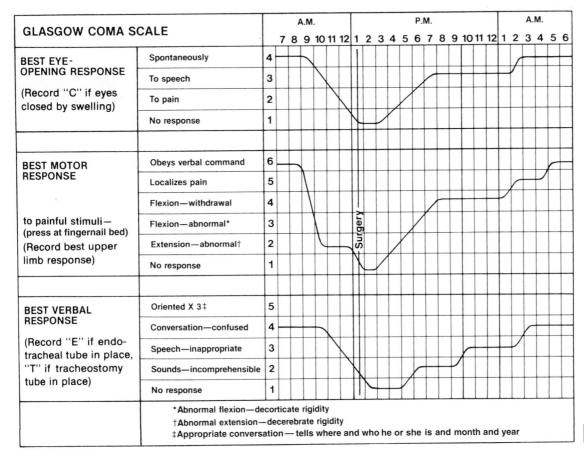

GLASGOW COMA SCALE		A.M. 7 8 9 10 11 12	P.M. 1 2 3 4 5 6 7 8 9 10 11 12	A.M. 1 2 3 4 5 6
BEST EYE-OPENING RESPONSE (Record "C" if eyes closed by swelling)	Spontaneously — 4			
	To speech — 3			
	To pain — 2			
	No response — 1			
BEST MOTOR RESPONSE to painful stimuli— (press at fingernail bed) (Record best upper limb response)	Obeys verbal command — 6			
	Localizes pain — 5			
	Flexion—withdrawal — 4			
	Flexion—abnormal* — 3			
	Extension—abnormal† — 2			
	No response — 1			
BEST VERBAL RESPONSE (Record "E" if endotracheal tube in place, "T" if tracheostomy tube in place)	Oriented X 3‡ — 5			
	Conversation—confused — 4			
	Speech—inappropriate — 3			
	Sounds—incomprehensible — 2			
	No response — 1			

*Abnormal flexion—decorticate rigidity
†Abnormal extension—decerebrate rigidity
‡Appropriate conversation — tells where and who he or she is and month and year

23–58

NORMAL RANGE OF FINDINGS   **ABNORMAL FINDINGS**

The scale is divided into three areas: eye opening, verbal response, and motor response. Each area is rated separately, and a number is given for the person's best response. The three numbers are added; the total score reflects the brain's functional level. A fully alert, normal person has a score of 15, whereas a score of 7 or less reflects coma. Serial assessments can be plotted on a graph to illustrate visually whether the person is stable, improving, or deteriorating.

The GCS assesses the functional state of the brain as a whole, not of any particular site in the brain. The scale is easy to learn and master, has good interrater reliability (Juarez and Lyons, 1995), and enhances interprofessional communication by providing a common language.

SUMMARY CHECKLIST: Neurologic Exam

Neurologic Screening Examination
1. **Mental status**
2. **Cranial nerves**
   II: Optic I
   III, IV, VI: Extraocular muscles
   V: Trigeminal
   VII: Facial mobility
3. **Motor function**
   Gait and balance
   Knee flexion—hop or shallow knee bend
4. **Sensory function**
   Superficial pain and light touch— arms and legs
   Vibration—arms and legs

5. **Reflexes**
   Biceps
   Triceps
   Patellar
   Achilles

Neurologic Complete Examination
1. **Mental status**
2. **Cranial nerves II through XII**
3. **Motor system**
   Muscle size, strength, tone
   Gait and balance
   Rapid alternating movements

4. **Sensory function**
   Superficial pain and light touch
   Vibration
   Position sense
   Stereognosis, graphesthesia, two-point discrimination
5. **Reflexes**
   DTRs: biceps, triceps, brachioradialis, patellar, Achilles
   Superficial: abdominal, plantar

Application and Critical Thinking

SAMPLE CHARTING

SUBJECTIVE

No unusually frequent or severe headaches, no head injury, dizziness or vertigo, seizures or tremors. No weakness, numbness or tingling, difficulty swallowing or speaking. Has no past history of stroke, spinal cord injury, meningitis, or alcoholism.

OBJECTIVE

Mental status: appearance, behavior, and speech appropriate; alert and oriented to person, place, and time; recent and remote memory intact.

Cranial nerves:

I: Identifies coffee and peppermint.

II: Vision 20/20 OS, 20/20 OD, peripheral fields intact by confrontation, fundi normal.

III, IV, VI: EOMs intact, no ptosis or nystagmus; pupils equal, round, react to light and accommodation (PERRLA).

V: Sensation intact and equal bilaterally, jaw strength equal bilaterally.

VII: Facial muscles intact and symmetric.

VIII: Hearing—whispered words heard bilaterally, Weber test—tone is heard midline without lateralization.

IX, X: Swallowing intact, gag reflex present, uvula rises in midline on phonation.

XI: Shoulder shrug, head movement intact and equal bilaterally.

XII: Tongue protrudes midline, no tremors.

Motor: no atrophy, weakness, or tremors. Gait smooth and coordinated, able to tandem walk, negative Romberg. Rapid alternating movements (RAM)—finger-to-nose smoothly intact.

Sensory: pinprick, light touch, vibration intact. Stereognosis—able to identify key.

Reflexes: normal abdominal, no Babinski's sign, DTRs 2+ and = bilaterally with downgoing toes, see drawing below:

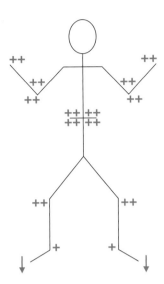

FOCUSED ASSESSMENT: CLINICAL CASE STUDY

J.T. is a 61-year-old white male carpenter with a large building firm who is admitted to the Rehabilitation Institute with a diagnosis of right hemiplegia and aphasia following a brain attack (CVA) 4 weeks PTA.

SUBJECTIVE

Because of J.T.'s speech dysfunction, history provided by wife.

4 weeks PTA—complaint of severe headache, then sudden onset of collapse and loss of consciousness while at work. Did not strike head as fell. Transported by ambulance to Memorial Hospital where admitting physician said J.T. "probably had a stroke." Right arm and leg were limp, and he remained unconscious. Admitted to critical care unit. Regained consciousness day 3 after admission, unable to move right side, unable to speak clearly or write. Remained in ICU 4 more days until "doctors were sure heart and breathing were steady."

3 weeks PTA—transferred to medical floor where care included physical therapy twice per day, and passive ROM 4 ×/day.

Now—some improvement in right motor function. Bowel control achieved with use of commode same time each day (after breakfast). Bladder control improved with some occasional incontinence, usually when cannot tell people he needs to urinate.

OBJECTIVE

Mental status: dressed in jogging suit, sitting in wheelchair, appears alert with appropriate eye contact, listening intently to history. Speech is slow, requires great effort, able to give one-word answers that are appropriate but lack normal tone. Seems to understand all language spoken to him. Follows requests appropriately, within limits of motor weakness.

Cranial nerves:

II: Acuity normal, fields by confrontation—right homonymous hemianopsia, fundi normal.

III, IV, VI: EOMs intact, no ptosis or nystagmus, PERRLA.

V: Sensation intact to pinprick and light touch. Jaw strength weak on right.

VII: Flat nasolabial fold on right, motor weakness on right lower face. Able to wrinkle forehead bilaterally, but unable to smile or bare teeth on right.

VIII: Hearing intact.

IX, X: Swallowing intact, gag reflex present, uvula rises midline on phonation.

XI: Shoulder shrug, head movement weaker on right.

XII: Tongue protrudes midline, no tremors.

Continued

Sensory: Pinprick and light touch present but diminished on right arm and leg. Vibration intact. Position sense impaired on right side. Stereognosis intact.

Motor: Right hand grip weak, right arm drifts, right leg weak, unable to support weight. Spasticity in right arm and leg muscles, limited range of motion on passive motion. Unable to stand up and walk unassisted. Unable to perform finger-to-nose or heel-to-shin on right side, left side smoothly intact.

Reflexes: Hyperactive 4+ with clonus, and upgoing toes in right leg. Abdominal and cremasteric reflexes absent on right.

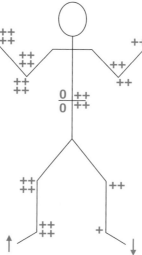

ASSESSMENT

Impaired verbal communication R/T effects of CVA
Impaired physical mobility R/T neuromuscular impairment
Disturbed body image R/T effects of loss of body function
Self-care deficits: feeding, bathing, toileting, dressing/grooming R/T muscular weakness
Disturbed sensory perception (absent right visual fields) R/T neurologic impairment
Risk for injury R/T visual field deficit

NURSING DIAGNOSES COMMONLY ASSOCIATED WITH NEUROLOGIC DISORDERS

RELATED FACTORS (Etiology)	DEFINING CHARACTERISTICS (Symptoms and Signs)
DIAGNOSIS: Disturbed Sensory perception: kinesthetic	
Effects of inner ear inflammation	Falling
Neurologic impairment	Vertigo
Side effects of tranquilizers, sedatives, muscle relaxants, or antihistamines	Stumbling
	Nausea
Sleep deprivation	Motion sickness
	Motor incoordination
	Alteration in posture
	Inability to sit or stand
DIAGNOSIS: Impaired verbal Communication	
Altered thought processes	Difficulty with phonation
Auditory impairment	Disorientation
Decreased circulation to the brain	Dyspnea
Effects of surgery or trauma	Flight of ideas
Physical barriers of	Impaired articulation
Intubation	Inability to
Tracheostomy	Find words
Inability to read or write	Identify objects
Language barrier	Modulate speech
Psychological barriers	Name words
Anxiety	Incessant verbalization
Fear	Lack of desire to speak
Inflammation	Loose association of ideas

RELATED FACTORS (Etiology)	DEFINING CHARACTERISTICS (Symptoms and Signs)

DIAGNOSIS: Impaired verbal Communication—cont'd

Mental retardation	Stuttering or slurring
Oral deformities	
Respiratory embarrassment	
Speech pattern dysfunction	

DIAGNOSIS: Reflex Incontinence

Neurologic impairment
    Cerebral loss
    Interruption of spinal nerve impulse above the level of S3
	Lack of awareness of
	    Being incontinent
	    Bladder filling
	Lack of urge to void or feelings of fullness
	Somewhat unpredictable voiding pattern
	Uninhibited bladder contractions and spasms at regular intervals
	Voiding in large amounts

DIAGNOSIS: Unilateral Neglect

Effects of disturbed perceptual abilities, e.g., hemianopsia, one-sided blindness Effects of neurologic illness or trauma	Does not look toward affected side Consistent inattention to stimuli on affected side Leaves food on plate on the affected side Inadequate self-care, positioning, and/or safety precautions in regard to affected side

OTHER RELATED NURSING DIAGNOSES

ACTUAL

Activity intolerance (see Chapter 18)
Anxiety
Disturbed Body image
Deficient Diversional activity
Dysreflexia
Fear
Hopelessness
Impaired Home maintenance
Total Incontinence
Impaired bed Mobility
Impaired physical Mobility (see Chapter 22)
Disturbed Sensory perception: tactile, visual
Sexual dysfunction
Social isolation
Disturbed Thought processes
Impaired Urinary elimination
Impaired Walking

RISK/WELLNESS

Risk
Risk for Aspiration
Risk for Autonomic dysreflexia
Risk for Caregiver role strain
Risk for Constipation
Risk for impaired Skin integrity (see Chapter 12)
Risk for Trauma (see Chapter 22)
Wellness
Improving Activity tolerance
Maintaining effective Communication

 ASSESSMENT VIDEO CRITICAL THINKING QUESTIONS

The Saunders *Physical Examination and Health Assessment* video "Neurologic System" will direct you to consider the following:

1. Which cranial nerve and sensory system assessments would you include in a neurologic screening examination?
2. Describe abnormal assessment findings that occur with lower motor neuron dysfunction of cranial nerve VII.
3. How would you modify your techniques when assessing an older adult's sensory system?

4. Which nursing diagnoses are appropriate for individuals with cranial nerve or sensory deficits?
5. Which motor system and reflex assessments would you include in a neurologic screening examination?
6. What abnormal findings may commonly be detected when assessing a child's gait?
7. What findings would you expect to see when assessing gait and balance in an older adult?
8. What techniques can you use to elicit deep tendon reflexes?

Abnormal Findings

TABLE 23–3: Abnormalities in Cranial Nerves

NERVE	TEST	ABNORMAL FINDINGS	POSSIBLE CAUSES
I: Olfactory	Identify familiar odors	Anosmia	Upper respiratory infection (temporary); tobacco or cocaine use; fracture of cribriform plate or ethmoid area; frontal lobe lesion; tumor in olfactory bulb or tract
II: Optic	Visual acuity	Defect or absent central vision	Congenital blindness, refractive error, acquired vision loss from numerous diseases (e.g., cerebrovascular accident, diabetes), trauma to globe or orbit (see discussion of cranial nerve III)
	Visual fields	Defect in peripheral vision, hemianopsia	
	Shine light in eye	Absent light reflex	
	Direct inspection	Papilledema	Increased intracranial pressure
		Optic atrophy	Glaucoma
		Retinal lesions	Diabetes
III: Oculomotor	Inspection	Dilated pupil, ptosis, eye turns out and slightly down	Paralysis in cranial nerve III from internal carotid aneurysm, tumor, inflammatory lesions, uncal herniation with increased intracranial pressure
	Extraocular muscle movement	Failure to move eye up, in, down	Ptosis from myasthenia gravis, oculomotor nerve palsy, Horner's syndrome
	Shine light in eye	Absent light reflex	Blindness, drug influence, increased intracranial pressure, CNS injury, circulatory arrest, CNS syphilis
IV: Trochlear	Extraocular muscle movement	Failure to turn eye down or out	Fracture of orbit, brain stem tumor
V: Trigeminal	Superficial touch—three divisions	Absent touch and pain, paresthesias	Trauma, tumor, pressure from aneurysm, inflammation, sequelae of alcohol injection for trigeminal neuralgia
	Corneal reflex	No blink	
	Clench teeth	Weakness of masseter or temporalis muscles	Unilateral weakness with cranial nerve V lesion; bilateral weakness with upper or lower motor neuron disorder
VI: Abducens	Extraocular muscle movement to right and left sides	Failure to move laterally, diplopia on lateral gaze	Brain stem tumor or trauma, fracture of orbit
VII: Facial	Wrinkle forehead, close eyes tightly	Absent or asymmetric facial movement	Bell's palsy (lower motor neuron lesion) causes paralysis of entire half of face
	Smile, puff cheeks	Loss of taste	Upper motor neuron lesions (cerebrovascular accident, tumor, inflammatory) cause paralysis of lower half of face, leaving forehead intact
	Identify tastes		Other lower motor neuron causes of paralysis: swelling from ear or meningeal infections

Continued

TABLE 23-3: Abnormalities in Cranial Nerves—cont'd

NERVE	TEST	ABNORMAL FINDINGS	POSSIBLE CAUSES
VIII: Acoustic	Hearing acuity	Decrease or loss of hearing	Inflammation, occluded ear canal, otosclerosis, presbycusis, drug toxicity, tumor
IX: Glossopharyngeal	Gag reflex	See cranial nerve X	
X: Vagus	Phonates "ahh"	Uvula deviates to side	Brain stem tumor, neck injury, cranial nerve X lesion
	Gag reflex	No gag reflex	Vocal cord weakness
	Note voice quality	Hoarse or brassy	Soft palate weakness
		Nasal twang	Unilateral cranial nerve X lesion
		Husky	
	Note swallowing	Dysphagia, fluids regurgitate through nose	Bilateral cranial nerve X lesion
XI: Spinal accessory	Turn head, shrug shoulders against resistance	Absent movement of sternomastoid or trapezius muscles	Neck injury, torticollis
XII: Hypoglossal	Protrude tongue	Deviates to side	Lower motor neuron lesion
	Wiggle tongue from side to side	Slowed rate of movement	Bilateral upper motor neuron lesion

TABLE 23-4: Abnormalities in Muscle Tone

CONDITION	DESCRIPTION	ASSOCIATED WITH
Flaccidity	Decreased muscle tone or hypotonia; muscle feels limp, soft, and flabby; muscle is weak and easily fatigued	Lower motor neuron injury (peripheral neuritis, poliomyelitis, Guillain-Barré syndrome). Early cerebrovascular accident and spinal cord injury are flaccid at first.
Spasticity	Increased tone; increased resistance to passive lengthening; then may suddenly give way (clasp-knife phenomenon)	Injury to corticospinal motor tract, e.g., paralysis with cerebrovascular accident (chronic stage)
Rigidity	Constant state of resistance; resists passive movement in any direction; dystonia	Injury to extrapyramidal motor tracts, e.g., parkinsonism
Cogwheel rigidity	Type of rigidity in which the increased tone is released by degrees during passive range of motion so it feels like small regular jerks	Parkinsonism

TABLE 23–5: Abnormalities in Muscle Movement

Paralysis

Decreased or loss of motor power due to problem with motor nerve or muscle fibers. Causes: acute—trauma, spinal cord injury, brain attack, poliomyelitis, polyneuritis, Bell's palsy; chronic—muscular dystrophy, diabetic neuropathy, multiple sclerosis; episodic—myasthenia gravis.

Patterns of paralysis: *hemiplegia*—spastic or flaccid paralysis of one side (right or left) of body and extremities; *paraplegia*—symmetric paralysis of both lower extremities; *quadriplegia*—paralysis in all four extremities; *paresis*—weakness of muscles rather than paralysis.

Fasciculation

Rapid, continuous twitching of resting muscle or part of muscle, without movement of limb, that can be seen or palpated. Types: fine—occurs with lower motor neuron disease, associated with atrophy and weakness; coarse—occurs with cold exposure or fatigue and is not significant.

Tic

Repetitive twitching of a muscle group at inappropriate times, e.g., wink, grimace, head movement, shoulder shrug; due to a neurologic cause, e.g., tardive dyskinesias; emotional cause; or may be under voluntary control.

Myoclonus

Rapid, sudden jerk or a short series of jerks at fairly regular intervals. A hiccup is a myoclonus of diaphragm. Single myoclonic arm or leg jerk is normal when the person is falling asleep; myoclonic jerks are severe with grand mal seizures.

Continued

TABLE 23–5: Abnormalities in Muscle Movement—cont'd

Tremor

Involuntary contraction of opposing muscle groups. Results in rhythmic, back-and-forth movement of one or more joints. May occur at rest or with voluntary movement. All tremors disappear while sleeping. Tremors may be slow (3 to 6 per second) or rapid (10 to 20 per second).

Rest Tremor

Coarse and slow (3 to 6 per second); partly or completely disappears with voluntary movement, e.g., "pill rolling" tremor of parkinsonism, with thumb and opposing fingers.

Intention Tremor

Rate varies; worse with voluntary movement. Occurs with cerebellar disease and multiple sclerosis.

Essential tremor (familial)—a type of intention tremor; most common tremor with older people. Benign (no associated disease) but causes emotional stress in business or social situations. Improves with the administration of sedatives, propranolol, alcohol, but use of alcohol is discouraged because of the risk of addiction.

Chorea

Sudden, rapid, jerky, purposeless movement involving limbs, trunk, or face.

Occurs at irregular intervals, not rhythmic or repetitive, more convulsive than a tic. Some are spontaneous, and some are initiated; all are accentuated by voluntary acts. Disappears with sleep. Common with Sydenham's and Huntington's disease.

Athetosis

Slow, twisting, writhing, continuous movement, resembling a snake or worm. Involves distal part of limb more than the proximal part. Occurs with cerebral palsy. Disappears with sleep. "Athetoid" hand—some fingers are flexed and some are extended.

TABLE 23–6: Abnormal Gaits

TYPE	CHARACTERISTIC APPEARANCE	POSSIBLE CAUSES
Spastic hemiparesis	Arm is immobile against the body, with flexion of the shoulder, elbow, wrist, fingers, and adduction of shoulder. The leg is stiff and extended and circumducts with each step (drags toe in a semicircle)	Upper motor neuron lesion of the corticospinal tract, e.g., cerebrovascular accident, trauma
Cerebellar ataxia	Staggering, wide-based gait; difficulty with turns; uncoordinated movement with positive Romberg sign	Alcohol or barbiturate effect on cerebellum; cerebellar tumor; multiple sclerosis
Parkinsonian (festinating)	Posture is stooped; trunk is pitched forward; elbows, hips, and knees are flexed. Steps are short and shuffling. Hesitation to begin walking, and difficult to stop suddenly. The person holds the body rigid. Walks and turns body as one fixed unit. Difficulty with any change in direction.	Parkinsonism
Scissors	Knees cross or are in contact, like holding an orange between the thighs. The person uses short steps, and walking requires effort	Paraparesis of legs, multiple sclerosis
Steppage or footdrop	Slapping quality—looks as if walking up stairs and finds no stair there. Lifts knee and foot high and slaps it down hard and flat to compensate for footdrop	Weakness of peroneal and anterior tibial muscles; due to lower motor neuron lesion at the spinal cord, e.g., poliomyelitis, Charcot-Marie-Tooth disease (an inherited peripheral neuropathy)

Continued

TABLE 23–6: Abnormal Gaits—cont'd

TYPE	CHARACTERISTIC APPEARANCE	POSSIBLE CAUSES
Waddling	Weak hip muscles—when the person takes a step, the opposite hip drops, which allows compensatory lateral movement of pelvis. Often, the person also has marked lumbar lordosis and a protruding abdomen	Hip girdle muscle weakness due to muscular dystrophy, dislocation of hips
Short leg	Leg length discrepancy >2.5 cm (1 in). Vertical telescoping of affected side, which dips as the person walks. Appearance of gait varies depending on amount of accompanying muscle dysfunction	Congenital dislocated hip; acquired shortening due to disease, trauma

TABLE 23–7: Characteristics of Upper and Lower Motor Neuron Lesions

	UPPER MOTOR NEURON LESION	LOWER MOTOR NEURON LESION
Weakness/ paralysis	In muscles corresponding to distribution of damage in pyramidal tract lesion; usually in hand grip, arm extensors, leg flexors	In specific muscles served by damaged spinal segment, ventral root, or peripheral nerve
Location	Descending motor pathways that originate in the motor areas of cerebral cortex and carry impulses to the anterior horn cells of the spinal cord	Nerve cells that originate in the anterior horn of spinal cord or in brain stem, and carry impulses by the spinal nerves or cranial nerves to the muscles, the "final common pathway"
Example	Brain attack or cerebrovascular accident	Poliomyelitis, herniated intervertebral disk
Muscle tone	Increased tone; spasticity	Loss of tone, flaccidity
Bulk	May have some atrophy from disuse; otherwise normal	Atrophy (wasting), may be marked
Abnormal movements	None	Fasciculations
Reflexes	Hyperreflexia, ankle clonus; diminished or absent superficial abdominal reflexes; positive Babinski's sign	Hyporeflexia or areflexia; no Babinski's sign, no pathologic reflexes
Possible nursing diagnoses	Risk for contractures; impaired physical mobility	Impaired physical mobility

TABLE 23–8: Common Patterns of Motor System Dysfunction

A—Cerebral palsy. Mixed group of paralytic neuromotor disorders of infancy and childhood; due to damage to cerebral cortex caused by a developmental defect, intrauterine meningitis or encephalitis, birth trauma, anoxia, or kernicterus.

B—Muscular dystrophy. Chronic, progressive wasting of skeletal musculature, which produces weakness, contractures, and in severe cases, respiratory dysfunction and death. Onset of symptoms occurs in childhood. Many types exist; the most severe is Duchenne's dystrophy, characterized by the waddling gait described in Table 23–6.

C—Hemiplegia. Damage to corticospinal tract. Initially flaccid when the lesion is acute; later, the muscles become spastic, and abnormal reflexes appear. Characteristic posture: arm—shoulder adducted, elbow flexed, wrist pronated, leg extended; face—weakness only in lower muscles. Hyperreflexia and possible clonus occur on the involved side; loss of corneal, abdominal, and cremasteric reflexes; positive Babinski's and Hoffman's reflexes.

D—Parkinsonism. Defect of extrapyramidal tracts, in the region of the basal ganglia, with loss of the neurotransmitter dopamine. Classic triad of symptoms: tremor, rigidity, akinesia. Also slower monotonous speech and diminutive writing. Body tends to stay immobile; facial expression is flat, staring, expressionless; excessive salivation occurs; reduced eye blinking. Posture is stooped; equilibrium is impaired; loses balance easily; gait is described in Table 23–6. Parkinsonian tremor; cogwheel rigidity on passive range of motion.

E—Cerebellar. A lesion in one hemisphere produces motor abnormalities on the ipsilateral side. Characterized by ataxia, lurching forward of affected side while walking, rapid alternating movements are slow and arrhythmic, finger-to-nose test reveals ataxia and tremor with overshoot or undershoot, and eyes display coarse nystagmus.

F—Paraplegia. Caused by spinal cord injury. A severe injury or complete transection initially produces "spinal shock," which is defined as no movement or reflex activity below the level of the lesion. Gradually, deep tendon reflexes reappear and become increased, flexor spasms of legs occur; and finally, extensor spasms of legs occur; these spasms lead to prevailing extensor tone.

TABLE 23–9: Common Patterns of Sensory Loss

TYPE	CHARACTERISTICS	POSSIBLE CAUSES
Peripheral neuropathy	Loss of sensation involves all modalities. Loss is most severe distally (feet and hands); response improves as stimulus is moved proximally (glove-and-stocking anesthesia). Anesthesia zone gradually merges into a hypoesthesia zone, then gradually becomes normal.	Metabolic disease, nutritional deficiency
Individual nerves or roots	Decrease or loss of all sensory modalities. Area of sensory loss corresponds to distribution of the involved nerve.	Trauma, vascular occlusion
Spinal cord hemisection (Brown-Séquard syndrome)	Loss of pain and temperature, contralateral side, starting one to two segments below the level of the lesion. Loss of vibration and position discrimination on the ipsilateral side, below the level of the lesion.	Meningioma, neurofibroma, cervical spondylosis, multiple sclerosis

Table continued on following page

TABLE 23–9: Common Patterns of Sensory Loss—cont'd

TYPE	CHARACTERISTICS	POSSIBLE CAUSES
Complete transection of the spinal cord 	Complete loss of *all* sensory modalities below the level of the lesion. Condition is associated with motor paralysis and loss of sphincter control.	Trauma, demyelinating disorders, tumor
Thalamus 	Loss of *all* sensory modalities on the face, arm, and leg on the side contralateral to the lesion.	Vascular occlusion
Cortex 	Since pain, vibration, and crude touch are mediated by thalamus, little loss of these sensory functions occurs with a cortex lesion. Loss of discrimination occurs on the contralateral side. Loss of graphesthesia, stereognosis, recognition of shapes and weights, finger finding.	Cerebral cortex, parietal lobe lesion

TABLE 23–10: Abnormal Postures

Decorticate Rigidity

Upper extremities—flexion of arm, wrist, and fingers; adduction of arm. Lower extremities—extension, internal rotation, plantar flexion. This indicates hemispheric lesion of cerebral cortex.

Decerebrate Rigidity

Upper extremities stiffly extended, adducted, internal rotation, palms pronated. Lower extremities stiffly extended, plantar flexion; teeth clenched; hyperextended back. More ominous than decorticate rigidity; indicates lesion in brain stem at midbrain or upper pons.

Flaccid Quadriplegia

Complete loss of muscle tone and paralysis of all four extremities, indicating completely nonfunctional brain stem.

Opisthotonos

Prolonged arching of the back, with head and heels bent backward. This indicates meningeal irritation.

TABLE 23–11: Pathologic Reflexes

Reflex	Method of Testing	Abnormal Response (Reflex Is Present)	Indications
Babinski	Stroke lateral aspect and across ball of foot	Extension of great toe, fanning of toes	Corticospinal (pyramidal) tract disease
Oppenheim	Stroke anterior medial tibial muscle	Same as above	Same
Gordon	Firmly squeeze calf muscles	Same as above	Same
Hoffman	Flick distal phalanx of middle or index finger	Clawing of fingers and thumb	Same
Kernig	Raise leg straight or flex thigh on abdomen, then extend knee	Resistance to straightening, pain down posterior thigh	Meningeal irritation
Brudzinski	Flex chin on chest, watch hips and knees	Resistance and pain in neck, with flexion of hips and knees	Meningeal irritation

TABLE 23–12: Frontal Release Signs

REFLEX

Snout

Method of Testing
Gently percuss oral region
Abnormal Response (Reflex Is Present)
Puckers lips
Indications
Frontal lobe disease, cerebral degenerative disease (Alzheimer's)

Sucking

Method of Testing
Touch oral region
Abnormal Response (Reflex Is Present)
Sucking movement of lips, tongue, jaw
Indications
Same as for snout reflex

Grasp

Method of Testing
Touch palm with your finger
Abnormal Response (Reflex Is Present)
Uncontrolled, forced grasping (grasp is usually last of these signs to appear, so its presence indicates severe disease)
Indications
Same as for snout reflex

BIBLIOGRAPHY

Beckerman BA: Nervous energy: conducting a neurologic assessment in the field, *Emerg Med Serv* 29(8):45–50, Aug 2000.

Bernstein S, Heimler R, Sasidharan P: Approaching the management of the neonatal intensive care unit graduate through history and physical assessment, *Pediatr Clin North Am* 45(1):79–105, Feb 1998.

Chasens ER, Umlauf MG: Post-polio syndrome, *Am J Nurs* 100(12):60–66, Dec 2000.

Fenichel GM: *Clinical pediatric neurology,* ed 4, Philadelphia, 2001, W.B. Saunders.

Fischer J, Mathieson C: The history of the Glasgow Coma Scale: implications for practice, *Crit Care Nurs Q* 23(4):52–58, Feb 2001.

Gawande A: The pain perplex, *The New Yorker* 74:86–94, Sep 21, 1998.

Goldsmith C: Parkinson's disease, *Am J Nurs* 99(2):46–47, Feb 1999.

Halper J, Holland N: Meeting the challenge of multiple sclerosis. Part I, *Am J Nurs* 98(10):26–31, Oct 1998.

Halper J, Holland N: Meeting the challenge of multiple sclerosis. Part II, *Am J Nurs* 98(11):39–45, Nov 1998.

Harrahill M: Glasgow Coma Scale: a quick review, *J Emerg Nurs* 22(1):81–83, Feb 1996.

Herf C, Nichols J, Fruh S: Meningococcal disease: recognition, treatment, and prevention, *Nurs Pract* 23(8):30–46, Aug 1998.

Hilton G: Acute head injury, *Am J Nurs* 101(9):51–52, Sep 2001.

Hobdell E: Infant neurologic assessment, *J Neurosci Nurs* 33(4):190–193, Aug 2001.

Jaweed MM, Monga TN: Neuromuscular function assessment, *Phys Med Rehabil* 11(1):205–237, Feb 1997.

Juarez VJ, Lyons M: Interrater reliability of the Glasgow Coma Scale, *J Neurosci Nurs* 27(5):283–286, Oct 1995.

Kuhlman KA, Hennessey WJ: Sensitivity and specificity of carpal tunnel syndrome signs, *Am J Phys Med Rehabil* 76(6):451–457, Nov–Dec 1997.

Lower J: Facing neuro assessment fearlessly, *Nursing* 32(2):58–65, Feb 2002.

Maher L: A quick neurologic examination, *Patient Care* 34(3):161–172, Feb 15, 2000.

O'Hanlon-Nichols T: Neurologic assessment, *Am J Nurs* 99(6):44–50, June 1999.

Orfanelli L: Neurologic examination of the toddler: how to assess for increased intracranial pressure following head trauma, *Am J Nurs* 101(12):24CC–FF, Dec 2001.

Petit J, Barkhaus PE: Evaluation and management of polyneuropathy: a practical approach, *Nurse Pract* 22(5):131–148, May 1997.

Pressman EK, Zeidman SM, Summers L: Comprehensive assessment of the neurologic system, *J Nurse Midwifery* 40(2):163–171, Mar–Apr 1995.

Richards KC, Hall KS, Shook D et al: Sleep-disordered breathing and stroke, *J Cardiovasc Nurs* 17(1):12–29, Oct 2002.

Riggio S, Jagoda A: The rapid neurologic examination, part 1: history, mental status, cranial nerves, *J Crit Illn* 14(6):325–331, Jun 1999.

Riggio S, Jagoda A: The rapid neurologic examination, part 2: movement, reflexes, sensation, balance, *J Crit Illn* 14(7):368–372, Jul 1999.

Schretzman D: Acute ischemic stroke, *Nurse Pract* 24(2):71–88, Feb 1999.

Tapper VJ: Pathophysiology, assessment, and treatment of Parkinson's disease, *Nurse Pract* 22(7):76–95, July 1997.

Umeh L, Wallhagen M, Nicologg N: Identifying diabetic patients at high risk for amputation, *Nurse Pract* 24(8):56–70, Aug 1999.

Waxman SG: *Correlative neuroanatomy,* ed 24, Stamford, CT, 1999, Appleton & Lange.

Male Genitalia

✿ Structure and Function

THE MALE GENITALIA

The male genital structures include the penis and scrotum externally and the testis, epididymis, and vas deferens internally. Glandular structures accessory to the genital organs (the prostate, seminal vesicles, and bulbourethral glands) are discussed in Chapter 25.

PENIS

The **penis** is composed of three cylindrical columns of erectile tissue: the two corpora cavernosa on the dorsal side and the corpus spongiosum ventrally (Fig. 24–1). At the distal end of the shaft, the corpus spongiosum expands into a cone of erectile tissue, the **glans.** The shoulder where the glans joins the shaft is the **corona.** The **urethra** transverses the corpus spongiosum, and its meatus forms a slit at the glans tip. Over the glans, the skin folds in and back on itself forming a hood or flap. This is the **foreskin** or **prepuce.** Often, it is surgically removed shortly after birth by circumcision. The **frenulum** is a fold of the foreskin extending from the urethral meatus ventrally.

SCROTUM

The **scrotum** is a loose protective sac, which is a continuation of the abdominal wall (Fig. 24–2). After adolescence, the scrotal skin is deeply pigmented and has large sebaceous follicles. The scrotal wall consists of thin skin lying in folds, or **rugae,** and the underlying cremaster muscle. The **cremaster muscle** controls the size of the scrotum by responding to ambient temperature. This is to keep the testes at 3° C below abdominal temperature, the best temperature for producing sperm. When it is cold, the muscle contracts, raising the sac and bringing the testes closer to the body to absorb heat necessary for sperm viability. As a result, the scrotal skin looks corrugated. When it is warmer, the muscle relaxes, the scrotum lowers, and the skin looks smoother.

Inside, a septum separates the sac into two halves. In each scrotal half is a **testis,** which produces sperm. The testis has a solid oval shape, which is compressed laterally and measures 4 to 5 cm long by 3 cm wide in the adult. The testis is suspended vertically by the spermatic cord. The left testis is lower than the right because the left spermatic cord is longer. Each testis is covered by a double-layered membrane, the tunica vaginalis, which separates it from the scrotal wall. The two layers are lubricated by fluid so that the testis can slide a little within the scrotum; this helps prevent injury.

Sperm are transported along a series of ducts. First, the testis is capped by the **epididymis,** which is a markedly coiled duct system and the main storage site of sperm. It is a comma-shaped structure, curved over the top and the posterior surface of the testis. Occasionally (in 6 to 7 percent of males), the epididymis is anterior to the testis.

The lower part of the epididymis is continuous with a muscular duct, the **vas deferens.** This duct approximates with other vessels (arteries and veins, lymphatics, nerves) to form the **spermatic cord.** The spermatic cord ascends along the posterior border of the testis and runs through the tunnel of

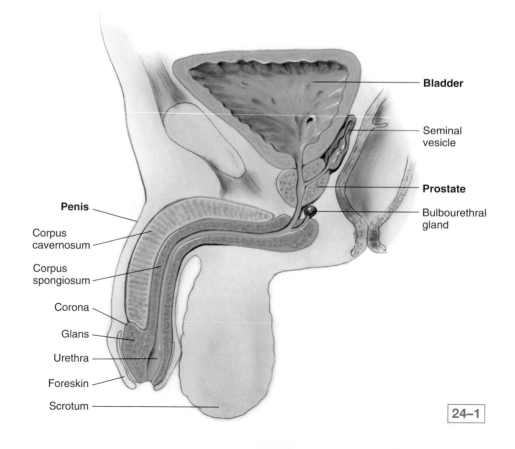

Bladder

Seminal vesicle

Prostate

Bulbourethral gland

Penis

Corpus cavernosum

Corpus spongiosum

Corona

Glans

Urethra

Foreskin

Scrotum

24–1

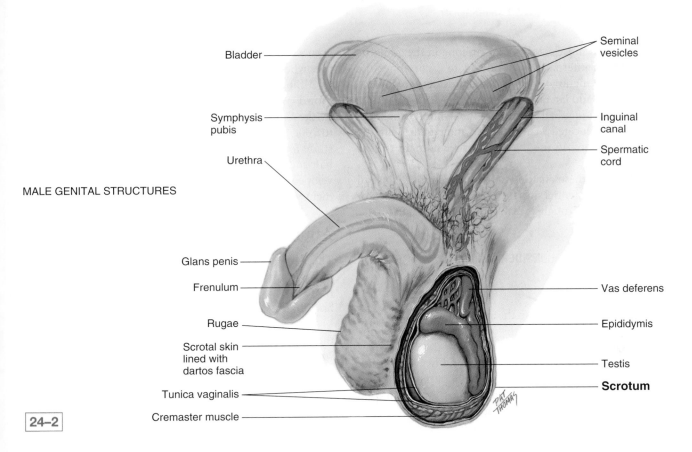

Bladder

Seminal vesicles

Symphysis pubis

Inguinal canal

Urethra

Spermatic cord

MALE GENITAL STRUCTURES

Glans penis

Frenulum

Vas deferens

Rugae

Epididymis

Scrotal skin lined with dartos fascia

Testis

Tunica vaginalis

Scrotum

Cremaster muscle

24–2

the inguinal canal into the abdomen. Here, the vas deferens continues back and down behind the bladder, where it joins the duct of the seminal vesicle to form the **ejaculatory duct.** This duct empties into the urethra.

The **lymphatics** of the penis and scrotal surface drain into the inguinal lymph nodes, whereas those of the testes drain into the abdomen. Abdominal lymph nodes are not accessible to clinical examination.

INGUINAL AREA

The **inguinal area,** or groin, is the juncture of the lower abdominal wall and the thigh (Fig. 24–3). Its diagonal borders are the anterior superior iliac spine and the symphysis pubis. Between these landmarks lies the **inguinal ligament** (Poupart's ligament). Superior to the ligament lies the **inguinal canal,** a narrow tunnel passing obliquely between lay-

Anterior superior iliac spine

Transversus abdominis m.

Inguinal ligament

Internal oblique m.

Inguinal lymph nodes

External oblique m.

Inguinal canal

Internal ring

External ring

Symphysis pubis

Femoral vein

Femoral artery

Femoral canal

STRUCTURES OF THE INGUINAL AREA

Spermatic cord

24–3

ers of abdominal muscle. It is 4 to 6 cm long in the adult. Its openings are an internal ring, located 1 to 2 cm above the midpoint of the inguinal ligament, and an external ring, located just above and lateral to the pubis.

Inferior to the inguinal ligament is the **femoral canal.** It is a potential space located 3 cm medial to and parallel with the femoral artery. You can use the artery as a landmark to find this space.

Knowledge of these anatomic areas in the groin is useful because they are potential sites for a hernia, which is a loop of bowel protruding through a weak spot in the musculature.

 DEVELOPMENTAL CONSIDERATIONS

INFANTS

Prenatally, the testes develop in the abdominal cavity near the kidneys. During the later months of gestation the testes migrate, pushing the abdominal wall in front of them and dragging the vas deferens, the blood vessels, and nerves behind. The testes descend along the inguinal canal into the scrotum before birth. At birth, each testis measures 1.5 to 2 cm long and 1 cm wide. Only a slight increase in size occurs during the prepubertal years.

ADOLESCENTS

Puberty begins sometime between the ages of $9\frac{1}{2}$ and $13\frac{1}{2}$. The first sign is enlargement of the testes. Next, pubic hair appears, then penis size increases. The stages of development are documented in Tanner's sexual maturity ratings (SMR) (Table 24–1).

The complete change in development from a preadolescent to an adult takes around 3 years, although the normal range is 2 to 5 years (Fig. 24–4). The chart shown in Figure 24–4 is useful in teaching a boy the expected sequence of

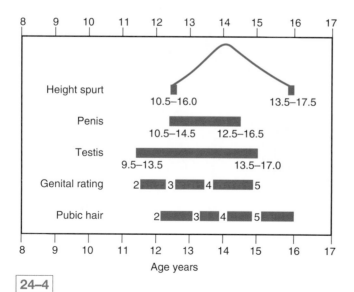

24–4

events and in reassuring him about the wide range of normal ages when these events are experienced.

Although Tanner's studies were based on data from post World War II British youth, Tanner's results are corroborated by the U.S. Health Examination Survey, which studied close to 7000 youth from 1966 to 1970 (Harlan et al., 1979). This study found concordance between Tanner's stages for pubic hair and genitalia. It also found that sexual characteristics developed similarly for black and white boys, and that development was not influenced by socioeconomic status.

ADULTS AND AGING ADULTS

The level of sexual development at the end of puberty remains constant through young and middle adulthood, with no further genital growth and no change in circulating sex hormone.

The male does not experience a definite end to fertility as the female does. Around age 40 years, the production of sperm begins to decrease, although it continues into the 80s and 90s. After age 55 to 60 years, testosterone production declines. This decline proceeds very gradually so that resulting physical changes are not evident until later in life. Aging changes also are due to decreased muscle tone, decreased subcutaneous fat, and decreased cellular metabolism.

In the aging male, the amount of pubic hair decreases, and the remaining hair turns gray. Penis size decreases. Due to decreased tone of the dartos muscle, the scrotal contents hang lower, the rugae decrease, and the scrotum looks pendulous. The testes decrease in size and are less firm to palpation. Increased connective tissue is present in the tubules, so these become thickened and produce less sperm.

In general, declining testosterone production leaves the older male with a slower and less intense sexual response. Although a wide range of individual differences can occur, the older male may find that an erection takes longer to develop and that it is less full or firm. Once obtained, the erection may be maintained for longer periods without ejaculation. Ejaculation is shorter and less forceful, and the volume of seminal fluid is less than when the man was younger. After ejaculation, rapid detumescence (return to the flaccid state) occurs, especially after 60 years of age. This occurs in a few seconds as compared with minutes or hours in the younger male. The refractory state (when the male is physiologically unable to ejaculate) lasts longer, from 12 to 24 hours as compared with 2 minutes in the younger male.

SEXUAL EXPRESSION IN LATER LIFE. Chronologic age by itself should not mean a halt in sexual activity. The above-mentioned physical changes need not interfere with the libido and pleasure from sexual intercourse. The older male is capable of sexual function as long as he is in reasonably good health and has an interested, willing partner. Even chronic illness does not mean a complete end to sexual desire or activity.

The danger is in the male misinterpreting normal age changes as a sexual failure. Once this idea occurs, it may demoralize the man and place undue emphasis on performance

TABLE 24–1: Sex Maturity Ratings (SMR) in Boys

DEVELOPMENTAL STAGE	PUBIC HAIR	PENIS	SCROTUM
1	No pubic hair. Fine body hair on abdomen (vellus hair) continues over pubic area	Preadolescent, size, and proportion the same as during childhood	Preadolescent, size, and proportion the same as during childhood
2	Few straight slightly darker hairs at base of penis. Hair is long and downy	Little or no enlargement	Testes and scrotum begin to enlarge. Scrotal skin reddens and changes in texture
3	Sparse growth over entire pubis. Hair darker, coarser, and curly	Penis begins to enlarge, especially in length	Further enlarged
4	Thick growth over pubic area but not on thighs. Hair coarse and curly as in adult	Penis grows in length and diameter, with development of glans	Testes almost fully grown, scrotum darker
5	Growth spread over medial thighs, although not yet up toward umbilicus*	Adult size and shape	Adult size and shape

*After puberty, pubic hair growth continues until the mid-20s, extending up the abdomen toward the umbilicus.
Adapted from Tanner JM: *Growth at adolescence*, Oxford, England, 1962, Blackwell Scientific Publications.

rather than on pleasure. In the absence of disease, a withdrawal from sexual activity may be due to

- Loss of spouse
- Depression
- Preoccupation with work
- Marital or family conflict
- Side effects of medications such as antihypertensives, psychotropics, antidepressants, antispasmodics, sedatives, tranquilizers or narcotics, and estrogens
- Heavy use of alcohol
- Lack of privacy (living with adult children or in a nursing home)
- Economic or emotional stress
- Poor nutrition
- Fatigue

 TRANSCULTURAL CONSIDERATIONS

CIRCUMCISION. Occasionally, during pregnancy or the immediate neonatal period, parents will ask you about whether or not to circumcise the male infant. Indications for circumcision include cultural reasons, the prevention of phimosis and inflammation of the glans penis and foreskin, decreasing the incidence of cancer of the penis, and slightly decreasing the incidence of urinary tract infections in infancy. However, there is no difference in risk of contracting sexually transmitted diseases (STDs) between circumcised and uncircumcised men (Laumann, Masi, and Zuckerman, 1997). Circumcision carries a very small but possible risk of complications, such as sepsis, amputation of the distal edge of the glans, removal of an excessive amount of foreskin, urethrocutaneous fistula (Behrman, 2000), and significant pain, about which the parents should know.

The decision to circumcise is culturally based. In the United States, 70 to 80 percent of newborn males are circumcised, while in Canada, Great Britain, Australia, and Sweden, circumcision is considered unnecessary, and less than 20 percent of newborn boys are circumcised (Cornell, 1997). Some groups, such as Jews and Muslims, practice circumcision as part of their religious value system. Other groups, such as Native Americans and Hispanics, have no tradition to practice circumcision. However, many parents in the United States who are not part of these groups also believe in circumcision because it conforms to dominant cultural values.

Subjective Data

1. Frequency, urgency, and nocturia	**5.** Past genitourinary history	**8.** Sexual activity and contraceptive use
2. Dysuria	**6.** Penis—pain, lesion, discharge	**9.** STD contact
3. Hesitancy and straining	**7.** Scrotum, self-care behaviors, lump	
4. Urine color		

EXAMINER ASKS	RATIONALE
1. Frequency, urgency, and nocturia. Urinating more often than usual?	**Frequency.** Average adult voids five to six times per day, varying with fluid intake, individual habits. Polyuria—excessive quantity. Oliguria—diminished quantity, <400 ml/24 hours.
 • Feel as if you cannot wait to urinate? • Awaken during the night because you need to urinate? How often? Is this a recent change?	**Urgency.** **Nocturia** occurs together with frequency and urgency in urinary tract disorders. Other origins: cardiovascular, habitual, diuretic medication.
2. Dysuria. Any pain or burning with urinating?	**Dysuria.** Burning is common with acute cystitis, prostatitis, urethritis.
3. Hesitancy and straining. Any trouble starting the urine stream? • Need to strain to start or maintain stream? • Any change in force of stream: narrowing, becoming weaker? • Dribbling, such that you must stand closer to the toilet? • Afterward, do you still feel you need to urinate? • Ever had any urinary tract infections?	**Hesitancy.** Straining. Loss of force and decreased caliber. Terminal dribbling. Sense of residual urine. Recurrent episodes of acute cystitis.

EXAMINER ASKS	RATIONALE
	Above-mentioned symptoms (i.e., hesitancy, and so on) suggest progressive prostatic obstruction.
4. Urine color. Is the usual **urine** clear or discolored, cloudy, foul-smelling, bloody?	As in urinary tract infection. Hematuria—a danger sign that warrants further workup.
5. Past genitourinary history. Any difficulty controlling your urine?	True incontinence—loss of urine without warning. Urgency incontinence—sudden loss, as with acute cystitis.
• Accidentally urinate when you sneeze, laugh, cough, or bear down?	Stress incontinence—loss of urine with physical strain due to weakness of sphincters.
• Any **history** of kidney disease, kidney stones, flank pain, urinary tract infections, prostate trouble?	
6. Penis. Any problem with penis—**pain, lesions?**	
• Any **discharge?** How much? Has that increased or decreased since start?	Urethral discharge occurs with infection.
• The color? Any odor? Discharge associated with pain or with urination?	
7. Scrotum, self-care behaviors. Any problem with the scrotum or testicles?	
• Do you perform testicular self-examination?	**Self-care behaviors.**
• Noticed any **lump** or **swelling** on testes?	
• Noted any change in size of the scrotum?	
• Noted any bulge or swelling in the scrotum? For how long? Ever been told you have a hernia? Any dragging, heavy feeling in scrotum?	Possible hernia.
8. Sexual activity and contraceptive use. Are you in a relationship involving sexual intercourse now?	Questions about **sexual activity** should be routine in review of body systems for these reasons:
• Are aspects of sex satisfactory to you and your partner?	• Communicates that you accept individual's sexual activity and believe it is important
• Are you satisfied with the way you and your partner communicate about sex?	• Your comfort with discussion prompts person's interest and possibly relief that topic has been introduced
• Occasionally a man notices a change in ability to have an erection when aroused. Have you noticed any changes?*	• Establishes a data base for comparisons with any future sexual activities
• Do you and your partner use a contraceptive? Which method? Is this satisfactory? Any questions about this method?	• Provides opportunity to screen sexual problems
• How many sexual partners have you had in the last 6 months?	Your questions should be objective and matter-of-fact.
• What is your sexual preference—relationship with a woman, a man, both?	Gay and bisexual men need to feel acceptance to discuss their health concerns.
9. STD contact. Any sexual contact with a partner having a sexually transmitted disease, such as gonorrhea, herpes, AIDS, chlamydia, venereal warts, syphilis?	
• When was this contact? Did you get the disease?	
• How was it treated? Any complications?	
• Do you use condoms to help prevent STDs?	
• Any questions or concerns about any of these diseases?	

*At times, phrase your questions so that it is all right for the person to acknowledge a problem.

EXAMINER ASKS	RATIONALE

Additional History For Infants and Children

1. Does your child have any problem urinating? Urine stream look straight?
- Any pain with urinating, crying, or holding the genitals?
- Any urinary tract infection?

2. (If child older than 2 to $2^1/_2$ years of age.) Has toilet training started? How is it progressing?
- Wet the bed at night? Is this a problem for child or for you (parents)? What have you done? How does the child feel about it?

3. Any problem with child's penis or scrotum: sores, swelling, discoloration?
- Told if his testes are descended?
- Ever had a hernia or hydrocele?
- Swelling in his scrotum during crying or coughing?

4. (Ask directly to preschooler or young school-age child.) Has anyone ever touched your penis or in between your legs and you did not want them to?

   Sometimes that happens to children and it's not okay. They should remember that they have not been bad. They should try to tell a big person about it. Can you tell me three different big people you trust who you could talk to?

Screen for sexual abuse. For prevention, teach the child that it's not okay for someone to look at or touch their private parts while telling them it's a secret. Naming three trusted adults will include someone outside the family—important, since most molestation is by a parent (Brown, 1997).

Additional History for Preadolescents and Adolescents

Use the following questions regarding sexual growth and development and sexual behavior. First
- Ask questions that seem appropriate for boy's age but be aware that norms vary widely. When you are in doubt, it is better to ask too many questions than to omit something. Children obtain information, often misinformation, from the media and from peers at surprisingly early ages. You may be sure your information will be more thoughtful and accurate.
- Ask direct, matter-of-fact questions. Avoid sounding judgmental.
- Start with a *permission statement.* "Often boys your age experience . . . " This conveys that it is normal and all right to think or feel a certain way.
- Try the *ubiquity approach,* "When did you . . . " rather than "Do you . . . " This method is less threatening because it implies that the topic is normal and unexceptional.
- Do not be concerned if a boy will not discuss sexuality with you or respond to your offers for more information. He may not wish to let on that he needs or wants more information. You do well to "open the door." The adolescent may come back at a future time.

1. Around age 12 to 13 years, but sometimes earlier, boys start to change and grow around the penis and scrotum. What changes have you noticed?

   Have you ever seen charts and pictures of normal growth patterns for boys? Let us go over these now.

   Who can you talk to about your body changes and about sex information? How do these talks go? Do you think you get enough information? What about sex education classes at school? How about your parents? Is there a favorite teacher, nurse, doctor, minister, or counselor to whom you can talk?

2. Boys around age 12 to 13 years (SMR3) have a normal experience of fluid coming out of the penis at night, called nocturnal emissions, or "wet dreams." Have you had this?

An occasional boy confuses this with a sign of STD or feels guilty.

EXAMINER ASKS	RATIONALE
3. Teenage boys have other normal experiences and wonder if they are the only ones who ever had them, like having an erection at embarrassing times, having sexual fantasies, or masturbating. Also, a boy might have a thought about touching another boy's genitals and wonder if this thought means he might be homosexual. Would you like to talk about any of these things?	A boy may feel guilty about experiencing these things if not informed that they are normal.

4. Often boys your age have questions about sexual activity. What questions do you have? How about things like birth control, or STDs such as gonorrhea or herpes? Any questions about these?
• Are you dating? Someone steady? Have you had intercourse? Are you using birth control? What kind?
 	
• What kind of birth control did you use the *last* time you had intercourse?
	Assess level of knowledge. Many boys will not admit they need more knowledge.
	  Avoid the term "having sex." It is ambiguous, and teens can take it to mean anything from foreplay to intercourse.
	  This particular question often reveals that the teen is not using any method of birth control.

5. Has a nurse or doctor ever taught you how to examine your own testicles to make sure they are healthy?	Assess knowledge of testicular self-examination.
6. Has anyone ever touched your genitals and you did not want them to? Another boy, or an adult, even a relative? Sometimes that happens to teenagers. They should remember it is not their fault. They should tell another adult about it.	

Additional History for the Aging Adult

1. Any difficulty urinating? Any hesitancy and straining? A weakened force of stream? Any dribbling? Or any incomplete emptying?	Early symptoms of enlarging prostate may be tolerated or ignored. Later symptoms are more dramatic: hematuria, urinary tract infection.
2. Do you need to get up at night to urinate? What medications are you taking? What fluids do you drink in the evening?	Nocturia may be due to diuretic medication, habit, or fluid ingestion 3 hours before bedtime, especially coffee and alcohol, which have a specific diuretic effect. Also, fluid retention from mild heart failure or varicose veins produces nocturia; recumbency at night mobilizes fluid.
3. A man in his 70s, 80s, or 90s may notice changes in his sexual relationship or in his sexual response and wonder if it is normal. For example, it is normal for an erection to develop slowly at this age. This is not a sign of impotence, but a man might wonder if it is.	Excluding physical illness, an older man is fully capable of sexual function. But some men assume normal changes mean that they are "old men" and voluntarily withdraw from sexual activity. The older person is not reluctant to discuss sexual activity, and most welcome the opportunity. Depressants to sexual desire and function include antihypertensives, sedatives, tranquilizers, estrogens, and alcohol. Alcohol decreases the sexual response even more dramatically in the older person.

PREPARATION

Position the male standing with undershorts down and appropriate draping. The examiner should be sitting. Alternatively, the male may be supine for the first part of the examination and stand to check for a hernia.

It is normal for a male to feel apprehensive about having his genitalia examined, especially by a female examiner. Younger adolescents usually have more anxiety than older adolescents. But any male may have difficulty dissociating a necessary, matter-of-fact step in the physical examination from the feeling this is an invasion of his privacy. His concerns are similar to those experienced by the female during the examination of the genitalia: modesty, fear of pain, cold hands, negative judgment, or memory of previously uncomfortable examinations. Additionally, he may fear comparison to others, or fear having an erection during the examination and that this would be misinterpreted by the examiner.

This normal apprehension becomes manifested in different behaviors. Many act resigned and embarrassed and avoid eye contact. An occasional man will laugh and make jokes to cover embarrassment. Also, a man may refuse examination by a female and insist on a male examiner.

Take time to consider these feelings, as well as to explore your own. It is normal for you to feel embarrassed and apprehensive too. You may worry about your age, lack of clinical experience, causing pain, or even that your movements might "cause" an erection. Some examiners feel guilty when this occurs. You need to accept these feelings and work through them so that you can examine the male in a professional way. Discussing these concerns in a group with other beginning examiners works best. Your demeanor is important. Your unresolved discomfort magnifies any discomfort the man may have.

Your demeanor should be *confident* and relaxed, unhurried yet businesslike. Do not discuss genitourinary history or sexual practices while you are performing the examination. This may be perceived as judgmental. Use a firm deliberate touch, not a soft, stroking one. If an erection does occur, do *not* stop the examination or leave the room. This only focuses more attention on the erection and increases embarrassment. Reassure the male that this is only a normal physiologic response to touch, just as when the pupil constricts in response to bright light. Proceed with the rest of the examination.

EQUIPMENT NEEDED

Gloves—Wear gloves during every male genitalia examination
Occasionally: glass slide for urethral specimen
Materials for cytology
Flashlight

NORMAL RANGE OF FINDINGS

INSPECT AND PALPATE THE PENIS

The skin normally looks wrinkled, hairless, and without lesions. The dorsal vein may be apparent (Fig. 24–5).

24–5

ABNORMAL FINDINGS

Inflammation.

Lesions: nodules, solitary ulcer (chancre), grouped vesicles or superficial ulcers, wartlike papules (see Table 24–2, p. 748).

NORMAL RANGE OF FINDINGS	ABNORMAL FINDINGS

The glans looks smooth and without lesions. Ask the uncircumcised male to retract the foreskin, or you retract it. It should move easily. Some cheesy smegma may have collected under the foreskin. After inspection, slide the foreskin back to the original position.

The urethral meatus is positioned just about centrally.

At the base of the penis, pubic hair distribution is consistent with age. Hair is without pest inhabitants.

Compress the glans anteroposteriorly between your thumb and forefinger (Fig. 24–6). The meatus edge should appear pink, smooth, and without discharge.

24–6

If you note urethral discharge, collect a smear for microscopic examination and a culture. If no discharge shows but the person gives a history of it, ask him to milk the shaft of the penis. This should produce a drop of discharge.

Palpate the shaft of the penis between your thumb and first two fingers. Normally, the penis feels smooth, semifirm, and nontender.

ABNORMAL FINDINGS

Inflammation. Lesions on glans or corona.

Phimosis—unable to retract the foreskin.

Paraphimosis—unable to return foreskin to original position.

Hypospadias—ventral location of meatus.

Epispadias—dorsal location of meatus (see Table 24–3).

Pubic lice or nits. Excoriated skin usually accompanies.

Stricture—narrowed opening.

Edges that are red, everted, edematous, along with purulent discharge, suggest urethritis (see Table 24–2).

Nodule or induration.
Tenderness.

NORMAL RANGE OF FINDINGS	ABNORMAL FINDINGS

INSPECT AND PALPATE THE SCROTUM

Inspect the scrotum as male holds the penis out of the way. Alternatively, you hold the penis out of the way with the back of your hand (Fig. 24–7). Scrotal size varies with ambient room temperature. Asymmetry is normal, with the left scrotal half usually lower than the right.

Scrotal swelling (edema) may be taut and pitting. This occurs with heart failure, renal failure, or local inflammation.

Lesions.

24–7

Spread rugae out between your fingers. Lift the sac to inspect the posterior surface. Normally, no scrotal lesions are present, except for the commonly found sebaceous cysts. These are yellowish, 1-cm nodules and are firm, nontender, and often multiple.

Palpate gently each scrotal half between your thumb and first two fingers (Fig. 24–8). The scrotal contents should slide easily. Testes normally feel oval, firm and rubbery, smooth, and equal bilaterally, and are freely movable and slightly tender to moderate pressure. Each epididymis normally feels discrete, softer than the testis, smooth, and nontender.

Inflammation.

Absent testis—may be a temporary migration or true cryptorchidism (see Table 24–4).

Atrophied testes—small and soft.

Fixed testes.

Nodules on testes or epididymides.

Marked tenderness.

An indurated, swollen, and tender epididymis indicates epididymitis.

24–8

NORMAL RANGE OF FINDINGS

Palpate each spermatic cord between your thumb and forefinger, along its length from the epididymis up to the external inguinal ring (Fig. 24–9). You should feel a smooth, nontender cord.

24–9

Normally, no other scrotal contents are present. If you do find a mass, note:

- Any tenderness?
- Is the mass distal or proximal to testis?
- Can you place your fingers over it?
- Does it reduce when person lies down?
- Can you auscultate bowel sounds over it?

TRANSILLUMINATION. Perform this maneuver if you note a swelling or mass. Darken the room. Shine a strong flashlight from behind the scrotal contents. Normal scrotal contents do not transilluminate.

INSPECT AND PALPATE FOR HERNIA

Inspect the inguinal region for a bulge as the person stands and as he strains down. Normally, none is present.

ABNORMAL FINDINGS

Thickened cord.

Soft, swollen, and tortuous—see the discussion of varicocele, Table 24–4.

Abnormalities in the scrotum: hernia, tumor, orchitis, epididymitis, hydrocele, spermatocele, varicocele (see Table 24–4).

Serous fluid does transilluminate and shows as a red glow, e.g., hydrocele, or spermatocele. Solid tissue and blood do not transilluminate, e.g., hernia, epididymitis, or tumor (see Table 24–4).

Bulge at external inguinal ring or at femoral canal. (A hernia may be present but easily reduced and may appear only intermittently with an increase in intraabdominal pressure.)

Palpate the inguinal canal (Fig. 24–10). For the right side, ask the male to shift his weight onto the left (unexamined) leg. Place your right index finger low on the right scrotal half. Palpate up the length of the spermatic cord, invaginating the scrotal skin as you go, to the external inguinal ring. It feels like a triangular slitlike opening, and it may or may not admit your finger. If it will admit your finger, gently insert it into the canal and ask the person to "bear down."* Normally, you feel no change. Repeat the procedure on the left side.

Palpate the femoral area for a bulge. Normally you feel none.

Palpable herniating mass bumps your fingertip or pushes against the side of your finger (see Table 24–5).

External inguinal ring

24–10

PALPATE INGUINAL LYMPH NODES

Palpate the horizontal chain along the groin inferior to the inguinal ligament and the vertical chain along the upper inner thigh.

It is normal to palpate an isolated node on occasion; it then feels small (<1 cm), soft, discrete, and movable (Fig. 24–11).

Enlarged, hard, matted, fixed nodes.

24–11

---

*Avoid the old direction, "turn your head and cough." For one thing, a brief cough does not give the steady, increased intraabdominal pressure you need. For another, the person is likely to cough right in your face.

NORMAL RANGE OF FINDINGS	ABNORMAL FINDINGS

SELF-CARE—TESTICULAR SELF-EXAMINATION (TSE)

Encourage self-care by teaching every male (from 13 to 14 years old through adulthood) how to examine his own testicles every month. The overall incidence of testicular cancer is still rare, but testicular cancer most commonly occurs in young men age 15 to 40 (American Cancer Society, 2002). Males with undescended testicles are at greatest risk, and white males are four times more likely to contract testicular cancer than nonwhites. This tumor has no early symptoms. If detected early by palpation and treated, the cure rate is almost 100 percent.

Early detection is enhanced if the male is familiar with his normal consistency. Points to include during health teaching are

- T = timing, once a month
- S = shower, warm water relaxes scrotal sac
- E = examine, check for changes, report changes immediately

Phrase your teaching something like this:

> *A good time to examine the testicles is during the shower or bath, when your hands are warm and soapy and the scrotum is warm. Cold hands stimulate a muscle (cremasteric) reflex, retracting the scrotal contents. The procedure is simple. Hold the scrotum in the palm of your hand and gently feel each testicle using your thumb and first two fingers. If it hurts, you are using too much pressure. The testicle is egg-shaped and movable. It feels rubbery with a smooth surface, like a hard-boiled egg. The epididymis is on top and behind the testicle; it feels a bit softer. If you ever notice a firm, painless lump, a hard area, or an overall enlarged testicle, call your physician for a further check.*

 DEVELOPMENTAL CONSIDERATIONS

Infants and Children

For an infant or toddler, perform this procedure right after the abdominal examination. In a preschool-age to young school-age child (3 to 8 years of age), leave underpants on until just before the examination. In an older school-age child or adolescent, offer an extra drape, as with the adult. Reassure child and parents of normal findings.

Inspect the penis and scrotum. Penis size is usually small in infants (2 to 3 cm) (Fig. 24–12) and in young boys until puberty. In the obese boy, the penis looks even smaller because of folds of skin covering the base.

Rarely, a very small penis may be an enlarged clitoris in a genetically female infant.
Enlarged penis—precocious puberty.
Redness, swelling, lesions.

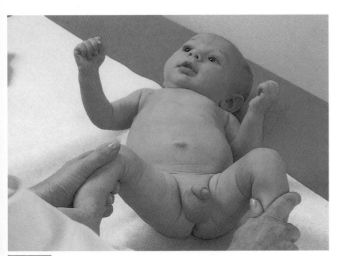

24–12

NORMAL RANGE OF FINDINGS	ABNORMAL FINDINGS
In the circumcised infant, the glans looks smooth with the meatus centered at the tip. While the child wears diapers, the meatus may become ulcerated from ammonia irritation. This is more common in circumcised infants.	Hypospadias, epispadias (see Table 24–3). Stricture—narrowed opening. Discharge. Occasionally, ulceration may produce a stricture, shown by a pinpoint meatus and a narrow stream. This increases the risk of urine obstruction.
If possible, observe the newborn's first voiding to assess strength and direction of stream.	Poor stream is significant, because it may indicate a stricture or neurogenic bladder.
If uncircumcised, the foreskin is normally tight during the first 3 months and should not be retracted because of the risk of tearing the membrane attaching the foreskin to the shaft. This leads to scarring and, possibly, to adhesions later in life. In infants older than 3 months of age, retract the foreskin gently to check the glans and meatus. It should return to its original position easily.	Phimosis—unable to retract the foreskin. Paraphimosis—the foreskin cannot be slipped forward once it is retracted. Dirt and smegma collecting under foreskin.

The scrotum looks pink in white infants and dark brown in dark-skinned infants. Rugae are well formed in the full-term infant. Size varies with ambient temperature, but overall, the infant's scrotum looks large in relation to the penis. No bulges, either constant or intermittent, are present.

Palpate the scrotum and testes. The cremasteric reflex is strong in the infant, pulling the testes up into the inguinal canal and abdomen from exposure to cold, touch, exercise, or emotion. Take care not to elicit the reflex: (1) Keep your hands warm and palpate from the external inguinal ring down; (2) block the inguinal canals with the thumb and forefinger of your other hand to prevent the testes from retracting (Fig. 24–13).

24-13

NORMAL RANGE OF FINDINGS	ABNORMAL FINDINGS

Normally, the testes are descended and are equal in size bilaterally (1.5 to 2 cm until puberty). It is important to document that you have palpated the testes. Once palpated, they are considered descended, even if they have retracted momentarily at the next visit.

Cryptorchidism: undescended testes (those that have never descended). Undescended testes are common in premature infants. They occur in 3 to 4 percent of term infants, although most have descended by 3 months of age. Age at which child should be referred differs among physicians (see Table 24–4).

If the scrotal half feels empty, search for the testes along the inguinal canal and try to milk them down. Ask the toddler or child to squat with the knees flexed up; this pressure may force the testes down. Or, have the young child sit cross-legged to relax the reflex (Fig. 24–14).

24–14

Migratory testes (physiologic cryptorchidism) are common because of the strength of the cremasteric reflex and the small mass of the prepubertal testes. Note that the affected side has a normally developed scrotum (with true cryptorchidism, the scrotum is atrophic) and that the testis can be milked down. These testes descend at puberty and are normal.

Palpate the epididymis and spermatic cord as described in the adult section. A common scrotal finding in the boy under 2 years of age is a *hydrocele,* or fluid in the scrotum. It appears as a large scrotum and transilluminates as a faint pink glow. It usually disappears spontaneously.

A hydrocele is a cystic collection of serous fluid in the tunica vaginalis, surrounding the testis. (See Table 24–4.)

Inspect the inguinal area for a bulge. If you do not see a bulge but the parent gives a positive history of one, try to elicit it by increasing intraabdominal pressure. Ask the boy to hold his breath and strain down or have him blow up a balloon.

If a hernia is suspected, palpate the inguinal area. Use your little finger to reach the external inguinal ring.

NORMAL RANGE OF FINDINGS	ABNORMAL FINDINGS

The Adolescent

The adolescent shows a wide variation in normal development of the genitals. Using the SMR charts, note: (1) enlargement of the testes and scrotum; (2) pubic hair growth; (3) darkening of scrotal color; (4) roughening of scrotal skin; (5) increase in penis length and width; and (6) axillary hair growth.

Be familiar with the normal sequence of growth.

The Aging Adult

In the older male, you may note thinner, graying pubic hair and the decreased size of the penis. The size of the testes may be decreased and may feel less firm. The scrotal sac is pendulous with less rugae. The scrotal skin may become excoriated if the man continually sits on it.

SUMMARY CHECKLIST: Male Genitalia Exam

1. Inspect and palpate the penis
2. Inspect and palpate the scrotum
3. If a mass exists, transilluminate it
4. Palpate for an inguinal hernia
5. Palpate the inguinal lymph nodes

 See Health Promotion Guide on CD

Application and Critical Thinking

SAMPLE CHARTING

SUBJECTIVE

Urinates four to five times/day, clear, straw-colored. No nocturia, dysuria, or hesitancy. No pain, lesions, or discharge from penis. Does not do testicular self-examination. No history of genitourinary disease. Sexually active in a monogamous relationship. Sexual life satisfactory to self and partner. Uses birth control via barrier method (partner uses diaphragm). No known STD contact.

OBJECTIVE

No lesions, inflammation, or discharge from penis. Scrotum—testes descended, symmetric, no masses. No inguinal hernia.

FOCUSED ASSESSMENT: CLINICAL CASE STUDY

SUBJECTIVE

R.C. is a 19-year-old student who 2 days PTA noted acute onset of painful urination, frequency, and urgency. Noted some thick penile discharge. States has no side pain, no abdominal pain, no fever, or genital skin rash. R.C. is concerned he has an STD because of episode of unprotected intercourse with a new partner 6 days PTA. Has no known allergies.

OBJECTIVE

Vital signs 37° C-72-16. No lesions or inflammation around penis or scrotum. Urethral meatus has mild edema with purulent urethral discharge. No pain on palpation of genitalia. Testes symmetric with no masses. No lymphadenopathy.

ASSESSMENT

Urethral discharge
Deficient knowledge about STD prevention R/T lack of information recall

NURSING DIAGNOSES COMMONLY ASSOCIATED WITH THE MALE GENITALIA AND RELATED DISORDERS

RELATED FACTORS (Etiology)	DEFINING CHARACTERISTICS (Symptoms and Signs)
DIAGNOSIS: Ineffective Sexuality patterns	
Effects of illness or medical treatment	Identification of sexual difficulties, limitations, or changes
Drugs	
Radiation	
Anomalies	
Extreme fatigue	
Obesity	
Pain	
Performance anxiety	
Deficient knowledge/skill about alternative responses to health-related transitions	
Pregnancy	
Surgery	
Recent childbirth	
Trauma	
Menopause	
Impaired relationship with a significant other	
Fear of pregnancy or of acquiring a sexually transmitted disease	
Conflicts with sexual orientation or variant preferences	
Ineffective or absent role models	
Loss of job or ability to work	
Separation from or loss of significant other	
DIAGNOSIS: Urinary retention	
Diminished or absent sensory and/or motor impulses	Bladder distention
Effects of medications	Diminished force of urinary stream
Anesthetics	Dribbling
Opiates	Dysuria
Psychotropics	Hesitancy
Strong sphincter	High residual urine
Urethral blockage associated with	Nocturia
Fecal impaction	Sensation of bladder fullness
Prostate hypertrophy	Small, frequent voiding or absence of urine output
Surgical swelling	
Postpartum edema	
Anxiety (fear of postoperative pain)	
DIAGNOSIS: Impaired Skin integrity	
Infection	Blisters
Allergy	Chafing
Chemical substances on skin	Disruption of skin surface or layers
Autoimmune dysfunction	Lesions
Decreased circulation	Pruritus
Edema	Bruising
Effects of aging or medications	Cyanosis
Excretions/secretions	Denuded skin
Immobility	Erythema
Insect bites	Induration
Parasites	
Pressure	
Radiation	
Shearing force	
Stress	
Surgery	

Continued

RELATED FACTORS (Etiology)   **DEFINING CHARACTERISTICS** (Symptoms and Signs)

OTHER RELATED NURSING DIAGNOSES

ACTUAL	RISK/WELLNESS
Anxiety	**Risk**
Delayed Growth and development	Risk for Infection
Incontinence	Risk for Trauma
Pain	**Wellness**
Rape trauma syndrome: compound reaction	Health-seeking behavior for instruction on testicular self-examination
Rape trauma syndrome (see Chapter 26)	
Rape trauma syndrome: silent reaction	
Sexual dysfunction (see Chapter 26)	
Ineffective Sexuality patterns	
Impaired Skin integrity	
Impaired Urinary elimination	
Urinary retention	

ASSESSMENT VIDEO CRITICAL THINKING QUESTIONS

The Saunders *Physical Examination and Health Assessment* video "Male Genitalia" will direct you to consider the following:

1. Which presenting symptoms are associated with abnormalities of the male genitalia?

2. What abnormal findings may be detected during inspection of the penis?

3. How do genitalia assessment findings in a male infant compare to those in a male adolescent?

Abnormal Findings

TABLE 24–2: Male Genital Lesions

Herpes Progenitalis

Clusters of small vesicles with surrounding erythema, which are often painful, erupt on the glans or foreskin. These rupture to form superficial ulcers. A sexually transmitted disease (STD), the initial infection lasts 7 to 10 days. The virus remains dormant indefinitely; recurrent infections last 3 to 10 days with milder symptoms.

Syphilitic Chancre

Begins within 2–4 weeks of infection, as a small, solitary, silvery papule that erodes to a red, round or oval, superficial ulcer with a yellowish serous discharge. Palpation reveals a nontender indurated base that can be lifted like a button between the thumb and the finger. Lymph nodes enlarge early but are nontender. This is an STD.

Reprinted from *Colour Atlas of Infectious Diseases,* 3rd edition, Emond, p. 173, 1995, by permission of the publisher Mosby.

◀ Condylomata Acuminata (Genital Warts)

Soft, pointed, moist, fleshy, painless papules may be single or multiple in a cauliflowerlike patch. Color may be gray, pale yellow, or pink in white males, and black or translucent gray-black in black males. They occur on shaft of penis, behind corona, or around the anus where they may grow into large grapelike clusters.

These are caused by the human papillomavirus (HPV) and are one of the most common STDs. The HPV infection is correlated with early onset of sexual activity, infrequent use of contraception, and multiple sexual partners.

Table continued on following page

TABLE 24-2: Male Genital Lesions—cont'd

Carcinoma

Begins as red, raised warty growth or as an ulcer, with watery discharge. As it grows, may necrose and slough. Usually painless. Almost always on glans or inner lip of foreskin and following chronic inflammation. Enlarged lymph nodes are common.

Urethritis (Urethral Discharge and Dysuria)

Infection of urethra causes painful burning urination. Meatus edges are reddened, everted, and swollen. Purulent urethral discharge is present. Urine is cloudy with discharge and mucous shreds. Cause determined by culture: (1) gonococcal urethritis has thick, profuse, yellow or gray-brown discharge; (2) nonspecific urethritis (NSU) may have similar discharge but often has scanty, mucoid discharge. Of these, about 50 percent are caused by chlamydia infection. This is important to differentiate because antibiotic treatment is different.

TABLE 24-3: Abnormalities on the Penis

Phimosis

Foreskin is advanced and fixed so tight it is impossible to retract over glans. May be congenital or acquired from adhesions secondary to infection. Poor hygiene leads to retained dirt and smegma, which increases risk of inflammation or calculus formation.

Paraphimosis

Foreskin is retracted and fixed. Once retracted behind glans, a tight or inflamed foreskin cannot return to its original position. Constriction impedes circulation, so glans swells. If untreated, it may compromise arterial circulation.

Continued

TABLE 24-3: Abnormalities on the Penis—cont'd

Epispadias

Meatus opens on the dorsal (upper) side of glans or shaft above a broad, spadelike penis. Rare; less common than hypospadias but more disabling because of associated urinary incontinence and separation of pubic bones.

Hypospadias

Urethral meatus opens on the ventral (under-) side of glans, shaft, or at the penoscrotal junction. A groove extends from the meatus to the normal location at the tip. This is a congenital defect that is important to recognize at birth. The newborn should not be circumcised because surgical correction may use foreskin tissue to extend urethral length.

Urethral Stricture (not illustrated)

Pinpoint, constricted opening at meatus or inside along urethra. Occurs congenitally or secondary to urethral injury. Gradual decrease in force and caliber of urine stream is most common symptom. Shaft feels indurated along ventral aspect at the site of the stricture.

Priapism (not illustrated)

Prolonged painful erection of penis without sexual desire. Rare condition occurs with sickle-cell trait or disease; leukemia where increased numbers of white blood cells produce engorgement; malignancy; or local trauma or spinal cord injuries with autonomic nervous system dysfunction.

Peyronie's Disease

Hard, nontender, subcutaneous plaques palpated on dorsal or lateral surface of penis. May be single or multiple and asymmetric. They are associated with painful bending of the penis during erection. Plaques are fibrosis of covering of corpora cavernosa. Usually occurs after 45 years. Its cause is unknown. Ten to 20 percent of those afflicted also have Dupuytren's contracture of the palm.

ABNORMAL FINDINGS

TABLE 24-4: Abnormalities in the Scrotum

DISORDER	CLINICAL FINDINGS	DISCUSSION
Absent Testis Cryptorchidism Empty scrotal half	S: Empty scrotal half O: Inspection—in true maldescent, atrophic scrotum on affected side Palpation—no testis A: Absent testis	True cryptorchidism—testes that have never descended. Incidence at birth is 3 to 4 percent, one-half of these descend in first month. Incidence with premature infants is 30 percent; in the adult 0.7 to 0.8 percent. True undescended testes have a histologic change by 6 years, causing decreased spermatogenesis and infertility.
Small Testis	S: (None) O: Palpation—small and soft (rarely may be firm) A: Small testis	Small and soft (<3.5 cm) indicates atrophy as with cirrhosis, hypopituitarism, following estrogen therapy, or as a sequelae of orchitis. Small and firm (<2 cm) occurs with Klinefelter's syndrome (hypogonadism).
Testicular Torsion	S: Excruciating pain in testicle of sudden onset, often during sleep or following trauma. May also have lower abdominal pain, nausea and vomiting, no fever O: Inspection—red, swollen scrotum, one testis (usually left) higher owing to rotation and shortening Palpation—cord feels thick, swollen, tender, epididymis may be anterior, cremasteric reflex is absent on side of torsion	Sudden twisting of spermatic cord. Occurs in late childhood, early adolescence, rare after age of 20 years. Torsion occurs usually on the left side. Faulty anchoring of testis on wall of scrotum allows testis to rotate. The anterior part of the testis rotates medially toward the other testis. Blood supply is cut off, resulting in ischemia and engorgement. This is an emergency requiring surgery; testis can become gangrenous in a few hours.
Epididymitis	S: Severe pain of sudden onset in scrotum, somewhat relieved by elevation (a positive Phren's sign); also rapid swelling, fever O: Inspection—enlarged scrotum; reddened Palpation—exquisitely tender; epididymis enlarged, indurated; may be hard to distinguish from testis. Overlying scrotal skin may be thick and edematous Laboratory—white blood cells and bacteria in urine A: Tender swelling of epididymis	Acute infection of epididymis commonly caused by prostatitis, after prostatectomy because of trauma of urethral instrumentation, or due to chlamydia, gonorrhea, or other bacterial infection. Often difficult to distinguish between epididymitis and testicular torsion.

S = subjective data; O = objective data; A = assessment.

TABLE 24–4: Abnormalities in the Scrotum—cont'd

DISORDER	CLINICAL FINDINGS	DISCUSSION
Spermatic Cord Varicocele 	S: Dull pain; constant pulling or dragging feeling; or may be asymptomatic O: Inspection—usually no sign. May show bluish color through light scrotal skin Palpation—when standing, feel soft, irregular mass posterior to and above testis; collapses when supine, refills when upright. Feels distinctive, like a "bag of worms" The testis on the side of the varicocele may be smaller owing to impaired circulation A: Soft mass on spermatic cord	A varicocele is dilated, tortuous varicose veins in the spermatic cord due to incompetent valves within the vein, which permit reflux of blood. Most often on left side, perhaps because left spermatic vein is longer and inserts at a right angle into left renal vein. Common in young males. Screen at early adolescence; early treatment important to prevent potential infertility when an adult. Treatment is relatively easy; surgical ligation of spermatic vein.
Spermatocele 	S: Painless, usually found on examination O: Inspection—does transilluminate higher in the scrotum than a hydrocele, and the sperm may fluoresce Palpation—round, freely movable mass lying above and behind testis. If large, feels like a third testis A: Free cystic mass on epididymis	Retention cyst in epididymis. Cause unclear but may be obstruction of tubules. Filled with thin, milky fluid that contains sperm. Most spermatoceles are small (<1 cm); occasionally, they may be larger and then mistaken for hydrocele.
Early Testicular Tumor 	S: Painless, found on examination O: Palpation—firm nodule or harder than normal section of testicle A: Solitary nodule	Most testicular tumors occur between the ages of 18 and 35. Practically all are malignant. Occur in whites; relatively rare in blacks, Mexican-Americans, and Asians. Must biopsy to confirm. Most important risk factor is undescended testis, even those surgically corrected. Early detection important in prognosis, but practice of testicular self-examination is currently low.
Diffuse Tumor 	S: Enlarging testis (most common symptom). When enlarges, has feel of increased weight O: Inspection—enlarged, does not transilluminate Palpation—enlarged, smooth, ovoid, firm. Important—firm palpation does *not* cause usual sickening discomfort as with normal testis A: Nontender swelling of testis	Diffuse tumor maintains shape of testis.

S = subjective data; O = objective data; A = assessment.

TABLE 24–4: Abnormalities in the Scrotum—cont'd

DISORDER	CLINICAL FINDINGS	DISCUSSION
Hydrocele Serous fluid Tunica vaginalis	S: Painless swelling, although person may complain of weight and bulk in scrotum O: Inspection—enlarged, mass does transilluminate with a pink or red glow (in contrast to a hernia) Palpation—nontender mass, able to get fingers above mass (in contrast to scrotal hernia) A: Nontender swelling of testis	Cystic. Circumscribed collection of serous fluid in tunica vaginalis, surrounding testis. May occur following epididymitis, trauma, hernia, tumor of testis, or spontaneously in the newborn.
Scrotal Hernia	S: Swelling, may have pain with straining O: Inspection—enlarged, may reduce when supine, does not transilluminate Palpation—soft mushy mass, palpating fingers cannot get above mass. Mass is distinct from testicle that is normal A: Nontender swelling of scrotum	Scrotal hernia usually due to indirect inguinal hernia (see Table 24–5).
Orchitis	S: Acute or moderate pain of sudden onset, swollen testis, feeling of weight, fever O: Inspection—enlarged, edematous, reddened; does not transilluminate Palpation—swollen, congested, tense, and tender; hard to distinguish testis from epididymis A: Tender swelling of testis	Acute inflammation of testis. Most common cause is mumps; can occur with any infectious disease. May have associated hydrocele that does transilluminate.
Scrotal Edema	S: Tenderness O: Inspection—enlarged, may be reddened (with local irritation) Palpation—taut with pitting Probably unable to feel scrotal contents A: Scrotal edema	Accompanies marked edema in lower half of body, e.g., congestive heart failure, renal failure, and portal vein obstruction. Occurs with local inflammation: epididymitis, torsion of spermatic cord. Also obstruction of inguinal lymphatics produces lymphedema of scrotum.

S = subjective data; O = objective data; A = assessment.

TABLE 24–5: Inguinal and Femoral Hernias

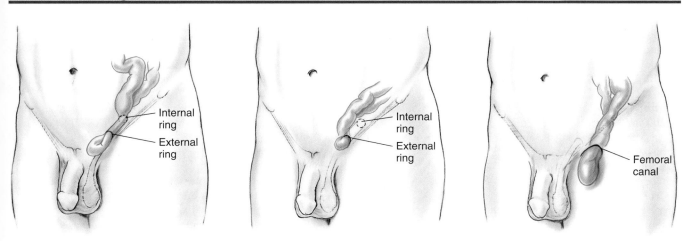

	INDIRECT INGUINAL	DIRECT INGUINAL	FEMORAL
Course	Sac herniates through internal inguinal ring; can remain in canal or pass into scrotum	Directly behind and through external inguinal ring, above inguinal ligament; rarely enters scrotum	Through femoral ring and canal, below inguinal ligament, more often on right side
Clinical Symptoms and Signs	Pain with straining; soft swelling that increases with increased intraabdominal pressure; may decrease when lying down	Usually painless; round swelling close to the pubis in area of internal inguinal ring; easily reduced when supine*	Pain may be severe, may become strangulated
Frequency	Most common; 60 percent of all hernias. More common in infants <1 year and in males 16 to 20 years of age	Less common, occurs most often in men >40, rare in women	Least common, 4 percent of all hernias; more common in women
Cause	Congenital or acquired	Acquired weakness; brought on by heavy lifting, muscle atrophy, obesity, chronic cough, or ascites	Acquired; due to increased abdominal pressure, muscle weakness, or frequent stooping

*__Reducible__—contents will return to abdominal cavity by lying down or gentle pressure. __Incarcerated__—herniated bowel cannot be returned to abdominal cavity. __Strangulated__—blood supply to hernia is shut off. Accompanied by nausea, vomiting, and tenderness.

BIBLIOGRAPHY

Adelman WP, Joffe A: Revisiting the adolescent male genital examination, *Patient Care* 34(4):83–93, Feb 29, 2000.

Allison L: Clinical effectiveness: testicular self-examination, *Prof Nurse* 15(11):710–713, Aug 2000.

American Cancer Society: http://www.cancer.org/eprise/ma/CRI_2_4_IX_What_is_testicular_cancer_41?sitearea=CR [Accessed 10/2002].

Behrman RE: *Nelson textbook of pediatrics,* ed 16, Philadelphia, 2000, WB Saunders.

Brown MS: Pediatric genital exam, *Nurse Pract* 22(7):160, July 1997.

Cornell S: Controversies in circumcision: examining a cultural norm, *Adv Nurs Pract* 5(10):49–52, Oct 1997.

Dufour JL: Assessing and treating epididymitis, *Nurse Pract* 26(3):23–24, Mar 2001.

Finan SL: Promoting healthy sexuality: guidelines for infancy through preschool, *Nurse Pract* 22(10):79–100, Oct 1997.

Finan SL: Promoting healthy sexuality: guidelines for early through older adulthood, *Nurse Pract* 22(10):54–64, Dec 1997.

Goldman BD: Common dermatoses of the male genitalia, *Postgrad Med* 108(4):89–96, Sep 15, 2000.

Harlan W et al: Secondary sex characteristics of boys 12 to 17 years of age: the U.S. Health Examination Survey, *J Pediatr* 95:293, 1979.

Klingman L: Assessing the male genitalia, *Am J Nurs* 99(7):47–50, July 1999.

Laumann EO, Masi CM, Zuckerman MA: Circumcision in the United States: prevalence, prophylactic effects, and sexual practice, *JAMA* 277(13):1052–1057, Apr 2, 1997.

Marshall W, Tanner J: Variations in the pattern of pubertal changes in boys, *Arch Dis Child* 45:13, 1970.

Miller KM: Testicular torsion, *Am J Nurs* 99(6):33, June 1999.

Nelson JA: Gay, lesbian, and bisexual adolescents: providing esteem-enhancing care to a battered population, *Nurse Pract* 22(2):94–109, Feb 1997.

Pasero C: Circumcision requires anesthesia and analgesia, *Am J Nurs* 101(9):22–23, Sep 2001.

Peck SA: The importance of the sexual health history in the primary care setting, *J Obstet Gynecol Nurs* 30(3):269–274, May/June 2001.

Ryan C, Futterman D, Stine K: Helping our hidden youth, *Am J Nurs* 98(12):37–41, Dec 1998.

Schoen EJ: Newborn circumcision decreases incidence and costs of urinary tract infections during the first year of life, *Pediatrics* 105(4):789–793, Apr 2000.

Tanner J: *Growth at adolescence,* ed 2, Oxford, England, 1962, Blackwell Scientific Publications.

Van Howe RS: Circumcision and infectious diseases revisited, *Pediatr Infect Dis J* 17(1):1–6, Jan 1998.

Warner PH, Rowe T, Whipple B: Shedding light on the sexual history, *Am J Nurs* 99(6):34–41, June 1999.

Wynd CA: Testicular self-examination in young adult men, *J Nurs Schol* 34(3):251–255, 2002.

CHAPTER 25

Anus, Rectum, and Prostate

Structure and Function

ANUS AND RECTUM

The **anal canal** is the outlet of the gastrointestinal tract, and it is about 3.8 cm long in the adult. It is lined with modified skin (having no hair or sebaceous glands) that merges with rectal mucosa at the anorectal junction. The canal slants forward toward the umbilicus, forming a distinct right angle with the rectum, which rests back in the hollow of the sacrum. Although the rectum contains only autonomic nerves, numerous somatic sensory nerves are present in the anal canal and external skin, so a person feels sharp pain from any trauma to the anal area.

The anal canal is surrounded by two concentric layers of muscle, the **sphincters** (Fig. 25–1). The internal sphincter is under involuntary control by the autonomic nervous system. The external sphincter surrounds the internal sphincter but also has a small section overriding the tip of the internal sphincter at the opening. It is under voluntary control. Except for the passing of feces and gas, the sphincters keep the anal canal tightly closed. The **intersphincteric groove** separates the internal and external sphincters and is palpable.

The **anal columns** (or columns of Morgagni) are folds of mucosa. These extend vertically down from the rectum and end in the **anorectal junction** (also called the mucocutaneous junction, pectinate, or dentate line). This junction is not palpable, but it is visible on proctoscopy. Each anal column contains an artery and a vein. Under conditions of chronic increased venous pressure, the vein may enlarge, forming a hemorrhoid. At the lower end of each column is a small crescent fold of mucous membrane, the **anal valve.** The space above the anal valve (between the columns) is a small recess, the **anal crypt.**

The **rectum,** which is 12 cm long, is the distal portion of the large intestine. It extends from the sigmoid colon, at the level of the third sacral vertebra, and ends at the anal canal.

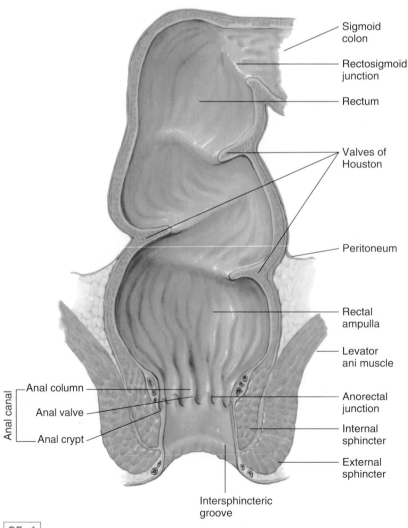

Sigmoid colon

Rectosigmoid junction

Rectum

Valves of Houston

Peritoneum

Rectal ampulla

Levator ani muscle

Anorectal junction

Internal sphincter

External sphincter

Anal canal

Anal column

Anal valve

Anal crypt

Intersphincteric groove

25–1

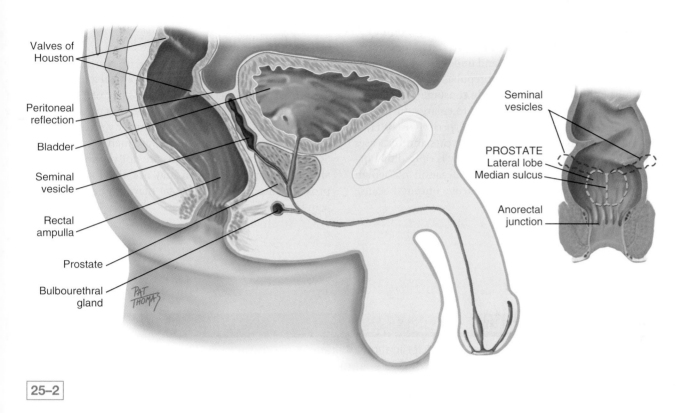

Seminal vesicles

PROSTATE
Lateral lobe
Median sulcus

Anorectal junction

Valves of Houston

Peritoneal reflection

Bladder

Seminal vesicle

Rectal ampulla

Prostate

Bulbourethral gland

PAT THOMAS

25–2

Just above the anal canal, the rectum dilates and turns posteriorly, forming the rectal ampulla. The rectal interior has three semilunar transverse folds called the **valves of Houston.** These cross one-half the circumference of the rectal lumen. Their function is unclear, but they may serve to hold feces as the flatus passes. The lowest is within reach of palpation, usually on the person's left side, and must not be mistaken for an intrarectal mass.

PERITONEAL REFLECTION. The peritoneum covers only the upper two-thirds of the rectum. In the male, the anterior part of the peritoneum reflects down to within 7.5 cm of the anal opening, forming the **rectovesical pouch** (Fig. 25–2) and then covers the bladder. In the female, this is termed the **rectouterine pouch,** and extends down to within 5.5 cm of the anal opening.

PROSTATE

In the male, the **prostate gland** lies in front of the anterior wall of the rectum and 2 cm behind the symphysis pubis. It surrounds the bladder neck and the urethra and has 15 to 30 ducts that open into the urethra. The prostate secretes a thin, milky alkaline fluid that helps sperm viability. It is a bilobed structure with a round or heart shape. It measures 2.5 cm long and 4 cm in diameter. The two lateral lobes are separated by a shallow groove called the **median sulcus.**

The two **seminal vesicles** project like rabbit ears above the prostate. The seminal vesicles secrete a fluid that is rich in fructose, which nourishes the sperm, and contains prostaglandins. The two **bulbourethral** (Cowper's) glands are each the size of a pea and are located inferior to the prostate on either side of the urethra (see Fig. 25–5). They secrete a clear, viscid mucus.

REGIONAL STRUCTURES

In the female, the uterine cervix lies in front of the anterior rectal wall and may be palpated through it.

The combined length of the anal canal and the rectum is about 16 cm in the adult. The average length of the examining finger is from 6 cm to 10 cm, bringing many rectal structures within reach.

The sigmoid colon is named from its S-shaped course in the pelvic cavity. It extends from the iliac flexure of the descending colon and ends at the rectum. It is 40 cm long and is accessible to examination only through the colonoscope. The flexible fiberoptic scope in current use provides a view of the entire mucosal surface of the sigmoid, as well as the colon.

 DEVELOPMENTAL CONSIDERATIONS

The first stool passed by the newborn is dark green meconium and occurs within 24 to 48 hours of birth, indicating anal patency. From that time on, the infant usually has a stool after each feeding. This response to eating is a wave of peristalsis called the gastrocolic reflex. It continues throughout life, although children and adults usually produce no more than one or two stools per day.

The infant passes stools by reflex. Voluntary control of the external anal sphincter cannot occur until the nerves supplying the area have become fully myelinated, usually around 1¹/₂ to 2 years of age. Toilet training usually starts after age 2 years.

At male puberty, the prostate gland undergoes a very rapid increase to more than twice its prepubertal size. During young adulthood its size remains fairly constant.

The prostate gland commonly starts to enlarge during the middle adult years. This *benign prostatic hypertrophy* (BPH) is present in 1 of 10 males at the age of 40 years and increases with age. It is thought that the hypertrophy is caused by hormonal imbalance that leads to the proliferation of benign adenomas. These gradually impede urine output because they obstruct the urethra.

 TRANSCULTURAL CONSIDERATIONS

Prostate cancer is more common in North America and northwestern Europe and is rare in Central and South America, Africa, and Asia. The incidence rates of prostate cancer are at least 50% higher for black American men than rates for men of other racial groups, and mortality rates are two times higher for black men than for white men (American Cancer Society, 2002). Reasons for this are not yet known. However, an inherited predisposition may account for 5% to 10% of prostate cancers, and dietary fat may also be a factor (American Cancer Society, 2002).

Subjective Data

1. Usual bowel routine
2. Change in bowel habits
3. Rectal bleeding, blood in the stool
4. Medications (laxatives, stool softeners, iron)
5. Rectal conditions (pruritus, hemorrhoids, fissure, fistula)
6. Family history
7. Self-care behaviors (diet of high-fiber foods, most recent examinations)

EXAMINER ASKS	RATIONALE
1. Usual bowel routine. Bowels move regularly? How often? Usual color? Hard or soft? Pain while passing a bowel movement?	Assess **usual bowel routine.** Dyschezia. Pain may be due to a local condition (hemorrhoid, fissure) or constipation.
2. Change in bowel habits. Any **change** in usual **bowel habits?** Loose stools, or diarrhea? When did this start? Is the diarrhea associated with nausea and vomiting, abdominal pain, something you ate recently?	Diarrhea occurs with gastroenteritis, colitis, irritable colon syndrome.
• Eaten at a restaurant recently? Anyone else in your group or family have the same symptoms?	Consider food poisoning.
• Traveled to a foreign country during the last 6 months?	Consider parasitic infection.
• Stools have a hard consistency? When did this start?	Constipation.
3. Rectal bleeding, blood in the stool. Ever had black or bloody stools? When did you first notice blood in the stools? What is the color, bright red or dark red-black? How much blood: spotting on the toilet paper or outright passing of blood with the stool? Do the bloody stools have a particular smell?	Melena. Black stools may be tarry due to occult blood (melena) from gastrointestinal bleeding, or nontarry from ingestion of iron medications. Red blood in stools occurs with gastrointestinal bleeding or localized bleeding around the anus, and also with colon and rectal cancer.
• Ever had clay-colored stools?	Clay color indicates absent bile pigment.
• Ever had mucus or pus in stool?	
• Frothy stool?	Steatorrhea is excessive fat in the stool as in malabsorption of fat.
• Need to pass gas frequently?	Flatulence.
4. Medications. What **medications** do you take—prescription and over-the-counter? Laxatives or stool softeners? Which ones? How often? Iron pills? Do you ever use enemas to move your bowels? How often?	

EXAMINER ASKS	RATIONALE
5. Rectal conditions. Any problems in rectal area: itching, pain or burning, hemorrhoids? How do you treat these? Any hemorrhoid preparations? Ever had a fissure, or fistula? How was this treated?	Pruritus.
• Ever had a problem controlling your bowels?	Fecal incontinence. Mucoid discharge and soiled under-wear occur with prolapsed hemorrhoids.
6. Family history. Any **family history:** polyps or cancer in colon or rectum, inflammatory bowel disease, prostate cancer?	Risk factors for colon cancer, rectal cancer, prostate cancer.
7. Self-care behaviors. What is the usual amount of **high-fiber foods** in your daily diet: cereals, apples or other fruits, vegetables, whole-grain breads? How many glasses of water do you drink each day?	High-fiber foods of the soluble type (beans, prunes, barley, carrots, broccoli, cabbage) have been shown to lower cholesterol, while insoluble fiber foods (cereals, wheat germ) reduce the risk of colon cancer. Also, fiber foods help fight obesity, stabilize blood sugar, and may help certain gastrointestinal disorders.
• Date last: digital rectal examination, stool blood test, colonoscopy, (for men) prostate-specific antigen blood test.	Early detection for cancer: digital rectal examination performed annually after age 50; fecal occult blood test annually after age 50; sigmoidoscopy every 5 years or colonoscopy every 10 years after age 50; prostate-specific antigen blood test annually for men over 50, except black men beginning at age 45 (American Cancer Society, 2002).

Additional History for Infants and Children

1. Have you ever noticed any irritation in your child's anal area: redness, raised skin, frequent itching?	In children, pinworms are a common cause of intense itching and irritated anal skin.

Objective Data

PREPARATION

Perform a rectal examination on all adults and particularly for those in middle and late years. Help the person assume one of the following positions (Fig. 25–3): Examine the male in the left lateral decubitus or standing position. Instruct the standing male to point his toes together; this relaxes the regional muscles, making it easier to spread the buttocks.

Place the female in the lithotomy position if examining genitalia as well; use the left lateral decubitus position for the rectal area alone.

EQUIPMENT NEEDED

Penlight
Lubricating jelly
Glove
Guaiac test container

Standing

Left lateral

Lithotomy

25–3

NORMAL RANGE OF FINDINGS

ABNORMAL FINDINGS

INSPECT THE PERIANAL AREA

Spread the buttocks wide apart and observe the perianal region. The anus normally looks moist and hairless, with coarse folded skin that is more pigmented than the perianal skin. The anal opening is tightly closed. No lesions are present.

Inspect the sacrococcygeal area. Normally, it appears smooth and even.

Instruct the person to hold the breath and bear down by performing a Valsalva maneuver. No break in skin integrity or protrusion through the anal opening should be present. Describe any abnormality in clock-face terms, with 12:00 as the anterior point toward the symphysis pubis and 6:00 toward the coccyx.

PALPATE THE ANUS AND RECTUM

Drop lubricating jelly onto your gloved index finger. Instruct the person that palpation is not painful but may feel like needing to move the bowels. Place the pad of your index finger gently against the anal verge (Fig. 25–4). You will feel the sphincter tighten, then relax. As it relaxes, flex the tip of your finger and slowly insert it into the anal canal in a direction toward the umbilicus. *Never* approach the anus at right angles with your index finger extended. Such a jabbing motion does not promote sphincter relaxation and is painful.

Inflammation. Lesions or scars. Linear split—fissure.

Flabby skin sac—hemorrhoid. Shiny blue skin sac—thrombosed hemorrhoid.

Small round opening in anal area—fistula (see Table 25–1).

Inflammation or tenderness, swelling, tuft of hair, or dimple at tip of coccyx may indicate pilonidal cyst (see Table 25–1).

Appearance of fissure, or hemorrhoids.

Circular red doughnut of tissue—rectal prolapse.

25–4

NORMAL RANGE OF FINDINGS

Rotate your examining finger to palpate the entire muscular ring. The canal should feel smooth and even. Note the intersphincteric groove circling the canal wall. To assess tone, ask the person to tighten the muscle. The sphincter should tighten evenly around your finger with no pain to the person.

Use a bidigital palpation with your thumb against the perianal tissue (Fig. 25–5). Press your examining finger toward it. This maneuver highlights any swelling or tenderness and helps assess the bulbourethral glands.

Bulbourethral gland

25–5

Above the anal canal, the rectum turns posteriorly, following the curve of the coccyx and sacrum. Insert your finger farther and explore all around the rectal wall. It normally feels smooth with no nodularity. Promptly report any mass you discover for further examination.

ABNORMAL FINDINGS

Decreased tone.
Increased tone occurs with inflammation and anxiety.

Tenderness.

Internal hemorrhoid above anorectal junction is not palpable unless thrombosed.

A soft, slightly movable mass may be a polyp.

A firm or hard mass with irregular shape or rolled edges may signify carcinoma (see Table 25–2).

NORMAL RANGE OF FINDINGS

PROSTATE GLAND. On the anterior wall in the male, note the elastic, bulging prostate gland (Fig. 25–6). Palpate the entire prostate in a systematic manner. Press *into* the gland at each location, because when a nodule occurs, it will not project into the rectal lumen. The surface should feel smooth and muscular; search for any distinct nodule or diffuse firmness. Note these characteristics:

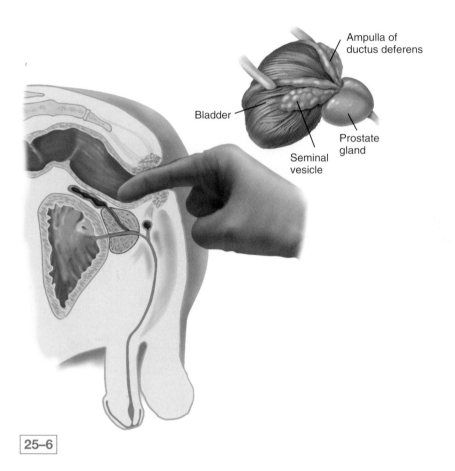

Ampulla of ductus deferens

Bladder

Seminal vesicle

Prostate gland

25–6

Size—2.5 cm long by 4 cm wide; should not protrude more than 1 cm into the rectum

Shape—heart shape, with palpable central groove

Surface—smooth

Consistency—elastic, rubbery

Mobility—slightly movable

Sensitivity—nontender to palpation

Enlarged, or atrophied gland.

Flat with no groove.

Nodular.

Hard; or boggy, soft, fluctuant.

Fixed.

Tender.

Enlarged, firm smooth gland with central groove obliterated suggests benign prostatic hypertrophy.

Swollen, exquisitely tender gland accompanies prostatitis.

Any stone-hard, irregular, fixed nodule indicates carcinoma (see Table 25–3).

In the female, palpate the cervix through the anterior rectal wall. It normally feels like a small round mass. You also may palpate a retroverted uterus or a tampon in the vagina. Do not mistake the cervix or a tampon for a tumor.

NORMAL RANGE OF FINDINGS	ABNORMAL FINDINGS

Withdraw your examining finger; normally, no bright red blood or mucus is on the glove. To complete the examination, offer the person tissues to remove the lubricant and help the person to a more comfortable position.

EXAMINATION OF STOOL. Inspect any feces remaining on the glove. Normally, the color is brown and the consistency is soft.

Jelly-like mucus shreds mixed in stool indicate inflammation.

Bright red blood on stool surface indicates rectal bleeding. Bright red blood mixed with feces indicates possible colonic bleeding.

Test any stool on the glove for **occult blood** using the specimen container that your agency directs. A negative response is normal. If the stool is *hematest* positive, it indicates occult blood. Note that a false-positive finding may occur if the person has ingested significant amounts of red meat within 3 days of the test.

Black tarry stool with distinct malodor indicates upper gastrointestinal bleeding with blood partially digested. (Must lose more than 50 cc from upper gastrointestinal tract to be considered melena.)

Black stool—also occurs with ingesting iron or bismuth preparations.

Gray, tan stool—absent bile pigment, e.g., obstructive jaundice.

Pale yellow, greasy stool—increased fat content (steatorrhea), as occurs with malabsorption syndrome.

Occult bleeding usually indicates cancer of colon.

 DEVELOPMENTAL CONSIDERATIONS

Infants and Children

For the newborn, hold the feet with one hand and flex the knees up onto the abdomen. Note the presence of the anus. Confirm a patent rectum and anus by noting the first meconium stool passed within 24 to 48 hours of birth. To assess sphincter tone, check the *anal reflex*. Gently stroke the anal area and note a quick contraction of the sphincter.

Imperforate anus.

For each infant and child, note that the buttocks are firm and rounded with no masses or lesions. Recall that the *mongolian spot* is a common variation of hyperpigmentation in black, Native American, Mediterranean, and Asian newborns (see Chapter 12).

Flattened buttocks in cystic fibrosis or celiac syndrome.

Coccygeal mass.

Meningocele (sac containing meninges that protrude through a defect in the bony spine).

Tuft of hair or pilonidal dimple.

Pustules indicate secondary infection of diaper rash.

The perianal skin is free of lesions. However, diaper rash is common in children younger than 1 year of age and is exhibited as a generalized reddened area with papules or vesicles.

Signs of physical or sexual abuse.

Fissure—common cause of constipation or rectal bleeding in child. (Painful, so the child does not defecate.)

Omit palpation unless the history or symptoms warrant. When internal palpation is needed, position the infant or child on the back with the legs flexed, and gently insert a gloved, well-lubricated finger into the rectum. Your fifth finger usually is long enough, and its smaller size is more comfortable for the in-

NORMAL RANGE OF FINDINGS	ABNORMAL FINDINGS

fant or child. However, you may need to use the index finger because of its better control and increased tactile sensitivity. On withdrawing the finger, scant bleeding or protruding rectal mucosa may occur.

Inspect the perianal region of the school-age child and adolescent during examination of the genitalia. Internal palpation is not performed routinely.

The Aging Adult

As an aging person performs the Valsalva maneuver, you may note relaxation of the perianal musculature and decreased sphincter control. Otherwise, the full examination proceeds as that described earlier for the younger adult.

SUMMARY CHECKLIST: Anus, Rectum, and Prostate Exam

1. Inspect anus and perianal area
2. Inspect during Valsalva maneuver
3. Palpate anal canal and rectum on all adults
4. Test stool for occult blood

 See Health Promotion Guide on CD

Application and Critical Thinking

SAMPLE CHARTING

SUBJECTIVE

Has one BM daily, soft, brown, no pain, no change in bowel routine. On no medications. Has no history of pruritus, hemorrhoids, fissure, or fistula. Diet includes one to two servings daily each of fresh fruits and vegetables but no whole-grain cereals or breads.

OBJECTIVE

No fissure, hemorrhoids, fistula, or skin lesions in perianal area. Sphincter tone good, no prolapse. Rectal walls smooth, no masses or tenderness. Prostate not enlarged, no masses or tenderness. Stool brown, hematest negative.

FOCUSED ASSESSMENT: CLINICAL CASE STUDY

SUBJECTIVE

C.M. is a 62-year-old white male with chronic obstructive pulmonary disease for 15 years, who today has "diarrhea for 3 days."

7 days PTA: C.M. seen at this agency for acute respiratory infection that was diagnosed as acute bronchitis and treated with oral ampicillin. Took medication as directed.

3 days PTA: symptoms of respiratory infection improved. Ingesting usual diet. Onset of four to five loose, unformed, brown stools a day. No abdominal pain or cramping. No nausea.

Now: diarrhea continues. No blood or mucus noticed in stool. No new foods or restaurant food in past 3 days. Wife not ill.

OBJECTIVE

Vital signs: 37° C-88-18. B/P 142/82.

Respiratory. Respirations unlabored. Barrel chest. Hyperresonant to percussion. Lung sounds clear but diminished. No crackles or rhonchi today.

Abdomen. Flat. Bowel sounds present. No organomegaly or tenderness to palpation.

Rectal. No lesions in perianal area. Sphincter tone good. Rectal walls smooth, no mass or tenderness. Prostate smooth and firm, no median sulcus palpable, no masses or tenderness. Stool brown, hematest negative.

ASSESSMENT

Diarrhea R/T effects of antibiotic medication

NURSING DIAGNOSES COMMONLY ASSOCIATED WITH ANAL AND RECTAL DISORDERS

RELATED FACTORS (Etiology)	DEFINING CHARACTERISTICS (Symptoms and Signs)

DIAGNOSIS: Constipation

Less than adequate dietary intake and bulk	Frequency less than usual pattern
Neuromuscular or musculoskeletal impairment	Hard, formed stools
Pain and discomfort on defecation	Palpable mass
Effects of	Straining at stool
Diagnostic procedures	Less than usual amount of stool
Pregnancy	Decreased bowel sounds
Aging	Gas pain and flatulence
Medication	Abdominal or back pain
Stress or anxiety	Reported feeling of abdominal or rectal fullness or pressure
Weak abdominal musculature	Impaired appetite
Immobility or less than adequate physical activity	Headache
Chronic use of laxatives and enemas	Nausea
Ignoring the urge to defecate	Irritability
Fear of rectal or cardiac pain	Palpable hard stool on rectal examination
Gastrointestinal lesions	

DIAGNOSIS: Bowel incontinence

Diarrhea	Involuntary passage of stool
Impaction	Lack of awareness of need to defecate
Impairment	Lack of awareness of passage of stool
Cognitive	Rectal oozing of stool
Neuromuscular	Urgency
Perceptual	
Large stool volume	
Depression	
Severe anxiety	
Physical or psychological barriers that prevent access to an acceptable toileting area	
Effects of medications	
Excessive use of laxatives	

OTHER RELATED NURSING DIAGNOSES

ACTUAL	RISK/WELLNESS
Perceived Constipation	**Risk**
Diarrhea (see Chapter 21)	Risk for Constipation
Impaired Skin integrity	Risk for Fluid imbalance
	Wellness
	Health-seeking behavior for information on high-fiber diet

ASSESSMENT VIDEO CRITICAL THINKING QUESTION

The Saunders *Physical Examination and Health Assessment* video "Male Genitalia" will direct you to consider the following:

1. Describe abnormal findings that may be noted on inspection of the perianal canal of an infant or child.

Abnormal Findings

TABLE 25–1: Abnormalities of the Anus and Perianal Region

Sinus tract

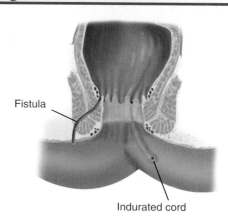

Fistula

Indurated cord

Pilonidal Cyst or Sinus

A hair-containing cyst or sinus located in the midline over the coccyx or lower sacrum. Often opens as a dimple with visible tuft of hair and, possibly, an erythematous halo. Or, may appear as a palpable cyst. When advanced, has a palpable sinus tract. Although it is a congenital disorder, the lesion is first diagnosed between the ages of 15 and 30 years.

Anorectal Fistula

A chronically inflamed gastrointestinal tract creates an abnormal passage from inner anus or rectum out to skin surrounding anus. Usually originates from a local abscess. The red, raised tract opening may drain serosanguineous or purulent matter when pressure is applied. Bidigital palpation may reveal an indurated cord.

Hypertrophic papilla

Fissure

Sentinel tag

◀ Fissure

A painful longitudinal tear in the superficial mucosa at the anal margin. Most fissures (>90%) occur in the posterior midline area. They are frequently accompanied by a papule of hyperplastic skin, called a *sentinel tag,* on the anal margin below. Fissures often result from trauma, e.g., passing a large, hard stool or from irritant diarrheal stools. The person has itching, bleeding, and exquisite pain. A resulting spasm in the sphincters makes the area painful to examine; local anesthesia may be indicated.

Continued

TABLE 25-1: Abnormalities of the Anus and Perianal Region—cont'd

Internal hemorrhoid

Thrombosed external hemorrhoid

◀ Hemorrhoids

These painless, flabby papules are due to a varicose vein of the hemorrhoidal plexus. An *external hemorrhoid* originates below the anorectal junction and is covered by anal skin. When *thrombosed*, it contains clotted blood and becomes a painful, swollen, shiny blue mass that itches and bleeds with defecation. When it resolves, it leaves a painless, flabby skin sac around the anal orifice. An *internal hemorrhoid* originates above the anorectal junction and is covered by mucous membrane. When the person performs a Valsalva maneuver, it may appear as a red mucosal mass. It is not palpable. All hemorrhoids result from increased portal venous pressure, as occurs with straining at stool, chronic constipation, pregnancy, obesity, chronic liver disease, or the low-fiber diet common in Western society.

Rectal Prolapse

The rectal mucous membrane protrudes through the anus, appearing as a moist red doughnut with radiating lines. When prolapse is incomplete, only the mucosa bulges. When complete, it includes the anal sphincters. Occurs following a Valsalva maneuver, such as straining at stool, or with exercise.

Pruritus Ani

Intense perianal itching is manifested by red, raised, thickened, excoriated skin around the anus. Common causes are pinworms in children and fungal infections in adults. The area is swollen and moist, and with a fungal infection, it appears dull grayish-pink. The skin is dry and brittle with psychosomatic itching.

TABLE 25–2: Abnormalities of the Rectum

Submucosal

Perianal   Ischiorectal

Abscess

A localized cavity of pus from infection in a pararectal space. Infection usually extends from an anal crypt. Characterized by persistent throbbing rectal pain. Termed by the space it occupies, e.g., a perianal abscess is superficial around the anal skin, and appears red, hot, swollen, indurated, and tender. An ischiorectal abscess is deep and tender to bidigital palpation. It occurs laterally between the anus and ischial tuberosity and is uncommon.

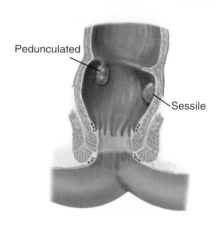

Pedunculated

Sessile

Rectal Polyp

A protruding growth from the rectal mucous membrane that is fairly common. The polyp may be *pedunculated* (on a stalk) or *sessile* (a mound on the surface, close to the mucosal wall). The soft nodule is difficult to palpate. Proctoscopy is needed as well as biopsy to screen for a malignant growth.

Fecal Impaction

A collection of hard, desiccated feces in the rectum. The obstruction often results from decreased bowel motility, in which more water is reabsorbed from the stool. Also occurs with retained barium from gastrointestinal x-ray examination. The person may complain of constipation or of diarrhea as a fecal stream passes around the impaction.

Rolled-edge neoplasm

Carcinoma

A malignant neoplasm in the rectum is asymptomatic, thus the importance of routine rectal palpation. An early lesion may be a single firm nodule. You may palpate an ulcerated center with rolled edges. As the lesion grows, it has an irregular cauliflower shape and is fixed and stone-hard. Refer a person with any rectal lesion for further study because about half are malignant.

TABLE 25–3: **Abnormalities of the Prostate Gland**

Benign Prostatic Hypertrophy (BPH)

S: Urinary frequency, urgency, hesitancy, straining to urinate, weak stream, intermittent stream, sensation of incomplete emptying, nocturia.

O: A symmetric nontender enlargement, commonly occurs in males beginning in the middle years. The prostate surface feels smooth, rubbery, or firm (like the consistency of the nose), with the median sulcus obliterated.

Prostatitis

S: Fever, chills, malaise, urinary frequency and urgency, dysuria, urethral discharge, dull, aching pain in perineal and rectal area.

O: An exquisitely tender enlargement is *acute* inflammation of the prostate gland yielding a swollen, slightly asymmetric gland that is quite tender to palpation.

With a chronic inflammation the signs can vary from tender enlargement with a boggy feel to isolated firm areas due to fibrosis. Or the gland may feel normal.

Carcinoma

S: Frequency, nocturia, hematuria, weak stream, hesitancy, pain or burning on urination, continuous pain in lower back, pelvis, thighs.

O: A malignant neoplasm often starts as a single hard nodule on the posterior surface, producing asymmetry and a change in consistency. As it invades normal tissue, multiple hard nodules appear, or the entire gland feels stone-hard and fixed. The median sulcus is obliterated.

S, Subjective data; *O,* objective data.

BIBLIOGRAPHY

Ahmed DS: Hidden factors in occult blood testing, *Am J Nurs* 100(12):25, Dec 2000.

American Cancer Society: Cancer Statistics, 2002. http://www.cancer.org/docroot/STT/stt_O.asp. Accessed October, 2002.

Chung-Park M: A look at colorectal cancer screening in women, *Nurs Pract* 27(6):43–48, June 2002.

Cydulka RK: Digital rectal examination for trauma: does every patient need one? *Ann Emerg Med* 39(4):462, Apr 2002.

Goolsby M: Screening, diagnosis, and management of prostate cancer: improving primary care outcomes, *Nurs Pract* 23(3):11–36, Mar 1998.

Macias DJ, Sarabia MH, Sklar DP: Male discomfort during the digital rectal examination: does examiner gender make a difference? *Am J Emerg Med* 18(6):676–678, Oct 2000.

Moul JW et al: Prostate-specific antigen values at the time of prostate cancer diagnosis in African-American men, *JAMA* 274(16):1277–1281, Oct 1995.

Pfenninger JL, Zainea GG: Common anorectal conditions, part I. Symptoms and complaints, *Am Fam Physician* 63(12):2391–2398, Jun 15, 2001.

Stern S, Altkorn D, Levinson W: Detection of prostate and colon cancer, *JAMA* 280(2):117–118, July 8, 1998.

Von Eschenback A et al: American Cancer Society guideline for the early detection of prostate cancer: update 1997, *CA Cancer J Clin* 47(5):261–264, Sep–Oct 1997.

Wright VC: When to suspect squamous cancer at colposcopy, *Nurs Pract* 26(9):50–61, Sep 2001.

Female Genitalia

Structure and Function

EXTERNAL GENITALIA

The external genitalia are called the **vulva,** or pudendum (Fig. 26–1). The **mons pubis** is a round, firm pad of adipose tissue covering the symphysis pubis. After puberty, it is covered with hair in the pattern of an inverted triangle. The **labia majora** are two rounded folds of adipose tissue extending from the mons pubis down and around to the perineum. After puberty, hair covers the outer surfaces of the labia, while the inner folds are smooth and moist, and contain sebaceous follicles.

Inside the labia majora are two smaller, darker folds of skin, the **labia minora.** These are joined anteriorly at the clitoris where they form a hood, or prepuce. The labia minora are joined posteriorly by a transverse fold, the **frenulum** or fourchette. The **clitoris** is a small, pea-shaped erectile body, homologous with the male penis and highly sensitive to tactile stimulation.

The labial structures encircle a boat-shaped space, or cleft, termed the **vestibule.** Within it are numerous openings. The **urethral meatus** appears as a dimple 2.5 cm posterior to the clitoris. Surrounding the urethral meatus are the tiny, multiple paraurethral (Skene's) glands. Their ducts are not visible but open posterior to the urethra at the 5 and 7 o'clock positions.

The **vaginal orifice** is posterior to the urethral meatus. It appears either as a thin median slit or as a large opening with irregular edges, depending on the presentation of the membranous **hymen.** The hymen is a thin, circular or crescent-shaped fold that may cover part of the vaginal orifice or may be absent completely. On either side and posterior to the vaginal orifice are two **vestibular (Bartholin's) glands,** which secrete a clear lubricating mucus during intercourse. Their ducts are not visible but open in the groove between the labia minora and the hymen.

INTERNAL GENITALIA

The internal genitalia include the **vagina,** a flattened, tubular canal extending from the orifice up and backward into the pelvis (Fig. 26–2). It is 9 cm long and sits between the rectum posteriorly and the bladder and urethra anteriorly. Its walls are in thick transverse folds, or **rugae,** enabling the vagina to dilate widely during child birth.

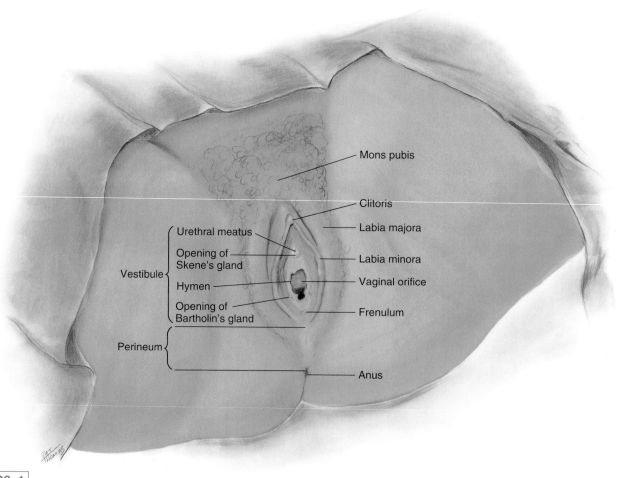

Mons pubis

Clitoris

Labia majora

Labia minora

Vaginal orifice

Frenulum

Anus

Vestibule
- Urethral meatus
- Opening of Skene's gland
- Hymen
- Opening of Bartholin's gland

Perineum

26–1

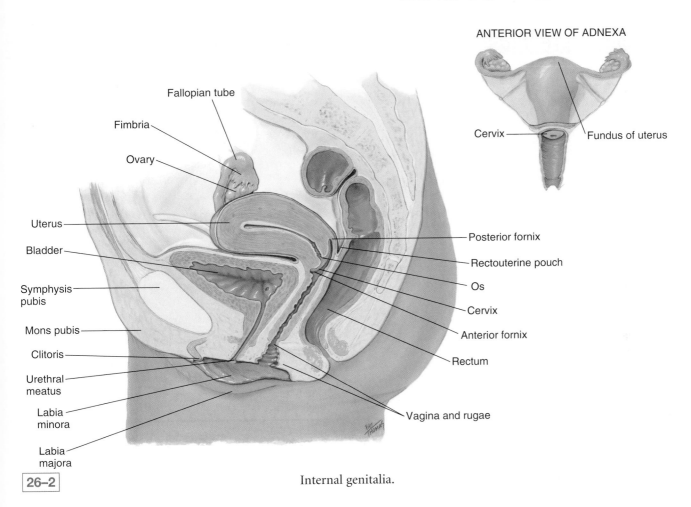

ANTERIOR VIEW OF ADNEXA

26–2 Internal genitalia.

At the end of the canal, the uterine **cervix** projects into the vagina. In the nulliparous female, the cervix appears as a smooth doughnut-shaped area with a small circular hole, or **os.** After childbirth, the os is slightly enlarged and irregular. The cervical epithelium is of two distinct types. The vagina and cervix are covered with smooth, pink, stratified squamous epithelium. Inside the os, the endocervical canal is lined with columnar epithelium that looks red and rough. The point where these two tissues meet is the **squamocolumnar junction** and is not visible.

A continuous recess is present around the cervix, termed the **anterior fornix** in front and the **posterior fornix** in back. Behind the posterior fornix, another deep recess is formed by the peritoneum. It dips down between the rectum and cervix to form the **rectouterine pouch,** or **cul-de-sac of Douglas.**

The **uterus** is a pear-shaped, thick-walled, muscular organ. It is flattened anteroposteriorly, measuring 5.5 to 8 cm long by 3.5 to 4 cm wide and 2 to 2.5 cm thick. It is freely movable, not fixed, and usually tilts forward and superior to the bladder (a position labeled as anteverted and anteflexed, see p. 785).

The **fallopian tubes** are two pliable, trumpet-shaped tubes, 10 cm in length, extending from the uterine fundus laterally to the brim of the pelvis. There, they curve posteriorly, their fimbriated ends located near the **ovaries.** The two ovaries are located one on each side of the uterus at the level of the anterior superior iliac spine. Each is oval shaped, 3 cm long by 2 cm wide by 1 cm thick, and serves to develop ova (eggs) as well as the female hormones.

 DEVELOPMENTAL CONSIDERATIONS

INFANTS AND ADOLESCENTS

At birth, the external genitalia are engorged because of the presence of maternal estrogen. The structures recede in a few weeks, remaining small until puberty. The ovaries are located in the abdomen during childhood. The uterus is small with a straight axis and no anteflexion.

At puberty, estrogens stimulate the growth of cells in the reproductive tract and the development of secondary sex characteristics. The first signs of puberty are breast and pubic hair development, beginning between the ages of 8½ and 13 years. These signs are usually concurrent, but it is not abnormal if they do not develop together. They take about 3 years to complete.

Menarche occurs during the latter half of this sequence, just after the peak of growth velocity. Irregularity of the menstrual cycle is common during adolescence because of the girl's occasional failure to ovulate. With menarche, the uterine body flexes on the cervix. The ovaries now are in the pelvic cavity.

TABLE 26–1: Sex Maturity Ratings (SMR) in Girls

Stage 1 Preadolescent. No pubic hair. Mons and labia covered with fine vellus hair as on abdomen.

Stage 2 Growth sparse and mostly on labia. Long, downy hair, slightly pigmented, straight or only slightly curly.

Stage 3 Growth sparse and spreading over mons pubis. Hair is darker, coarser, curlier.

Stage 4 Hair is adult in type but over smaller area; none on medial thigh.

Stage 5 Adult in type and pattern; inverse triangle. Also on medial thigh surface.

Tanner's table on the five stages of pubic hair development (sex maturity rating [SMR]) is helpful in teaching girls the expected sequence of sexual development (Table 26–1).

These data are derived from Tanner's study of white British females and may not necessarily generalize to all other racial groups. For example, mature Asian women normally have fine sparse pubic hair. However, the U.S. Health Examination Survey (Harlan et al., 1980) studied girls representative of the contemporary United States population. Its findings correlate closely with Tanner's SMR results. One significant difference is that black girls tend to develop breasts and pubic hair earlier than white girls of the same age.

THE PREGNANT FEMALE

Shortly after the first missed menstrual period in the pregnant female, the genitalia show signs of the growing fetus. The cervix softens (*Goodell's sign*) at 4 to 6 weeks, and the vaginal mucosa and cervix look cyanotic (*Chadwick's sign*) at 8 to 12 weeks. These changes occur because of increased vascularity and edema of the cervix and hypertrophy and hyperplasia of the cervical glands. The isthmus of the uterus softens (*Hegar's sign*) at 6 to 8 weeks.

The greatest change is in the uterus itself. It increases in capacity by 500 to 1000 times its nonpregnant state, at first because of hormone stimulation, and then because of the increasing size of its contents (Cunningham et al., 2001). The nonpregnant uterus has a flattened pear shape. Its early growth encroaches on the space occupied by the bladder, which produces the symptom of urinary frequency. By 10 to 12 weeks' gestation, the uterus becomes globular in shape and is too large to stay in the pelvis. At 20 to 24 weeks, the uterus has an oval shape. It rises almost to the liver, displacing the intestines superiorly and laterally.

A clot of thick, tenacious mucus forms in the spaces of the cervical canal (the mucus plug), which protects the fetus from infection. The mucus plug dislodges when labor begins at the end of term, producing a sign of labor called "bloody show." Cervical and vaginal secretions increase during pregnancy and are thick, white, and more acidic. The increased acidity occurs because of the action of *Lactobacillus acidophilus*, which changes glycogen into lactic acid. The acidic pH keeps pathogenic bacteria from multiplying in the vagina, but the increase in glycogen increases the risk of candidiasis (commonly called a yeast infection) during pregnancy.

THE AGING FEMALE

In contrast to the slowly declining hormones in the aging male, the female's hormonal milieu decreases rapidly. *Menopause* is cessation of the menses. Usually this occurs around the ages of 48 to 51 years, although a wide normal variation of ages from 35 to 60 years exists. The stage of menopause includes the preceding 1 to 2 years of decline in ovarian function, shown by irregular menses that gradually become farther apart and produce a lighter flow than usual. The ovaries stop producing progesterone and estrogen. Since cells in the reproductive tract are estrogen dependent, decreased estrogen levels during menopause bring dramatic physical changes.

The uterus shrinks in size because of its decreased myometrium. The ovaries atrophy to 1 to 2 cm and are not palpable after menopause. Ovulation still may occur sporadically after menopause. The sacral ligaments relax, and the pelvic musculature weakens, so the uterus droops. Sometimes it may protrude, or prolapse, into the vagina. The cervix shrinks and looks paler with a thick, glistening epithelium.

The vagina becomes shorter, narrower, and less elastic because of increased connective tissue. Without sexual activity, the vagina atrophies to one half its former length and width. The vaginal epithelium atrophies, becoming thinner, drier, and itchy. This results in a fragile mucosal surface that is at risk for bleeding and vaginitis. Decreased vaginal secretions leave the vagina dry and at risk for irritation and pain with intercourse (dyspareunia). The vaginal pH becomes more alkaline, and a decreased glycogen content occurs from the decreased estrogen. These factors also increase the risk of vaginitis because they create a suitable medium for pathogens.

Externally, the mons pubis looks smaller because the fat pad atrophies. The labia and clitoris gradually decrease in size. Pubic hair becomes thin and sparse.

Declining estrogen levels produce some physiologic changes in the female sexual response cycle (Table 26–2). However, these changes do not affect sexual pleasure and function. Sexual desire and the need for full sexual expression continue. As with the male, the older female is capable of sexual function given reasonably good health and an interested partner. The problem for many older women is finding a socially acceptable sexual partner. Aging women greatly outnumber their male counterparts, and aging women are more likely to be single while males their same age are more likely to be married.

TABLE 26–2: Aging Changes in Sexual Response Cycle

PHASE	PHYSIOLOGIC CHANGE
Excitement	Reduced amount of vaginal secretion and lubrication
Plateau	Less expansion of vagina
	Labia majora do not elevate against perineum
	No color change in labia minora (was from pink to cardinal-red or dark red)
	Size of clitoris decreases after age 60
Orgasm	Shorter duration
Resolution	Occurs more rapidly

Data from Masters WH, Johnson VE: *Human sexual response,* Boston, 1966, Little, Brown, and Company.

Subjective Data

1. Menstrual history	**6.** Vaginal discharge	**10.** Sexually transmitted disease (STD) contact
2. Obstetric history	**7.** Past history	**11.** STD risk reduction
3. Menopause	**8.** Sexual activity	
4. Self-care behaviors	**9.** Contraceptive use	
5. Urinary symptoms		

EXAMINER ASKS	RATIONALE
1. Menstrual history. Tell me about your menstrual periods:	**Menstrual history** is usually nonthreatening, thus it is a good place to start history.
• Date of your last menstrual period? • Age at first period?	LMP—last menstrual period. Menarche—onset between 12 and 14 years indicates normal growth; onset between 16 and 17 years suggests an endocrine problem.
• How often are your periods?	Cycle—normally varies every 18 to 45 days. Amenorrhea—absent menses.
• How many days does your period last? • Usual amount of flow: light, medium, heavy? How many pads or tampons do you use each day or hour? • Any clotting?	Duration—average 3 to 7 days. Menorrhagia—heavy menses. Clotting indicates heavy flow or vaginal pooling.
• Any pain or cramps before or during period? How do you treat it? Interfere with daily activities? Any other associated symptoms: bloating, cramping, breast tenderness, moodiness? Any spotting between periods?	Dysmenorrhea.

EXAMINER ASKS	RATIONALE
2. Obstetric history. Have you ever been pregnant? • How many times? • How many babies have you had? • Any miscarriage or abortion? • For each pregnancy, describe: duration, any complication, labor and delivery, baby's sex, birth weight, condition. • Do you think you may be pregnant now? What symptoms have you noticed?	**Obstetric history.** Gravida—number of pregnancies. Para—number of births. Abortions—interrupted pregnancies, including elective abortions and spontaneous miscarriages.
3. Menopause. Have your periods slowed down or stopped? • Any associated symptoms of menopause, e.g., hot flash, numbness and tingling, headache, palpitations, drenching sweats, mood swings, vaginal dryness, itching? Any treatment? • If hormone replacement, how much? How is it working? Any side effects? • How do you feel about going through menopause?	**Menopause**—cessation of menstruation. Perimenopausal period, from 40 to 55 years of age, has hormone shifts, resulting in vasomotor instability. Side effects of estrogen replacement therapy include fluid retention, breast pain or enlargement, vaginal bleeding. Although this is a normal life stage, reaction varies from acceptance to feelings of loss.
4. Self-care behaviors. How often do you have a gynecologic checkup? • Last Papanicolaou smear? Results? • Has your mother ever mentioned taking hormones while pregnant with you?	Assess **self-care behaviors.** Maternal ingestion of DES (diethylstilbestrol) causes cervical and vaginal abnormalities in female offspring requiring frequent follow-up.
5. Urinary symptoms. Any problems with urinating? Frequently and small amounts? Cannot wait to urinate? • Any burning or pain on urinating? • Awaken during night to urinate? • Blood in the urine? • Urine dark, cloudy, foul smelling? • Any difficulty controlling urine or wetting yourself? • Urinate with a sneeze, laugh, cough, bearing down?	**Urinary symptoms.** Frequency. Urgency. Dysuria. Nocturia. Hematuria. Bile in urine or urinary tract infection. True incontinence—loss of urine without warning. Urgency incontinence—sudden loss, as with acute cystitis. Stress incontinence—loss of urine with physical strain due to muscle weakness.
6. Vaginal discharge. Any unusual **vaginal discharge**? Increased amount? • Character or color: white, yellow-green, gray, curdlike, foul smelling? • When did this begin? • Is the discharge associated with vaginal itching, rash, pain with intercourse? • Taking any medications?	Normal discharge is small, clear or cloudy, and always nonirritating. Suggests vaginal infection; character of discharge often suggests causative organism (see Table 26–6). Acute versus chronic problem. Occurs secondary to irritation from discharge. Dyspareunia occurs with vaginitis of any cause. Factors that increase risk of vaginitis: • Oral contraceptives increase glycogen content of vaginal epithelium, providing fertile medium for some organisms.

EXAMINER ASKS

RATIONALE

- Family history of diabetes?
- What part of your menstrual cycle are you in now?

- Use a vaginal douche? How often?
- Use feminine hygiene spray?
- Wear nonventilating underpants, pantyhose?
- Treated the discharge with anything? Result?

- Broad-spectrum antibiotics alter balance of normal flora.
- Diabetes increases glycogen content.
- Menses, postpartum, menopause have a more alkaline vaginal pH.
- Frequent douching alters pH.
- Spray has risk of contact dermatitis.
- Local irritation.

7. Past history. Any other problems in the genital area? Sores or lesions—now or in the past? How were these treated?
- Any abdominal pain?
- Any past surgery on uterus, ovaries, vagina?

Assess feelings. Some fear loss of sexual response following hysterectomy, which may cause problems in intimate relationships.

8. Sexual activity. Often women have a question about their **sexual relationship** and how it affects their health. Do you?
- Are you in a relationship involving sex now?
- Are aspects of sex satisfactory to you and your partner?
- Satisfied with the way you and partner communicate about sex?
- Satisfied with your ability to respond sexually?
- Do you have more than one sexual partner?

Begin with open-ended question to assess individual needs. Include appropriate questions as a routine part of history:

- Communicates that you accept individual's sexual activity and believe it is important.
- Your comfort with discussion prompts person's interest and possibly relief that the topic has been introduced.
- Establishes a data base for comparison with any future sexual activities.
- Provides opportunity to screen sexual problems.

- What is your sexual preference: relationship with a man, with a woman, both?

Lesbians and bisexual women need to feel acceptance to discuss their health concerns.

9. Contraceptive use. Currently planning a pregnancy, or avoiding pregnancy?
- Do you and your partner use a **contraceptive?** Which method? Is this satisfactory? Do you have any questions about method?
- Which methods have you used in the past? Have you and partner discussed having children?
- Have you ever had any problems becoming pregnant?

If oral contraceptives are used, assess smoking history. Cigarettes increase cardiovascular side effects of oral contraceptives.

Infertility is considered after 1 year of engaging in unprotected sexual intercourse without conceiving.

10. Sexually transmitted disease (STD) contact. Any sexual contact with partner having a sexually transmitted disease, such as gonorrhea, herpes, AIDS, chlamydial infection, venereal warts, syphilis? When? How was this treated? Were there any complications?

11. STD risk reduction. Any precautions to reduce risk of STDs? Use condoms at each episode of sexual intercourse?

EXAMINER ASKS	RATIONALE

Additional History for Infants and Children

1. Does your child have any problem urinating? Pain with urinating, crying, holding genitals? Urinary tract infection?
  - (If the child is older than 2 to 2½ years of age) Has toilet training started? How is it progressing?
  - Does the child wet bed at night? Is this a problem for child or you (parents)? What have you (parents) done?

2. Problem with genital area: itching, rash, vaginal discharge?

Occurs with poor perineal hygiene or insertion of foreign body in vagina.

3. (To child) Has anyone ever touched you in between your legs and you did not want them to? Sometimes that happens to children. They should remember they have not been bad. They should try to tell a big person about it. Can you tell me three different big people you trust who you could talk to?

Screen for sexual abuse. For prevention, teach the child that it's not okay for someone to look at or touch their private parts while telling them it's a secret. Naming three trusted adults will include someone outside the family—important since most molestation is by a parent (Brown, 1997).

Additional History for Preadolescents and Adolescents

Use the following questions, as appropriate, to assess sexual growth and development and sexual behavior. First

  - Ask questions that seem appropriate for girl's age but be aware that norms vary widely. When in doubt, it is better to ask too many questions than to omit something. Children obtain information, often misinformation, from the media and from peers at surprisingly early ages. You can be sure your information will be more thoughtful and accurate.
  - Ask direct, matter-of-fact questions. Avoid sounding judgmental.
  - Start with a *permission statement,* "Often girls your age experience . . . " This conveys that it is normal to think or feel a certain way.
  - Try the open-ended, "When did you . . . " rather than "Do you . . . " This is less threatening because it implies that the topic is normal and unexceptional.

1. Around age 11, but sometimes earlier, girls start to develop breasts and pubic hair. Have you ever seen charts and pictures of normal growth patterns for girls? Let us go over these now.

2. Have your periods started? How did you feel? Were you prepared or surprised?

Assess attitude of girl and parents. Note inadequate preparation or attitude of distaste.

3. Who in your family do you talk to about your body changes and about sex information? How do these talks go? Do you think you get enough information? What about sex education classes at school? Is there a teacher, a nurse or doctor, a minister, a counselor to whom you can talk?

  Often girls your age have questions about sexual activity. Do you have questions? Are you dating? Someone steady?

  Do you and your boyfriend have intercourse? Are you using condoms? What method of protection did you use the last time you had sex?

Avoid the term "sexually active," which is ambiguous.

EXAMINER ASKS	RATIONALE
4. Has anyone ever talked to you about sexually transmitted diseases, such as herpes, gonorrhea, or AIDS?	Teach STD risk reduction.
5. Sometimes it happens that a person touches a girl in a way that she does not want them to. Has that ever happened to you? If that happens, the girl should remember it is not her fault. She should tell another adult about it.	Screen for sexual abuse.

Additional History for the Aging Adult

1. After menopause, noted any vaginal bleeding?	Postmenopausal bleeding warrants further workup and referral.
2. Any vaginal itching, discharge, pain with intercourse?	Associated with atrophic vaginitis.
3. Any pressure in genital area, loss of urine with cough or sneeze, back pain, or constipation?	Occurs with weakened pelvic musculature and uterine prolapse.
4. Are you in a relationship involving sex now? Are aspects of sex satisfactory to you and your partner? Is there adequate privacy for a sexual relationship?	

Objective Data

PREPARATION

Assemble the equipment before helping the woman into position. Arrange within easy reach. Familiarize yourself with the vaginal speculum before the examination. Practice opening and closing the blades, locking them into position, and releasing them. Try both metal and plastic types. Note that the plastic speculum locks and unlocks with a resounding click that can be alarming to the uninformed woman.

A

B

26–3

EQUIPMENT NEEDED

Gloves
Protective clothing for examiner
Goose-necked lamp with a strong light
Vaginal speculum of appropriate size
  (Fig. 26–3)
  Graves' speculum—useful for most
    adult women, available in varying
    lengths and widths
  Pederson speculum—narrow blades,
    useful for young or postmenopausal
    women with narrowed introitus
Large cotton-tipped applicators (rectal
  swabs)
Materials for cytologic study:
  Glass slide with frosted end
  Sterile Cytobrush or cotton-tipped
    applicator
  Ayre's spatula
  Spray fixative
  Specimen container for gonorrhea
    culture (GC)/*Chlamydia*
  Small bottle of normal saline, potas-
    sium hydroxide (KOH), and acetic acid
    (white vinegar)
Lubricant

POSITION

Initially, the woman should be sitting up. An equal status position is important to establish trust and rapport before the vaginal examination.

For the examination, the woman should be placed in the lithotomy position, with the examiner sitting on a stool. Help the woman into lithotomy position, with the body supine, feet in stirrups and knees apart, and buttocks at edge of examining table (Fig. 26–4). Ask the woman to lift her hips as you guide them to the edge of the table. Some women prefer to leave their shoes or socks on. Or, you can place an exam glove over each of the stirrups to warm the stirrups and keep her feet from slipping.

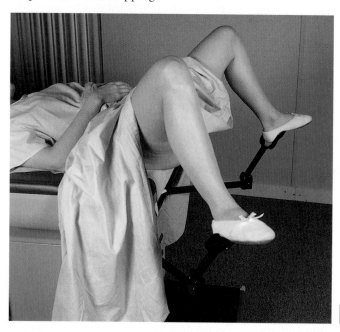

26–4

The arms should be at the woman's sides or across the chest, not over the head, because this position only tightens the abdominal muscles. The traditional mode is to drape the woman fully, covering the stomach and legs, exposing only the vulva to your view. Be sure to push down the drape between the woman's legs so that you can see her face.

The lithotomy position leaves many women feeling helpless and vulnerable. Indeed, many women tolerate the pelvic examination because they consider it basic for health care, yet they find it embarrassing and uncomfortable. Previous examinations may have been painful, or the previous examiner's attitude hurried and patronizing.

The examination need not be this way. You can help the woman relax, decrease her anxiety, and retain a sense of control by employing these measures:

- Have her empty the bladder before the examination.
- Position the exam table so that her perineum is not exposed to an inadvertent open door.
- Ask if she would like a friend, family member, or chaperone present. Position this person by the woman's head to maintain privacy.
- Elevate her head and shoulders to a semi-sitting position to maintain eye contact.
- Place the stirrups so the legs are not abducted too far.
- Explain each step in the examination before you do it.
- Assure the woman she can stop the examination at any point should she feel any discomfort.
- Use a gentle, firm touch, and gradual movements.
- Communicate throughout the examination. Maintain a dialogue to share information.

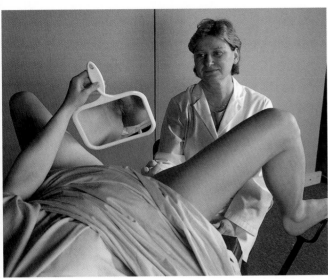

26–5

- Use the techniques of the *educational* or *mirror pelvic examination* (Fig. 26–5). This is a routine examination with some modifications in attitude, position, and communication. First, the woman is considered an active participant, one who is interested in learning and in sharing decisions about her own health care. The woman props herself up on one elbow, or the head of the table is raised. Her other hand holds a mirror between her legs, above the examiner's hands. The woman can see all that the examiner is doing and has a full view of her genitalia.

The mirror works well for teaching normal anatomy and its relation to sexual behavior. Even women who are in a sexual relationship or who have had children may be surprisingly uninformed about their own anatomy. You will find the woman's enthusiasm on seeing her own cervix is rewarding too.

The mirror pelvic examination also works well when abnormalities arise because the woman can see the rationale for treatment and can monitor progress at the next appointment. She is more willing to comply with treatment when she shares in the decision.

NORMAL RANGE OF FINDINGS	ABNORMAL FINDINGS

EXTERNAL GENITALIA

Inspection
Note:
- Skin color (Fig. 26–6).

Refer any suspicious pigmented lesion for biopsy.

26–6

NORMAL RANGE OF FINDINGS

ABNORMAL FINDINGS

- Hair distribution is in the usual female pattern of inverted triangle, although it normally may trail up the abdomen toward the umbilicus.

Consider delayed puberty if no pubic hair or breast development has occurred by age 13.

Nits or lice at the base of pubic hair.

Swelling.

- Labia majora normally are symmetric, plump, and well formed. In the nulliparous woman, labia meet in the midline; following a vaginal delivery, the labia are gaping and slightly shriveled.
- No lesions should be present, except for occasional sebaceous cysts. These are yellowish, 1-cm nodules that are firm, nontender, and often multiple.

Excoriation, nodules, rash, or lesions (see Table 26–3).

With your gloved hand, separate the labia majora to inspect:

- Clitoris (Fig. 26–7).
- Labia minora are dark pink and moist, usually symmetric.

Inflammation or lesions.

26–7

- Urethral opening appears stellate or slitlike and is midline.
- Vaginal opening, or introitus, may appear as a narrow vertical slit or as a larger opening.
- Perineum is smooth. A well-healed episiotomy scar, midline or mediolateral, may be present following a vaginal birth.
- Anus has coarse skin of increased pigmentation (see Chapter 25 for assessment).

Polyp.

Foul-smelling, irritating discharge.

Palpation

Assess the urethra and Skene's glands (Fig. 26–8). Dip your gloved finger in a bowl of warm water to lubricate. Then insert your index finger into the vagina, and gently milk the urethra by applying pressure up and out. This procedure should produce no pain. If any discharge appears, culture it.

Tenderness.

Induration along urethra.

Urethral discharge.

NORMAL RANGE OF FINDINGS	ABNORMAL FINDINGS

26–8

Assess Bartholin's glands. Palpate the posterior parts of the labia majora with your index finger in the vagina and your thumb outside (Fig. 26–9). Normally, the labia feel soft and homogeneous.

Swelling (see Table 26–3).

Induration.

Pain with palpation.

Erythema around or discharge from duct opening.

26–9

Assess the support of pelvic musculature by using these maneuvers:

1. Palpate the perineum. Normally, it feels thick, smooth, and muscular in the nulliparous woman, and thin and rigid in the multiparous woman.
2. Ask the woman to squeeze the vaginal opening around your fingers; it should feel tight in the nulliparous woman and have less tone in the multiparous woman.
3. Using your index and middle fingers, separate the vaginal orifice and ask the woman to strain down. Normally, no bulging of vaginal walls or urinary incontinence occurs.

Tenderness.
Paper-thin perineum.
Absent or decreased tone may diminish sexual satisfaction.

Bulging of the vaginal wall indicates cystocele, rectocele, or uterine prolapse (see Table 26–4).
Urinary incontinence.

INTERNAL GENITALIA

Speculum Examination

Select the proper-sized speculum. Warm and lubricate the speculum under warm running water. Avoid gel lubricant at this point because it is bacteriostatic and would distort cells in the cytology specimen you will collect.

A good technique is to dedicate one hand to the patient and the other hand to picking up equipment in the room. For example, hold the speculum in your left hand (the equipment hand), with the index and the middle fingers surrounding the blades and your thumb under the thumbscrew. This prevents the blades from opening painfully during insertion. With your right index and middle fingers (the patient hand), push the introitus down and open to relax the pubococcygeal muscle (Fig. 26–10). Tilt the width of the blades obliquely and insert the speculum past your right fingers, applying any pressure downward. This avoids pressure on the sensitive urethra above it.

26–10

Ease insertion by asking the woman to bear down. This method relaxes the perineal muscles and opens the introitus. (With experience, you can combine speculum insertion with assessing the support of the vaginal muscles.) As the blades pass your right fingers, withdraw your fingers. Now change the hand holding the speculum to your right hand and turn the width of the blades horizontally. Continue to insert in a 45-degree angle downward toward the small of the woman's back (Fig. 26–11). This matches the natural slope of the vagina.

NORMAL RANGE OF FINDINGS	ABNORMAL FINDINGS

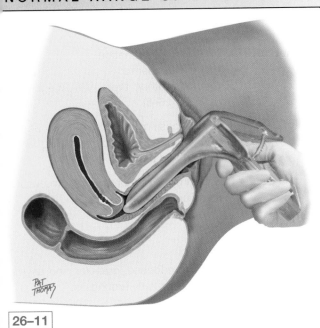

26–11

After the blades are fully inserted, open them by squeezing the handles together (Fig. 26–12). The cervix should be in full view. Sometimes this does not occur (especially with beginning examiners), because the blades are angled above the location of the cervix. Try closing the blades, withdrawing about halfway, and reinserting in a more *downward* plane. Then slowly sweep upward. Once you have the cervix in full view, lock the blades open by tightening the thumbscrew.

26–12

NORMAL RANGE OF FINDINGS

ABNORMAL FINDINGS

Inspect the cervix and its os

Note:

- **Color.** Normally the cervical mucosa is pink and even. During the 2nd month of pregnancy it looks blue (Chadwick's sign), and after menopause it is pale.

- **Position.** Midline, either anterior or posterior. Projects 1 to 3 cm into the vagina.

- **Size.** Diameter is 2.5 cm (1 inch).

- **Os.** This is small and round in the nulliparous woman. In the parous woman, it is a horizontal irregular slit and also may show healed lacerations on the sides (Fig. 26–13).

- **Surface.** This is normally smooth, but **cervical eversion,** or ectropion, may occur normally after vaginal deliveries. The endocervical canal is everted or "rolled out." It looks like a red, beefy halo inside the pink cervix surrounding the os. It is difficult to distinguish this normal variation from an abnormal condition (e.g., erosion, or carcinoma), and biopsy may be needed.

Redness, inflammation.
Pallor with anemia.
Cyanotic other than with pregnancy (see Table 26–5).

Lateral position may be due to adhesion or tumor. Projection of more than 3 cm may be a prolapse.

Hypertrophy of more than 4 cm occurs with inflammation or tumor.

Surface reddened, granular, and asymmetric, particularly around os.

Friable, bleeds easily.

Any lesions: white patch on cervix; strawberry spot.

Refer any suspicious red, white, or pigmented lesion for biopsy (see erosion, ulceration, and carcinoma, Table 26–5).

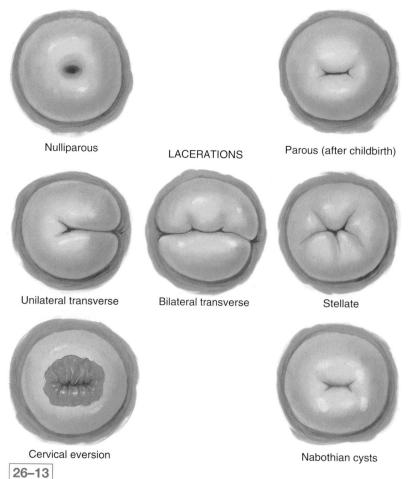

NORMAL VARIATIONS OF THE CERVIX

Nulliparous

LACERATIONS

Parous (after childbirth)

Unilateral transverse

Bilateral transverse

Stellate

Cervical eversion

Nabothian cysts

26–13

NORMAL RANGE OF FINDINGS

Nabothian cysts are benign growths that commonly appear on the cervix after childbirth. They are small, smooth, yellow nodules that may be single or multiple. Less than 1 cm, they are retention cysts due to obstruction of cervical glands.

- **Note the cervical secretions.** Depending on the day of the menstrual cycle, secretions may be clear and thin, or thick, opaque, and stringy. Always they are odorless and nonirritating.

If secretions are copious, swab the area with a thick-tipped rectal swab. This method sponges away secretions, and you have a better view of the structures.

Obtain cervical smears and cultures

The Papanicolaou, or Pap, smear screens for cervical cancer. Do not obtain during the woman's menses or if a heavy infectious discharge is present. Instruct the woman not to douche, have intercourse, or put anything into the vagina within 24 hours before collecting the specimens. Obtain the Pap smear before other specimens so you will not disrupt or remove cells. Laboratories may vary in method, but usually the test consists of three specimens:

VAGINAL POOL. Gently rub the blunt end of an Ayre spatula over the vaginal wall under and lateral to the cervix (Fig. 26–14). Wipe the specimen on a slide and spray with fixative immediately. If the mucosa is very dry (as in a postmenopausal woman), moisten a sterile swab with normal saline to collect this specimen.

26–14

CERVICAL SCRAPE (**Fig. 26–15**). Insert the bifid end of the Ayre spatula into the vagina with the more pointed bump into the cervical os. Rotate it 360 to 720 degrees, using firm pressure. The rounded cervix fits snugly into the spatula's groove. The spatula scrapes the surface of the squamocolumnar junction and cervix as you turn the instrument. Spread the specimen from both sides of the spatula onto a glass slide. Use a single stroke to thin out the specimen, not a back-and-forth motion. This specimen is important for the adolescent whose endocervical cells have not yet migrated into the endocervical canal.

ABNORMAL FINDINGS

Cervical polyp—bright red growth protruding from the os (see Table 26–5).

Foul-smelling, irritating, with yellow, green, white, or gray discharge (see Table 26–6).

26–15

NORMAL RANGE OF FINDINGS

ENDOCERVICAL SPECIMEN (Fig. 26–16). Insert a Cytobrush (instead of a cotton applicator) into the os. A Cytobrush gives a higher yield of endocervical cells at the squamocolumnar junction, or SCJ, and safety for use during pregnancy has been shown (Stillson, Knight, and Elswick, 1997). The woman may feel a slight pinch with the brush and scant bleeding may occur. For this reason, collect the endocervical specimen last so that bleeding will not obscure cytologic evaluation.

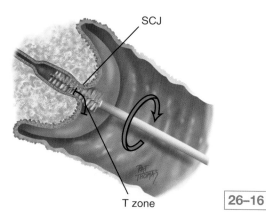

26–16

Rotate the brush 720 degrees in ONE direction in the endocervical canal, either clockwise or counterclockwise. Then rotate the brush gently on a slide to deposit all the cells. Rotate in the opposite direction from the one in which you obtained the specimen. Avoid leaving a thick specimen that would be hard to read under the microscope. Immediately (within 2 seconds) spray the slide with fixative to avoid drying.

For the woman following hysterectomy whose cervix has been removed, collect a scrape from the end of the vagina and a vaginal pool.

Immediately spray the slides with fixative. The frosted ends of the slides should be labeled with the woman's name. Send these to the laboratory with the following necessary data:

- Date of specimen
- Woman's date of birth
- Date of last menstrual period
- Hormone administration if any
- If pregnant, with estimated date of delivery
- Known infections
- Prior surgery or radiation
- Prior abnormal cytology
- Abnormal findings on physical examination

These data are important for accurate interpretation; e.g., a specimen may be interpreted as positive unless the laboratory technicians know the woman has had prior radiation treatment.

To screen for STDs, or if you note any abnormal vaginal discharge, obtain the following samples:

SALINE MOUNT, OR "WET PREP." Spread a sample of the discharge onto a glass slide and add one drop of normal saline and a coverslip.

KOH PREP. To a sample of the discharge on a glass slide, add one drop potassium hydroxide and a coverslip.

GONORRHEA (GC)/CHLAMYDIA CULTURE. Insert a sterile cotton applicator into the os, rotate it 360 degrees, and leave it in place 10 to 20 seconds for complete saturation. Insert into specimen container and label immediately. Note that

NORMAL RANGE OF FINDINGS	ABNORMAL FINDINGS

newer specimen containers from many laboratories combine the GC/*Chlamydia* culture and do not require incubation.

ANAL CULTURE. Insert a sterile cotton swab into the anal canal about 1 cm. Rotate it, and move it side to side. Leave in place 10 to 20 seconds. If the swab collects feces, discard it and begin again. Insert into specimen container.

FIVE PERCENT ACETIC ACID WASH. Acetic acid (white vinegar) screens for asymptomatic human papilloma virus (HPV), which causes genital warts. After all other specimens are gathered, soak a thick-tipped cotton rectal swab with acetic acid and "paint" the cervix. Acetic acid dissolves mucus and temporarily causes intracellular dehydration and coagulation of protein. A normal response (indicating no HPV infection) is no change in the cervical epithelium.

Rapid acetowhitening or blanching, especially with irregular borders, suggests HPV infection (see Table 26–3).

Inspect the vaginal wall
Loosen the thumbscrew but continue to hold the speculum blades open. Slowly withdraw the speculum, rotating it as you go, to fully inspect the vaginal wall. Normally, the wall looks pink, deeply rugated, moist and smooth, and is free of inflammation or lesions. Normal discharge is thin and clear, or opaque and stringy, but always odorless.

Inflammation or lesions.

Leukoplakia, appears as spot of dried white paint.

Vaginal discharge: thick, white, and curd-like with candidiasis; profuse, watery, gray-green, and frothy with trichomoniasis; or any gray, green-yellow, white, or foul-smelling discharge (see Table 26–6).

When the blade ends near the vaginal opening, let them close, but be careful not to pinch the mucosa or catch any hairs. Turn the blades obliquely to avoid stretching the opening. Place the metal speculum in a basin to be cleaned later and soaked in a sterilizing and disinfecting solution; discard the plastic variety. Discard your gloves and wash hands.

Bimanual Examination
Rise to a stand, and have the woman remain in lithotomy position. Drop lubricant onto the first two fingers of your gloved intravaginal hand (Fig. 26–17). Assume the "obstetric" position with the first two fingers extended, the last two flexed onto the palm, and the thumb abducted. Insert your fingers into the vagina, with any pressure directed posteriorly. Wait until the vaginal walls relax, then insert your fingers fully.

26–17

NORMAL RANGE OF FINDINGS

You will use both hands to palpate the internal genitalia to assess their location, size, and mobility, and to screen for any tenderness or mass. One hand is on the abdomen while the other (often the dominant, more sensitive hand) inserts two fingers into the vagina (Fig. 26–18). It does not matter which you choose as the intravaginal hand; try each way, and settle on the most comfortable method for you.

26-18

Palpate the vaginal wall. Normally, it feels smooth and has no area of induration or tenderness.

Nodule.
Tenderness.

CERVIX. Locate the cervix in the midline, often near the anterior vaginal wall. The cervix points in the opposite direction of the fundus of the uterus. Palpate using the palmar surface of the fingers. Note these characteristics of a normal cervix:

• **Consistency**—feels smooth and firm, as the consistency of the tip of the nose. It softens and feels velvety at 5 to 6 weeks of pregnancy (Goodell's sign).

Hard with malignancy.
Nodular.

• **Contour**—evenly rounded.

Irregular.

• **Mobility**—With a finger on either side, move the cervix gently from side to side. Normally, this produces no pain (Fig. 26–19).

Immobile with malignancy.

26-19

NORMAL RANGE OF FINDINGS

Palpate all around the fornices; the wall should feel smooth.

Next, use your abdominal hand to push the pelvic organs closer for your intravaginal fingers to palpate. Place your hand midway between the umbilicus and the symphysis; push down in a slow, firm manner, fingers together and slightly flexed. Brace the elbow of your pelvic arm against your hip, and keep it horizontal. The woman must be relaxed.

UTERUS. With your intravaginal fingers in the anterior fornix, assess the uterus. Determine the position, or *version*, of the uterus (Fig. 26–20). This compares the long axis of the uterus with the long axis of the body. In many women, the uterus is anteverted; you palpate it at the level of the pubis with the cervix pointing posteriorly. Two other positions occur normally (midposition and retroverted), as well as two aspects of flexion, where the long axis of the uterus is not straight but is flexed.

ABNORMAL FINDINGS

Painful with inflammation or ectopic pregnancy.

Anteverted

Midposition

Anteflexed

Retroflexed

Retroverted

26–20

Palpate the uterine wall with your fingers in the fornices. Normally, it feels firm and smooth, with the contour of the fundus rounded. It softens during pregnancy. Bounce the uterus gently between your abdominal and intravaginal hand. It should be freely movable and nontender.

Enlarged uterus (see Table 26–7).

Lateral displacement.

Nodular mass. Irregular, asymmetric uterus. Fixed and immobile.

Tenderness.

NORMAL RANGE OF FINDINGS

ADNEXA. Move both hands to the right to explore the adnexa. Place your abdominal hand on the lower quadrant just inside the anterior iliac spine and your intravaginal fingers in the lateral fornix (Fig. 26–21). Push the abdominal hand in and try to capture the ovary. Often, you cannot feel the ovary. When you can, it normally feels smooth, firm, and almond shaped, and is highly movable, sliding through the fingers. It is slightly sensitive but not painful. The fallopian tube is not palpable normally. No other mass or pulsation should be felt.

Enlarged adnexa. Nodules or mass in adnexa.

Immobile.

Markedly tender (see Table 26–8).

Pulsation or palpable fallopian tube suggests ectopic pregnancy; this warrants immediate referral.

26–21

A note of caution—Normal adnexal structures often are not palpable. Be careful not to mistake an abnormality for a normal structure. To be safe, consider abnormal any mass that you cannot *positively* identify, and refer the woman for further study.

Move to the left to palpate the other side. Then, withdraw your hand and check secretions on the fingers before discarding the glove. Normal secretions are clear or cloudy and odorless.

Rectovaginal Examination

Use this technique to assess the rectovaginal septum, posterior uterine wall, cul-de-sac, and rectum. Change gloves to avoid spreading any possible infection. Lubricate the first two fingers. Instruct the woman that this may feel uncomfortable and will mimic the feeling of moving her bowels. Ask her to bear down as you insert your index finger into the vagina and your middle finger gently into the rectum (Fig. 26–22).

NORMAL RANGE OF FINDINGS	ABNORMAL FINDINGS

Uterus retroflexed

RECTOVAGINAL PALPATION

 26–22

While pushing with the abdominal hand, repeat the steps of the bimanual examination. Try to keep the intravaginal finger on the cervix so the intrarectal finger does not mistake the cervix for a mass. Note:

- Rectovaginal septum should feel smooth, thin, firm, and pliable.
- Rectovaginal pouch, or cul-de-sac, is a potential space and usually not palpated.
- Uterine wall and fundus feel firm and smooth.

Rotate the intrarectal finger to check the rectal wall and anal sphincter tone. (See Chapter 25 for assessment of anus and rectum.) Check your gloved finger as you withdraw; test any adherent stool for occult blood.

Give the woman tissues to wipe the area and help her up. Remind her to slide her hips back from the edge before sitting up so she will not fall.

DEVELOPMENTAL CONSIDERATIONS

Infants and Children

PREPARATION

- **Infant**—place on examination table.
- **Toddler/preschooler**—place on parent's lap.
  Frog-leg position—hips flexed, soles of feet together and up to bottom.
  Preschool child may want to separate her own labia.
  No drapes—the young girl wants to see what you are doing.
- **School-age child**—place on examination table, frog-leg position, no drapes.

During childhood, a routine screening is limited to inspection of the external genitalia to determine that (1) the structures are intact, (2) the vagina is present, and (3) the hymen is patent.

Nodular or thickened.

NORMAL RANGE OF FINDINGS

ABNORMAL FINDINGS

The newborn's genitalia are somewhat engorged. The labia majora are swollen, the labia minora are prominent and protrude beyond the labia majora, the clitoris looks relatively large, and the hymen appears thick. Because of transient engorgement, the vaginal opening is more difficult to see now than it will be later. Place your thumbs on the labia majora. Push laterally while pushing the perineum down, and try to note the vaginal opening above the hymenal ring. Do not palpate the clitoris because it is very sensitive.

A sanguineous vaginal discharge and/or leukorrhea (mucoid discharge) are normal during the first few weeks because of the maternal estrogen effect. (This also may cause transient breast engorgement and secretion.) During the early weeks, the genital engorgement resolves, and the labia minora atrophy and remain small until puberty (Fig. 26–23).

Ambiguous genitalia are rare but are suggested by a markedly enlarged clitoris, fusion of the labia (resembling scrotum), and palpable mass in fused labia (resembling testes) (see Table 26–9).

Imperforate hymen warrants referral.

Lesions, rash.

26–23

Between the ages of 2 months and 7 years, the labia majora are flat, the labia minora are thin, the clitoris is relatively small, and the hymen is tissue-paper thin. Normally, no irritation or foul-smelling discharge is present.

In the young school-age girl (7 to 10 years), the mons pubis thickens, the labia majora thicken, and the labia minora become slightly rounded. Pubic hair appears beginning around age 11, although sparse pubic hair may occur as early as age 8 years. Normally, the hymen is perforate.

Almost always in these age groups, an external examination will suffice. If needed, an internal pelvic examination is best performed by a pediatric gynecologist using specialized instruments.

The Adolescent

The adolescent girl has special needs during the genitalia examination. Examine her alone, without the mother present. Assure her of privacy and confidentiality. Allow plenty of time for health education and discussion of pubertal progress. Assess her growth velocity and menstrual history, and use the SMR charts to teach breast and pubic hair development. Assure her that increased vaginal fluid (physiologic *leukorrhea)* is normal because of the estrogen effect.

Poor perineal hygiene.
Pest inhabitants. Excoriations.
During and after toddler age, foul-smelling discharge occurs with lodging of foreign body, pinworms, or infection.

Absence of pubic hair by 13 years indicates delayed puberty.
Amenorrhea in adolescent, together with bluish and bulging hymen, indicates imperforate hymen and warrants referral.

NORMAL RANGE OF FINDINGS	ABNORMAL FINDINGS

A pelvic examination is indicated when contraception is desired, when the girl's sexual activity includes intercourse, or at age 18 years in virgins. Periodic Pap smears also are started when intercourse begins. Although the techniques of the examination are listed in the adult section, you will need to provide additional time and psychological support for the adolescent having her first pelvic examination.

The experience of the first pelvic examination determines how the adolescent will approach future care. Your accepting attitude and gentle, unhurried approach are important. You have a unique teaching opportunity here. Take the time to teach, using the girl's own body as illustration. Your frank discussion of anatomy and sexual behavior communicates that these topics are acceptable to discuss and not taboo with health care providers. This affirms the girl's self-concept.

During the bimanual examination, note that the adnexa are not palpable in the adolescent.

Pelvic or adnexal mass.

The Pregnant Female

Depending on the week of gestation of the pregnancy, inspection shows the enlarging abdomen (see Fig. 27–1 in the following chapter). The height of the fundus ascends gradually as the fetus grows. At 16 weeks, the fundus is palpable halfway between the symphysis and umbilicus; at 20 weeks, at the lower edge of the umbilicus; at 28 weeks, halfway between the umbilicus and the xiphoid; and at 34 to 36 weeks, almost to the xiphoid. Then close to term, the fundus drops as the fetal head engages in the pelvis.

The external genitalia show hyperemia of the perineum and vulva because of increased vascularity. Varicose veins may be visible in the labia or legs. Hemorrhoids may show around the anus. Both are caused by interruption in venous return from the pressure of the fetus.

Internally, the walls of the vagina appear violet or blue (Chadwick's sign) because of hyperemia. The vaginal walls are deeply rugated and the vaginal mucosa thickens. The cervix looks blue, feels velvety, and feels softer than in the nonpregnant state, making it a bit more difficult to differentiate from the vaginal walls.

During bimanual examination, the isthmus of the uterus feels softer and is more easily compressed between your two hands (Hegar's sign). The fundus balloons between your two hands; it feels connected to, but distinct from, the cervix because the isthmus is so soft.

Search the adnexal area carefully during early pregnancy. Normally, the adnexal structures are not palpable.

An ectopic pregnancy has serious consequences (see Table 26–8).

The Aging Adult

Natural lubrication is decreased; to avoid a painful examination, take care to lubricate instruments and the examining hand adequately. Use the Pedersen speculum (rather than the Graves) because its narrower, flatter blades are more comfortable in women with vaginal stenosis or dryness.

Menopause and the resulting decrease in estrogen production cause numerous physical changes. Pubic hair gradually decreases, becoming thin and sparse in later years. The skin is thinner and fat deposits decrease, leaving the mons pubis smaller and the labia flatter. Clitoris size also decreases after age 60.

Internally, the rugae of the vaginal walls decrease, and the walls look pale pink because of the thinned epithelium. The cervix shrinks and looks pale and glistening. It may retract, appearing to be flush with the vaginal wall. In some, it is hard to distinguish the cervix from the surrounding vaginal mucosa. Alternately, the cervix may protrude into the vagina if the uterus has prolapsed.

Refer any suspicious red, white, or pigmented lesion for biopsy.

Vaginal atrophy increases the risk of infection and trauma.

With the bimanual examination, you may need to insert only one gloved finger if vaginal stenosis exists. The uterus feels smaller and firmer, and the ovaries are not palpable normally.

Refer any mass for prompt evaluation.

NORMAL RANGE OF FINDINGS	ABNORMAL FINDINGS

Prior surgery for hysterectomy does not preclude the need for routine gynecologic care, including the Pap smear. The Pap smear can help detect gynecologic malignancies even when the cervix has been removed. Be aware that older women may have special needs and will appreciate the following plans of care: for those with arthritis, taking a mild analgesic or antiinflammatory before the appointment may ease joint pain in positioning; schedule appointment times when joint pain or stiffness is at its least; allow extra time for positioning and "unpositioning" after the examination; and be careful to maintain dignity and privacy.

SUMMARY CHECKLIST: Female Genitalia Exam

1. Inspect external genitalia
2. Palpate labia, Skene's and Bartholin's glands
3. Using vaginal speculum, inspect cervix and vagina
4. Obtain specimens for cytologic study
5. Perform bimanual examination: cervix, uterus, adnexa
6. Perform rectovaginal examination
7. Test stool for occult blood

 See Health Promotion Guide on CD

Application and Critical Thinking

SAMPLE CHARTING

SUBJECTIVE

Menarche age 12, cycle usually q 28 days, duration 5 days, flow moderate, no dysmenorrhea, LMP April 3. Grav O/Para O/Ab O. Gyne checkups yearly. Last Pap test 1 year PTA, negative.

No urinary problems, no irritating or foul-smelling vaginal discharge, no sores or lesions, no history pelvic surgery. Satisfied with sexual relationship with husband, uses vaginal diaphragm for birth control, no plans for pregnancy at this time. Aware of no STD contact to self or husband.

OBJECTIVE

External genitalia—no swelling, lesions, or discharge. No urethral swelling or discharge. Internal—vaginal walls have no bulging or lesions, cervix pink with no lesions, scant clear mucoid discharge.

Bimanual—no pain on moving cervix, uterus anteflexed and anteverted, no enlargement or irregularity. Adnexa—ovaries not enlarged. Rectal—no hemorrhoids, fissures or lesions, no masses or tenderness, stool brown with guaiac test negative.

FOCUSED ASSESSMENT: CLINICAL CASE STUDY 1

J.K., 27-year-old, white, married newspaper reporter, Grav O/Para O/Ab O. Presents at clinic with "urinary burning, vaginal itching, and discharge × 4 days."

SUBJECTIVE

3 weeks PTA: treated at clinic for bronchitis with erythromycin. Improved within 5 days.

4 to 5 days PTA: noted burning on urination, intense vaginal itching, thick, white, "smelly" discharge. Warm water douche—no relief.

No previous history vaginal infection, urinary tract infection, or pelvic surgery. Monogamous sexual relationship, has used low-estrogen birth control pills for 3 years with no side effects.

OBJECTIVE

Vulva and vagina erythematous and edematous. Thick, white, curdlike discharge clinging to vaginal walls. Cervix pink, no lesions. Bimanual examination—no pain on palpating cervix, uterus not enlarged, ovaries not enlarged.

Specimens: Pap smear, GC/Chlamydia to lab. KOH prep shows mycelia and spores of Candida albicans.

ASSESSMENT

Candida vaginitis
Pain R/T infectious process

FOCUSED ASSESSMENT: CLINICAL CASE STUDY 2

Brenda, 17-year-old, white high school student, comes to clinic for pelvic examination.

SUBJECTIVE

Menarche 12 years, cycle q 30 days, duration 6 days, mild cramps relieved by acetaminophen. LMP March 10. No dysuria, vaginal discharge, vaginal itching. Relationship involving intercourse with one boyfriend for 8 months PTA. For birth control, boyfriend uses condoms "sometimes." Wants to start birth control pills. Never had pelvic examination. No knowledge of breast self-examination. No knowledge of STDs except AIDS. Smokes cigarettes, 1/2 PPD, started age 11.

OBJECTIVE

Breasts—symmetric, no lesions or discharge, palpation reveals no mass or tenderness.
   External genitalia—no redness, lesions, or discharge. Internal genitalia—vaginal walls and cervix pink with no lesions or discharge. Specimens obtained. Acetic acid wash shows no acetowhitening.
   Bimanual—no tenderness to palpation, uterus anteverted with no enlargement, ovaries not enlarged. Rectum—no masses, fissure, or tenderness. Stool brown and guaiac test negative.
   Specimens—GC, Chlamydia, Pap smear to lab.

ASSESSMENT

Breast and pelvic structures appear healthy.
   Deficient knowledge regarding: breast self-examination; birth control measures; STD prevention; cigarette smoking R/T lack of exposure

NURSING DIAGNOSES COMMONLY ASSOCIATED WITH THE FEMALE GENITALIA AND RELATED DISORDERS

RELATED FACTORS (Etiology)	DEFINING CHARACTERISTICS (Symptoms and Signs)
DIAGNOSIS: Sexual dysfunction	
Depression	Decreased or absent sexual desire
Disturbance in self-esteem or body image	Impotence
Lack of significant other	Delayed development of secondary sex characteristics
Lack of privacy	Sexual promiscuity
Effects of actual or perceived limitation imposed by disease and/or therapy	Exhibitionism
	Guilt
Substance abuse	Alterations in achieving perceived sex role or sexual satisfaction
Physical or psychosocial abuse	Verbalization about the problem
Dysfunctional interpersonal relationships	Conflicts involving values
Ineffective or absent role models	Changes in interest in self and others
Failure to identify satisfactorily with same-sex parent	Seeking confirmation of desirability
Cultural norms regarding male/female roles	Voyeurism
Values conflict	Transsexualism
Knowledge deficit	Transvestism
	Masochism/sadism

DIAGNOSIS: Functional Incontinence	
Deficits	Unpredictable voiding pattern
Cognitive	Unrecognized signals of bladder fullness
Motor	Urge to void or bladder contractions sufficiently strong to
Sensory	result in loss of urine before reaching an appropriate site
Altered environment	or receptacle

Continued

RELATED FACTORS (Etiology)	DEFINING CHARACTERISTICS (Symptoms and Signs)

DIAGNOSIS: Rape-trauma syndrome

Rape event

Acute Phase
Emotional reactions
  Anger
  Crying
  Overcontrol
  Panic
  Denial
  Self-blame
  Emotional shock
  Embarrassment
  Fear of being alone
  Humiliation
  Fear of physical violence and death
  Mistrust of the opposite sex
  Desire for revenge
  Change in sexual behavior
Multiple physical symptoms
  Muscle tension
  Pain
  Sleep pattern disturbance
  Gastrointestinal irritability
  Genitourinary discomfort
Long-Term Phase
Mentally reliving rape
Depression
Loss of self-confidence
Changes in lifestyle
  Changes in residence
  Dealing with repetitive nightmares and phobias
Anxiety
Ambivalence about own sexuality

OTHER RELATED NURSING DIAGNOSES

ACTUAL	RISK/WELLNESS
Ineffective Sexuality patterns (see Chapter 24)	**Risk**
Impaired Skin integrity (see Chapters 12 and 24)	Risk for urinary urge incontinence
Pain	Risk for infection
Stress Incontinence	Risk for post-trauma syndrome
Reflex Incontinence	**Wellness**
Total Incontinence	Health seeking behavior for information on STD risk
Urge Incontinence	reduction

 ASSESSMENT VIDEO CRITICAL THINKING QUESTIONS

The Saunders *Physical Examination and Health Assessment* video "Female Genitalia" will direct you to consider the following:

1. What presenting complaint would lead you to assess the female genitalia?
2. How may you adapt the female genitalia assessment to allow for health education?
3. How do normal genitalia assessment findings differ between nulliparous women and parous women who gave birth vaginally?
4. What normal and abnormal assessment findings may commonly be detected by a rectovaginal examination?

Abnormal Findings

TABLE 26–3: Abnormalities of the External Genitalia

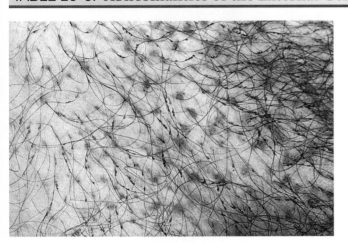

Pediculosis Pubis (Crab Lice)

S: Severe perineal itching.
O: Excoriations and erythematous areas. May see little dark spots (lice are small), nits (eggs) adherent to pubic hair near roots. Usually localized in pubic hair, occasionally in eyebrows or eyelashes.

Herpes Simplex Virus—Type 2 (Herpes Genitalis)*

S: Episodes of local pain, dysuria, fever.
O: Clusters of small, shallow vesicles with surrounding erythema; erupt on genital areas and inner thigh. Also, inguinal adenopathy, edema. Vesicles on labia rupture in 1 to 3 days, leaving painful ulcers. Initial infection lasts 7 to 10 days. Virus remains dormant indefinitely; recurrent infections last 3 to 10 days with milder symptoms.

Syphilitic Chancre*

O: Begins as a small, solitary silvery papule that erodes to a red, round or oval, superficial ulcer with a yellowish serous discharge. Palpation—nontender indurated base; can be lifted like a button between thumb and finger. Nontender inguinal lymphadenopathy.

Reprinted from *Colour Atlas of Infectious Diseases,* 3rd edition, Emond, p. 161, 1995, by permission of the publisher Mosby.

Red Rash—Contact Dermatitis

S: History of skin contact with allergenic substance in environment, intense pruritus.
O: Primary lesion—red, swollen, vesicles. Then may have weeping of lesions, crusts, scales, thickening of skin, excoriations from scratching. May result from reaction to feminine hygiene spray or synthetic underclothing.

*This condition is a sexually transmitted disease (STD). The classic term, *venereal disease,* a disease transmitted only by sexual intercourse, now is obsolete. A broader category, STDs, includes all conditions that are *usually* or *can be* transmitted during sexual intercourse or intimate sexual contact with an infected partner. Although not inclusive of all STDs, the conditions described in this table encompass more common conditions.

S, Subjective data; O, objective data.

Table continued on following page

TABLE 26–3: Abnormalities of the External Genitalia—cont'd

Genital Human Papillomavirus (HPV, Condylomata Acuminata, Genital Warts)*

S: Painless warty growths, may be unnoticed by woman.
O: Pink or flesh-colored, soft, pointed, moist, warty papules. Single or multiple in a cauliflowerlike patch. Occur around vulva, introitus, anus, vagina, cervix.

HPV infection is common among sexually active women, especially adolescents, regardless of ethnicity or socioeconomic status. Risk factors include early age at menarche and multiple sexual partners. The long incubation period (6 weeks to 8 months) makes it difficult to establish history of exposure. A strong association of HPV infection and abnormal cervical cytology exists.

Abscess of Bartholin's Gland

S: Local pain, can be severe.
O: Overlying skin red and hot. Posterior part of labia swollen; palpable fluctuant mass and tenderness. Mucosa shows red spot at site of duct opening; can express purulent discharge. Often secondary to gonococcal infection.*

Reprinted from *Colour Atlas of Infectious Diseases,* 3rd edition, Emond, p. 161, 1995, by permission of the publisher Mosby.

Urethritis (not illustrated)

S: Dysuria.
O: Palpation of anterior vaginal wall shows erythema, tenderness, induration along urethra, purulent discharge from meatus. Caused by *Neisseria gonorrhoeae, Chlamydia,* or *Staphylococcus* infection.

Urethral Caruncle

S: Tender, painful with urination, urinary frequency, hematuria, dyspareunia, or asymptomatic.
O: Small, deep red mass protruding from meatus; usually secondary to urethritis or skenitis; lesion may bleed on contact.

*This condition is a sexually transmitted disease (STD). The classic term, *venereal disease,* a disease transmitted only by sexual intercourse, now is obsolete. A broader category, STDs, includes all conditions that are *usually* or *can be* transmitted during sexual intercourse or intimate sexual contact with an infected partner. Although not inclusive of all STDs, the conditions described in this table encompass more common conditions.

S, Subjective data; *O,* objective data.

TABLE 26–4: Abnormalities of the Pelvic Musculature

Cystocele (with prolapse)

S: Feeling of pressure in vagina, stress incontinence.

O: With straining or standing, note introitus widening and the presence of a soft, round anterior bulge. The bladder, covered by vaginal mucosa, prolapses into vagina, in this case with a uterine prolapse.

Rectocele

S: Feeling of pressure in vagina, possibly constipation.

O: With straining or standing, note introitus widening and the presence of a soft, round bulge from posterior. Here, part of the rectum, covered by vaginal mucosa, prolapses into vagina.

◀ Uterine Prolapse

O: With straining or standing, uterus protrudes into vagina. Prolapse is graded: first degree, cervix appears at introitus with straining; second degree, cervix bulges outside introitus with straining; third degree (in this case), whole uterus protrudes even without straining—essentially, uterus is inside out.

S, Subjective data; *O,* objective data.

ABNORMAL FINDINGS

TABLE 26–5: **Abnormalities of the Cervix**

Bluish Cervix—Cyanosis

O: Bluish discoloration of the mucosa occurs normally in pregnancy (Chadwick's sign at 6 to 8 weeks' gestation) and with any other condition causing hypoxia or venous congestion, e.g., heart failure, pelvic tumor.

Erosion

O: Cervical lips inflamed and eroded. Reddened granular surface is superficial inflammation, with no ulceration (loss of tissue). Usually secondary to purulent or mucopurulent cervical discharge. Biopsy needed to distinguish erosion from carcinoma; cannot rely on inspection.

Human Papillomavirus (HPV, Condylomata)

O: Virus can appear in various forms when affecting cervical epithelium. Here warty growth appears as abnormal thickened white epithelium. Visibility of lesion is enhanced by acetic acid (vinegar) wash, which dissolves mucus and temporarily causes intracellular dehydration and coagulation of protein.

Polyp

S: May have mucoid discharge or bleeding.
O: Bright red, soft, pedunculated growth emerges from os. It is a benign lesion, but this must be determined by biopsy. May be lined with squamous or columnar epithelium.

◀ Diethylstilbestrol (DES) Syndrome

S: Prenatal exposure to DES causes cervical and vaginal abnormalities.
O: Red, granular patches of columnar epithelium extend beyond normal squamocolumnar junction onto cervix and into fornices (vaginal adenosis). Also cervical abnormalities: circular groove, transverse ridge, protuberant anterior lip, "cocks-comb" formation. Warrants monitoring by physician.

S, Subjective data; *O,* objective data.

Continued

TABLE 26–5: Abnormalities of the Cervix—cont'd

◀ Carcinoma

S: Bleeding between menstrual periods or after menopause, unusual vaginal discharge.

O: Chronic ulcer and induration are early signs of carcinoma, although the lesion may or may not show on the exocervix. (Here, lesion is mostly around the external os.) Diagnosed by Papanicolaou smear and biopsy. Risk factors for cervical cancer are early age at first intercourse, multiple sex partners, cigarette smoking, certain sexually transmitted diseases.

S, Subjective data; *O,* objective data.

TABLE 26–6: Vulvovaginal Inflammations

Atrophic Vaginitis

S: Postmenopausal vaginal itching, dryness, burning sensation, dyspareunia, mucoid discharge (may be flecked with blood).

O: Pale mucosa with abraded areas that bleed easily; may have bloody discharge.

An opportunistic infection related to chronic estrogen deficiency.

Candidiasis (Moniliasis)

S: Intense pruritus, thick whitish discharge.

O: Vulva and vagina are erythematous and edematous. Discharge is usually thick, white, curdy, "like cottage cheese." Diagnose by microscopic examination of discharge on potassium hydroxide wet mount.

Predisposing causes—use of oral contraceptives or antibiotics, more alkaline vaginal pH (as with menstrual periods, postpartum, menopause), also pregnancy from increased glycogen and diabetes.

*This condition is considered an STD.
S, Subjective data; *O,* objective data.

Table continued on following page

TABLE 26–6: Vulvovaginal Inflammations—cont'd

Trichomoniasis*

S: Pruritus, watery and often malodorous vaginal discharge, urinary frequency, terminal dysuria. Symptoms are worse during menstruation when the pH becomes optimal for the organism's growth.

O: Vulva may be erythematous. Vagina diffusely red, granular, occasionally with red raised papules and petechiae ("strawberry" appearance). Frothy, yellow-green, foul-smelling discharge. Microscopic examination of saline wet mount specimen shows characteristic flagellated cells.

Bacterial Vaginosis (*Gardnerella vaginalis, Haemophilus vaginalis,* or Nonspecific Vaginitis)*

S: Profuse discharge, "constant wetness" with "foul, fishy, rotten" odor.

O: Thin, creamy, gray-white, malodorous discharge. No inflammation on vaginal wall or cervix because this is a surface parasite. Microscopic view of saline wet mount specimen shows typical "clue cells."

Chlamydia*

S: (Mimics gonorrhea.) Three of four infected women have no symptoms. May have urinary frequency, dysuria, or vaginal discharge, postcoital bleeding.

O: May have yellow or green mucopurulent discharge, friable cervix, cervical motion tenderness. Signs are subtle, easily mistaken for gonorrhea. The two are important to distinguish because antibiotic treatment is different; if the wrong drug is given or if the condition is untreated, chlamydia can ascend the reproductive tract to cause pelvic inflammatory disease (PID), and result in infertility. This is the most common STD in the United States; the highest prevalence is among sexually active adolescent girls, with an incidence of almost 30 percent in some settings (Burstein et al., 1998). Clinicians are urged to screen all sexually active girls every 6 months, regardless of symptoms or risk.

Gonorrhea*

S: Variable: vaginal discharge, dysuria, abnormal uterine bleeding, abscess in Bartholin's or Skene's glands; the majority of cases are asymptomatic.

O: Often no signs are apparent. May have purulent vaginal discharge. Diagnose by positive culture of organism. If the condition is untreated, it may progress to acute salpingitis, pelvic inflammatory disease (PID).

*This condition is considered an STD.
S, Subjective data; *O*, objective data.

TABLE 26–7: Conditions of Uterine Enlargement

Pregnancy

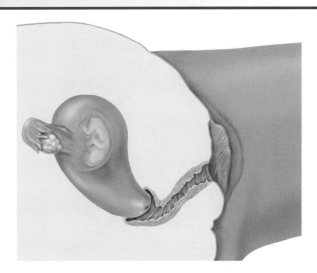

Obviously a normal condition, pregnancy is included here for comparison.

S: Amenorrhea, fatigue, breast engorgement, nausea, change in food tolerance, weight gain.

O: Early signs: cyanosis of vaginal mucosa and cervix (Chadwick's sign). Palpation—soft consistency of cervix, enlarging uterus with compressible fundus and isthmus (Hegar's sign at 10 to 12 weeks).

Myomas (Leiomyomas, Uterine Fibroids)

S: Varies, depending on size and location. Often no symptoms. When symptoms do occur, include vague discomfort, bloating, heaviness, pelvic pressure, dyspareunia, urinary frequency, backache, or hypermenorrhea if myoma disturbs endometrium. Heavy bleeding produces anemia.

O: Uterus irregularly enlarged, firm, mobile, and nodular with hard, painless nodules in the uterine wall.

They are usually benign. Highest incidence between the ages of 30 and 45 years and in blacks. Myomas are estrogen dependent; after menopause, the lesions usually regress but do not disappear. Surgery may be indicated.

Carcinoma of the Endometrium

S: Abnormal and intermenstrual bleeding before menopause; postmenopausal bleeding or mucosanguineous discharge. Pain and weight loss occur late in the disease.

O: Uterus may be enlarged.

The Pap smear is rarely effective in detecting endometrial cancer. Women at high risk should have an endometrial tissue sample evaluated at menopause and periodically thereafter (American Cancer Society, 1998). Risk factors for endometrial cancer are early menarche, late menopause, history of infertility, failure to ovulate, tamoxifen, unopposed estrogen therapy (which continually stimulates the endometrium, causing hyperplasia), and obesity (which increases endogenous estrogen).

S, Subjective data; *O,* objective data.

Table continued on following page

TABLE 26–7: Conditions of Uterine Enlargement—cont'd

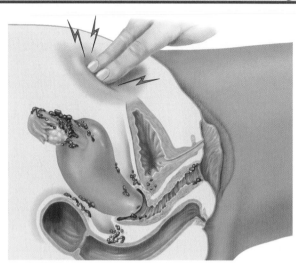

◀ Endometriosis

S: Cyclic or chronic pelvic pain, occurring as dysmenorrhea, or dyspareunia, low backache. Also may have irregular uterine bleeding or hypermenorrhea or may be asymptomatic.

O: Uterus fixed, tender to movement. Small, firm nodular masses tender to palpation on posterior aspect of fundus, uterosacral ligaments, ovaries, sigmoid colon. Ovaries often enlarged.

Masses are aberrant growths of endometrial tissue scattered throughout pelvis due to transplantation of tissue by retrograde menstruation. Ectopic tissue responds to hormone stimulation; builds up between periods, sloughs during menstruation. May cause infertility due to pelvic adhesions, tubal obstruction, decreased ovarian function.

S, Subjective data; *O*, objective data.

TABLE 26–8: Adnexal Enlargement

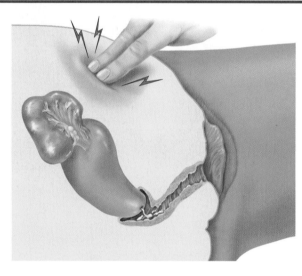

◀ Fallopian Tube Mass—Acute Salpingitis (Pelvic Inflammatory Disease [PID])

S: Sudden fever >38° C or 100.4° F, suprapubic pain and tenderness.

O: Acute—rigid boardlike lower abdominal musculature. May have purulent discharge from cervix. Movement of uterus and cervix causes intense pain. Pain in lateral fornices and adnexa. Bilateral adnexal masses difficult to palpate because of pain and muscle spasm. Chronic—bilateral, tender, fixed adnexal masses.

Complications include ectopic pregnancy, infertility, and reinfection. PID usually caused by *Neisseria gonorrhoeae* and *Chlamydia trachomatis.*

◀ Fallopian Tube Mass—Ectopic Pregnancy

S: Amenorrhea or irregular vaginal bleeding, pelvic pain.

O: Softening of cervix and fundus; movement of cervix and uterus causes pain; palpable tender pelvic mass, which is solid, mobile, unilateral.

This has potential for serious sequelae; seek gynecologic consultation immediately before the mass ruptures or shows signs of acute peritonitis.

S, Subjective data; *O*, objective data.

Continued

TABLE 26–8: Adnexal Enlargement—cont'd

Fluctuant Ovarian Mass—Ovarian Cyst

S: Usually asymptomatic.

O: Smooth, round, fluctuant, mobile, nontender mass on ovary. Some cysts resolve spontaneously within 60 days but must be followed closely.

S, Subjective data; *O*, objective data.

Solid Ovarian Mass—Ovarian Cancer

S: Usually asymptomatic. May have abdominal enlargement from fluid accumulation.

O: Solid tumor palpated on ovary. Heavy, solid, fixed, poorly defined mass suggests malignancy; benign mass may feel mobile and solid.

Biopsy necessary to distinguish the two types of masses. The Pap smear does not detect ovarian cancer. Women over age 40 should have a thorough pelvic examination every year.

TABLE 26–9: Abnormalities in Pediatric Genitalia

Ambiguous Genitalia

Female pseudohermaphroditism is a congenital anomaly resulting from hyperplasia of the adrenal glands, which exposes the female fetus to excess amounts of androgens. This causes masculinized external genitalia, here shown as enlargement of the clitoris and fusion of the labia. Ambiguous means the enlarged clitoris here may look like a small penis with hypospadias, and the fused labia look like an incompletely formed scrotum with absent testes. Other forms of intersexual conditions occur, and the family must be referred for diagnostic evaluation.

Vulvovaginitis in Child

This infection is caused by *Candida albicans* in a diabetic child. Symptoms include pruritus and burning when urine touches excoriated area. Examination shows red, shiny, edematous vulva, vaginal discharge, excoriated area from scratching.

Other, more common causes of vulvovaginitis in the prepubertal child include infection from a respiratory or bowel pathogen, sexually transmitted disease, or presence of a foreign body.

BIBLIOGRAPHY

American Cancer Society: *Cancer facts and figures—1998,* Atlanta, GA, 1998, American Cancer Society.

Andrews WC: Approaches to taking a sexual history, *J Women's Health & Gender Based Med* 9(suppl 1):S21–S24, 2000.

Arvidson CR: Primary care approaches: the adolescent gynecologic exam, *Pediatr Nurs* 25(1):71–74, Jan-Feb 1999.

Brown MS: Pediatric genital exam, *Nurs Pract* 22(7):160, July 1997.

Burstein GR et al: Incident *Chlamydia trachomatis* infection among inner-city adolescent females, *JAMA* 280(6):521-526, Aug 12, 1998.

Castellsague X et al: Circumcised men have a significantly lower risk of acquiring genital HPV infection, *N Engl J Med* 346(15):1105–1112, 2002.

Corwin EJ: Endometriosis: pathophysiology, diagnosis, and treatment, *Nurs Pract* 22(10):35–51, Oct 1997.

Cunningham FG, Gant NF, Leveno KJ: *Williams' obstetrics,* ed 21, Stamford, CT, 2001, Appleton & Lange.

Daley AM, Cromwell PF: How to perform a pelvic exam for the sexually active adolescent, *Nurs Pract* 27(9):28–45, Sept 2002.

Dealy MF: Dysfunctional uterine bleeding in adolescents, *Nurs Pract* 23(5):12–25, May 1998.

Elliott KA: Managing patients with vulvovaginal candidiasis, *Nurs Pract* 23(3):44–53, Mar 1998.

Gingerich P, Ricciardi R: Markers for sexual abuse in the adolescent pelvic examination, *Nurse Pract Forum* 12(2):79–80, Jun 2001.

Goodman L et al: Cervical dysplasia in women with HIV, *Nurs Pract* 24(8):79–85, Aug 1999.

Harlan WR, Harlan EA, Grillo GP: Secondary sex characteristics of girls 12 to 17 years of age—The U.S. Health Examination Survey, *J Pediatr* 96:1074–1078, 1980.

Harris LL: Ovarian cancer: screening for early detection, *Am J Nurs* 102(10):46–53, Oct 2002.

Hennigen L, Kollar LM, Rosenthal SL: Methods for managing pelvic examination anxiety, *J Pediatr Health Care* 14(1):9–12, Jan/Feb 2000.

Hubbaard HS: Gynecologic examination of adolescents, *Am J Nurs* 101(3):24AAA–24DDD, Mar 2001.

Ivey JB: The adolescent with pelvic inflammatory disease: assessment and management, *Nurs Pract* 22(2):78–93, Feb 1997.

Kahn JA et al: Prevalence and correlates of pelvic examinations in sexually active female adolescents, *Ambulatory Pediatr* 2(3):212–217, May/Jun 2002.

Khosla RK: Detecting sexually transmitted disease: a new role for urinalysis in the preparticipation exam? *Phys Sports Med* 23(1):77–104, Jan 1995.

Kimble-Haas SL: The intrauterine device: dispelling the myths, *Nurs Pract* 23(11):58–73, Nov 1998.

Klingman L: Assessing the female reproductive system, *Am J Nurs* 99(8):37–43, Aug 1999.

Marantides D: Management of polycystic ovary syndrome, *Nurs Pract* 22(12):34–41, Dec 1997.

Marshall WA, Tanner JM: Variations in pattern of pubertal changes in girls, *Arch Dis Child* 44:291–303, 1969.

McCartney PR: Vaginal and speculum self-examination: it's OK to peek, *MCN* 25(5):274, Sep/Oct 2000.

McConkey TE, Sale M, Holcomb L: Assessing the female sexual assault survivor, *Nurs Pract* 26(7):28–41, July 2001.

Miller KE, Graves JC: Update on the prevention and treatment of sexually transmitted diseases, *Am Fam Physician* 61(2):379–386, Jan 15, 2000.

Moran G: Diagnosing STDs: Part 1. Ulcerating diseases, *Emerg Med* 29(1):58–70, Jan 1997.

Moran G: Diagnosing STDs: Part 2. Lesionless disorders, *Emerg Med* 29(2):20–31, Feb 1997.

Muscari ME: The first gynecologic exam, *Am J Nurs* 99(1 part 1):66–68, Jan 1999.

Orr DP: Urine-based diagnosis of sexually transmitted infections using amplified DNA techniques: a shift in paradigms? *J Adol Health* 20(1):3–5, Jan 1997.

Orr DP et al: Subsequent sexually transmitted infection in urban adolescents and young adults, *Arch Pediatr Adolesc Med* 155(8):947–953, Aug 2001.

Penn C et al: Assessment of urinary incontinence, *J Gerontol Nurs* 2(1):8–19, Jan 1996.

Ricciardi R: First pelvic examination in the adolescent, *Nurse Pract Forum* 11(3):161–169, Sep 2000.

Sandhaus S: Genital herpes in pregnant and nonpregnant women, *Nurs Pract* 26(4):15–35, Apr 2001.

Sharts-Hopko NC: Hysterectomy for nonmalignant conditions, *Am J Nurs* 101(9):32–41, Sep 2001.

Stewart FH et al: Clinical breast and pelvic examination requirements for hormonal contraception, *JAMA* 285:2232–2239, 2001.

Stillson T, Knight AL, Elswick RK: The effectiveness and safety of two cervical cytologic techniques during pregnancy, *J Fam Pract* 45(2):159–163, Aug 1997.

Ugarriza DN, Klinger S, O'Brien S: Premenstrual syndrome: diagnosis and intervention, *Nurs Pract* 23(9):40–58, Sep 1998.

Wan J: Sexually transmitted diseases in the adolescent male, *Contemp Urol* 11(4):71–76, Apr 1999.

Wright TC, Cox JT, Massad LS: Abnormal Pap smears: critical new guidelines, *Clin Review* 12(8):54–59, Aug 2002.

The Pregnant Female

Structure and Function

PREGNANCY AND THE ENDOCRINE PLACENTA

The first day of the menses is day 1 of the menstrual cycle. For the first 14 days of the cycle, one or more follicles in the ovary develop and mature. One follicle grows faster than the others, and on day 14 of the menstrual cycle, this dominant follicle ruptures and ovulation occurs. If the ovum meets viable sperm, fertilization occurs somewhere in the oviduct (fallopian tube). The remaining cells in the follicle form the **corpus luteum,** or "yellow body," which makes important hormones. Chief among these is progesterone, which prevents the sloughing of the endometrial wall, ensuring a rich vascular network into which the fertilized ovum will implant.

The fertilized ovum, now called the **blastocyst,** continues to divide, differentiate, and grow rapidly. Specialized cells in the blastocyst produce human chorionic gonadotropin (hCG), which stimulates the corpus luteum to continue making progesterone. Between days 20 and 24, the blastocyst implants into the wall of the uterus, which may cause a small amount of vaginal bleeding. A specialized layer of cells around the blastocyst becomes the **placenta.** The placenta starts to produce progesterone to support the pregnancy at 7 weeks, and takes over this function completely from the corpus luteum at about 10 weeks.

The placenta functions as an endocrine organ and produces several hormones. These hormones help in the growth and maintenance of the fetus, and they direct changes in the woman's body to prepare for birth and lactation. The hCG stimulates the rise in progesterone during pregnancy. Progesterone maintains the endometrium around the fetus, increases the alveoli in the breast, and keeps the uterus in a quiescent state. Estrogen stimulates the duct formation in the breast, increases the weight of the uterus, and increases certain receptors in the uterus that are important at birth.

The average length of pregnancy is 280 days from the first day of the last menstrual period (LMP), which is equal to 40 weeks, 10 lunar months, or 9 calendar months. Note that this includes the 2 weeks when the follicle was maturing but before conception actually occurred. Pregnancy is divided into three trimesters: (1) the first 12 weeks; (2) from 13 to 27 weeks; and (3) from 28 weeks to delivery. A woman who is pregnant for the first time is called a **primigravida.** After she delivers, she is called a **primipara.** The **multigravida** is a pregnant woman who has previously carried a fetus to the point of viability. She is a **multipara** after delivery. Any pregnant woman might be called a gravida.

CHANGES DURING NORMAL PREGNANCY

Pregnancy is diagnosed by three types of signs and symptoms. **Presumptive signs** are those the woman experiences, such as amenorrhea, breast tenderness, nausea, fatigue, and increased urinary frequency. **Probable signs** are those detected by the examiner, such as an enlarged uterus. **Positive signs** of pregnancy are those that are direct evidence of the fetus, such as the auscultation of fetal heart tones (FHTs) or positive cardiac activity on ultrasound (US).

FIRST TRIMESTER

Conception occurs on approximately the 14th day of the menstrual cycle. The blastocyst (developing fertilized ovum) implants in the uterus 6 to 10 days after conception, sometimes accompanied by a small amount of painless bleeding, which may be interpreted as a menstrual period (Cunningham et al., 2001). The serum hCG becomes positive after implantation. The following menstrual period is missed. At the time of the missed menses, hCG can be detected in the urine. Breast tingling and tenderness begin as the rising estrogen levels promote mammary growth and development of the ductal system; progesterone stimulates the alveolar system as well as the mammary growth. Chorionic somatomammotropin (also called human placental lactogen or hPL), also produced by the placenta, stimulates breast growth and exerts lactogenic properties (Varney, 1997). More than half of all pregnant women experience nausea and vomiting. The cause is unclear but may involve the hormonal changes of pregnancy, low blood sugar, gastric overloading, slowed peristalsis, an enlarging uterus, and emotional factors. Fatigue is common and may be related to the initial fall in metabolic rate that occurs in early pregnancy (Varney, 1997).

Estrogen, and possibly progesterone, cause hypertrophy of the uterine muscle cells, and uterine blood vessels and lymphatics enlarge. The uterus becomes globular in shape, softens, and flexes easily over cervix (**Hegar's sign**). This causes compression of the bladder, which results in urinary frequency. Increased vascularity, congestion, and edema cause the cervix to soften (**Goodell's sign**) and become bluish purple (**Chadwick's sign**).

Early first-trimester blood pressures reflect prepregnancy values. In the 7th gestational week, blood pressure begins to drop as a result of falling peripheral vascular resistance. Systemic vascular resistance decreases due to the vasodilatory effect of progesterone and prostaglandins, and possibly because of the low resistance of the placental bed (Creasy and Resnick, 1999).

At the end of 9 weeks, the embryonic period ends and the fetal period begins, at which time major structures are present (Varney, 1997). FHTs can be heard by Doppler ultrasound between 9 and 12 weeks. The uterus may be palpated just above the symphysis pubis at approximately 12 weeks. See Figure 27–1 for growth of the uterine fundus during the first trimester.

SECOND TRIMESTER

By weeks 12 to 16, the nausea, vomiting, fatigue, and urinary frequency of the first trimester improve. The woman recognizes fetal movement ("quickening") at approximately 18 to

20 weeks (the multigravida earlier). As breast enlargement continues, the veins of the breast enlarge and are more visible through the skin of lightly pigmented women. **Colostrum,** the precursor of milk, may be expressed from the nipples. Colostrum is yellow in color, and contains more minerals and protein but less sugar and fat than mature milk. Colostrum also contains antibodies, which are protective for the newborn during its first days of life until mature milk production begins (Cunningham et al., 2001). The areola and nipples darken, it is thought, because estrogen and progesterone have a melanocyte-stimulating effect, and melanocyte-stimulating hormone levels escalate from the 2nd month of pregnancy until delivery. For the same reason, the midline of the abdominal skin becomes pigmented and is called the **linea nigra. Striae gravidarum** ("stretch marks") may be noted on the breast, abdomen, and areas of weight gain.

During the second trimester, systolic blood pressure may be 2 to 8 mm Hg lower and diastolic blood pressure 5 to 15 mm Hg lower than prepregnancy levels (Cunningham et al., 2001). This drop is most pronounced at 20 weeks, and may cause symptoms of dizziness and faintness, particularly after rising quickly. Stomach displacement due to the enlarging uterus, and altered esophageal sphincter and gastric tone as a result of progesterone, predispose the woman to heartburn. Intestines are also displaced by the growing uterus, and tone and motility are decreased due to the action of progesterone, often causing constipation. The gallbladder, possibly due to

the action of progesterone on its smooth muscle, empties sluggishly and may become distended. The stasis of bile, together with the increased cholesterol saturation of pregnancy, predisposes some women to gallstone formation.

Progesterone and, to a lesser degree, estrogen cause increased respiratory effort during pregnancy by increasing tidal volume. Hemoglobin, and therefore oxygen carrying capacity, also increases. Increased tidal volume causes a slight drop in partial pressure of arterial carbon dioxide ($PaCO_2$), causing the woman to occasionally experience dyspnea (Cunningham et al., 2001).

The high level of estrogen during pregnancy causes an increase in the major thyroxine transport protein, thyroxine-binding globulin. Several thyroidal stimulating factors of placental origin are produced. The thyroid gland enlarges due to hyperplasia and increased vascularity.

Cutaneous blood flow is augmented during pregnancy due to decreased vascular resistance, presumably helping to dissipate heat generated by increased metabolism. Gums may hypertrophy and bleed easily. This condition is called **gingivitis** or **epulis of pregnancy,** and occurs due to growth of the capillaries of the gums (Cunningham et al., 1997). For the same reason, nosebleeds may occur more frequently than usual.

FHTs are audible by fetoscope (as opposed to Doppler) at approximately 17 to 19 weeks. The fetal outline is palpable through the abdominal wall at approximately 20 weeks. A multicenter study lists the following expected survival rates: 15.5% of neonates born at 25 weeks' gestation survive; 54.7% at 26 weeks; 67% at 27 weeks; 77.4% at 28 weeks; and 85.2% at 29 weeks, increasing slowly to 33 weeks, when 97.9% of the neonates survive (Creasy and Resnick, 1999). Figure 27–1 illustrates the growth of the uterine fundus during the second trimester.

THIRD TRIMESTER

Blood volume, which increased rapidly during the second trimester, peaks in the middle of the third trimester at approximately 45% greater than the prepregnancy level and plateaus thereafter (Creasy and Resnick, 1999). Erythrocyte mass increases by 20 to 30% (caused by an increase in erythropoiesis, mediated by progesterone, estrogen, and placental chorionic somatomammotropin), while plasma volume increases slightly more, causing a slight hemodilution and a small drop in hematocrit. Blood pressure slowly rises again to approximately the prepregnant level (Cunningham et al., 2001).

Uterine enlargement causes the diaphragm to rise and the shape of the rib cage to widen at the base. Decreased space for lung expansion may cause a sense of shortness of breath. The rising diaphragm displaces the heart up and to the left. Cardiac output, stroke volume, and force of contraction are increased. The pulse rate rises 15 to 20 beats per minute (Creasy and Resnick, 1999). Due to the increase in blood volume, a functional systolic murmur, grade ii/iv or less, can be heard in more than 95% of pregnant women (Creasy and Resnick, 1999).

HEIGHT OF FUNDUS AT WEEKS OF GESTATION

27–1

Edema of the lower extremities may occur due to the enlarging fetus impeding venous return and due to lower colloid osmotic pressure. The edema worsens with dependency, such as prolonged standing. Varicosities, for which many women have a familial tendency, may form or enlarge due to progesterone-induced vascular relaxation as well as engorgement caused by the weight of the full uterus compressing the inferior vena cava and the vessels of the pelvic area, resulting in venous congestion in the legs, vulva, and rectum. Hemorrhoids are varicosities of the rectum that are worsened by constipation, which occurs due to relaxation of the large bowel by progesterone.

Progressive lordosis occurs to compensate for the shifting center of balance caused by the anteriorly bulging uterus, predisposing the woman to backaches. Slumping of the shoulders and anterior flexion of the neck secondary to the increasing weight of the breasts may cause aching and numbness of the arms and hands due to compression of the median and ulnar nerves in the arm (Varney, 1997).

Approximately 2 weeks before going into labor, the primigravida experiences engagement (also called "lightening" or "dropping"), when the fetal head moves down into the pelvis. Symptoms include a lower-appearing and smaller-measuring fundus, urinary frequency, increased vaginal secretions due to increased pelvic congestion, and increased lung capacity. In the multigravida, the fetus may move down at any time in late pregnancy or often not until labor. The cervix, in preparation for labor, begins to thin (efface) and open (dilate). A thick **mucous plug,** formed in the cervix as a mechanical barrier during pregnancy, is expelled at variable times before or during labor. Between 37 and 42 weeks, the pregnancy is considered full term. After 42 weeks, the pregnancy is considered postdates.

DETERMINING WEEKS OF GESTATION

The **expected date of confinement** (EDC) (also less commonly known as the expected date of delivery, or EDD), being 280 days from the first day of the LMP, may be calculated by using **Nägele's rule.** That is, determine the first day of the last normal menstrual period (normal in timing, length, premenstrual symptoms, and amount of flow and cramping). Using the first day of the LMP, add 7 days and subtract 3 months. This date is the EDC. This date can then be used with a pregnancy wheel, on which the EDC arrow is set, then the present date will be pointing to the present week's gestation (Fig. 27–2). The number of weeks of gestation also can be estimated by physical exam, by measurement of the maternal serum hCG, by ultrasound, and by signs such as the first perceived fetal movement.

WEIGHT GAIN IN PREGNANCY

The amount of weight gained by term represents a baby, amniotic fluid, placenta, increased uterine size, increased blood volume, increased extravascular fluid, maternal fat stores, and increased breast size. In 1990, the National Academy of Science made the following recommendation for weight gain

during pregnancy, which was later accepted by the American College of Obstetricians and Gynecologists: 28 to 40 lb for underweight women, 25 to 35 lb for normal weight women, 15 to 25 lb for overweight women, and 35 to 45 lb for twin gestation. A healthy outcome may be expected within a great range of weight gain (Cunningham et al., 2001).

DEVELOPMENTAL CONSIDERATIONS

In industrialized countries, the risks for the adolescent who is pregnant are largely psychosocial. This young woman is at risk for the downward cycle of poverty beginning with an incomplete education, failure to limit family size, and continuing with failure to establish a vocation and become independent. She may be unprepared emotionally to be a mother. Her social situation may be stressful. She may not have the support of her family, her partner, or his family. Medical risks for the pregnant adolescent are generally related to poverty, inadequate nutrition, substance abuse, sexually transmitted diseases, and poor health before pregnancy. The adolescent is also at risk for preeclampsia and for bearing a low-birth-weight infant, and it is unclear whether this is due to biologic or social factors (Cunningham et al., 2001). The adolescent, for social reasons, often seeks health care later, and early prenatal care has been shown to provide optimal management. In developing countries, maternal mortality for pregnant teenagers is a major concern due to hypertension, embolism, ectopic pregnancy, and complications from pregnancy termination where abortion is illegal (Cunningham et al., 2001).

Since many baby boomers have delayed childbearing, and since the advent of assisted conception, more women older than age 35 are now becoming pregnant. Primigravidae pregnant after the age of 35 years have been referred to as **"elderly primigravidae,"** though many clinicians now consider this to

27–2

be an unfortunate term. Women over 35 are often more prepared emotionally and financially to parent; however, they are more at risk for infertility. Female fertility declines with maternal age due to ovulation and atresia of follicles, causing anovulation to occur with increasing frequency after the age of 40 (Kennedy, Griffin, and Frishman, 1998; Rousseau, 1998). Once conception is achieved, the older woman is at increased risk for congenital anomalies, particularly Down syndrome, which occurs much more frequently after age 35 (Cunningham et al., 2001).

Women 35 years and older are offered genetic counseling and prenatal screening such as maternal serum screening and ultrasound as well as **chorionic villi sampling (CVS)** and **amniocentesis**. For these tests, fetal material is removed from the uterus and analyzed for genetic make-up. Another first trimester screening tool that may be used is that of fetal nuchal translucency screening (FNT). This ultrasound testing done between 10 and 14 weeks assesses for an abnormal fluid collection at the nape of the fetal neck and is most accurate when done in conjunction with maternal serum beta-hCG and pregnancy-associated plasma protein (PAPP-A).

Because the incidence of chronic diseases increases with age, women over age 35 who are pregnant more often suffer medical complications such as diabetes, obesity and hypertension (Cunningham et al., 2001). The increased incidence of hypertension causes an increase in placental abruption and pregnancy-induced hypertension. Hypertension, in turn, increases intrauterine growth restriction (IUGR). More women of advanced maternal age experience placenta previa, placental abruption, and uterine rupture. They experience more spontaneous abortions, in part because of the increase in genetically abnormal embryos. A Centers for Disease Control and Prevention study found that maternal mortality for women older than 35 was two times that of women aged 20 to 24 (CDC, 2001). Advanced maternal age (≥35) itself is considered a risk factor for maternal death. There are still wide variances in maternal deaths between white and nonwhite populations. There also exists a geographic difference where maternal deaths are higher in the South and lowest in the Western states. Again, the racial differences in each region play a role. Women over the age of 35 more often deliver by cesarean section due to factors that include increased risk for pregnancy-induced hypertension (PIH), diabetes, preterm labor (PTL), and placental accidents. More than 80% of maternal deaths worldwide are due to hemorrhage, sepsis, unsafe abortion, obstructed labor, and hypertensive disease of pregnancy (UNFPA, 2001).

TRANSCULTURAL CONSIDERATIONS

Some complications of pregnancy occur more frequently among some racial groups than others. Women who live in underdeveloped nations do not have the advantages of advanced technology. Every minute, a woman somewhere dies in pregnancy or childbirth. This adds up to 1400 women dying each day and more than 500,000 each year from pregnancy-related causes (UNFPA, 2001). About 95% of these deaths occur in developing countries (Gabbe et al., 2002). According to the CDC in 1997, the Hispanic, Asian/Pacific Islander, and American Indian/Alaska Native population represented 16% of all reproductive age women (ages 15 to 49) in the United States but accounted for only 23.5% of all live births (CDC, 2001). Nonwhite pregnant women have an increased risk of gestational diabetes mellitus (GDM), pregnancy-induced hypertension (PIH), and preterm labor and birth (PTL/PTD).

Pregnancy, however, is not only a medical event, but also one with profound psychological and social meaning for the woman and also for her family and community. All cultures are unique and recognize pregnancy as a period in a woman's life that surrounds special customs and beliefs that have been developed throughout the ages. The spiritual practices and beliefs either provide her with or without support. Understanding what role these beliefs and practices play in the woman's pregnancy helps the health care provider to acknowledge the cultural differences. Pregnancy is intensely personal, and involves such charged issues as sexuality, relationships, contraceptive, nutritional practices, maternal weight gain, and abortion. You must be sensitive to these issues. You may begin by inquiring whether the woman and/or her significant others have any special requests. This communicates your intention to respect cultural differences and preferences. A continuing rapport will help enable the woman to bring up issues as they develop.

A woman's resistance to an action or a suggestion by the clinician may represent a cultural issue. Such issues may also be held differently by the woman and one or more of her significant others, and such situations must be handled with care. Examples of culturally charged issues are dietary practices, sexuality during and after pregnancy, preference for gender of care provider, preference for gender of infant, and contraceptive usage. Use your skill to understand such preferences within a cultural context and accept rather than judge the person. Whenever safe and possible, respect such wishes. This enhances the success of the birth in its psychological and social dimensions.

Subjective Data

1. Menstrual history	**4.** Present pregnancy	**7.** Review of systems
2. Gynecologic history	**5.** Past medical history	**8.** Nutritional history
3. Obstetric history	**6.** Family history	**9.** Environment/hazards

EXAMINER ASKS	RATIONALE
1. Menstrual history • When was the first day of your last menstrual period that was normal in timing, premenstrual symptoms, length, amount of flow, cramping?	Using Nägele's rule, calculate the EDC using this date. With a pregnancy wheel, determine the present number of weeks of gestation.
2. Gynecologic history • Ever had surgery of the cervix? Uterus?	Cervical surgery may affect the integrity of the cervix during pregnancy and, during labor, may impede cervical dilation. Uterine surgery may place the woman at risk for uterine rupture during pregnancy and labor.
• Any history of genital herpes?	Onset during pregnancy is potentially *teratogenic,* i.e., causing physical defects in the developing fetus, and a lesion at delivery precludes vaginal birth.
• When your mother was pregnant with you, did she ever take a drug called diethylstilbesterol (DES)?	Prenatal exposure to DES may cause vaginal, cervical, and/or uterine abnormalities in the daughter, which may increase the risk of spontaneous abortion or affect the integrity of the cervix during pregnancy.
3. Obstetric history • In earlier pregnancies, any history of hypertension, diabetes, β-hemolytic streptococcus infection, intrauterine growth restriction, congenital anomalies, premature labor, postpartum hemorrhage, or postpartum depression?	The woman who has experienced these complications in the past is at increased risk for them in subsequent pregnancies.
• How did you experience previous pregnancies and deliveries?	The subjective quality of previous experiences tells a great deal about the woman's emotions regarding the present pregnancy.
• Ever had a cesarean section? If so, what was the indication? At how many centimeters of dilation, if any, was the surgery performed? What type of uterine incision was made? (Confirming records of this surgery must be obtained.)	The woman who has had surgery on her uterus is at risk for uterine rupture during pregnancy and labor. The vertical, or "classical," incision carries a higher risk of rupture, and mandates that all subsequent deliveries be by cesarean section. The "low transverse," or horizontal incision carries a low risk, and subsequent deliveries may be vaginal. Note that the direction of the skin scar does not necessarily tell how the uterus was incised.
• Tell me the weights of your babies at birth.	A small infant may indicate prematurity or intrauterine growth restriction—complications that the woman is at risk to repeat. A large infant may indicate gestational diabetes (also repeatable). Conversely, birth weights of other children may indicate a "constitutional size"—e.g., the tendency of a couple to conceive smaller but normal children. Also, the woman's pelvis has been "proven" to the weight of the largest baby born vaginally; bear this number in mind as labor begins, estimating and comparing the weight of the baby about to be born.

EXAMINER ASKS	RATIONALE
• Did you breastfeed the previously born infants? How was that experience for you?	The woman's experience and knowledge base will shape the practitioner's teaching and support.

4. Present pregnancy. [Having calculated the present number of weeks of gestation, you can reassess the probable accuracy of that date when eliciting the following history]

EXAMINER ASKS	RATIONALE
• What method of contraceptive did you use most recently, and when did you discontinue it?	Recent use of birth control pills or other hormonal contraceptives may have caused delayed ovulation and irregular menses, which must be considered when establishing the EDC. An intrauterine device (IUD) that is still in place requires removal and threatens the pregnancy. Also, this opens topic of whether pregnancy was planned.
• Was the pregnancy planned? How do you feel about it?	Even a planned pregnancy represents loss for the woman—perhaps a loss of freedom, compromise of goals, loss of time with other children or partner. The first trimester is known as the "trimester of ambivalence," and encouraging acceptance and expression of these feelings facilitates resolution.
• How does the baby's father feel about the pregnancy? Other family members?	The woman may need assistance in gathering together her support group. Inviting significant others to future visits affirms their importance and supports their involvement.
• Experienced any vaginal bleeding? When? How much? What color? Accompanied by any pain?	Vaginal bleeding may indicate threatened abortion, cervicitis, or other complications, and must be investigated.
• Experienced abdominal pain? When? Where in your abdomen? Accompanied by vaginal bleeding?	The most common causes of abdominal pain in early pregnancy are spontaneous abortion, ectopic pregnancy, urinary tract infection, and round ligament discomfort. Later in pregnancy, premature labor must be ruled out. Also consider other medical and surgical causes for abdominal pain.
• Experienced any illnesses since being pregnant? Had any x-rays? Taken any medications? Used any recreational drugs or alcohol? Do you smoke cigarettes?	The potential effect of any teratogenic exposure must be discussed with the woman. Refer for expert counseling if necessary.
• Experiencing any visual changes such as the new onset of blurred vision or spots before your eyes?	In the third trimester, this may be a sign of preeclampsia. Evaluate for other signs and symptoms of preeclampsia (see Table 27–2).
• Experiencing any edema? Where and under what circumstances?	In the third trimester, differentiate the normal weight-dependent edema of pregnancy from the edema of preeclampsia.
• Any burning, frequency, or burning with urination? Any blood in your urine? Do you void in small amounts?	Differentiate the normal urinary frequency of the first and third trimesters from urinary tract infection, for which pregnant women are at increased risk. Findings are confirmed by urinalysis.

EXAMINER ASKS	RATIONALE
• Any vaginal burning or itching? Any foul-smelling or colored discharge? Large amount of discharge?	Rule out vaginal infection. If symptoms exist, add cultures or a wet mount to the pelvic examination. Discuss partner treatment if necessary. Educate the woman to the normal increase in vaginal secretions during pregnancy.
• What date did you first feel the baby move?	This sign is compared with the EDC in evaluation of the accuracy of that date. Tell the woman who has not experienced movement to note and report that event at the following prenatal visit.
• How does the baby move on a daily basis?	Fetal movement is an excellent indicator of fetal health. Many clinicians assign women to count fetal movements starting at 28 weeks of pregnancy.
• Do you have cats in the home?	Educate the woman about toxoplasmosis, a teratogenic disease transmitted through cat feces. To avoid exposure, another person should empty cat litter at frequent intervals.
• Do you plan to breastfeed this baby?	Arrange reading, classes, and other support for the woman who is breastfeeding for the first time, or for the woman with an unsuccessful earlier experience.

5. Past medical history

EXAMINER ASKS	RATIONALE
• Ever had German measles (rubella)?	This mild childhood disease is highly teratogenic, especially during the first trimester. Instruct the woman who has not had rubella to avoid small children who are ill. Check immunity status in the serum prenatal panel as well. The nonimmune woman will be offered immunization after delivery.
• Ever had chickenpox?	Rarely, varicella causes congenital anomalies. The nonimmune woman should avoid exposure.
• Any injury to the back or another weight-bearing part?	The localized and overall weight gain of pregnancy as well as the joint-softening property of progesterone causes lordosis and will aggravate such injuries with increasing gestation.
• Have you been tested for HIV? When? What was the result? Ever had a blood transfusion? Used intravenous drugs? Had a sexual partner who had any HIV risk factors? Are you and your partner mutually monogamous?	HIV status must be addressed to promote the health of the gravida as well as to consider therapies that can decrease the risk of transmission of the virus across the placenta to the fetus. Breastfeeding is contraindicated for the HIV-positive mother because the virus is present in the breast milk. Educate the gravida who practices high-risk activities.
• Do you smoke cigarettes? How many? For how many years? Ever tried to quit? Drink any alcohol? How much of what type? Use any street drugs?	Educate the woman regarding the danger of these substances in pregnancy. Smoking increases the risk of ectopic pregnancy, spontaneous abortion, low

EXAMINER ASKS	RATIONALE
	birth weight, prematurity, preterm premature rupture of membranes, pregnancy-induced hypertension, placental abruption, and sudden infant death syndrome. Alcohol increases the risk to the fetus of fetal alcohol syndrome (see Table 13–3). Cocaine use during pregnancy is associated with a number of congenital anomalies, a fourfold increased risk for abruptio placenta and the risk of fetal addiction. Narcotic-addicted infants may experience developmental delays or behavioral disturbances (Cunningham et al., 2001). Consider referral to a counseling/support program and periodic toxicology screening.
• Do you take any prescribed medications?	Screen all medications to establish safety during pregnancy.
6. Family history. Anyone in your family have hypertension?	Increases the risk of chronic hypertension and of preeclampsia.
• Diabetes? If so, of juvenile or adult onset? Insulin dependent?	Increases risk of gestational diabetes. A heavy family history might prompt early screening and dietary interventions.
• Mental illness?	Increases risk for postpartum depression (Cunningham et al., 2001).
• Kidney disease?	Increases risk for renal disease, hypertension, and preeclampsia.
• Fraternal twins?	The tendency to ovulate twice in one month is familial, and thus the incidence of twinning is increased.
• Anyone in your family, or in the family of the baby's father, had congenital anomalies?	Some anomalies, such as heart conditions, are familial. Offer genetic counseling if needed.
• Is your racial descent Mediterranean? Black? Ashkenazi Jewish? Irish?	Increased risk for β-thalassemia. Increased risk for sickle-cell disease. Increased risk for Tay-Sachs disease. Increased risk for spinal malformations.
7. Review of systems	
• Your weight before pregnancy?	Baseline needed to evaluate changes.
• Wear glasses?	A transient change in visual correction may occur during pregnancy.
• When did you last see the dentist? Need any dental work?	Gums may be puffy and bleed easily during pregnancy, predisposing the woman to caries. Encourage careful dental hygiene. Suggest any dental care be done, if possible, during the second trimester, and to notify the dentist that she is pregnant.
• Been exposed to tuberculosis (TB)?	Consider TB screening using the tine test.
• Any cardiovascular disease, such as vascular disease, or disease of a heart valve?	The woman with cardiac disease who becomes pregnant must be monitored

EXAMINER ASKS	RATIONALE
	carefully for signs of cardiac compromise. Blood volume increases by 40 percent, and the demand on the heart is significantly increased.
• Any anemia? What kind? When? Was it treated? How? Did it improve?	Pregnancy worsens any preexisting anemia, as iron is utilized extensively by the fetus. Identify the need for early supplementation. Sickle-cell anemia may worsen during pregnancy, while sickle-cell carriers experience more urinary tract infections. Screen the latter periodically for bacteriuria.
• Had a thrombophlebitis?	Pregnancy itself is a hypercoagulable state due to increases in coagulation factors I, VII, VIII, IX, and X. This increases the risk of phlebitis (Cunningham et al., 2001).
• Have you had hypertension or kidney disease?	The woman with renal disease or with chronic hypertension is at increased risk for preeclampsia. Know the baseline BP and renal function to evaluate any changes.
• Ever had hepatitis?	Confirm this with serum testing. Treatment for mother and/or baby when born may be appropriate. Breastfeeding may be contraindicated in some cases.
• Have you had urinary tract infections?	The hormonal milieu of pregnancy predisposes the woman to urinary tract infections (UTIs), so a history of infection before pregnancy may indicate periodic screening. Pregnancy may also mask the symptoms of UTIs. Further, a serious UTI may cause irritability of the uterus, threatening the pregnancy. Educate the woman in measures to prevent such infections.
• Have you experienced depression or any other mental illness?	This woman will be at risk for postpartum depression. Assist her to prepare a support network. Counseling may help her successfully navigate the developmental challenges of becoming a mother.
• Do you have diabetes? Did you have diabetes during a previous pregnancy?	Diabetes is carefully managed during pregnancy to avoid serious complications, such as a macrosomic infant and operative delivery. Consider early screening and nutritional interventions.
8. Nutritional history	
• Do you follow a special diet?	A special diet may put the woman at nutritional risk. Help achieve adequate nutrition within the confines of her diet.

EXAMINER ASKS	RATIONALE
• Any food intolerance?	A food intolerance might affect the woman's and fetus's nutrition, such as lactose intolerance limiting calcium intake.
• Do you crave nonfoods such as ice, paint chips, dirt, or clay?	Craving for ice and/or dirt is called pica and is associated with anemia.
9. Environment/hazards • What is your occupation? What are the physical demands of the work? Are you exposed to any strong odors, chemicals, radiation, or other harmful substances?	Hazards? Possible teratogenic exposures? The woman who is rubella nonimmune may be advised not to continue working in a day care center. Suitability for pregnancy? The woman whose job requires long hours of standing may be disabled early if signs of preterm labor occur.
• Do you consider your food and housing adequate?	If appropriate, refer for state and federal programs to assist with food, housing, or other needs.
• Do you have a regular exercise program? What type?	Regular exercise in pregnancy may reduce risk of pregnancy-induced hypertension.
• How do you wear your seat belt when driving?	For maternal and fetal safety, instruct the woman to place the lap belt below the uterus and to use the shoulder strap simultaneously.
• Other questions or concerns?	Encourage the woman to write down questions between visits.

 # Objective Data

PREPARATION

The initial exam for pregnancy is often a woman's first pelvic exam, and many women are extremely anxious. Alternatively, the woman may not know for certain if she is pregnant, and she may be anxious about the findings. Verbally prepare the woman for what will happen during the exam before touching her. Save the pelvic exam for last—By that time the woman will be more comfortable with your gentle, informing manner. Communicate all findings as you go along to demonstrate your respectful affirmation of her control and responsibility in her own health and health care and that of her child's.

Ask the woman to empty her bladder before the exam, reserving a specimen for dipping for protein and glucose, and for urinalysis, if required. Ask her to weigh herself before the exam on the office scale.

Give the woman a gown and drape. Begin the examination with the woman sitting on the exam table, wearing the gown, her lap covered by a drape. During the breast exam, help her to lie down. She remains recumbent for the abdominal and extremity exam. Use the lithotomy position for the pelvic exam (see Chapter 26). Help her to a seated position to check her BP at the end of the exam, when, it is hoped, she will be most relaxed.

EQUIPMENT NEEDED

Stethoscope BP cuff
Centimeter measuring tape
Fetoscope and Doppler sonometer
Reflex hammer
Urine collection containers
Chemostix for checking urine for glucose and protein
Equipment needed for pelvic exam as noted in Chapter 26.

NORMAL RANGE OF FINDINGS

GENERAL SURVEY

Observe the woman's state of nourishment, and her grooming, posture, mood, and affect, which reflect her mental state. Throughout the exam, observe her maturity and ability to attend and learn in order to plan your teaching of the information she needs to successfully complete a healthy pregnancy.

Undernourished; or obesity.

Poor grooming, a slumped posture, and a flat affect may be signs of depression and risk for postpartum depression. Poor grooming may reflect a lack of resources and a need for a social service referral.

A lack of attention may indicate some preoccupation with a concern. The woman who has had learning difficulties may benefit from written and verbal information, special classes, as well as a support person to accompany her. A flat, unclear affect may indicate depression or the influence of drugs.

SKIN

Note any scars (particularly those of previous cesarean section). Many women experience skin changes during pregnancy that may spontaneously resolve after the pregnancy, such as acne or skin tags. Vascular spiders may be present on the upper body. Some women develop **chloasma,** known as the "mask of pregnancy," which is a butterfly-shaped pigmentation of the face. Note the presence of the **linea nigra,** a hyperpigmented line that begins at the sternal notch and extends down the abdomen through the umbilicus to the pubis (Fig. 27–3). Also note **striae,** or stretch marks, in areas of weight gain, particularly on the abdomen and breasts of multiparous women. These marks are bright red when they first form, but they will shrink and lighten to a silvery color (in the lightly pigmented woman) after the pregnancy (see Fig. 27–3).

Multiple bruises may suggest physical abuse.

Tracks (scars along easily accessed veins) may indicate intravenous drug use.

Palmar erythema in the first trimester may indicate hepatitis, but thereafter is not clinically significant (Varney, 1997).

27–3

MOUTH

Mucous membranes should be red and moist. Gum hypertrophy (surface looks smooth and stippling disappears) may occur normally during pregnancy (pregnancy gingivitis). Bleeding gums may be from estrogen stimulation, which causes increased vascularity and fragility.

Pale mucous membranes are indicative of anemia.

Poor dental hygiene during pregnancy may lead to preterm delivery or low birth weight infants.

NORMAL RANGE OF FINDINGS	ABNORMAL FINDINGS

NECK

The thyroid may be palpable and feel full but smooth during the normal pregnancy of a euthyroid woman.

Solitary nodules indicate neoplasm; multiple nodules usually indicate inflammation or a multinodular goiter. Significant diffuse enlargement occurs with hyperthyroidism, thyroiditis, and hypothyroidism.

BREASTS

The breasts are enlarged (Fig. 27–4), perhaps with resulting striae and may be very tender. The areolae and nipples enlarge and darken in pigmentation, the nipples become more erect, and "secondary areolae" (mottling around the areolae) may develop. The blood vessels of the breast enlarge, and may shine blue through a seemingly more translucent than usual chest wall. When auscultating, blood flow through these blood vessels can be heard and may be mistaken for a cardiac murmur. This sound is called the mammary souffle (SOO-FL). Montgomery's tubercles, located around the areola and responsible for skin integrity of the areola, enlarge. Colostrum, a thick yellow fluid, may be expressed from the nipples.

27–4

The breast tissue feels nodular as the mammary alveoli hypertrophy. Take this opportunity to teach or reinforce breast self-exam (BSE). The woman should expect changes in the breast tissue during the pregnancy. Due to the lack of menses, instruct her to perform BSE according to the calendar on a monthly basis, on a date familiar to her such as her birth date.

Recall that some women have an embryologic remnant called a supernumerary nipple, which may or may not have breast tissue beneath it. Possibly mistaken previously for a mole, these occur under the arm or in a line directly underneath each nipple on the abdominal wall (see Chapter 17). This nipple and breast tissue may show the same changes of pregnancy. Instruct the woman to check these areas as well during breast self-examination.

Refer any unusual breast lump for further study.

HEART

The pregnant woman often develops a functional, soft, blowing, systolic murmur, which occurs due to increased volume. The murmur requires no treatment and will resolve after pregnancy.

Note any other murmur and refer. Valvular disease may necessitate the use of prophylactic antibiotics at delivery. Pregnancy places a large hemodynamic burden on the heart, and the woman with cardiac disease is managed closely.

LUNGS

The lungs are clear bilaterally to auscultation with no crackles or wheezing. Shortness of breath is common in the 3rd trimester due to pressure on the diaphragm from the enlarged uterus.

Women with asthma exacerbations during pregnancy may have expiratory (and possibly inspiratory) wheeze.

NORMAL RANGE OF FINDINGS	ABNORMAL FINDINGS

PERIPHERAL VASCULATURE

The legs may show diffuse, bilateral pitting edema, particularly if the exam is occurring later in the day when the woman has been on her feet and in the third trimester. Varicose veins in the legs are common in the third trimester. The Homans' sign is negative.

Edema, together with increased BP and proteinuria, is a sign of preeclampsia. The pregnant woman is at risk for thrombophlebitis—Carefully evaluate any redness, or red, hot, tender swelling to rule out phlebitis. Varicosities increase the risk of thrombophlebitis, and she should not wear restrictive clothing or sit without moving legs for a long period. Varicosities will worsen with the weight and volume of pregnancy, and support hose help to minimize them.

NEUROLOGIC

Using the reflex hammer, check the biceps, patellar, and ankle deep tendon reflexes (DTRs). Normally these are 1+ to 2+ and equal bilaterally.

Brisk or greater than 2+ DTRs and clonus may be associated with elevated BP and cerebral edema in the preeclamptic woman.

INSPECT AND PALPATE THE ABDOMEN

Observe the shape and contours of the abdomen to discern signs of fetal position. As the woman lifts her head, you may see the **diastasis recti,** the separation of the abdominal muscles, which occurs during pregnancy, with the muscles returning together after pregnancy with abdominal exercise. When palpating, note the abdominal muscle tone, which grows more relaxed with each subsequent pregnancy. Note any tenderness; the uterus is normally nontender.

The fundus should be palpable abdominally from 12 weeks' gestation on. Use the side of your hand and begin palpating centrally on the abdomen higher than you expect the uterus to be. Palpate down until you feel the fundus. Alternatively, stand at the woman's right side facing her head (Fig. 27–5). Place the palm of your right hand on the curve of the uterus in the left lower quadrant; and your left palm on the curve of the uterus in the right lower quadrant. Moving from hand to hand, allowing the curve of the uterus to guide you, "walk" your hands to where they meet centrally at the fundus.

Note the fundal location by landmarks and fingerbreadths, as described in Figure 27–1. Note that individual women's variations in location of landmarks as well as examiner's variations in finger width makes this measurement inexact. It is more accurate to use the centimeter measuring tape and measure the height of the fundus in centimeters from the superior border of the symphysis to the fundus (Fig. 27–6). After 20 weeks, the number of centimeters should approximate the number of weeks of gestation.

Beginning at 20 weeks, you may feel fetal movement, and the fetus's head can be ballotted. A gentle, quick palpation with the fingertips can locate a head that is not only hard when you push it away, but is hard as it bobs or bounces back against your fingers.

If you suspect the woman to be in labor, palpate for uterine contractions. Palpate the uterus over its entire surface to familiarize yourself with its "indentability." Then rest your hand lightly on the uterus with fingers opened. When the uterus contracts, it rises and pulls together, drawing your fingers closer together.

A lagging fundal height ≥2 cm may indicate intrauterine growth restriction, transverse lie, or oblique presentation of the fetus.

NORMAL RANGE OF FINDINGS	ABNORMAL FINDINGS

27–5

27–6

During the contraction, notice that the uterus is less "indentable." When the uterus relaxes, your fingers relax open again. In this way, contractions can be monitored for frequency (from the beginning of one contraction to the beginning of the next), length, and quality. Note that a mild contraction feels like the firmness of the tip of your nose; a moderate contraction feels like your chin; and a hard contraction feels like a forehead. (Make allowance for the amount of soft tissue between your fingers and the uterus.)

An abnormal uterine contraction is dystonic in nature; the contraction begins in the lower uterine segment and may delay cervical dilation.

Leopold's Maneuvers

In the third trimester, perform Leopold's maneuvers to determine fetal lie, presentation, attitude, position, variety, and engagement. **Fetal lie** is the orientation of the fetal spine to the maternal spine and may be longitudinal, transverse, or oblique. **Presentation** describes the part of the fetus that is entering the pelvis first. **Attitude** is the position of fetal parts in relation to each other, and may be flexed, military (straight), or extended. **Position** designates the location of a fetal part to the right or left of the maternal pelvis. **Variety** is the location of the fetal back to the anterior, lateral, or posterior part of the maternal pelvis. **Engagement** occurs when the widest diameter of the presenting part has descended into the pelvic inlet—specifically, to the imagined plane at the level of the ischial spines.

Leopold's first maneuver is performed by facing the gravida's head, and placing your fingertips around the top of the fundus (Fig. 27–7). Note its size, consistency, and shape. Imagine what fetal part is in the fundus. The breech feels large and firm. Moving it between the thumb and fingers of the hand, because it is attached to the fetus at the waist, results in moving it slowly and with difficulty. In contrast, the fetal head feels large, round, and hard. When it is ballotted, it feels hard as you push it away and hard again as it bobs back against your fingers in an "answer." Note that the "bobbing" or "ballotting" sensation of the movement occurs because the head is attached at the neck and moves easily. If there is no part in the fundus, the fetus is in the transverse lie.

27–7   Leopold's first maneuver.

For **Leopold's second maneuver,** move your hands to the sides of the uterus (Fig. 27–8). Note whether small parts or a long, firm surface are palpable on the woman's left or right side. The long, firm surface is the back. Note whether the back is anterior, lateral, or out of reach (posterior). The small parts, or limbs, indicate a posterior position when they are palpable all over the abdomen.

| 27–8 | Leopold's second maneuver. |

Leopold's third maneuver, also called Pawlik's maneuver, requires the woman to bend her knees up slightly (Fig. 27–9). Grasp the lower abdomen just above the symphysis pubis between the thumb and fingers of one hand and, as you did at the fundus during the first maneuver, determine what part of the fetus is there. If the presenting part is beginning to engage, it will feel "fixed." With this maneuver alone, it may be difficult to differentiate the shoulder from the vertex.

| 27–9 | Leopold's third maneuver. |

The **fourth maneuver** assists in determining engagement and, in the vertex presentation, to differentiate shoulder from vertex (Fig. 27–10). The woman's knees are still bent. Facing her feet, place your palms, with fingers pointing toward the feet, on either side of the lower abdomen. Pressing your fingers firmly, move slowly down toward the pelvic inlet. If your fingers meet, the presenting part is not engaged. If your fingers diverge at the pelvic rim meeting a hard prominence on one side, this prominence is the occiput. This indicates the vertex is presenting with a deflexed head (the face presenting). If your fingers meet hard prominences on both sides, the vertex is engaged in either a military or a flexed position. If your fingers come to the pelvic brim diverged but with no prominences palpable, the vertex is "dipping" into the pelvis, or is engaged. In this case, the firm object felt above the symphysis pubis in the third maneuver is the shoulder.

27–10 Leopold's fourth maneuver.

See Figure 27–11 for various fetal positions and where to auscultate the fetal heart tones for each. At the end of pregnancy, 96% of fetal presentations are vertex, 3.5% are breech, 0.3% are face, and 0.4% are shoulder (Cunningham et al., 2001).

RSA and LSA = right and left sacral anterior (breech)
RMA and LMA = right and left mentum anterior (face)
ROA and LOA = right and left occiput anterior (vertex)
ROP and LOP = right and left occiput posterior (vertex)

27–11 Location of FHTs for various fetal positions.

NORMAL RANGE OF FINDINGS	ABNORMAL FINDINGS

AUSCULTATE THE FETAL HEART TONES

FHTs are a positive sign of pregnancy. They can be heard with the Doppler ultrasound at 8 to 10 weeks' gestation and with a fetoscope at 20 weeks. This use of the fetoscope assists in dating the pregnancy. FHTs are auscultated best over the shoulder of the fetus. After identifying the position of the fetus (see Fig. 27–11), use the heart tones to confirm your findings. Count the FHTs for 15 seconds and multiply by 4 to obtain the rate (Fig. 27–12). The normal rate is between 120 and 160 beats per minute. Spontaneous accelerations of FHTs indicate fetal well-being.

If no FHTs are heard, verify fetal cardiac activity with ultrasound.

Further investigate any decelerations of FHTs.

27–12

Differentiate the FHTs from the slower rate of the maternal pulse, and the uterine souffle (the soft, swishing sound of the placenta receiving the pulse of maternal arterial blood) by palpating the mother's pulse while you listen. Also, distinguish FHTs from the funic souffle (blood rushing through the umbilical arteries at the same rate as the FHTs). The FHTs are a double sound, like the tick-tock of a watch under a pillow, whereas the funic souffle is a sharp, whistling sound that is heard only 15% of the time (Cunningham et al., 2001).

All of the abdominal findings are of interest to the woman—Share them with her. Often she will want to listen to FHTs with her significant others.

PELVIC EXAMINATION

Genitalia

Use the procedure for the pelvic examination described in Chapter 26. Note the following characteristics. You may note a bluish-purple discoloration of the external genitalia, **Chadwick's sign** of pregnancy. The enlargement of the labia minora is common in multiparous women. Labial varicosities may be present. The perineum may be scarred from a previous episiotomy or from lacerations. Note the presence of any hemorrhoids of the rectum.

Speculum Examination

When examining the vagina, again you may see **Chadwick's sign,** the bluish-purplish discoloration of the vaginal wall and cervix due to increased vascularity and engorgement (Fig. 27–13). Note the vaginal discharge. Vaginal discharge in pregnancy may be heavier in amount, but should be similar in description to the woman's nonpregnant discharge, and should not be associated with itching, burning, or an unusual odor (except that, occasionally, chapping of the vaginal area may be seen due to excessive moisture). Perform a wet mount or culture of the discharge when you are uncertain of its normalcy.

Note whether the cervix appears open. Note whether it is the smooth, round cervix with a dotlike external os of the nulliparous woman, or the irregular multiparous cervix with an external os that appears more like a crooked line, the result of cervical dilation and possibly lacerations in a previous pregnancy.

A friable cervix bleeds easily when touched with a cotton swab, cytobrush, or speculum, and may be due to cervicitis. Obtain cultures.

27–13

Bimanual Examination

As described in Chapter 26, palpate the uterus between your internal and external hands. Note its position. The pregnant uterus may be rotated toward the right side as it rises out of the pelvis due to the presence of the descending colon on the left. This is called **dextrorotation.** Irregular enlargement of the uterus may be noted at 8 to 10 weeks and occurs when implantation occurs close to a cornual area of the uterus. This is called **Piskacek's sign.** Also you may note **Hegar's sign,** when the enlarged uterus bends forward on its softened isthmus.

Note the size and consistency of the uterus. The 6-week gestation uterus may seem only slightly enlarged and softened. The 8-week gestation uterus is approximately the size of an avocado, approximately 7 to 8 cm across the fundus. The 10-week gestation uterus is about the size of a grapefruit and may reach to the pelvic brim, but is narrow and does not fill the pelvis from side to side; the 12-week gestation uterus will fill the pelvis. After 12 weeks, the uterus is sized from the abdomen. The multigravid uterus may be larger initially, and early sizing of this uterus may be less reliable for dating.

Softening of the cervix is called **Goodell's sign.** When examining the cervix, note its position (anterior, midposition, or posterior); degree of effacement (or thinning, expressed in percentages assuming a ≥2-cm long cervix initially); dilation (opening, expressed in centimeters); consistency (soft or firm); and the station of the presenting part (centimeters above or below the ischial plane) (Fig. 27–14).

A shortened cervix is <2 cm.

NORMAL RANGE OF FINDINGS

ABNORMAL FINDINGS

A

Internal os

Cavity of cervix with mucous plug

External os

B

Dilating, effacing cervix

External os

C

-5 cm
-4
-3
-2
-1
0 cm
+1
+2
+3
+4
+5 cm

Ischial spine

27–14 **A,** Cervix before labor. **B,** Cervix begins to efface and dilate. **C,** Station height of presenting part in relation to ischial spines.

The ovaries rise with the growing uterus. Always examine the adnexae to rule out the presence of a mass, such as an ectopic pregnancy.

Ask the woman to squeeze your fingers as they rest in the vagina to determine tone. Take this opportunity to teach Kegel exercise, the squeezing of the vagina, which the woman can do to prepare for and to recover from birth. (The woman can also identify the exercise of these muscles by stopping the flow of urine midstream, although she should only do this once, and should usually let urine flow freely.) Direct the woman to squeeze slowly to a peak at the count of eight and then release slowly to the count of eight. You can prescribe this exercise to be performed 50 to 100 times a day.

The woman will often appreciate palpating her own uterus from the abdomen. If the uterus is small, you can lift it up internally.

Adnexal enlargement and pain with palpation occurs with ectopic pregnancy or ovarian mass.

Pelvimetry

Assess the bones of the pelvis for shape and size. The dimensions may indicate the favorableness of the bony structure for vaginal delivery. However, the relaxation of the pelvic joints, the widening of the pelvis in the squatting position, and the capacity of the fetal head to mold to the shape of the pelvis, may enable a vaginal birth despite seemingly unfavorable measurements.

To aid in visualizing the pelvis, imagine three planes: the pelvic inlet (from the sacral promontory to the upper edge of the pubis), the midpelvis, and the pelvic outlet (from the coccyx to the lower edge of the pubis) (Fig. 27–15). Assessment of each of these pelvic planes, as described in the following techniques, allows you to estimate the adequacy of the pelvis for vaginal delivery.

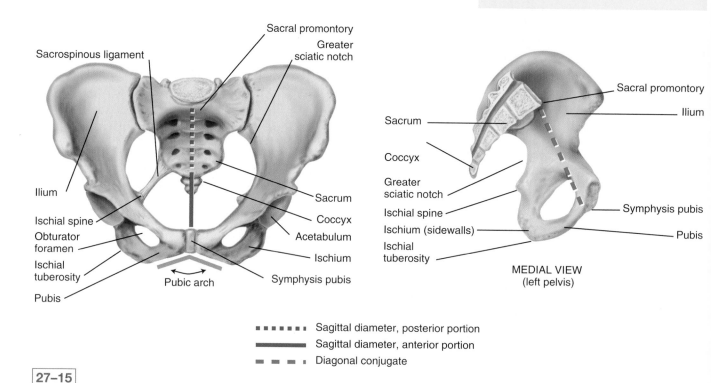

Sacral promontory
Greater sciatic notch
Sacrospinous ligament
Ilium
Ischial spine
Obturator foramen
Ischial tuberosity
Pubis
Pubic arch
Sacrum
Coccyx
Acetabulum
Ischium
Symphysis pubis

Sacrum
Coccyx
Greater sciatic notch
Ischial spine
Ischium (sidewalls)
Ischial tuberosity
Sacral promontory
Ilium
Symphysis pubis
Pubis

MEDIAL VIEW
(left pelvis)

- - - - - - - Sagittal diameter, posterior portion
————— Sagittal diameter, anterior portion
— — — Diagonal conjugate

27–15

There are four general types of pelves: gynecoid, anthropoid, android, and platypelloid (Table 27–1). Most commonly, a woman's pelvis will be an "intermediate" or "mixed" type. You may postpone examination of the bony pelvis until the third trimester when the vagina is more distensible. With your two fingers still in the vagina, note the shape and width of the pubic arch (a 90-degree arch, or 2 fingerbreadths, is desirable). If you are right-handed, move your hand to the woman's right pelvis. If you are left-handed, move it to the left side of the woman's pelvis. Assess the inclination and curve of the side walls, and the prominence of the ischial spine (refer back to Fig. 27–15 for location of these landmarks). Move your fingers back and forth between the spines to get an impression of the transverse diameter—10 cm is desirable. Sweep your fingers down the sacrum, noting its shape and inclination (hollow, J-shaped, or straight). Assess the coccyx for prominence and mobility. From the sacrum, locate the sacrospinous ligament. Assess the length of the ligament—2½ to 3 fingerbreadths is adequate. Assess the shape and width of the sacrospinous notch. Shift to the other side of the pelvis and assess it for similarity to the first.

TABLE 27-1: The Four Pelvic Types

THE GYNECOID PELVIS

GYNECOID

Inlet round or oval.
Posterior sagittal diameter of inlet only slightly less than anterior sagittal diameter.
Pubic arch wide (90 degrees or more).
Spines are not prominent, allowing a transverse diameter at spines 10 cm or more.
Sacrosciatic notch round and wide.
Straight side walls.
Posterior pelvis is round and wide.

Sacrum is parallel with the symphysis pubis; hollow and concave.

Favors vaginal delivery.
Seen in 50% of all women.

THE ANDROID PELVIS

ANDROID

Inlet heart-shaped.
Posterior sagittal diameter of inlet less than the anterior sagittal diameter.
Pubic arch narrow (less than 90 degrees).
Spines are prominent, decreasing transverse diameter at spines.

Sacrosciatic notch is narrow and highly arched.
Side walls converge.
Posterior sagittal diameter decreases from inlet to outlet as sacrum inclines forward.
Sacrum is straight and prominent; coccyx may be prominent.
Anterior of pelvis is narrow and triangular.
The "male" pelvis.
Poor prognosis for vaginal delivery.
Seen more frequently in Caucasian women.

THE ANTHROPOID PELVIS

ANTHROPOID

Inlet oval in shape.
Pubic arch may be somewhat narrow.
Spines usually prominent but not encroaching because of the spaciousness of the posterior segment.
Sacrosciatic notch average height but wide (about 4 fingerbreadths).
Side walls somewhat convergent.
Sacrum posteriorly inclined, with posterior sagittal diameters long throughout the pelvis.
Occurs in 40.5% nonwhite women; 23.5% white women.
If pelvis somewhat large, adequate for vaginal delivery since posterior pelvis is generous.

THE PLATYPELLOID PELVIS

PLATYPELLOID

Inlet shaped like a flattened gynecoid pelvis.
Pubic arch wide.
Spines usually prominent but not encroaching because of the already wide interspinous diameter.
Sacrosciatic notch wide and flat.
Side walls slightly convergent.
Sacrum inclined posteriorly and hollow, making a short and shallow pelvis.
Occurs in less than 3% of all women.
Not conducive to vaginal delivery.

Data from Varney H: *Varney's midwifery*, ed 3, Sudbury, MA, 1997, Jones and Bartlett.

The pelvic inlet cannot be reached by clinical examination, but you can estimate it by the measure of the **diagonal conjugate,** which indicates the anteroposterior diameter of the pelvic inlet. Having measured the length of the second and third fingers of your examining hand, with your fingers still in the vagina, point these fingers toward the sacral promontory (Fig. 27–16). If you cannot reach the promontory, note the measurement as being greater than the centimeters of length of your examining fingers. A measurement of 11.5 to 12.0 cm is desirable.

■ ■ ■ Diagonal conjugate

27–16   Diagonal conjugate.

Remove your fingers from the vagina. Having previously measured the width of your own hand across the knuckles, form your hand into a closed fist and place it across the perineum between the ischial tuberosities. Estimate this diameter, which is the **biischial diameter** (also known as the intertubous diameter and the transverse diameter of the pelvic outlet). A measurement greater than 8 cm is generally adequate (Fig. 27–17).

When describing pelvimetry, note all of the above measurements and state the pelvic type. The pelvis may be described as being "proven" to the number of pounds of the largest vaginally born infant. Alternatively, to describe a small pelvis, you may make the assessment, for example, "adequate for a 7-lb baby."

NORMAL RANGE OF FINDINGS

ABNORMAL FINDINGS

| 27–17 | Biischial diameter. |

Blood Pressure

After the exam, take the blood pressure when the woman is the most relaxed, in the semi-Fowler's or upright position. An elevated pressure should be rechecked on the right arm with the woman resting on her left side.

Chronic hypertension: a documented history of high blood pressure prior to pregnancy or a persistent elevation of at least 140/90 mm Hg on two occasions more than 24 hours apart before the 20th week of gestation (Gabbe et al., 2002).

ROUTINE LABORATORY AND RADIOLOGIC IMAGING STUDIES

At the onset of pregnancy, order a routine prenatal panel, which usually includes a complete blood count, serology, rubella antibodies, hepatitis B screening, blood type and Rhesus factor, and an antibody screening. Some providers screen for herpes simplex virus (HSV) I and II. Sickle cell screening may be indicated. For some populations, a PPD/TINE test may be indicated to rule out active or exposure to tuberculosis. Offer the woman HIV screening. Obtain Pap smear at the initial visit along with cervical cultures.

Collect a clean-catch urinalysis at the initial prenatal visit to rule out cystitis. At each prenatal visit, check the urine for protein and glucose. A clean-catch specimen is ideal for this dip because a random specimen may include vaginal secretions, which contain protein, skewing the results.

Each agency has a policy regarding the frequency of ultrasound (US) examinations. Some providers prefer to do an ultrasound for dating at the time of the maternal serum Alphafetoprotein or "quad" screening is drawn, since accurate dating is essential. Others will do it later (11 to 14 weeeks' gestation), when measuring for fetal translucency (another fetal risk screening tool), which is best done at this gestation. Some providers utilize ultrasound only when there is a medical indication; others routinely order US to confirm dates and fetal normalcy (insofar as ultrasound is able to determine normalcy), as well as for any specific medical indication, such as the fundus measuring small or large for dates. The US shows placental and fetal location and fetal gender.

SUMMARY CHECKLIST: The Pregnant Female

1. Collect historical information.
2. Determine EDC and present number of weeks of gestation.
3. Instruct the woman to undress and empty her bladder, saving her urine to dip it for protein and glucose.
4. Measure weight.
5. Perform a physical examination, starting with general survey.
6. Inspect skin for pigment changes, scars.
7. Check oral mucous membranes.
8. Palpate thyroid gland.
9. Inspect breast changes and palpate.
10. Auscultate breath sounds, heart sounds, heart rate, and any murmurs.
11. Check lower extremities for edema, varicosities, and reflexes.
12. The abdomen: Measure fundus height, perform Leopold's maneuvers, auscultate FHTs.
13. The pelvic exam: Note signs of pregnancy, the condition of the cervix, and the size and position of the uterus.
14. Perform pelvimetry.
15. Measure the blood pressure.

Application and Critical Thinking

SAMPLE CHARTING

SUBJECTIVE

Rosa Gutierrez is a 27-year-old Hispanic Gravida 2/Para 1 who presents with her husband and daughter for her first prenatal visit. She is a full-time homemaker who completed 2 years of college. Last normal menstrual period (LNMP) was April 4 of this year (certain of date), with an expected date of confinement (EDC) of January 11 of next year, making her 10 weeks' gestation today. Her obstetric history includes a normal spontaneous vaginal delivery (NSVD) 3 years ago of a viable 7 lb 12 oz female infant after an 8-hour labor without anesthesia, midline episiotomy. No complications of pregnancy, delivery, or the postpartum. She breastfed this daughter, Ana, for 1 year. Present pregnancy was planned, and Rosa and her husband are pleased. Rosa is having breast tenderness, and nausea on occasion, which resolves with crackers. No past medical or surgical conditions are present. She denies allergies. Family history is significant only for diet-controlled adult-onset diabetes in two maternal aunts.

OBJECTIVE

General: appears well nourished and is carefully groomed. English is second language, and Rosa is fluent. Skin: light tan in color, surface smooth with no lesions, small tattoo noted on left forearm. Mouth: good dentition and oral hygiene. Oral mucosa pink, no gum hypertrophy. Thyroid gland small and smooth.

Chest expansion equal, respirations effortless. Lung sounds clear bilaterally with no adventitious sounds. No CVA tenderness.

Heart: rate 76 bpm, regular rhythm, S_1 and S_2 are normal, not accentuated or diminished, with soft, blowing systolic murmur Gr ii/vi at 2nd left interspace.

Breasts: tender, without masses, with supple, everted nipples. Breast self-exam reviewed.

Abdomen: no masses, bowel sounds present. No hepatosplenomegaly. Uterus nonpalpable. No inguinal lymphadenopathy noted.

Extremities: no varicosities, redness, or edema. Homans' sign negative. DTRs 2+ and equal bilaterally. BP 110/68 in semi-Fowler's.

Pelvic: Bartholin's, urethra, and Skene's glands (BUS) negative for discharge. Vagina: pink, with white, creamy, nonodorous discharge. Cervix: pink, closed, multiparous, 2 cm long, firm.

Uterus: 10-week size, consistent with dates, nontender, dextrorotated. FHTs heard with Doppler, rate 140s.

Pelvis: pubic arch wide; side walls straight, spines blunt, interspinous diameter >10 cm.

Sacrum hollow; coccyx mobile. Sacrospinous ligament 3 fingerbreadths (FBs) wide. Diagonal conjugate >12 cm, bituberous diameter >8 cm. Spacious gynecoid pelvis proven to 7 lb 12 oz.

ASSESSMENT

Intrauterine pregnancy 10 weeks by good dates, size = dates.
Rosa and husband happy with pregnancy; she feels well.

PLAN

Begin prenatal vitamins.
Prenatal blood screen and urinalysis.
HIV offered and accepted.
Reviewed comfort measures for nausea.
Return visit in 4 weeks.

NURSING DIAGNOSES COMMONLY ASSOCIATED WITH PREGNANCY

RELATED FACTORS (Etiology)	DEFINING CHARACTERISTICS (Symptoms and Signs)
DIAGNOSIS: Impaired Parenting	
Ineffective role model	Verbalizes disappointment in gender or physical characteristics of infant
Effects of physical and psychosocial abuse	Verbalizes resentment toward infant
Unmet social/emotional maturational needs of parenting figure	Verbalizes role inadequacy
Interruption in bonding process	Verbalizes frustration
Unrealistic expectations for self, infant, partner	Lack of parental attachment behaviors
Multiple pregnancies	Inattention to infant's/child's needs
Physical or mental handicaps	Noncompliance with health appointments
Acute/chronic mental or physical illnesses	History of child abuse by primary caretaker
Limited cognitive functioning	Compulsively seeks role approval from others
Lack of support from significant others	
Lack of knowledge	
Lack of role identity	
Perceived threat to own survival, physical and emotional	
Presence of stress (financial, legal, cultural move)	

OTHER RELATED NURSING DIAGNOSES

ACTUAL	RISK/WELLNESS
Disturbed Body image (see Chapter 13)	**Risk**
Impaired Comfort	Risk for imbalanced Nutrition: less than body requirements
Constipation	Risk for imbalanced Nutrition: more than body requirements
Compromised family Coping	Risk for ineffective Sexual patterns
Fatigue	**Wellness**
Ineffective Health maintenance	Potential for effective Health management
Noncompliance	Potential for effective Nutritional-metabolic pattern
Disturbed Sleep pattern	Potential for positive Role-relationship pattern

ASSESSMENT VIDEO CRITICAL THINKING QUESTIONS

The Saunders *Physical Examination and Health Assessment* video "The Pregnant Woman" will direct you to consider the following:

1. What information does an obstetric history provide and how is it used?
2. Why should you document the patient's position when taking her blood pressure?
3. When is edema in the legs a danger sign in a pregnant patient?
4. Why are the external genitalia examined?
5. Why are pelvic measurements important to a prenatal assessment?
6. What is the significance of a fundal height that is higher or lower than expected for the patient's weeks of gestation?

TABLE 27–2: Preeclampsia

Preeclampsia is a condition specific to pregnancy that is rarely seen before 20 weeks of gestation except in the presence of a molar (gestational trophoblastic) pregnancy. The etiology remains unknown, but theories include coagulation abnormalities, vascular endothelial damage, cardiovascular maladaptation, immunologic phenomena, dietary deficiencies or excess, and genetic predisposition. Predisposing conditions include a family or personal history of preeclampsia, nulliparity, obesity, multifetal gestation, preexisting medical-genetic conditions such as chronic hypertension, renal disease, type 1 (insulin-dependent) diabetes, factor V Leiden, and thrombophelias such as antiphospholipid antibody syndrome (Gabbe, 2002).

The classic symptoms are elevated blood pressure and proteinuria. Edema is common in pregnancy, and is the least reliable symptom that is no longer considered a part of the diagnosis of preeclampsia (Gabbe et al., 2002). However, when edema of the face is of sudden onset and is associated with sudden weight gain, one must consider preeclampsia. Proteinuria is a late development in preeclampsia and is an indicator of the severity of the disease. The BP should be compared with the woman's first prenatal BP (before 20 weeks' gestation). An increase of 15 mm Hg diastolic over the baseline or a BP greater than 140 systolic or 90 diastolic is considered hypertension. Hypertension is necessary for the diagnosis of preeclampsia, but preeclampsia may be seen without the edema or proteinuria.

Onset and worsening symptoms may be sudden. Subjective signs may include headaches and visual changes (spots, blurring or flashing lights) due to cerebral edema, and/or right upper quadrant (RUQ)/epigastric pain due to liver enlargement where it becomes enlarged, necrotic, and hemorrhagic. Liver enzymes become elevated. Hematocrit usually

increases and the platelets drop. Serum creatinine and BUN elevate. Hemolysis occurs, in part at least, as a result of vasospasm. A serious variant of preeclampsia, the **HELLP** syndrome, involves Hemolysis, Elevated Liver enzymes, and Low Platelets, and represents an ominous clinical picture. Untreated preeclampsia may progress to eclampsia, which is manifested by generalized tonic-clonic seizures. Eclampsia may develop as late as 10 days postpartum.

Before the syndrome becomes clinically manifested, it is affecting the placenta through vasospasm and a series of small infarctions. The placenta's capacity to deliver oxygen and nutrients may be seriously diminished, and fetal growth may be restricted.

TABLE 27–3: Fetal Size Inconsistent with Dates

Size Small for Dates
Fundal height measures smaller than expected for dates.

Inaccuracy of Dates
Conception may have occurred later than originally thought. Reconsider the woman's menstrual history, sexual history, contraceptive use, early pregnancy testing, early sizing of the uterus, ultrasound results, timing of pregnancy symptoms, including the date of quickening, and the fundal height measurements. If, after this review, the expected date of delivery is correct, than further investigation is required.

Premature Labor
When premature labor engages the presenting part of the fetus into the pelvis for delivery, the fundus may shorten. Premature or preterm birth occurs before 37 weeks' gestation, which happens 9.9% for whites, 11.2% for Hispanic, and 17.6% for African-American women in the United States (Gabbe et al., 2002). Risk indicators for preterm birth include abdominal surgery during the current pregnancy, age of <18 years or >35 years, chronic urinary tract infections, conization of the cervix, hydramnios, hypertensive disorders, low socioeconomic status, low pre-pregnancy weight, African-American race, multiple gestation, woman was herself a preterm infant, poor nutrition, previous preterm delivery, cigarette smoking, strenuous work, substance/drug abuse (especially cocaine and alcohol), two or more second trimester terminations, uterine anomalies, and uterine infections (Swenson, 2001).

Continued

TABLE 27–3: Fetal Size Inconsistent with Dates—cont'd

Intrauterine Growth Retardation (IUGR) or Fetal Growth Restriction	IUGR, a syndrome where the neonate fails to meet its growth potential, is associated with an increase in fetal and neonatal mortality and morbidity. Its origin may be feto-placental, as with chromosomal abnormalities, genetic syndromes, congenital malformations, infectious diseases, and placental pathology. Or its origin may be maternal, as with decreased uteroplacental blood flow as seen with hypertensive disorders, poor maternal weight gain, poor maternal nutrition, and a previous pregnancy with an IUGR infant. Other factors include infectious diseases (rubella, cytomegalovirus); multiple gestation; and environmental toxins such as smoking, maternal drug ingestion, and alcohol.
Fetal Position	Fetal position varies until about 34 weeks, when the vertex should settle into the pelvis and remain there. The fetus occupying a transverse lie, or shoulder presentation, results in the maternal abdomen's widening from side to side and the fundal height's diminishing. Fetal malposition may occur with lax maternal abdominal musculature (simply not holding the baby in close), an abnormality in the fetus (e.g., the enlarged head of the hydrocephalic infant), placenta previa (the placenta being implanted over the cervix, blocking fetal descent), or a restricted maternal pelvis.
Size Large for Dates	Fundal height measures larger than expected for dates.
Inaccuracy of Dates	Review the same findings as listed above.
Hydatidiform mole	Also termed *gestational trophoblastic neoplasia* (GTN), it is a result of abnormal proliferation of trophoblastic tissue associated with pregnancy. In 50% of cases, uterine size is excessive; in these cases the gestational age and uterine size do not coincide.
Multiple fetuses	The frequency of multiple fetuses increases with advanced maternal age and is enhanced by the increasing use of fertility drugs. The uterus enlarges where the fundal height may be beyond the calculated/expected gestational age. Ultrasound examination confirms the diagnosis.
Polyhydramnios	An amniotic fluid volume is a maximum volume pocket (MVP) above 8.0 cm or an AFI above the 95th percentile. The cause is usually idiopathic, but may be in part due to fetal anomalies, insulin-dependent diabetes, gestational diabetes, and multiple fetuses (Creasy, 1997).
Leiomyoma (Myoma or "Fibroids")	These are preexisting benign tumors of the uterine wall, which then are stimulated to enlarge by the estrogen levels of pregnancy. Myomata may be located anywhere in the uterine wall (see Table 26–7). When they grow in the outer uterine wall, the myometrium, they may affect the clinician's judgment of where the fundus of the uterus should be measured. A myoma may grow just underneath the endometrial surface into the uterine cavity, displacing the fetus or preventing its descent into the pelvis.
Fetal macrosomia	This is a condition where the infant's weight is beyond 4000 g or 4500 g, regardless of the gestational age. 1998 data from the National Center for Health Statistics showed that 10% of all live born infants in the United States weighed more than 4000 g (ACOG Compendium, 2002). Maternal risk factors for macrosomia include a prior history of a macrosomic infant, maternal obesity, weight gain during the pregnancy, multiparity, male fetus, gestational age >40 weeks, ethnicity, maternal birth weight, maternal height, maternal age <17 years and a positive 50 g glucose screen with a negative 3 hour GTT. Birth risks to the mother include labor abnormalities, an increased incidence for cesarean section, bladder trauma, and vaginal tissue trauma. Fetal risks include birth trauma such as fractured clavicle and brachial plexus nerve damage due to shoulder dystocia, depressed Apgar scores, extended hospitalizations, and possible fetal mortality.

ABNORMAL FINDINGS

TABLE 27–4: Disorders of Pregnancy

DISORDER/CONDITION	DESCRIPTION
Vaginal bleeding	Some women will have bright red, pink or dark brown spotting at some time during the first trimester. This is not always a sign of pending pregnancy loss but may be from a blighted ovum, friable cervix, ectopic pregnancy, perigestational hemorrhage, or cervical lesions. In the second and third trimester, vaginal bleeding may be indicative of abruptio placentae, placenta previa, uterine rupture, cervical dilation, or a friable cervix. Risk factors for increased risk of vaginal bleeding include pregnancy-induced hypertension (PIH), chronic hypertension (CHTN), cocaine use, abdominal trauma, uterine anomalies, prolonged premature rupture of membranes, and prior placental abruption.
Incompetent cervix	Cervical incompetence is marked by gradual and painless premature dilation and effacement of the cervix that can lead to fetal loss if undetected early enough to have a cervical cerclage placed. Its cause may be congenital, as seen in some women after diethylstilbestrol (DES) exposure, and/or it may be acquired after cervical trauma or a cone biopsy.
Hyperemesis	Hyperemesis is excessive vomiting in pregnancy that may last well into the second trimester and beyond. It can interfere with electrolytes, acid base balance, and nutritional status. Dehydration and starvation may ensue and lead to fetal IUGR. Nausea and vomiting are not uncommon in pregnancy and usually resolve between weeks 16 and 20 and may be controlled with dietary and lifestyle changes or oral antiemetics. Hyperemesis is the extreme of vomiting and may require home infusion therapy or hospitalization. Risk factors include a previous history of hyperemesis, molar pregnancy, multiple gestation, emotional stress, history of GI reflux, uncontrolled thyroid disease, primigravida, and obesity.
Preterm labor	Preterm labor is labor occurring after 20 weeks and before completion of 37 weeks' gestation. Preterm labor is a major factor for fetal morbidity and mortality. Some risk factors include: chronic urinary tract infections (UTIs), polyhydramnios, multiple gestation, previous preterm labor and/or delivery, smoking, substance abuse, poor prenatal care, poor weight gain after 20 weeks' gestation, history of cervical conization, low socioeconomic status, nonwhite race, uterine infections, and cases where the patient herself was a preterm infant.
Decreased fetal movement	Fetal movement is one indicator of fetal well-being and should begin from 28 weeks' gestation. There are various methods used; the important thing is to be consistent and count every day. A decrease in fetal movement should be reported and followed by a non-stress test (fetal monitoring). Cessation of fetal movement may be indicative of fetal distress or impending fetal demise.

TABLE 27–5: Malpresentations

Vertex (for comparison)

Complete breech

Footling breech

Frank breech

Transverse lie and
shoulder presentation

Face presentation

Brow presentation

Compound presentation

Malpresentations may be detected by the hands of an experienced examiner, confirmed by the FHT location, and further confirmed by ultrasound. Before 34 weeks' gestation, any position is normal. The vertex presentation is desirable thereafter, because spontaneous turning becomes less likely as the fetus grows in proportion to the amount of space and fluid in the uterus and pelvis.

BIBLIOGRAPHY

American College of Obstetricians and Gynecologists: *Antepartum Fetal Surveillance,* Washington, DC, October 1999, The Association (Technical Bulletin No. 9).

American College of Obstetricians and Gynecologists: *Fetal Macrosomia,* Washington, DC, November 2000, The Association (Technical Bulletin No. 22).

American College of Obstetricians and Gynecologists: *Special Problems of Multiple Gestation,* Washington, DC, November 1998, The Association (Educational Bulletin No. 253).

American College of Obstetricians and Gynecologists: *Thyroid Disease in Pregnancy,* Washington, DC, November 2001, The Association (Technical Bulletin No. 32).

Bastian LA, Piscitelli JT: Is this patient pregnant? Can you reliably rule in or out early pregnancy by clinical examination? *JAMA* 18:586–591, Aug 20, 1997.

Beamer LC: Fetal nuchal translucency: a prenatal screening tool, *JOGNN* 30(4):376–385, 2001.

Burrow GN, Duffy TP, editors: *Medical complications during pregnancy,* ed 4, Philadelphia, 1999, WB Saunders.

Burton J, Reyes M: Breath in, breath out: controlling asthma during pregnancy, *Lifelines* 5:1, 25–30, 2001.

Callister LC: Culturally competent care of women and newborns: knowledge, attitude, and skills, *JOGNN* 30(2):209–215, 2001.

Centers for Disease Control and Prevention: *Morbidity and Mortality Weekly Report (MMWR)* 50(18), May 11, 2001.

Centers for Disease Control and Prevention: *Morbidity and Mortality Weekly Report (MMWR)* 47(34), September 4, 1998.

Chin HG: *On call obstetrics and gynecology,* ed 2, Philadelphia, 2001, WB Saunders.

Creasy RK, Resnick R: *Maternal-fetal medicine,* ed 4, Philadelphia, 1999, WB Saunders.

Cunningham FG et al: *Williams obstetrics,* ed 21, Stamford, CT, 2001, Appleton & Lange.

Gabbe SG, Niebyl JR, Simpson JL: *Obstetrics: normal and problem pregnancies,* ed 4, New York, 2002, Churchill Livingstone.

Kennedy HP, Griffin M, Frishman G: Enabling conception and pregnancy: midwifery care of women experiencing infertility, *J Nurse Midwifery* 43(3):190–207, 1998.

Lowe SW, Pruitt RH, Smart PT, Dooley RL: Routine use of ultrasound during pregnancy, *Nurse Pract* 23(10):60–71, Oct 1998.

Mattson S: Working toward cultural competence, making the first steps through cultural assessment, *Lifelines* 4(4):41–43, 2000.

National Center for Chronic Disease Prevention & Health Promotion: *CDC Press Release, CDC report highlights selected racial and ethnic pregnancy-related death rates,* Atlanta, May 11, 2001, CDC.

O'Day MP: Cardio-respiratory physiological adaptation of pregnancy, *Semin Perinatol* 21(4):268–275, Aug 1997.

Rousseau ME: Women's midlife health, *J Nurse Midwifery* 43(3):208–223, 1998.

Star WL et al: *Ambulatory obstetrics,* ed 3, San Francisco, 1999, UCSF Nursing Press.

Swenson D: *Telephone triage for the obstetric patient: a nursing guide,* Philadelphia, 2001, WB Saunders.

United Nations Population Fund: *Fast facts on maternal health and morbidity,* UNFPA, 2001.

Varney H: *Varney's midwifery,* ed 3, Sudbury, MA, 1997, Jones and Bartlett.

CHAPTER 28

The Complete Health Assessment:
Putting It All Together

The choreography of the complete history and physical examination is the art of arranging all the separate steps you have learned so far. Your first examination may seem awkward and contrived; you may have to pause and think of what comes next rather than just gather data. Repeated rehearsals will make the choreography smoother. You will come to the point at which the procedure flows naturally, and even if you forget a step, you will be able to insert it gracefully into the next logical place.

The following examination sequence is one suggested route. It is intended to minimize the number of position changes for the patient and for you. With experience, you may wish to adapt this and arrange a sequence that feels natural for you. Perform all the steps listed here for a complete examination. With experience, you will learn to strike a balance between which steps you must retain to be thorough and which corners you may safely cut when time is pressing.

Have all equipment prepared and accessible before the examination. Review Chapter 9, "Assessment Techniques and the Clinical Setting," for the list of necessary equipment, the setting, the patient's emotional state, your demeanor, and the preparation of the patient considering his or her age.

SEQUENCE	**SELECTED PHOTOS**

The patient walks into the room, sits; the examiner sits facing the patient; the patient is in street clothes.

THE HEALTH HISTORY

Collect the history, complete or limited as visit warrants. While obtaining the history and throughout the examination, note data on the person's general appearance.

GENERAL APPEARANCE

1. Appears stated age
2. Level of consciousness
3. Skin color
4. Nutritional status
5. Posture and position comfortably erect
6. Obvious physical deformities
7. Mobility
   Gait
   Use of assistive devices
   Range of motion (ROM) of joints
   No involuntary movement
8. Facial expression
9. Mood and affect
10. Speech: articulation, pattern, content appropriate, native language
11. Hearing
12. Personal hygiene

MEASUREMENT

1. Weight
2. Height
3. Skinfold thickness, if indicated
4. Vision using Snellen's eye chart

The rules are to show position change for the patient or examiner.

SEQUENCE	SELECTED PHOTOS

Ask the person to empty the bladder (save specimen, if needed), disrobe except for underpants, and put on a gown. The person sits with legs dangling off side of the bed or table; you stand in front of the person.

SKIN

1. Examine both hands and inspect the nails.
2. For the rest of the examination, examine skin with corresponding regional examination.

VITAL SIGNS

1. Radial pulse
2. Respirations
3. Blood pressure
4. Temperature (if indicated)

HEAD AND FACE

1. Inspect and palpate scalp, hair, and cranium.
2. Inspect face: expression, symmetry (cranial nerve VII).
3. Palpate the temporal artery, then the temporomandibular joint as the person opens and closes the mouth.
4. Palpate the maxillary sinuses and the frontal sinuses; if tender, transilluminate the sinuses.

EYE

1. Test visual fields by confrontation (cranial nerve II).
2. Test extraocular muscles: corneal light reflex, six cardinal positions of gaze (cranial nerves III, IV, VI).
3. Inspect external eye structures.
4. Inspect conjunctivae, sclerae, corneas, irides.
5. Test pupil: size, response to light and accommodation.

   Darken room.

6. Using an ophthalmoscope, inspect ocular fundus: red reflex, disc, vessels, and retinal background.

EAR

1. Inspect the external ear: position and alignment, skin condition, and auditory meatus.
2. Move auricle and push tragus for tenderness.
3. Using an otoscope, inspect the canal, then the tympanic membrane for color, position, landmarks, and integrity.
4. Test hearing: voice test; tuning fork tests—Weber and Rinne.

SEQUENCE	SELECTED PHOTOS

NOSE

1. Inspect the external nose: symmetry, lesions.
2. Test the patency of each nostril.
3. Using a speculum, inspect the nares: nasal mucosa, septum, and turbinates.

MOUTH AND THROAT

1. Using a penlight, inspect the mouth: buccal mucosa, teeth and gums, tongue, floor of mouth, palate, and uvula.
2. Grade tonsils, if present.
3. Note mobility of uvula as the person phonates "ahh," and test gag reflex (cranial nerves IX, X).
4. Ask the person to stick out the tongue (cranial nerve XII).
5. With a gloved hand, bimanually palpate the mouth, if indicated.

NECK

1. Inspect the neck: symmetry, lumps, and pulsations.
2. Palpate the cervical lymph nodes.
3. Inspect and palpate the carotid pulse, one side at a time. If indicated, listen for carotid bruits.
4. Palpate the trachea in midline.
5. Test ROM and muscle strength against your resistance: head forward and back, head turned to each side, and shoulder shrug (cranial nerve XI).

Step behind the person, taking your stethoscope, ruler, and marking pen with you.
  6. Palpate thyroid gland.

Open the person's gown to expose all of the back for examination of the thorax, but leave gown on shoulders and anterior chest.

CHEST, POSTERIOR AND LATERAL

1. Inspect the posterior chest: configuration of the thoracic cage, skin characteristics, and symmetry of shoulders and muscles.
2. Palpate: symmetric expansion; tactile fremitus; lumps or tenderness.
3. Palpate length of spinous processes.
4. Percuss over all lung fields, percuss diaphragmatic excursion.
5. Percuss costovertebral angle, noting tenderness.
6. Auscultate breath sounds; note adventitious sounds.

SEQUENCE	SELECTED PHOTOS

Move around to face the patient; the patient remains sitting. For a female breast examination, ask permission to lift gown to drape on the shoulders, exposing the anterior chest; for a male, lower the gown to the lap.

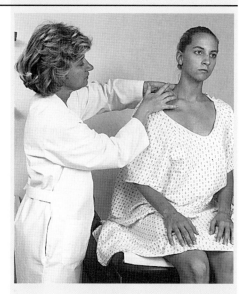

CHEST, ANTERIOR

1. Inspect: respirations and skin characteristics.
2. Palpate: tactile fremitus, lumps, or tenderness.
3. Percuss lung fields.
4. Auscultate breath sounds.

HEART

1. Ask the person to lean forward and exhale briefly; auscultate cardiac base for any murmurs.

UPPER EXTREMITIES

1. Test ROM and muscle strength of hands, arms, and shoulders.
2. Palpate the epitrochlear nodes.

FEMALE BREASTS

1. Inspect for symmetry, mobility, and dimpling as the woman lifts arms over the head, pushes the hands on the hips, and leans forward.
2. Inspect supraclavicular and infraclavicular areas.

Help the woman to lie supine with head at a 30- to 45-degree angle. Stand at the person's *right* side. Drape the gown up across shoulders and place an extra sheet across lower abdomen.

3. Palpate each breast, lifting the same side arm up over head. Include the tail of Spence and areola.
4. Palpate each nipple for discharge.
5. Support the person's arm and palpate axilla and regional lymph nodes.
6. Teach breast self-examination.

MALE BREASTS

1. Inspect and palpate while palpating the anterior chest wall.
2. Supporting each arm, palpate the axilla and regional nodes.

NECK VESSELS

1. Inspect each side of neck for a jugular venous pulse, turning the person's head slightly to the other side.
2. Estimate jugular venous pressure, if indicated.

SEQUENCE	SELECTED PHOTOS

HEART

1. Inspect the precordium for any pulsations and/or heave (lift).
2. Palpate the apical impulse and note the location.
3. Palpate precordium for any abnormal thrill.
4. Auscultate apical rate and rhythm.
5. Auscultate with the diaphragm of the stethoscope to study heart sounds, inching from the apex up to the base, or vice versa.
6. Auscultate the heart sounds with the bell of the stethoscope, again inching through all locations.
7. Turn the person over to left side while again auscultating apex with the bell.

_____

The person should be supine, with the bed or table flat; arrange drapes to expose the abdomen from the chest to the pubis.

ABDOMEN

1. Inspect: contour, symmetry, skin characteristics, umbilicus, and pulsations.
2. Auscultate bowel sounds.
3. Auscultate for vascular sounds over the aorta and renal arteries.
4. Percuss all quadrants.
5. Percuss height of the liver span in right midclavicular line.
6. Percuss the location of the spleen.
7. Palpate: light palpation in all quadrants, then deep palpation in all quadrants.
8. Palpate for liver, spleen, kidneys, and aorta.
9. Test the abdominal reflexes, if indicated.

INGUINAL AREA

1. Palpate each groin for the femoral pulse and the inguinal nodes. Lift the drape to expose the legs.

SEQUENCE	SELECTED PHOTOS

LOWER EXTREMITIES

1. Inspect: symmetry, skin characteristics, and hair distribution.
2. Palpate pulses: popliteal, posterior tibial, dorsalis pedis.
3. Palpate for temperature and pretibial edema.
4. Separate toes and inspect.
5. Test ROM and muscle strength of hips, knees, ankles, and feet.

Ask the person to sit up and to dangle the legs off the bed or table. Keep the gown on and the drape over the lap.

MUSCULOSKELETAL

1. Note muscle strength as person sits up.

NEUROLOGIC

1. Test sensation in selected areas on face, arms, hands, legs, and feet: superficial pain, light touch, and vibration.
2. Test position sense of finger, one hand.
3. Test stereognosis.
4. Test cerebellar function of the upper extremities using finger-to-nose test or rapid-alternating-movements test.
5. Test the cerebellar function of the lower extremities by asking the person to run each heel down the opposite shin.
6. Elicit deep tendon reflexes: biceps, triceps, brachioradialis, patellar, and Achilles.
7. Test the Babinski's reflex.

SEQUENCE	**SELECTED PHOTOS**

Ask the person to stand with the gown on. Stand close to the person.

LOWER EXTREMITIES

1. Inspect legs for varicose veins.

MUSCULOSKELETAL

1. Ask the person to walk across the room in his or her regular walk, turn, then walk back toward you, in heel-to-toe fashion.
2. Ask the person to walk on the toes for a few steps, then to walk on the heels for a few steps.
3. Stand close and check Romberg's sign.
4. Ask the person to hold the edge of the bed and to perform a shallow knee bend, one for each leg.
5. Stand behind and check the spine as the person touches the toes.
6. Stabilize the pelvis and test the ROM of the spine as the person hyperextends, rotates, and laterally bends.

Sit on a stool in front of a male. The person stands.

MALE GENITALIA

1. Inspect the penis and scrotum.
2. Palpate the scrotal contents. If a mass exists, transilluminate.
3. Check for inguinal hernia.
4. Teach testicular self-examination.

For an adult male, ask him to bend over the examination table, supporting the torso with forearms on the table. Assist the bedfast male to a left lateral position, with the right leg drawn up.

MALE RECTUM

1. Inspect the perianal area.
2. With a gloved lubricated finger, palpate the rectal walls and prostate gland.
3. Save a stool specimen for an occult blood test.

SEQUENCE	SELECTED PHOTOS

Assist the female back to the examination table, and help her assume the lithotomy position. Drape her appropriately. You sit on a stool at the foot of the table, then stand.

FEMALE GENITALIA

1. Inspect the perineal and perianal areas.
2. Using a vaginal speculum, inspect the cervix and vaginal walls.
3. Procure specimens.
4. Perform a bimanual examination; cervix, uterus, and adnexa.
5. Continue the bimanual examination, checking the rectum and rectovaginal walls.
6. Save a stool specimen for an occult blood test.
7. Provide tissues for the female to wipe the perineal area, and help her up to a sitting position.

Tell the patient you are finished with the examination and that you will leave the room as he or she gets dressed. Return to discuss the examination and further plans and to answer any questions. Thank the person for his or her time.

For the hospitalized person, return the bed and any room equipment to the way you found it. Make sure the call light and telephone are in easy reach.

THE NEONATE AND INFANT

Review Chapter 9, "Assessment Techniques and Approach to the Clinical Setting," for the steps on preparation and positioning and on developmental principles of the infant. The 1-minute and 5-minute Apgar results will give important data on the neonate's immediate response to extrauterine life. The following sequence will expand these data. You may reorder this sequence as the infant's sleep and wakefulness state or physical condition warrants.

The infant is supine on a warming table or examination table with an overhead heating element. The infant may be nude except for a diaper over a boy.

Vital Signs
Note pulse, respirations, and temperature.

Measurement
Weight, length, and head circumference are measured and plotted on growth curves for the infant's age.

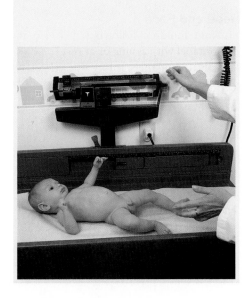

SEQUENCE	SELECTED PHOTOS

General Appearance

1. Body symmetry, spontaneous position, flexion of head and extremities, and spontaneous movement.
2. Skin color and characteristics, any obvious deformities.
3. Symmetry and positioning of the facial features.
4. Alert, responsive affect.
5. Strong, lusty cry.

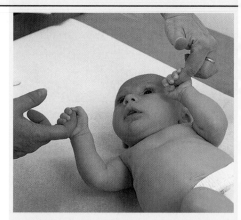

Chest and Heart

1. Inspect the skin condition over the chest and abdomen, chest configuration, and nipples and breast tissue.
2. Note movement of the abdomen with respirations, and any chest retraction.
3. Palpate: apical impulse and note its location; chest wall for thrills; tactile fremitus if the infant is crying.
4. Auscultate: breath sounds, heart sounds in all locations, and bowel sounds in the abdomen and in the chest.

Abdomen

1. Inspect the shape of the abdomen and skin condition.
2. Inspect the umbilicus; count vessels; note condition of cord or stump, any hernia.
3. Palpate skin turgor.
4. Palpate lightly for muscle tone, liver, spleen tip, and bladder.
5. Palpate deeply for kidneys, any mass.
6. Palpate femoral pulses, inguinal lymph nodes.
7. Percuss all quadrants.

Head and Face

1. Note molding following delivery, any swelling on cranium, bulging of fontanel with crying or at rest.
2. Palpate fontanels, suture lines, and any swellings.
3. Inspect positioning and symmetry of facial features at rest and while the infant is crying.

SEQUENCE	SELECTED PHOTOS

To open the neonate's eyes, support the head and shoulders and gently lower the baby backward, or ask the parent to hold the baby over his or her shoulder while you stand behind the parent.

Eyes

1. Inspect the lids (edematous in the neonate), palpebral slant, conjunctivae, any nystagmus, and any discharge.
2. Using a penlight: elicit the pupillary reflex, blink reflex, and corneal light reflex; assess tracking of moving light.
3. Using an ophthalmoscope, elicit the red reflex.

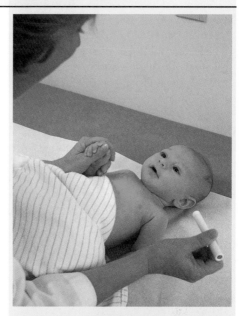

Ears

1. Inspect size, shape, alignment of auricle, patency of auditory canals, any extra skin tags or pits.
2. Note the startle reflex in response to a loud noise.
3. Palpate flexible auricles.
   (Defer otoscopic examination until the end of the complete examination.)

Nose

1. Determine the patency of the nares.
2. Note the nasal discharge, sneezing, and any flaring with respirations.

Mouth and Throat

1. Inspect the lips and gums, high-arched intact palate, buccal mucosa, tongue size, and frenulum of tongue; note absent or minimal salivation in neonate.
2. Note the rooting reflex.
3. Insert a gloved little finger, note the sucking reflex, and palpate palate.

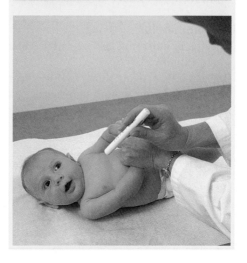

SEQUENCE	SELECTED PHOTOS

Neck

1. Lift the shoulders and let the head lag to inspect the neck: Note midline trachea, any skinfolds, and any lumps.
2. Palpate the lymph nodes, the thyroid, and any masses.
3. While the infant is supine, elicit the tonic neck reflex; note a supple neck with movement.

Upper Extremities

1. Inspect and manipulate, noting ROM, muscle tone, and absence of scarf sign (elbow should not reach midline).
2. Count fingers, count palmar creases, and note color of hands and nail beds.
3. Place your thumbs in the infant's palms to note the grasp reflex, then wrap your hands around infant's hands to pull up and note the head lag.

Lower Extremities

1. Inspect and manipulate the legs and feet, noting ROM, muscle tone, and skin condition.
2. Note alignment of feet and toes, look for flat soles, and count toes; note any syndactyly.
3. Test Ortolani's sign for hip stability.

Genitalia

1. Females. Inspect labia and clitoris (edematous in the newborn), vernix caseosa between labia, and patent vagina.
2. Males. Inspect position of urethral meatus (do not retract foreskin), strength of urine stream if possible, and rugae on scrotum.
3. Palpate the testes in the scrotum.

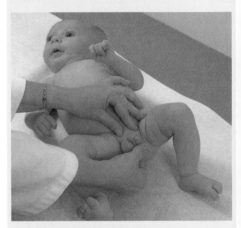

Lift the infant under the axillae, and hold the infant facing you at eye level.

Neuromuscular

1. Note shoulder muscle tone and the infant's ability to stay in your hands without slipping.
2. Rotate the neonate slowly side to side; note the doll's eye reflex.
3. Turn the infant around so his or her back is to you; elicit the stepping reflex and the placing reflex against the edge of the examination table.

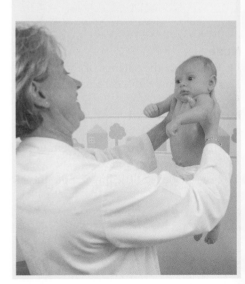

SEQUENCE	SELECTED PHOTOS

Turn the infant over and hold him or her prone in your hands, or place the infant prone on the examination table.

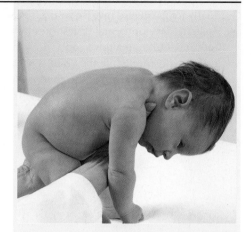

Spine and Rectum
1. Inspect the length of the spine, trunk incurvation reflex, and symmetry of gluteal folds.
2. Inspect intact skin; note any sinus openings, protrusions, or tufts of hair.
3. Note patent anal opening. Check for passage of meconium stool during the first 24 to 48 hours.

Final Procedures
1. Using an otoscope, inspect the auditory canal and the tympanic membrane.
2. Elicit the Moro reflex by letting the infant's head and trunk drop back a short way, by jarring crib sides, or by making a loud noise.

THE YOUNG CHILD

Review the developmental considerations in preparing for an examination of the toddler and the young child in Chapter 9, "Assessment Techniques and the Clinical Setting." A young child during this time is beset with independence and dependence needs on the parent, is aware of and fearful of a new environment, has a fear of invasive procedures, dislikes being restrained, and may be attached to a security object.

Focus on the parent as the child plays with a toy.

The Health History
1. Collect the history, including developmental data.
   During the history, note data on general appearance.

General Appearance
1. Note child's ability to amuse himself or herself while the parent speaks.
2. Note parent and child interaction.
3. Note gross motor and fine motor skills as the child plays with toys.

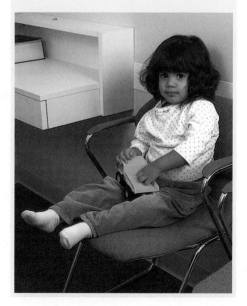

SEQUENCE	SELECTED PHOTOS

Gradually focus on and involve yourself with the child, at first in a "play" period.

4. Evaluate developmental milestones by using a Denver II test: gait, jumping, hopping, building a tower, and throwing a ball.
5. Evaluate posture while the child is sitting and standing. Evaluate alignment of the legs and feet while the child is walking.
6. Evaluate speech acquisition.
7. Evaluate vision, hearing ability.
8. Evaluate social interaction.

Ask the parent to undress the child to the diaper or the underpants. Position the older infant and young child, 6 months to 2 or 3 years, in the parent's lap. Move your chair to sit knee-to-knee with the parent. A 4- or 5-year-old child usually feels comfortable on the examination table.

Measurement

Height, weight, head circumference (may need to defer head circumference until later in the examination).

Chest and Heart

1. Auscultate breath sounds and heart sounds in all locations, count respiratory rate, count heart rate, and auscultate bowel sounds.
2. Inspect size, shape, and configuration of chest cage. Assess respiratory movement.
3. Inspect pulsations on the precordium. Note nipple and breast development.
4. Palpate: apical impulse and note location, chest wall for thrills, any tactile fremitus.

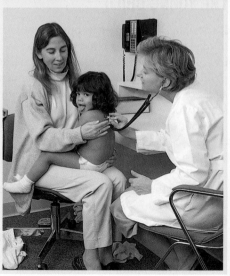

SEQUENCE	SELECTED PHOTOS

The child should be sitting up in the parent's lap or on the examination table, diaper or underpants in place.

Abdomen
1. Inspect shape of abdomen, skin condition, and periumbilical area.
2. Palpate skin turgor, muscle tone, liver edge, spleen, kidneys, and any masses.
3. Palpate the femoral pulses. Compare strength with radial pulses.
4. Palpate inguinal lymph nodes.

Genitalia
1. Inspect the external genitalia.
2. On males, palpate the scrotum for testes. If masses are present, transilluminate.

Lower Extremities
1. Test Ortolani's sign for hip stability.
2. Note alignment of legs and skin condition.
3. Note alignment of feet. Inspect toes and longitudinal arch.
4. Palpate the dorsalis pedis pulse.
5. Gain cooperation with reflex hammer. Elicit plantar, Achilles, and patellar reflexes.

The child should be sitting up in the parent's lap or on the examination table, diaper or underpants in place.

Upper Extremities
1. Inspect arms and hands for alignment, skin condition; inspect fingers and note palmar creases.
2. Palpate and count the radial pulse.
3. Test biceps and triceps reflexes with a reflex hammer.
4. Measure blood pressure.

SEQUENCE	SELECTED PHOTOS

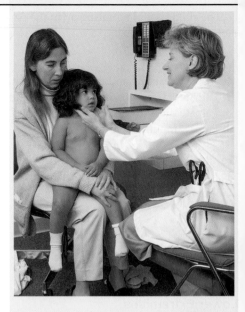

Head and Neck
1. Inspect the size and shape of the head and symmetry of facies.
2. Palpate the fontanels and cranium. Palpate the cervical lymph nodes, trachea, and thyroid gland.
3. Measure the head circumference.

Eyes
1. Inspect the external structures. Note any palpebral slant.
2. Using a penlight, test the corneal light and pupillary light reflexes.
3. Direct a moving penlight for cardinal positions of gaze.
4. If indicated, perform the cover test, covering the eye with your thumb in a young child, or use an index card.
5. Inspect conjunctivae and sclerae.
6. Using an ophthalmoscope, check the red reflex. Inspect the fundus as much as possible.

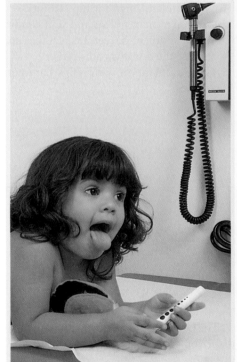

Nose
1. Inspect the external nose and skin condition.
2. Using a penlight, inspect the nares for foreign body, mucosa, septum, and turbinates.

Mouth and Throat
1. Using a penlight, inspect the mouth, buccal mucosa, teeth and gums, tongue, palate, and uvula in midline. Use a tongue blade as the last resort.

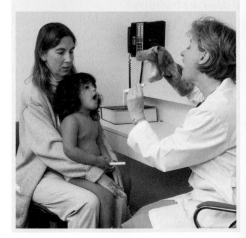

SEQUENCE	**SELECTED PHOTOS**

Ears

1. Inspect and palpate the auricle. Note any discharge from the auditory meatus. Check for any foreign body.
2. Using an otoscope, inspect the ear canal and tympanic membrane. Gain co-operation through the use of a puppet, encouraging the child to handle the equipment or to look in the parent's ear as you hold the otoscope. You may need to have the parent help restrain the child.

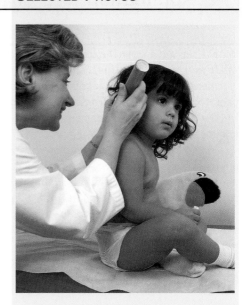

THE SCHOOL-AGE CHILD, THE ADOLESCENT, AND THE AGING ADULT

The sequence of the examination for people in these age groups is the head-to-toe format described in the adult section. However, you should be aware of differences in approach and timing and special developmental considerations. Review Chapter 9, "Assessment Techniques and the Clinical Setting," for a full discussion of these factors.

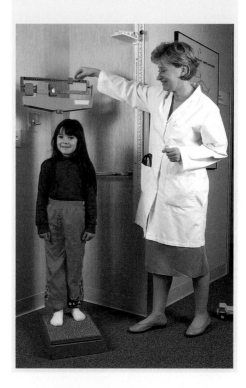

Application and Critical Thinking

RECORDING THE DATA

Record the data from the history and physical examination as soon after the event as possible. Memory fades as the day develops, especially when you are responsible for the care of more than one person.

It is difficult to strike a balance between recording too much data and recording too little. It is important to remember that, from a legal perspective, if it is not documented, it was not done. Data important for the diagnosis and treatment of the person's health should be recorded, as well as data that contribute to your decision-making process. This includes charting relevant normal or negative findings.

On the other hand, a listing of every assessment parameter described in this text yields an unwieldy, unworkable record. One way to keep your record complete yet succinct is to study your writing style. Use short, clear phrases. Avoid redundant introductory phrases such as, "The patient states that . . . " Avoid redundant descriptions such as "no inguinal, femoral, or umbilical hernias." Just write, "no hernias."

Use simple line drawings to describe your findings. You do not need artistic talent; draw a simple sketch of a tympanic membrane, breast, abdomen, or cervix and mark your findings on it. A clear picture is worth many sentences of words.

Study the following complete history and physical examination for a sample write-up. Note that the subject is the same young woman introduced in Chapter 1 of this text.

HEALTH HISTORY

BIOGRAPHICAL DATA

Name: Ellen K.   Birth date: 1/18/
Address: 123 Center St.   Birthplace: Springfield
Marital Status: single   Race: white

Ellen K. is a 23-year-old, single, white, female cashier at a tavern, currently unemployed for 6 months.

Source. Ellen, seems reliable.

Reason for Seeking Care. "I'm coming in for alcohol treatment."

History of Present Illness. First alcoholic drink, age 16. First intoxication, age 17, drinking one to two times per week, a 6-pack per occasion. Attending high school classes every day, but grades slipping from A−/B+ average to C− average. At age 20, drinking two times per week, six to nine beers per occasion. At age 22, drinking two times per week, a 12-pack per occasion, and occasionally a 6-pack the next day to "help with the hangover." During this year, experienced blackouts, failed attempts to cut down on drinking, being physically sick the morning after drinking, and being unable to stop drinking once started. Also, incurred three driving-under-the-influence (DUI) legal offenses. Last DUI 1 month PTA, last alcohol use just before DUI, 18 beers that occasion. Abstinent since that time.

PAST HEALTH

Childhood Illnesses. Chickenpox at age 6. No measles, mumps, croup, pertussis. No rheumatic fever, scarlet fever, or polio.

Accidents. 1. Auto accident, age 12, father driving, Ellen thrown from car, right leg crushed. Hospitalized at Memorial, surgery for leg pinning to repair multiple compound fracture. 2. Auto accident, age 21, head hit dashboard, no loss of consciousness, treated and released at Memorial Hospital ED. 3. Auto accident, age 23, "car hit median strip," no injuries, not seen at hospital.

Chronic Illnesses. None.

Hospitalizations. Age 12, Memorial Hospital, surgery to repair right leg as described, Dr. M.J. Carlson, surgeon.

Obstetric History. Gravida 0/Para 0/Abortion 0.

Immunizations. Childhood immunizations up to date. Last tetanus "probably high school." No TB skin test.

Last Examinations. Yearly pelvic examinations at Health Department since age 15, told "normal." High school sports physical as sophomore. Last dental examination as high school junior; last vision test for driver's license age 16, never had ECG, chest x-ray study.

Allergies. No known allergies.

Current Medications. Birth control pills, low-estrogen type, 1/day, for 5 years. No other prescription or over-the-counter medications.

FAMILY HISTORY

Ellen is second youngest child, parents divorced 8 years, father has chronic alcoholism. See Family genogram below.

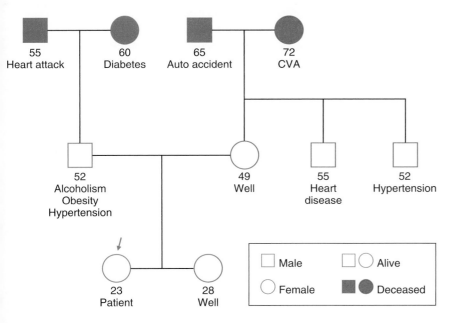

REVIEW OF SYSTEMS

General Health. Reports usual health "OK." No recent weight change, no fatigue, weakness, fever, sweats.

Skin. No change in skin color, pigmentation, or nevi. No pruritus, rash, lesions. Has bruise now over right eye, struck by boyfriend 1 week PTA. No history skin disease. Hair, no loss, change in texture. Nails, no change. Self-care. Stays in sun "as much as I can." No use of sunscreen. Goes to tanning beds at hair salon twice/week during winter.

Head. No unusually frequent or severe headaches, no head injury, dizziness, syncope, or vertigo.

Eyes. No difficulty with vision or double vision. No eye pain, inflammation, discharge, lesions. No history glaucoma or cataracts. Wears no corrective lenses.

Ears. No hearing loss or difficulty. No earaches, infections now or as child, no discharge, tinnitus, or vertigo. Self-care. No exposure to environmental noise, cleans ears with washcloth.

Nose. No discharge, has two to three colds per year, no sinus pain, nasal obstruction, epistaxis, or allergy.

Mouth and Throat. No mouth pain, bleeding gums, toothache, sores or lesions in mouth, dysphagia, hoarseness, or sore throat. Has tonsils. Self-care. Brushes teeth twice/day, no flossing.

Neck. No pain, limitation of motion, lumps, or swollen glands.

Breast. No pain, lump, nipple discharge, rash, swelling, or trauma. No history breast disease in self, mother, or sister. No surgery. Self-care. Does not do breast self-examination.

Respiratory. No past history lung disease, no chest pain with breathing, wheezing, shortness of breath. Colds sometimes "go to my chest," treats with over-the-counter cough medicine and aspirin. Occasional early morning cough, nonproductive. Smokes cigarettes 2 PPD ×2 years, prior use 1 PPD ×4 years. Never tried to quit. Works in poorly ventilated tavern, "everybody smokes."

Cardiovascular. No chest pain, palpitation, cyanosis, fatigue, dyspnea with exertion, orthopnea, paroxysmal nocturnal dyspnea, nocturia, edema. No history of heart murmur, hypertension, coronary artery disease, or anemia.

Peripheral Vascular. No pain, numbness or tingling, swelling in legs. No coldness, discoloration, varicose veins, infections, or ulcers. Legs are unequal in length as sequelae of accident age 12. Self-care. Usual work as cashier involves standing for 8-hour shifts, no support hose.

Gastrointestinal. Appetite good with no recent change. No food intolerance, heartburn, indigestion, pain in abdomen, nausea, or vomiting. No history of ulcers, liver or gallbladder disease, jaundice, appendicitis, or colitis. Bowel movement 1/day, soft, brown, no rectal bleeding or pain. Self-care. No use of vitamins, antacids, laxatives. Diet recall—see Functional Assessment.

Continued

Urinary. No dysuria, frequency, urgency, nocturia, hesitancy, or straining. No pain in flank, groin, suprapubic region. Urine color yellow, no history kidney disease.

Genitalia. Menarche age 11. Last menstrual period April 18. Cycle usually q 28 days, duration 4 to 5 days, flow moderate, no dysmenorrhea. No vaginal itching or discharge, sores or lesions.

Sexual health. In relationship now that includes intercourse. This boyfriend has been her only sexual partner for 2 years, had one other partner before that. Uses birth control pills to prevent pregnancy, partner uses no condoms. Concerned that boyfriend may be having sex with other women but has not confronted him. Aware of no STD contact. Never been tested for AIDS. Past history of sexual abuse by father from ages 12 to 16 years, abuse did not include intercourse. Ellen is unwilling to discuss further at this time.

Musculoskeletal. No past history arthritis, gout. No joint pain, stiffness, swelling, deformity, limitation of motion. No muscle pain, or weakness. Bone trauma at age 12, has sequela of unequal leg lengths, right leg shorter, walks with limp. Self-care. No walking or running for sport or exercise "because of leg." Able to stand as cashier. Uses lift pad in right shoe to equalize leg length.

Neurologic. No history of seizure disorder, stroke, fainting. Has had blackouts with alcohol use. No weakness, tremor, paralysis, problems with coordination, difficulty speaking or swallowing. No numbness or tingling. Not aware of memory problem, nervousness or mood change, depression. Had counseling for sexual abuse in the past. Denies any suicidal ideation or intent during adolescent years or now.

Hematologic. No bleeding problems in skin, excessive bruising. Not aware of exposure to toxins, never had blood transfusion, never used needles to shoot drugs.

Endocrine. Paternal grandmother with diabetes. No increase in hunger, thirst, or urination; no problems with hot or cold environments; no change in skin, appetite, or nervousness.

FUNCTIONAL ASSESSMENT

Self-Concept. Graduated from high school. Trained "on-the-job" as bartender, also worked as cashier in tavern. Unemployed now, on public aid, does not perceive she has enough money for daily living. Lives with older sister. Raised as Presbyterian, believes in God, does not attend church. Believes self to be "honest, dependable." Believes limitations are "smoking, weight, drinking."

Activity-Exercise. Typical day: arises 9:00 AM, light chores or TV, spends day looking for work, running errands, with friends, bedtime at 11:00 PM. No sustained physical exercise. Believes self able to perform all ADLs; limp poses no problem in bathing, dressing, cooking, household tasks, mobility, driving a car, or work as cashier. No mobility aids. Hobbies are fishing, boating, snowmobiling, although currently has no finances to engage in most of these.

Sleep-Rest. Bedtime 11:00 PM. Sleeps 8 to 9 hours. No sleep aids.

Nutrition. 24-hour recall: breakfast, none; lunch, bologna sandwich, chips, diet soda; dinner, hamburger, french fries, coffee; snacks, peanuts, pretzels, potato chips, "bar food." This menu is typical of most days. Eats lunch at home alone. Most dinners at fast-food restaurants or in tavern. Shares household grocery expenses and cooking chores with sister. No food intolerances.

Alcohol. See present illness. Denies use of street drugs. Cigarettes, smokes 2 PPD ×2 years, prior use 1 PPD ×4 years. Never tried to quit. Boyfriend smokes cigarettes.

Interpersonal Relationships. Describes family life growing up as chaotic. Father physically abusive toward mother and sexually abusive toward Ellen. Parents divorced because of father's continual drinking. Few support systems currently. Estranged from mother, "didn't believe me about my father." Father estranged from entire family. Gets along "OK" with sister. Relationship with boyfriend chaotic, has hit her twice in the past. Ellen has never pressed legal charges. No close women friends. Most friends are "drinking buddies" at tavern.

Coping and Stress Management. Believes housing adequate, adequate heat and utilities, and neighborhood safe. Believes home has no safety hazards. Does not use seat belts. No travel outside 60 miles of hometown.

Identifies current stresses to be drinking, legal problems with DUIs, unemployment, financial worries. Considers her drinking to be problematic.

PERCEPTION OF HEALTH

Identifies alcohol as a health problem for herself, feels motivated for treatment. Never been interested in physical health and own body before, "Now I think it's time I learned." Expects health care providers to "Help me with my drinking. I don't know beyond that." Expects to stay at this agency for 6 weeks, "Then, I don't know what."

PHYSICAL EXAMINATION

Height: 163 cm (5'4") Weight: 68.6 kg (151 lb)
B/P: 142/100 right arm, sitting
140/96 right arm, lying
138/98 left arm, lying
Temp: 37° C Pulse 76, regular   Respirations: 16, unlabored

General Survey. Ellen K. is a 23-year-old white female, not currently under the influence of alcohol or other drugs, who articulates clearly, ambulates without difficulty, and is in no distress.

Skin. Uniformly tan-pink in color, warm, dry, intact, turgor good. No lesions, birthmarks, edema. Resolving 2-cm yellow-green hematoma present over right eye, no swelling, ocular structures not involved. Hair, normal distribution and texture, no pest inhabitants. Nails, no clubbing, biting, or discolorations. Nail beds pink and firm with prompt capillary refill.

Head. Normocephalic, no lesions, lumps, scaling, parasites, or tenderness. Face, symmetric, no weakness, no involuntary movements.

Eyes. Acuity by Snellen chart O.D. 20/20, O.S. 20/20−1. Visual fields full by confrontation. EOMs intact, no nystagmus. No ptosis, lid lag, discharge, or crusting. Corneal light reflex symmetric, no strabismus. Conjunctivae clear. Sclera white, no lesion or redness. PERRLA. Fundi: discs flat with sharp margins. Vessels present in all quadrants without crossing defects. Background has even color, no hemorrhage or exudates.

Ears. Pinna no mass, lesions, scaling, discharge, or tenderness to palpation. Canals clear. Tympanic membrane pearly gray, landmarks intact, no perforation. Whispered words heard bilaterally. Weber test—tone heard midline with lateralization. Rinne test—AC > BC and = bilaterally.

Nose. No deformities or tenderness to palpation. Nares patent. Mucosa pink, no lesions. Septum midline, no perforation. No sinus tenderness.

Mouth. Mucosa and gingivae pink, no lesions or bleeding. Right lower 1st molar missing, multiple dark spots on most teeth, gums receding on lower incisors. Tongue symmetric, protrudes midline, no tremor. Pharynx pink, no exudate. Uvula rises midline on phonation. Tonsils 1+. Gag reflex present.

Neck. Neck supple with full ROM. Symmetric, no masses, tenderness, lymphadenopathy. Trachea midline. Thyroid nonpalpable, not tender. Jugular veins flat @ 45 degrees. Carotid arteries 2+ and = bilaterally, no bruits.

Spine and Back. Normal spinal profile, no scoliosis. No tenderness over spines, no CVA tenderness.

Thorax and Lungs. AP < transverse diameter. Chest expansion symmetric. Tactile fremitus equal bilaterally. Lung fields resonant. Diaphragmatic excursion 4 cm and = bilaterally. Breath sounds diminished. Expiratory wheeze in posterior chest at both bases, scattered rhonchi in posterior chest at both bases, do not clear with coughing.

Breasts. Symmetric; no retraction, discharge, or lesions. Contour and consistency firm and homogeneous. No masses or tenderness, no lymphadenopathy.

Heart. Precordium, no abnormal pulsations, no heaves. Apical impulse at 5th ics in left MCL, no thrills. S_1–S_2 are not diminished or accentuated, no S_3 or S_4. Systolic murmur, grade ii/vi, loudest at left lower sternal border, no radiation, present supine and sitting.

Abdomen. Flat, symmetric. Skin smooth with no lesions, scars, or striae. Bowel sounds present, no bruits. Tympany predominates in all quadrants. Liver span 7 cm in right MCL. Abdomen soft, no organomegaly, no masses or tenderness, no inguinal lymphadenopathy.

Extremities. Color tan-pink, no redness, cyanosis, lesions other than surgical scar. Scar right lower leg, anterior, 28 cm × 2 cm wide, well healed. No edema, varicosities. No calf tenderness. All peripheral pulses present, 2+ and = bilaterally. Asymmetric leg length, right leg 3 cm shorter than left.

Musculoskeletal. Temporomandibular joint no slipping or crepitation. Neck full ROM, no pain. Vertebral column no tenderness, no deformity or curvature. Full extension, lateral bending, rotation. Arms symmetric, legs measure as above, extremities have full ROM, no pain or crepitation. Muscle strength, able to maintain flexion against resistance and without tenderness.

Neurologic. Mental status. Appearance, behavior, speech appropriate. Alert and oriented to person, place, time. Thought coherent. Remote and recent memories intact. Cranial nerves II through XII intact. Sensory: pinprick, light touch, vibration intact. Stereognosis, able to identify key. Motor: no atrophy, weakness, or tremors. Gait has limp, able to tandem walk with shoes on. Negative Romberg's sign. Cerebellar, finger-to-nose smoothly intact. DTRs (see stick gram).

DTRs

Continued

Genitalia. External genitalia has no lesion, discharge. Internal genitalia: vaginal walls pink, no lesion. Cervix pink, nulliparous os, no lesions, small amount nonodorous clear discharge. Specimens for Pap test, GC/chlamydia, trichomoniasis, moniliasis obtained. Swabbing mucosa with acetic acid shows no acetowhitening.

Bimanual, no pain on moving cervix, uterus midline, no enlargement, masses, or tenderness. Adnexa, ovaries not enlarged, no tenderness. Anus, no hemorrhoids, fissures, or lesions. Rectal wall intact, no masses or tenderness. Stool soft, brown; Hematest negative.

ASSESSMENT

Alcohol dependence, severe, with physiologic dependence
Nicotine dependence with physiologic dependence
Elevated blood pressure
Systolic heart murmur
Ineffective airway clearance R/T tracheobronchial secretions and obstruction
Right orbital contusion (resolving)
Risk for trauma
Self-care deficit: oral hygiene R/T lack of motivation
Deficient knowledge about alcoholism disease process, treatment options, support systems R/T lack of exposure
Deficient knowledge about balanced diet R/T lack of exposure and substance abuse
Dysfunctional family processes: alcoholism
Chronic low self-esteem R/T effects of alcoholism, sexual abuse, physical abuse

ASSESSMENT VIDEO CRITICAL THINKING QUESTIONS

The Saunders *Physical Examination and Health Assessment* video "Head-to-Toe Examination" will direct you to consider the following:

ADULT

1. What information can be gained about the patient's mental status during the health history interview?
2. How would you adapt breast inspection for a woman with pendulous breasts?
3. If you detect a heart murmur during auscultation, what should you do?
4. If the patient were to have abdominal distention, how would you assess his liver span?
5. What alternative techniques might you use to palpate the liver and spleen?
6. If the popliteal pulse is difficult to find, what technique might you use to palpate it?
7. What techniques can you use to elicit a deep tendon reflex if it does not appear at first?

NEONATE

8. What vital information about a neonate can you obtain from the maternal history?
9. What information can you gain from the gestational age assessment? Why is it important to know the neonate's age at the time of the examination?
10. Why is nasal patency so important to the neonate's health? What other techniques can you use to assess it?
11. What effects can maternal hormone levels have on a neonate's assessment findings?
12. What is an innocent murmur and why is it common in neonates?

13. Which developmental reflexes are commonly present in neonates? Why are they tested?

CHILD

14. When assessing a child's general appearance, what findings would cause concern?
15. What mistakes may commonly occur when assessing a child's height and weight?
16. What condition should an examiner of a child expect if pain results from pulling on the auricle?
17. What abnormal findings may be found when assessing respirations in a child?
18. Name one common illness in which a child's spleen typically is enlarged?
19. What is the difference between pigeon toes (pes varus) and metatarsus adductus?

AGING ADULT

20. During the health history, how would you assess an older adult patient's risk factors and functional status?
21. What strategies can you use to assess an older adult's understanding of prescribed medications, medication use, and compliance with the prescribed regimen?
22. During an older adult's physical examination, how would you screen for risk factors?
23. How could you adapt the physical examination for an older adult with arthritis?
24. Which assessment findings may indicate a prostate disorder?
25. What physiologic changes occur in the female genitalia as a result of menopause?

Appendix A: NANDA-Approved Nursing Diagnoses

Activity Intolerance
Activity Intolerance, Risk for
Adjustment, Impaired
Airway Clearance, Ineffective
Allergy Response, Latex
Allergy Response, Risk for Latex
Anxiety
Anxiety, Death
Aspiration, Risk for
Attachment, Risk for Impaired Parent/Infant/Child
Autonomic Dysreflexia
Autonomic Dysreflexia, Risk for
Body Image, Disturbed
Body Temperature, Risk for Imbalanced
Bowel Incontinence
Breastfeeding, Effective
Breastfeeding, Ineffective
Breastfeeding, Interrupted
Breathing Pattern, Ineffective
Cardiac Output, Decreased
Caregiver Role Strain
Caregiver Role Strain, Risk for
Communication, Impaired Verbal
Communication, Readiness for Enhanced
Conflict, Decisional
Conflict, Parental Role
Confusion, Acute
Confusion, Chronic
Constipation
Constipation, Perceived
Constipation, Risk for
Coping, Ineffective
Coping, Ineffective Community
Coping, Readiness for Enhanced
Coping, Readiness for Enhanced Community
Coping, Defensive
Coping, Compromised Family
Coping, Disabled Family
Coping, Readiness for Enhanced Family
Denial, Ineffective
Dentition, Impaired
Development, Risk for Delayed
Diarrhea
Disuse Syndrome, Risk for
Diversional Activity, Deficient
Energy Field, Disturbed
Environmental Interpretation Syndrome, Impaired
Failure to Thrive, Adult
Falls, Risk for
Family Processes, Dysfunctional: Alcoholism
Family Processes, Interrupted
Family Processes, Readiness for Enhanced
Fatigue
Fear
Fluid Balance, Readiness for Enhanced
Fluid Volume, Deficient
Fluid Volume, Excess
Fluid Volume, Risk for Deficient
Fluid Volume, Risk for Imbalanced
Gas Exchange, Impaired

Grieving, Anticipatory
Grieving, Dysfunctional
Growth and Development, Delayed
Growth, Risk for Disproportionate
Health Maintenance, Ineffective
Health-Seeking Behaviors
Home Maintenance, Impaired
Hopelessness
Hyperthermia
Hypothermia
Identity, Disturbed Personal
Incontinence, Functional Urinary
Incontinence, Reflex Urinary
Incontinence, Stress Urinary
Incontinence, Total Urinary
Incontinence, Urge Urinary
Incontinence, Risk for Urge Urinary
Infant Behavior, Disorganized
Infant Behavior, Risk for Disorganized
Infant Behavior, Readiness for Enhanced Organized
Infant Feeding Pattern, Ineffective
Infection, Risk for
Injury, Risk for
Injury, Risk for Perioperative-Positioning
Intracranial Adaptive Capacity, Decreased
Knowledge, Deficient
Knowledge, Readiness for Enhanced
Loneliness, Risk for
Memory, Impaired
Mobility, Impaired Bed
Mobility, Impaired Physical
Mobility, Impaired Wheelchair
Nausea
Neglect, Unilateral
Noncompliance
Nutrition, Imbalanced: Less than Body Requirements
Nutrition, Imbalanced: More than Body Requirements
Nutrition, Readiness for Enhanced
Nutrition, Risk for Imbalanced: More than Body Requirements
Oral Mucous Membrane, Impaired
Pain, Acute
Pain, Chronic
Parenting, Impaired
Parenting, Readiness for Enhanced
Parenting, Risk for Impaired
Peripheral Neurovascular Dysfunction, Risk for
Poisoning, Risk for
Post-Trauma Syndrome
Post-Trauma Syndrome, Risk for
Powerlessness
Powerlessness, Risk for
Protection, Ineffective
Rape-Trauma Syndrome
Rape-Trauma Syndrome: Compound Reaction
Rape-Trauma Syndrome: Silent Reaction
Relocation Stress Syndrome
Relocation Stress Syndrome, Risk for
Role Performance, Ineffective
Self-Care Deficit, Bathing/Hygiene
Self-Care Deficit, Dressing/Grooming

From NANDA International (2002). NANDA: *Nursing Diagnoses: Definitions and Classification 2003-2004,* Philadelphia: NANDA.

Self-Care Deficit, Feeding
Self-Care Deficit, Toileting
Self-Concept, Readiness for Enhanced
Self-Esteem, Chronic Low
Self-Esteem, Situational Low
Self-Esteem, Risk for Situational Low
Self-Mutilation
Self-Mutilation, Risk for
Sensory Perception, Disturbed
Sexual Dysfunction
Sexuality Patterns, Ineffective
Skin Integrity, Impaired
Skin Integrity, Risk for Impaired
Sleep Deprivation
Sleep Pattern, Disturbed
Sleep, Readiness for Enhanced
Social Interaction, Impaired
Social Isolation
Sorrow, Chronic
Spiritual Distress
Spiritual Distress, Risk for
Spiritual Well-Being, Readiness for Enhanced
Sudden Infant Death Syndrome, Risk for
Suffocation, Risk for

Suicide, Risk for
Surgical Recovery, Delayed
Swallowing, Impaired
Therapeutic Regimen Management, Effective
Therapeutic Regimen Management, Ineffective
Therapeutic Regimen Management, Ineffective Community
Therapeutic Regimen Management, Ineffective Family
Therapeutic Regimen Management, Readiness for Enhanced
Thermoregulation, Ineffective
Thought Processes, Disturbed
Tissue Integrity, Impaired
Tissue Perfusion, Ineffective
Transfer Ability, Impaired
Trauma, Risk for
Urinary Elimination, Impaired
Urinary Elimination, Readiness for Enhanced
Urinary Retention
Ventilation, Impaired Spontaneous
Ventilatory Weaning Response, Dysfunctional
Violence, Risk for Other-Directed
Violence, Risk for Self-Directed
Walking, Impaired
Wandering

Appendix B: Recommended Childhood and Adolescent Immunization Schedule—United States, 2003

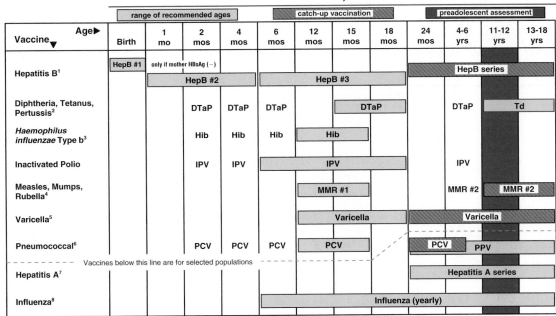

	range of recommended ages				catch-up vaccination				preadolescent assessment			
Vaccine ▼ Age ►	**Birth**	**1 mo**	**2 mos**	**4 mos**	**6 mos**	**12 mos**	**15 mos**	**18 mos**	**24 mos**	**4-6 yrs**	**11-12 yrs**	**13-18 yrs**
Hepatitis B[1]	HepB #1	only if mother HBsAg (−)									HepB series	
			HepB #2			HepB #3						
Diphtheria, Tetanus, Pertussis[2]			DTaP	DTaP	DTaP		DTaP			DTaP	Td	
Haemophilus influenzae Type b[3]			Hib	Hib	Hib	Hib						
Inactivated Polio			IPV	IPV		IPV				IPV		
Measles, Mumps, Rubella[4]						MMR #1				MMR #2	MMR #2	
Varicella[5]						Varicella				Varicella		
Pneumococcal[6]			PCV	PCV	PCV	PCV			PCV	PPV		
Hepatitis A[7]										Hepatitis A series		
Influenza[8]						Influenza (yearly)						

Vaccines below this line are for selected populations

This schedule indicates the recommended ages for routine administration of currently licensed childhood vaccines, as of December 1, 2002, for children through age 18 years. Any dose not given at the recommended age should be given at any subsequent visit when indicated and feasible. ▓ Indicates age groups that warrant special effort to administer those vaccines not previously given. Additional vaccines may be licensed and recommended during the year. Licensed combination vaccines may be used whenever any components of the combination are indicated and the vaccine's other components are not contraindicated. Providers should consult the manufacturers' package inserts for detailed recommendations.

1. Hepatitis B vaccine (HepB). All infants should receive the first dose of hepatitis B vaccine soon after birth and before hospital discharge; the first dose may also be given by age 2 months if the infant's mother is HBsAg-negative. Only monovalent HepB can be used for the birth dose. Monovalent or combination vaccine containing HepB may be used to complete the series. Four doses of vaccine may be administered when a birth dose is given. The second dose should be given at least 4 weeks after the first dose, except for combination vaccines which cannot be administered before age 6 weeks. The third dose should be given at least 16 weeks after the first dose and at least 8 weeks after the second dose. The last dose in the vaccination series (third or fourth dose) should not be administered before age 6 months.

Infants born to HBsAg-positive mothers should receive HepB and 0.5 mL Hepatitis B Immune Globulin (HBIG) within 12 hours of birth at separate sites. The second dose is recommended at age 1-2 months. The last dose in the vaccination series should not be administered before age 6 months. These infants should be tested for HBsAg and anti-HBs at 9-15 months of age.

Infants born to mothers whose HBsAg status is unknown should receive the first dose of the HepB series within 12 hours of birth. Maternal blood should be drawn as soon as possible to determine the mother's HBsAg status; if the HBsAg test is positive, the infant should receive HBIG as soon as possible (no later than age 1 week). The second dose is recommended at age 1-2 months. The last dose in the vaccination series should not be administered before age 6 months.

2. Diphtheria and tetanus toxoids and acellular pertussis vaccine (DTaP). The fourth dose of DTaP may be administered as early as age 12 months, provided 6 months have elapsed since the third dose and the child is unlikely to return at age 15-18 months. **Tetanus and diphtheria toxoids (Td)** is recommended at age 11-12 years if at least 5 years have elapsed since the last dose of tetanus and diphtheria toxoid-containing vaccine. Subsequent routine Td boosters are recommended every 10 years.

3. Haemophilus influenzae type b (Hib) conjugate vaccine. Three Hib conjugate vaccines are licensed for infant use. If PRP-OMP (PedvaxHIB® or ComVax®[Merck]) is administered at ages 2 and 4 months, a dose at age 6 months is not required. DTaP/Hib combination products should not be used for primary immunization in infants at ages 2, 4 or 6 months, but can be used as boosters following any Hib vaccine.

4. Measles, mumps, and rubella vaccine (MMR). The second dose of MMR is recommended routinely at age 4-6 years but may be administered during any visit, provided at least 4 weeks have elapsed since the first dose and that both doses are administered beginning at or after age 12 months. Those who have not previously received the second dose should complete the schedule by the 11-12 year old visit.

5. Varicella vaccine. Varicella vaccine is recommended at any visit at or after age 12 months for susceptible children, i.e. those who lack a reliable history of chickenpox. Susceptible persons aged ≥13 years should receive two doses, given at least 4 weeks apart.

6. Pneumococcal vaccine. The heptavalent **pneumococcal conjugate vaccine (PCV)** is recommended for all children age 2-23 months. It is also recommended for certain children age 24-59 months. **Pneumococcal polysaccharide vaccine (PPV)** is recommended in addition to PCV for certain high-risk groups. See MMWR 2000;49(RR-9);1-38.

7. Hepatitis A vaccine. Hepatitis A vaccine is recommended for children and adolescents in selected states and regions, and for certain high-risk groups; consult your local public health authority. Children and adolescents in these states, regions, and high risk groups who have not been immunized against hepatitis A can begin the hepatitis A vaccination series during any visit. The two doses in the series should be administered at least 6 months apart. See MMWR 1999;48(RR-12);1-37.

8. Influenza vaccine. Influenza vaccine is recommended annually for children age ≥6 months with certain risk factors (including but not limited to asthma, cardiac disease, sickle cell disease, HIV, diabetes, and household members of persons in groups at high risk; see MMWR 2002;51(RR-3);1-31), and can be administered to all others wishing to obtain immunity. In addition, healthy children age 6-23 months are encouraged to receive influenza vaccine if feasible because children in this age group are at substantially increased risk for influenza-related hospitalizations. Children aged ≤12 years should receive vaccine in a dosage appropriate for their age (0.25 mL if age 6-35 months or 0.5 mL if aged ≥3 years). Children aged ≤8 years who are receiving influenza vaccine for the first time should receive two doses separated by at least 4 weeks.

For additional information about vaccines, including precautions and contraindications for immunization and vaccine shortages, please visit the National Immunization Program Website at www.cdc.gov/nip or call the National Immunization Information Hotline at 800-232-2522 (English) or 800-232-0233 (Spanish).

Approved by the Advisory Committee on Immunization Practices (www.cdc.gov/nip/acip), the American Academy of Pediatrics (www.aap.org), and the American Academy of Family Physicians (www.aafp.org).

Appendix C: Recommended Dietary Intakes

For more than 50 years, nutrition experts have produced a set of nutrient and energy standards known as the Recommended Dietary Allowances (RDA). A major revision is currently underway to replace the RDA. The revised recommendations are called Dietary Reference Intakes (DRI) and reflect the collaborative efforts of both the United States and Canada. Until 1997, the RDA were the only standards available and they will continue to serve health professionals until DRI can be established for all nutrients. For this reason, both the 1989 RDA and the 1997 DRI for selected nutrients are presented here.

1989 RECOMMENDED DIETARY ALLOWANCES (RDA)

Age (yr)	(kcal) Energy	(g) Protein	(μg RE) Vitamin A	(mg α-TE) Vitamin E	(μg) Vitamin K	(mg) Vitamin C	(mg) Thiamin	(mg) Riboflavin	(mg NE) Niacin	(mg) Vitamin B$_6$	(μg) Folate	(μg) Vitamin B$_{12}$	(mg) Iron	(mg) Zinc	(μg) Iodine	(μg) Selenium
INFANTS																
0.0–0.5	650	13	375	3	5	30	0.3	0.4	5	0.3	25	0.3	6	5	40	10
0.5–1.0	850	14	375	4	10	35	0.4	0.5	6	0.6	35	0.5	10	5	50	15
CHILDREN																
1–3	1300	16	400	6	15	40	0.7	0.8	9	1.0	50	0.7	10	10	70	20
4–6	1800	24	500	7	20	45	0.9	1.1	12	1.1	75	1.0	10	10	90	20
7–10	2000	28	700	7	30	45	1.0	1.2	13	1.4	100	1.4	10	10	120	30
MALES																
11–14	2500	45	1000	10	45	50	1.3	1.5	17	1.7	150	2.0	12	15	150	40
15–18	3000	59	1000	10	65	60	1.5	1.8	20	2.0	200	2.0	12	15	150	50
19–24	2900	58	1000	10	70	60	1.5	1.7	19	2.0	200	2.0	10	15	150	70
25–50	2900	63	1000	10	80	60	1.5	1.7	19	2.0	200	2.0	10	15	150	70
51+	2300	63	1000	10	80	60	1.2	1.4	15	2.0	200	2.0	10	15	150	70
FEMALES																
11–14	2200	46	800	8	45	50	1.1	1.3	15	1.4	150	2.0	15	12	150	45
15–18	2200	44	800	8	55	60	1.1	1.3	15	1.5	180	2.0	15	12	150	50
19–24	2200	46	800	8	60	60	1.1	1.3	15	1.6	180	2.0	15	12	150	55
25–50	2200	50	800	8	65	60	1.1	1.3	15	1.6	180	2.0	15	12	150	55
51+	1900	50	800	8	65	60	1.0	1.2	13	1.6	180	2.0	10	12	150	55
PREGNANT	+300	60	800	10	65	70	1.5	1.6	17	2.2	400	2.2	30	15	175	65
LACTATING																
1st 6 mo.	+500	65	1300	12	65	95	1.6	1.8	20	2.1	280	2.6	15	19	200	75
2nd 6 mo.	+500	62	1200	11	65	90	1.6	1.7	20	2.1	260	2.6	15	16	200	75

1997 DIETARY REFERENCE INTAKES (DRI)

AGE (YR)	(μg) VITAMIN D	(mg) CALCIUM	(mg) PHOSPHORUS	(mg) MAGNESIUM	(mg) FLUORIDE
INFANTS					
0.0–0.5	5	210	100	30	0.01
0.5–1.0	5	270	275	75	0.5
CHILDREN					
1–3	5	500	460	80	0.7
4–8	5	800	500	130	1.1
MALES					
9–13	5	1300	1250	240	2.0
14–18	5	1300	1250	410	3.2
19–30	5	1000	700	400	3.8
31–50	5	1000	700	420	3.8
51–70	10	1200	700	420	3.8
71+	10	1200	700	420	3.8
FEMALES					
9–13	5	1300	1250	240	2.0
14–18	5	1300	1250	360	2.9
19–30	5	1000	700	310	3.1
31–50	5	1000	700	320	3.1
51–70	10	1200	700	320	3.1
71+	10	1200	700	320	3.1
PREGNANT			*	+40	
LACTATING	*	*	*	*	

*Values are the same as for older women of comparable age.

Appendix D: Pattern of Normal Prenatal Weight Gain

WEIGHT CATEGORY BASED ON BMI*	TOTAL WEIGHT GAIN†		1ST TRIMESTER GAIN		2ND AND 3RD TRIMESTER WEEKLY GAIN	
TABLE D: Recommended Weight Gain for Pregnant Women Based on Body Mass Index	(LB)	(KG)	(LB)	(KG)	(LB)	(KG)
Underweight (BMI < 19.8)	28–40	12.5–18	5	2.3	1.07	0.49
Normal weight (BMI = 19.8–2.6)	25–35	11.5–16	3.5	1.6	0.97	0.44
Overweight (BMI > 26–29)	15–25	7–11.5	2	0.9	0.67	0.3
Obese (BMI > 29)	≥15	6				

*Body mass index (BMI).

†Young adolescents and black women should strive for gains at the upper end of the recommended range. Short women (<62 in or <157 cm) should strive for gains at the lower end of the range.

Data from Subcommittee on Nutritional Status and Weight Gain During Pregnancy and Subcommittee on Dietary Intake and Nutrient Supplements During Pregnancy, Food and Nutrition Board, National Academy of Sciences: *Nutrition during pregnancy,* Parts I and II. Washington, DC, 1990, National Academy Press. From Mahan LK, Escott-Stump S: *Krause's food nutrition & diet therapy,* ed 10, Philadelphia, 2000, W.B. Saunders, p. 169.

The Weighting Game Weight Graph

YOUR BEGINNING WEIGHT _____ lb.

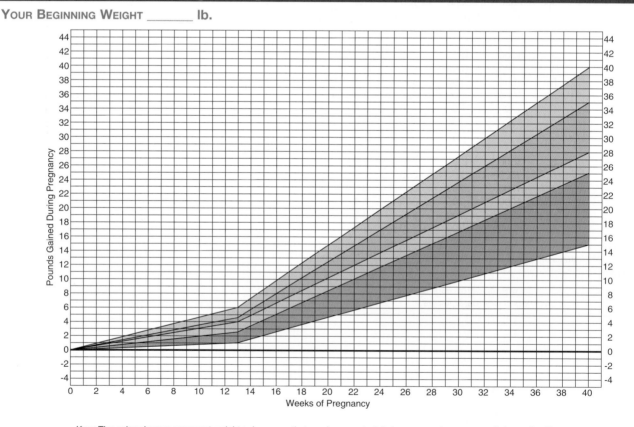

Key : The colored areas represent weight gain ranges that can be expected during a normal pregnancy. Ask your health care provider in which category you belong. This is not the time to lose weight. Try to gain weight at a steady pace. Report any sudden and/or unexplained weight changes to your health care provider.

If your weight was normal before you became pregnant, try to keep your weight in the yellow/orange range.

If you were underweight before you became pregnant, your weight gain should be in the orange/pink range.

If your weight was much higher than ideal, your weight gain should be in the blue-green range.

Appendix E: Body Mass Index Table

BMI	19	20	21	22	23	24	25	26	27	28	29	30	31	32	33	34	35
HEIGHT (INCHES)							BODY WEIGHT (POUNDS)										
58	91	96	100	105	110	115	119	124	129	134	138	143	148	153	158	162	167
59	94	99	104	109	114	119	124	128	133	138	143	148	153	158	163	168	173
60	97	102	107	112	118	123	128	133	138	143	148	153	158	163	168	174	179
61	100	106	111	116	122	127	132	137	143	148	153	158	164	169	174	180	185
62	104	109	115	120	126	131	136	142	147	153	158	164	169	175	180	186	191
63	107	113	118	124	130	135	141	146	152	158	163	169	175	180	186	191	197
64	110	116	122	128	134	140	145	151	157	163	169	174	180	186	192	197	204
65	114	120	126	132	138	144	150	156	162	168	174	180	186	192	198	204	210
66	118	124	130	136	142	148	155	161	167	173	179	186	192	198	204	210	216
67	121	127	134	140	146	153	159	166	172	178	185	191	198	204	211	217	223
68	125	131	138	144	151	158	164	171	177	184	190	197	203	210	216	223	230
69	128	135	142	149	155	162	169	176	182	189	196	203	209	216	223	230	236
70	132	139	146	153	160	167	174	181	188	195	202	209	216	222	229	236	243
71	136	143	150	157	165	172	179	186	193	200	208	215	222	229	236	243	250
72	140	147	154	162	169	177	184	191	199	206	213	221	228	235	242	250	258
73	144	151	159	166	174	182	189	197	204	212	219	227	235	242	250	257	265
74	148	155	163	171	179	186	194	202	210	218	225	233	241	249	256	264	272
75	152	160	168	176	184	192	200	208	216	224	232	240	248	256	264	272	279
76	156	164	172	180	189	197	205	213	221	230	238	246	254	263	271	279	287

BMI	36	37	38	39	40	41	42	43	44	45	46	47	48	49	50	51	52	53	54
58	172	177	181	186	191	196	201	205	210	215	220	224	229	234	239	244	248	253	258
59	178	183	188	193	198	203	208	212	217	222	227	232	237	242	247	252	257	262	267
60	184	189	194	199	204	209	215	220	225	230	235	240	245	250	255	261	266	271	276
61	190	195	201	206	211	217	222	227	232	238	243	248	254	259	264	269	275	280	285
62	196	202	207	213	218	224	229	235	240	246	251	256	262	267	273	278	284	289	295
63	203	208	214	220	225	231	237	242	248	254	259	265	270	278	282	287	293	299	304
64	209	215	221	227	232	238	244	250	256	262	267	273	279	285	291	296	302	308	314
65	216	222	228	234	240	246	252	258	264	270	276	282	288	294	300	306	312	318	324
66	223	229	235	241	247	253	260	266	272	278	284	291	297	303	309	315	322	328	334
67	230	236	242	249	255	261	268	274	280	287	293	299	306	312	319	325	331	338	344
68	236	243	249	256	262	269	276	282	289	295	302	308	315	322	328	335	341	348	354
69	243	250	257	263	270	277	284	291	297	304	311	318	324	331	338	345	351	358	365
70	250	257	264	271	278	285	292	299	306	313	320	327	334	341	348	355	362	369	376
71	257	265	272	279	286	293	301	308	315	322	329	338	343	351	358	365	372	379	386
72	265	272	279	287	294	302	309	316	324	331	338	346	353	361	368	375	383	390	397
73	272	280	288	295	302	310	318	325	333	340	348	355	363	371	378	386	393	401	408
74	280	287	295	303	311	319	326	334	342	350	358	365	373	381	389	396	404	412	420
75	287	295	303	311	319	327	335	343	351	359	367	375	383	391	399	407	415	423	431
76	295	304	312	320	328	336	344	353	361	369	377	385	394	402	410	418	426	435	443

Source: National Institutes of Health: *The practical guide: identification, evaluation, and treatment of overweight and obesity in adults* [Monograph], Washington, DC, 2000, NHLBI Obesity Education Initiative.

Appendix F: Selected Percentiles of Triceps Skinfold Thickness and Bone-Free Upper Arm Area by Height in U.S. Men, Age 25 to 54 Years, with Small, Medium, and Large Frames

Height (in)	Height (cm)	Triceps (mm) 5	10	15	50	85	90	95	Bone-Free MAMA (cm²) 5	10	15	50	85	90	95
Small frame															
62	157				11							52			
63	160			6	10	17					32	48	54		
64	163		5	5	10	16	18			37	38	49	58	63	
65	165	4	5	6	11	17	19	21	31	35	37	47	60	63	71
66	168	5	6	6	11	18	18	20	31	36	38	49	60	62	71
67	170	5	6	6	11	18	20	22	35	39	41	49	58	60	62
68	173	5	6	6	10	15	16	20	33	37	40	49	59	62	69
69	175		6	6	11	17	20			36	40	58	61	63	
70	178			7	10	17					35	48	57		
71	180			7	10	16					39	47	52		
72	183				10							45			
73	185														
74	188														
Medium frame															
62	157				15							58			
63	160				11							55			
64	163		6	6	12	18	20			43	47	56	67	71	
65	165	5	7	8	12	20	22	25	40	43	45	56	67	69	70
66	168	5	6	7	11	16	18	22	38	42	44	55	69	72	78
67	170	5	7	7	13	21	23	28	39	42	44	53	66	69	73
68	173	4	5	7	11	18	20	24	41	44	45	55	67	71	76
69	175	5	6	7	12	18	20	24	38	41	44	54	66	69	73
70	178	5	6	7	12	18	20	23	39	42	43	55	65	68	72
71	180	4	5	7	12	19	21	25	37	41	44	54	67	68	73
72	183	5	7	7	12	20	22	26	40	42	44	56	65	67	74
73	185	6	7	8	12	20	24	27	39	42	43	55	67	69	73
74	188		6	9	13	21	23			43	43	55	62	63	
Large frame															
62	157														
63	160														
64	163														
65	165				14							62			
66	168			9	14	30					48	58	76		
67	170		7	7	11	23	27			50	52	61	73	78	
68	173		9	10	14	22	23			51	53	65	78	86	
69	175	6	7	8	15	25	29	31	46	48	49	61	73	78	83
70	178	7	7	7	14	23	25	30	43	47	50	61	75	77	86
71	180	6	8	10	15	25	27	31	47	48	50	62	75	81	83
72	183	5	6	7	12	20	22	25	45	48	50	61	77	80	86
73	185	5	6	7	13	19	22	31	47	49	51	66	79	83	86
74	188			8	12	19					53	66	78		

MAMA, Mid-arm muscle area.
Adapted from Frisancho AR: New standards of weight and body composition by frame size and height for assessment of nutritional status of adults and the elderly, *Am J Clin Nutr* 40:808–819, 1984 © American Society for Clinical Nutrition.

Appendix G: Selected Percentiles of Triceps Skinfold Thickness and Bone-Free Upper Arm Area by Height in U.S. Women, Age 25 to 54 Years, with Small, Medium, and Large Frames

Height		Triceps (mm)							Bone-Free MAMA (cm^2)						
in	cm	5	10	15	50	85	90	95	5	10	15	50	85	90	95
Small frame															
58	147		12	13	24	30	33			22	24	29	36	44	
59	150	8	11	14	21	29	36	37	17	20	22	28	38	39	43
60	152	8	11	12	21	28	29	33	19	21	22	28	36	40	44
61	155	11	12	14	21	28	31	34	20	21	23	28	28	39	42
62	157	10	12	14	20	28	31	34	20	21	21	27	33	35	37
63	160	10	11	13	20	27	30	36	20	21	22	27	33	35	38
64	163	10	13	13	20	28	30	34	22	23	23	28	34	38	42
65	165	12	13	14	22	29	31	34	21	22	23	28	37	39	47
66	168			12	19	30					23	27	35		
67	170				18							26			
68	173				20							25			
69	175														
70	178														
Medium frame															
58	147			20	25	40					24	35	42		
59	150	15	19	21	30	37	40	40	23	24	26	33	43	45	49
60	152	14	15	17	26	35	37	41	22	25	25	32	42	45	49
61	155	11	14	15	25	34	36	42	21	24	25	31	42	45	51
62	157	12	14	16	24	34	36	40	21	23	25	31	40	43	48
63	160	12	13	15	24	33	35	38	22	23	25	32	41	43	50
64	163	11	14	15	23	33	36	40	21	23	24	31	40	43	48
65	165	12	14	15	22	31	34	38	21	23	24	31	40	43	49
66	168	11	13	14	22	31	33	37	21	23	24	30	39	41	44
67	170	12	13	15	21	29	30	35	22	24	25	30	40	43	48
68	173	10	14	15	22	31	32	36	22	24	25	30	37	38	39
69	175		11	12	19	29	31			23	24	30	36	39	
70	178				19							32			
Large frame															
58	147														
59	150				36							45			
60	152				38							44			
61	155		25	26	36	48	50			29	33	41	62	74	
62	157	16	19	22	34	48	48	50	26	28	31	44	56	63	72
63	160	18	20	22	34	48	48	50	27	30	32	43	60	65	77
64	163	16	20	21	32	43	45	49	26	28	29	39	50	55	63
65	165	17	20	21	31	43	46	48	27	28	29	39	56	59	67
66	168	13	17	18	27	40	43	45	23	24	27	35	49	53	69
67	170	13	16	17	30	41	43	49	25	28	30	37	50	53	55
68	173		16	20	29	37	40			28	30	38	51	54	
69	175			21	30	42					27	35	49		
70	178				20							37			

MAMA, Mid-arm muscle area.

Adapted from Frisancho AR: New standards of weight and body composition by frame size and height for assessment of nutritional status of adults and the elderly, *Am J Clin Nutr* 40:808–819, 1984 © American Society for Clinical Nutrition.

Appendix H: Percentiles of Upper Arm Circumference (mm) and Estimated Upper Arm Muscle Circumference (mm)

AGE (YR)	ARM CIRCUMFERENCE (mm)							ARM MUSCLE CIRCUMFERENCE (mm)						
	5	10	25	50	75	90	95	5	10	25	50	75	90	95
Males														
1–1.9	142	146	150	159	170	176	183	110	113	119	127	135	144	147
2–2.9	141	145	153	162	170	178	185	111	114	122	130	140	146	150
3–3.9	150	153	160	167	175	184	190	117	123	131	137	143	148	153
4–4.9	149	154	162	171	180	186	192	123	126	133	141	148	156	159
5–5.9	153	160	167	175	185	195	204	128	133	140	147	154	162	169
6–6.9	155	159	167	179	188	209	228	131	135	142	151	161	170	177
7–7.9	162	167	177	187	201	223	230	137	139	151	160	168	177	190
8–8.9	162	170	177	190	202	220	245	140	145	154	162	170	182	187
9–9.9	175	178	187	200	217	249	257	151	154	161	170	183	196	202
10–10.9	181	184	196	210	231	262	274	156	160	166	180	191	209	221
11–11.9	186	190	202	223	244	261	280	159	165	173	183	195	205	230
12–12.9	193	200	216	232	254	282	303	167	171	182	195	210	223	241
13–13.9	194	211	228	247	263	286	301	172	179	196	211	226	238	245
14–14.9	220	226	237	253	283	303	322	189	199	212	223	240	260	264
15–15.9	222	229	244	264	284	311	320	199	204	218	237	254	266	272
16–16.9	244	248	262	278	303	324	343	213	225	234	249	269	287	296
17–17.9	246	253	267	285	308	336	347	224	231	245	258	273	294	312
18–18.9	245	260	276	297	321	353	379	226	237	252	264	283	298	324
19–24.9	262	272	288	308	331	355	372	238	245	258	273	289	309	321
25–34.9	271	282	300	319	342	362	375	243	250	264	279	298	314	326
35–44.9	278	287	305	326	345	363	374	247	255	269	286	302	318	327
45–54.9	267	281	301	322	342	362	376	239	249	265	281	300	315	326
55–64.9	258	273	296	317	336	355	269	236	245	260	278	295	310	320
65–74.9	248	263	285	307	325	344	355	223	235	251	268	284	298	306
Females														
1–1.9	138	142	148	156	164	172	177	105	111	117	124	132	139	143
2–2.9	142	145	152	160	167	176	184	111	114	119	126	133	142	147
3–3.9	143	150	158	167	175	183	189	113	119	124	132	140	146	152
4–4.9	149	154	160	169	177	184	191	115	121	128	136	144	152	157
5–5.9	153	157	165	175	185	203	211	125	128	134	142	151	159	165
6–6.9	156	162	170	176	187	204	211	130	133	138	145	154	166	171
7–7.9	164	167	174	183	199	216	231	129	135	142	151	160	171	176
8–8.9	168	172	183	195	214	247	261	138	140	151	160	171	183	194
9–9.9	178	182	194	211	224	251	260	147	150	158	167	180	194	198
10–10.9	174	182	193	210	228	251	265	148	150	159	170	180	190	197
11–11.9	185	194	208	224	248	276	303	150	158	171	181	196	217	223
12–12.9	194	203	216	237	256	282	294	162	166	180	191	201	214	220
13–13.9	202	211	223	243	271	301	338	169	175	183	198	211	226	240
14–14.9	214	223	237	252	272	304	322	174	179	190	201	216	232	247
15–15.9	208	221	239	254	279	300	322	175	178	189	202	215	228	244
16–16.9	218	224	241	258	283	318	334	170	180	190	202	216	234	249
17–17.9	220	227	241	264	295	324	350	175	183	194	205	221	239	257
18–18.9	222	227	241	258	281	312	325	174	179	191	202	215	237	245
19–24.9	221	230	247	265	290	319	345	179	185	195	207	221	236	249
25–34.9	233	240	256	277	304	342	368	183	188	199	212	228	246	264
35–44.9	241	251	267	290	317	356	378	186	192	205	218	236	257	272
45–54.9	242	256	274	299	328	362	384	187	193	206	220	238	260	274
55–64.9	243	257	280	303	335	367	385	187	196	209	225	244	266	280
65–74.9	240	252	274	299	326	356	373	185	195	208	225	244	264	279

From Frisancho AR: New norms of upper limb fat and muscle areas for assessment of nutritional status, *Am J Clin Nutr* 30:2540–2548, 1981 © American Society for Clinical Nutrition.

Appendix I: Frame Size by Elbow Breadth of Male and Female Adults in the United States

AGE (YR)	FRAME SIZE (CM)		
	SMALL	MEDIUM	LARGE
Males			
18–24	≤6.6	>6.6 and <7.7	≥7.7
25–34	≤6.7	>6.7 and <7.9	≥7.9
35–44	≤6.7	>6.7 and <8.0	≥8.0
45–54	≤6.7	>6.7 and <8.1	≥8.1
55–64	≤6.7	>6.7 and <8.1	≥8.1
65–74	≤6.7	>6.7 and <8.1	≥8.1
Females			
18–24	≤5.6	>5.6 and <6.5	≥6.5
25–34	≤5.7	>5.7 and <6.8	≥6.8
35–44	≤5.7	>5.7 and <7.1	≥7.1
45–54	≤5.7	>5.7 and <7.2	≥7.2
55–64	≤5.8	>5.8 and <7.2	≥7.2
65–74	≤5.8	>5.8 and <7.2	≥7.2

From Frisancho AR: New standards of weight and body composition by frame size and height for assessment of nutritional status of adults and the elderly, *Am J Clin Nutr* 40:808–819, 1984, 1981 © American Society for Clinical Nutrition.

Appendix J-1: Standard Precautions

SYNOPSIS OF TYPES OF PRECAUTIONS AND PATIENTS REQUIRING THE PRECAUTIONS

STANDARD PRECAUTIONS

Use Standard Precautions for the care of all patients

AIRBORNE PRECAUTIONS

In addition to Standard Precautions, use Airborne Precautions for patients known or suspected to have serious illnesses transmitted by airborne droplet nuclei. Examples of such illnesses include:

1. Measles
2. Varicella (including disseminated zoster)*
3. Tuberculosis†

DROPLET PRECAUTIONS

In addition to Standard Precautions, use Droplet Precautions for patients known or suspected to have serious illnesses transmitted by large-particle droplets. Examples of such illnesses include:

1. Invasive *Haemophilus influenzae* type b disease, including meningitis, pneumonia, epiglottitis, and sepsis
2. Invasive *Neisseria meningitidis* disease, including meningitis, pneumonia, and sepsis
3. Other serious bacterial respiratory infections spread by droplet transmission, including:
   a) Diphtheria (pharyngeal)
   b) Mycoplasma pneumonia
   c) Pertussis
   d) Pneumonic plague
   e) Streptococcal pharyngitis, pneumonia, or scarlet fever in infants and young children

Continued

4. Serious viral infections spread by droplet transmission, including:
   a) Adenovirus*
   b) Influenza
   c) Mumps
   d) Parvovirus B19
   e) Rubella

CONTACT PRECAUTIONS

In addition to Standard Precautions, use Contact Precautions for patients known or suspected to have serious illnesses easily transmitted by direct patient contact or by contact with items in the patient's environment. Examples of such illnesses include:

1. Gastrointestinal, respiratory, skin, or wound infections or colonization with multi-drug–resistant bacteria judged by the infection control program, based on current state, regional, or national recommendations, to be of special clinical and epidemiologic significance
2. Enteric infections with a low infectious dose or prolonged environmental survival, including:
   a) *Clostridium difficile*
   b) For diapered or incontinent patients: enterohemorrhagic *Escherichia coli* O157:H7, *Shigella* hepatitis A, or rotavirus
3. Respiratory syncytial virus, parainfluenza virus, or enteroviral infections in infants and young children
4. Skin infections that are highly contagious or that may occur on dry skin, including:
   a) Diphtheria (cutaneous)
   b) Herpes simplex virus (neonatal or mucocutaneous)
   c) Impetigo
   d) Major (noncontained) abscesses, celllulitis, or decubiti
   e) Pediculosis
   f) Scabies
   g) Staphylococcal furunculosis in infants and young children
   h) Zoster (disseminated or in the immunocompromised host)*
5. Viral/hemorrhagic conjunctivitis
6. Viral hemorrhagic infections (Ebola, Lassa, or Marburg)

*Certain infections require more than one type of precaution.
†See CDC "Guidelines for Preventing the Transmission of Tuberculosis in Health-Care Facilities."
Adapted from Garner JS: *Guidelines for isolation precautions in hospitals,* Atlanta, 1996, Public Health Service, U.S. Department of Health and Human Services, Centers for Disease Control and Prevention.

Appendix J-2: Transmission-Based Precautions

AIRBORNE PRECAUTIONS

In addition to Standard Precautions, use Airborne Precautions, or the equivalent, for patients known or suspected to be infected with microorganisms transmitted by airborne droplet nuclei (small-particle residue [5 μm or smaller in size] of evaporated droplets containing microorganisms that remain suspended in air and that can be dispersed widely by air currents within a room or over a long distance).

A. PATIENT PLACEMENT

Place the patient in a private room that has (1) monitored negative air pressure in relation to the surrounding areas, (2) 6 to 12 air changes per hour, and (3) appropriate discharge of air outdoors or monitored high-efficiency filtration of room air before the air is circulated to other areas in the hospital. Keep the room door closed and the patient in the room. When a private room is not available, place the patient in a room with a patient who has active infection with the same microorganism, unless otherwise recommended, but with no other infection.

B. RESPIRATORY PROTECTION

Wear respiratory protection when entering the room of a patient with known or suspected infectious pulmonary tuberculosis. Susceptible persons should not enter the room of patients known or suspected to have measles (rubeola) or varicella (chickenpox) if other immune caregivers are available. If susceptible persons must enter the room of a patient known or suspected to have measles (rubeola) or varicella, they should wear respiratory protection. Persons immune to measles (rubeola) or varicella need not wear respiratory protection.

C. PATIENT TRANSPORT

Limit the movement and transport of the patient from the room to essential purposes only. If transport or movement is necessary, minimize patient dispersal of droplet nuclei by placing a surgical mask on the patient, if possible.

D. ADDITIONAL PRECAUTIONS FOR PREVENTING TRANSMISSION OF TUBERCULOSIS

Consult CDC "Guidelines for Preventing the Transmission of Tuberculosis in Health-Care Facilities" for additional prevention strategies.

DROPLET PRECAUTIONS

In addition to Standard Precautions, use Droplet Precautions, or the equivalent, for a patient known or suspected to be infected with microorganisms transmitted by droplets (large-particle droplets [larger than 5 μm in size] that can be generated by the patient during coughing, sneezing, talking, or the performance of procedures).

A. PATIENT PLACEMENT

Place the patient in a private room. When a private room is not available, place the patient in a room with a patient who has active infection with the same microorganism but with no other infection (cohorting). When a private room is not available and cohorting is not achievable, maintain spatial separation of at least 3 ft between the infected patient and other patients and visitors. Special air handling and ventilation are not necessary, and the door may remain open.

B. MASK

In addition to Standard Precautions, wear a mask when working within 3 ft of the patient. (Logistically, some hospitals may want to implement the wearing of a mask to enter the room.)

C. PATIENT TRANSPORT

Limit the movement and transport of the patient from the room to essential purposes only. If transport or movement is necessary, minimize patient dispersal of droplets by masking the patient, if possible.

CONTACT PRECAUTIONS

In addition to Standard Precautions, use Contact Precautions, or the equivalent, for specified patients known or suspected to be infected or colonized with epidemiologically important microorganisms that can be transmitted by direct contact with the patient (hand or skin-to-skin contact that occurs when performing patient-care activities that require touching the patient's dry skin) or indirect contact (touching) with environmental surfaces or patient-care items in the patient's environment.

A. PATIENT PLACEMENT

Place the patient in a private room. When a private room is not available, place the patient in a room with a patient who has active infection with the same microorganism but with no other infection (cohorting). When a private room is not available and cohorting is not achievable, consider the epidemiology of the microorganisms and the patient population when determining patient placement.

B. GLOVES AND HANDWASHING

In addition to wearing gloves as outlined under Standard Precautions, wear gloves (clean, nonsterile gloves are adequate) when entering the room. During the course of providing care for a patient, change gloves after having contact with infective material that may contain high concentrations of microorganisms (fecal material and wound drainage). Remove gloves before leaving the patient's environment and wash hands immediately with an antimicrobial agent or a waterless antiseptic agent. After glove removal and handwashing, ensure that hands do not touch potentially contaminated environmental surfaces or items in the patient's room to avoid transfer of microorganisms to other patients or environments.

C. GOWN

In addition to wearing a gown as outlined under Standard Precautions, wear a gown (a clean, nonsterile gown is adequate) when entering the room if you anticipate that your clothing will have substantial contact with the patient, environmental surfaces, or items in the patient's room, or if the patient is incontinent or has diarrhea, an ileostomy, a colostomy, or wound drainage not contained by a dressing. Remove the gown before leaving the patient's environment. After gown removal, ensure that clothing does not contact potentially contaminated environmental surfaces to avoid transfer of microorganisms to other patients or environments.

D. PATIENT TRANSPORT

Limit the movement and transport of the patient from the room to essential purposes only. If the patient is transported out of the room, ensure that precautions are maintained to minimize the risk of transmission of microorganisms to other patients and contamination of environmental surfaces or equipment.

E. PATIENT-CARE EQUIPMENT

When possible, dedicate the use of noncritical patient-care equipment to a single patient (or cohort of patients infected or colonized with the pathogen requiring precautions) to avoid sharing between patients. If use of common equipment or items is unavoidable, then adequately clean and disinfect them before use for another patient.

F. ADDITIONAL PRECAUTIONS FOR PREVENTING THE SPREAD OF VANCOMYCIN RESISTANCE

Consult the HICPAC report on preventing the spread of vancomycin resistance for additional prevention strategies.

Adapted from Garner JS, Hospital Infection Control Practices Advisory Committee: *Guideline for isolation precautions in hospitals*, Atlanta, 1996, Public Health Service, US Department of Health and Human Services, Centers for Disease Control and Prevention.

Appendix K: Sample Growth Charts for Girls and Boys (Height and Weight)

Birth to 36 months: Girls
Length-for-age and Weight-for-age percentiles

Name _____

Record # _____

Published May 30, 2000 (modified 4/20/01).
Source: Developed by the National Center for Health Statistics incollaboration with
    the National Center for Chronic Disease Prevention and Health Promotion (2000).
    http://www.cdc.gov/growthcharts

Birth to 36 months: Girls
Head circumference-for-age and
Weight-for-length percentiles

NAME _____

RECORD # _____

AGE (MONTHS)

Birth 3 6 9 12 15 18 21 24 27 30 33 36

HEAD CIRCUMFERENCE

95
90
75
50
25
10
5

LENGTH

| cm | 64 66 68 70 72 74 76 78 80 82 84 86 88 90 92 94 96 98 100 |
| in | 26 27 28 29 30 31 32 33 34 35 36 37 38 39 40 41 |

WEIGHT

95
90
75
50
25
10
5

Date	Age	Weight	Length	Head Circ.	Comment

| cm | 46 48 50 52 54 56 58 60 62 |
| in | 18 19 20 21 22 23 24 |

Published May 30, 2000 (modified 10/16/00).
SOURCE: Developed by the National Center for Health Statistics in collaboration with
the National Center for Chronic Disease Prevention and Health Promotion (2000).
http://www.cdc.gov/growthcharts

SAFER · HEALTHIER · PEOPLE™

2 to 20 years: Girls
Stature-for-age and Weight-for-age percentiles

NAME _____

RECORD # _____

Date	Age	Weight	Stature	BMI*

*To Calculate BMI: Weight (kg) ÷ Stature (cm) ÷ Stature (cm) x 10,000
or Weight (lb) ÷ Stature (in) ÷ Stature (in) x 703

Published May 30, 2000 (modified 11/21/00).
SOURCE: Developed by the National Center for Health Statistics in collaboration with
the National Center for Chronic Disease Prevention and Health Promotion (2000).
http://www.cdc.gov/growthcharts

SAFER · HEALTHIER · PEOPLE™

Birth to 36 months: Boys
Length-for-age and Weight-for-age percentiles

Name _____

Record # _____

Age (months)

Birth   3   6   9   12   15   18   21   24   27   30   33   36

Length

95
90
75
50
25
10
5

95
90
75
50
25
10
5

Weight

Age (months)

| | 12 | 15 | 18 | 21 | 24 | 27 | 30 | 33 | 36 | kg | lb |

Mother s stature_____
Father s stature_____

Gestational
Age:_____ Weeks

Comment

Date	Age	Weight	Length	Head circ.			
	Birth						

Weight

lb   kg

Birth   3   6   9

Published May 30, 2000 (modified 4/20/01).
Source: Developed by the National Center for Health Statistics incollaboration with
the National Center for Chronic Disease Prevention and Health Promotion (2000).
http://www.cdc.gov/growthcharts

SAFER · HEALTHIER · PEOPLE™

**Birth to 36 months: Boys
Head circumference-for-age and
Weight-for-length percentiles**

Name _____

Record # _____

Source: Developed by the National Center for Health Statistics incollaboration with
the National Center for Chronic Disease Prevention and Health Promotion (2000).
http://www.cdc.gov/growthcharts
Published May 30, 2000 (modified 4/20/01).

SAFER · HEALTHIER · PEOPLE™

2 to 20 years: Boys
Stature-for-age and Weight-for-age percentiles

NAME _____

RECORD # _____

Mother s Stature _____		Father s Stature _____		
Date	Age	Weight	Stature	BMI*

*To Calculate BMI: Weight (kg) ÷ Stature (cm) ÷ Stature (cm) x 10,000
or Weight (lb) ÷ Stature (in) ÷ Stature (in) x 703

AGE (YEARS)
12 13 14 15 16 17 18 19 20

STATURE

cm   in
190   76
185   74
180   72
175   70
170   68
165   66
160   64
155   62
150   60

in cm   3   4   5   6   7   8   9 10 11

STATURE

62 160
60 155
58 150
56 145
54 140
52 135
50 130
48 125
46 120
44 115
42 110
40 105
38 100
36 95
34 90
32 85
30 80

95
90
75
50
25
10
5

WEIGHT

105 230
100 220
95   210
90   200
85   190
80   180
75   170
70   160
65   150
60   140
55   130
50   120
45   110
40   100
35   90
30   80

WEIGHT

80 35
70 30
60 25
50 20
40 15
30
     10

lb kg   AGE (YEARS)   kg lb

2   3   4   5   6   7   8   9 10 11 12 13 14 15 16 17 18 19 20

Published May 30, 2000 (modified 11/21/00).
SOURCE: Developed by the National Center for Health Statistics in collaboration with
the National Center for Chronic Disease Prevention and Health Promotion (2000).
http://www.cdc.gov/growthcharts

SAFER · HEALTHIER · PEOPLE™

Appendix L-1: Maturational Assessment of Gestational Age (New Ballard Score)

NAME _____ SEX _____

HOSPITAL NO. _____ BIRTH WEIGHT _____

RACE _____ LENGTH _____

DATE/TIME OF BIRTH _____ HEAD CIRC. _____

DATE/TIME OF EXAM _____ EXAMINER _____

AGE WHEN EXAMINED _____

APGAR SCORE: 1 MINUTE _____ 5 MINUTES _____ 10 MINUTES _____

NEUROMUSCULAR MATURITY

NEUROMUSCULAR MATURITY SIGN	SCORE							RECORD SCORE HERE
	-1	0	1	2	3	4	5	
POSTURE								
SQUARE WINDOW (Wrist)	>90°	90°	60°	45°	30°	0°		
ARM RECOIL		180°	140°-180°	110°-140°	90°-110°	<90°		
POPLITEAL ANGLE	180°	160°	140°	120°	100°	90°	<90°	
SCARF SIGN								
HEEL TO EAR								

TOTAL NEUROMUSCULAR MATURITY SCORE

PHYSICAL MATURITY

PHYSICAL MATURITY SIGN	SCORE							RECORD SCORE HERE
	-1	0	1	2	3	4	5	
SKIN	sticky friable transparent	gelatinous red translucent	smooth pink visible veins	superficial peeling &/or rash, few veins	cracking pale areas rare veins	parchment deep cracking no vessels	leathery cracked wrinkled	
LANUGO	none	sparse	abundant	thinning	bald areas	mostly bald		
PLANTAR SURFACE	heel-toe 40-50 mm:-1 <40 mm:-2	>50 mm no crease	faint red marks	anterior transverse crease only	creases ant. 2/3	creases over entire sole		
BREAST	imperceptible	barely perceptible	flat areola no bud	stippled areola 1-2 mm bud	raised areola 3-4 mm bud	full areola 5-10 mm bud		
EYE/EAR	lids fused loosely: -1 tightly: -2	lids open pinna flat stays folded	sl. curved pinna; soft; slow recoil	well-curved pinna; soft but ready recoil	formed & firm instant recoil	thick cartilage ear stiff		
GENITALS (Male)	scrotum flat, smooth	scrotum empty faint rugae	testes in upper canal rare rugae	testes descending few rugae	testes down good rugae	testes pendulous deep rugae		
GENITALS (Female)	clitoris prominent & labia flat	prominent clitoris & small labia minora	prominent clitoris & enlarging minora	majora & minora equally prominent	majora large minora small	majora cover clitoris & minora		

TOTAL PHYSICAL MATURITY SCORE

Reference
Ballard JL, Khoury JC, Wedig K, et al: New Ballard Score, expanded to include extremely premature infants. *J Pediatr* 1991; 119:417-423. Reprinted by permission of Dr. Ballard and Mosby.

SCORE

Neuromuscular _____

Physical _____

Total _____

MATURITY RATING

score	weeks
-10	20
-5	22
0	24
5	26
10	28
15	30
20	32
25	34
30	36
35	38
40	40
45	42
50	44

GESTATIONAL AGE (weeks)

By dates _____

By ultrasound _____

By exam _____

Appendix L-2: Classification of Newborns (Both Sexes) by Intrauterine Growth and Gestational Age

NAME _____   DATE OF EXAM _____   LENGTH _____

HOSPITAL NO. _____   SEX _____   HEAD CIRC. _____

RACE _____   BIRTH WEIGHT _____   GESTATIONAL AGE _____

DATE OF BIRTH _____

CLASSIFICATION OF INFANT*	Weight	Length	Head Circ.
Large for Gestational Age (LGA) (>90th percentile)			
Appropriate for Gestational Age (AGA) (10th to 90th percentile)			
Small for Gestational Age (SGA) (<10th percentile)			

*Place an "X" in the appropriate box (LGA, AGA or SGA) for weight, for length and for head circumference.

References
1. Battaglia FC, Lubchenco LO: A practical classification of newborn infants by weight and gestational age. J Pediatr 1967; 71:159-163.
2. Lubchenco LO, Hansman C, Boyd E: Intrauterine growth in length and head circumference as estimated from live births at gestational ages from 26 to 42 weeks. Pediatrics 1966; 37:403-408.

A service of **SIMILAC® WITH IRON** Infant Formula

The Ross Hospital Formula System

A5860(0.05)/JULY 1993

ROSS ROSS PRODUCTS DIVISION ABBOTT LABORATORIES COLUMBUS, OHIO 43215-1724

LITHO IN USA

Appendix M-1: Blood Pressure Levels for the 90th and 95th Percentiles of Blood Pressure for Girls Age 1 to 17 Years by Percentiles of Height

AGE (YR)	BLOOD PRESSURE PERCENTILE*	SYSTOLIC BLOOD PRESSURE BY PERCENTILE OF HEIGHT (mm Hg)†							DIASTOLIC BLOOD PRESSURE BY PERCENTILE OF HEIGHT (mm Hg)†)						
		5%	10%	25%	50%	75%	90%	95%	5%	10%	25%	50%	75%	90%	95%
1	90th	97	98	99	100	102	103	104	53	53	53	54	55	56	56
	95th	101	102	103	104	105	107	107	57	57	57	58	59	60	60
2	90th	99	99	100	102	103	104	105	57	57	58	58	59	60	61
	95th	102	103	104	105	107	108	109	61	61	62	62	63	64	65
3	90th	100	100	102	103	104	105	106	61	61	61	62	63	63	64
	95th	104	104	105	107	108	109	110	65	65	65	66	67	67	68
4	90th	101	102	103	104	106	107	108	63	63	64	65	65	66	67
	95th	105	106	107	108	109	111	111	67	67	68	69	69	70	71
5	90th	103	103	104	106	107	108	109	65	66	66	67	68	68	69
	95th	107	107	108	110	111	112	113	69	70	70	71	72	72	73
6	90th	104	105	106	107	109	110	111	67	67	68	69	69	70	71
	95th	108	109	110	111	112	114	114	71	71	72	73	73	74	75
7	90th	106	107	108	109	110	112	112	69	69	69	70	71	72	72
	95th	110	110	112	113	114	115	116	73	73	73	74	75	76	76
8	90th	108	109	110	111	112	113	114	70	70	71	71	72	73	74
	95th	112	112	113	115	116	117	118	74	74	75	75	76	77	78
9	90th	110	110	112	113	114	115	116	71	72	72	73	74	74	75
	95th	114	114	115	117	118	119	120	75	76	76	77	78	78	79
10	90th	112	112	114	115	116	117	118	73	73	73	74	75	76	76
	95th	116	116	117	119	120	121	122	77	77	77	78	79	80	80
11	90th	114	114	116	117	118	119	120	74	74	75	75	76	77	77
	95th	118	118	119	121	122	123	124	78	78	79	79	80	81	81
12	90th	116	116	118	119	120	121	122	75	75	76	76	77	78	78
	95th	120	120	121	123	124	125	126	79	79	80	80	81	82	82
13	90th	118	118	119	121	122	123	124	76	76	77	78	78	79	80
	95th	121	122	123	125	126	127	128	80	80	81	82	82	83	84
14	90th	119	120	121	122	124	125	126	77	77	78	79	79	80	81
	95th	123	124	125	126	128	129	130	81	81	82	83	83	84	85
15	90th	121	121	122	124	125	126	127	78	78	79	79	80	81	82
	95th	124	125	126	128	129	130	131	82	82	83	83	84	85	86
16	90th	122	122	123	125	126	127	128	79	79	79	80	81	82	82
	95th	125	126	127	128	130	131	132	83	83	83	84	85	86	86
17	90th	122	123	124	125	126	128	128	79	79	79	80	81	82	82
	95th	126	126	127	129	130	131	132	83	83	83	84	85	86	86

Reproduced with permission from *Pediatrics,* Vol. 98, Pages 649-667, Tables 2 and 3, Copyright 1996.
*Blood pressure percentile was determined by a single reading.
†Height percentile was determined by standard growth curves.

Appendix M-2: Blood Pressure Levels for the 90th and 95th Percentiles of Blood Pressure for Boys Age 1 to 17 Years by Percentiles of Height

AGE (YR)	BLOOD PRESSURE PERCENTILE*	SYSTOLIC BLOOD PRESSURE BY PERCENTILE OF HEIGHT (mm Hg)†							DIASTOLIC BLOOD PRESSURE BY PERCENTILE OF HEIGHT (mm Hg)†						
		5%	10%	25%	50%	75%	90%	95%	5%	10%	25%	50%	75%	90%	95%
1	90th	94	95	97	98	100	102	102	50	51	52	53	54	54	55
	95th	98	99	101	102	104	106	106	55	55	56	57	58	59	59
2	90th	98	99	100	102	104	105	106	55	55	56	57	58	59	59
	95th	101	102	104	106	108	109	110	59	59	60	61	62	63	63
3	90th	100	101	103	105	107	108	109	59	59	60	61	62	63	63
	95th	104	105	107	109	111	112	113	63	63	64	65	66	67	67
4	90th	102	103	105	107	109	110	111	62	62	63	64	65	66	66
	95th	106	107	109	111	113	114	115	66	67	67	68	69	70	71
5	90th	104	105	106	108	110	112	112	65	65	66	67	68	69	69
	95th	108	109	110	112	114	115	116	69	70	70	71	72	73	74
6	90th	105	106	108	110	111	113	114	67	68	69	70	70	71	72
	95th	109	110	112	114	115	117	117	72	72	73	74	75	76	76
7	90th	106	107	109	111	113	114	115	69	70	71	72	72	73	74
	95th	110	111	113	115	116	118	119	74	74	75	76	77	78	78
8	90th	107	108	110	112	114	115	116	71	71	72	73	74	75	75
	95th	111	112	114	116	118	119	120	75	76	76	77	78	79	80
9	90th	109	110	112	113	115	117	117	72	73	73	74	75	76	77
	95th	113	114	116	117	119	121	121	76	77	78	79	80	80	81
10	90th	110	112	113	115	117	118	119	73	74	74	75	76	77	78
	95th	114	115	117	119	121	122	123	77	78	79	80	80	81	82
11	90th	112	113	115	117	119	120	121	74	74	75	76	77	78	78
	95th	116	117	119	121	123	124	125	78	79	79	80	81	82	83
12	90th	115	116	117	119	121	123	123	75	7	76	77	78	78	79
	95th	119	120	121	123	125	126	127	79	79	80	81	82	83	83
13	90th	117	118	120	122	124	125	126	75	76	76	77	78	79	80
	95th	121	122	124	126	128	129	130	79	80	81	82	83	83	84
14	90th	120	121	123	125	126	128	128	76	76	77	78	79	80	80
	95th	124	125	127	128	130	132	132	80	81	81	82	83	84	85
15	90th	123	124	125	127	129	131	131	77	77	78	79	80	81	81
	95th	127	128	129	131	133	134	135	81	81	83	83	84	85	86
16	90th	125	126	128	130	132	133	134	79	79	80	81	82	82	83
	95th	129	130	132	134	136	137	138	83	83	84	85	86	87	87
17	90th	128	129	131	133	134	136	136	81	81	82	83	84	85	85
	95th	132	133	135	136	138	140	140	85	85	86	87	88	89	89

*Blood pressure percentile was determined by a single measurement.
†Height percentile was determined by standard growth curves.

Illustration Credits

Spanish/English assessment tool is modified from Black JM, Matassarin-Jacobs E: *Luckmann and Sorensen's medical-surgical nursing: a psychophysiologic approach,* ed 4, Philadelphia, 1993, Saunders. Adapted from *Taber's cyclopedic dictionary,* ed 16, Philadelphia, 1989, F.A. Davis.

CHAPTER 1

Figure 1-1: From Alfaro-LeFevre R: *Critical thinking in nursing: a practical approach,* ed 2, Philadelphia, 1999, Saunders.
Figure 1-2: From Alfaro-LeFevre R: *Critical thinking in nursing: a practical approach,* ed 2, Philadelphia, 1999, Saunders.
Figure 1-3: From U.S. Bureau of the Census (pie charts); Michael D. Hoefer, Immigration and Naturalization Service (1998 World Map, 1996-98 U.S. Maps, Graphs); Carl Haub, Population Reference Bureau, National Geographic Maps.

CHAPTER 2

Figure 2-1: From Gorrie TM, McKinney ES, Murray SS: *Foundations of maternal-newborn nursing,* ed 2, Philadelphia, 1998, Saunders.
Figure 2-6: From Rick Brady, Riva, MD.
Figure 2-10: From Rick Brady, Riva, MD.
Figure 2-12: From Rick Brady, Riva, MD.

CHAPTER 4

Figure 4-2: From Potter PA, Perry AG: *Fundamentals of nursing,* ed 5, St Louis, 2001, Mosby.

CHAPTER 5

Figure 5-1: From Nursing Research Consortium on Violence and Abuse (NRCVA), 1988.
Figure 5-2: From Family Violence Prevention Fund (http://endabuse.org/), 1999.
Figure 5-3: Courtesy Daniel J. Sheridan, PhD, RN, CNS, Hanover, MD.
Figure 5-4: Courtesy Daniel J. Sheridan, PhD, RN, CNS, Hanover, MD.
Figure 5-5: Courtesy Daniel J. Sheridan, PhD, RN, CNS, Hanover, MD.
Figure 5-6: Courtesy Daniel J. Sheridan, PhD, RN, CNS, Hanover, MD.
Figure 5-7: Courtesy Daniel J. Sheridan, PhD, RN, CNS, Hanover, MD.
Figure 5-8: Courtesy Daniel J. Sheridan, PhD, RN, CNS, Hanover, MD.
Figure 5-9: Courtesy Daniel J. Sheridan, PhD, RN, CNS, Hanover, MD.
Figure 5-10: Courtesy Jacquelyn C. Campbell, PhD, RN, © 1985, 1988, 2001.

CHAPTER 8

Figure 8-1: Courtesy of *The Pantagraph,* Bloomington, IL, July 15, 2001.
Figure 8-2: From Nutrition Screening Initiative: *Implementing nutrition screening and intervention strategies,* Washington, DC, 1993, Nutrition Screening Initiative. (Reprinted with permission by the Nutrition Screening Initiative, a project of the American Academy of Family Physicians, the American Dietetic Association, and the National Council on Aging, Inc., and funded in part by a grant from Ross Products Divisions, Abbott Laboratories.)
Art for Table 8-7: (marasmus) from Hall R, Evered DC: *Color atlas of endocrinology,* ed 2, London, 1990, Mosby.
Art for Table 8-8: (pellagra) from Latham MC et al: *Scope manual on nutrition,* Kalamazoo, 1980, The Upjohn Company, copyright by Thomas Spies, MD; (follicular hyperkeratosis) from Taylor KB,

Anthony LE: *Clinical nutrition,* New York, 1983, McGraw-Hill, copyright by Harold H. Sandstead; (scorbutic gums) from Taylor KB, Anthony LE: *Clinical nutrition,* New York, 1983, McGraw-Hill, copyright by The Upjohn Company; (kwashiorkor) from Hall R, Evered DC: *Color atlas of endocrinology,* ed 2, London, 1990, Mosby; (Bitot's spots) from Taylor KB, Anthony LE: *Clinical nutrition,* New York, 1983, McGraw-Hill, copyright by Helen Keller International, Inc; (rickets) from Latham MC et al: *Scope manual on nutrition,* Kalamazoo, 1980, The Upjohn Company, copyright by Rosa Lee Nemir, MD; (magenta tongue) from McLaren DS: *Color atlas of nutritional disorders,* London, 1981, Wolfe Medical, copyright by C.E. Butterworth, Jr; (HIV infection discordant twins) from Friedman-Kien AE: *Color atlas of AIDS,* Philadelphia, 1989, Saunders.

CHAPTER 9

Figure 9-14: Courtesy of *The Pantagraph,* Bloomington, IL, August 10, 1998.

CHAPTER 10

Figure 10-16: From Rossman I: *Clinical geriatrics,* ed 3, Philadelphia, 1986, Lippincott.
Art for Table 10-6: (hypopituitary dwarfism) from Hall R, Evered DC: *Color atlas of endocrinology,* ed 2, London, 1990, Mosby; (gigantism) from Hall R, Evered DC: *Color atlas of endocrinology,* ed 2, London, 1990, Mosby; (acromegaly [hyperpituitarism]) Reprinted from the Clinical Slide Collection on the Rheumatic Diseases. © 1991, 1995, 1997. Used by permission of the American College of Rheumatology; (achondroplastic dwarfism) from Jones A, Owen R: *Color atlas of clinical orthopedics,* ed 2, London, 1995, Mosby; (anorexia nervosa) Courtesy of George D. Comerci, MD; (Marfan's syndrome) from Manusov EG, Martucci E: The Marfan syndrome, *Arch Fam Med* 3:824, 1994. Copyrighted 1994, American Medical Association; (endogenous obesity—Cushing's syndrome) from Wenig BM, Heffess CS, Adair CF: *Atlas of endocrine pathology,* Philadelphia, 1997, Saunders.

CHAPTER 11

Figure 11-4: From McCaffery M, Pasero C: *Pain: clinical manual,* ed 2, St Louis, 1999, Mosby.
Figure 11-5: From McCaffery M, Pasero C: *Pain: clinical manual,* ed 2, St Louis, 1999, Mosby.
Figure 11-6: From McCaffery M, Pasero C: *Pain: clinical manual,* ed 2, St Louis, 1999, Mosby.
Figure 11-7: From Wong DL et al: *Wong's essentials of pediatric nursing,* ed 6, St Louis, 2001, Mosby.
Figure 11-8: From Rick Brady, Riva, MD.
Figure 11-9: From Krechel SW, Bildner J: CRIES: a new neonatal postoperative pain measurement score: initial testing of validity and reliability, *Pediatr Anesth* 5:53-61, 1995.

CHAPTER 12

Figure 12-4, *A*: From Hurwitz S: *Clinical pediatric dermatology: a textbook of skin disorders of childhood and adolescence,* ed 2, Philadelphia, 1993, Saunders.
Figure 12-4, *B*: From Hurwitz S: *Clinical pediatric dermatology: a textbook of skin disorders of childhood and adolescence,* ed 2, Philadelphia, 1993, Saunders.

Figure 12-4, *C:* From Lookingbill DP, Marks JG: *Principles of dermatology,* ed 2, Philadelphia, 1993, Saunders.

Figure 12-6: From Lookingbill DP, Marks JG: *Principles of dermatology,* ed 2, Philadelphia, 1993, Saunders.

Figure 12-9: From Callen JP et al: *Color atlas of dermatology,* Philadelphia, 1993, Saunders.

Figure 12-10: From Hurwitz S: *Clinical pediatric dermatology: a textbook of skin disorders of childhood and adolescence,* ed 2, Philadelphia, 1993, Saunders.

Figure 12-12: Courtesy Jane Deacon, RNC, MS, NNP, The Children's Hospital, Denver, CO.

Figure 12-13: From Bowden VR, Dickey SB, Greenburg CS: *Children and their families: the continuum of care,* Philadelphia, 1998, Saunders.

Figure 12-14: From Hurwitz S: *Clinical pediatric dermatology: a textbook of skin disorders of childhood and adolescence,* ed 2, Philadelphia, 1993, Saunders.

Figure 12-15: From Hurwitz S: *Clinical pediatric dermatology: a textbook of skin disorders of childhood and adolescence,* ed 2, Philadelphia, 1993, Saunders.

Figure 12-16: From Gorrie TM, McKinney ES, Murray SS: *Foundations of maternal-newborn nursing,* ed 2, Philadelphia, 1998, Saunders.

Figure 12-17: From Hurwitz S: *Clinical pediatric dermatology: a textbook of skin disorders of childhood and adolescence,* ed 2, Philadelphia, 1993, Saunders.

Figure 12-18: From Gorrie TM, McKinney ES, Murray SS: *Foundations of maternal-newborn nursing,* ed 2, Philadelphia, 1998, Saunders.

Figure 12-19, *A:* From Habif TP et al: *Skin disease: diagnosis and treatment,* ed 3, St Louis, 2001, Mosby.

Figure 12-19, *B:* From Habif TP et al: *Skin disease: diagnosis and treatment,* ed 3, St Louis, 2001, Mosby.

Figure 12-20: From Lookingbill DP, Marks JG: *Principles of dermatology,* ed 2, Philadelphia, 1993, Saunders.

Figure 12-21: From Lookingbill DP, Marks JG: *Principles of dermatology,* ed 2, Philadelphia, 1993, Saunders.

Figure 12-22: From Lookingbill DP, Marks JG: *Principles of dermatology,* ed 2, Philadelphia, 1993, Saunders.

Figure 12-23: From Lookingbill DP, Marks JG: *Principles of dermatology,* ed 2, Philadelphia, 1993, Saunders.

Figure 12-24: From Callen JP et al: *Color atlas of dermatology,* Philadelphia, 1993, Saunders.

Art for Table 12-4: (urticaria [hives]) from Fireman P: *Atlas of allergies,* ed 2, London, 1996, Mosby.

Art for Table 12-6: (port-wine stain [nevus flammeus]) from Hurwitz S: *Clinical pediatric dermatology: a textbook of skin disorders of childhood and adolescence,* ed 2, Philadelphia, 1993, Saunders; (strawberry mark [immature hemangioma]) from Lookingbill DP, Marks JG: *Principles of dermatology,* ed 2, Philadelphia, 1993, Saunders; (cavernous hemangioma [mature]) from Habif TP et al: *Skin disease: diagnosis and treatment,* ed 3, St Louis, 2001, Mosby; (spider or star angioma) from Hurwitz S: *Clinical pediatric dermatology: a textbook of skin disorders of childhood and adolescence,* ed 2, Philadelphia, 1993, Saunders; (venous lake) from Habif TP et al: *Skin disease: diagnosis and treatment,* ed 3, St Louis, 2001, Mosby; (petechiae) from Dockery GL: *Cutaneous disorders of the lower extremity,* Philadelphia, 1997, Saunders; (purpura) from Hurwitz S: *Clinical pediatric dermatology: a textbook of skin disorders of childhood and adolescence,* ed 2, Philadelphia, 1993, Saunders.

Art for Table 12-7: (diaper dermatitis) from Hurwitz S: *Clinical pediatric dermatology: a textbook of skin disorders of childhood and adolescence,* ed 2, Philadelphia, 1993, Saunders; (intertrigo [candidiasis]) from Hurwitz S: *Clinical pediatric dermatology: a textbook of skin disorders of childhood and adolescence,* ed 2, Philadelphia, 1993, Saunders; (impetigo) from Hurwitz S: *Clinical pediatric dermatology: a textbook of skin disorders of childhood and adolescence,* ed 2, Philadelphia, 1993, Saunders; (atopic dermatitis [eczema]) from Hurwitz S: *Clinical pediatric dermatology: a textbook of skin disorders of childhood and adolescence,* ed 2, Philadelphia, 1993, Saunders; (measles [rubeola] in dark skin) from Feigin RD, Cherry JD: *Textbook of pediatric infectious diseases,* ed 4, Philadelphia, 1998, Saunders; (measles [rubeola] in light skin) from Hurwitz S: *Clinical pediatric dermatology: a textbook of skin disorders of childhood and adolescence,* ed 2, Philadelphia, 1993, Saunders; (German measles [rubella]) from Hurwitz S: *Clinical pediatric dermatology: a textbook of skin disorders of childhood and adolescence,* ed 2, Philadelphia, 1993, Saunders; (chickenpox [varicella]) from Callen JP et al: *Color atlas of dermatology,* Philadelphia, 1993, Saunders.

Art for Table 12-8: (primary contact dermatitis) from Lookingbill DP, Marks JG: *Principles of dermatology,* ed 2, Philadelphia, 1993, Saunders; (allergic drug reaction) from Lookingbill DP, Marks JG: *Principles of dermatology,* ed 2, Philadelphia, 1993, Saunders; (tinea corporis [ringworm of the body]) from Hurwitz S: *Clinical pediatric dermatology: a textbook of skin disorders of childhood and adolescence,* ed 2, Philadelphia, 1993, Saunders; (tinea pedis [ringworm of the foot]) from Feigin RD, Cherry JD: *Textbook of pediatric infectious diseases,* ed 4, Philadelphia, 1998, Saunders; (psoriasis) from Lookingbill DP, Marks JG: *Principles of dermatology,* ed 2, Philadelphia, 1993, Saunders; (tinea versicolor) from Lookingbill DP, Marks JG: *Principles of dermatology,* ed 2, Philadelphia, 1993, Saunders; (labial herpes simplex [cold sores]) from Hurwitz S: *Clinical pediatric dermatology: a textbook of skin disorders of childhood and adolescence,* ed 2, Philadelphia, 1993, Saunders; (herpes zoster [shingles]) from Hurwitz S: *Clinical pediatric dermatology: a textbook of skin disorders of childhood and adolescence,* ed 2, Philadelphia, 1993, Saunders; (erythema migrans of Lyme disease) from Swartz MH: *Textbook of physical diagnosis: history and examination,* ed 4, Philadelphia, 2002, Saunders.

Art for Table 12-9: (basal cell carcinoma) from Lookingbill DP, Marks JG: *Principles of dermatology,* ed 2, Philadelphia, 1993, Saunders; (squamous cell carcinoma) from Lookingbill DP, Marks JG: *Principles of dermatology,* ed 2, Philadelphia, 1993, Saunders; (malignant melanoma) from Lookingbill DP, Marks JG: *Principles of dermatology,* ed 2, Philadelphia, 1993, Saunders.

Art for Table 12-10: (epidemic Kaposi's sarcoma: patch stage) from Friedman-Kien AE: *Color atlas of AIDS,* Philadelphia, 1989, Saunders; (epidemic Kaposi's sarcoma: advanced disease) from Friedman-Kien AE: *Color atlas of AIDS,* Philadelphia, 1989, Saunders; (epidemic Kaposi's sarcoma: plaque stage) from Friedman-Kien AE: *Color atlas of AIDS,* Philadelphia, 1989, Saunders.

Art for Table 12-11: (anthrax) from Ishak KG et al: *Tumors of the liver, atlas of tumor pathology, third series,* Washington, DC, 2001, Armed Forces Institute of Pathology/American Registry of Pathology; (smallpox [variola major]) from Fenner F et al: *Smallpox and its eradication,* Geneva, 1988, World Health Organization.

Art for Table 12-12: (seborrheic dermatitis [cradle cap] from Hurwitz S: *Clinical pediatric dermatology: a textbook of skin disorders of childhood and adolescence,* ed 2, Philadelphia, 1993, Saunders; (tinea capitis [scalp ringworm]) from Lookingbill DP, Marks JG: *Principles of dermatology,* ed 2, Philadelphia, 1993, Saunders; (toxic alopecia) from Hurwitz S: *Clinical pediatric dermatology: a textbook of skin disorders of childhood and adolescence,* ed 2, Philadelphia, 1993, Saunders; (alopecia areata) from Hurwitz S: *Clinical pediatric dermatology: a textbook of skin dis-*

orders of childhood and adolescence, ed 2, Philadelphia, 1993, Saunders; (traumatic alopecia: traction alopecia) from Hurwitz S: *Clinical pediatric dermatology: a textbook of skin disorders of childhood and adolescence*, ed 2, Philadelphia, 1993, Saunders; (trichotillomania) from Callen JP et al: *Color atlas of dermatology*, Philadelphia, 1993, Saunders; (pediculosis capitis [head lice]) from Callen JP et al: *Color atlas of dermatology*, Philadelphia, 1993, Saunders; (hirsutism) from Wenig BM, Heffess CS, Adair CF: *Atlas of endocrine pathology*, Philadelphia, 1997, Saunders; (furuncle and abscess) from Lookingbill DP, Marks JG: *Principles of dermatology*, ed 2, Philadelphia, 1993, Saunders.

Art for Table 12-13: (koilonychias [spoon nails]) from Callen JP et al: *Color atlas of dermatology*, Philadelphia, 1993, Saunders; (paronychia) from Lookingbill DP, Marks JG: *Principles of dermatology*, ed 2, Philadelphia, 1993, Saunders; (Beau's line) from Callen JP et al: *Color atlas of dermatology*, Philadelphia, 1993, Saunders; (splinter hemorrhages) from Callen JP et al: *Color atlas of dermatology*, Philadelphia, 1993, Saunders; (late clubbing) Reprinted from the Clinical Slide Collection on the Rheumatic Diseases. © 1991, 1995, 1997. Used by permission of the American College of Rheumatology; (onycholysis) from Arndt KA et al: *Primary care dermatology*, Philadelphia, 1997, Saunders; (pitting) from Lookingbill DP, Marks JG: *Principles of dermatology*, ed 2, Philadelphia, 1993, Saunders; (habit-tic dystrophy) from Hurwitz S: *Clinical pediatric dermatology: a textbook of skin disorders of childhood and adolescence*, ed 2, Philadelphia, 1993, Saunders.

CHAPTER 13

Figure 13-16: From Gorrie TM, McKinney ES, Murray SS: *Foundations of maternal-newborn nursing*, ed 2, Philadelphia, 1998, Saunders.

Figure 13-17, *A*: From Gorrie TM, McKinney ES, Murray SS: *Foundations of maternal-newborn nursing*, ed 2, Philadelphia, 1998, Saunders.

Figure 13-19: From Behrman RE, Vaughn VC: *Nelson textbook of pediatrics*, ed 14, Philadelphia, 1992, Saunders.

Art for Table 13-1: (hydrocephalus) from Bowden VR, Dickey SB, Greenburg CS: *Children and their families: the continuum of care*, Philadelphia, 1998, Saunders; (Paget's disease of bone [osteitis deformans]) Reprinted from the Clinical Slide Collection on the Rheumatic Diseases. © 1991, 1995, 1997. Used by permission of the American College of Rheumatology; (acromegaly) from Damjanov I: *Pathology for the health-related professions*, Philadelphia, 1996, Saunders.

Art for Table 13-2: (torticollis [wryneck]) from Liebert PS: *Color atlas of pediatric surgery*, ed 2, Philadelphia, 1996, Saunders; (thyroid—multiple nodules) from Swartz MH: *Textbook of physical diagnosis: history and examination*, ed 4, Philadelphia, 2002, Saunders; (pilar cyst [Wen]) from Callen JP et al: *Color atlas of dermatology*, Philadelphia, 1993, Saunders; (parotid gland enlargement) from Swartz MH: *Textbook of physical diagnosis: history and examination*, ed 4, Philadelphia, 2002, Saunders.

Art for Table 13-3: (fetal alcohol syndrome) Photo from Streissguth AP, Landesman-Dwyer S, Martin JC et al: Teratogenic effects of alcohol in humans and laboratory animals, *Science* 209:353-361, 1980. Illustration from Streissguth AP, Little RE: "Unit 5: Alcohol, Pregnancy, and the Fetal Alcohol Syndrome: Second Edition," Project Cork Institute Medical School Curriculum ("slide lecture series") on Biomedical Education: Alcohol Use and Its Medical Consequences, produced by Dartmouth Medical School; (congenital hypothyroidism) from Zitelli BJ, Davis HW: *Atlas of pediatric physical diagnosis*, ed 4, St Louis, 2002, Mosby,

courtesy of Dr. Thomas P. Foley, Jr.; (Down syndrome) from Zitelli BJ, Davis HW: *Atlas of pediatric physical diagnosis*, ed 4, St Louis, 2002, Mosby; (atopic [allergic] facies) from Hawke M: *Diagnostic handbook of otorhinolaryngology*, London, 1998, Martin Dunitz; (allergic salute and crease) from Zitelli BJ, Davis HW: *Atlas of pediatric physical diagnosis*, ed 4, St Louis, 2002, Mosby.

Art for Table 13-4: (Cushing's syndrome) from Braverman IM: *Skin signs of systemic disease*, ed 3, Philadelphia, 1998, Saunders; (hyperthyroidism) from Swartz MH: *Textbook of physical diagnosis: history and examination*, ed 4, Philadelphia, 2002, Saunders; (myxedema [hypothyroidism]) from Hall R, Evered DC: *Color atlas of endocrinology*, ed 2, London, 1990, Mosby; (Bell's palsy [right side]) from Swartz MH: *Textbook of physical diagnosis: history and examination*, ed 4, Philadelphia, 2002, Saunders; (scleroderma) Reprinted from the Clinical Slide Collection on the Rheumatic Diseases. © 1991, 1995, 1997. Used by permission of the American College of Rheumatology.

CHAPTER 14

Figure 14-23: Courtesy Heather Boyd-Monk and Wills Eye Hospital, Philadelphia.

Figure 14-24: Courtesy Heather Boyd-Monk and Wills Eye Hospital, Philadelphia.

Figure 14-29: From Zitelli BJ, Davis HW: *Atlas of pediatric physical diagnosis*, ed 4, St Louis, 2002, Mosby.

Figure 14-30: From Albert DM, Jakobiec FA: *Principles and practice of ophthalmology*, Philadelphia, 1994, Saunders.

Figure 14-31: From Friedman N, Pineda R: *The Massachusetts eye and ear infirmary illustrated manual of ophthalmology*, Philadelphia, 1998, Saunders.

Figure 14-32: From Swartz MH: *Textbook of physical diagnosis: history and examination*, ed 4, Philadelphia, 2002, Saunders.

Figure 14-33: From Albert DM, Jakobiec FA: *Principles and practice of ophthalmology*, vol 3, Philadelphia, 1994, Saunders.

Figure 14-34: From Friedman N, Pineda R: *The Massachusetts eye and ear infirmary illustrated manual of ophthalmology*, Philadelphia, 1998, Saunders.

Art in Table 14-2: (pseudostrabismus) from Zitelli BJ, Davis HW: *Atlas of pediatric physical diagnosis*, ed 4, St Louis, 2002, Mosby; (L esotropia) from Zitelli BJ, Davis HW: *Atlas of pediatric physical diagnosis*, ed 4, St Louis, 2002, Mosby; (R exotropia) from Zitelli BJ, Davis HW: *Atlas of pediatric physical diagnosis*, ed 4, St Louis, 2002, Mosby.

Art in Table 14-3: (periorbital edema) from Ibsen OAC, Phelan JA: *Oral pathology for the dental hygienist*, ed 2, Philadelphia, 1992, Saunders; (exophthalmos [protruding eye]) from Scheie HG, Albert DM: *Textbook of opthalmology*, ed 9, Philadelphia, 1977, Saunders; (ptosis [drooping upper lip]) Courtesy Heather Boyd-Monk and Wills Eye Hospital, Philadelphia; (upward palpebral slant) from Zitelli BJ, Davis HW: *Atlas of pediatric physical diagnosis*, ed 4, St Louis, 2002, Mosby; (ectropion) from Albert DM, Jakobiec FA: *Principles and practice of ophthalmology*, vol 3, Philadelphia, 1994, Saunders; (entropion) from Albert DM, Jakobiec FA: *Principles and practice of ophthalmology*, vol 3, Philadelphia, 1994, Saunders.

Art in Table 14-4: (blepharitis [inflammation of the eyelids]) from Friedman N, Pineda R: *The Massachusetts eye and ear infirmary illustrated manual of ophthalmology*, Philadelphia, 1998, Saunders; (chalazion) Courtesy Heather Boyd-Monk and Wills Eye Hospital, Philadelphia; (hordeolum [stye]) from Albert DM, Jakobiec FA: *Principles and practice of ophthalmology*, vol 3, Philadelphia, 1994, Saunders; (dacryocystitis [inflammation of the lacrimal sac]) from Friedman N, Pineda R: *The Massachusetts eye and ear* *infirmary illustrated manual of ophthalmology*, Philadelphia, 1998, Saunders; (basal cell carcinoma) from Scheie HG, Albert DM: *Textbook of opthalmology*, ed 9, Philadelphia, 1977, Saunders.

Art in Table 14-5: (conjunctivitis) from Albert DM, Jakobiec FA: *Principles and practice of ophthalmology*, vol 1, Philadelphia, 1994, Saunders; (subconjunctival hemorrhage) Courtesy Heather Boyd-Monk and Wills Eye Hospital, Philadelphia; (iritis [circum-corneal redness]) from Scheie HG, Albert DM: *Textbook of opthalmology*, ed 9, Philadelphia, 1977, Saunders; (acute glaucoma) from Scheie HG, Albert DM: *Textbook of opthalmology*, ed 9, Philadelphia, 1977, Saunders.

Art in Table 14-6: (pterygium) from Albert DM, Jakobiec FA: *Principles and practice of ophthalmology,* vol 1, Philadelphia, 1994, Saunders; (corneal abrasion) Courtesy Heather Boyd-Monk and Wills Eye Hospital, Philadelphia; (hyphema) from Scheie HG, Albert DM: *Textbook of opthalmology*, ed 9, Philadelphia, 1977, Saunders; (hypopyon) from Scheie HG, Albert DM: *Textbook of opthalmology*, ed 9, Philadelphia, 1977, Saunders.

Art in Table 14-8: (central gray opacity – nuclear cataract) from Friedman N, Pineda R: *The Massachusetts eye and ear infirmary illustrated manual of ophthalmology*, Philadelphia, 1998, Saunders; (star-shaped opacity—cortical cataract) from Friedman N, Pineda R: *The Massachusetts eye and ear infirmary illustrated manual of ophthalmology*, Philadelphia, 1998, Saunders.

Art in Table 14-9: (optic atrophy [disc pallor]) from Friedman N, Pineda R: *The Massachusetts eye and ear infirmary illustrated manual of ophthalmology*, Philadelphia, 1998, Saunders; (papilledema [choked disc]) Courtesy Heather Boyd-Monk and Wills Eye Hospital, Philadelphia; (excessive cup-disc ratio) from Friedman N, Pineda R: *The Massachusetts eye and ear infirmary illustrated manual of ophthalmology*, Philadelphia, 1998, Saunders.

Art in Table 14-10: (arteriovenous crossing) from Friedman N, Pineda R: *The Massachusetts eye and ear infirmary illustrated manual of ophthalmology*, Philadelphia, 1998, Saunders; (narrowed arteries) from Friedman N, Pineda R: *The Massachusetts eye and ear infirmary illustrated manual of ophthalmology*, Philadelphia, 1998, Saunders; (microaneurysms) from Friedman N, Pineda R: *The Massachusetts eye and ear infirmary illustrated manual of ophthalmology*, Philadelphia, 1998, Saunders.

CHAPTER 15

Figure 15-8: From Adams GL, Bois LR, Hilger PA: *Boies fundamentals of otolaryngology: a textbook of ear, nose, and throat diseases*, ed 6, Philadelphia, 1989, Saunders.

Art for Table 15-1: (frostbite) Reprinted from the Clinical Slide Collection on the Rheumatic Diseases. © 1991, 1995, 1997. Used by permission of the American College of Rheumatology; (otitis externa—swimmer's ear) from Habif TP et al: *Skin disease: diagnosis and treatment*, ed 3, St Louis, 2001, Mosby; (branchial remnant and ear deformity) from Liebert PS: *Color atlas of pediatric surgery*, ed 2, Philadelphia, 1996, Saunders.

Art for Table 15-2: (sebaceous cyst) from Liebert PS: *Color atlas of pediatric surgery*, ed 2, Philadelphia, 1996, Saunders; (tophi) Reprinted from the Clinical Slide Collection on the Rheumatic Diseases. © 1991, 1995, 1997. Used by permission of the American College of Rheumatology; (chondrodermatitis nodularis helicis) from Habif TP et al: *Skin disease: diagnosis and treatment*, ed 3, St Louis, 2001, Mosby; (keloid) from Liebert PS: *Color atlas of pediatric surgery*, ed 2, Philadelphia, 1996, Saunders; (carcinoma) from Callen JP et al: *Color atlas of dermatology*, Philadelphia, 1993, Saunders.

Art for Table 15-5: (retracted drum) from Adams GL, Bois LR, Hilger PA: *Boies fundamentals of otolaryngology: a textbook of ear, nose,*

and throat diseases, ed 6, Philadelphia, 1989, Saunders; (serous otitis media) from Swartz MH: *Textbook of physical diagnosis: history and examination*, ed 4, Philadelphia, 2002, Saunders; (acute purulent otitis media—early stage) from Adams GL, Bois LR, Hilger PA: *Boies fundamentals of otolaryngology: a textbook of ear, nose, and throat diseases*, ed 6, Philadelphia, 1989, Saunders; (acute purulent otitis media—later stage) from Adams GL, Bois LR, Hilger PA: *Boies fundamentals of otolaryngology: a textbook of ear, nose, and throat diseases*, ed 6, Philadelphia, 1989, Saunders; (perforation) from Swartz MH: *Textbook of physical diagnosis: history and examination*, ed 4, Philadelphia, 2002, Saunders; (insertion of tympanostomy tubes) from Fireman P: *Atlas of allergies*, ed 2, London, 1996, Mosby; (cholesteatoma) from Swartz MH: *Textbook of physical diagnosis: history and examination*, ed 4, Philadelphia, 2002, Saunders; (bullous myringitis) from Swartz MH: *Textbook of physical diagnosis: history and examination*, ed 4, Philadelphia, 2002, Saunders.

CHAPTER 16

Figure 16-9: From Fireman P: *Atlas of allergies*, ed 2, London, 1996, Mosby.

Figure 16-15: From Ibsen OAC, Phelan JA: *Oral pathology for the dental hygienist*, ed 2, Philadelphia, 1996, Saunders.

Figure 16-16: From Ibsen OAC, Phelan JA: *Oral pathology for the dental hygienist*, ed 2, Philadelphia, 1996, Saunders.

Figure 16-22: From Zitelli BJ, Davis HW: *Atlas of pediatric physical diagnosis*, ed 4, St Louis, 2002, Mosby.

Art for Table 16-1: (foreign body) from Fireman P: *Atlas of allergies*, ed 2, London, 1996, Mosby; (perforated septum) from Hawke M: *Diagnostic handbook of otorhinolaryngology*, London, 1998, Martin Dunitz; (acute rhinitis) from Fireman P: *Atlas of allergies*, ed 2, London, 1996, Mosby; (allergic rhinitis) from Fireman P: *Atlas of allergies*, ed 2, London, 1996, Mosby; (polyps) from Fireman P: *Atlas of allergies*, ed 2, London, 1996, Mosby; (carcinoma) from Hawke M: *Diagnostic handbook of otorhinolaryngology*, London, 1998, Martin Dunitz.

Art for Table 16-2: (cleft lip) from Ibsen OAC, Phelan JA: *Oral pathology for the dental hygienist*, ed 2, Philadelphia, 1996, Saunders; (herpes simplex 1) from Callen JP et al: *Color atlas of dermatology*, Philadelphia, 1993, Saunders; (angular chelitis [stomatitis, perleche]) from Callen JP et al: *Color atlas of dermatology*, Philadelphia, 1993, Saunders; (squamous cell carcinoma) from Hawke M: *Diagnostic handbook of otorhinolaryngology*, London, 1998, Martin Dunitz; (retention "cyst" [mucocele]) from Hawke M: *Diagnostic handbook of otorhinolaryngology*, London, 1998, Martin Dunitz.

Art for Table 16-3: (baby bottle tooth decay) Courtesy of F. Ferguson, Department of Children's Dentistry, School of Dental Medicine, SUNY at Stony Brook, Stony Brook, NY 11733; (dental caries) Courtesy of A. McWhorter, Pediatric Dentistry, Baylor College of Dentistry, The Texas A & M University System, Dallas, TX; (epulis) from Ibsen OAC, Phelan JA: *Oral pathology for the dental hygienist*, ed 2, Philadelphia, 1996, Saunders; (gingival hyperplasia) from Ibsen OAC, Phelan JA: *Oral pathology for the dental hygienist*, ed 2, Philadelphia, 1996, Saunders; (gingivitis) from Callen JP et al: *Color atlas of dermatology*, Philadelphia, 1993, Saunders.

Art for Table 16-4: (aphthous ulcers) from Sleisinger MH, Fordtran JS: *Gastrointestinal diseases: pathophysiology, diagnosis, and management*, vol 1, ed 5, Philadelphia, 1993, Saunders; (Koplik's spots) from Feigin RD, Cherry JD: *Textbook of pediatric infectious diseases*, ed 4, Philadelphia, 1998, Saunders; (leukoplakia) from Sleisinger MH, Fordtran JS: *Gastrointestinal diseases: pathophysi-*

ology, diagnosis, and management, vol 1, ed 5, Philadelphia, 1993, Saunders; (candidiasis or monilial infection) from Callen JP et al: *Color atlas of dermatology,* Philadelphia, 1993, Saunders.

Art for Table 16-5: (ankyloglossia) from Ibsen OAC, Phelan JA: *Oral pathology for the dental hygienist,* ed 2, Philadelphia, 1996, Saunders; (fissured or scrotal tongue) from Callen JP et al: *Color atlas of dermatology,* Philadelphia, 1993, Saunders; (geographic tongue [migratory glossitis]) from Callen JP et al: *Color atlas of dermatology,* Philadelphia, 1993, Saunders; (smooth, glossy tongue [atrophic glossitis]) from Adams GL, Bois LR, Hilger PA: *Boies fundamentals of otolaryngology: a textbook of ear, nose, and throat diseases,* ed 6, Philadelphia, 1989, Saunders; (black hairy tongue) from Callen JP et al: *Color atlas of dermatology,* Philadelphia, 1993, Saunders; (enlarged tongue [macroglossia]) from Zitelli BJ, Davis HW: *Atlas of pediatric physical diagnosis,* ed 4, St Louis, 2002, Mosby, courtesy of Dr. Christine Williams; (carcinoma) from Wenig BM, Heffess CS, Adair CF: *Atlas of endocrine pathology,* Philadelphia, 1997, Saunders.

Art for Table 16-6: (cleft palate) from Zitelli BJ, Davis HW: *Atlas of pediatric physical diagnosis,* ed 4, St Louis, 2002, Mosby, Courtesy of Dr. Michael Sherlock; (bifid uvula) from Hawke M: *Diagnostic handbook of otorhinolaryngology,* London, 1998, Martin Dunitz; (oral Kaposi's sarcoma) from Friedman-Kien AE: *Color atlas of AIDS,* Philadelphia, 1989, Saunders; (acute tonsillitis) from Hawke M: *Diagnostic handbook of otorhinolaryngology,* London, 1998, Martin Dunitz.

CHAPTER 17

Figure 17-6: Redrawn from Tanner JM: *Growth at adolescence,* Oxford, 1962, Blackwell Scientific.

Figure 17-8: From Callen JP et al: *Color atlas of dermatology,* Philadelphia, 1993, Saunders.

Figure 17-21: From Moore KL, Persaud TN: *Before we are born: essentials of embryology and birth defects,* ed 5, Philadelphia, 1998, Saunders.

Art for Table 17-3: (dimpling) from Evans AJ et al: *Atlas of breast disease management: 50 illustrative cases,* Philadelphia, 1998, Saunders; (edema [peau d'orange]) from Mansel R: *Color atlas of breast diseases,* London, 1995, Mosby; (fixation) from Mansel R: *Color atlas of breast diseases,* London, 1995, Mosby; (deviation in nipple pointing) from Mansel R: *Color atlas of breast diseases,* London, 1995, Mosby.

Art for Table 17-6: (mammary duct ectasia) from Mansel R: *Color atlas of breast diseases,* London, 1995, Mosby; (carcinoma) from Evan AJ set al: *Atlas of breast disease management: 50 illustrative cases,* Philadelphia, 1998, Saunders; (intraductal papilloma) from Mansel R: *Color atlas of breast diseases,* London, 1995, Mosby; (Paget's disease [intraductal carcinoma]) from Mansel R: *Color atlas of breast diseases,* London, 1995, Mosby.

Art for Table 17-7: (breast abscess) from Mansel R: *Color atlas of breast diseases,* London, 1995, Mosby; (mastitis) from Mansel R: *Color atlas of breast diseases,* London, 1995, Mosby.

Art for Table 17-8: (gynecomastia) from Evans AJ et al: *Atlas of breast disease management: 50 illustrative cases,* Philadelphia, 1998, Saunders; (carcinoma) from Haagensen CD: *Diseases of the breast,* ed 3, Philadelphia, 1986, Saunders.

CHAPTER 18

Figure 18-12: From Nichols FH, Zwelling E: *Maternal-newborn nursing: theory and practice,* Philadelphia, 1997, Saunders.

CHAPTER 19

Figure 19-15: From Lakatta EG: Cardiovascular function in later life, *Cardiovasc Med* 10:37-40, 1985.

Figure 19-16: From Office of Minority Health, Washington, DC, 1990.

CHAPTER 20

Figure 20-7: From Behrman RE, Vaguhn VC: *Nelson textbook of pediatrics,* ed 14, Philadelphia, 1992, Saunders.

Figure 20-20, *B:* From Bloom A, Watkins PH, Ireland J: *Color atlas of diabetes,* ed 2, St Louis, 1992, Mosby.

Art for Table 20-2: (Raynaud's syndrome) from Walker JM, Helewa A: *Physical therapy in arthritis,* Philadelphia, 1996, Saunders; (lymphedema) from Swartz MH: *Textbook of physical diagnosis: history and examination,* ed 4, Philadelphia, 2002, Saunders.

Art for Table 20-4: (arteriosclerosis—ischemic ulcer) from Dockery GL: *Cutaneous disorders of the lower extremity,* Philadelphia, 1997, Saunders; (venous [stasis] ulcer) from Lookingbill DP, Marks JG: *Principles of dermatology,* ed 2, Philadelphia, 1993, Saunders; (superficial varicose veins) from Dockery GL: *Cutaneous disorders of the lower extremity,* Philadelphia, 1997, Saunders; (deep vein thrombophlebitis) from Dockery GL: *Cutaneous disorders of the lower extremity,* Philadelphia, 1997, Saunders.

CHAPTER 21

Art for Table 21-4: (umbilical hernia) from Zitelli BJ, Davis HW: *Atlas of pediatric physical diagnosis,* ed 4, St Louis, 2002, Mosby, courtesy of Dr. Thomas P. Foley, Jr.

CHAPTER 22

Figure 22-33, *C:* From Dieppe PA, Cooper C, McGill N: *Arthritis and rheumatism in practice,* London, 1991, Gower Medical Publishing.

Figure 22-34, *B:* From Dieppe PA, Cooper C, McGill N: *Arthritis and rheumatism in practice,* London, 1991, Gower Medical Publishing.

Figure 22-50: From Zitelli BJ, Davis HW: *Atlas of pediatric physical diagnosis,* ed 4, St Louis, 2002, Mosby.

Figure 22-54: From Rossman I: *Clinical geriatrics,* ed 3, Philadelphia, 1986, Lippincott.

Art for Table 22-4: (atrophy) from Bunker T, Schranz PJ: *Clinical challenges in orthopaedics: the shoulder,* London, 1998, Martin Dunitz; (dislocated shoulder) from Bunker T, Schranz PJ: *Clinical challenges in orthopaedics: the shoulder,* London, 1998, Martin Dunitz; (joint effusion) from Bunker T, Schranz PJ: *Clinical challenges in orthopaedics: the shoulder,* London, 1998, Martin Dunitz; (tear of rotator cuff) from Polley HF, Hunder GG: *Physical examination of the joints,* ed 2, Philadelphia, 1978, Saunders; (frozen shoulder—adhesive capsulitis) from Polley HF, Hunder GG: *Physical examination of the joints,* ed 2, Philadelphia, 1978, Saunders.

Art for Table 22-5: (olecranon bursitis) from Dieppe PA, Cooper C, McGill N: *Arthritis and rheumatism in practice,* London, 1991, Gower Medical Publishing; (gouty arthritis) from Polley HF, Hunder GG: *Physical examination of the joints,* ed 2, Philadelphia, 1978, Saunders; (subcutaneous nodules) from Callen JP et al: *Color atlas of dermatology,* Philadelphia, 1993, Saunders; (epicondylitis—tennis elbow) from Jones A, Owen R: *Color atlas of clinical orthopedics,* ed 2, London, 1995, Mosby.

Art for Table 22-6: (ganglion cyst) from Callen JP et al: *Color atlas of dermatology,* Philadelphia, 1993, Saunders; (carpal tunnel syndrome with atrophy of thenar eminence) Reprinted from the

Clinical Slide Collection on the Rheumatic Diseases. © 1991, 1995, 1997. Used by permission of the American College of Rheumatology; (ankylosis) from Polley HF, Hunder GG: *Physical examination of the joints*, ed 2, Philadelphia, 1978, Saunders; (swan-neck and boutonnière deformity) from Clinical Slide Collection on the Rheumatic Diseases, 1991, 1995, 1997; (ulnar deviation or drift) from Walker JM, Helewa A: *Physical therapy in arthritis*, Philadelphia, 1996, Saunders; (degenerative joint disease or osteoarthritis) from Walker JM, Helewa A: *Physical therapy in arthritis*, Philadelphia, 1996, Saunders; (syndactyly) from Liebert PS: *Color atlas of pediatric surgery*, ed 2, Philadelphia, 1996, Saunders; (polydactyly) from Liebert PS: *Color atlas of pediatric surgery*, ed 2, Philadelphia, 1996, Saunders.

Art for Table 22-7: (mild synovitis) from Dieppe PA, Cooper C, McGill N: *Arthritis and rheumatism in practice*, London, 1991, Gower Medical Publishing; (prepatellar bursitis) from Dieppe PA, Cooper C, McGill N: *Arthritis and rheumatism in practice*, London, 1991, Gower Medical Publishing; (swelling of menisci) from Jones A, Owen R: *Color atlas of clinical orthopedics*, ed 2, London, 1995, Mosby.

Art for Table 22-8: (achilles tenosynovitis) from Dieppe PA, Cooper C, McGill N: *Arthritis and rheumatism in practice*, London, 1991, Gower Medical Publishing; (tophi with chronic gout) from Dockery GL: *Cutaneous disorders of the lower extremity*, Philadelphia, 1997, Saunders; (acute gout) from Dieppe PA, Cooper C, McGill N: *Arthritis and rheumatism in practice*, London, 1991, Gower Medical Publishing; (hallux valgus with bunion and hammer toes) from Walker JM, Helewa A: *Physical therapy in arthritis*, Philadelphia, 1996, Saunders.

Art for Table 22-9: (scoliosis) from Zitelli BJ, Davis HW: *Atlas of pediatric physical diagnosis*, ed 4, St Louis, 2002, Mosby; (herniated nucleus pulposus) from Polley HF, Hunder GG: *Physical examination of the joints*, ed 2, Philadelphia, 1978, Saunders.

Art for Table 22-10: (congenital dislocated hip) from Zitelli BJ, Davis HW: *Atlas of pediatric physical diagnosis*, ed 4, St Louis, 2002, Mosby; (talipes equinovarus [clubfoot]) from A.E. Chudley, MD; (spina bifida) from Walsh PC et al: *Campbell's urology*, ed 5, Philadelphia, 1986, Saunders.

CHAPTER 23

Figure 23-52, B: From Fenichel GM: *Clinical pediatric neurology*, Philadelphia, 1988, Saunders.

Figure 23-58: From Hickey JV: *Neurological and neurosurgical nursing*, ed 2, Philadelphia, 1986, Lippincott.

CHAPTER 24

Figure 24-4: Redrawn from Marshall WA, Tanner JM: Variations in the pattern of pubertal changes in boys, *Arch Dis Child* 45:22, 1970.

Art for Table 24-2: (herpes progenitalis) Courtesy of Pfizer Laboratories Division, Pfizer Inc, New York. From "A close look at VD: a slide presentation produced as a public service"; (syphilitic chancre) from Emond RT, Rowl HAK, Welsby P: *Color atlas of infectious diseases*, ed 3, London, 1995, Mosby; (condylomata acuminate [genital warts]) from Habif TP et al: *Skin disease: diagnosis and treatment*, ed 3, St Louis, 2001, Mosby; (carcinoma) from Callen JP et al: *Color atlas of dermatology*, Philadelphia, 1993, Saunders; (urethritis [urethral discharge and dysuria])

from Emond RT, Rowl HAK, Welsby P: *Color atlas of infectious diseases*, ed 3, London, 1995, Mosby.

Art for Table 24-3: (phimosis) from Liebert PS: *Color atlas of pediatric surgery*, ed 2, Philadelphia, 1996, Saunders; (hypospadias) from Liebert PS: *Color atlas of pediatric surgery*, ed 2, Philadelphia, 1996, Saunders; (epispadias) from Zitelli BJ, Davis HW: *Atlas of pediatric physical diagnosis*, ed 4, St Louis, 2002, Mosby; (Peyronie's disease) Courtesy of Dr. Hans Stricker, Department of Urology, Henry Ford Hospital, Detroit, MI.

CHAPTER 26

Art for Table 26-3: (pediculosis pubis [crab lice]) from Callen JP et al: *Color atlas of dermatology*, Philadelphia, 1993, Saunders; (herpes simplex virus—type 2 [herpes genitalis]) from Callen JP et al: *Color atlas of dermatology*, Philadelphia, 1993, Saunders; (red rash—contact dermatitis) Courtesy of Pfizer Laboratories Division, Pfizer Inc, New York. From "A close look at VD: a slide presentation produced as a public service"; (syphilitic chancre) from Emond RT, Rowl HAK, Welsby P: *Color atlas of infectious diseases*, ed 3, London, 1995, Mosby; (genital human papillomavirus [HPV, condylomata, acuminata, genital warts]) from Habif TP et al: *Skin disease: diagnosis and treatment*, ed 3, St Louis, 2001, Mosby; (abscess of Bartholin's gland) from Emond RT, Rowl HAK, Welsby P: *Color atlas of infectious diseases*, ed 3, London, 1995, Mosby; (urethral caruncle) from Rimsza ME: An illustrated guide to adolescent gynecology, *Pediatr Clin North Am* 36(3):641, 1989.

Art for Table 26-4: (cystocele) from Symonds EM, McPherson MBA: *Color atlas of obstetrics and gynecology*, London, 1994, Mosby; (rectocele) from Huffman JW: *Gynecology and obstetrics*, Philadelphia, 1962, Saunders; (uterine prolapse) from Symonds EM, McPherson MBA: *Color atlas of obstetrics and gynecology*, London, 1994, Mosby.

Art for Table 26-5: (human papilloma virus infection) from Symonds EM, McPherson MBA: *Color atlas of obstetrics and gynecology*, London, 1994, Mosby; (polyp) from Symonds EM, McPherson MBA: *Color atlas of obstetrics and gynecology*, London, 1994, Mosby; (carcinoma) from Symonds EM, McPherson MBA: *Color atlas of obstetrics and gynecology*, London, 1994, Mosby.

Art for Table 26-6: (gonorrhea) Courtesy of Pfizer Laboratories Division, Pfizer Inc, New York. From "A close look at VD: a slide presentation produced as a public service."

Art for Table 26-9: (ambiguous genitalia) from Moore KL, Persaud TN: *Before we are born: essentials of embryology and birth defects*, ed 5, Philadelphia, 1998, Saunders; (vulvovaginitis in child) from Feigin RD, Cherry JD: *Textbook of pediatric infectious diseases*, ed 4, Philadelphia, 1998, Saunders.

CHAPTER 27

Figure 27-4: From Symonds EM, McPherson MBA: *Color atlas of obstetrics and gynecology*, London, 1994, Mosby.

Figure 27-13: From Symonds EM, McPherson MBA: *Color atlas of obstetrics and gynecology*, London, 1994, Mosby.

Art for Table 27-2: (preeclampsia) from Symonds EM, McPherson MBA: *Color atlas of obstetrics and gynecology*, London, 1994, Mosby.

Art for Table 27-3: (fetal macrosomia) from Symonds EM, McPherson MBA: *Color atlas of obstetrics and gynecology*, London, 1994, Mosby.

Index

Page numbers with "t" denote tables, and those with "f" denote figures.

887

ASSESSMENT TERMS: ENGLISH AND SPANISH

ENGLISH	SPANISH	ENGLISH	SPANISH
HISTORY TAKING			
How do you feel?	¿Cómo se siente?	Since when has your eyesight failed you?	¿Desde cuándo ha disminuido su visión?
Good	Bien	Do you sometimes see things double?	¿Ve las cosas doble algunas veces?
Bad	Mal	Tell me what number it is.	Digame qué número es éste.
Let me see . . .	Déjeme ver . . .	Tell me what letter it is.	Dígame qué letra es ésta.
Let me feel your pulse.	Déjeme tomarle el pulso.	Do you see things through a mist?	¿Ve las cosas nubladas?
How does your head feel?	¿Cómo siente la cabeza?	Can you see clearly?	¿Puede ver claramente?
Your memory	Su memoria	Better at a distance?	¿Mejor a cierta distancia?
Is it good?	¿Es buena?	Nausea	Náusea
Have you any pain in the head?	¿Le duele la cabeza?	Does eating make you vomit?	¿El comer le hace vomitar?
Did you fall and how did you fall?	¿Se cayó, y cómo se cayó?	How are your stools?	¿Cómo son sus defecaciones?
Did you faint?	¿Se desmayó?	Are they regular?	¿Son regulares?
Have you ever had fainting spells?	¿Ha tenido desmayos alguna vez?	Have you noticed their color?	¿Se ha fijado en el color?
Have you slept well?	¿Ha dormido bien?	Are you constipated?	¿Está estreñido?
Have you any difficulty in breathing?	¿Tiene dificultad al respirar?	Do you have diarrhea?	¿Tiene diarrea?
Since when do you cough?	¿Desde cuándo tose Ud?	Have you any difficulty passing water?	¿Tiene dificultad en orinar?
You cough a little?	¿Tose poco?	Do you pass water involuntarily?	¿Orina sin querer?
Do you expectorate much?	Escupe mucho?	Are any of your limbs swollen?	¿Están hinchados algunos de sus miembros?
What is the color of your expectorations?	De qué color es el esputo?	How long have they been swollen like this?	¿Desde cuándo están hinchados así?
The hearing	El oído		
Is it affected?	¿Está afectado?		
Do you have ringing in the ears?	¿Le Zumban los oídos?		